Anesthesia for Obstetrics

THIRD EDITION

Anesthesia for Obstetrics

THIRD EDITION

EDITED BY

Sol M. Shnider, M.D.

Professor of Anesthesia
Obstetrics, Gynecology and Reproductive Sciences
Vice Chairman, Department of Anesthesia
University of California, San Francisco
School of Medicine
San Francisco, California

Gershon Levinson, M.D.

California Pacific Medical Center
Associate Clinical Professor of Anesthesia
University of California, San Francisco
School of Medicine
San Francisco, California

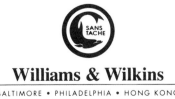

Williams & Wilkins

BALTIMORE • PHILADELPHIA • HONG KONG
LONDON • MUNICH • SYDNEY • TOKYO

A WAVERLY COMPANY

Editor: Timothy H. Grayson
Project Manager: Victoria Rybicki Vaughn
Copy Editor: Kathy Lumpkin
Designer: Jo Anne Janowiak
Illustration Planner: Lorraine Wrzosek
Cover Designer: Wilma E. Rosenberger
Cover Illustration: Mother and Child
    Eskimo Sculpture by Peter Anoutak

Copyright © 1993
Williams & Wilkins
428 East Preston Street
Baltimore, Maryland 21202, USA

Accurate indications, adverse reactions, and dosage schedules for drugs are provided in this book, but it is possible that they may change. The reader is urged to
review the package information data of the manufacturers of the medications
mentioned.

Printed in the United States of America

First Edition 1979
Second Edition 1987

Library of Congress Cataloging in Publication Data

Anesthesia for obstetrics / edited by Sol M. Shnider, Gershon
  Levinson. — 3rd ed.
      p.   cm.
    Includes bibliographical references and index.
    ISBN 0-683-07751-1
    1. Anesthesia in obstetrics.   I. Shnider, Sol M., 1929–
II. Levinson, Gershon, 1943–   .
    [DNLM: 1. Anesthesia, Obstetrical.   WO 450 A5787]
RG732.A553   1993
617.9'682--dc20
DNLM/DLC
for Library of Congress   92-49993
                                                            CIP

93 94 95 96
3 4 5 6 7 8 9 10

To
Beatrice, Ethel, Earl and Allan,
and
Jean, Charles, Jonathan and Celia
for their patience and love

Preface to Third Edition

Anesthesia for Obstetrics has become the standard textbook in obstetric anesthesia. Various editions have been translated into Spanish, French, Portuguese, and German, making the textbook a valuable international clinical guide and reference source for students and practitioners.

Since 1987, changes and advances in the field of obstetric anesthesia have been occurring rapidly, necessitating the current revision and updating of each chapter. The chapters dealing with spinal and epidural opiates, regional anesthesia for vaginal delivery, anesthesia for cesarean section, the impact of obstetric anesthesia on uterine activity and labor, perinatal pharmacology, preterm labor, and neurologic complications of regional anesthesia have received especially extensive revisions. The chapter on resuscitation of the newborn has been revised to include the new recommendations of the American Heart Association.

Since publication of the second edition, the global tragedy of human immunodeficiency disease with resulting perinatal AIDS has become a widespread problem. Anesthetic implications for the mother, fetus, newborn, and health care worker are discussed in a new chapter. The increasing problem of maternal substance abuse has also necessitated the addition of a new chapter. The continued rise in the number of lawsuits in the area of perinatal medicine has led to a new section detailing available information on obstetric anesthesia malpractice lawsuits, in addition to the section on general considerations and recommendations regarding obstetric anesthesia and lawsuits.

The new edition now includes 34 authors, seven of whom are new to this edition. Many of the authors are internationally recognized authorities in anesthesiology, perinatology, and law. We believe the third edition will be an even more valuable standard reference textbook than the previous editions.

We wish to express our gratitude to the many people who made this book a reality. First, of course, we wish to thank each of the contributors for their valuable time and efforts. The extensive use of figures would not have been possible without the kind permission of the many publishers of scientific journals and books who allowed us to reproduce previously published figures. We would also like to thank Doctor Craig Fong for valuable editorial assistance and for his unselfish expertise in performing a variety of editorial services.

This edition would never have seen the light of day without the tireless efforts of Judy Johnson. Without her encouragement, enthusiasm, dedication, and competence in pursing the myriad details necessary for a publication of this magnitude, the project could never have proceeded so smoothly. Her editorial professionalism was a major contribution to the ultimate quality of this book.

Preface to First Edition

Anesthesia for Obstetrics is a textbook covering all aspects of obstetric anesthesia. Physiologic, pharmacologic and clinical aspects have been integrated to provide a sound basis for the safe practice of obstetric anesthesia.

The editors—together with 17 distinguished authorities in the fields of anesthesiology, obstetrics, neonatology and law—have provided an up-to-date review of anesthesia for vaginal delivery and cesarean section, anesthesia for complicated obstetrics, anesthetic applications and evaluation and resuscitation of the fetus and neonate. We have oriented this textbook to practitioners and students of anesthesia. The comprehensive and concise coverage and authoritative nature of this publication should appeal to all health care providers of pregnant women. Skill-ful application of the information in this volume will help provide optimum care for the mother and her newborn.

We wish to express our gratitude to all of our contributors as well as to the many publishers of scientific journals and books who permitted us to reproduce their previously published figures.

We are deeply appreciative of the efforts of Anita Edgecombe in the preparation of the manuscript and of Karen Olson and Doctors E. I. Eger II, W. K. Hamilton, P. L. Wilkinson, and R. K. Creasy, who provided valuable advice in the editing of this book. We also thank Merrilyn Jones and Judy Johnson for help in proofreading and preparing the index and Mary Briscoe for her original illustrations.

Contributors

Gerard M. Bassell, M.D., B.S.
Professor of Anesthesiology, Obstetrics and Gynecology, University of Kansas School of Medicine; Vice Chairman, Department of Anesthesiology, Director of Obstetric Anesthesia, Wesley Women's Hospital, Wichita, Kansas

Diane R. Biehl, M.D.
Professor, Department of Perinatology, University of Manitoba; Head, Department of Anaesthesia, St. Boniface General Hospital, Winnipeg, Manitoba, Canada

Philip R. Bromage, M.B., B.S. (Lond), F.F.A.R.C.S., F.R.C.P.C.
Scientist-in-Residence, Department of Anesthesiology, Christiana Hospital, Medical Center of Delaware, Newark, Delaware

H. S. Chadwick, M.D.
Associate Professor of Anesthesiology, Director of Obstetrical Anesthesia, Department of Anesthesiology, University of Washington, Seattle, Washington

Theodore G. Cheek, M.D.
Associate Professor of Anesthesia, Obstetrics and Gynecology, Director of Obstetrical Anesthesia, Hospital of the University of Pennsylvania, Philadelphia, Pennsylvania

David H. Chestnut, M.D.
Professor of Anesthesia, Obstetrics and Gynecology, University of Iowa College of Medicine; Director of Obstetric Anesthesia, University of Iowa Hospital and Clinics, Iowa City, Iowa

Sheila E. Cohen, M.B., Ch.B., F.F.A.R.C.S.
Professor of Anesthesia, Director of Obstetric Anesthesia, Stanford University School of Medicine, Stanford, California

Ermelando V. Cosmi, M.D., L.D.
Professor of Obstetrics, Gynecology and Anesthesiology, University of Rome, Rome, Italy

Marrs A. Craddick, LL.B., J.D.
Attorney-at-Law, Danville, California

Patricia A. Dailey, M.D.
Staff Anesthesiologist, Mills Hospital, San Mateo; Assistant Clinical Professor of Anesthesia, University of California, San Francisco, San Francisco, California

Sanjay Datta, M.D.
Professor of Anesthesia, Harvard Medical School; Director of Obstetrical Anesthesia, Brigham and Women's Hospital, Boston, Massachusetts

Jay S. DeVore, M.D.
Staff Anesthesiologist, Major Hospital, Shelbyville, Indiana

Edward A. Eisler, M.D.
Staff Anesthesiologist, Director of Obstetrical Anesthesia, California Pacific Medical Center, Pacific Campus; Clinical Instructor, Department of Anesthesia, University of California, San Francisco, San Francisco, California

Mieczyslaw Finster, M.D.
Professor of Anesthesia, Obstetrics and Gynecology, College of Physicians and Surgeons of Columbia University, New York, New York

Craig J. Fong, M.D.
Research Fellow, Obstetrical Anesthesia, Department of Anesthesia, University of California, San Francisco, San Francisco, California

George A. Gregory, M.D.
Professor of Anesthesia and Pediatrics, Department of Anesthesia and Cardiovascular Research Institute, University of California, San Francisco, San Francisco, California

Brett B. Gutsche, M.D.
Professor of Anesthesiology, Obstetrics and Gynecology, Hospital of the University of Pennsylvania, Philadelphia, Pennsylvania

Stephen Halpern, M.D., F.R.C.P.C.
Assistant Professor, Department of Anaesthesia, University of Toronto; Director of Obstetrical Anaesthesia, Women's College Hospital, Toronto, Ontario, Canada

Samuel C. Hughes, M.D.
Associate Professor of Clinical Anesthesia, Department of Anesthesia, Director of Obstetrical Anesthesia, San Francisco General Hospital, University of California, San Francisco, San Francisco, California

David Karp, M.A.
Loss Prevention Manager, Medical Insurance Exchange of California, Oakland, California

Dennis M. Kotelko, M.D., F.R.C.P.C.
Research Director of Obstetric Anesthesia, Cedars-Sinai Medical Center, Los Angeles, California

Russell K. Laros, Jr., M.D.
Professor and Vice Chairman, Department of Obstetrics, Gynecology and Reproductive Sciences, University of California, San Francisco, San Francisco, California

Gershon Levinson, M.D.
Staff Anesthesiologist, California Pacific Medical Center, California Campus; Associate Clinical Professor of Anesthesia, University of California, San Francisco, San Francisco, California

Dennis T. Mangano, Ph.D., M.D.
Professor and Vice Chairman, Department of Anesthesia, Veterans Affairs Medical Center, University of California, San Francisco, San Francisco, California

Gertie F. Marx, M.D.
Professor of Anesthesiology, Albert Einstein College of Medicine, Bronx, New York

Anthony C. Miller, M.D.
Clinical Director of Obstetrical Anesthesia, Northeast Anesthesia PA, Eastern Maine Medical Center, Bangor, Maine

Julian T. Parer, M.D., Ph.D.
Professor of Obstetrics, Gynecology and Reproductive Sciences, Associate Staff, Cardiovascular Research Institute, University of California, San Francisco, San Francisco, California

Hilda Pederson, M.B., Ch.B., F.F.A.R.C.S.
Professor of Clinical Anesthesia, College of Physicians and Surgeons of Columbia University, New York, New York

David H. Ralston, M.D.
Staff Anesthesiologist, South Coast Medical Center, South Laguna, California

Stephen H. Rolbin, M.D.C.M., F.R.C.P.(C)
Department of Anaesthesia, Director of Obstetric Anaesthesia, Assistant Professor, University of Toronto, Toronto, Ontario, Canada

Mark A. Rosen, M.D.
Associate Professor of Clinical Anesthesia, Obstetrics, Gynecology and Reproductive Sciences, University of California, San Francisco, San Francisco, California

Sol M. Shnider, M.D.
Professor and Vice Chairman, Department of Anesthesia; Professor of Obstetrics, Gynecology and Reproductive Sciences, University of California, San Francisco, San Francisco, California

Jan D. Vertommen, M.D.
Staff Anesthesiologist, University Hospitals, Katholieke Universiteit, Leuven, Belgium

Richard G. Wright, M.D.
Assistant Clinical Professor of Anesthesia, University of California, Davis; Staff Anesthesiologist, Sutter Community Hospital, Sacramento, California

Contents

SECTION ONE.
OBSTETRIC PHYSIOLOGY AND PHARMACOLOGY

SECTION TWO.
ANESTHESIA FOR VAGINAL DELIVERY

SECTION FIVE.
NONOBSTETRIC DISORDERS DURING PREGNANCY

SECTION SIX.
FETUS AND NEWBORN

APPENDIX

OBSTETRIC PHYSIOLOGY AND PHARMACOLOGY

CHAPTER 1

Maternal Physiologic Alterations During Pregnancy

Theodore G. Cheek, M.D.
Brett B. Gutsche, M.D.

Pregnancy, labor, and delivery profoundly alter maternal physiology and the response to medical therapies, such as anesthesia. Pregnancy has been described as the only physiologic state in which most physiologic parameters are abnormal. These changes are seen in the common physical complaints of pregnancy. Breathlessness and frequent upper respiratory tract infections reflect increased respiratory drive and airway swelling. Ankle edema, leg varices, and hemorrhoids indicate lower extremity venous engorgement and stasis. Heartburn, nausea, and vomiting imply decreased gastric emptying, increased gastric acidity, and decreased gastroesophageal junction tone. Back pain accompanies increased lumbar vertebral lordosis and weight-bearing strain. Urinary frequency and infection is evidence of the decreased capacity of the bladder. Early in pregnancy, rising levels of progesterone, estrogen, human chorionic gonadotropin, and prostaglandin play a primary role in the anatomic and physiologic changes of pregnancy. As pregnancy progresses the enlarging uterus assumes a more important role in the alteration of respiratory, circulatory, gastrointestinal, renal, and skeletal functions. This chapter contains a review of these physiologic changes and a discussion of the implications for anesthesia care of the parturient. Familiarity with this subject will contribute to the best possible anesthetic outcome. Thoughtful and well-conceived recent reviews on maternal physiologic changes (1–3) and their anesthetic implications (4–6) are available for further study.

RESPIRATORY CHANGES DURING PREGNANCY

The respiratory changes that occur during pregnancy are of special significance to the anesthetist (Table 1.1). Ventilation increases during and after the first trimester of pregnancy, and shortness of breath may occur during the latter months of pregnancy. Capillary engorgement of the mucosa throughout the respiratory tract causes swelling of the nasal and oral pharynx, larynx, and trachea. As a result the parturient frequently appears to have symptoms of upper respiratory tract infection and laryngitis, with nasal congestion and voice change (7). These changes may be markedly exacerbated by a mild upper respiratory tract infection, fluid overload (8), or the edema associated with pre-

Table 1.1
Changes in the Respiratory System at Term[a]

Variable	Direction of Change	Average Change
Minute ventilation	⇑	+50%
Alveolar ventilation	⇑	+70%
Tidal volume	⇑	+40%
Respiratory rate	⇑	+15%
Arterial P_{O_2}	⇑	+10 torr
Inspiratory lung capacity	⇑	+5%
Oxygen consumption	⇑	+20%
Dead space	⇔	No change
Lung compliance (alone)	⇔	No change
Arterial pH	⇔	No change
Vital capacity	⇔	No change
FEV 1	⇔	No change
Diffusing capacity	⇔	No change
Maximum breathing capacity	⇔	No change
Closing volume	⇓ or	No change
Airway resistance	⇓	−36%
Total pulmonary resistance	⇓	−50%
Total compliance	⇓	−30%
Chest wall compliance (alone)	⇓	−45%
Arterial P_{CO_2}	⇓	−10 torr
Serum bicarbonate	⇓	−4 mEq/L
Total lung capacity	⇓	−0–5%
Functional residual capacity	⇓	−20%
Expiratory reserve volume	⇓	−20%
Residual volume	⇓	−20%

[a] Adapted from references 11–13, 17, 21, 22, and 25–31.

eclampsia-eclampsia, which occasionally leads to a severely compromised airway (9).

Manipulation of the upper airway requires special care. Suctioning, the placement of airways, and careless laryngoscopy may result in trauma and bleeding. Manipulation of the nasal airway usually is associated with a brisk epistaxis. Upper airway obstruction may occur early in anesthetic induction. When endotracheal intubation is performed, a 6- to 7-mm cuffed endotracheal tube is recommended because the area of the glottis is often decreased by swelling of the false vocal cords. Attempts to intubate the parturient with an 8-mm cuffed tube, normally suitable for the adult female, may result in trauma and an inability to pass the endotracheal catheter. Breast engorgement can interfere with laryngoscopy, making the use of a short-handled blade necessary (10).

Minute ventilation (VE) is increased by 30% at the seventh week of pregnancy and about 50% at term primarily as a result of an increased tidal volume with little change (or at most a slight increase) in respiratory rate (11–13). This is caused by progesterone-induced increased sensitivity to carbon dioxide and an increased metabolic rate (14).

As a result of this increased alveolar ventilation at term, maternal $PaCO_2$ is usually decreased to about 32 torr, but little maternal alkalosis occurs because of a compensatory renal excretion of serum bicarbonate of about 4 mEq/liter (from 26 to 22 mEq/liter). During labor, particularly in the latter first stage and second stage as pain becomes severe, maternal minute ventilation may be increased as much as 300% compared with the nonpregnant state, with the development of marked maternal hypocarbia ($PaCO_2$ 20 torr or less) alkalemia (pH greater than 7.55) (Fig. 1.1) (15). This marked respiratory alkalosis may cause hypoventilation between painful contractions (Fig. 1.2) and a leftward shift of the oxyhemoglobin curve, causing oxygen to be more tightly bound to maternal hemoglobin, thus compromising its availability to the fetus (16). It has been demonstrated that effective epidural analgesia alone can markedly diminish maternal hyperventilation and oxygen consumption (Fig. 1.3) (15, 17–20), which indicates that hyperventilation in part is due to the pain of labor (19, 20).

Lung volumes and lung capacities are not greatly changed by pregnancy. Changes are primarily limited to the functional residual capacity, which is decreased 15 to 20% in the gravida at term (Fig. 1.4). It has been shown that most of this decrease is due to a reduction in the expiratory reserve volume secondary to an increase in tidal volume. Vital capacity, taken in the upright position, remains essentially unchanged throughout pregnancy because of an increase in inspiratory reserve. A significant decrease

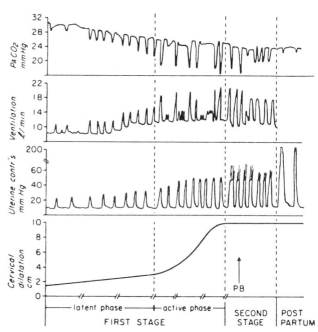

Figure 1.1. The progressive hyperventilation and hypocapnia experienced by the unmedicated woman during successive stages of labor is caused by increasing intensity of painful uterine contractions. Painful expulsion efforts during the second stage result in ventilation nearly double that of early labor, which can be partially relieved by pudendal block (Reprinted by permission from Bonica JJ: *Obstetric Analgesia and Anesthesia*. World Federation of Societies of Anaesthesiologists, Amsterdam, 1980.)

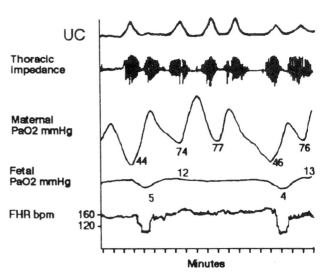

Figure 1.2. Maternal and fetal hypoxia during hypoventilation between contractions is caused by excessive maternal hyperventilation. (Reprinted with permission by Bonica JJ: Labour pain. In *Textbook of Pain*. PD Wall, R Melzack, eds. Churchill Livingstone, Edinburgh, 1984, as redrawn from Huch A, Huch R, Schneider H, Rooth G: Continuous transcutaneous monitoring of fetal oxygen tension during labour. Br J Obstet Gynaecol 84(suppl):1–39, 1977.)

in vital capacity during pregnancy may indicate pulmonary or cardiovascular dysfunction. Earlier data (21) have indicated that total lung capacity at term is decreased about 5% as a result of a 4-cm elevation of the diaphragm caused by the gravid uterus. A later study disputes these findings and indicates there is a 5- to 7-cm increase in chest circumference that compensates for the elevation of the diaphragm (22). Contrary to early reports, the diaphragm is not splinted at term but moves freely (23). Radiographs taken during normal pregnancy show increased lung markings that may simulate mild pulmonary edema (24).

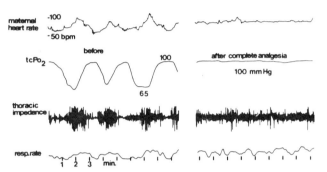

Figure 1.3. Maternal hyperventilation during painful uterine contractions results in hypoventilation between contractions with a corresponding decrease in transcutaneous oxygen tension (tc Po_2) to 65 to 70 mm Hg. After effective epidural analgesia to Po_2 is maintained at a stable 100 mm Hg. (Reprinted by permission from Huch R, Huch A, Lubbers DW: *Transcutaneous PO₂*. Thieme-Stratton, New York, 1981, p 139.)

The supine position markedly impairs respiratory function in late pregnancy. Measurements of closing volume (lung volume during expiration at which airways begin to close in the dependent zones of the lungs) have shown that, in one-third to one-half of supine pregnant women, closing capacity will exceed functional residual capacity (FRC). This means that in the supine position the mother is at risk for hypoxemia as well as impaired organ perfusion (25, 26). One would also expect the pregnant woman to be more susceptible to atelectasis and to develop an increased oxygen alveolar-arterial (A-a) gradient more readily. Although this concept has been challenged (27), most studies in normal parturients demonstrate a wide variability in A-a gradient and dead space to tidal volume ratio (V_D/V_T) (28, 29), which highlights the risk of the supine position. In the upright position, measurements of small airway function (closing volume and flow-volume loops) are similar to nonpregnant values.

Oxygen uptake in pregnancy is markedly increased both at rest (about 20%) and during exercise (30, 31) at term as compared with the nonpregnant state. This is due to an increased maternal metabolism and the increased work required in breathing. Oxygen consumption is increased an additional 63% with painful uterine contractions. Regional analgesia during the first and second stage of labor eliminates this additional increase in oxygen consumption (20). Flow-volume loops, timed forced expiratory volume,

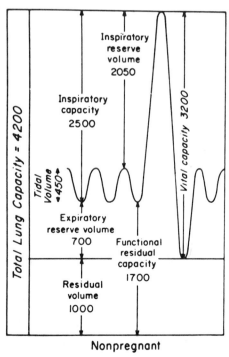

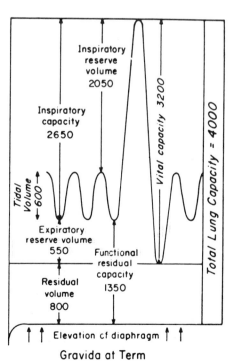

Figure 1.4. Pulmonary volumes and capacities during pregnancy, labor, and postpartum period. (Reprinted by permission from Bonica JJ: *Principles and Practice of Obstetric Analgesia and Anesthesia*, Davis, Philadelphia, 1967.)

and other flow characteristics during pregnancy are little changed from the nonpregnant state (27).

Changes of respiratory function during pregnancy are important to the anesthetist. The decrease in functional residual capacity combined with the increased minute ventilation increases the rapidity of induction with inhalation anesthetics. The decrease in functional residual capacity will increase the uptake of the more insoluble inhalation drugs, whereas the increased minute ventilation hastens the uptake of the more soluble inhalation drugs. In addition, the minimum alveolar concentration (MAC) of potent inhalation drugs was found to be decreased in pregnancy by 24 to 40% in animal studies (32, 33). The above factors combine to increase the parturient's sensitivity to inhalation anesthetic agents. Low concentrations of inhalation gases administered for analgesia may produce general anesthesia with loss of protective airway reflexes. Higher doses, which are safe in the nonpregnant patient, may produce overdosage with cardiopulmonary depression in the parturient.

The decrease in functional residual capacity, increased oxygen consumption, and increased A-a gradient lower the maternal oxygen reserve and make the pregnant patient in labor more vulnerable to hypoxia. This justifies an increased F_{IO_2} in high-risk parturients either in labor or under general anesthesia. Induction of anesthesia with endotracheal intubation in the parturient breathing air, in contrast to the nonparturient, is associated with a more precipitous decrease of PaO_2 after 1 min of apnea (Fig. 1.5) (34). The tendency for rapid development of hypoxia is aggravated by increased oxygen consumption during labor. The risk of hypoxia on induction can be decreased with 2 to 3 min of 100% mask oxygen (35) or by several deep breaths of 100% oxygen before induction of general anesthesia (36). An excellent review of the history and understanding of maternal respiratory and metabolic changes is available (11). The anesthetic significance of the respiratory changes is summarized in Table 1.2.

CARDIOVASCULAR CHANGES DURING PREGNANCY

During pregnancy, numerous changes occur in the cardiovascular system that provide for the needs of the fetus and prepare the mother for delivery (Table 1.3). The diaphragmatic rise shifts the position of the heart leftward and may cause an enlarged appearance on radiographic examination (Fig. 1.6). When compared to nonpregnant women, Doppler and M-mode echocardiography at 38 weeks of gestation indicate an increase in end-diastolic chamber size (4.86 vs. 4.67 cm respectively) and an increase in total left

ventricular wall thickness (2.01 vs. 1.69 cm respectively) (37). Asymptomatic pericardial effusion has been reported in some parturients by echocardiographic examination (38). An innocent grade I to II systolic heart murmur caused by increased blood flow and vasodilation may be heard. The electrocardiogram (ECG) may show an increase in benign dysrhythmia; reversible ST, T, and Q wave changes; and some left axis deviation. These normal findings must

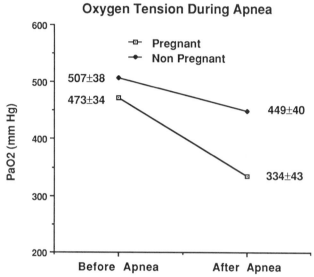

Figure 1.5. Decrease in arterial P_{O_2} after 1 min of apnea in pregnant and nonpregnant patients. (Graph developed from data in Archer GW Jr, Marx GF: Arterial oxygen tension during apnea in parturient women. Br J Anaesth 46:358–360, 1974.)

Table 1.2
Respiratory Changes: Anesthetic Significance

A. Airway management is more challenging
  1. Weight gain and breast engorgement hinder laryngoscopy
  2. Swollen mucosa bleeds easily; avoid intranasal manipulation
  3. Use smaller endotracheal tube (6–7 mm)
B. Response to anesthetics
  1. MAC decreased
  2. Decreased FRC results in faster induction with insoluble agents
  3. Increased VE speeds induction with soluble agents
  4. Rapid overdose with loss of airway reflexes
C. Greater risk of hypoxemia
  1. Decreased FRC means less oxygen reserve
  2. Increased oxygen consumption
  3. Rapid airway obstruction
D. Excessive mechanical hyperventilation ($P_{ET}CO_2 < 24$) may reduce maternal cardiac output and uterine blood flow
E. Maternal and fetal hypoxemia is associated with pain-induced hyper- and hypoventilation; can be avoided with effective analgesia

be differentiated from those indicating heart disease, which include (a) systolic murmur greater than grade III, (b) any diastolic murmur, (c) severe arrhythmias, and (d) unequivocal cardiac enlargement on radiographic examination (24, 39).

Much of the average 28-lb weight gain in pregnancy is attributed to the increase in intravascular and extravascular fluid (Table 1.4). Maternal blood volume markedly increases during pregnancy (Fig. 1.7) (40–42). Plasma volume increases from 40 to 70 ml/kg, and red blood cell volume from 25 to 30 ml/kg. The plasma volume increase may be mediated by

Table 1.3
Changes in Cardiovascular System[a]

Variable	Direction of Change	Average Change
Blood volume	⇑	+35
Plasma volume	⇑	+45%
Red blood cell volume	⇑	+20%
Cardiac output	⇑	+40%
Stroke volume	⇑	+30%
Heart rate	⇑	+15%
Femoral (uterine?) venous pressure	⇑	+15 torr
Total peripheral resistance	⇓	−15%
Mean arterial blood pressure	⇓	−15 torr
Systolic blood pressure	⇓	−0–15 torr
Diastolic blood pressure	⇓	−10–20 torr
Central venous pressure	⇔	No change

[a] Adapted from references 41–51.

a resetting of the osmotic threshold for thirst and vasopressin secretion (43). The increase in maternal blood volume begins in the first trimester, has its maximum rate of increase in the second trimester, and continues to increase at a slower rate early in the third trimester. Contrary to earlier studies conducted with subjects in the supine position, maternal blood volume decreases only slightly, if at all, late in the third trimester (41). Near term there is about a 35 to 40% expansion of the blood volume by 1000 to 1500 ml compared with the nonpregnant state. Much of this increased blood volume perfuses the gravid uterus, and with contractions 300 to 500 ml may be forced from the uterus into the maternal vascular system (42, 44). An average blood loss of less than 500 ml occurs in a normal vaginal delivery. With the uncomplicated vaginal delivery of twins or with cesarean section, maternal blood loss exceeding 1000 ml is rare. The normal nonpregnant blood volume is not reached until 7 to 14 days postpartum (42).

Red blood cell mass increases with pregnancy, but at a slower rate than plasma volume, which accounts for the relative anemia of pregnancy (40). Nevertheless, a hemoglobin of less than 11 g or hematocrit of 33% at any time during pregnancy represents maternal anemia, usually secondary to iron deficiency.

The normal parturient is well prepared to lose considerable blood at the time of delivery and rarely will require transfusion unless blood loss exceeds 1500 ml. Not only does the parturient have an increased

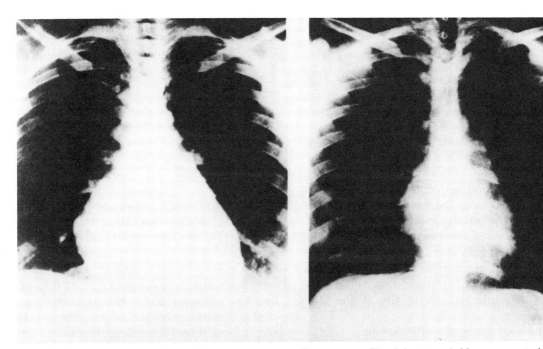

Figure 1.6. Chest radiograph of a woman during pregnancy (*left*) and postpartum (*right*). (Reprinted with permission from Burwell CS, McAnulty JH, Ueland K, eds. *Heart Disease in*

Pregnancy: Physiology and Management. Little, Brown, Boston, 1986, pp 60–63.)

Table 1.4
Distribution of Weight Gain During Pregnancy[a]

Tissue Fluid	Increase in Weight in Grams (and Pounds) up to			
	10 wk	20 wk	30 wk	40 wk
Fetus	5 (0.01)	300 (0.7)	1500 (3.3)	3400 (7.5)
Placenta	20 (0.04)	170 (0.4)	430 (0.9)	650 (1.4)
Amniotic Fluid	30 (0.07)	350 (0.8)	750 (1.7)	800 (1.8)
Uterus	140 (0.3)	320 (0.7)	600 (1.3)	70 (2.1)
Breasts	45 (0.1)	180 (0.4)	360 (0.8)	405 (0.9)
Blood	100 (0.2)	600 (1.3)	1300 (2.9)	1250 (2.8)
Extracellular extravascular fluid (no edema present)	0 (0)	30 (0.06)	80 (0.2)	1680 (3.7)
Subtotal	340 (0.7)	1950 (4.3)	5020 (11.1)	9115 (20.2)
Maternal Reserves	310 (0.7)	2050 (4.5)	3480 (7.7)	3345 (7.4)
Total Weight Gain	650 (1.4)	4000 (8.8)	8500 (18.7)	12,500 (27.5)

[a] Reprinted with permission from Hytten F, Chamberlain G: *Clinical Physiology in Obstetrics*. Blackwell Scientific, Oxford, 1980, p 217.

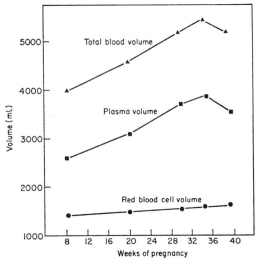

Figure 1.7. Changes in total blood volume, plasma volume, and red blood cell volume in normal pregnancy. Note the continued increase in red blood cell volume and plasma volume late in the third trimester. (Reprinted by permission from Moir DD, Carty MJ: *Obstetric Anesthesia, and Analgesia*. Williams & Wilkins, Baltimore, 1977.)

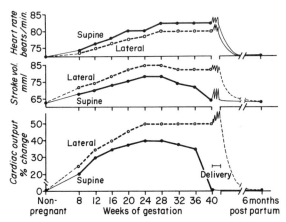

Figure 1.8. Changes in maternal heart rate, stroke volume, and cardiac output during pregnancy with the gravida in the supine and lateral position. These curves are based on data derived from several studies by Ueland (41). (Reprinted by permission from Bonica JJ, ed. *Obstetric Analgesia and Anesthesia*. World Federation of Societies of Anaesthesiologists, Amsterdam, 1980.)

blood volume, but at the time of delivery the uterus contracts, essentially giving an autotransfusion in excess of 500 ml of blood (44). The contracted uterus also effectively decreases the vascular space by the same volume. However, the gravida with hypertension, whether essential or pregnancy induced, usually has a diminished blood volume at term that may be less than that of her normal nonpregnant counterpart (see Chapter 17) (45). Blood loss in these patients is not well tolerated, especially by the fetus before delivery.

During the first trimester of pregnancy, cardiac output is increased approximately 30 to 40%. An additional slight increase occurs during the second trimester. Earlier studies indicate that cardiac output

then falls toward nonpregnant values during the third trimester. These earlier studies, however, were done with the gravid patient supine. Lees et al. (46, 47) and Ueland et al. (48) showed that the pronounced decrease in cardiac output after 28 weeks that occurs in the supine position was due primarily to obstruction of the inferior vena cava. Ueland et al. (48) found a decrease in cardiac output in the sitting and lateral position as the patient approached term, but this decrease was of a much smaller magnitude than that seen in the supine position (Fig. 1.8). Recent invasive human studies agree with these results (Fig. 1.9) (49).

During labor, cardiac output increases with uterine contractions 15% during the latent phase, 30% during the active phase, and 45% during the expulsive stage, compared with prelabor values (50). This increase in cardiac output is due to an increase in

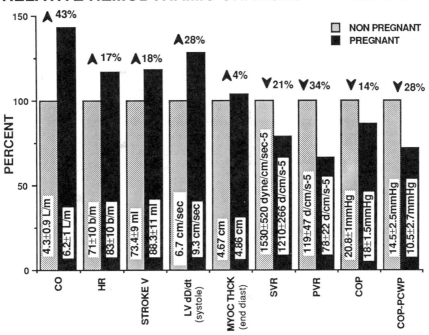

Figure 1.9. Hemodynamic changes of pregnancy from echocardiographic and pulmonary artery catheter monitors in healthy women. *CO* indicates cardiac output; *HR*, heart rate; *Stroke V*, stroke volume; *LV dD/dt (systole)*, left ventricle change (diameter/time); *MYOC THCK (end diastole), myocardial thickness; SVR*, systemic vascular resistance; *PVR*, pulmonary vascular resistance; *COP*, colloid oncotic pressure; *COP – PCWP*, colloid oncotic pressure minus pulmonary capillary wedge pressure. (Data extracted from Robson SC, Hunter S, Moore M, Dunlop W: Haemodynamic changes during the puerperium: A Doppler and M-mode echocardiographic study. Br J Obstet Gynaecol 94:1028–1039, 1987 and Clark SL, Cotton DB, Lee W, Bishop C, Hill T, Southwick J, Pivarnik J, Spillman T, DeVore G, Phelan J, Hankins G, Benedetti TJ, Tolley D: Central hemodynamic assessment of normal term pregnancy. Am J Obstet Gynecol 161:1439–1442, 1989.)

both heart rate and stroke volume (51, 52). Each uterine contraction increases cardiac output an additional 10 to 25% (51). The greatest increase occurs immediately after delivery when the cardiac output is an average of 80% above prelabor values (52); this is attributed to autotransfusion and the increased venous return associated with uterine involution. Cardiac output then gradually declines (52, 53) to nonpregnant levels by 2 weeks after delivery. A detailed review of the endocrinologic influence over the relationship between cardiac output and blood volume is available (54).

Blood pressure is not increased during normal pregnancy because of a 21% and 34% decrease in systemic and pulmonary vascular resistance, respectively. The reported decrease in vessel tone may be mediated in part by α- and β-receptor down-regulation and prostacyclin changes that result in increased renal, uterine, and extremity blood flow (55–58). This may also explain the decreased maternal chronotropic response after the administration of test doses of epinephrine and isoproterenol (59, 60). These changes serve to improve oxygen delivery and dis-

sipate heat generated by increased maternal and fetoplacental metabolism. Despite a general decrease in vascular tone, there is a greater maternal dependence on vasomotor response to maintain hemodynamic stability (61). This explains in part the 50% decrease in maternal blood pressure observed in studies of complete sympathectomy (62). These observations underscore the importance of fluid administration before regional block in pregnancy—a subject that is discussed in greater detail in Chapter 12, on cesarean section. During labor each uterine contraction is associated with a 5 to 20% increase in blood pressure (Fig. 1.10) (44).

Aortocaval Compression

Up to 15% of pregnant patients near term develop signs of shock—including hypotension, pallor, sweating, nausea, vomiting, and changes in cerebration—when they assume the supine position. Howard and co-workers (63) described the syndrome and named it the "supine hypotension syndrome." By injection of radiopaque dye in a femoral vein, Kerr and co-workers (64) showed that the inferior vena

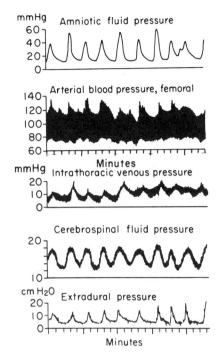

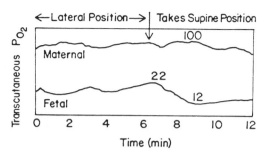

Figure 1.11. Continuous monitoring of maternal and fetal transcutaneous P_{O_2} during labor. Fetal P_{O_2} was monitored using a fetal scalp transcutaneous oxygen electrode. When mother turned from the lateral to the supine position, fetal P_{O_2} promptly decreased. (Modified from Huch A, Huch R, Schneider H, Rooth G: Continuous transcutaneous monitoring of fetal oxygen tension during labour. Br J Obstet Gynaecol 84(suppl):1–39, 1977.)

Figure 1.10. Hemodynamic effects of uterine contractions. Note the increase in arterial blood pressure and central venous pressure, which is reflected in cerebrospinal fluid and extradural pressures. (Reprinted by permission from Bonica JJ: *Obstetric Analgesia and Anesthesia*. World Federation of Societies of Anaesthesiologists, Amsterdam, 1980.)

cava was totally obstructed by the gravid uterus in the supine position. In part, blood from below the obstructed inferior vena cava returned to the heart via the paravertebral (epidural) veins emptying into the azygos system. Turning the gravid patient on her side partially relieved the obstruction of the vena cava. The maternal symptoms of supine hypotension were attributed to lack of venous return to the heart. Compression of the inferior vena cava is most common late in pregnancy before the presenting fetal part becomes fixed in the pelvis. This compression produces pooling of venous blood and increased venous pressure in the lower torso and lower extremities, which may explain the tendency toward phlebitis and the development of venous varicosities in pregnancy. The increase in uterine venous pressure may affect the well-being of the fetus through a resultant decrease in uterine blood flow. Blood flow to the uterus is directly related to the perfusion pressure, that is, uterine artery minus venous pressure. In the supine position, even without arterial hypotension, uterine perfusion pressure decreases as a result of the increased uterine venous pressure.

Bieniarz and co-workers (65) produced serial radiographs of the aorta in 70 subjects after injection of radiopaque dye in the femoral arteries and found the aorta to be partially occluded when the gravid subject

was supine. Compression of the aorta is not associated with maternal symptoms but causes arterial hypotension in the lower extremities and uterine arteries, which can further decrease uterine blood flow and result in fetal asphyxia and fetal distress (66). Hence, even with normal upper extremity maternal blood pressure, uteroplacental perfusion may decrease in the supine position. Kauppila et al (67) found that turning the mother at term from the left lateral to the supine position decreased the intervillous blood flow by 20%. Similarly Huch and co-workers (16) demonstrated a 40% decrease in transcutaneous fetal oxygen tension when the mother was turned from the lateral to the supine position (Fig. 1.11).

It is imperative that the anesthetist appreciate the importance of the syndrome now called aortocaval compression and realize that anesthesia may augment its signs and symptoms. The ill effects of aortocaval compression on the mother and fetus may manifest as early as the 20th week of gestation. Drugs causing vasodilation, such as halothane and thiopental, or techniques causing sympathetic blockade, such as subarachnoid or epidural block, will further decrease venous return to the heart in the presence of vena caval obstruction. The sympathetic block impairs the parturient's ability to compensate for the decreased venous return by vasoconstriction. Thus arterial hypotension is much more common and severe during anesthesia in pregnancy compared with the nonpregnant state (62).

Prevention of aortocaval compression is preferred to treatment. The gravida at term should never be allowed to assume the supine position (Fig. 1.12). Abnormal fetal heart rate patterns indicating uteroplacental insufficiency are frequently observed in parturients placed in the supine position, particularly in the presence of major conduction or general

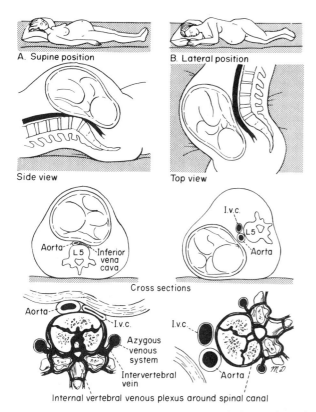

Figure 1.12. Lateral and cross-sectional views of uterine aortocaval compression in the supine position and its resolution by lateral positioning of the pregnant woman. (Reprinted by permission from Bonica JJ: *Obstetric Analgesia and Anesthesia.* World Federation of Societies of Anaesthesiologists, Amsterdam, 1980.)

anesthesia. Prevention of aortocaval compression consists of left uterine displacement (LUD), which can be accomplished by manual displacement of the uterus in which the uterus is lifted and displaced to the left. Alternatively, the patient may be positioned on her left side either by tipping the operating or delivery table 15 degrees to the left or by using sheets, a foam rubber wedge, or an inflatable bag to elevate the right buttock and back 10 to 15 cm. Stationary left uterine displacers such as the one designed by Colon-Morales (68), which is placed under the patient's right hip, are effective. In about 10% of women, right uterine displacement is more effective than LUD. This is demonstrated if maternal vital signs or the fetal heart rate pattern are more favorable in the right uterine displaced position. Placing the patient in the Trendelenburg position without LUD is an inappropriate means of prophylaxis and may actually worsen the condition by shifting the uterus further back onto the vena cava and aorta. An unusually large uterus, such as seen with twins or polyhydramnios, may require as much as 30 degrees of uterine displacement to avoid aortocaval compression (69). Intense

bearing down during the second stage of labor has also been shown to cause aortocaval compression (70). During cesarean section, neonates from mothers with uterine displacement had less frequent and less severe depression by Apgar score and less acidosis than those from mothers in the supine position (71). If hypotension develops in the gravid patient near term, one should immediately suspect inferior vena caval occlusion and displace the uterus to the left without delay.

Oxygen transport during pregnancy is increased. Although a lower hematocrit decreases oxygen-carrying capacity from 19.5 to 16.0 vol/100 ml, this is overcome by other compensatory changes. Increased ventilation in pregnancy results in arterial oxygen tensions averaging 103 torr. Increased cardiac output, vasodilation of the uterus and kidneys, and hemodilution increase blood flow to important target organs. Kambam and co-workers (72) have shown that the maternal oxyhemoglobin dissociation P_{50} is shifted to the right from 26.7 to 30.2 mm Hg at term. This increases the available oxygen at the tissue level.

There is a 14% decline in plasma colloid oncotic pressure (COP) (20.8 ± 1 mm Hg to 18 ± 1.5 mm Hg) that may favor mild edema formation in late pregnancy (55). A reported 28% decline in plasma colloid oncotic pressure to pulmonary capillary wedge pressure gradient (14.5 ± 2.5 to 10.5 ± 2.7 mm Hg) (Fig. 1.9) implies a tendency to develop pulmonary edema in the presence of altered pulmonary capillary permeability or markedly increased cardiac preload (49). After delivery COP often decreases further. Combined with sustained high cardiac output, women with severe preeclampsia or who have recently received β-agonist therapy are at particular risk for pulmonary edema in the postpartum period. In a recent series, radiolabeled interstitial lung water increased in 7 of 20 normal pregnant women. This was not associated with an increased incidence of pulmonary edema (73).

The clotting factor substrate increases as gestation progresses. Thus the pregnant woman becomes hypercoagulable as gestation progresses. This, combined with rapid myometrial contraction during placental separation, avoids excessive maternal blood loss at delivery. These changes also place the pregnant woman at greater risk for deep vein thrombosis. Factors VII, VIII, and X and, particularly, plasma fibrinogen are markedly increased after the third month of gestation (Table 1.5). A 20% decline in the platelet count seen at term does not influence bleeding time (74). Fibrinolysis, formerly thought to be depressed in pregnancy, has been shown to be normal, but levels of plasminogen activator are depressed as a result of sequestration at sites of fibrin deposition (75). Leukocyte

Table 1.5
Coagulation Factors and Inhibitors during Normal Pregnancy[a]

Factor	Nonpregnant	Late Pregnancy
Factor I (fibrinogen)	200–450 mg/dL	400–650 mg/dL
Factor II (prothrombin)	75–125%	100–125%
Factor V	75–125%	100–150%
Factor VII	75–125%	150–250%
Factor VIII	75–150%	200–500%
Factor IX	75–125%	100–150%
Factor X	75–125%	150–250%
Factor XI	5–125%	50–100%
Factor XII	75–125%	100–200%
Factor XIII	75–125%	35– 75%
Antithrombin III	85–110%	75–100%
Antifactor Xa	85–110%	75–100%

[a] Reprinted by permission from Hathaway WE, Bonnar J: Coagulation in pregnancy. In *Perinatal Coagulation*. WE Hathaway, J Bonnar, eds. Grune & Stratton, New York, 1978.

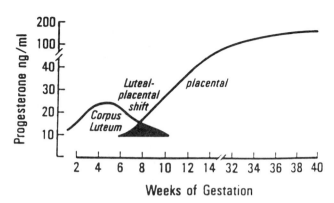

Figure 1.13. A shift of progesterone production from the corpus luteum to the placenta occurs at approximately the eighth to ninth week of gestation. The black area represents the estimated duration for this functional transition. (Reprinted by permission from Yen SCC: Endocrine and other evaluations of the fetal environment. In *Maternal-Fetal Medicine: Principles and Practice*. 2nd ed. RK Creasy, R Resnik, eds. WB Saunders, Philadelphia, 1989, p 376.)

Table 1.6
Cardiovascular Changes: Anesthetic Significance

A. Venodilation may increase the incidence of accidental epidural vein puncture.

B. Healthy parturient will tolerate up to 1500 ml blood loss; transfusion rarely required (hemorrhage at delivery remains an important risk).

C. Oxytocin with a free water IV infusion may lead to fluid overload.

D. High hemoglobin level (>14) indicates low-volume state caused by preeclampsia, hypertension, or inappropriate diuretics.

E. Cardiac output remains high in first few hours postpartum; women with cardiac or pulmonary disease remain at risk after delivery.

F. Epidural block reduces cardiac work during labor and may be beneficial in some cardiac disease states.

G. Maternal blood pressure of <90 to 95 torr during regional block should be of concern because it may be associated with a proportional decrease in uterine blood flow.

H. ALWAYS AVOID AORTOCAVAL COMPRESSION: 70 to 80% of supine parturients with a T4 sympathectomy develop significant hypotension.

levels increase during pregnancy to a high of 12,000 to 21,000/ml during the third trimester; this has been attributed to increases in plasma-free cortisol and estrogen levels (74). An excellent review of the history of maternal cardiovascular physiology research is available (24). The anesthetic significance of the cardiovascular changes is summarized in Table 1.6.

NERVOUS SYSTEM CHANGES DURING PREGNANCY

Anesthetic requirement (MAC) for inhalation agents is decreased up to 40% during pregnancy, as measured

in animals (32, 33). Thus concentrations of inhalation agents that would not produce loss of consciousness in the surgical patient may cause unconsciousness in the parturient patient, thereby subjecting her to the dangers of airway obstruction, vomiting, and aspiration. The mechanism for the decrease in MAC is uncertain, but hormonal, serotonergic, and endogenous opiate changes during pregnancy may be responsible. Progesterone, the levels of which increases 10-to 20-fold (Fig. 1.13) during late pregnancy (76, 77), has a sedative activity (78) and in large doses induces loss of consciousness in humans (79).

The role of endorphins in pregnancy is incompletely understood. Maternal β-endorphin blood levels become increased during gestation (80–82). They increase significantly in most parturients during labor and delivery; the increase is proportional to the frequency and duration of uterine contractions, which reflects the stress of labor (82–86). Cesarean section performed with the patient under general anesthesia is associated with a marked increase of β-endorphin levels (87). Lumbar epidural analgesia itself is not associated with an increase in β-endorphin and blocks its elevation in labor, vaginal delivery, and cesarean section. This indicates that major conduction analgesia decreases the stress of labor, which might be an advantage in the high-risk parturient. The effects of physiologic increases in β-endorphines on the subjective responses to the pain of parturition or MAC is unclear (83, 86, 88).

Gintzler (88) found that, during pregnancy in rats, a progressive increase in pain tolerance can be abolished by a long-term administration of a narcotic antagonist. Steinbrook found that, whereas plasma β-endorphin levels increased in pregnancy and during labor, cerebrospinal fluid (CSF) levels remained unchanged (82). Guistino and co-workers (89) reported that women who exercised in pregnancy, when compared with controls, had 34% higher plasma β-endorphin levels at the end of labor (~59 pg vs. ~44 pg) and lower visual analog pain scores (60 vs. 85). Although this was statistically significant, one must question the clinical difference in terms of discomfort levels. Intrathecal administration of β-endorphin in higher than physiologic concentrations produces effective analgesia during labor (90). Thus a pregnancy-induced activation of the endorphin system may contribute to a decreased anesthetic requirement.

Circulatory changes within the vertebral column have important effects on subarachnoid and epidural techniques of regional analgesia. As a result of increased intraabdominal pressure, epidural veins become engorged, making accidental intravascular injection during lumbar epidural or caudal epidural block common. Baseline extradural pressures are higher ($+1$ cm H_2O) in full-term parturients than in nonpregnant women (-1 cm H_2O). As labor progresses this pressure increases steadily to reach 4 to 10 cm H_2O at the conclusion of the first stage of labor (Fig. 1.10). Second-stage bearing-down efforts can raise the extradural pressure to 60 cm H_2O (91) as a result of progressive venous engorgement and the muscle activity of bearing down. CSF pressures in the second stage of labor may reach 70 cm H_2O during contractions and bearing-down efforts. The use of the hanging drop technique to identify the epidural space and entering the space during a contraction may increase the hazard of dural puncture. Although injection of local anesthetics into the epidural space during a contraction in the first stage of labor has been shown to have no effect on the resulting level of anesthetic block (92), such injections in the subarachnoid space during contractions may produce increased upward spread of the block, especially if the mother strains.

The gravid patient requires less local anesthetic to produce the same level of spinal or epidural block than does her nonpregnant counterpart (93–95). Some authors suggest that the epidural volume dose for patients during cesarean section is no different than for nonpregnant surgery patients (96, 97). However, in one study (96) the nonpregnant group was unusually obese and not a valid control. Close inspection of the second study (97) shows a small but evident decrease in epidural dose requirements for cesarean section. In the past this decrease in local anesthesia requirement was explained completely by the engorgement of epidural veins, which decreased the volume of the epidural space and prevented loss of local anesthetic solution through the intervertebral foramina (98, 99). More recently it has been suggested that acid-base changes in CSF (94, 100) and/or hormonal changes such as high progesterone levels may increase nerve sensitivity to local anesthetics (101–103). Datta and co-workers have shown an increase in human CSF progesterone levels in pregnant (122 ± 8 ng) compared with nonpregnant women (61 ± 2.3 ng) (104). Lidocaine blockade of the median nerve was faster in pregnant (4 min) compared with nonpregnant (11.5 min) patients (105). However, progesterone applied directly to nerve-conduction preparations does not affect local anesthesia conduction blockade (106). It is suggested that the increased sensitivity to conduction blockade seen with chronic progesterone treatment in animals (102) is an indirect effect that requires some time. Likewise, the 30 to 50% reduction of local anesthetic required to produce a similar level of subarachnoid block in the gravid patient may be explained by (a) swelling of the epidural veins, which decreases the volume of CSF in the vertebral column; (b) labor-induced increases in CSF pressure (80); and (c) increased neurosensitivity to local anesthetics. Although CSF protein binding of local anesthetics does not appear to be altered in pregnancy (98, 99), the increased lumbar lordosis of pregnancy may enhance cephalad spread of local anesthetic solutions placed in the CSF. Several studies have shown that the duration and maximal level of block obtained with both epidural and subarachnoid analgesia begin to decline in the first 3 postpartum days (108–110).

GASTROINTESTINAL CHANGES DURING PREGNANCY

Pregnancy is associated with a shift in the position of the stomach caused by the gravid uterus, which changes the angle of the gastroesophageal junction (111). This frequently results in incompetence of the gastroesophageal pinchcock mechanism, which allows gastric reflux and production of esophagitis and heartburn in 45 to 70% of pregnant women (112). It makes the parturient prone to silent regurgitation, active vomiting, and aspiration during general anesthesia or impaired consciousness from any cause. Although the decrease in gastric motility and emptying time in pregnancy has been debated in recent years (113), there is general agreement that stomach emptying time is prolonged in pregnancy and this increases the parturient's risk of pulmonary aspiration (114, 115). The enlarged uterus displaces the pylorus upward and backward and may retard gastric emptying. The hormone gastrin produced by the placenta raises the acid, chloride, and enzyme content of the stomach to levels above normal (116–118).

Investigations by Roberts and Shirley (117, 118) indicated that approximately 25% of parturients undergoing elective cesarean section after an overnight fast were considered at risk for aspiration because they had a gastric volume in excess of 25 ml with a pH of less than 2.5. Another study of women shortly after delivery found a gastric pH of less than 2.5 in all and a gastric volume of 25 ml in 60% (119). Intragastric pressure is increased during the last weeks of pregnancy and may reach levels exceeding 40 cm H_2O in cases of obesity, multiple gestation, and hydramnios (120). Epidural analgesia has minimal effects on gastric emptying (121). Narcotics delay stomach-emptying time (122), and narcotics and anticholinergics decrease lower gastroesophageal tone (123–126). All parturients must be considered at risk for pulmonary aspiration of both acid material, causing the acid aspiration syndrome of Mendelson (127), and solid material, associated with atelectasis, lung abscess, and mechanical obstruction. The magnitude and prevention of this problem are considered in Chapter 23.

RENAL CHANGES DURING PREGNANCY

Renal plasma flow (RPF) and glomerular filtration rate (GFR) increases rapidly to 50 to 60% above nonpregnant values by the fourth month of gestation (128). Increased aldosterone levels contribute to increased total body water and sodium. The threshold for antidiuretic hormone (ADH) secretion may be reset, which contributes to decreased plasma osmolality and slightly lower plasma sodium levels. During the third trimester RPF and GFR slowly return toward normal. Compression of the aorta caused by the gravid uterus in the supine patient may decrease renal blood flow to levels below those preceding pregnancy. The high RPF and GFR result in an increase in creatinine clearance. The upper limits of normal for blood urea nitrogen (BUN) and serum creatinine values are lower in the pregnant woman. There is a 40% reduction in BUN to 8 or 9 mg/dl^{-1} and in creatinine to 0.46 mg/dl^{-1} during a normal pregnancy. Tubular reabsorption of electrolytes and water increases in proportion to the GFR; therefore no loss or accumulation of electrolytes occurs. Plasma renin activity is increased, as is the renin substrate angiotensin to which the normal gravid patient has decreased sensitivity (129, 130). Glucosuria of 1 to 10 g/day and proteinuria of up to 300 mg/day are common and may not be associated with any pathologic condition (131).

Renal calyces, pelves, and ureters dilate after the third month of gestation. Early dilation is due to progesterone production, which induces atony of the calyces and ureters (132). Later the ureters are com-

pressed at the pelvic brim by the enlarging uterus, further contributing to this dilation. The resulting urinary stasis contributes to the frequency of urinary tract infections during pregnancy.

HEPATIC AND ENDOCRINE CHANGES DURING PREGNANCY

Increased serum glutamic-oxaloacetic transaminase, lactic dehydrogenase, alkaline phosphatase, and cholesterol levels are common during pregnancy and labor, with 80% of parturients having an abnormal bromsulfopthalein excretion test result (133, 134). These abnormal liver function test results do not necessarily indicate hepatic disease. Serum bilirubin and hepatic blood flow are unaltered. Both total protein and the albumin-to-globulin ratio are decreased in pregnancy (135). Decreased serum albumin levels may result in higher free blood levels of some substances that are highly protein bound.

Average serum cholinesterase activity is reduced 24% before delivery and 33% at 3 days postpartum, returning to normal by 2 to 6 weeks postpartum (136, 137). Despite these lower levels of activity, prolonged respiratory impairment rarely occurs following appropriate doses of succinylcholine (136, 138). This may be due to a larger volume of distribution for serum cholinesterase at term and agrees with the prolonged succinylcholine block seen in the first postpartum days as this volume rapidly contracts (139). Prolonged neuromuscular impairment, rarely lasting more than 20 min, has been reported in 2 to 6% of parturients having genotypically normal but often low levels of serum pseudocholinesterase (136–144). Dehydration, acidosis, diabetes mellitus, electrolyte abnormalities, and magnesium, trimethaphan, and cholinesterase inhibitors may depress or interact with serum cholinesterase activity (137, 140). These conditions have been associated with prolonged recovery from succinylcholine. Monitoring muscle twitch with a nerve stimulator when succinylcholine is used in the gravid patient is useful in preventing prolonged muscle weakness (145). The hydrolysis of 2-chloroprocaine, which requires serum pseudocholinesterase, appears normal in the parturient (146).

Although pregnancy is associated with mild thyroid gland hypertrophy, free thyroxine and triiodothyronine levels remain normal (6). Profound alterations in gestational hormones are thoroughly reviewed by Cunningham and co-authors (147).

References

1. Hytten F, Chamberlain G: *Clinical Physiology in Obstetrics*, 2nd ed. Blackwell Scientific Publications, Oxford, 1980.
2. Metcalfe J, Stock MK, Barron DH: Maternal physiology dur-

ing gestation. In *The Physiology of Reproduction*. K Knobil, L Ewing, eds. Raven Press, New York, 1988, pp 2145–2176.

3. Weinberger SE, Weiss ST, Cohen WR, Weiss JW, Johnson TS: Pregnancy and the lung. Am Rev Respir Dis 121:559–581, 1980.

4. Conklin K: Maternal physiological adaptations during gestation, labor and the puerperium. Semin Anesth 10:221–234, 1991.

5. Camann WR, Ostheimer GW: Physiological adaptations during pregnancy. Int Anesth Clin 28:2–10, 1990.

6. Cohen S: Physiologic alterations of pregnancy: Anesthetic implications. In ASA Refresher Course Lectures. San Francisco, JB Lippincott, Hagerstown, MD, 1991, No 211.

7. Mackenzie AI: Laryngeal oedema complicating obstetric anaesthesia. Anaesthesia 33:271, 1978.

8. Procter AJM, White JB: Laryngeal edema in pregnancy. Anaesthesia 38:167, 1983.

9. Heller PJ, Scheider EP, Marx GF: Pharyngolaryngeal edema as a presenting symptom in pre-eclampsia. Obstet Gynecol 62:523–527, 1983.

10. Datta S, Briwa J: Modified laryngoscope for endotracheal intubation of obese patients. Anesth Analg 60:120–122, 1981.

11. Prowse CM, Gaensler EA: Respiratory acid base changes during pregnancy. Anesthesiology 26:381–392, 1965.

12. Pernoll ML, Metcalf J, Kovach PA, Wachtel R, Dunham MJ: Ventilation during rest and exercise in pregnancy and postpartum. Resp Physiol 25:295–310, 1975.

13. Clapp JF II, Seaward BL, Sleamaker RH, Hiser J: Maternal physiologic adaptations to early human pregnancy. Am J Obstet Gynecol 159:1456–1460, 1988.

14. Lyons HA, Antonio R: The sensitivity of the respiratory center in pregnancy and after the administration of progesterone. Trans Assoc Amer Physicians 72:173–180, 1959.

15. Bonica JJ: Labour pain. In *Textbook of Pain*. PD Wall, R Melzack, eds. Churchill Livingstone, Edinburgh, 1984, pp 377–392.

16. Huch A, Huch R, Schneider H, Rooth G: Continuous transcutaneous monitoring of fetal oxygen tension during labour. Br J Obstet Gynaecol (suppl) 84:1–39, 1977.

17. Fisher A, Prys-Roberts C: Maternal pulmonary gas exchange: A study during normal labor and extradural blockade. Anaesthesia 23:350–356, 1968.

18. Peabody JL: Transcutaneous oxygen measurement to evaluate drug effects. Clin Perinatol 6:109–121, 1979.

19. Sangoul F, Fox GS, Houle GL: Effect of regional analgesia on maternal oxygen consumption during the first stage of labor. Am J Obstet Gynecol 121:1080–1083, 1975.

20. Hagerdal M, Morgan CW, Sumner AE, Gutsche BB: Minute ventilation and oxygen consumption during labor with epidural analgesia. Anesthesiology 59:425–427, 1983.

21. Cugell DW, Frank NR, Gaensler EA: Pulmonary function in pregnancy. I. Serial observations in normal women. Am Rev Tuberc 67:568–599, 1953.

22. Leontic EA: Respiratory disease in pregnancy. Med Clin North Am 61:111–128, 1977.

23. McGinty AP: The comparative effects of pregnancy and phrenic nerve interruption on the diaphragm and their relation to pulmonary tuberculosis. Am J Obstet Gynecol 35:237–248, 1938.

24. Metcalf J, McAnulty JH, Ueland K: Burwell and Metcalfe's Heart Disease and Pregnancy: Physiology and Management. 2nd ed. Boston, Little, Brown, 1986, p 25.

25. Bevan DR, Holdcroft A, Loh L, MacGregor WG, O'Sullivan JC: Closing volume and pregnancy. Br Med J 1:13–15, 1974.

26. Russell IF, Chambers WA: Closing volume in normal pregnancy. Br J Anaesth 53:1043–1047, 1981.

27. Baldwin GR, Moorthi DS, Whelton JA, MacDonnell K: New lung functions and pregnancy. Am J Obstet Gynecol 127:235–239, 1977.

28. Awe RJ, Nicotra MB, Newsom TD, Viles R: Arterial oxygenation and alveolar-arterial gradients in term pregnancy. Obstet Gynecol 53:182–186, 1979.

29. Lyons G, Tunstall GL: Maternal blood gas tensions (PAO$_2$-PaO$_2$) physiological shunt and VD/VT during general anaesthesia for caesarean section. Br J Anaesth 51:1059–1062, 1979.

30. Clapp JF, III: Oxygen consumption during treadmill exercise before, during and after pregnancy. Am J Obstet Gynecol 161:1458–1464, 1989.

31. McMurray RG, Katz VL, Berry MJ, Cefalo RC: The effect of pregnancy on metabolic responses during rest, immersion, and aerobic exercise in the water. Am J Obstet Gynecol 158:481–486, 1988.

32. Palahniuk RJ, Shnider SM, Eger EI II: Pregnancy decreases the requirements for inhaled anesthetic agents. Anesthesiology 41:82–83, 1974.

33. Datta S, Migliozzi RP, Flanagan HL, Krieger NR: Chronically administered progesterone decreases halothane requirements in rabbits. Anesth Analg 68:46–50, 1989.

34. Archer GW Jr, Marx GF: Arterial oxygen tension during apnea in parturient women. Br J Anaesth 46:358–360, 1974.

35. Byrne F, Oduro-Dominah A, Kipling R: The effect of pregnancy on pulmonary nitrogen washout. Anaesthesia 42:148–150, 1987.

36. Norris MC, Kirkland MR, Torjman MC, Goldberg ME: Denitrogenation in pregnancy. Can J Anaesth 36:523–525, 1989.

37. Robson SC, Hunter S, Moore M, Dunlop W: Haemodynamic changes during the puerperium: A doppler and M-mode echocardiographic study. Br J Obstet Gynaecol 94:1028–1039, 1987.

38. Enein M, Zina AA, Kassem M, el-Tabbakh G: Echocardiography of the pericardium in pregnancy. Obstet Gynecol 69:851–853, 1987.

39. Elkayam U, Gleicher N: Hemodynamics and cardiac function during normal pregnancy and the puerperium. In *Cardiac Problems in Pregnancy*. U Elkayam, N Gleicher, eds. Alan R Liss, New York, 1990, pp 5–24.

40. Assali NS, Brinkman CR III: Disorders of maternal cirulatory and respiratory adjustments. In *Pathophysiology of Gestation: Maternal Disorders, Vol 1*. NS Assali, CR Brinkman III, eds. Academic, New York, 1972, pp 278–285.

41. Ueland K: Maternal cardiovascular dynamics. VII. Intrapartum blood volume changes. Am J Obstet Gynecol 126:671–677, 1976.

42. Pritchard JA: Changes in blood volume during pregnancy and delivery. Anesthesiology 26:393–399, 1965.

43. Lindheimer MD, Barron WM, Durr J, Davison JM: Water homeostasis and vasopressin release during rodent and human gestation. Am J Kidney Dis 9:270–275, 1987.

44. Hendricks CH: Hemodynamics of a uterine contraction. Am J Obstet Gynecol 76:968–982, 1958.

45. Goodlin RC, Dobry CA, Anderson JC, Woods RE, Quaile M: Clinical signs of normal volume expansion during pregnancy. Am J Obstet Gynecol 145:1001–1009, 1983.

46. Lees MM, Taylor SH, Scott DB: A study of cardiac output at rest throughout pregnancy. J Obstet Gynaecol Br Commonw 74:319–328, 1967.

47. Lees MM, Scott DB, Kerr MG: The circulatory effects of recumbent postural change in late pregnancy. Clin Sci 32:453–465, 1967.

48. Ueland K, Novy MJ, Peterson EN: Maternal cardiovascular dynamics. IV. The influence of gestational age on the maternal cardiovascular response to posture and exercise. Am J Obstet Gynecol 104:856–864, 1969.

49. Clark SL, Cotton DB, Lee W, Bishop C, Hill T, Southwick J, Pivarnik J, Spillman T, DeVore G, Phelan J, Hankins G, Benedetti TJ, Tolley D: Central hemodynamic assessment of normal term pregnancy. Am J Obstet Gynecol 161:1439–1442, 1989.

50. Ueland K, Hansen JM: Maternal cardiovascular dynamics. III. Labor and delivery under local and caudal analgesia. Am J Obstet Gynecol 103:8–18, 1969.

51. Ueland K, Hansen JM: Maternal cardiovascular dynamics. II. Posture and uterine contractions. Am J Obstet Gynecol 103:1–7, 1969.

52. Hansen JM, Ueland K: The influence of caudal analgesia on cardiovascular dynamics during labour and delivery. Acta Anaesthesiol Scand 23(suppl):449–452, 1966.

53. Walters WAW, McGregor WG, Hills M: Cardiac output at rest, during pregnancy and the puerperium. Clin Sci 30:1–11, 1966.

54. Longo LD: Maternal blood volume and cardiac output during pregnancy: A hypothesis of enocrinologic control. Am J Physiol 245:R720–R729, 1983.

55. Oian P, Maltau JM, Noddeland H, Fadnes HO: Oedema: Preventing mechanisms in subcutaneous tissue of normal pregnant women. Br J Obstet Gynaecol 92:1113–1119, 1985.

56. Goodman RP, Killom AP, Brash AR, Branch RA: Prostacyclin production during pregnancy: Comparison of production during normal pregnancy and pregnancy complicated by hypertension. Am J Obstet Gynecol 142:817–822, 1982.

57. Ylikorkala O, Jouppila P, Kirkinen P, Viinikka L: Maternal prostacyclin, thromboxane, and placental blood flow. Am J Obstet Gynecol 145:730–732, 1983.

58. Clark KE, Austin JE, Seeds AE: Effect of bisenoic prostaglandins and arachidonic acid on the uterine vasculature of pregnant sheep. Am J Obstet Gynecol 142:261–268, 1982.

59. DeSimone CA, Leighton BL, Norris MC, Chayen B, Menduke H: The chronotropic effect of isoproteronol is reduced in term pregnant women. Anesthesiology 69:626–628, 1988.

60. Paller MS: Decreased pressor responsiveness in pregnancy: Studies in experimental animals. Am J Kidney Dis 9:308–311, 1987.

61. Goodlin RC: Venous reactivity and pregnancy abnormalities. Acta Obstet Gynecol Scand 65:345–348, 1986.

62. Assali NS, Prystowsky H: Studies on autonomic blockade. I. Comparison between the effects of tetraethyl ammonium chloride (TEAC) and high selective spinal anesthesia on the blood pressure of normal and toxemic pregnancy. J Clin Invest 29:1354–1366, 1950.

63. Howard BK, Goodson JH, Mengert WF: Supine hypotension syndrome in late pregnancy. Obstet Gynecol 1:371–377, 1953.

64. Kerr MG, Scott DB, Samule E: Studies of the inferior vena cava in late pregnancy. Br Med J 1:532–533, 1964.

65. Bieniarz I, Crottogini JJ, Curachet E: Aortocaval compression by the uterus in late human pregnancy. Am J Obstet Gynecol 100:203–217, 1968.

66. Marx GF: Aortocaval compression: Incidence and prevention. Bull NY Acad Med 50:443–446, 1974.

67. Kauppila A, Kokinen M, Puolakka J, Tuimala R, Kuikka J: Decreased intervillous and unchanged myometrial blood flow in supine recumbency. Obstet Gynecol 55:203–205, 1980.

68. Colon-Morales MA: A self-supporting device for continuous left uterine displacement during cesarean section. Anesth Analg 49:223–224, 1970.

69. Kim YI, Chandra P, Marx GF: Successful management of severe aortocaval compression in twin pregnancy. Obstet Gynecol 46:362–364, 1975.

70. Bassell GM, Humayun SG, Marx GF: Maternal bearing down efforts—another fetal risk? Obstet Gynecol 56:39–41, 1980.

71. Crawford JS: Anesthesia for section: Further refinements of a technique. Br J Anaesth 45:726–731, 1973.

72. Kambam JR, Handte RE, Brown WU Jr, Smith BE: Effect of normal and preeclamptic pregnancies on the oxyhemoglobin dissociation curve. Anesthesiology 65:426–427, 1986.

73. Maclennan FM, MacDonald AF, Campbell DM: Lung water during the puerperium. Anaesthesia 42:141–147, 1987.

74. Pitkin RM, Witte DL: Platelet and leukocyte counts in pregnancy. JAMA 242:2696–2698, 1979.

75. Fletcher AP, Alkjaersig NK, Burstein R: The influence of pregnancy upon blood coagulation and plasma fibrinolytic function. Am J Obstet Gynecol 134:743–751, 1979.

76. Yannone ME, McCurcy JR, Goldfein A: Plasma progesterone levels in normal pregnancy, labor and the puerperium. II. Clinical data. Am J Obstet Gynecol 101:1058–1061, 1968.

77. Datta S, Hurley RJ, Naulty SJ, Stern P, Lambert D, Concepcion M, Tulchinsky D, Weiss J, Ostheimer GW: Plasma and cerebrospinal fluid progesterone levels in pregnant and nonpregnant women. Anesth Analg 65:950–954, 1986.

78. Selye H: Studies concerning the anesthetic action of steroid hormones. J Pharmacol Exp Ther 73:127–141, 1941.

79. Merryman W: Progesteron "anesthesia" in human subjects. J Clin Endocrinol Metab 14:1567–1569, 1954.

80. Houck JC, Kimball C, Chang C, Pedigo NW, Yamamura HI: Placental β-endorphin-like peptides. Science 207:78–80, 1980.

81. Csontos K, Rust M, Halt V, Mahr W, Kromer W, Teschemacher HJ: Elevated plasma β-endorphin levels in pregnant women and their neonates. Life Sci 25:835–844, 1979.

82. Steinbrook RA, Carr DB, Datta S, Naulty JS, Lee C, Fisher J: Dissociation of plasma and cerebrospinal fluid beta-endorphin immunoreactivity levels during pregnancy and parturition. Anesth Analg 61:893–897, 1982.

83. Pilkington JW, Nemeroff CB, Mason GA, Prange AJ: Increase in plasma β-endorphin like immunoreactivity at parturition in normal women. Am J Obstet Gynecol 145:111–113, 1983.

84. Facchinetti F, Centini G, Parrini D, Petraglia F, D'Antona N, Cosmi EV, Genazzani AR: Opioid plasma levels during labour. Gynecol Obstet Invest 13:155–163, 1982.

85. Fletcher JE, Thomas TA, Hill RG: β-endorphins and parturition. Lancet 1:310, 1980.

86. Thomas TA, Fletcher JE, Hill RG: Influence of medication, pain and progress in labour on plasma β-endorphin-like immunoreactivity. Br J Anaesth 54:401–408, 1982.

87. Abboud TK, Noueihid R, Khoo S, Hoffman DI, Varakian L, Henriksen E, Goebelsmann U: Effect of induction of general and regional anesthesia for cesarean section and maternal plasma β-endorphin levels. Am J Obstet Gynecol 146:927–930, 1983.

88. Gintzler AR: Endorphin-mediated increases in pain threshold during pregnancy. Science 210:193–195, 1980.

89. Guistino V, Bazzano C, Edwards WT: Effects of physical activity on maternal plasma β-endorphin levels and perception of labor pain. Am J Obstet Gynecol 160:707–712, 1989.

90. Oyama T, Akitoma M, Takeo T, Ling N, Guillemin R: Beta-endorphin in obstetric analgesia. Am J Obstet Gynecol 137:613–616, 1980.

91. Galbert MW, Marx GF: Extradural pressures in the parturient patient. Anesthesiology 40:499–502, 1974.

92. Sivakumaran C, Ramanathan S, Chalon J, Turndorf H: Uterine contractions and the spread of local anesthetics in the epidural space. Anesth Analg 61:127–129, 1982.

93. Bonica JJ: Maternal physiologic and psychologic alterations. In *Obstetric Anesthesia and Perinatology*. E Cosmi, ed. Appleton-Century-Crofts, New York, 1981, pp 28–29.

94. Fagraeus L, Urban B, Bromage P: Spread of epidural analgesia in early pregnancy. Anesthesiology 58:184–187, 1983.

95. Bromage P: Physiology and pharmacology of epidural analgesia. Anesthesiology 28:592–622, 1967.

96. Grundy EM, Zamora AM, Winnie AP: Comparison of spread of epidural anesthesia in pregnant and nonpregnant women. Anesth Analg 57:544–546, 1978.

97. Sharrock NE, Greenidge J: Epidural dose responses in pregnant and nonpregnant patients. Anesthesiology 51:S298, 1978.

98. Bromage PR: Continuous lumbar epidural analgesia for obstetrics. Can Med Assoc J 85:1136–1140, 1961.

99. Marx GF, Bassell GM: Physiologic considerations of the mother. In *Obstetric Analgesia and Anaesthesia*. GF Marx, GM Bassell, eds. Elsevier Publications, New York, 1980, p 35.

100. Dautenhahn DL, Fagraeus L: Acid-base changes of spinal fluid during pregnancy. Anesth Analg 63:204, 1984.

101. Datta S, Lambert DH, Gregus J, Gissen AJ, Covino BG: Differential sensitivities of mammalian nerve fibers during pregnancy. Anesth Analg 62:1070–1072, 1983.

102. Flanagan HL, Datta S, Lambert DH, Gissen AJ, Covino B: Effect of pregnancy on bupivacaine-induced conduction blockade in the isolated rabbit vagus nerve. Anesth Analg 66:123–126, 1987.

103. Sevarino FB, Gilbertson LI, Gugino LD, Courtney MA, Datta S: The effect of pregnancy on the nervous system response to sensory stimulation. Anesthesiology 69:A695, 1988.

104. Datta S, Hurley R, Naulty SJ, Stern P, Lambert DH, Concepcion M, Tulchinsky D, Weiss JB, Ostheimer GW: Plasma and cerebrospinal fluid progesterone concentrations in pregnant and nonpregnant women. Anesth Analg 65:950–954, 1986.
105. Butterworth JF, Walker FO, Lyzak SZ: Pregnancy increases median nerve susceptibility to lidocaine. Anesthesiology 72:962–965, 1990.
106. Bader AM, Datta S, Moller B, Covino BG: Acute progesterone treatment has no effect on bupivacaine-induced conduction blockade in the isolated rabbit vagus nerve. Anesth Analg 71:541–544, 1990.
107. Marx GF, Oka Y, Orkin LR: Cerebrospinal fluid pressures during labor. Am J Obstet Gynecol 84:213–219, 1967.
108. Crawford JS: Principles and Practice of Obstetric Anaesthesia, 4th ed. Blackwell Scientific Publications, Oxford, 1972.
109. Marx GF: Regional analgesia in obstetrics. Anaesthetist 21:84–91, 1972.
110. McCausland AM, Hyman C, Winsor T, Trotter AD: Venous distensibility during pregnancy. Am J Obstet Gynecol 81:472–479, 1961.
111. Marx GF: Physiology of pregnancy. In ASA Refresher Courses, Anesthesiology, Vol 3. SC Hershey, ed. Lippincott, Philadelphia, 1975, pp 117–128.
112. Hart DM: Heartburn in pregnancy. J Int Med Res 6(suppl):1–5, 1978.
113. O'Sullivan GM, Sutton AJ, Thompson SA, Carrie LE, Bullingham MB: Noninvasive measurement of gastric emptying in obstetric patients. Anesth Analg 66:505–511, 1987.
114. Christofides ND, Ghatei MA, Bloom SR, Borberg C, Gillmer MD: Decreased plasma motilin concentration in pregnancy. Br Med J 285:1453–1454, 1982.
115. Davison JS, Davison MC, Hay DM: Gastric emptying time in late pregnancy and labour. J Obstet Gynaecol Br Commonw 77:37–41, 1970.
116. Attia RR, Ebeid AM, Fischer JE, Goudsouzian NG: Maternal-fetal and placental gastrin concentrations. Anaesthesia 37:18–21, 1982.
117. Roberts RB, Shirley MB: Reducing the risk of acid aspiration during cesarean section. Anesth Analg 53:859–868, 1974.
118. Roberts RB, Shirley MB: The obstetrician's role in reducing the risk of aspiration pneumonitis with particular reference to the use of oral antacids. Am J Obstet Gynecol 124:611–617, 1976.
119. James CF, Gibbs CP, Banner TE: Post-partum perioperative risk of aspiration pneumonia. Anesthesiology 61:756–759, 1984.
120. Spence AA, Moir DD, Finlay WEI: Observations on intragastric pressure. Anaesthesia 22:249–256, 1967.
121. Wilson J: Gastric emptying in labor: Some recent findings and their clinical significance. J Int Med Res 6(suppl):54–62, 1978.
122. Nimmo WS, Wilson J, Prescott LF: Narcotic analgesics and delayed gastric emptying in labour. Lancet 1:890–893, 1975.
123. Hall AW, Moosa AR, Clark J, Cooley GR, Skinner DB: The effect of premedication drugs on the lower esophageal high pressure zone and reflux status in rhesus monkeys and man. Gut 16:347–352, 1975.
124. Brock-Utne JG, Rubin J, Downing JW, Dimopoulos GE, Mishal MG, Naicker M: The administration of metoclopramide with atropine. Anaesthesia 31:1186–1190, 1976.
125. Brock-Utne JG, Rubin J, Welmas S, Dimopoulos GE, Mishal MG, Downing JW: The action of commonly used anti-emetics on the lower esophageal sphincter. Br J Anaesth 50:295–298, 1978.
126. Brock-Utne JG, Rubin J, Welman S, Dimopoulos GE, Mishal MG, Downing JW: The effect of glycopyrrolate (Robinul) on the lower esophageal sphincter. Can Anaesth Soc J 25:144–146, 1978.
127. Mendelson CL: The aspiration of stomach contents into the lungs during obstetric anesthesia. Am J Obstet Gynecol 52:191–206, 1946.
128. Dignam WJ, Titus P, Assali NS: Renal function in human pregnancy. I. Changes in glomerular filtration rate and renal plasma flow. Proc Soc Exp Biol Med 97:512–514, 1958.
129. Sundsfjord JA, Aakvaag A: Plasma renin activity, plasma renin substrate and urinary aldosterone excretion in the menstrual cycle in relation to the concentration of progesterone and oestrogens in the plasma. Acta Endocrinol 71:519–529, 1972.
130. Talledo OE, Chesley LC, Zuspan FP: Renin-angiotensin system in normal and toxemic pregnancies. III. Differential sensitivity to angiotensin II and norepinephrine in toxemia at pregnancy. Am J Obstet Gynecol 100:218–221, 1968.
131. Toback FG, Hall PW, Lindheimer MD: Effect of posture on urinary protein patterns in nonpregnant, pregnant and toxemic women. Obstet Gynecol 35:765–768, 1970.
132. Van Wagenen G, Jenkins RH: An experimental examination of factors causing ureteral dilation of pregnancy. J Urol 42:1010–1020, 1939.
133. Smith BE, Moya F, Shnider SM: The effects of anesthesia on liver function during labor. Anesth Analg 41:24–31, 1962.
134. Yip DM, Baker AL: Liver diseases in pregnancy. Clin Perinatol 12:683–694, 1985.
135. McNair RD, Jaynes RV: Alterations in liver function during normal pregnancy. Am J Obstet Gynecol 80:500–505, 1960.
136. Shnider SM: Serum cholinesterase activity during pregnancy, labor and puerperium. Anesthesiology 26:335–339, 1965.
137. Weissman DB, Ehrenwerth J: Prolonged neuromuscular blockade in a parturient associated with succinylcholine. Anesth Analg 62:444–446, 1983.
138. Blitt CD, Petty WC, Alberternst EE, Wright BJ: Correlation of plasma cholinesterase activity and duration of action of succinylcholine during pregnancy. Anesth Analg 56:78–83, 1977.
139. Leighton BL, Cheek TG, Gross JB, Apfelbaum JL, Shantz BB, Gutsche BB, Rosenberg H: Succinylcholine pharmacodynamics in peripartum patients. Anesthesiology 64:202–205, 1986.
140. Ravindran RS, Cummins DF, Pantazis KL, Strausberg BJ, Baenziger JC: Unusual aspects of low levels of pseudocholinesterase in a pregnant patient. Anesth Analg 61:953–955, 1982.
141. Kuhnert BR, Philipson EH, Pimental R, Kuhnert PM: A prolonged chloroprocaine epidural block in a postpartum patient with abnormal pseudocholinesterase. Anesthesiology 56:477–478, 1982.
142. Whittaker M: Plasma cholinesterase variants and the anaesthetist. Anaesthesia 35:174–197, 1980.
143. Viby-Mogenson J: Correlation of succinylcholine duration of action with plasma cholinesterase activity in subjects with the genotypically normal enzyme. Anesthesiology 53:517–520, 1980.
144. Kambam JR, Naukam RJ, Parris W, Franks JJ, Perry SM, Sastry BVR, Smith BE: Effects of progesterone, estriol and prostaglandin on pseudocholinesterase activity. Anesthesiology 71:A883, 1989.
145. Viegas O: Guest discussion: Correlation of plasma cholinesterase activity and duration of action of succinylcholine during pregnancy. Anesth Analg 56:81–82, 1977.
146. O'Brien J, Abbey V, Hinsvark O, Perel J, Finster M: Metabolism and measurement of chloroprocaine: An ester type local anesthetic. J Pharm Sci 68:75–78, 1979.
147. Cunningham FG, MacDonald PC, Gant NF: Human pregnancy: Overview, organization and diagnosis. In Williams Obstetrics, 18th ed. Appleton & Lange, Norwalk, 1989, pp 7–85.

CHAPTER 2

Uteroplacental Circulation and Respiratory Gas Exchange

Julian T. Parer, M.D., Ph.D.

The placenta is a union of maternal and fetal tissues for purposes of physiologic exchange. Because most stillbirths and depressed fetuses are the result of intrauterine asphyxia, the factors responsible for adequacy of placental function, particularly respiratory gas exchange, assume great importance.

PLACENTAL ANATOMY AND CIRCULATION

The human placenta is described as a villous hemochorial type. The villi are projections of fetal tissue surrounded by chorion that are exposed to circulating maternal blood. The chorion is the outermost fetal tissue layer. At term the human placenta weighs about 500 g and is disc shaped, with a diameter of approximately 20 cm and a thickness of 3 cm. The fetal-to-placental weight ratio is normally approximately 6:1 at term. Before this the placenta is relatively heavier and the ratio is less (e.g., 3:1 at 30 weeks' gestation).

Circulation of blood through the placenta is illustrated in Figure 2.1. The maternal blood is carried initially in the uterine arteries, and these ultimately divide into spiral arteries in the basal plate. Blood is spurted, probably under arterial pressure, from these arteries into the intervillous space. It traverses upward toward the chorionic plate, passing fetal villi, and finally drains back to veins in the basal plate. It is likely that, throughout this passage past the villi, the maternal blood is exchanging substances with fetal blood within the villi. The fetal circulation within the placenta is quite different. Blood is carried into the placenta by two umbilical arteries that successively divide into smaller vessels within the fetal villi. Ultimately, capillaries traverse the tips of the fetal villi, and it is at this point that exchange occurs with maternal blood within the intervillous space. The blood is finally collected into a single umbilical vein in the umbilical cord, and this carries the nutrient-rich and waste-poor blood to the fetus.

Fetal and maternal blood are separated by three microscopic tissue layers in the human placenta. The first layer is the fetal trophoblast, which consists of cytotrophoblast and syncytiotrophoblast. The syncytiotrophoblast is the metabolically active part of the placenta, where much of the endocrine function of the placenta occurs. The other tissue layers are fetal connective tissue, which serves to support the villi, and the endothelium of fetal capillaries (Fig. 2.2).

The quantitative relationship of fetal and maternal blood flow and relative concentrations of substances at any one point in the human placenta are quite complex. The relative rates of blood flow in various areas of the placenta are quite variable, and there is a continually changing concentration of nutrients and waste materials in various areas of the placenta as exchange occurs (1).

MECHANISMS OF EXCHANGE

Substances are exchanged across the placental membrane by five mechanisms (2).

1. Diffusion

This is a physicochemical process in which no energy is required and substances pass from one area to another on the basis of a concentration gradient. The respiratory gases, oxygen and carbon dioxide, the fatty acids, and the smaller ions (e.g., Na^+ and Cl^-) are transported by this mechanism (2).

Facilitated diffusion describes the mechanism of passage of glucose and some other carbohydrates. With this mechanism, substances still pass down a concentration gradient, but the rate of passage is greater than can be explained by the gradient alone. Possibly carrier molecules are involved, and there may be need for energy expenditure.

2. Active Transport

This mechanism allows for the passage of substances in a direction against the concentration gradient. Energy is required; carrier molecules are involved; and active transport is subject to inhibition by certain metabolites. The amino acids, water-

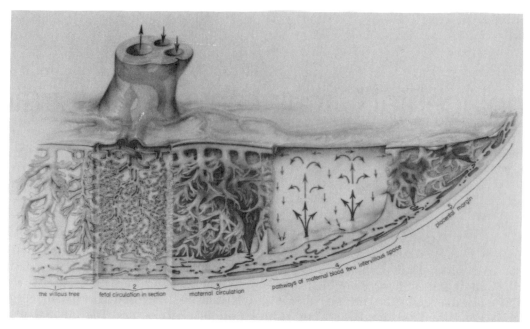

Figure 2.1. The circulation of blood in the primate placenta. Fetal circulation is shown in the *two panels at left* and the umbilical cord (*above*). The *right panels* show the maternal blood spurting from spiral arteries in the basal area through the intervillous space. The blood passes fetal villi, exchanges substances with fetal blood within the villi, and ultimately drains into veins in the basal area. (Drawing by Ranice W. Crosby for Dr. Elizabeth M. Ramsey. Reprinted by courtesy of the Carnegie Institution of Washington, D.C.)

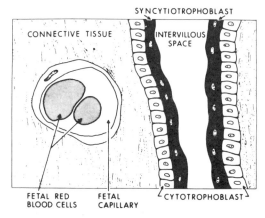

Figure 2.2. Drawing from an electron micrograph of cross-section through parts of two fetal villi, showing tissue layers that separate fetal and maternal blood in the human placenta. The cytotrophoblastic layer is much less distinct in the third trimester than is depicted here. (Reprinted by courtesy of Berkeley Bio-Engineering, Inc., Berkeley, CA.)

soluble vitamins and some of the larger ions (e.g., Ca^{++} and Fe^{++}) are transported by this mechanism.

3. Bulk Flow

This describes the passage of substances resulting from a hydrostatic or osmotic gradient. Water is transported by this mechanism and may also carry some solutes with it under the influence of this mechanism.

4. Pinocytosis

Some large molecules such as the immune globulins appear to be transported by being enclosed in small vesicles consisting of cell membranes. These are pinched off on one side of the placenta and traverse to the other side, where their contents are released.

5. Breaks

The delicate, filmy villi may at times break off within the intervillous space, and the contents may be extruded into the maternal circulation. It is also thought that maternal intravascular contents may be taken up by the fetal circulation at times. The most important result of this is seen when fetal Rh-positive red blood cells are deposited in the vascular system of an Rh-negative mother, resulting in isoimmunization and subsequent erythroblastosis fetalis.

DIFFUSION

When limitations of placental transfer occur in the human, they usually are first recognized as limitations of those substances that are exchanged by diffusion. For example, an acute decrease in placental function limits passage of oxygen to and carbon dioxide from the fetus, resulting in fetal asphyxia. A more chronic decrease in placental function may result in limitation of substances necessary for growth (e.g., carbohydrates), thus giving rise to a fetus that is growth retarded. Hence, the process of diffusion is examined in some detail.

Fick's diffusion equation describes the physico-chemical process:

$$\text{Rate of transfer} = \frac{\text{concentration gradient} \times \text{area} \times \text{permeability}}{\text{membrane thickness}}$$

Each of the factors determining rate of passage of substances by diffusion is considered in turn.

Concentration Gradient

The concentration gradient of a substance across the placenta is equal to the difference between the mean maternal blood concentration and the mean fetal blood concentration within each of the exchanging areas. As noted above, however, it is most unlikely that this gradient is constant throughout the placenta because of the placenta's peculiar circulatory anatomy. It probably varies from place to place and also from time to time in any particular area. However, by considering a simplified exchanging membrane with blood flowing in from each side, each of the factors that would affect the concentration gradient can be conceptually discussed (Fig. 2.3). These factors are:

1. *Concentration of substance in maternal arterial blood.*
2. *Concentration of substance in fetal arterial blood.*
3. *Maternal intervillous space blood flow.*
4. *Fetal-placental blood flow.*
5. *Diffusing capacity of the placenta for the substance.*
6. *Ratio of maternal to fetal blood flow in exchanging areas.* This is analogous to ventilation perfusion ratios as applied to the lung. Inequalities in the ratio give rise to decreased efficiency of transfer. Exchange of substances is optimal if the flows are evenly matched.
7. *Binding of substances to molecules and dissociation rates.* Depending on the rate of dissociation, this reaction time could limit the transfer of a substance. This does not appear to be limiting with regard to the dissociation of oxygen and hemoglobin.
8. *Geometry of exchanging surfaces with respect to blood flow.* If blood flows are traveling in the same direction during exchange the system is called concurrent. If the blood flows are traveling in opposite directions the system is called countercurrent. This latter system is the most efficient from the

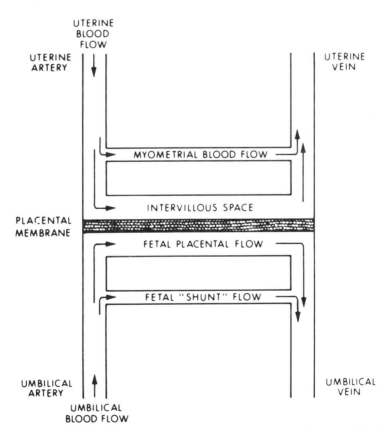

Figure 2.3. Simplified diagram of pattern of circulation through the placenta. (Reprinted by courtesy of Berkeley Bio-Engineering, Inc., Berkeley, CA.)

exchange point of view. As can be seen in Figure 2.1, in the human placenta it is unlikely that either of these simplified concepts holds. The human pattern has been described as the multivillous stream system (1). The evaluation of the mean concentration gradient of any nutrient in this system becomes extremely complex.

9. The metabolism of the substance. If a substance is consumed within the placenta, its rate of passage across the placenta will not be reflected by the concentration gradient. For example, oxygen is consumed in considerable quantities by the trophoblast and the rate of passage appears to be relatively inefficient when based on oxygen tension gradients alone.

Area of the Placenta

The villous surface area of the human term placenta (3) is approximately 11 m^2. In comparison, the lung has an alveolar surface area of 70 m^2. The area of actual exchange, the vasculosyncytial membrane—that is, the area where fetal capillaries approach closely enough to the surface to exchange materials with maternal blood—is 1.8 m^2.

Placental area is decreased in a number of clinical situations. An acute decrease occurs with abruptio placentae. With part of the placenta separated, the fetus does not necessarily expire through asphyxia. Its ability to survive depends on the placental reserve that existed before the episode of abruption. Some placentas, particularly those in cases of maternal hypertension or those that have infarcted fibrotic areas, have a reduced area available for exchange and, hence, lowered reserve. Thus the placenta of a mother with long-term hypertension is likely to be smaller than expected, as is the fetus. The infarctions are thought to be caused by maternal arteriolar deficiencies giving rise to devitalization of certain cotyledonary areas, resulting in fibrosis of the villi. Additionally, in certain cases of intrauterine infection or congenital defects, the placentas are decreased in size and area. Large placentas are found in certain diabetics and in erythroblastosis fetalis. In the former case it is not certain whether the increased area improves the transfer of nutrients to the fetus. In the latter case, most of the increased placental mass is thought to be hydropic in origin and, hence, is unlikely to improve the exchange characteristics of the placenta.

Permeability of the Placental Membrane

The permeability of a membrane to a substance depends on characteristics both of the membrane and of the substance that is being exchanged. The units for permeability can be found by a transposition of

Fick's diffusion equation. There are three major determinants of permeability.

1. Molecular size. A molecular weight of 1000 is a rough dividing line between those substances that cross the placenta by diffusion and those that are relatively impermeable by diffusion. Below a molecular weight of 1000 the rate of passage of the molecule is related to its weight unless other properties (see the following) prevent or hasten rate of passage. A common clinical example is found in cases in which it is necessary to anticoagulate a pregnant woman. If one uses heparin, with a molecular weight above 6000, one does not concomitantly heparinize the fetus. However, with the use of warfarin (Coumadin), with a molecular weight of 330, the fetus will also be anticoagulated. This is considered undesirable, particularly in the intrapartum period when fetal bleeding may occur. Also, warfarin may have some teratogenic effects in the first trimester.

2. Lipid solubility. A lipid-soluble substance traverses the placenta more rapidly than one that is not lipid soluble.

3. Electrical charge. This deters the passage of a substance across the placenta. For example, succinylcholine, commonly used during balanced anesthesia, is highly ionized and is poorly diffusable across the placenta despite its molecular weight of 361. Thiopental, with a molecular weight of 264, is lipid soluble, relatively unionized, and moves very rapidly into the fetal circulation.

Substances are classified into those in which the rate of passage is either "permeability limited" or "flow limited" (4). A substance that has poor permeability is limited in its rate of passage across the placenta by permeability and not by rates of blood flow. Hence, increasing the rate of blood flow will not improve its rate of passage much at all. The majority of biologic molecules are limited in their rate of passage across the placenta by resistance to diffusion. However, substances that are highly permeable are limited by the rate of blood flow. Oxygen and carbon dioxide are examples of this. Decreasing the rate of blood flow decreases the rate of exchange considerably.

Diffusion Distance

The average distance for diffusion across the placenta (3) has been measured as approximately 3.5 μ. This contrasts with the much smaller distance from alveolus to pulmonary capillary in the lung (0.5 μ). The diffusion distance decreases as the placenta matures, but it is not clear whether this improves the placenta's characteristics for exchange. The distance is increased in several conditions, such as erythroblastosis fetalis and congenital syphilis. This increased distance probably is due to villous edema and presumably decreases the organ's efficiency for exchange. Fibrous or calcific deposits in the placental vasculature, such as are found in diabetes melitus or preeclampsia, presumably increase diffusion distance.

UTERINE BLOOD FLOW

Because uterine blood flow is one of the prime determinants of passage of a number of critical substances across the placenta, its characteristics and the factors affecting it are discussed. A detailed discussion of the effects of obstetric anesthesia on uterine blood flow can be found in Chapter 3.

Uterine blood flow rises progressively throughout pregnancy and in the term fetus is approximately 700 ml/min (Fig. 2.4). This represents about 10% of the cardiac output. Approximately 70 to 90% of the uterine blood flow passes through the intervillous space, and the remainder largely supplies the myometrium.

The uterine vascular bed is thought to be almost maximally dilated under normal conditions, with little capacity to dilate further (5). It is not autoregu-

lated, so flow is proportional to the mean perfusion pressure. However, it is capable of marked vasoconstriction by α-adrenergic action. It is not responsive to changes in respiratory gas tensions. The uterine blood flow is determined by the following relationship:

$$\text{Uterine blood flow} = \frac{\begin{array}{c}\text{uterine arterial pressure}\\ -\text{ uterine venous pressure}\end{array}}{\text{uterine vascular resistance}}$$

Hence, any factor affecting either of the three values on the right side of the above relationship will alter uterine blood flow. A number of causes of decreased uterine blood flow are shown in Table 2.1.

Uterine contractions decrease uterine blood flow as a result of increased uterine venous pressure brought about by increased intramural pressure of the uterus. There may also be a decrease in uterine arterial pressure with contractions. Uterine hypertonus causes a decreased uterine blood flow through the same mechanism.

In sheep it has been shown that, if uterine arterial perfusion pressure is altered without changing the resistance of the uterine vascular bed, there is a direct relationship between uterine blood flow and the pressure (5). Hence, hypotension through any of the mechanisms noted in Table 2.1 will cause a decrease in blood flow.

In the case of maternal arterial hypertension it is likely that there is a concomitant increased vascular resistance that is shared by the uterine vascular bed. This therefore results in a decrease in uterine blood flow. Either endogenous or exogenous vasoconstriction results in decreased blood flow because of increased uterine vascular resistance.

There are few useful means of increasing uterine blood flow in cases in which it is known to be less

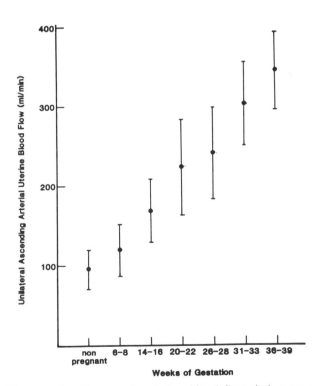

Figure 2.4. Changes in uterine blood flow during pregnancy. Assuming equal flow in both uterine arteries, total uterine blood flow as measured by a transvaginal duplex Doppler ultrasound would be about 700 ml/minute. (Reprinted by permission from Thaler I, Manor D, Itskovitz J, Rottem S, Levit N, Timor-Tritsch I, Brandes JM: Changes in uterine blood flow during human pregnancy. Am J Obstet Gynecol 162:121–125, 1990.)

Table 2.1
Factors Causing Decreased Uterine Blood Flow

Uterine contractions
Hypertonus
Abruptio placentae
Tetanic contraction
Overstimulation with oxytocin
Hypotension
Sympathetic block
Hypovolemic shock
Supine hypotensive syndrome
Hypertension
Essential
Preeclamptic
Vasoconstriction, endogenous
Sympathetic discharge
Adrenal medullary activity
Vasoconstrictors, exogenous
Most sympathomimetics (α-adrenergic effects)
Exception is ephedrine (primarily β-adrenergic effect)

than optimal. The most important clinical considerations are the avoidance or correction of factors responsible for an acute decrease in blood flow (e.g., excessive uterine activity or maternal hypotension).

Some of the β-mimetic agents that are used as uterine relaxants for preterm labor may increase uterine blood flow, but this effect, if it occurs, is small and may only be a result of decreased uterine tonus. There are a number of experimental means of increasing uterine blood flow, sometimes transiently, but these have no real clinical use. Examples of such treatments include estrogens, acetylcholine, nitroglycerine, cyanide, ischemia, and mild hypoxia, the latter either acute or chronic (6).

Clinically, it has been known for many years that maternal bed rest may improve the outcome in suspected fetal growth retardation. There is some evidence that bed rest does improve fetal growth, as evidenced by increasing estriol excretion (7).

UMBILICAL BLOOD FLOW

The umbilical blood flow in the undisturbed fetus at term is about 120 ml/kg/min or 360 ml/min. Such measurements have been obtained by noninvasive methods using ultrasound techniques (8). This is somewhat higher than values obtained immediately after birth, but the latter are probably affected by cord manipulation during the birth process. The measurements have not yet found clinical applicability, but the same technique can be used to calculate the peak systolic-to-diastolic ratio, which is a reflection of vascular resistance distal to the point of measurement.

The umbilical blood flow in the human is considerably less than that of the sheep, where it is approximately 200 ml/kg/min (9). The differences may be explained by the somewhat higher metabolic rate of the sheep (body temperature 39°C) and differences in hemoglobin concentrations (sheep, 10 g/dl vs. human, 15 g/dl). It is important to recognize this species difference because the bulk of our information regarding fetal circulatory physiology comes from the chronically instrumented sheep fetus. In sheep, the umbilical blood flow is approximately 45% of the combined ventricular output (9) and about 20% of this blood flow is "shunted," that is, it does not exchange with maternal blood (1). It is either carried through actual vascular shunts within the fetal side of the placenta or else it does not approach closely enough to maternal blood for exchange with it.

Umbilical blood flow is unaffected by acute moderate hypoxia but is decreased by severe hypoxia (10). Whether the umbilical cord is innervated is still in question; however, umbilical blood flow decreases with the administration of catecholamines. It is also decreased by acute cord occlusion. There are no known means of increasing umbilical flow in patients in whom it is thought to be decreased chronically. However, certain fetal heart rate patterns (i.e., variable decelerations), have been ascribed to transient umbilical cord compression in the fetus during labor. Manipulation of maternal position either to the lateral or Trendelenburg position can sometimes abolish these patterns, the implication being that cord compression has been relieved.

Blood Flow Studies in the Human Fetus

Blood Velocity Wave Forms. Real-time directed Doppler ultrasound has been used to investigate human fetal, placental, and uterine blood flows (11). Doppler ultrasound allows for measurement of velocity waveforms of red blood cells traveling in vessels. The velocity data can be used to make inferences about blood flow, vascular resistance, and myocardial contractility. Blood flow velocity waveforms have a characteristic appearance that varies from vessel to vessel (see Fig. 3.3). The observed waveform shape is affected by the pumping ability of the heart, the heart rate, the elasticity of the vessel wall, the outflow impedance, and the blood viscosity. Waveforms in arteries supplying low-resistance vascular beds have a characteristically high forward velocity during diastole, whereas absent or reverse diastolic flow is seen in arteries supplying high-resistance vascular beds. These observations prompted the definition of indices of flow that could be related to the vascular resistance of a downstream vascular bed. The most commonly used indices are:

Pulsatility Index: $PI = V_{max} - V_{min}/V_{mean}$
Pourcelot Ratio: $PR = V_{max} - V_{min}/V_{max}$
AB(SD) Ratio: $AB = V_{max} - /V_{min}$

where V_{max} = Point of maximal blood flow velocity/cardiac cycle
V_{min} = Point of minimal blood flow velocity/cardiac cycle
V_{mean} = Mean blood flow velocity/cardiac cycle.

Blood Flow. Doppler ultrasound permits the estimation of blood flows in the human fetus. Blood flow is calculated using the formula:
$$Q = (V \times A)/\cos \theta$$

where V = mean velocity as averaged over many cardiac cycles (cm/s)
A = estimated cross-sectional area of the vessel (cm²)
θ = angle between the Doppler beam and the direction of flow of the blood

This calculation (Fig. 2.5) is complicated by the variation in the velocity of blood cells across a vascular lumen. Cells flow faster in the center of the vessel and slower near the vessel wall. The overall flow in

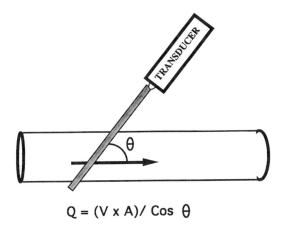

$$Q = (V \times A)/ \cos \theta$$

Figure 2.5. The blood flow (*Q*) through a vessel is quantitated as the product of mean velocity (*V*) of red blood cells and cross-sectional area (*A*) of the vessel, divided by the cosine of the angle of insonation of the vessel (cos θ). (Modified from Copel JA, Grannum PA, Hobbins JC, Cunningham FG: Doppler ultrasound in obstetrics. In *Williams' Obstetrics* 16th ed. Appleton & Lange, Norwalk, CT, 1988.)

a vessel is the sum of the different flows across the lumen. For this reason, satisfactory volume flow measurements can best be made on large vessels (4 to 10 mm in diameter) with appropriate Doppler angles (30 to 60 degrees). The two-dimensional echo Doppler provides a means of estimating fetal cardiac output by quantifying blood flow volume at the atrioventricular valve orifices. The estimated cardiac output of the human fetus (553 ml/min/kg) is higher than that of the sheep (450 ml/min/kg). In addition, the right and left ventricular outputs are more similar in the human, as compared with the sheep. The ratio of right-to-left ventricular outputs decreases with advancing gestation from 1.3 at 15 weeks to 1.1 at 40 weeks. In normal pregnancy, high forward velocity levels in the umbilical artery are maintained throughout diastole. A lowered diastolic flow, as seen in severe intrauterine growth retardation, may reflect raised placental resistance (12). Marx and colleagues used Doppler ultrasound waveform analysis to demonstrate a significant reduction in umbilical artery vascular resistance (systolic/diastolic ratio) with epidural analgesia in healthy laboring women (13). Youngstrom et al. (14) investigated the effect of more extensive epidural anesthesia (and maternal sympathetic blockade) on umbilical artery flow velocity waveforms in healthy, nonlaboring women undergoing elective cesarean section. They found no statistically significant change in umbilical artery resistance (S/D ratio).

OXYGEN TRANSFER TO THE FETUS

As mentioned previously, it is likely that most stillbirths and cases of fetal depression are the result of inadequate exchange of the respiratory gases. Oxygen has the lowest storage-to-utilization ratio of all nutrients in the fetus. From animal experimentation it can be calculated that in a term fetus the quantity of oxygen is approximately 42 ml and the normal oxygen consumption is approximately 21 ml/min (10). This means that, in theory, the fetus has a 2-min supply of oxygen. However, fetuses do not consume the total quantity of oxygen in their body within 2 min, nor do they expire after this time. In fact, irreversible brain damage does not occur until about 10 min have elapsed (15). This is because the fetus has a number of important compensatory mechanisms that enable it to survive on a lesser quantity of oxygen for longer periods. Clinical situations in which there is total cessation of oxygen delivery are rare. These include sudden total abruption of the placenta or complete umbilical cord compression, generally after prolapse of the cord.

It is known from animal experimentation that the compensations that occur in the hypoxic fetus are: (*a*) redistribution of blood flow to vital organs including heart, brain, and placenta; (*b*) decreased total oxygen consumption (e.g., with moderate hypoxia the fetal oxygen consumption drops to 50% of the normal level); and (*c*) dependence of certain vascular beds on anaerobic metabolism. These compensatory mechanisms appear to be initiated with mild hypoxia and result in the maintenance of O_2 supply to vital organs during times of O_2 limitation (10).

It is of value to examine the factors that determine oxygen transfer from mother to fetus (Table 2.2). Because the transfer of oxygen to the fetus depends on rates of blood flow and not limitations to diffusion, the respective blood flow on each side of the placenta assumes major importance for maintenance of fetal oxygenation. Animal work suggests that in the normal placenta there is a "safety factor" of approximately 50% in the uterine blood flow. That is, the uterine blood flow will drop to half its normal value before severe fetal acidosis becomes evident (16) and oxygen uptake declines (17). This only applies to the normal situation with normal placental reserve and is unlikely to be the case in pathologic situations, such as in the infant of a hypertensive mother. In such situations the placental function may be adequate for oxygenation but not for fetal growth, and a growth-retarded infant may result from such a pregnancy. Furthermore, with superimposition of uterine contractions on such a fetus, there may be transient inadequacy of uterine blood flow during the uterine contractions; this may be recognized by responses of the fetal heart rate (i.e., late decelerations).

Additional important determinants of fetal oxygenation include oxygen tension in maternal arterial and fetal arterial blood. In general, maternal arterial oxygen tension depends on adequate ventilation and pulmonary integrity. Disruptions of this function are relatively rare in obstetrics, although they can occur with pulmonary diseases such as asthma, with congestive heart failure, or in mothers with congenital cardiac defects. The oxygen affinity and oxygen capacity of maternal and fetal bloods are also important determinants of fetal oxygen transfer. At a given oxygen tension the quantity of oxygen carried by blood depends on the oxygen capacity, which depends on the hemoglobin concentration, and on the oxygen affinity. The oxygen affinity of fetal blood is greater than that of maternal blood (Fig. 2.6). That is, the oxygen dissociation curve of the fetus is to the left of that of the mother. In addition, the hemoglobin concentration of fetal blood is approximately 15 g/100 ml in the term fetus, whereas that of the mother is approximately 12 g/100 ml. Both of these factors, an increased oxygen affinity and higher oxygen capacity, confer advantages to the fetus for oxygen uptake across the placenta (Fig. 2.7). Probable values of the oxygen content and oxygen tension in umbilical vessels and maternal uterine artery and vein is illustrated in Figure 2.8.

Because most measurements have been made in the human fetus during or after labor, the values of oxygen saturation, oxygen tension, and pH are generally depressed compared with those of the mother. In fact, investigations on chronically instrumented animals have shown that the oxygen saturation and content of fetal blood and acid-base status is very close to that of maternal blood; only the P_{O_2} is lower. The arteriovenous oxygen differences across each side of the placenta are also illustrated in Figure 2.8. Notice that the quantity of oxygen delivered or taken up by each 100 ml of circulating blood in the placenta is approximately equal in the mother and fetus. This further suggests approximate equality of blood flows on each side of the placenta. A number of additional miscellaneous factors determine the rate of oxygen transfer across the placenta; they are listed in Table 2.2 as the last six determinants. They appear to be relatively minor compared with the major factors already outlined.

CARBON DIOXIDE AND ACID-BASE BALANCE

Carbon dioxide crosses the placenta even more readily than does oxygen. In general the determinants for oxygen transfer also apply to carbon dioxide transfer across the placenta. It is limited by rate of blood flow and not by resistance to diffusion. The carbon dioxide tension in fetal blood in the undisturbed state is close to 40 mm Hg (1). It is well known that the maternal arterial carbon dioxide tension is approximately 34 mm Hg, and the mother is in a state of compensated respiratory alkalosis. The pH of fetal blood under undisturbed conditions is probably close to 7.4, and the bicarbonate concentration is close to that in maternal blood.

Table 2.2
Factors Affecting Oxygen Transfer from Mother to Fetus

Intervillous blood flow
Fetal-placental blood flow
Oxygen tension in maternal arterial blood
Oxygen tension in fetal arterial blood
Oxygen affinity of maternal blood
Oxygen affinity of fetal blood
Hemoglobin concentration or oxygen capacity of maternal blood
Hemoglobin concentration or oxygen capacity of fetal blood
Maternal and fetal blood pH and P_{CO_2} (Bohr effect)
Placental diffusing capacity
Placental vascular geometry
Ratio of maternal to fetal blood flow in exchanging areas
Shunting around exchange sites
Placental oxygen consumption

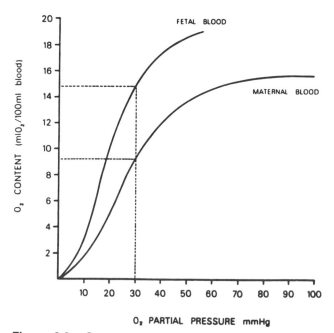

Figure 2.6. Oxygen dissociation curves of maternal and fetal blood. The *vertical broken line* illustrates the higher oxygen affinity of fetal blood—fetal blood is more highly saturated with oxygen than is maternal blood at the same oxygen partial pressure. (Reprinted by permission from Parer JT: Uteroplacental physiology and exchange. In *Handbook of Fetal Heart Rate Monitoring*. WB Saunders, Philadelphia, 1963, p 26.)

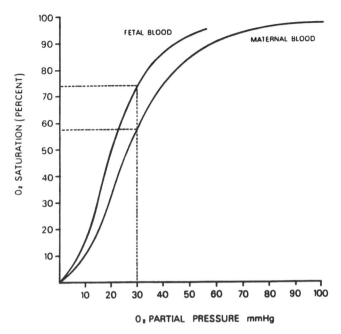

Figure 2.7. Oxygen dissociation curves relating oxygen content of blood to oxygen partial pressure in maternal and fetal blood. This relationship illustrates the even greater oxygen content of fetal blood when the greater hemoglobin content of fetal blood is taken into account. (Reprinted by permission from Parer JT: Uteroplacental physiology and exchange. In *Handbook of Fetal Heart Rate Monitoring*. WB Saunders, Philadelphia, 1963, p 27.)

Bicarbonate and the fixed acids cross the placenta much more slowly than does carbon dioxide; that is, equilibration takes a matter of hours rather than seconds. There is a situation analogous to "respiratory acidosis" that occurs in the fetus when blood flow, either uterine or umbilical, is acutely compromised. In such cases, the pH drops and CO_2 tension is elevated, but the metabolic acid-base status remains unchanged. This occurs during severe or profound fetal decelerations (called variable decelerations) in association with certain uterine contractions, especially during the second stage of labor. These acid-base changes are generally rapidly resolved with cessation of the contraction and the bradycardia. However, as noted earlier, if there is a significant oxygen lack that is unrelieved, the fetus will decrease its oxygen consumption, redistribute blood flow, and depend partly on anaerobic metabolism to supply its energy needs, albeit with decreased efficiency. Under these conditions, lactate (an end product of anaerobic metabolism) is produced, resulting in a metabolic acidosis. The acidosis may also be aggravated by a combined respiratory acidosis because of retained carbon dioxide. Unlike carbon dioxide, lactate is lost slowly from the fetus.

CLINICAL IMPLICATIONS

Fetal compromise results from a disruption of normal placental exchange mechanisms. With a knowl-

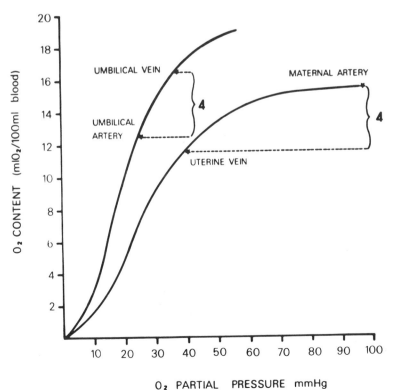

Figure 2.8. Oxygen contents and tensions, and arteriovenous oxygen concentration differences (*brackets*), on fetal and maternal side of the placenta. These are probable values in the undisturbed human, although use has been made of data from many sources, including experimental animals.

edge of the components involved in exchange of nutrients and waste materials across the placenta, potential problems can be recognized and corrections can be made.

The most important components of placental exchange are the rates of blood flow on each side of the placenta and the area available for exchange. Uterine blood flow will decline in the presence of factors causing decreased perfusion pressure or increased uterine vascular resistance. Common clinical occurrences are hypotension, hypertension, endogenous or exogenous vasoconstriction, and possibly severe psychologic stress. The uterine vascular bed, as previously noted, is not autoregulated and has little capacity to dilate further. During labor, it is most likely that the rate of uterine blood flow is the limiting factor in cases of fetal compromise because of the intermittent decline in uterine blood flow with each uterine contraction. In addition, transient or persistent umbilical cord compression may cause fetal asphyxia.

References

1. Metcalfe J, Bartels H, Moll W: Gas exchange in the pregnant uterus. Physiol Rev 47:782–838, 1967.
2. Longo LD: Placental transfer mechanisms: An overview. In *Obstetrics and Gynecology Annual.* RM Wynn, ed. Appleton-Century-Crofts, New York, 1972, pp 103–138.
3. Aherne W, Dunnill MS: Morphometry of the human placenta. Br Med Bull 22:5–8, 1966.
4. Meschia G: Physiology of transplacental diffusion. In *Obstetrics and Gynecology Annual.* RM Wynn, ed. Appleton-Century-Crofts, New York, 1976, pp 21–38.
5. Assali NS, Brinkman CR III: The uterine circulation and its control. In *Respiratory Gas Exchange and Blood Flow in the Placenta.* LD Longo, H Bartels, eds. US Department of Health, Education and Welfare, Washington, DC, 1972, pp 121–141.
6. Greiss F Jr: Concepts of uterine blood flow. In *Obstetrics and Gynecology Annual.* RM Wynn, ed. Appleton-Century-Crofts, New York, 1973, pp 55–83.
7. Beischer NA, Drew JH, Kenny JM, O'Sullivan EF: The effect of rest and intravenous infusion of hypertonic dextrose on subnormal estriol excretion in pregnancy. In *Clinics in Perinatology.* A Milunsky, ed. WB Saunders, Philadelphia, 1974, pp 253–272.
8. Gill RW, Trudinger BJ, Garrett WJ, Kossoff G, Warren PS: Fetal umbilical venous flow measured in utero by pulsed Doppler and B-mode ultrasound. Am J Obstet Gynecol 139:720–725, 1981.
9. Heymann MA: Fetal cardiovascular physiology. In *Maternal-Fetal Medicine: Principles and Practice.* RK Creasy, R Resnik, eds. WB Saunders, Philadelphia, 1984, pp 259–273.
10. Court DJ, Parer JT: Experimental studies in fetal asphyxia and fetal heart rate interpretation. In *Research in Perinatal Medicine, Vol 1.* PW Nathanielsz, JT Parer, eds. Perinatology Press, Ithaca, NY, 1985, pp 114–164.
11. Trudinger BJ, Giles WB, Cook CM: Flow velocity wave-forms in the maternal uteroplacental and fetal placental circulation. Am J Obstet Gynecol 152:155–163, 1985.
12. Fleischer A, Schulman H, Farmakides G, Bracero L, Blattner P, Randolph G: Umbilical velocity wave ratios in intrauterine growth retardation. Am J Obstet Gynecol 151:502–505, 1985.
13. Marx GF, Patel S, Berman JA, Farmakides G, Schulman H: Umbilical blood flow velocity waveforms in different maternal positions and with epidural analgesia. Obstet Gynecol 68:61–64, 1986.
14. Youngstrom P, Veille JC, Kanaan C, Wilson B: Umbilical artery flow velocity waveforms before and during epidural anesthesia for cesarean section. Anesthesiology 69:A704, 1988.
15. Myers RE: Two patterns of perinatal brain damage and their conditions of occurrence. Am J Obstet Gynecol 112:246–276, 1972.
16. Parer JT, Behrman RE: The influence of uterine blood flow on the acid-base status of the rhesus monkey. Am J Obstet Gynecol 107:1241–1249, 1970.
17. Wilkening RB, Meschia G: Fetal oxygen uptake, oxygenation and acid-base balance as a function of uterine blood flow. Am J Physiol 24:H749–H755, 1983.

CHAPTER 3

Obstetric Anesthesia and Uterine Blood Flow

Sol M. Shnider, M.D.

Gershon Levinson, M.D.

Ermelando V. Cosmi, M.D., L.D.

Obstetric anesthesia and analgesia may directly affect uterine blood flow or may alter the response of the uteroplacental circulation to noxious stimuli and to various pharmacologic agents. As stated in Chapter 2, uterine blood flow varies directly with the perfusion pressure, (i.e., uterine arterial minus uterine venous pressure) and inversely with uterine vascular resistance. Obstetric anesthesia may affect uterine blood flow by (a) changing the perfusion pressure, that is, altering the uterine arterial or venous pressure; or (b) changing uterine vascular resistance either directly through changes in vascular tone or indirectly by altering uterine contractions or uterine muscle tone.

Direct measurement of human uterine blood flow is not usually possible because of the relative inaccessibility of the human uteroplacental circulation. Changes in uterine blood flow are usually assessed from fetal and neonatal acid-base and heart rate status. In the late 1970s a group of Finnish investigators developed a quantitative method for measuring both the intervillous and myometrial components of human uterine blood flow based upon the clearance of xenon-133 given intravenously (1). Because it is unconventional in the United States to use even the smallest amounts of radioactive injectates in pregnant women, this technique (using less than 1 mrad) has not become popular in this country. Nonetheless, a variety of common obstetric anesthetic techniques and adjuvants have been examined using this technique and thus it is described in some detail.

Placental blood flow is measured immediately before and at various times after the drug is administered. Radioactive xenon-133 (2 mCi) in physiologic saline is injected rapidly into the antecubital vein followed immediately by 10 ml of saline. Since xenon-133 is freely diffusible, it is cleared completely from the circulation during passage through the lungs. However, when the patient holds her breath for about 20 sec after injection, the radioisotope enters the systemic circulation as a small bolus and reaches both the uterus and the placenta. The clearance of the isotope is measured with a scintillation detector over the placenta. In order to use this technique the placenta must be on the anterior uterine wall as determined by sonography and the diameter of the measuring area at the level of the placenta must be 10 cm. A bi-exponential curve $(A_1e^{-k1t} + A_2e^{-k2t})$ is obtained (Fig. 3.1). The component with the longer half-life represents myometrial blood flow, and the component with the shorter half-life represents flow through the intervillous space. The *myometrial blood flow* (F_2) is calculated from the equation $F_2 = \Delta k_2$, where Δ is the partition coefficient of xenon between blood and the myometrial tissue (0.70). The *intervillous flow* (F_1) is obtained from the equation $F_1 = 100(k_1)$. This method has been shown to be highly reproducible (Fig. 3.2) (2).

Currently, the most popular technique for assessing uteroplacental circulation is by a Doppler ultrasound system which displays blood flow velocity-time waveforms. The basic principle behind this technique is the Doppler effect. Sound at a fixed frequency (usually 3 to 5 mHz) is directed toward a blood vessel. When the sound is returned, the frequency is different from the original. This change, called the ***Doppler shift,*** depends on the velocity of the red blood cells in the vessel, the angle between the ultrasound beam and the vessel, and the speed of sound in tissue. This principle can be used to directly or indirectly determine changes of blood flow within uterine vessels.

Actual measurements of blood flow require precise measurement of the cross-sectional areas of the

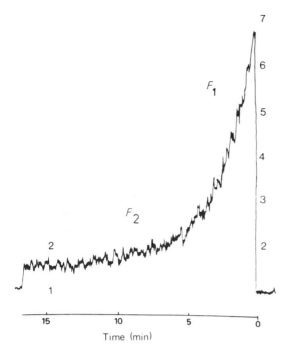

Figure 3.1. Typical bi-exponential curve obtained from a scintillation counter placed over the placenta and myometrium. F_1 corresponds to intervillous blood flow and F_2 to myometrial blood flow. (Reprinted by permission from Jouppila R, Jouppila P, Hollmén A, Kuikka J: Effect of segmental extradural analgesia on placental blood flow during normal labour. Br J Anaesth 50:563–567, 1978.)

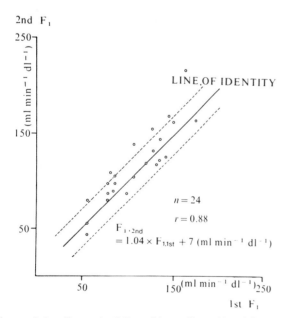

Figure 3.2. Reproducibility of intervillous blood flow measurements in 24 patients during the last few weeks of pregnancy. The *dashed lines* indicate ±20 ml/min/dl. (Reprinted by permission from Jouppila R, Jouppila P, Kuikka J, Hollmén A: Placental blood flow during caesarean section under lumbar extradural analgesia. Br J Anaesth 50:275–278, 1978.)

vessel. An additional problem in converting velocity measurements to actual flows is the difficulty in precisely measuring the angle between the ultrasound beam and the vessel. Describing the relationship between the Doppler waveform during systole and diastole—that is, the systolic/diastolic ratio (S/D ratio)—allows one to study relative changes without actually measuring absolute flow.

Doppler arterial waveforms in most vessels typically show high systolic velocity and little or no diastolic velocity. During pregnancy, maternal uteroplacental vessels show continuous diastolic flow (Fig. 3.3). Any decrease, absence, or reversal of end-diastolic flow velocity is considered abnormal. Details of the technique for measuring uteroplacental arterial flow velocity waveforms may be found in reviews by McFarland et al. (3), Trudinger et al. (4), and Copel et al. (5).

The vast majority of direct information on the effects of anesthesia on uteroplacental circulation has been derived mainly from animal experiments, recognizing that, because of species differences, extrapolation of these data to the human pregnancy must be done with caution. The development of chronic maternal-fetal animal preparations has allowed precise measurement of changes in uterine and placental blood flow and of the effect of these changes on fetal cardiovascular and acid-base status (Fig. 3.4). Uterine blood flow can be measured directly by placing an electromagnetic flow probe on a branch of the uterine artery (6) or indirectly using a steady-state diffusion technique (Fick's principle) with either antipyrine (7), tritiated water (8), or nitrous oxide (9). Distribution of blood flow within the uterus to the placenta, myometrium, and endometrium can be measure by the injection of radioactive microspheres into the maternal left ventricle (10). Details of these techniques may be found in review articles by Schenk and Race (11) and Lewis (12). This chapter reviews the effects of commonly used anesthetic agents, techniques, and adjuvants and of anesthetic complications on uterine blood flow.

INTRAVENOUS INDUCTION AGENTS

Barbiturates

Ultrashort-acting barbiturates are most commonly used for induction of anesthesia and are usually followed by endotracheal intubation and nitrous oxide maintenance. Palahniuk and Cumming (13) studied this sequence and reported that uterine blood flow fell 20% after induction of anesthesia without a significant fall in maternal arterial blood pressure. Fetal oxygen saturation and pH also fell. They postulated that the increase in uterine vascular resistance was

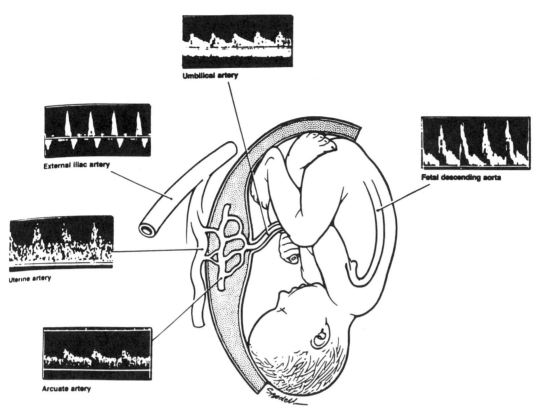

Figure 3.3. Doppler waveforms from normal pregnancy. Shown clockwise are normal waveforms from the maternal arcuate, uterine, and external iliac arteries and from the fetal umbilical artery and descending aorta. Reversed end-diastolic flow velocity is apparent in the external iliac artery, whereas continuous diastolic flow characterizes the uterine and ar- cuate vessels. Finally, note the greatly diminished end-dia- stolic flow in the fetal descending aorta. (Modified from Copel JA, Grannum PA, Hobbins JC, Cunningham FG: Doppler ultrasound in obstetrics. In *Williams Obstetrics* (Suppl No 16). Appleton & Lange, Norwalk, CT, 1988.)

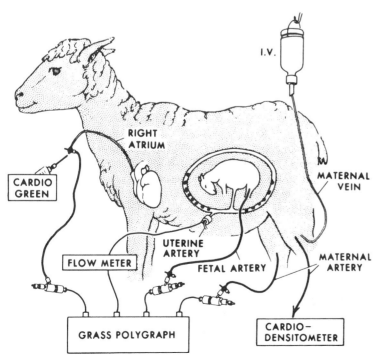

Figure 3.4. Diagram of sheep experimental preparation with chronically implanted maternal and fetal intravascular catheters and an electromag- netic flow probe around a branch of uterine artery. (Reprinted by permission from Ralston DH, Shni- der SM, deLorimier AA: Effects of equipotent ephedrine, metaraminol, mephentermine and methoxamine on uterine blood flow in the pregnant ewe. Anesthesiology 40:354–370, 1974.)

due to maternal catecholamine release during light anesthesia.

Shnider et al. (14) reported that, in sheep, intravenous induction of anesthesia with thiopental and succinylcholine followed by direct laryngoscopy and endotracheal intubation resulted in an increase in arterial plasma norepinephrine of 89% from control. Blood pressure rose 65%, uterine vascular resistance rose 42%, and uterine blood flow fell 24%. These acute cardiovascular changes quickly diminished with the termination of airway manipulation. Recently, Alon et al. (15), also studying pregnant sheep, reported that uterine blood flow decreased about 40% during thiopental induction and endotracheal intubation, then rapidly increased significantly to a point approximately 28 ± 27% above baseline values during anesthetic maintenance with isoflurane (Fig. 3.5). Jouppila et al. (16), using the radioactive xenon technique, corroborated these findings in humans. During the induction of general anesthesia for cesarean section, they found a marked decrease in placental blood flow with a mean reduction of 35% (Fig. 3.6).

Propofol

In contrast to thiopental, uterine blood flow demonstrated no change during induction of anesthesia with propofol (2 mg/kg) despite a significant increase in mean arterial blood pressure. Unlike the uterine blood flow response during maintenance of anesthesia with isoflurane, maintenance of anesthesia with infusions of propofol at either 150, 300, or 450 μg/kg/min (15) did not change uterine blood flow from preinduction baseline values, and it remained stable throughout anesthesia (Fig. 3.7).

Diazepam

In pregnant sheep diazepam in doses as high as 0.5 mg/kg did not alter maternal and fetal cardiovascular function and uteroplacental blood flow (17). However, larger doses produced an 8 to 12% decrease in arterial pressure with an equivalent decrease in uterine blood flow. Fetal oxygenation was not affected. Cosmi (18) also observed that the bolus injection of diazepam to the ewe in doses of 0.18 mg/kg has no deleterious effects on maternal and fetal blood pressure or acid-base status.

Ketamine

Ketamine usually increases arterial blood pressure. Studies by Greiss and Van Wilkes (19) and Ralston et al. (20) have shown that drugs that cause increases in maternal arterial blood pressure as a re-

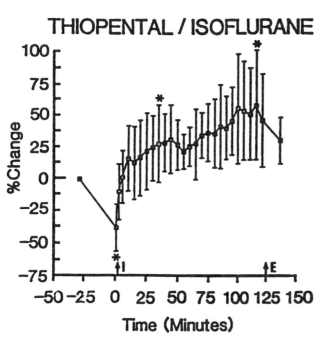

Figure 3.5. Changes in uterine blood flow following induction with thiopental, 5 mg/kg, succinylcholine, 1.5 mg/kg, endotracheal intubation, and maintenance with 1% isoflurane and N$_2$O, 50% (inspired concentration) in oxygen. *I* = intubation; *E* = extubation; *asterisk* = statistically significant differences from control values (*P* < 0.05). (Reprinted by permission from Alon E, Rosen MA, Shnider SM, Ball RH, Parer JT: Maternal and fetal effects of propofol anesthesia in the ewe. Anesthesiology 75:A1077, 1991.)

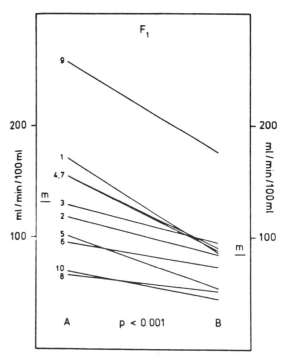

Figure 3.6. The individual intervillous flow changes: *A* = before anesthesia; *B* = immediately following induction of anesthesia with thiopental, 4 mg/kg, and succinylcholine, 1 mg/kg. m̲ = mean value. (Reprinted by permission from Jouppila P, Kuikka J, Jouppila R, Hollmén A: Effect of induction of general anesthesia for cesarean section on intervillous blood flow. Acta Obstet Gynecol Scand 58:249–253, 1979.)

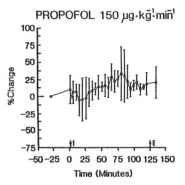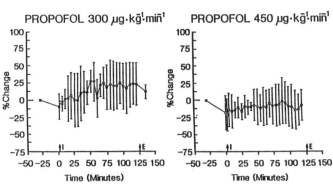

Figure 3.7. Changes in uterine blood flow following induction with propofol, 2 mg/kg, succinylcholine, 1.5 mg/kg, endotracheal intubation, and infusion of varying doses of propofol with N₂O, 50% (inspired concentration) and oxygen. *I* = intubation; *E* = extubation. (Reprinted by permission from Alon E, Rosen MA, Shnider SM, Ball RH, Parer JT: Maternal and fetal effects of propofol anesthesia in the ewe. Anesthesiology 75:A1077, 1991.)

sult of vasoconstriction may lead to a decrease in uterine blood flow with consequent fetal hypoxia and acidosis. Levinson and co-workers (21) administered 5 mg/kg of ketamine to a group of pregnant ewes near term. They found a 15% increase in mean maternal blood pressure and a 10% increase in uterine blood flow. Eng and co-workers (22) reported similar results in monkeys. Craft et al. (23) administered 0.7 mg/kg of ketamine to pregnant sheep and found similar results. Maternal effects consisted of a slight increase in blood pressure and cardiac output (up to 16%) and a moderate increase in uterine resting tone, whereas uterine blood flow remained relatively constant (Fig. 3.8).

Cosmi (24) evaluated the effects of ketamine in pregnant sheep not in labor and during labor. In the ewes not in labor (condition resembling that of elective cesarean section), the drug was administered intravenously in doses of 1.8 to 2.2 mg/kg. Anesthesia was maintained with nitrous oxide and oxygen, and ventilation was controlled. Under these conditions ketamine produced increases in mean maternal blood pressure and heart rate and in uterine blood flow without significant changes in fetal cardiovascular and acid-base status. However, when ketamine in doses of 0.9 to 5 mg/kg was given to the ewes in labor, Cosmi observed a marked increase of maternal ventilation as well as increases in uterine tone and in frequency and intensity of uterine contractions and a slight decrease of uterine blood flow. These changes were dose related and accompanied by fetal tachycardia and acidosis. Similarly, Galloon (25) reported a dose-related increase in uterine muscle tone after ketamine administration in patients undergoing therapeutic abortion during the second trimester.

Therefore there appears to be some variability in the maternal circulatory response to ketamine related in part to the presence or absence of labor, the dosage,

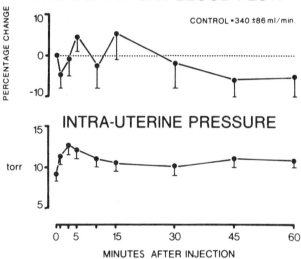

Figure 3.8. Percentage change from control (±SE) of uterine artery blood flow and absolute values of intrauterine pressure following intravenous ketamine, 0.7 mg/kg. Intrauterine pressure increased significantly (*P* < 0.01). (Reprinted by permission from Craft JR Jr, Coaldrake LA, Yonekura ML, Dao SD, Co EG, Roizen MF, Mazel P, Gilman R, Shokes L, Trevor AJ: Ketamine, catecholamines, and uterine tone in pregnant ewes. Am J Obstet Gynecol 146:429–434, 1983.)

and the stage of gestation. It would appear, however, that ketamine in the usual clinical doses (0.25–1 mg/kg) does not adversely affect uterine blood flow. Several studies report normal neonatal clinical and acid-base conditions after the administration of ketamine in doses up to 1 mg/kg for vaginal and abdominal delivery (24, 26–29).

INHALATION AGENTS

The effect of inhalation analgesia-anesthesia on the uteroplacental circulation and on the fetus is still a controversial matter. Some authors (30, 31) report fetal asphyxia, whereas others (32, 33) indicate that well-conducted inhalation anesthesia produces no effects on the fetus and the uteroplacental circulation.

Halothane

Halothane has a unique and specific place in obstetric anesthesia because of its potent uterine relaxant properties. Hence, it is the agent of choice when uterine relaxation is required—for example, for version and extraction, breech delivery, retained placenta, tetanic contractions, and surgical manipulations (34–36). Recent attempts to improve fetal oxygenation by increasing maternal inspired oxygen concentration (37) have stimulated interest in the use of halothane with lower concentrations of nitrous oxide for cesarean section (38). In addition, its use has also been recommended to improve fetal oxygenation in case of fetal distress caused by uterine tetany (39).

Several investigators have studied the effect of halothane on uterine blood flow. Palahniuk and Shnider (40) found that in the pregnant ewe during light and moderately deep anesthesia (1 and 1.5 minimum alveolar concentration [MAC]) maternal blood pressure was slightly depressed (less than 20% from control), but uterine vasodilation occurred and uteroplacental blood flow was maintained. Neither fetal hypoxemia nor metabolic acidosis occurred (see Fig. 11.1). Deep levels of anesthesia (2 MAC) produced greater reductions in maternal blood pressure and cardiac output. Despite uterine vasodilation, uterine blood flow decreased and the fetuses became hypoxic and acidotic. Similar results have been reported by Carenza and Cosmi (41) in pregnant sheep and by Eng et al. (42) in pregnant monkeys. Furthermore, Cosmi (30) has reported that in humans light to moderate planes of halothane anesthesia (i.e., 0.5 to 1 vol/100 ml) did not alter either maternal cardiovascular function or fetal acid-base status. In contrast, deep planes (i.e., 1.5 vol/100 ml or greater) produced maternal hypotension and fetal acidosis.

Shnider and co-workers (14) studied the effects in pregnant ewes of halothane 0.5% inspired combined with 50% N_2O and oxygen. They reported a 22% increase in uterine blood flow during the 1-hr administration period. Thus it seems that low concentrations of halothane do not adversely affect uteroplacental circulation and, in fact, produce uterine vasodilation. Increasing concentrations produce progressive decreases in the uterine blood flow due to maternal hypotension.

Isoflurane

Studies by Palahniuk and Shnider (40) indicate that isoflurane is essentially indistinguishable from halothane in its effects on maternal and fetal cardiovascular and acid-base status. Light planes of anesthesia do not decrease uterine blood flow, but deep planes do. Similarly, Alon et al. (15) reported that, in pregnant ewes, light anesthesia produced by inhalation of isoflurane 1% combined with 50% N_2O and oxygen produced a 25% increase in uterine blood flow (Fig. 3.5).

Methoxyflurane

Smith and co-workers (43) reported that, in contrast to halothane, light anesthesia (1 and 1.5 MAC) with methoxyflurane did not produce uterine vasodilation. Slight to moderate falls in maternal arterial pressure produced comparable falls in uterine blood flow. No serious fetal deterioration was seen. Deep levels of methoxyflurane anesthesia (2 MAC) produced marked falls in maternal blood pressure, cardiac output, and uterine blood flow. Fetal hypoxemia and acidosis developed.

Enflurane

Carenza and Cosmi (41) have studied the effect of enflurane in pregnant sheep and found that light to moderate planes of anesthesia (i.e., 0.4 to 0.8 vol/ml) did not alter maternal and fetal cardiovascular performance, uteroplacental blood flow, and fetal acid-base status. Shnider and co-workers (14) administered 1 vol/100 ml enflurane to healthy pregnant ewes for 1 hr and found no significant changes in blood pressure, uterine blood flow, maternal plasma norepinephrine levels, or fetal cardiovascular or acid-base variables.

Fluroxene

Eng et al. (44) studied the effect of fluroxene in the pregnant primate and found that inhalation of 4 vol/100 ml of fluroxene combined with nitrous oxide and oxygen did not affect uteroplacental circulation or fetal and maternal cardiovascular and acid-base status. In contrast, at 8 vol/100 ml, fluroxene produced a decrease of maternal blood pressure and uterine artery blood flow, fetal hypoxia, and acidosis. Because of its flammability, this agent is no longer used.

LOCAL ANESTHETICS

Gibbs and Noel (45) and Cibils (46) demonstrated a vasoconstricting effect of both lidocaine and mepivacaine using an in vitro preparation of human uterine artery segments obtained from cesarean hysterectomy specimens. The concentrations of local anesthetics ranged from 400 to 1000 μg/ml, concentrations well above levels achieved during clinical use. Uterine vasoconstriction was not seen with lower concentrations nor in uterine arteries taken from nonpregnant hysterectomy specimens, indicating that the response was dose related and occurred only during pregnancy. Pretreatment of the strips with phenoxybenzamine (an α-adrenergic blocker) did not abolish the vasoconstrictive response.

Greiss et al. (47), injecting 20-, 40-, and 80-mg boluses of either lidocaine or mepivacaine into the dorsal aorta of eight anesthetized pregnant ewes, found a dose-related, transient (2 to 3 min) decrease in uterine blood flow and a simultaneous increase in intrauterine pressure (Fig. 3.9). Uterine arterial blood levels were not measured. These investigators also infused lidocaine, mepivacaine, bupivacaine, and procaine directly into the uterine artery of nonpregnant ewes (Fig. 3.10). The following uterine arterial concentrations reduced mean uterine blood flow by 40%: bupivacaine 5 μg/ml, mepivacaine 40 μg/ml, procaine 40 μg/ml, and lidocaine 200 μg/ml. Such enormously high concentrations could not occur during epidural anesthesia in the absence of an intravenous injection.

Subsequent studies in the pregnant ewe by Fishburne et al. (48) and Pue et al. (49) produced similar findings of uterine vasoconstriction occurring only at very high blood levels, which might be found in the uterine vasculature during paracervical blocks (close proximity of the injected drugs to the uterine arteries) or during systemic toxic reactions. Morish-

ima et al. (50) found that, during lidocaine-induced maternal convulsions in the pregnant ewe, uterine blood flow was reduced 55 to 71% of control values. The lack of uterine vasoconstriction with low blood levels of lidocaine was demonstrated by Biehl et al. (51). These investigators infused the local anesthetic intravenously to produce blood levels (2 to 4 μg/ml) in the pregnant ewe comparable to those usually found in the human parturient undergoing epidural anesthesia during the first and second stages of labor. They found that a 2-hr exposure to these low concentrations of lidocaine did not significantly decrease uterine blood flow or increase intraamniotic pressure. Similarly, lidocaine in a dose of 0.4 mg/kg or chloroprocaine in doses up to 2 mg/kg administered intravenously to guinea pigs did not significantly decrease uterine blood flow velocity (52, 53).

Cocaine is a potent local anesthetic with unique vasoconstrictive properties. Aside from its well-known widespread drug abuse potential, it is an ideal agent for anesthetizing the nasopharynx prior to nasotracheal intubation or upper airway surgical procedures. Studies on the effect of intravenous cocaine on uterine blood flow have shown that cocaine in doses between 0.5 mg/kg and 2.8 mg/kg produced a dose-related fall in uterine blood flow (Fig. 3.11) (54–56). In addition, these workers reported that placental transfer of cocaine occurred within 3 min and the ratio of maternal-fetal arterial drug concentrations at 5 min was 1:1.2. These studies indicate that cocaine may significantly decrease uterine blood flow and thus should be administered cautiously and sparingly to human parturients.

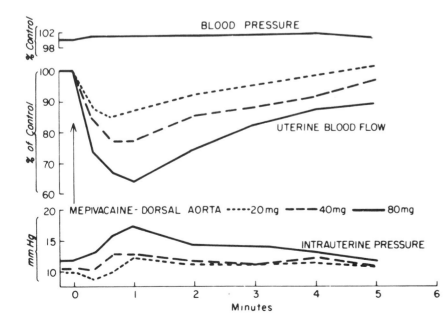

Figure 3.9. Effects of increasing intraaortic doses of mepivacaine on uterine blood flow and intrauterine pressure in pregnant ewes near term. Note the progressive decrease in uterine blood flow with similar inverse changes in intrauterine pressure. (Reprinted by permission from Greiss FC Jr, Still JG, Anderson SG: Effects of local anesthetic agents on the uterine vasculatures and myometrium. Am J Obstet Gynecol 124:889–899, 1976.)

Figure 3.10. Dose-response curves with four local anesthetics in nonpregnant ewes illustrating comparative responses. (Reprinted by permission from Greiss FC Jr, Still JG, Anderson SG: Effects of local anesthetic agents on the uterine vasculatures and myometrium. Am J Obstet Gynecol 124:889–899, 1976.)

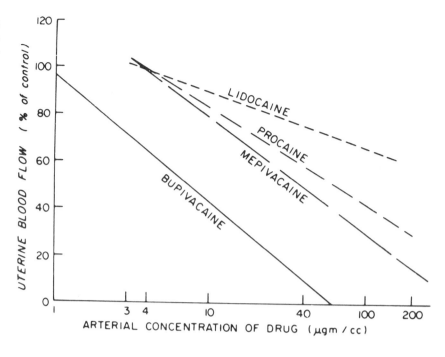

Figure 3.11. Responses of maternal mean arterial pressure (*top*), total uterine blood flow (*middle*), and uterine vascular resistance (*bottom*) to maternal administrations of cocaine. Single asterisks indicate $P < .001$. (Reprinted by permission from Woods JR Jr, Plessinger MA, Clark KE: Effect of cocaine on uterine blood flow and fetal oxygenation. JAMA 257:957–961, 1987.)

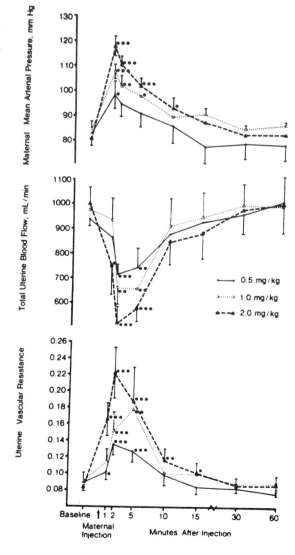

REGIONAL ANESTHESIA

The most frequent complication of spinal, lumbar epidural, and caudal anesthesia is systemic hypotension. The decrease in mean arterial blood pressure reduces uterine blood flow proportionately (57, 58). On the other hand, epidural anesthesia uncomplicated by arterial hypotension is associated with no alterations in uterine blood flow (59).

Brotanek et al. (60) found that epidural anesthesia with mepivacaine did not change uterine blood flow in pregnant women in labor provided the blood pressure did not fall. These studies, performed with a heated thermistor probe, allowed only a qualitative estimate of the changes in flow. No fetal cardiovascular or acid-base data were obtained.

Wallis et al. (59) measured uterine blood flow and percentage of uterine blood flow distributed to the placenta during lumbar epidural anesthesia in the pregnant ewe. Chloroprocaine with and without epinephrine was used. Blood pressure was maintained by intravenous fluid infusion. Except for a transient 14% decrease in uterine blood flow in the ewes receiving chloroprocaine with epinephrine, uterine blood flow remained near control values and was sufficient at all times to maintain stable fetal acid-base and blood gas values (Fig. 3.12). The percentage of uterine blood flow distributed to the placenta in the absence of uterine contractions was not altered

by epidural anesthesia or by addition of epinephrine to the anesthetic solution.

Jouppila and coworkers (2, 61–63) and Hollmén and co-workers (64, 65) have studied extensively the effect of regional anesthesia for labor or cesarean section on uteroplacental perfusion. Studies in healthy women not in labor undergoing cesarean section indicated that neither epidural (2) nor spinal (63) anesthesia, uncomplicated by hypotension, is associated with changes in intervillous blood flow. However, women with preeclampsia showed an improvement in intervillous blood flow following initiation of the block. All parturients in these studies were prehydrated with Ringer's lactate solution (1500 to 2000 ml) prior to the block.

Healthy women in labor showed a 35% increase in intervillous blood flow following the administration of either 10 ml of 0.25% bupivacaine or 2% chloroprocaine (Fig. 3.13) (64). In patients with preeclampsia the epidural injection of 10 ml of 0.25% bupivacaine resulted in a much more significant improvement in intervillous blood flow; the increase amounted to 77% (62). These investigators (61, 64), using smaller volumes of drug (e.g., 4 ml of 0.5% bupivacaine with or without epinephrine 1:200,000), found no improvement in placental blood flow. The authors postulated that the more widespread sympathectomy obtained with larger volumes, together

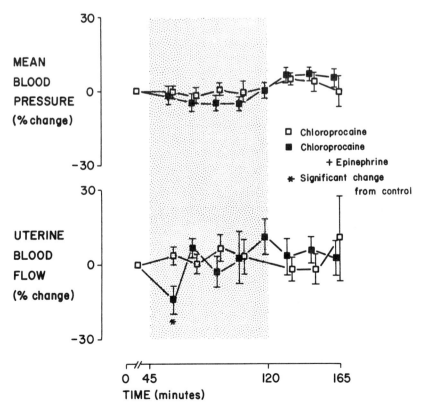

Figure 3.12. Effects of epidural anesthesia (*shaded area*) on mean maternal blood pressure and uterine blood flow. All values subsequent to each control value are given as mean percentage changes with standard errors. (Reprinted by permission from Wallis KL, Shnider SM, Hicks JS, Spivey HT: Epidural anesthesia in the normotensive pregnant ewe: Effects on uterine blood flow and fetal acid-base status. Anesthesiology 44:481–487, 1976.)

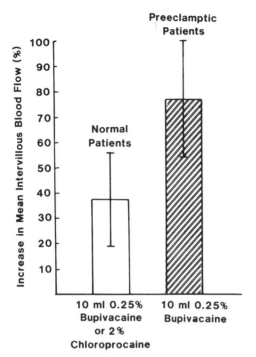

Figure 3.13. Percentage increase in mean intervillous blood flow values (±SE) after epidural anesthesia for labor in normal and preeclamptic patients. (Redrawn by permission from Hollmén A, Jouppila R, Jouppila P, Koivula A, Vierola H: Effect of extradural analgesia using bupivacaine and 2-chloroprocaine on intervillous blood flow during normal labour. Br J Anaesth 54:837–842, 1982; and Jouppila P, Jouppila R, Hollmén A, Koivula A: Lumbar epidural analgesia to improve intervillous blood flow during labor in severe preeclampsia. Obstet Gynecol 59:158–161, 1982.)

with the relief of pain and anxiety, tends to restore uterine blood flow to its normal nonstressed basal condition.

Recent studies using Doppler ultrasound to measure uteroplacental arterial flow velocity waveforms have confirmed with rare exception (66) the lack of deleterious effects of epidural anesthesia on uterine blood flow (67–70). These studies involved women receiving epidural blocks to T3–T5 dermatome levels for elective cesarean sections. These women were all prehydrated with 1 to 2 liters of balanced salt solution, positioned with left uterine tilt, and received either lidocaine 2% or bupivacaine 0.5%, both with and without epinephrine 1:200,000.

CATECHOLAMINES AND STRESS

Adrenergic stimulation produced by either exogenous or endogenous catecholamines can constrict uterine vessels and reduce uterine blood flow. Exogenous catecholamines (primarily epinephrine) are administered with local anesthetics to produce vasoconstriction at the site of injection. Endogenous cat-

echolamines (both epinephrine and norepinephrine) are released during anxiety and pain. Vasopressors are frequently used to prevent or treat spinal or epidural hypotension.

Epinephrine

Epinephrine has significant effects on both α- and β-adrenergic receptors. High epinephrine blood levels achieved by accidental intravascular injection of epinephrine-containing local anesthetics produce α-adrenergic effects, including hypertension, increased total peripheral resistance, uterine vasoconstriction, increased uterine activity, and decreased uterine blood flow. In ewes given 0.10 to 1 μg/kg/min of epinephrine, maternal pressure rose 65% above control and uterine blood flow fell 55 to 75% (71). Injection of epinephrine 20 μg in pregnant ewes decreased uterine blood flow 40% for about 60 sec (72). Similarly, injections of epinephrine 0.2 to 1 μg/kg in the pregnant guinea pig produced transient dose-related decreases in uterine artery blood flow velocities (52, 73).

Low blood levels of epinephrine, such as occur from systemic absorption during caudal or epidural block, have been shown to produce a generalized β-adrenergic response that becomes maximal 15 min after epidural injection (74). A number of studies on the β-adrenergic effects of epinephrine on the uterine vessels have produced conflicting results.

Rosenfeld and colleagues (75) infused 50 to 100 μg of epinephrine intravenously over a 5-min period into pregnant ewes and produced a generalized β-adrenergic effect with tachycardia and increased cardiac output and blood flow to skeletal muscles. However, although blood pressure did not change, uterine blood flow decreased almost 50%. These investigators postulated that the uterine artery in the pregnant ewe may be more sensitive to the α-adrenergic effects of epinephrine while vasculature of skeletal muscle, adipose tissue, or other visceral organs may be more sensitive to the β-adrenergic effects. In contrast, deRosayro et al. (76) studied the effects of epidural epinephrine (100 μg) *without* local anesthetic drugs on the cardiovascular system of anesthetized pregnant ewes. Except for slight tachycardia there were no significant cardiovascular changes. Uterine blood flow remained stable. Wallis et al. (59) did find a transient 14% reduction in uterine blood flow in pregnant ewes who received epidural epinephrine (60 to 80 μg) combined with 1.5% chloroprocaine. These ewes had decreases in total peripheral resistance and increases in cardiac output, although blood pressure did not change. Because uterine blood flow did not change in animals who received only chloroprocaine, the decrease in uterine blood flow was possibly due to the combination of epinephrine absorbed from the epidural space and sympathectomy produced by the local anesthetic.

Albright et al. (77) did not corroborate these latter findings. These investigators reported that epidural chloroprocaine 10 ml with epinephrine 1:200,000 did not alter *human* intervillous blood flow during epidural anesthesia for labor despite a reduction in mean blood pressure of 11 torr. Levinson et al. (76) compared 2% lidocaine alone to 2% lidocaine with 1:200,000 epinephrine administered for epidural anesthesia for cesarean section. They found no adverse effects of epinephrine on the mother or neonate as ascertained by the incidence of hypotension, low Apgar scores, or abnormal fetal acid-base status.

In summary, there may be transient fluctuations in uterine blood flow after epidural anesthesia with epinephrine-containing solutions. However, these have little effect on the healthy fetus.

Stress

Myers (79) reported that maternal stress and anxiety in the pregnant rhesus monkey produced fetal asphyxia, likely due to uterine vasoconstriction as a consequence of maternal catecholamine release. Shnider et al. (80) found that stress sufficient to produce maternal hypertension resulted in a precipitous

fall in uterine blood flow and increase in plasma norepinephrine in pregnant ewes. Similarly, Martin and Gingerick (81) found a marked reduction in uterine blood flow in response to severe stress in the pregnant rhesus monkey.

Lederman et al. (82, 83) have reported that both primiparous and multiparous parturients who are very anxious during labor have increased circulating epinephrine blood levels and a higher incidence of abnormal fetal heart rate patterns compared to those who are less anxious. Again, we would presume that these findings are due to uterine hypoperfusion.

Vasopressors

Vasopressors with predominant α-adrenergic activity reduce uterine blood flow and may adversely affect the fetus (84, 85). Methoxamine, phenylephrine, angiotensin, or norepinephrine treatment of spinal hypotension in animals diminishes uterine blood flow and leads to fetal asphyxia (85–87). Ephedrine, mephentermine, and metaraminol restore uterine blood flow toward normal (Fig. 3.14) (88–90).

Studies of treatment of spinal or epidural hypotension using either low dose phenylephrine (20 to 100 μg), or ephedrine (10 to 15 mg) in elective cesarean sections have not confirmed the animal data

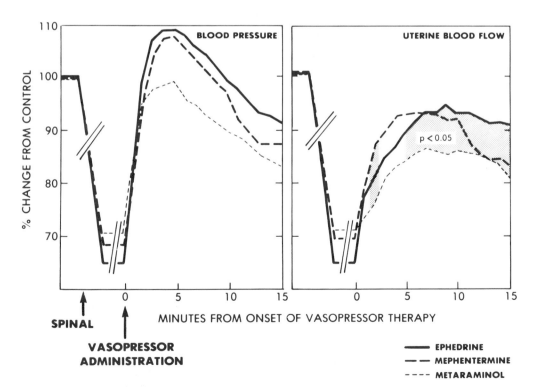

Figure 3.14. Average response patterns to ephedrine and slow infusions of mephentermine and metaraminol after hypotension induced by spinal anesthesia. After 4 min, uterine blood flow was significantly higher with ephedrine and me-

phentermine than with metaraminol therapy. (Reprinted by permission from James FM III, Greiss FC Jr, Kemp RA: An evaluation of vasopressor therapy for maternal hypotension during spinal anesthesia. Anesthesiology 33:25–34, 1970.)

(91, 92). Using an impedance cardiograph to measure stroke volume (SV), ejection fraction (EF), and end-diastolic volume (EDV), Ramanathan and Grant (91) showed that both ephedrine and phenylephrine produce venoconstriction to a greater degree than arterial constriction, improve venous return (cardiac preload), increase cardiac output, and likely restore uterine perfusion (Fig. 3.15).

Prophylactic vasopressor administration has also been studied. Eng et al. (85) reported that methoxamine infusion in pregnant primates decreased uterine blood flow and produced fetal asphyxia. Infusion of ephedrine, a predominantly β-adrenergic-stimulating drug, had no discernible effect on uterine blood flow or fetal acid-base status during the infusion. In normotensive pregnant ewes, Ralston et al. (20) found that infusion of methoxamine or metaraminol decreased uterine blood flow at all dose levels. On the other hand, doses of ephedrine that raised blood pressure to even 50% above control had no detrimental effect on uterine blood flow or fetal acid-base status (Fig. 3.16). Hollmén et al. (65) reported that there were no adverse effects of prophylactic ephedrine on human intervillous blood flow during cesarean section performed under epidural anesthesia. Therefore it seems that drugs such as ephedrine or mephentermine, which support maternal blood pressure augmenting venous return and by central adrenergic stimulation (positive inotropic and chronotropic activity), have minimal effects on uterine blood flow in the normotensive mother and restore uterine blood flow when used to treat spinal or epidural hypotension. Human studies, as reported above, suggest that carefully titrated doses of phenylephrine may also produce beneficial hemodynamic effects without adversely affecting the fetus and may be useful in selected patients. For the overwhelming majority of patients, ephedrine remains the vasopressor of choice.

Dopamine, a catecholamine that stimulates dopaminergic and α- and β-adrenergic receptors, has been studied in normotensive and hypotensive pregnant sheep. In normotensive animals, Callender et al. (93) reported that doses that increase maternal blood pressure and cardiac output decrease uterine blood flow. Rolbin et al. (94) reported that dopamine, when used to treat spinal hypotension, corrected maternal blood pressure but resulted in a further fall in uterine blood flow. This was due to a significant increase in uterine vascular resistance despite minimal changes in total peripheral resistance. Conflicting results were reported by Cabalum et al. (95), who found that dopamine infusion in doses similar to those used by Rolbin restored uterine blood flow with the correction of hypotension. A possible explanation for the differences found in these studies is that Cabalum et al. did not place the flow probe around a branch of the uterine artery, but rather the internal iliac artery, and thus their flow signal may not reflect that of the uterine circulation (96). A vasoconstrictive effect on uterine blood vessels has been reported with β-adrenergic drugs such as isoxsuprine (97), ritodrine (72, 98), and terbutaline (99). The effects of dopamine on the uterine vessels likely represent an increased sensitivity of these vessels to dopamine's α-adrenergic stimulation.

ANTIHYPERTENSIVE AGENTS

Hypertensive disorders of pregnancy frequently require therapy. Ideally, drugs used to treat maternal hypertension should reduce blood pressure and uterine vascular resistance so that uterine blood flow is either unchanged or increased.

Hydralazine

Hydralazine, a slow-acting antihypertensive drug, is used widely in the treatment of gestational hypertension. The effects of hydralazine on uterine blood

Figure 3.15. Stroke volume (*SV*), end-diastolic volume (*EDV*), and systemic vascular resistance (*SVR*) before anesthesia (*1*), during hypotension (*2*), after therapy with ephedrine or phenylephrine and (*3*), *Asterisk* = significant difference from 1 and 3 (*P* < .01). Measurements in the control group were obtained before anesthesia and T6 sensory level. (Reprinted by permission from Ramanathan S, Grant GJ: Vasopressor therapy for hypotension due to epidural anesthesia for cesarean section. Acta Anaesthesiol Scand 32:559–565, 1988.)

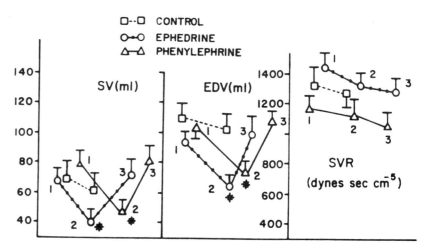

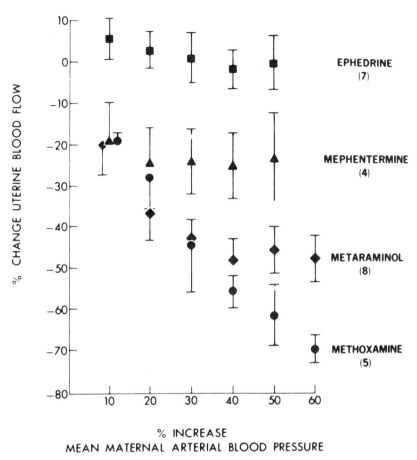

Figure 3.16. Mean changes in uterine blood flow at equal elevations of mean arterial blood pressure after vasopressor administration. (Reprinted by permission from Ralston DH, Shnider SM, deLorimier AA: Effects of equipotent ephedrine, metaraminol, mephentermine and methoxamine on uterine blood flow in the pregnant ewe. Anesthesiology 40:354–370, 1974.)

flow in the hypertensive pregnant ewe have been studied by Brinkman and Assali (100). These investigators induced severe hypertension and reduction in uterine blood flow by placing a modified Goldblatt clamp around one renal artery and removing the contralateral kidney. Hydralazine, in this preparation, reduced blood pressure while increasing uterine blood flow. Similarly, in a study by Ring et al. (101) on phenylephrine-induced hypertension, hydralazine slowly lowered the blood pressure while significantly increasing uterine blood flow, although uterine blood flow did not return to normal (Fig. 3.17). During cocaine-induced hypertension in the pregnant ewe, hydralazine did not restore uterine blood flow as maternal blood pressure returned to normal (Fig. 3.18) (102). In humans the effects of intravenously infused hydralazine (incremental doses up to 125 μg/min during 60 min) were studied by Jouppila et al. (103) in 10 women with acute or superimposed severe preeclampsia. The intervillous and umbilical vein blood flow were measured before and during hydralazine infusion with the xenon-133 method and with a combination of real-time and Doppler ultrasonic equipment, respectively. Maternal blood pressure decreased and pulse rate in-

creased during the infusion. Hydralazine did not change the intervillous blood flow but increased the blood flow in the umbilical vein. The results indicated that hydralazine affected the placental and fetal circulations differently.

Nitroglycerin

Craft et al. (104) found that a nitroglycerin infusion administered to pregnant ewes during phenylephrine-induced hypertension resulted in a reduction in blood pressure associated with an improvement in uterine blood flow.

Nitroprusside

Nitroprusside, a rapidly acting antihypertensive is popular in the management of nonobstetric hypertensive emergencies. Similar to hydralazine, the drug causes a decrease in total peripheral resistance and an increase in coronary and mesenteric blood flow (105–107). Ring et al. (101) reported that, although nitroprusside decreased total peripheral resistance, it failed to correct the fall in uterine blood flow (Fig. 3.17). In contrast, using isolated uterine arteries from pregnant patients (obtained during cesarean-hysterectomy), Nelson and Suresh (108) demonstrated that,

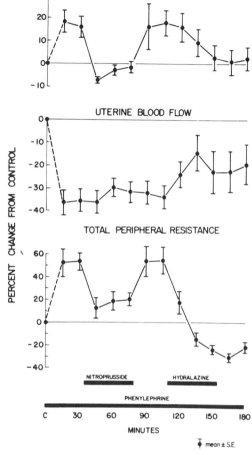

Figure 3.17. Percentage change from control of maternal mean arterial blood pressure, uterine blood flow, and total peripheral resistance during phenylephrine-induced hypertension and correction of hypertension with nitroprusside and hydralazine. Hydralazine, but not nitroprusside, resulted in a significant increase in uterine blood flow ($P < 0.05$). (Reprinted by permission from Ring G, Krames E, Shnider SM, Wallis KL, Levinson G: Comparison of nitroprusside and hydralazine in hypertensive pregnant ewes. Obstet Gynecol 50:598–602, 1977.)

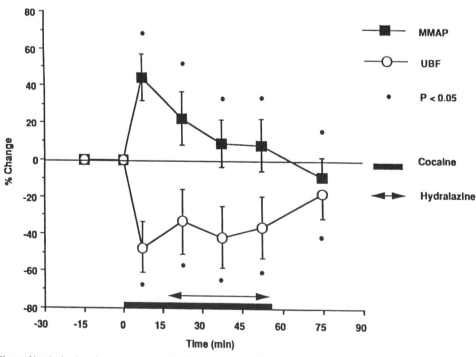

Figure 3.18. Effect of hydralazine therapy on cocaine-induced maternal hypertension. Percentage change in maternal mean arterial pressure (MMAP) and uterine blood flow (UBF) during cocaine administration and hydralazine therapy ($n = 10$). The arrow represents the time of hydralazine treatment. Both drugs were discontinued at 55 min. Values are expressed as ±SD. Changes are compared to baseline values with sig- nificance noted (*asterisk = $P < 0.05$*). (Reprinted by per- mission from Vertommen JD, Hughes SC, Rosen MA, Shnider SM, Espinoza MI, Messer CP, Johnson JL, Parer JT: Hy- dralazine does not restore uterine blood flow during cocaine-induced hypertension in the pregnant ewe. Anesthesiology 76:580–587, 1992.)

although both nitroprusside and hydralazine inhibited norepinephrine-induced uterine artery contraction, nitroprusside had a greater potency compared to hydralazine in producing direct vasodilation of the uterine arteries from pregnant humans.

For maternal indications, nitroprusside has been administered because of its rapid action as a vasodilator to reduce arterial blood pressure. This hypotensive action may prevent serious complications such as cerebrovascular accidents or acute heart failure. Preeclamptic patients undergoing general anesthesia may be exposed to these complications due to the acute hypertension associated with laryngoscopy and intubation. Thus short-term use of nitroprusside during induction of anesthesia might attenuate this pressor response.

However, the fetal safety of nitroprusside has been questioned. Naulty et al. (109) reported that, in pregnant normotensive ewes receiving an infusion of nitroprusside for 1 hr, maternal arterial and umbilical venous levels of nitroprusside were identical. In some animals fetal cyanide toxicity and death occurred. On the other hand, Ellis et al. (110) performed a similar study on hypertensive (norepinephrine induced) ewes. As used in this animal model, the clinical doses of nitroprusside did not result in high fetal or maternal cyanide levels. There were no fetal deaths associated with the study. The authors postulated that nitroprusside could be used safely at induction of general anesthesia in the preeclamptic patient to attenuate the pressor response to laryngoscopy and intubation. However, they recommended that the use of nitroprusside be restricted to the period immediately prior to induction of general anesthesia in order to limit the exposure of the fetus to cyanide.

Labetalol

Labetalol is a combined α- and β-adrenergic blocking agent. It is used orally to decrease blood pressure in preeclamptic women (111–113). It is also used intravenously to rapidly decrease blood pressure in severely preeclamptic women and to attenuate the hemodynamic response to tracheal intubation (114). Intravenously administered labetalol does not alter uterine blood flow in preeclamptic women at rest (115), nor does intravenously administered labetalol alter placental perfusion in pregnant hypertensive rats (116). In the near-term pregnant ewe, intravenous bolus administration of labetalol ameliorated the effects of increased circulating norepinephrine on maternal arterial pressure and uterine blood flow and produced less adrenergic blockade in the fetus than in the mother (117).

CALCIUM CHANNEL-BLOCKING DRUGS

Calcium channel-blocking drugs are potentially useful in obstetrics. They produce arteriolar vaso-

dilatation and may be effective agents in the management of preeclampsia. They slow atrioventricular conduction and may have a role in maternal and fetal supraventricular tachyarrhythmias. They inhibit uterine contractility and thus may be useful in the treatment of preterm labor.

Murad and co-workers (118) studied the hemodynamic effects of *verapamil* in the awake pregnant ewe. Verapamil (0.2 mg/kg) administered intravenously over 3 min resulted in a variety of maternal cardiovascular changes: a transient (2 to 5 min) decrease in systolic, diastolic, and mean blood pressures, and increase in central venous, mean pulmonary artery, and pulmonary capillary wedge pressures. These results are consistent with the negative inotropic and peripheral vasodilating effects of verapamil. Cardiac output, systemic peripheral vascular resistance, and pulmonary vascular resistance were unaffected. Uterine blood flow decreased 25% at 2 min, then remained slightly below control levels for 30 min after drug injection. Thus the effects of verapamil on uterine blood flow suggest that the drug should be used with caution in cases of uteroplacental insufficiency.

Studies of *nicardipine* in rabbits (119) and monkeys (120) and *nifedipine* in sheep (121) have all shown that these drugs decrease uteroplacental blood flow. On the other hand, studies in humans using Doppler ultrasound have shown that short-term *oral* administration does not significantly alter uteroplacental circulation (122, 123).

MAGNESIUM SULFATE

Since its first use in obstetrics reported in 1925 by Lazard (124) and Dorsett (125), magnesium sulfate has been used parenterally as an adjunct in the management of certain hypertensive diseases of pregnancy, especially preeclampsia and eclampsia. Its effects on the central and peripheral nervous systems and on neuromuscular transmission are discussed in Chapters 17 and 18. Its action on the maternal and fetal cardiovascular systems and uteroplacental circulation has been investigated in pregnant normotensive and hypertensive ewes (126, 127).

Magnesium sulfate was administered to the mother in amounts sufficient to produce a constant serum concentration of between 5 and 12 mEq/liter in a study by Dandavino et al. (126) and between 5 and 7 mEq/liter in a study by Krames et al. (127). Dandavino and co-workers found that magnesium sulfate produced a fall in the systemic arterial blood pressure both in hypertensive and normotensive animals. However, this effect was transient, lasting less than 10 min. The uteroplacental blood flow increased by about 10%. Administration of high doses of magnesium sulfate (a 4-g bolus injection followed by a 2 to

4 g/hr infusion) produced an initial and transitory decrease of maternal arterial pressure that was greater in the hypertensive than in the normotensive animals. However, 5 to 10 min after the start of the infusion, the mean arterial pressure in both groups had returned to control values. The uteroplacental blood flow increased an average of 13.5% in the normotensive and 7.7% in the hypertensive animals. Krames et al. found that magnesium sulfate produced a decrease in mean arterial blood pressure of 7% with a 7% rise in uterine vascular conductance, thereby resulting in no change in uterine blood flow.

The results of these studies suggest that magnesium sulfate has only a mild and transient effect on maternal arterial pressure and uterine blood flow.

EPIDURAL OPIATES

Epidural opiates are widely used for the treatment of labor pain. Studying pregnant ewes near term, Rosen and co-workers (128) administered 20 mg of morphine into the epidural space. These investigators found no significant changes in uterine blood flow nor, indeed, in any maternal or fetal cardiovascular or acid-base variable during a 2-hr study period. Craft et al. (129) confirmed these findings. They found no significant deleterious effects on uterine blood flow or maternal and fetal hemodynamic and acid-base parameters following the administration to the awake pregnant ewe of 50, 75, or 100 μg fentanyl (129, 130, 131) or 10 or 20 μg of sufentanil (Craft JB Jr, unpublished data).

CLONIDINE

Clonidine is used orally as an antihypertensive, intravenously to rapidly control hypertensive emergencies, and epidurally to produce analgesia by an opiate-independent mechanism. It acts primarily by stimulation of α_2-adrenergic receptors, although in high concentrations it will stimulate other receptor subtypes. It causes constriction of human uterine arteries in vitro by a mixed α_1- and α_2-adrenergic mechanism (132).

The effects on uterine blood flow of orally administered clonidine have not been studied, but it has been used safely for many years without apparent adverse maternal, fetal, or neonatal effects (133–136). In normotensive pregnant ewes, intravenous clonidine increases intraamniotic pressure and decreases uterine blood flow without altering maternal or fetal blood pressure (Fig. 3.19) (137). The effect on uterine blood flow of intravenous clonidine in a hypertensive animal model has not been studied. Epidurally administered clonidine did not affect uterine blood flow nor did it alter maternal or fetal blood pressure (138).

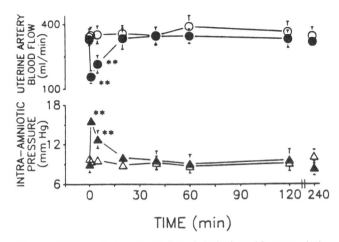

Figure 3.19. Uterine blood flow (*circles*) and intraamniotic pressures (*triangles*) after maternal intravenous injection of saline solution ($\triangle$ $\bigcirc$) or clonidine, 300 μg ($\blacktriangle$ $\bullet$). Each point represents mean $\pm$ SEM of six to eight animals. (** = $P <$ .01 versus saline solution.) (Reprinted by permission from Eisenach JC, Castro MI, Dewan DM, Rose JC, Grice SC: Intravenous clonidine hydrochloride toxicity in pregnant ewes. Am J Obstet Gynecol 160:471–476, 1988.)

Intravenously administered α_2-adrenergic agonists such as clonidine have also been shown to have other adverse effects. These include rapid placental transfer (136, 137), maternal and fetal hypoxemia (139, 140), hyperglycemia (137), and decreased heart rate. The mechanism of the hypoxemia is not well understood since it is not a result of respiratory or cardiovascular depression or pulmonary vasoconstriction (140). The hyperglycemia is the result of inhibition of insulin release (141). Despite numerous side effects of *intravenous* clonidine, *epidural* clonidine may be safe and has the advantage of not inducing pruritus, nausea, vomiting or respiratory depression.

DANTROLENE

Dantrolene is currently indispensable in the treatment of malignant hyperthermia, although infrequent malignant hyperthermia has been reported during labor and delivery (142–147). Pretreatment of susceptible patients with oral dantrolene before induction of labor or a cesarean section is controversial. Recommended regimens include dantrolene (25 mg orally four times a day) for 5 days before delivery, then for 3 days after delivery in progressively decreasing doses (day 1, 25 mg three times; day 2, 25 mg twice; day 3, 25 mg once) (148). Dantrolene crosses the placenta with a fetal/maternal ratio between 0.18 and 0.4 and no apparent adverse effects in the infants (148, 149). Craft et al. (149) studied 1.2 mg/kg and 2.4 mg/kg of dantrolene administered intravenously to awake pregnant ewes and demonstrated the drug's maternal and fetal safety. Maternal blood pressure and cardiac output increased slightly, but no significant changes were observed in maternal heart rate, central venous pressure, or uterine blood flow. Fetal heart rate decreased 25% by 3 min but returned to normal by 10 min. No clinically significant changes in maternal or fetal acid-base status were noted.

RESPIRATORY GASES

Contrary to earlier beliefs, *moderate* hypoxia, hypercapnia, and hypocapnia do not affect uteroplacental blood flow (151, 152). On the other hand, marked changes in respiratory gases decrease placental perfusion. Dilts et al. (153) measured uterine blood flow in pregnant sheep during severe maternal hypoxia induced by ventilating the lungs with 6 or 12% oxygen gas mixtures. When the lungs were ventilated with a gas mixture containing 6% oxygen, there was an increase in cardiac output and a decrease in maternal systemic vascular resistance. Uteroplacental vascular resistance increased, and uterine blood flow decreased markedly (Fig. 3.20). Milder

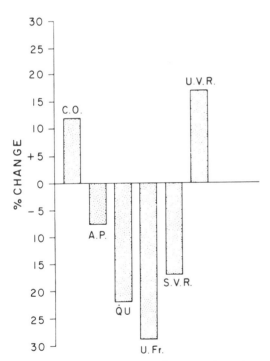

Figure 3.20. Percentage change in systemic and uteroplacental hemodynamics during experimental hypoxia induced by ventilating the ewe with a gas mixture containing 6% oxygen. Note the increase in cardiac output (*C.O.*) and in the uterine vascular resistance (*U.V.R.*) and the marked fall in uterine blood flow (*QU*), uterine fraction of cardiac output (*U.Fr.*), systemic vascular resistance (*S.V.R.*), and arterial pressure (*A.P.*). (Reprinted by permission from Dilts PV Jr, Brinkman CR III, Kirschbaum TH, Assali NS: Uterine and systemic hemodynamic interrelationships and their response to hypoxia. Am J Obstet Gynecol 103:138–157, 1969.)

hypoxia induced with 12% oxygen produced changes that were qualitatively smaller. These investigators attributed these hemodynamic changes to the enhanced output of catecholamines induced by hypoxia. When the mother was made hypoxic by reducing arterial PO_2 to 40 torr, the fetus also became hypoxic.

Effects of maternal **hypercapnia** on the uteroplacental circulation are variable. An increase (154), decrease (155), and no changes (7, 156) have been reported. Walker et al. (157), using chronic unanesthetized sheep preparations, found that by increasing the arterial PCO_2 to 60 torr, uterine blood flow increased. Mean arterial pressure rose while uterine vascular resistance was unchanged. However, at $PaCO_2$ levels above 60 torr, uterine vascular resistance increased progressively and uterine blood flow fell, despite further increases in mean arterial pressure (Fig. 3.21).

Maternal **hypocapnia** is a frequent phenomenon in pregnant women. It may occur spontaneously as a result of painful uterine contractions, anxiety and apprehension during labor, or improperly performed Lamaze technique. Controlled ventilation during anesthesia may also accidently produce severe maternal alkalemia. Controversy still exists regarding its effects on the fetus and the uteroplacental circulation. Some investigators have reported that marked hyperventilation ($PaCO_2$ of 17 torr or less) causes uteroplacental vasoconstriction, decreases uteroplacental blood flow, and induces fetal hypoxia, acidosis, and neonatal depression (158, 159). Others have denied that maternal hyperventilation, even of marked degree, is harmful to the fetus. These investigators found minimal changes in the acid-base status of the fetus and no significant effect on uteroplacental blood flow (160, 161). Levinson et al. (155) studied changes in uterine blood flow and fetal oxygenation in unanesthetized pregnant ewes during mechanical hyperventilation. In order to evaluate separately the effects of maternal hypocapnia and positive pressure ventilation, CO_2 was added to the inspired air during mechanical hyperventilation to produce normocapnia and hypercapnia. Uterine blood flow decreased approximately 25% during all hyperventilation periods (Fig. 3.22). Because the reduction in uterine blood flow was unrelated to changes in maternal $PaCO_2$ (range 17 to 64 torr) or pH (range 7.74 to 7.24), the decrease probably was caused by the mechanical effect of positive pressure ventilation.

Metabolic alkalosis may also be detrimental to the fetus as a result of decreased uteroplacental blood flow and displacement of the maternal oxygen-hemoglobin dissociation curve to the left, resulting in increased affinity of maternal hemoglobin for ox-

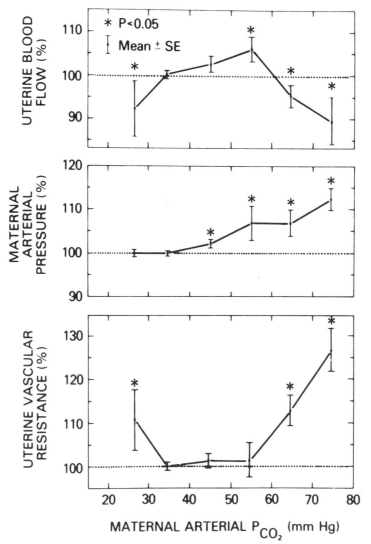

Figure 3.21. Percentage change of uterine blood flow, maternal arterial pressure, and uterine vascular resistance during progressive increases of arterial P_{CO_2} induced in conscious pregnant ewes by adding CO_2 to inspired gas mixture. (Reprinted by permission from Walker AM, Oakes GK, Ehrenkranz R, McLaughlin M, Chez RA: Effects of hypercapnia on uterine and umbilical circulations in conscious pregnant sheep. J Appl Physiol 41:727–733, 1976.)

ygen and decreased release at the placenta (159, 162–164). In the pregnant ewe, Cosmi (18) found that maternal metabolic alkalosis induced by intravenous infusion of trihydroxymethylaminomethane (THAM) caused maternal bradycardia and hypotension, decreased uterine blood flow, and induced fetal hypoxia and acidosis. Ralston et al. (163) produced maternal alkalemia with the infusion of sodium bicarbonate in normal pregnant ewes and found a 16% reduction in uterine blood flow with a concomitant decrease in fetal oxygenation and pH. On the other hand, in Cosmi's study (18), the infusion of small doses of sodium bicarbonate (e.g., 100 mEq over 12

min) to the acidotic ewe did not alter uterine blood flow.

SUMMARY

Intravenous induction agents, inhalation and local anesthetics, endogenous and exogenous catecholamines and vasopressors, antihypertensive agents and magnesium sulfate, respiratory gases, and metabolic alkalosis can all alter uterine blood flow. Their net effects on uterine blood flow ultimately depend on how these agents alter uterine perfusion pressure relative to uterine vascular resistance.

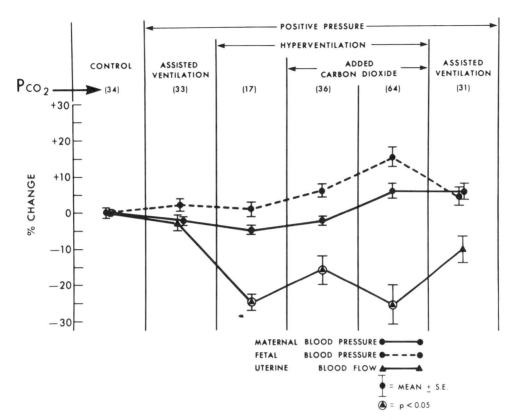

Figure 3.22. Changes from control values in mean maternal and fetal arterial blood pressure and uterine blood flow during five periods of positive pressure ventilation. Mean maternal Pa_{CO_2} during each period is indicated at the *top* of the figure.

(Reprinted by permission from Levinson G, Shnider SM, deLorimier AA, Steffenson JL: Effects of maternal hyperventilation on uterine blood flow and fetal oxygenation and acid-base status. Anesthesiology 40:340–347, 1974.)

References

1. Rekonen A, Luotola H, Pitkanen M, Kuikka J, Pyorala T: Measurement of intervillous and myometrial blood flow by an intravenous ^{133}Xe method. Br J Obstet Gynaecol 83:723–728, 1976.
2. Jouppila R, Jouppila P, Kuikka J, Hollmén A: Placental blood flow during caesarean section under lumbar extradural analgesia. Br J Anaesth 50:275–278, 1988.
3. McParland P, Pearce JM: Doppler blood flow in pregnancy: Review article. Placenta 9:427–450, 1988.
4. Trudinger BJ, Giles WB, Cook CM: Uteroplacental blood flow velocity: Time waveforms in normal and complicated pregnancy. Br J Obstet Gynaecol 92:39–45, 1985.
5. Copel JA, Grannum PA, Hobbins JC, Cunningham FG: Doppler ultrasound in obstetrics. In *Williams' Obstetrics*, Suppl No 16. Appleton & Lange, Norwalk, CT, 1988.
6. Greiss FC Jr: The uterine vascular bed: Effect of adrenergic drug stimulation. Obstet Gynecol 21:295–301, 1963.
7. Huckabee WE: Uterine blood flow. Am J Obstet Gynecol 84:1623–1633, 1962.
8. Parer JT, Lannoy CW, Behrman RE: Uterine blood flow and oxygen consumption in rhesus monkeys with retained placentas. Am J Obstet Gynecol 100:806–812, 1968.
9. Assali NS, Rauramo L, Peltonen T: Measurement of uterine blood flow and uterine metabolism. VIII. Uterine and fetal blood flow and oxygen consumption in early human pregnancy. Am J Obstet Gynecol 79:86–98, 1960.
10. Makowski EL, Meschia G, Droegemueller W, Battaglia FC: Distribution of uterine blood flow in the pregnant sheep. Am J Obstet Gynecol 101:409–412, 1968.
11. Schenk WG Jr, Race D: Methods of measurement of blood flow: A current appraisal. J Surg Res 6:361–371, 1966.

12. Lewis BV: Uterine blood flow. Obstet Gynecol Surv 24:1211–1233, 1969.
13. Palahniuk RJ, Cumming M: Foetal deterioration following thiopentone-nitrous oxide anaesthesia in the pregnant ewe. Can Anaesth Soc J 24:361–370, 1977.
14. Shnider SM, Wright RG, Levinson G, Roizen MF, Rolbin SH, Biehl D, Johnson J, Jones M: Plasma norephinephrine and uterine blood flow changes during endotracheal intubation and general anesthesia in the pregnant ewe. In *Abstracts of Scientific Papers*, American Society of Anesthesiologists, Chicago, 1978, p 115.
15. Alon E, Rosen MA, Shnider SM, Ball RH, Parer JT: Maternal and fetal effects of propofol anesthesia in the ewe. Anesthesiology 75:A1077, 1991.
16. Jouppila P, Kuikka J, Jouppila R, Hollmén A: Effect of induction of general anesthesia for cesarean section on intervillous blood flow. Acta Obstet Gynecol Scand 58:249–253, 1979.
17. Mofid M, Brinkman CR III, Assali NS: Effects of diazepam on uteroplacental and fetal hemodynamics and metabolism. Obstet Gynecol 41:364–368, 1973.
18. Cosmi EV: Fetal homeostasis. In *Pulmonary Physiology of the Fetus, Newborn and Child*. EM Scarpelli, PAM Auld, eds. Lea & Febiger, Philadelphia, 1975, p 61.
19. Griess FC Jr, Van Wilkes D: Effects of sympathomimetic drugs and angiotensin on the uterine vascular bed. Obstet Gynecol 23:925–930, 1964.
20. Ralston DH, Shnider SM, deLorimier AA: Effects of equipotent ephedrine, metaraminol, mephentermine and methoxamine on uterine blood flow in the pregnant ewe. Anesthesiology 40:354–370, 1974.
21. Levinson G, Shnider SM, Gildea JE, deLorimier AA: Maternal and foetal cardiovascular and acid-base changes during ke-

tamine anaesthesia in pregnant ewes. Br J Anaesth 45:1111–1115, 1973.

22. Eng M, Berges PU, Bonica JJ: The effects of ketamine on uterine blood flow in the monkey. In *Abstracts of Scientific Papers*, Society for Gynecological Investigation, Atlanta, 1973, p 48.

23. Craft JB Jr, Coaldrake LA, Yonekura JL, Dao SD, Co EF, Roizen MF, Mazel P, Gilman R, Shokes L, Trevor AJ: Ketamine, catecholamines, and uterine tone in pregnant ewes. Am J Obstet Gynecol 146:429–434, 1983.

24. Cosmi EV: Effetti della ketamina sulla madre e sul feto. Studio sperimentale e clinico. Minerva Anestesiol 43:379, 1977.

25. Galloon S: Ketamine for obstetric delivery. Anesthesiology 44:522–524, 1976.

26. Chodoff P, Stella JG: Use of Cl-581-A phencyclidine derivative for obstetrical anesthesia. Anesth Analg 45:527–530, 1966.

27. Meer FM, Downing JW, Coleman AJ: An intravenous method of anesthesia for caesarean section. II. Ketamine. Br J Anaesth 45:191–196, 1973.

28. Akamatsu TJ, Bonica JJ, Rehmet R, Eng M, Ueland K: Experiences with the use of ketamine for parturition. I. Primary anesthetic for vaginal delivery. Anesth Analg 53:284–287, 1974.

29. Hodgkinson R, Marx GF, Kim SS, Miclat NM: Neonatal neurobehavioral tests following vaginal delivery under ketamine, thiopental and extradural anesthesia. Anesth Analg 56:548–553, 1977.

30. Cosmi EV, Marx GF: The effect of anesthesia on the acid-base status of the fetus. Anesthesiology 30:238–242, 1969.

31. Brann AW Jr, Myers RE, DiGiacomo R: The effect of halothane-induced maternal hypotension in the fetus. In *Medical Primatology 1970*. Proceedings of the 2nd Conference on Experimental Medicine and Surgery in Primates, New York, 1969. S Karger, Basel, 1971, p 637.

32. Moir DD: Anaesthesia for caesarean section. An evaluation of a method using low concentrations of halothane and 50 per cent of oxygen. Br J Anaesth 42:136–142, 1970.

33. Bonica JJ: Halothane in obstetrics. In *The Anesthesiologist, Mother and Newborn*. SM Shnider, F Moya, eds. Williams & Wilkins, Baltimore, 1974, pp 114–121.

34. Allard E, Guimond C: L'halothane en obstetrique. Can Anaesth Soc J 11:38–87, 1964.

35. Stoelting VK: Fluothane in obstetric anesthesia. Anesth Analg 43:243–246, 1964.

36. Crawford JS: The place of halothane in obstetrics. Br J Anaesth 34:386–390, 1962.

37. Marx GF, Mateo CV: Effects of different oxygen concentrations during general anesthesia for elective cesarean section. Can Anaesth Soc J 18:587–593, 1971.

38. Galbert MW, Gardner AE: Use of halothane in a balanced technique for cesarean section. Anesth Analg 51:701–704, 1972.

39. Phillips JM, Evans JA: Acute anesthetic and obstetric management of patients with severe abruptio-placenta. Anesth Analg 49:998–1004, 1970.

40. Palahniuk RJ, Shnider SM: Maternal and fetal cardiovascular and acid-base changes during halothane and isoflurane anesthesia in the pregnant ewe. Anesthesiology 41:462–472, 1974.

41. Carenza L, Cosmi EV: Analgo-anetesia in travaglio nel parto: Valutazione des metodi e dei farmaci. In *58th Congress of the Italian Society of Obstetrics and Gynecology*. Mattioli Publ, Fidenza, Italy, 1977, p 286.

42. Eng M, Bonica JJ, Akamatsu TJ, Berges PU, Der Yuen D, Ueland K: Maternal and fetal responses to halothane in pregnant monkeys. Acta Anaesth Scand 19:154–158, 1975.

43. Smith JB, Manning FA, Palahniuk RJ: Maternal and foetal effects of methoxyflurane anaesthesia in the pregnant ewe. Can Anaesth Soc J 22:449–459, 1975.

44. Eng M, Berges PU, Der Yuen D, Bonica JJ, Ueland K: A comparison of the effects of the inhalation of 4% and 8% fluoroxene in the pregnant primate. Acta Anaesth Scand 20:183–188, 1976.

45. Gibbs CP, Noel SC: Human uterine artery responses to lidocaine. Am J Obstet Gynecol 126:313–315, 1976.

46. Cibils LA: Response of human uterine arteries to local anesthetics. Am J Obstet Gynecol 126:202–210, 1976.

47. Greiss FC Jr, Still JG, Anderson SG: Effects of local anesthetic agents on the uterine vasculatures and myometrium. Am J Obstet Gynecol 124:889–899, 1976.

48. Fishburne JI, Hopkinson RB, Greiss FC Jr: Responses of gravid uterine vasculature to arterial levels of local anesthetic agents. In *Abstracts of Scientific Papers*, Society for Obstetric Anesthesia and Perinatology, Seattle, 1977, p 37.

49. Pue AF, Plumer MH, Resnik R, Brink GW: Effects of local anesthetics on uterine blood flow in pregnant sheep. In *Abstracts of Scientific Papers*. Society for Obstetric Anesthesia and Perinatology, Seattle, 1977, p 47.

50. Morishima HO, Gutsche BB, Keenaghan JB, Barkus BS, Covino BG: The effect of lidocaine-induced maternal convulsions on the fetal lamb. In *Abstracts of Scientific Papers*. American Society of Anesthesiologists, New Orleans, 1977, p 293.

51. Biehl D, Shnider SM, Levinson G, Callender K: The direct effects of circulating lidocaine on uterine blood flow and foetal well-being in the pregnant ewe. Can Anaesth Soc J 24:445–451, 1977.

52. Chestnut DH, Weiner CP, Martin JG, Herrig JE, Wang JP: Effect of intravenous epinephrine on uterine artery blood flow velocity in the pregnant guinea pig. Anesthesiology 65:633–636, 1986.

53. Chestnut DH, Weiner CP, Herrig JE: The effect of intravenously administered 2-chloroprocaine upon uterine artery blood flow velocity in gravid guinea pigs. Anesthesiology 70:305–308, 1989.

54. Foutz SE, Kotelko DM, Shnider SM, Thigpen JW, Rosen MA, Brookshire GL, Koike M, Levinson G, Elias-Baker B: Placental transfer and effects of cocaine on uterine blood flow and the fetus. Anesthesiology 59:A422, 1983.

55. Moore TR, Sorg J, Key TC, Resnik R: Effects of intravenous cocaine on uterine blood flow and cardiovascular parameters in the pregnant ewe. In *Abstracts of Scientific Papers*. Society for Gynecological Investigation, Phoenix, 1985, p 175.

56. Woods JR Jr, Plessinger MA, Clark KE: Effect of cocaine on uterine blood flow and fetal oxygenation. JAMA 257:957–961, 1987.

57. Greiss FC Jr, Crandell DL: Therapy for hypotension induced by spinal anesthesia during pregnancy. JAMA 191:793–796, 1965.

58. Greiss FC Jr: Pressure-flow relationship in the gravid uterine vascular bed. Am J Obstet Gynecol 96:41–47, 1966.

59. Wallis KL, Shnider SM, Hicks JS, Spivey HT: Epidural anesthesia in the normotensive pregnant ewe: Effects on uterine blood flow and fetal acid-base status. Anesthesiology 44:481–487, 1976.

60. Brotanek V, Vasicka A, Santiago A, Brotanek JD: The influence of epidural anesthesia on uterine blood flow. Obstet Gynecol 42:276–282, 1973.

61. Jouppila R, Jouppila P, Hollmén A, Kuikka J: Effects of segmental extradural analgesia on placental blood flow during normal labour. Br J Anesth 50:563–567, 1978.

62. Jouppila P, Jouppila R, Hollmén A, Koivula A: Lumbar epidural analgesia to improve intervillous blood flow during labor in severe preeclampsia. Obstet Gynecol 59:158–161, 1982.

63. Jouppila P, Jouppila R, Barinoff T, Koivula A: Placental blood flow during caesarean section performed under subarachnoid blockade. Br J Anaesth 56:1379–1382, 1984.

64. Hollmén A, Jouppila R, Jouppila P, Koivula A, Vierola H: Effect of extradural analgesia using bupivacaine and 2-chloroprocaine on intervillous blood flow during normal labour. Br J Anaesth 54:837–842, 1982.

65. Hollmén AI, Jouppila R, Albright GA, Jouppila P, Vierola H, Koivula A: Intervillous blood flow during caesarean section with prophylactic ephedrine and epidural anaesthesia. Acta Anaesthesiol Scand 28:396–400, 1984.

66. Baumann H, Alon E, Atanassoff P, Pasch TH, Huch A, Huch R: Effect of epidural anesthesia for cesarean delivery on maternal femoral arterial and venous, uteroplacental, and umbilical blood flow velocities and waveforms. Obstet Gynecol 75:194–198, 1990.

67. Giles W, Lah F, Trudinger B: The effect of epidural anaesthesia for caesarean section on maternal uterine and fetal umbilical artery blood flow velocity waveforms. Br J Obstet Gynaecol 94:55–59, 1987.

68. Petrikovsky B, Cohen M, Tancer M: Uterine and umbilical blood flow during caesarean section under epidural anaesthesia. Acta Obstetrica Gynaecologica Scand 67:737–739, 1988.

69. Morrow RJ, Rolbin SH, Ritchie JWK, Haley S: Epidural anaesthesia and blood flow velocity in mother and fetus. Can J Anaesth 36:519–522, 1989.

70. Turner GA, Newnham JP, Johnson C, Westmore M: Effects of extradural anaesthesia on umbilical and uteroplacental arterial flow velocity waveforms. Br J Anaesth 67:306–309, 1991.

71. Barton MD, Kilam AP, Meschia G: Response of ovine uterine blood flow to epinephrine and norepinephrine. Proc Soc Exp Biol Med 145:996–1003, 1974.

72. Hood DD, Dewan DM, James FM II: Maternal and fetal effects of epinephrine in gravid ewes. Anesthesiology 64:610–613, 1986.

73. Chestnut DH, Ostman LG, Weiner CP, Hdez MJ, Wang JP: The effect of vasopressor agents upon uterine artery blood flow velocity in the gravid guinea pig subjected to ritodrine infusion. Anesthesiology 68:363–366, 1988.

74. Bonica JJ, Akamatsu TJ, Berges PU, Morikawa K, Kennedy WF Jr: Circulatory effects of peridural block. II. Effects of epinephrine. Anesthesiology 34:514–522, 1972.

75. Rosenfeld CR, Barton MD, Meschia G: Effects of epinephrine on distribution of blood flow in the pregnant ewe. Am J Obstet Gynecol 124:156–163, 1976.

76. deRosayro AM, Nahrwold ML, Hill AB: Cardiovascular effects of epidural epinephrine in the pregnant sheep. Reg Anesth 6:4, 1981.

77. Albright GA, Jouppila R, Hollmén AI, Jouppila P, Vierola H, Koivula A: Epinephrine does not alter human intervillous blood flow during epidural anesthesia. Anesthesiology 54:131–135, 1981.

78. Levinson G, Shnider SM, Krames E, Ring G: Epidural anesthesia for cesarean section: Effects of epinephrine in the local anesthetic solution. In Abstracts of Scientific Papers. American Society of Anesthesiologists, Chicago, 1975, p 285.

79. Myers RE: Maternal psychological stress and fetal asphyxia: A study in the monkey. Am J Obstet Gynecol 122:47–59, 1975.

80. Shnider SM, Wright RG, Levinson G, Roizen MF, Wallis KL, Rolbin SH, Craft JB Jr: Uterine blood flow and plasma norepinephrine changes during maternal stress in the pregnant ewe. Anesthesiology 50:524–527, 1979.

81. Martin CB Jr, Gingerick B: Uteroplacental physiology. JOGNN 5(suppl):16–25, 1976.

82. Lederman RP, Lederman E, Work BA Jr, McCann DS: The relationship of maternal anxiety, plasma catecholamines and plasma cortisol to progress in labor. Am J Obstet Gynecol 132:495–500, 1978.

83. Lederman RP, Lederman E, Work B, McCann DS: Anxiety and epinephrine in multiparous labor: Relationship to duration of labor and fetal heart rate pattern. Am J Obstet Gynecol 153:870–877, 1985.

84. Adamsons K, Mueller-Heubach E, Myers RE: Production of fetal asphyxia in the rhesus monkey by administration of catecholamines to the mother. Am J Obstet Gynecol 109:248–262, 1971.

85. Eng M, Berges PU, Ueland K, Bonica JJ, Parer JT: The effects of methoxamine and ephedrine in normotensive pregnant primates. Anesthesiology 35:354–360, 1971.

86. Shnider SM, deLorimier AA, Asling JH, Morishima HO: Vasopressors in obstetrics. II. Fetal hazards of methoxamine administration during obstetric spinal anesthesia. Am J Obstet Gynecol 106:680–686, 1970.

87. Greiss FC Jr, Gobble FL Jr: Effect of sympathetic nerve stimulation on the uterine vascular bed. Am J Obstet Gynecol 97:962–967, 1967.

88. James FM III, Greiss FC Jr, Kemp RA: An evaluation of vasopressor therapy for maternal hypotension during spinal anesthesia. Anesthesiology 33:25–34, 1970.

89. Eng M, Berges PU, Parer JT, Bonica JJ, Ueland K: Spinal anesthesia and ephedrine in pregnant monkeys. Am J Obstet Gynecol 115:1095–1099, 1973.

90. Shnider SM, deLorimier AA, Steffenson JL: Vasopressors in obstetrics. III. Fetal effects of metaraminol infusion during obstetric spinal hypotension. Am J Obstet Gynecol 108:1017–1022, 1970.

91. Ramanathan S, Grant GJ: Vasopressor therapy for hypotension due to epidural anesthesia for cesarean section. Acta Anaesthesiol Scand 32:559–565, 1988.

92. Moran DH, Perillo M, Bader AM, Datta S: Phenylephrine in treating maternal hypotension secondary to spinal anesthesia. Anesthesiology 71:A857, 1989.

93. Callender K, Levinson G, Shnider SM, Feduska N, Biehl DR, Ring G: Dopamine administration in the normotensive pregnant ewe. Obstet Gynecol 51:586–589, 1978.

94. Rolbin SH, Levinson G, Shnider SM, Biehl DR, Wright R: Dopamine treatment of spinal hypotension decreases uterine blood flow in the pregnant ewe. Anesthesiology 51:36–40, 1978.

95. Cabalum T, Zugaib M, Lieb S, Nuwayhid B, Brinkman CR III, Assali NS: Effect of dopamine on hypotension induced by spinal anesthesia. Am J Obstet Gynecol 133:630–634, 1979.

96. Tabsh K, Nuwayhid B, Erkkola R, Zugaib M, Lieb S, Ushioda E, Brinkman CR III, Assali NS: Hemodynamic responses of the pelvic vascular bed to vasoactive stimuli in pregnant sheep. Biol Neonate 39:52–60, 1981.

97. Ehrenkranz RA, Hamilton LA, Bennan SC, Oakes GK, Walker AM, Chez RA: Effects of salbutamol and isoxsuprine on uterine and umbilical blood flow in pregnant sheep. Am J Obstet Gynecol 128:287–293, 1977.

98. Enrenkranz RA, Walker AM, Oakes GK, McLaughlin MK, Chez RA: Effect of ritodrine infusion on uterine and umbilical blood flow in pregnant sheep. Am J Obstet Gynecol 126:343–349, 1976.

99. Chestnut DH, Weiner CP, Wang JP, Herrig JE, Martin JG: The effect of ephedrine upon uterine artery blood flow velocity in the pregnant guinea pig subjected to terbutaline infusion and acute hemorrhage. Anesthesiology 66:508–512, 1987.

100. Brinkman CR III, Assali NS: Uteroplacental hemodynamic response to antihypertensive drugs in hypertensive pregnant sheep. In Hypertension in Pregnancy. MD Lindhimer, AL Katz, FP Zuspan, eds. John Wiley, New York, 1976, pp 363–375.

101. Ring G, Krames E, Shnider SM, Wallis KL, Levinson G: Comparison of nitroprusside and hydralazine in hypertensive pregnant ewes. Obstet Gynecol 50:598–602, 1977.

102. Vertommen JD, Hughes SC, Rosen MA, Shnider SM, Espinoza MI, Messer CP, Johnson JL, Parer JT: Hydralazine does not restore uterine blood flow during cocaine-induced hypertension in the pregnant ewe. Anesthesiology 76:580–587, 1992.

103. Jouppila P, Kirkinen P, Koivula A, Ylikorkala O: Effects of dihydralazine infusion on the fetoplacental blood flow and maternal prostanoids. Obstet Gynecol 65:115–118, 1985.

104. Craft JB Jr, Co EG, Yonekura ML, Gilman RM: Nitroglycerin therapy for phenylephrine-induced hypertension in pregnant ewes. Anesth Analg 59:494–499, 1980.

105. Schlant RC, Tsagaris TS, Robertson RJ Jr: Studies on the acute cardiovascular effects of intravenous sodium nitroprusside. Am J Cardiol 9:51–59, 1972.

106. Styles MB, Coleman AJ, Leary WP: Some hemodynamic effects of sodium nitroprusside. Anesthesiology 38:173–176, 1973.

107. Ross G, Cole PV: Cardiovascular actions of sodium nitro-prusside in dogs. Anaesthesia 28:400–406, 1973.
108. Nelson SH, Suresh MS: Comparison of nitroprusside and hydralazine in isolated uterine arteries from pregnant and nonpregnant patients. Anesthesiology 68:541–547, 1988.
109. Naulty JS, Cefalo R, Rodkey FL: Placental transfer and fetal toxicity of sodium nitroprusside. In *Abstracts of Scientific Papers*. American Society of Anesthesiologists, San Francisco, 1976, p 543.
110. Ellis SC, Wheeler AS, James FM III, Rose JC, Meis PH, Greiss FC, Urban RB, Shihabi Z: Sodium nitroprusside for hypertension in gravid ewes. Anesthesiology 55:A302, 1981.
111. Mabie WC, Gonzalez AR, Sibai BM, Amon E: Comparative trial of labetalol and hydralazine in the acute management of severe hypertension complicating pregnancy. Obstet Gynecol 70:328–333, 1987.
112. Pickles CJ, Symonds EM, Pipkin FB: The fetal outcome in a randomized double-blind controlled trial of labetalol versus placebo in pregnancy-induced hypertension. Br J Obstet Gynaecol 96:38–43, 1989.
113. Plouin P-F, Breart G, Maillard F, Papiernik E, Relier J-P: Comparison of antihypertensive efficacy and perinatal safety of labetalol and methyldopa in the treatment of hypertension in pregnancy: A randomized controlled trial. Br J Obstet Gynaecol 95:868–876, 1988.
114. Ramanathan J, Sibai BM, Mabie WC, Chauhan D, Ruiz AG: The use of labetalol for attenuation of the hypertensive response to endotracheal intubation in preeclampsia. Am J Obstet Gynecol 159:650–654, 1988.
115. Joupilla P, Kirkinen P, Koivula A, Ylikorkala O: Labetalol does not alter the placental and fetal blood flow or maternal prostanoids in pre-eclampsia. Br J Obstet Gynaecol 93:543–547, 1986.
116. Ahokas RA, Mabie WC, Sibai BM, Anderson GD: Labetalol does not decrease placental perfusion in the hypertensive term-pregnant rat. Am J Obstet Gynecol 160:480–484, 1989.
117. Eisenach JC, Mandell G, Dewan DM: Maternal and fetal effects of labetalol in pregnant ewes. Anesthesiology 74:292–297, 1991.
118. Murad SHN, Tabsh KMA, Shilyanski G, Kapur PA, Ma C, Lee C, Conklin KA: Effects of verapamil on uterine blood flow and maternal cardiovascular function in the awake pregnant ewe. Anesth Analg 64:7–10, 1985.
119. Lirette M, Holbrook RH, Katz M: Cardiovascular and uterine blood flow changes during nicardipine HCl tocolysis in the rabbit. Obstet Gynecol 69:79–82, 1987.
120. Ducsay CA, Thompson JS, Wu AT, Novy MJ: Effects of calcium entry blocker (nicardipine) tocolysis in rhesus macaques: Fetal plasma concentrations and cardiorespiratory changes. Am J Obstet Gynecol 157:1482–1486, 1987.
121. Harake B, Gilbert RD, Ashwal S, Power GG: Nifedipine: Effects on fetal and maternal hemodynamics in pregnant sheep. Am J Obstet Gynecol 157:1003–1008, 1987.
122. Mari G, Kirshon B, Moise KJ, Lee W, Cotton DB: Doppler assessment of the fetal and uteroplacental circulation during nifedipine therapy for preterm labor. Am J Obstet Gynecol 161:1514–1518, 1989.
123. Pirhonen JP, Erkkola RU, Erblad UU, Nyman L: Single dose of nifedipine in normotensive pregnancy: Nifedipine concentrations, hemodynamic responses, and uterine and fetal flow velocity waveforms. Obstet Gynecol 76:807–811, 1990.
124. Lazard EM: A preliminary report on the intravenous use of magnesium sulfate in puerperial eclampsia. Am J Obstet Gynecol 9:178–188, 1925.
125. Dorsett L: The intramuscular injection of magnesium sulfate for the control of convulsions in eclampsia. Am J Obstet Gynecol 11:227–231, 1926.
126. Dandavino A, Woods JR Jr, Murayama L, Brinkman CR III, Assali NS: Circulatory effects of magnesium sulfate in normotensive and renal hypertensive pregnant sheep. Am J Obstet Gynecol 127:769–774, 1977.
127. Krames E, Ring G, Wallis KL, Levinson G, Shnider SM: The effect of magnesium sulfate on uterine blood flow and fetal

well-being in the pregnant ewe. In *Abstracts of Scientific Papers*. American Society of Anesthesiologists, Chicago, 1975, p 287.
128. Rosen MA, Hughes SC, Curtis JD, Norton M, Levinson G, Shnider SM: Effects of epidural morphine on uterine blood flow and acid-base status in the pregnant ewe. Anesthesiology 57:A383, 1982.
129. Craft JB Jr, Bolan JC, Coaldrake LA, Mondino M, Mazel P, Gilman RM, Shikes LK, Woolf WA: The maternal and fetal cardiovascular effects of epidural morphine in the sheep model. Am J Obstet Gynecol 142:835–839, 1982.
130. Craft JB Jr, Robichaux AG, Kim HS, Thorpe DH, Mazel P, Woolf WA, Stolte A: The maternal and fetal cardiovascular effects of epidural fentanyl in the sheep model. Am J Obstet Gynecol 148:1098–1104, 1984.
131. Craft JB Jr, Coaldrake LA, Bolan JC, Mondino M, Mazel P, Gilman RM, Shokes LK, Woolf WA: Placental passage and uterine effects of fentanyl. Anesth Analg 62:894–898, 1983.
132. Ribeiro CAF, Macedo TA: Pharmacological characterization of the postsynaptic alpha-adrenoceptors in human uterine artery. J Pharm Pharmacol 38:600–605, 1986.
133. Horvath JS, Phippard A, Korda A, Henderson-Smart DJ, Child A, Tiller J: Clonidine hydrochloride: A safe and effective antihypertensive agent in pregnancy. Obstet Gynecol 66:634–638, 1985.
134. Hartikaninen-Sorri A-L, Heikkinen JE, Koivisto M: Pharmacokinetics of clonidine during pregnancy and nursing. Obstet Gynecol 69:598–600, 1987.
135. Tuimala R, Punnonen R, Kauppila E: Clonidine in the treatment of hypertension during pregnancy. Ann Chir Gynaecol 74(suppl):47–50, 1985.
136. Huisjes HJ, Hadders-Algra M, Touwen BCL: Is clonidine a behavioral teratogen in the human? Early Hum Dev 14:43–48, 1986.
137. Eisenach JC, Castro MI, Dewan DM, Rose JC, Grice SC: Intravenous clonidine hydrochloride toxicity in pregnant ewes. Am J Obstet Gynecol 160:471–476, 1988.
138. Eisenach JC, Rose JC, Dewan DM, Grice SC: Effects of epidural clonidine in pregnant ewes. Anesthesiology 67:A448, 1987.
139. Jansen CAM, Lowe KC, Nathanielsz PW: The effects of xylazine on uterine activity, fetal and maternal oxygenation, cardiovascular function, and fetal breathing. Am J Obstet Gynecol 148:386–390, 1984.
140. Eisenach JC: Intravenous clonidine produces hypoxemia by a peripheral alpha$_2$-adrenergic mechanism. J Pharmacol Exp Ther 244:247–252, 1988.
141. Metz SA, Halter JB, Robertson RP: Induction of defective insulin secretion and impaired glucose tolerance by clonidine: Selective stimulation of metabolic alpha-adrenergic pathways. Diabetes 27:554–562, 1978.
142. Wadhwa RK: Obstetric anesthesia for a patient with malignant hyperthermia susceptibility. Anesthesiology 46:63–64, 1977.
143. Willatts SM: Malignant hyperthermia susceptibility: Management during pregnancy and labour. Anaesthesia 34:41–46, 1979.
144. Lips FJ, Newland M, Dutton G: Malignant hyperthermia triggered by cyclopropane during cesarean section. Anesthesiology 56:144–146, 1982.
145. Cupryn JP, Kennedy A, Byrick RJ: Malignant hyperthermia in pregnancy. Am J Obstet Gynecol 150:327–328, 1984.
146. Gibbs JM: Unexplained hyperpyrexia during labor (letter). Anaesth Intensive Care 12:375, 1984.
147. Doublas MJ, McMorland GH: The anaesthetic management of the malignant hyperthermia susceptible parturient. Can Anaesth Soc J 33:371–378, 1986.
148. Shime J, Gare D, Andrews J, Britt B: Dantrolene in pregnancy: Lack of adverse effects on the fetus and newborn infant. Am J Obstet Gynecol 159:831–834, 1988.
149. Morison DH: Placental transfer of dantrolene (letter). Anesthesiology 59:265, 1983.
150. Craft JB Jr, Goldberg NH, Lim M, Landsberger E, Mazel P,

Abramson FP, Stolte AL, Braswell ME Jr, Farina JP: Cardiovascular effects and placental passage of dantrolene in the maternal-fetal sheep model. Anesthesiology 68:68–72, 1988.

151. Greiss FC Jr, Anderson SG, King LC: Uterine vascular bed: Effects of acute hypoxia. Am J Obstet Gynecol 113:1057–1064, 1972.

152. Makowski EL, Hertz RH, Meschia G: Effect of acute maternal hypoxia and hyperoxia on the blood flow to the pregnant uterus. Am J Obstet Gynecol 115:624–629, 1973.

153. Dilts PV Jr, Brinkman CR III, Kirschbaum TH, Assali NS: Uterine and systemic hemodynamic interrelationships and their response to hypoxia. Am J Obstet Gynecol 103:138–157, 1969.

154. Assali NS, Holm LW, Sehgal N: Hemodynamic changes in fetal lamb in utero in response to asphyxia, hypoxia and hypercapnia. Circ Res 11:423–430, 1962.

155. Levinson G, Shnider SM, deLorimier AA, Steffenson JL: Effects of maternal hyperventilation on uterine blood flow and fetal oxygenation and acid-base status. Anesthesiology 40:340–347, 1974.

156. Wolkoff AS, McGee JA, Flowers CE, Bawden JW: Alterations in uterine blood flow in the pregnant ewe. I. Associated changes in blood gases. Obstet Gynecol 23:636–637, 1964.

157. Walker AM, Oakes GK, Ehrenkranz R, McLaughlin M, Chez RA: Effects of hypercapnia on uterine and umbilical circulation in conscious pregnant sheep. J Appl Physiol 41:727–733, 1976.

158. Morishima HO, Daniel SS, Adamsons K Jr, James LS: Effects of positive pressure ventilation of the mother upon the acid-base state of the fetus. Am J Obstet Gynecol 93:269–273, 1965.

159. Motoyama EK, Rivard G, Acheson F, Cook CD: Adverse effect of maternal hyperventilation on the foetus. Lancet 1:286–288, 1966.

160. Lumley J, Renou P, Newman W, Wood C: Hyperventilation in obstetrics. Am J Obstet Gynecol 103:847–855, 1969.

161. Parer JT, Eng M, Aoba H, Ueland K: Uterine blood flow and oxygen uptake during maternal hyperventilation in monkeys at cesarean section. Anesthesiology 32:130–135, 1970.

162. Johnson GH, Brinkman CR III, Assali NS: Effects of acid and base infusion on umbilical hemodynamics. Am J Obstet Gynecol 112:1122–1128, 1972.

163. Ralston DH, Shnider SM, deLorimier AA: Uterine blood flow and fetal acid-base changes after bicarbonate administration to the pregnant ewe. Anesthesiology 40:348–353, 1974.

164. Buss DD, Bisgard EG, Rawlings CA, Rankin JHG: Uteroplacental blood flow during alkalosis in the sheep. Am J Physiol 228:1497–1500, 1975.

Effects of Anesthesia on Uterine Activity and Labor

Anthony C. Miller, M.D.
Jay S. DeVore, M.D.
Edward A. Eisler, M.D.

The conduct of an obstetric anesthetic and the progress and management of labor are inextricably bound together. Without question, the course of a parturient's labor affects the management of her obstetric anesthesia and analgesia. However, despite years of investigations into the subject, the effects of anesthesia on labor are still controversial; there is little consensus; and much of the discussion between obstetricians and obstetric anesthetists centers on this topic.

DEFINITIONS

Uterine activity is defined in terms of the frequency of contraction of the uterus and the pressure generated by these contractions. Such activity can be monitored indirectly by a tocodynamometer applied to the maternal abdomen or directly by an intrauterine pressure catheter (IUPC) inserted into the uterine cavity. The tocodynamometer is triggered by the changing shape of the uterus during a contraction. Because it is externally applied, the data are quantitative only with respect to the frequency of contractions. The intraamniotic catheter, however, also measures both the intrauterine pressure during contractions and resting uterine tone, that is, the lowest pressure recorded between contractions.

Several systems have been devised for describing uterine activity. One of the earliest and still most commonly used was developed by Caldeyro-Barcia (1). With this system, the number of contractions in a 10-min period is multiplied by the force of these contractions (peak amplitude minus resting tone in millimeters of mercury). The result is stated in *Montevideo units*. Another method calculates the area under the uterine pressure curve and yields a result that is expressed in torr-minutes or *uterine activity units* (2). Yet another system simply records the mean peak amplitude of contractions over a 10-min period.

All of these methods have been used in assessing the effect of drugs on uterine activity.

Progress of labor refers to increasing cervical dilation and effacement and the descent of the presenting fetal part in the pelvis as originally described by Friedman (Fig. 4.1) (3). The *first stage of labor* refers to the period from the beginning of cervical dilation and effacement (onset of regular, painful contractions) to its completion (4). It is divided into the *latent* and *active phases*, which are distinguished by the rate of cervical dilation (Fig. 4.1). The *second stage of labor* extends from complete cervical dilation until delivery of the infant, and the *third stage* from then until the placenta is delivered (4).

Abnormal progress of labor is defined by the following patterns (Table 4.1): *prolonged latent phase, slow slope (protracted) active phase, active phase arrest, protracted descent, and arrest of descent* (4). During the latent phase, incoordinate uterine contraction and, possibly, excessive sedation or anesthesia that decrease uterine activity (see "Regional Anesthesia and Analgesia" in the following) are common causes for labor prolongation (5). During the active phase or second stage of labor, cephalopelvic disproportion, malposition, and malpresentation are the most common etiologic factors (5). Diagnosis and treatment of abnormal labor are crucial because it is associated with increased perinatal morbidity and mortality (5).

Uterine relaxation is defined as diminution or cessation of uterine contractions and a decrease in resting uterine tone.

INHALATION AGENTS

Many inhalation anesthetics have a direct and dose-related effect on uterine activity. Naftalin et al. (6, 7), using in vitro preparations of both rat and human myometrium, demonstrated a dose-related reduction

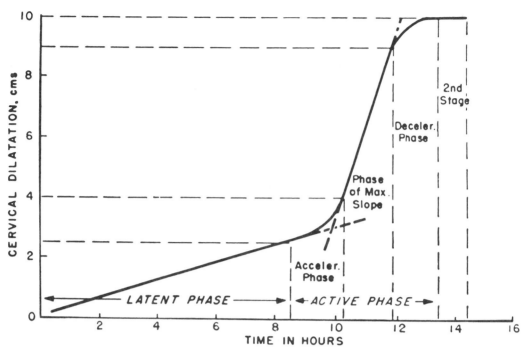

Figure 4.1. The mean labor curve (cervical dilation vs. time) based on a graphicostatistical analysis of 500 primigravidas at term. (Reprinted by permission from Friedman EA: Pri-migravid labor: A graphicostatistical analysis. Obstet Gynecol 6:567–589, 1955.)

Table 4.1
Prolonged Labor: Diagnostic Features

	Prolonged Latent Phase	Slow Slope (Protracted) Active Phase	Active Phase Arrest	Protracted Descent of Fetus	Arrest of Descent
Nulliparas	>20 h	<1.2 cm/h	No cervical dilation for 2 h	<1 cm/h	No descent for 1 h
Multiparas	>14 h	<1.5 cm/h		<2 cm/h	

in both resting tone and peak tension with halothane (Fig. 4.2). Similar findings have been reported by Munson et al. (8) for diethyl ether, halothane, enflurane, and isoflurane using myometrial strips from pregnant and nonpregnant women. Vasicka and Kretchmer (9) showed that analgesic doses of halothane markedly diminish uterine activity, whereas anesthetic amounts nearly abolish it. However, they did not precisely measure the concentrations they were administering. Abadir et al. (10) concluded that isoflurane reduces both the frequency of contractions and the interval between them in uterine specimens from gravid patients. Concentrations of isoflurane from 0.5 to 1.5% significantly reduced uterine activity, and a concentration of 1.4% inactivated 50% of the myometrial strips (10). In one study equipotent doses of the halogenated agents halothane, enflurane, and isoflurane produced equal uterine relaxation (11). In another study equipotent concentrations of inhaled

anesthetics were found to depress uterine activity in the following order of increasing potency: cyclopropane, methoxyflurane, diethyl ether, halothane, isoflurane, and enflurane (12) (Fig. 4.3). However, there should be no important clinical difference in the profound relaxation produced by the latter three agents (12). Nitrous oxide has little or no effect on the uterus (8, 9, 12), whereas methoxyflurane is capable of producing profound relaxation only in high concentrations (12).

General anesthesia can be used to rapidly and reliably produce uterine relaxation to dissipate a tetanic contraction or facilitate intrauterine manipulations. Concentrations of halothane, enflurane, or isoflurane from 1.5 to 2 times the minimum alveolar concentration will adequately relax the uterus. Alveolar concentrations (MAC) of halothane, enflurane, or isoflurane of 1.5 to 2.0% will relax the uterus. Any of the three can be used, although isoflurane may be

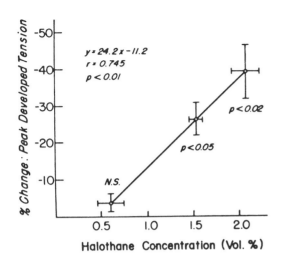

Figure 4.2. Effect of halothane on isometric developed tension in pregnant rat myometrium. *Brackets* include standard errors of the mean. P values refer to changes in developed tension from control. (Reprinted by permission from Naftalin NJ, Phear WPC, Goldberg AH: Halothane and isometric contractions of isolated pregnant rat myometrium. Anesthesiology 42:458–463, 1975.)

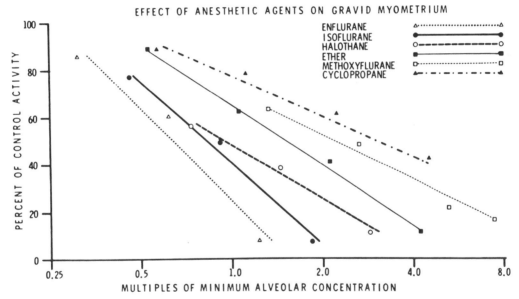

Figure 4.3. The relative effect of anesthetics on isolated human gravid uterine muscle. (Reprinted by permission from Tjeuw MTB, Yao F, Poznak AV: Depressant effects of anesthetics on isolated human gravid and nongravid uterine muscle. Chin Med J 99:235–242, 1986.)

the most desirable because its low solubility allows the most rapid changes in concentration.

Drugs that relax the uterus may increase blood loss after delivery, but if the concentration of the inhaled agent is decreased rapidly, and an uterotonic agent is administered, the uterus will contract and bleeding from the placental bed will stop. The response of the uterus to oxytocin during halothane or enflurane anesthesia is related to the dose of the anesthetic (13).

At high concentrations, halothane (1.6 vol/100 ml) and enflurane (3 vol/100 ml) will block the uterine response to oxytocin. At lower doses, halothane (1 vol/100 ml) and enflurane (2 vol/100 ml), while relaxing the uterus, will not block the response to 10 mU of oxytocin. The relaxation produced by concentrations of isoflurane up to 1.5% is reversed by oxytocin (10).

Inhalation analgesia for vaginal delivery with low-dose methoxyflurane, enflurane, or isoflurane has minimal effects on uterine activity, duration of labor, or postpartum blood loss. Similarly, investigators have found no additional maternal bleeding during anesthesia for cesarean section with low doses of halothane or enflurane (14–16). Marx and co-workers (13), studying parturients in the immediate postpartum period, found that inhalation of 0.5% halothane or 1% enflurane did not decrease uterine tone or contractility and did not alter the uterine response to oxytocin. As stated above, isoflurane does not inhibit oxytocin's uterotonic effect (10).

In summary, nitrous oxide does not affect uterine activity, yet volatile agents suppress it in a dose-dependent manner. Oxytocin negates the uterine relaxation caused by low clinical doses of inhaled anesthetics.

PARENTERAL AGENTS

DeVoe et al. (17) reported that meperidine (100 mg) administered intravenously during the active phase of labor produced either no change or an increase in uterine activity in 42 of 45 patients. However, 38 of the patients were receiving oxytocin augmentation, and there were no controls; therefore any increase may have been due to the natural course of labor. Similarly, Filler et al. (18) noted increases in Montevideo units after meperidine, pentazocine, or low spinal anesthesia. Both studies concluded that the decrease in pain provided by the analgesia reduces maternal epinephrine secretion, and this reduction in β-adrenergic stimulation improves uterine contractility.

On the other hand, Petrie et al. (19), after measuring uterine activity units, reported that total uterine activity in unmedicated labor increases with the passage of time. They observed the effect of several systemic analgesics and hypnotics by comparing the total uterine activity units in a 30-min control period with a 30-min period after intravenous administration of the drug. They also compared the slope of the plot of uterine activity vs. time in the preinjection and postinjection periods (Fig. 4.4). They found that with the narcotics meperidine, morphine, and alphaprodine the total number of uterine activity units before and after injection was not significantly different, but the postinjection uterine activity slope changed from the expected positive to negative. The same was true for the tranquilizing agents hydroxyzine and promethazine. These results imply that the agents studied could somewhat slow the course of labor, although the authors cautioned that their investigations did not include direct measurement of the progress of labor. Some studies suggest that the inhibitory effects of parenteral narcotics on uterine

contractility may occur only during the latent phase (20).

Rayburn et al. (21) compared intravenously administered fentanyl (50 to 100 μg/hour) with intravenously administered meperidine (25 to 50 mg/2 to 3 hours) in a randomized, non–blinded study. There was no difference between the groups with respect to efficacy of the analgesics, duration of labor, or mode of delivery. However, the fentanyl-treated group had a lesser incidence of vomiting and prolonged maternal sedation, and the neonates of this group required less naloxone. Barbiturates cause dose-related inhibition of uterine contractility (20). In contrast, the benzodiazepine diazepam has no such effect (20).

The anesthetic agent ketamine has received considerable attention in obstetrics. Oats et al. (22) demonstrated that, during second trimester abortions 2 mg/kg ketamine caused an increase in intrauterine pressure equal to ergometrine, whereas in cesarean section the same dose caused no change (see Figs. 8.18 and 8.19). Marx et al. (23), studying postpartum uterine pressures with different doses of ketamine, failed to demonstrate an increase in uterine tone, although uterine activity increased briefly.

In summary, parenteral narcotics and tranquilizers have little effect on uterine contractility. However, any heavy sedation caused by these drugs might prolong the latent phase. Barbiturates do inhibit uterine contractions in a dose-dependent fashion.

REGIONAL ANESTHESIA AND ANALGESIA

The greatest controversy in obstetric anesthesia involves the effects of regional analgesia on the progress and outcome of labor.

Very few studies have examined the effects of intrathecal narcotics on labor. Abouleish et al. reported that subarachnoid morphine injection prolongs the first stage of labor (23a).

Although some studies purport to demonstrate differences in the labors of women receiving epidural analgesia, firm conclusions are difficult to make. Patients who receive epidural analgesia are often different from other parturients to whom they are compared: Women who receive epidural analgesia come to the hospital at an earlier stage of labor and already have prolonged labors before the block is begun (24–26). Similarly, they are more likely to have induction or augmentation of their labors (25, 27). Women who receive conduction analgesia are often those who have failed to receive adequate pain relief from some other method (28, 29). Using radiographic pelvimetry, Floberg et al. (30) showed that patients who request epidural analgesia are more likely to have small pelvic outlet capacity. In some studies (31, 32), the group

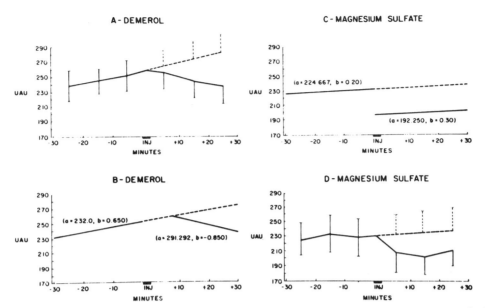

Figure 4.4. Results of administration of meperidine (Demerol) and magnesium sulfate. A and D, mean uterine activity units (UAU ± SE) per 10-min segment of labor in the preinjection and postinjection periods is contrasted with the expected (----) UAU for the study period. B and C, regression line for the preinjection period is contrasted with the observed postinjection values. (Reprinted by permission from Petrie RH, Wu R, Miller FC, Sacks DA, Sugarman R, Paul RH, Hon EH: The effect of drugs on uterine activity. Obstet Gynecol 48:431–435, 1976.)

receiving epidurals contained a disproportion of primigravidas, who are more likely to have long labors and operative deliveries. In many older studies, patients often received epidural analgesia because of coexisting medical or obstetric complications (33–36). Some studies included in their statistics patients who received the conduction block to undergo an instrumental delivery (37, 38).

All of these confounding variables make it nearly impossible to discern the precise effects of epidural analgesia per se. Nevertheless, some conclusions can be drawn. First, local anesthetics can have a direct effect on the uterus. The high concentrations that might be achieved with an accidental intravascular injection or paracervical block can increase uterine tone (39); very high concentrations can lead to tetanic contractions (Fig. 4.5). When Greiss et al. (40) injected local anesthetics directly into the uterine artery of pregnant ewes, a dose-related increase in uterine tone was noted. In vitro studies of uterine muscle strips demonstrate that local anesthetics increase tone but decrease the rate and strength of contractions (41), and this effect is antagonized by calcium (42). Jenssen (43) found that paracervical block increases the rate of contraction and decreases the rate of relaxation.

More important are the effects of local anesthetic concentrations usually achieved clinically. To examine these effects, it is best to consider the stages of labor separately.

First Stage of Labor

It has generally been taught that regional anesthesia administered in the latent phase will significantly prolong labor, whereas the same technique applied when labor is well established will have little or no effect. This idea first appeared as an aside in two early series evaluating caudal analgesia for labor (44, 45). Friedman and Sachtleben (33, 46) studied the effects of caudal analgesia on the first stage of labor and concluded that conduction analgesia begun in the latent phase will lengthen labor substantially. Current dogma about not beginning epidural analgesia until the active phase of labor is based on these investigations. However, in the first study (33), the authors themselves admit that their own data do not support the conclusion. In the second study the authors compared women who were experiencing prolongation of the latent phase with normal controls, and they concluded that the analgesia was the cause of the dysfunctional labor in 5.9% (46). Yet, as explained above, patients who receive regional analgesia are often not comparable to women with normal labor patterns. Vasicka et al. (9, 47) showed that conduction anesthesia caused, at most, a transient (10 to 20 min) decrease in uterine contractility, provided hypotension was avoided. Furthermore, the effect of oxytocin was not impeded by the anesthesia (9). In many cases the spinal or epidural anesthetic in Vasicka's studies was begun in the latent phase. Two studies randomized women *before* labor to receive

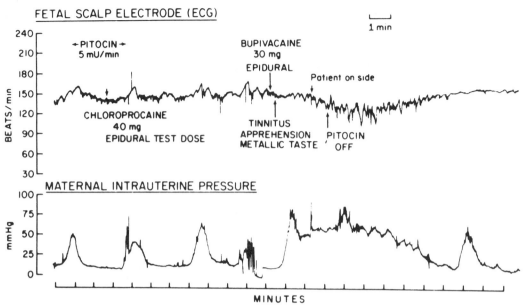

Figure 4.5. Tetanic uterine contraction occurring after inadvertant intravenous injection of bupivacaine. (Reprinted by permission from Greiss FC Jr, Still JG, Anderson SG: Effects of local anesthetic agents on the uterine vasculatures and myometrium. Am J Obstet Gynecol 124:889–899, 1976.)

epidural bupivacaine or intramuscular meperidine when they requested pain relief (48, 49). In both studies no difference in the length of the first stage of labor was detected between the groups. In one (49), most of the epidural catheters were placed in the latent phase. Nevertheless, the idea of avoiding regional analgesia in the latent phase became well established, and subsequent studies have focused mostly on the active phase.

Several nonrandomized studies also suggest that epidural analgesia has a minimal effect on the first stage of labor. In a retrospective study, Crawford (50) noted no difference in the duration of the first stage of labor regardless of parity or use of oxytocin. Jouppila et al. (51), using a case-control study design, matched women receiving epidural analgesia with control patients for parity and spontaneous or induced labor. They determined that, although the total length of the first stage was greater in primigravidas receiving epidural analgesia, once the analgesia was begun the remainder of the first stage was the same duration as that for the controls with equivalent cervical dilation. In multigravidas, no difference in the first-stage duration was detected. Phillips and coworkers (52) reported no difference in the length of the first stage when they compared the labors of women receiving epidural analgesia with standard labor curves. Cowles (53) made a similar comparison and found no difference for multigravidas but shorter first stages for primigravidas who had received epidural analgesia. Studd and his colleagues (24) found that women in unaugmented labor who were given epi-

dural blocks had longer first stages than did parturients not receiving blocks. However, the rate of cervical dilation was no different between the groups; the epidural group merely had been admitted while at a lesser cervical dilation. Women whose labors were augmented exhibited no effects of epidural analgesia on the duration of the first stage. Moir and Willocks (54) found that the rate of cervical dilation was increased in 70% and unchanged in another 18.6% of women when epidural analgesia was established. Other clinicians report enhanced and more effective uterine contractility following epidural (53–56) or caudal (57–60) anesthesia and recommended conduction analgesia for parturient patients with incoordinate uterine activity, (54, 55, 61–63), multiple gestation (64), or breech presentation (65, 66).

On the other hand, some studies have indicated that the first stage of labor is longer in women who receive epidural analgesics. In a retrospective study Schussman et al. (27) found longer first stages in low-risk parturients who had received epidurals, even when those who required induction of labor were excluded. Kilpatrick and Laros (38) examined the records of 6991 women who did not require induction or augmentation of labor and concluded that the use of conduction anesthesia is associated with a longer first stage. Read et al. (67) and Willdeck-Lund et al. (68) have also reported statistically significant decreases in uterine contractions and cervical dilation after commencement of epidural analgesia.

Many studies have examined the effects of variations in technique of conduction analgesia on the progress in labor. The choice of local anesthetic could be important: Lowensohn et al. (69) observed a significant depression of uterine activity lasting approximately 30 min after lidocaine injection through lumbar epidural catheters but did not make a similar observation after prilocaine administration (Fig. 4.6). (Prilocaine is now seldom used because of its propensity to cause methemoglobinemia.) Zador and Nilsson (70, 71) reported a similar transient decrease in uterine activity after the epidural injection of lidocaine. Crawford (72), Schellenberg (73), and Tyack et al. (74) all investigated epidural anesthesia with bupivacaine and noticed no decrease in uterine activity after injection.

Although the studies noted above suggest a difference between local anesthetics with regard to their effects on uterine contractility, others have failed to find a difference. Gal et al. (75) found that bupivacaine, lidocaine, and chloroprocaine used epidurally had little effect on uterine activity. Similarly, Abboud and colleagues (76, 77) detected no difference in the duration of the first stage or in uterine activity among patients who received epidural bupivacaine, chloroprocaine, or lidocaine by intermittent bolus injection or continuous infusion.

Many of the studies mentioned above, as well as others (78–80), have detected a transient decrease in uterine activity after the establishment of an epidural block. However, perhaps it is not the block itself that is responsible for this phenomenon: Cheek and co-workers (81) showed that women who received a 1000-ml intravenous fluid bolus exhibited a decrease in uterine activity for 20 min, yet those who received a 500 ml bolus or maintenance fluid only did not demonstrate any change in activity. The establishment of an epidural block did not affect uterine contractions in any of the groups. In fact, in the group receiving maintenance fluids but no bolus, uterine activity increased once epidural analgesia was established. One hypothesis offered to explain this phenomenon is that the fluid bolus inhibits antidiuretic hormone release from the posterior pituitary gland. Since this organ also releases oxytocin, the production of that hormone might also be transiently suppressed. This may partially explain the transient changes in uterine contractility observed in association with epidural analgesia. Nevertheless, the benefits of hydration before the administration of an epidural block are well established and should not be avoided because of concern that uterine activity might be transiently depressed.

Craft et al. (78) demonstrated that the decreased uterine activity associated with epidural analgesia did not occur when the patient was in the lateral position. Schellenberg (73), analyzing uterine activity before and after top-up doses of bupivacaine during epidural block, also concluded that aortocaval compression—and *not* local anesthetic dose—was

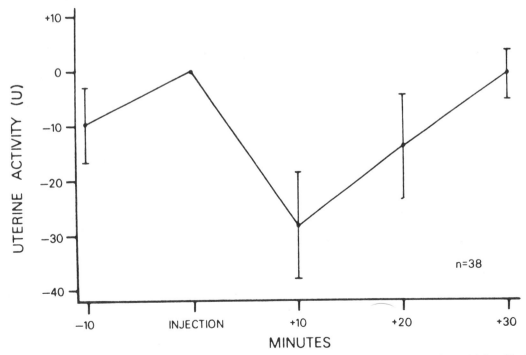

Figure 4.6. Uterine activity in patients receiving lidocaine (±2 SE). (Reprinted by permission from Lowensohn RI, Paul R, Fales S, Yeh S, Hon EH: Intrapartum epidural anesthesia: An evaluation of effects on uterine activity. Obstet Gynecol 44:388–393, 1974.)

the apparent reason for decreased uterine activity. This suggests that decreased uterine perfusion can occur in the absence of demonstrable hypotension.

With regard to other aspects of the epidural technique, the following have been shown not to affect the duration of the first stage of labor: intermittent bolus injection vs. continuous infusion (82–84); the addition of fentanyl (85, 86), alfentanil (87), or sufentanil (88, 132); and the administration of pain relief by patient-controlled epidural analgesia (89, 90).

In summary, provided that uterine displacement is maintained and hypotension avoided, epidural analgesia appears to have little effect on the progress of labor during the first stage. A transient decrease in uterine activity—possibly related to the intravenous fluid bolus—may occur after the establishment of the block, but normal activity resumes within 30 min. With regard to uterine activity, there appears to be little difference among the various drugs administered epidurally or in their method of administration. Although traditional wisdom dictates the avoidance of epidural analgesia during the latent phase of the first stage, the data supporting this assertion are not strong. Moreover, the alternative parenteral analgesics also may prolong the latent phase (20). Furthermore, any deleterious effect that analgesia might have on contractility could be easily reversed by oxytocin. We and others believe that it is more appropriate to provide pain relief to a woman who complains of uncomfortable contractions than to deny her comfort until an arbitrary cervical dilation has been attained (91).

Second Stage of Labor and Mode of Delivery

Some studies (24, 92) have indicated that patients receiving epidural analgesia have longer second stages, yet others (37, 93–95) have failed to find a difference. Epidural block has been reported to affect not only the duration of the second stage of labor, but also the frequency of instrumental delivery. With regard to the latter, investigators report an incredible range in frequency of operative vaginal deliveries in association with conduction block: Jouppila et al. (51) reported no vacuum deliveries in multiparas who received epidural analgesia. Hollmén and associates (36) similarly described an instrumental delivery rate of 7.4% in epidural patients. However, Browne and Catton (96) found an operative vaginal delivery rate of 84.2% in parturients who had received epidural blockade.

Because women who receive epidural analgesia can be so different from other parturients, it may be inappropriate to presume that the high rates of instrumental delivery observed for these patients are a result of the analgesia. Several studies have at-

tempted to resolve this issue by examining the effect of the arrival of an epidural analgesia service on the overall rate of operative delivery in an obstetric department. Two such retrospective investigations (97, 98) describe no change in the frequency of forceps deliveries when conduction analgesia became available. However, another similar study found an increase in instrumental deliveries after the arrival of the epidural analgesia (99).

A change in the technique of epidural analgesia may also affect the incidence of operative delivery (100). For example, the incidence of operative vaginal deliveries and cesarean sections was examined following a major change in the technique of epidural management in one busy obstetric suite (100). Instead of using intermittent boluses of a relatively high concentration of lidocaine during the first stage of labor with no administration during the second stage, low concentrations of bupivacaine with fentanyl were administered by continuous infusion until delivery. Although the fraction of patients receiving epidural analgesia increased, the overall number of operative vaginal deliveries and cesarean sections both decreased.

Very few studies of the effects of epidural analgesia have randomized women to receive epidural block or another method of pain relief. Philipsen et al. (49) and Robinson et al. (48) randomized women to be given epidural block or intramuscular meperidine once they requested analgesia. The former investigation found no difference in the duration of the second stage or the rate of instrumental delivery, but no epidural injections were given during the second stage, and only 44% of patients received more than one dose. The latter study, which used 0.5% bupivacaine, found that the patients receiving epidural analgesia had longer second stages and more forceps deliveries. In both studies, the epidural block provided superior analgesia.

There are several reasons why conduction analgesia might affect the length of the second stage and the mode of delivery. Some authorities have proposed that distension of the lower vagina by the fetal presenting part leads to an increase in the release of oxytocin, and this *Ferguson reflex* might be interrupted by epidural blockade (101). However, it is uncertain whether this reflex exists in humans; a clear correlation between a rise in the serum concentration of oxytocin and spontaneous delivery cannot be demonstrated (101). Furthermore, tremendous variation exists among parturients in the serum concentration of oxytocin necessary to produce adequate uterine contractility (102). A prospective, randomized, double-blind study showed that routine oxytocin infusion during the second stage for women receiving epidural analgesia led to a briefer second stage, a shorter period of expulsive effort, and fewer nonrotational instrumental deliveries (103).

Epidural blockade can affect the adequacy of the maternal expulsive effort. Nearly 50% of patients given 0.25% bupivacaine by bolus injections lose the urge to bear down, and this can be associated with instrumental delivery (50). Motor block and loss of the bearing-down reflex are associated with increasing concentrations of bupivacaine (0.5% vs. 0.25%) and not with increasing volumes of injection (26, 104). On the other hand, increasing volume is associated with better analgesia (26, 104).

Several studies report an increase in persistent occiput posterior position and the use of rotational forceps in patients who received epidural analgesics. Studd et al. (24) found a 20-fold increase in rotational forceps deliveries in such women. Hoult et al. (35) have reported a fivefold increase in instrumental delivery and a threefold increase in fetal malposition (i.e., persistent occiput posterior) when parturients given epidural analgesics were compared with those given pethidine or no anesthesics. They suggested that the malposition may result from relaxation of the pelvic muscles caused by the conduction block (35). Of note in this study was a self-imposed time limit for the second stage and the use of high concentrations of bupivacaine (0.5%). Other studies also found a marked increase in forceps deliveries in women who received epidural analgesics (53, 105). However, some prospective studies failed to demonstrate any increase in malposition in parturients receiving epidural analgesics (26, 106). In a randomized, prospective trial, Phillips et al. (107) showed that patients who were not given further epidural analgesics once the fetal head reached the ischial spine were *more* likely to deliver from the occiput posterior or transverse position than women who did receive analgesics until delivery. Floberg and associates (30) demonstrated that small pelvic outlet capacity is associated with both persistent occiput posterior position and the use of epidural analgesia, but the epidural blockade is not independently associated with malposition.

Some authorities (24, 108) suggested that the high rate of forceps deliveries, especially rotational forceps, associated with epidural analgesia might be lowered if the second stage of labor were allowed to proceed for a longer time. Others (109, 110) further suggested that the presenting fetal part rotates later in labor and lower in the pelvis when epidural analgesics are employed. Because it was noted that neonatal mortality was associated with longer labor (111), older obstetric teaching dictated operative delivery of the fetus if the second stage persisted beyond 1

Table 4.2
ACOG Definitions for Prolonged Second Stage of Labor[a]

Primigravida
  More than 2 hours without regional analgesia
  More than 3 hours with regional analgesia

Multigravida
  More than 1 hour without regional analgesia
  More than 2 hours with regional analgesia

[a] Based upon Committee on Obstetrics: Maternal and Fetal Medicine: ACOG Committee Opinion No. 59. Obstetric Forceps, 1988.

(112) or 2 (111) hours. Thus many of the labors in the early studies may have been terminated by rotational, midcavity forceps delivery because an arbitrary amount of time had elapsed. However, with the advent of electronic fetal heart rate monitoring, it is no longer necessary to intervene at any particular time as long as the heart rate pattern is reassuring (113). The American College of Obstetricians and Gynecologists (ACOG) now recommends that, if electronic monitoring indicates fetal well-being, the second stage should not be considered prolonged for women receiving epidural analgesics until 2 hours have passed for multigravidas or 3 hours for primigravidas (114) (Table 4.2). Now that duration of the second stage alone is no longer considered an indication for the termination of labor, the issue of malposition as a result of epidural analgesia seems to have disappeared from the literature.

Three studies have shown that delaying maternal expulsive effort until the fetal head is below the level of the ischial spines (107), visible at the introitus (112), or until 1 hour has passed since attainment of complete cervical dilation (115) reduces the incidence of forceps delivery.

With regard to parity, the vast majority of studies have shown that nulliparous women who receive epidural analgesics are more likely to have an instrumental delivery than multiparous women receiving the same pain relief (24, 25, 34, 36, 37, 50, 51, 104, 106, 116–121). One study (122) indicated the reverse, and another (123) suggested no difference between primigravidas and multigravidas.

Another area of investigation concerns whether the continuation of epidural analgesia throughout the second stage and the provision of the "perineal dose" (a bolus of local anesthetic given with the patient in the sitting position to block the sacral roots) increase the duration of the second stage and the incidence of instrumental delivery. Hoult et al. (35) suggested that allowing the analgesia to wear off during the expulsive effort might improve the chance of spontaneous delivery. Similarly, Walton and Reynolds

(118) indicated that the use of sitting top-up doses in the first stage increases the likelihood of operative vaginal delivery. However, a study by Phillips et al. (107) does not support these conclusions: Patients whose epidural analgesia was continued until delivery did not have longer second stages or higher rates of instrumental delivery than parturients whose analgesia was allowed to dissipate. In fact, for women over 25 years of age, those given epidural blocks were *less* likely to have an instrumental delivery.

Three prospective, randomized, double-blind studies by Chestnut et al. (92, 94, 95) attempted to resolve these issues. In all three studies, the women were randomized to have their epidural infusions continued during the second stage or be converted to saline infusions. When 0.75% lidocaine was used, there was no difference in the length of the second stage or in the incidence of instrumental delivery (95). However, analgesia was not significantly different, either. This confirms many anesthesiologists impressions that dilute lidocaine is not an effective labor analgesic. When the local anesthetic was 0.125% bupivacaine, the group whose infusions were continued had significantly increased numbers of low forceps and midvacuum deliveries, longer second stages, and more motor block (92). The analgesia was significantly better for these women. Parturients for whom continuous infusion of 0.0625% bupivacaine plus 0.0002% fentanyl (2 μg/ml) was maintained until delivery had superior analgesia compared with women whose infusions were changed to saline (94). There was no difference in the duration of the second stage or in the rate of instrumental deliveries between the groups (94). A prospective trial by Johnsrud et al. (124) showed that a continuous infusion of 0.25% bupivacaine during the second stage did not affect its duration or the incidence of operative vaginal delivery if routine intravenous oxytocin infusions were employed. In another prospective study, Gal et al. (75) compared 3% chloroprocaine administered epidurally to local perineal infiltration of 1% lidocaine for patients who all had epidural bupivacaine in the first stage. There was no difference in the length of the second stage, but the epidural group had six times more low forceps deliveries.

Thus it seems that the particular kind of local anesthetic and its concentration may be important in determining the effect of the epidural analgesic on the second stage of labor and on the mode of delivery. The results of other studies are divided on this question. Abboud et al. (77) concluded that patients who received 0.125% bupivacaine infusions were less likely to have spontaneous deliveries than those who received 0.75% chloroprocaine or 0.75% lidocaine in-

fusions. Feiss and colleagues (125) detected no difference in the incidence of forceps deliveries between women who received 0.25% bupivacaine or 2% chloroprocaine. The analgesia was superior in the bupivacaine group.

Study results conflict with regard to the effects of continuous epidural infusions as opposed to intermittent bolus injections. Smedstad and Morison (126) showed that there was no difference in the length of the second stage or in the quality of analgesia between groups of women who received 0.25% bupivacaine by bolus or infusion. However, the infusion group had significantly more outlet forceps deliveries. The length of the second stage per se was not used as an indication for the operative delivery. Li et al. (82) compared 0.25% bupivacaine bolus injections with infusions of 0.0625% or 0.125% bupivacaine at various rates and found no difference in duration of the second stage, motor block, mode of delivery, or quality of analgesia. In an investigation comparing local anesthetic plus narcotic given either as boluses of 0.25% bupivacaine plus 36–45 μg fentanyl or as infusions of 0.25% bupivacaine with fentanyl 4.5 μg/ml at 3 ml/hr, D'Athis et al. (83) found better analgesia in the infusion group but no difference in the mode of delivery. (The length of the second stage was not reported.) Bogod and associates (84) compared 0.5% bupivacaine injections with infusions of the 0.125% concentration of the same agent. They reported no difference in mode of delivery or maternal satisfaction. They did detect significantly more motor block and a nonsignificant increase in the duration of the second stage in the infusion group.

Two studies compared continuous epidural infusions with patient-controlled epidural analgesia (PCEA) and found no difference in the length of the second stage or outcome of labor (90, 127). In addition, both studies concluded that there is no benefit to PCEA.

Many investigations have compared a variety of epidural analgesic recipes using the narcotics fentanyl, sufentanil, and alfentanil added to bupivacaine, and most show no effect on the duration of the second stage or on the mode of delivery (85–88, 128–131). In a prospective, randomized, double-blind study, Vertommen et al. (132) showed that the addition of 10-μg sufentanil to intermittent bolus injections of 0.125% bupivacaine plus epinephrine 1:800,000 up to a maximum of 30 μg sufentanil did not affect the length of the second stage or incidence of cesarean section and reduced the incidence of operative vaginal delivery. The women who received sufentanil required less bupivacaine and had less motor block. One study with a small number of patients detected a higher rate of instrumental deliveries and cesarean sections in patients whose epidural analgesic contained fentanyl (90). However, the nonnarcotic group mixed patients receiving continuous infusion and PCEA, whereas the fentanyl group exclusively used PCEA. Furthermore, the overall rate of operative vaginal and abdominal deliveries was not changed from the institution's norm, and the authors concluded that their result probably reflected "random variation" (90). A report by Naulty et al. (100) showed that the incidence of forceps deliveries and cesarean sections declined when the epidural analgesic technique was changed from intermittent boluses of lidocaine or bupivacaine to infusions of bupivacaine plus fentanyl.

One prospective study by Thorp et al. (133) suggested that epidural analgesia may be associated with an increased frequency of cesarean section for dystocia in nulliparas. However, the epidural analgesia group had more women who received oxytocin, and the duration of oxytocin use, maximum oxytocin dose, and birth weights were greater than for the nonepidural group. Nevertheless, the authors maintain that the increase in cesarean sections was still associated with epidural analgesia when the other factors were controlled by multivariate analysis. A retrospective study by Gribble and Meier showed that the arrival of an epidural analgesia service did not affect the rate of cesarean section for all indications, including dystocia (133a). Other factors beyond analgesia, such as obstetric management, can affect the rate of abdominal delivery. Neuhoff et al. (134) showed that cesarean section of dystocia was much more common for private patients than clinic patients, even though the two groups received epidural analgesics with the same frequency. One sobering suggestions for why Thorp's study detected an increase in cesarean section for patients with epidurals in contrast to many earlier investigations was offered by the authors (133): Perhaps the medicolegal climate in the United States is leading to a conversion from forceps or vacuum extractions to abdominal deliveries, which might be perceived by some to be safer.

In summary, there are many unanswered questions with regard to the effects of conduction analgesia on the second stage of labor and mode of delivery. Nevertheless, some conclusions can be drawn. Epidural analgesics are safe and provide unparalleled analgesia. Patients who request epidural block are often different from other patients with whom they may be compared: They are likely to have more painful, dysfunctional labors. The length of the second stage can probably be increased by the use of epidural analgesia, but using more dilute concentrations of local anesthetics (perhaps in combination with narcotics) appears to minimize this problem. Furthermore, when epidural analgesia is employed, less fetal acidosis develops during a prolonged first or second stage (70, 71, 135–138).

The greater incidence of rotational forceps delivery formerly associated with epidural analgesia is avoided if arbitrary limits on the length of the second stage are avoided. The frequency of low and outlet instrumental deliveries may be increased in women, especially nulliparas, who receive epidural blockade. However, several studies have demonstrated that such low-station operative vaginal procedures do not lead to increased neonatal morbidity (111, 139–142). Finally, many other factors, most notably obstetric management, have at least as great an effect as epidural analgesia. For example, having the parturient patient assume a sitting position significantly shortens the duration of the second stage (143). Using multivariate analysis, Pipes et al. demonstrated that the use of epidural analgesia, active phase duration, parity, patient height, birth weight, and station at complete cervical dilation could account for less than 25% of the variance in second-stage duration (143a). The remaining variance is unexplained.

In light of the uncertainty, what should we tell our patients? We can emphasize the effectiveness and safety of epidural analgesia. Women can be told that they may spend more time in an expulsive effort if they choose an epidural block, but they should be more comfortable than they might be with other methods of pain relief. With regard to operative delivery, it would be reasonable to advise women who ask about this issue that epidural analgesia could increase the possibility of a low forceps delivery, although the topic is very controversial. One should then stress that there is no evidence that such a delivery is more dangerous for the neonate. Furthermore, in one study epidural analgesia was not associated with an increased incidence or severity of birth-canal trauma (143b).

What should be our goals for labor analgesia? First, strive for analgesia, not anesthesia. Totally painless labor and a dense motor block may not be in the parturient's best interest. Second, the patient's happiness is more important than the anesthesiologist's. Many women prefer to maintain some sensation, even if it is mildly uncomfortable, rather than receive a dense motor block. Finally, analgesia should be maintained until delivery unless there is a strong indication that such a course is not in the patient's or fetus' interest. If requested to allow a block to subside, before taking such an action, consider the following: Has the women been coached to bear down properly? Would the use of an oxytocin infusion be helpful? Would decreasing the rate or concentration of the epidural infusion be a better course? Does the patient believe that more sensation would be helpful?

VASOPRESSORS

A major side effect of regional anesthesia in obstetrics is hypotension, and occasionally vasopressors must be used to restore blood pressure. The effect of these agents on uterine blood flow is discussed in Chapter 3. They may also have direct effects on uterine muscle. There are both α- and β-adrenergic receptors in uterine muscle: α-receptor stimulation leads to uterine hypertonus, whereas β-receptor stimulation causes a decrease in uterine tone and contractility (144). Methoxamine was used in the past to counteract the hypotension of regional anesthesia, but its use in obstetrics should be avoided. It has a direct constricting effect on the uterine artery, and its α-receptor agonism has been reported to cause tetanic uterine contractions (47) (Fig. 4.6). Ephedrine, the vasopressor of choice in obstetrics, seems to have little effect on uterine activity.

Epinephrine is sometimes added to local anes-

thetics to augment their analgesia, prolong their duration, and decrease their circulating blood level. These effects are all mediated by α-receptor agonism. The β-receptor stimulation of this small dose of epinephrine may affect uterine activity and the course of labor.

Gunther and Bauman (145) and Gunther and Bellville (146) showed that the first stage of labor was prolonged in parturients receiving lidocaine or mepivacaine with epinephrine, compared with patients receiving those agents without epinephrine during continuous caudal anesthesia. In addition, almost twice as many women required oxytocin augmentation when solutions containing epinephrine were used (146). The doses of epinephrine, which ranged between 100 and 125 μg, are larger than those commonly used today. Craft et al. (78) compared lidocaine with and without epinephrine for lumbar epidural anesthesia and found that, although patients receiving the epinephrine-containing solution had a slight decrease in uterine activity, the overall progress of labor was not significantly affected (Table 4.3). Abboud and colleagues (147–149) demonstrated that the addition of epinephrine 1:300,000 to 0.5% bupivacaine and 1.5% lidocaine or 1:200,000 epineph-

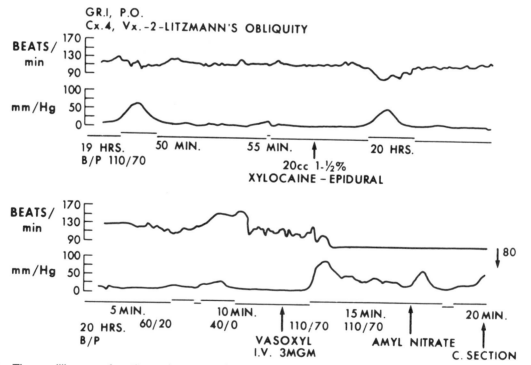

Figure 4.7. Three milligrams of methoxamine were administered to treat maternal hypotension following epidural anesthesia. The *upper tracing* (fetal heart rate) shows a severe fetal bradycardia; the *lower tracing* (intraamniotic pressure) shows the tetanic uterine contraction that resulted from meth-

oxamine. (Reprinted by permission from Vasicka A, Hutchinson HT, Eng M, Allen CR: Spinal and epidural anesthesia, fetal and uterine response to acute hypo- and hypertension. Am J Obstet Gynecol 90:800–810, 1964.)

Table 4.3
Effect of Local Analgesic on Cervical Dilation and Uterine Forces[a]

Drug	Measurement	
	First 20 min	Second 20 min
	Cervical dilation, cm[b]	
1.5% lidocaine with 1:200,000 epinephrine	+0.7 ± 0.6	+1.6 ± 0.4 (p < .001)
1.5% lidocaine (plain)	+0.8 ± 0.3 (p < 0.05)	+2.0 ± 0.4 (p < .001)
	Uterine forces, M.U.[c]	
1.5% lidocaine with 1:200,000 epinephrine	−47.8 ± 17.6 (p < .02)	+1.9 ± 19.6
1.5% lidocaine (plain)	+ 6.2 ± 18.1	+30.8 ± 26

[a] Reprinted with permission from Craft JB, Epstein BS, Coakley CS: Effect of lidocaine with epinephrine versus lidocaine (plain) on induced labor. Anesth Analg 51:243–246, 1972.
[b] All changes are related to the baseline period and are tabulated for the first period and then for the total of both periods.
[c] All changes are related to the baseline period and are tabulated for *each* 20-min period.

rine to 2% chloroprocaine did not affect uterine activity in Montevideo units, the duration of the first or second stages, or the mode of delivery. Eisenach et al. (150, 151) similarly reported no effects on the duration of labor from the addition of epinephrine 1:300,000 to 0.25% bupivacaine with or without fentanyl.

Zador and Nilsson (70, 71) demonstrated that adding epinephrine to lidocaine administered intermittently or by continuous infusion accentuates and prolongs the transient decrease in uterine activity, which they observed following the initiation of epidural analgesia. However, this depressant effect resolved within 90 min, and in the patients receiving a continuous infusion, there was no effect on the duration of the first or second stage of labor (71). (It was not possible to determine effects on the length of the first stage in the intermittent bolus group because their labors were already prolonged before the establishment of the epidural block [70].)

In summary, most studies suggest that epinephrine added in concentrations no greater than 1:200,000 to local anesthetic administered epidurally does not affect the course of labor significantly. Beyond this, however, is the question of the need for epinephrine beyond a test dose. Bupivacaine, now commonly used in obstetrics, is long acting, and epinephrine may or may not affect its duration (152–154). Moreover, the popularity of continuous infusions for epidural labor analgesia has made the issue of analgesia duration after bolus injection almost moot. Chloroprocaine is also popular, and adding epinephrine to it seems to be illogical: One of the advantages of this local anesthetic is its short duration of action, and one would not want to prolong it by the addition of epinephrine. Furthermore, its very rapid metabolism in plasma negates the need for epinephrine to decrease its toxicity.

CONCLUSION

The course of labor is quite unpredictable because it is influenced by so many factors. Maternal discomfort, the size of the pelvic outlet, the size of the baby, and obstetric management all affect progress of labor just as much as the provision of analgesia. Anesthetic techniques can and do affect uterine activity and the course of fetal descent and delivery, but judicious management by both anesthesiologist and obstetrician can result in maternal comfort without significantly prolonging labor or increasing the risk to mother or baby.

References

1. Alvarez H, Caldeyro-Barcia R: Contractility of the human uterus recorded by new methods. Surg Gynecol Obstet 91:1–13, 1950.
2. Hon EH, Paul RH: Quantitation of uterine activity. Obstet Gynecol 42:368–370, 1973.
3. Friedman EA: Primigravid labor: A graphicostatical analysis. Obstet Gynecol 6:567–589, 1955.
4. Cunningham FG, MacDonald PC, Gant NF: Parturition: Biomolecular and physiological processes. In *Williams Obstetrics*, 18th ed. Appleton & Lange, Norwalk, CT, 1989, p 213.
5. Cunningham FG, MacDonald PC, Gant NF: Dystocia due to abnormalities of the expulsive forces and precipitate labor. In *Williams Obstetrics*, 18th ed. Appleton & Lange, Norwalk, CT, 1989, pp 341–348.
6. Naftalin NJ, Phear WPC, Goldberg AH: Halothane and isometric contractions of isolated pregnant rat myometrium. Anesthesiology 42:458–463, 1975.
7. Naftalin NJ, McKay DM, Phear WPC, Goldberg AH: The effects of halothane on pregnant and nonpregnant human myometrium. Anesthesiology 46:15–19, 1977.
8. Munson ES, Maier WR, Caton D: Effects of halothane, cyclopropane and nitrous oxide on isolated human uterine muscle. J Obstet Gynaecol Br Commonw 76:27–33, 1969.
9. Vasicka A, Kretchmer H: Effect of conduction and inhalation anesthesia on uterine contractions: Experimental study of the influence of anesthesia on intraamniotic pressures. Am J Obstet Gynecol 82:600–611, 1961.
10. Abadir AR, Humayen SG, Calvello D, Gintautas J: Effects of isoflurane and oxytocin on gravid human uterus *in vitro*. Anesth Analg 66:S1, 1987.
11. Munson ES, Embro WJ: Enflurane, isoflurane, and halothane

and isolated human uterine muscle. Anesthesiology 46:11–14, 1977.

12. TJeuw MTB, Yao F, Van Poznak A: Depressant effects of anesthetics on isolated human gravid and non-gravid uterine muscle. Chin Med J 99:235–242, 1986.

13. Marx GF, Kim YO, Lin CC, Halery S, Schulman H: Postpartum uterine pressures under halothane or enflurane anesthesia. Obstet Gynecol 51:695–698, 1978.

14. Moir DD: Anaesthesia for caesarean section. An evaluation of a method using low concentrations of halothane and 50 per cent oxygen. Br J Anaesth 42:136–142, 1970.

15. Galbert MW, Gardner AE: Use of halothane in a balanced technique for cesarean section. Anesth Analg 51:701–704, 1972.

16. Coleman AJ, Downing JW: Enflurane anesthesia for cesarean section. Anesthesiology 43:354–357, 1975.

17. DeVoe SJ, DeVoe K Jr, Rigsby WC, McDaniels BA: Effect of meperidine on uterine contractility. Am J Obstet Gynecol 105:1004–1007, 1969.

18. Filler WW Jr, Hall WC, Filler NW: Analgesia in obstetrics. Am J Obstet Gynecol 98:832–846, 1967.

19. Petrie RH, Wu R, Miller FC, Sacks DA, Sugarman R, Paul RH, Hon EH: The effect of drugs on uterine activity. Obstet Gynecol 48:431–435, 1976.

20. Friedman EA: Effects of drugs on uterine contractility. Anesthesiology 26:409–422, 1965.

21. Rayburn WF, Smith CV, Parriott JE, Woods RE: Randomized comparison of meperidine and fentanyl during labor. Obstet Gynecol 14:604–606, 1989.

22. Oats JN, Vasey DP, Waldron BA: Effects of ketamine on the pregnant uterus. Br J Anaesth 51:1163–1166, 1979.

23. Marx GF, Hwang HS, Chandra P: Post-partum uterine pressures with different doses of ketamine. Anesthesiology 50:163–166, 1979.

23a. Abouleish E, Rawal N, Shaw J, Lorenz T, Rashad MN: Intrathecal morphine 0.2 mg versus epidural bupivacaine 0.125% or their combination: Effects on parturients. Anesthesiology 74:711–716, 1991.

24. Studd JWW, Crawford JS, Duignan NM, Rowbotham CJF, Hughes AO: The effect of lumbar epidural analgesia on the rate of cervical dilatation and the outcome of labour of spontaneous onset. Br J Obstet Gynaecol 87:1015–1021, 1980.

25. Willdeck-Lund G, Lindmark G, Nilsson BA: Effect of segmental epidural block on the course of labour and the condition of the infant during the neonatal period. Acta Anaesth Scand 23:301–311, 1979.

26. Thornburn J, Moir DD: Extradural analgesia: The influence of volume and concentration of bupivacaine on the mode of delivery, analgesic efficacy and motor block. Br J Anaesth 53:933–939, 1981.

27. Schussman LC, Woolley FR, Larsen LC, Hoffman RO: Epidural anesthesia in low-risk obstetrical patients. J Fam Pract 14:851–858, 1982.

28. Moore J, Murnaghan GA, Lewis MA: A clinical evaluation of the maternal effects of lumbar extradural analgesia for labour. Anaesthesia 29:537–544, 1974.

29. Raabe N, Belfrage P: Lumbar epidural analgesia in labour: A clinical analysis. Acta Obstet Gynecol Scand 55:125–129, 1976.

30. Floberg J, Belfrage P, Ohlsén H: Influence of the pelvic outlet capacity on fetal head presentation at delivery. Acta Obstet Gynecol Scand 66:127–130, 1987.

31. Moir DD: Local anaesthetic techniques in obstetrics. Br J Anaesth 58:747–759, 1986.

32. Morgan B, Bulpitt CJ, Clifton P, Lewis PJ: Effectiveness of pain relief in labour: Survey of 1000 mothers. Br Med J 285:689–690, 1982.

33. Friedman EA, Sachtleben MR: Caudal anesthesia: The factors that influence its effect on labor. Obstet Gynecol 13:442–450, 1959.

34. Brown SE, Vass ACR: An extradural service in a district general hospital. Br J Anaesth 49:243–246, 1977.

35. Hoult J, MacLennan AH, Carrie LES: Lumbar epidural analgesia in labour: Relation to fetal malposition and instrumental delivery. Br Med J 1:14–16, 1977.

36. Hollmén A, Jouppila R, Pihlajaniemi R, Karvonen P, Sjöstedt E: Selective lumbar epidural block in labour: A clinical analysis. Acta Anaesth Scand 21:174–181, 1977.

37. Cox SM, Bost JE, Faro S, Carpenter RJ: Epidural anesthesia during labor and the incidence of forceps delivery. Tex Med J 83:45–47, 1987.

38. Kilpatrick SJ, Laros RK: Characteristics of normal labor. Obstet Gynecol 74:85–87, 1989.

39. Evans JA, Chastain GM, Philips JM: The use of local anesthetic agents in obstetrics. South Med J 62:519–524, 1969.

40. Greiss FC Jr, Still JG, Anderson SC: Effects of local anesthetic agents on the uterine vasculatures and myometrium. Am Obstet Gynecol 124:889–899, 1976.

41. McCaughey HS Jr, Corey EL, Eastwood D, Thornton WN: Effects of synthetic anesthetics on the spontaneous motility of human uterine muscles in vitro. Obstet Gynecol 19:233–240, 1962.

42. Feinstein MB: Inhibition of contraction and Ca^{++} exchangeability in rat uterus by local anesthetics. J Pharmacol Exp Ther 152:516–524, 1966.

43. Jenssen H: The shape of the amniotic pressure curve before and after paracervical block during labour. Acta Obstet Gynecol Scand 42:(Suppl)1–29, 1975.

44. Siever JM, Mousel LH: Continuous caudal anesthesia in three hundred unselected obstetric cases. JAMA 122:424–426, 1943.

45. Ritmiller LF, Rippmann ET: Caudal analgesia in obstetrics: Report of thirteen years' experience. Obstet Gynecol 9:25–28, 1957.

46. Friedman EA, Sachtleben MR: Dysfunctional labor. I. Prolonged latent phase in the nullipara. Obstet Gynecol 17:135–148, 1961.

47. Vasicka A, Hutchinson HT, Eng M, Allen CR: Spinal and epidural anesthesia, fetal and uterine response to acute hypo- and hypertension. Am J Obstet Gynecol 90:800–810, 1964.

48. Robinson JO, Rosen M, Evans JM, Revill SI, David H, Rees GAD: Maternal opinion about analgesia for labour: A controlled trial between epidural block and intramuscular pethidine combined with inhalation. Anaesthesia 35:1173–1181, 1980.

49. Philipsen T, Jensen N-H: Epidural block or parenteral pethidine as analgesic in labour: A randomized study concerning progress in labour and instrumental deliveries. Eur J Obstet Gynecol Reprod Biol 30:27–33, 1989.

50. Crawford JS: The second thousand epidural blocks in an obstetric hospital practice. Br J Anaesth 44:1277–1286, 1972.

51. Jouppila R, Jouppila P, Karinen J-M, Hollmén A: Segmental epidural analgesia in labour: Related to the progress of labour, fetal malposition and instrumental delivery. Acta Obstet Gynecol Scand 58:135–139, 1979.

52. Phillips JC, Hochberg CJ, Petrakis JK, Van Winkle JD: Epidural analgesia and its effects on the "normal" progress of labor. Am J Obstet Gynecol 129:316–323, 1977.

53. Cowles GT: Experiences with lumbar epidural block. Obstet Gynecol 26:734–739, 1965.

54. Moir DD, Willocks J: Management of incoordinate uterine action under continuous epidural analgesia. Br Med J 2:396–400, 1967.

55. Ruppert H: The influence of extradural spinal anesthesia on the motility of the gravid uterus. In Proceedings of the First World Congress of Anesthesiologists. Burgess, Minneapolis, 1956.

56. Akamatsu TJ: Advances in obstetric anesthesiology during the period 1960–1970. In Clinical Anesthesiology: A Decade of Clinical Progress. LW Fabian, ed. Davis, Philadelphia, 1971.

57. Reynolds SRM, Harris JS, Kaiser IH: Clinical Measurement of Uterine Forces in Pregnancy and Labor. Charles C Thomas, Springfield, IL, 1954, p 232.

58. Alvarez H, Poseiro JJ, Pose SV: Effects of the anesthetic block-

age of the spinal cord on the contractility of the pregnant human uterus. XXI International Congress of Physiological Sciences, Buenos Aires, 1959.

59. Cibils LA, Spackman TJ: Caudal analgesia in first-stage labor: Effect on uterine activity and the cadiovascular system. Am J Obstet Gynecol 84:1042–1050, 1962.

60. Hunter CA: Uterine motility studies during labor: Observations on bilateral sympathetic nerve block in the normal and abnormal first stage of labor. Am J Obstet Gynecol 85:681–685, 1963.

61. Climie GR: The place of continuous lumbar epidural analgesia in the management of abnormally prolonged labour. Med J Aust 2:447–450, 1964.

62. Moir DD, Willocks J: Continuous epidural analgesia in incoordinate uterine action. Acta Anaesthesiol Scand 23:(Suppl)144–153, 1966.

63. Mercer WH, Simons EG, Philpott RH: The use of lumbar epidural analgesia during the first stage of labour in high risk pregnancies. South Afr Med J 48:774–779, 1974.

64. Crawford JS: An appraisal of lumbar epidural blockade in labour in patients with multiple pregnancy. Br J Obstet Gynaecol 82:929–935, 1975.

65. Crawford JS: An appraisal of lumbar epidural blockade in patients with a singleton fetus presenting by the breech. J Obstet Gynaecol Br Commonw 81:867–872, 1974.

66. Donnai P, Nicholas AD: Epidural analgesia, fetal monitoring and the condition of the baby at birth with breech presentation. Br J Obstet Gynaecol 82:360–365, 1975.

67. Read MD, Hunt LP, Anderson JM, Leiberman BA: Epidural block and the progress and outcome of labor. J Obstet Gynaecol 4:35–39, 1983.

68. Willdeck-Lund G, Lindmark G, Nilsson BA: Effect of segmental epidural analgesia upon the uterine activity with special reference to the use of different local anaesthetic agents. Acta Anaesth Scand 23:519–528, 1979.

69. Lowensohn RI, Paul R, Fales S, Yeh S, Hon EH: Intrapartum epidural anesthesia: An evaluation of effects on uterine activity. Obstet Gynecol 44:388–393, 1974.

70. Zador C, Nilsson BA: Low dose intermittent epidural anaesthesia with lidocaine for vaginal delivery. II. Influence on labour and foetal acid-base status. Acta Obstet Gynecol Scand 34:(Suppl)17–30, 1974.

71. Zador G, Nilsson BA: Continuous drip lumbar epidural anaesthesia with lidocaine for vaginal delivery. II. Influence on labour and foetal acid-base status. Acta Obstet Gynecol Scand 34:(Suppl)41–49, 1974.

72. Crawford JS: Patient management during extradural anaesthesia for obstetrics. Br J Anaesth 47:273–277, 1975.

73. Schellenberg JS: Uterine activity during lumbar epidural analgesia with bupivacaine. Am J Obstet Gynecol 127:26–31, 1977.

74. Tyack AJ, Parsons RJ, Miller DR, Nicholas ADC: Uterine activity and plasma bupivacaine levels after caudal epidural analgesia. J Obstet Gynaecol Br Commonw 80:896–901, 1973.

75. Gal D, Choudhy R, Ung K-A, Abadir A, Tancer ML: Segmental epidural analgesia for labor and delivery. Acta Obstet Gynecol Scand 58:429–431, 1979.

76. Abboud TK, Khoo SS, Miller F, Doan T, Henriksen EH: Maternal, fetal, and neonatal responses after epidural anesthesia with bupivacaine, 2-chloroprocaine, or lidocaine. Anesth Analg 61:638–644, 1982.

77. Abboud TK, Afrasiabi A, Sarkis F, Daftarian F, Nagappala S, Noueihid R, Kuhnert BR, Miller F: Continuous infusion epidural analgesia in parturients receiving bupivacaine, chloroprocaine, or lidocaine: Maternal, fetal, and neonatal effects. Anesth Analg 63:421–428, 1984.

78. Craft JB, Epstein BS, Coakley CS: Effect of lidocaine with epinephrine versus lidocaine (plain) or induced labor. Anesth Analg 51:243–246, 1972.

79. Jouppila P, Jouppila R, Kaar K, Merila M: Fetal heart patterns and uterine activity after segmental epidural analgesia. Br Obstet Gynaecol 84:481–486, 1977.

80. Matadial L, Cibils LA: The effect of epidural anesthesia on uterine activity and blood pressure. Am J Obstet Gynecol 125:846–854, 1976.

81. Cheek TG, Samuels P, Tobin M, Gutsche BB: Rapid intravenous saline infusion decreases uterine activity in labor: Epidural analgesia does not. Anesthesiology 71:A884, 1989.

82. Li DF, Rees GAD, Rosen M: Continuous extradural infusion of 0.0625% or 0.125% bupivacaine for pain relief in primigravid labour. Br J Anaesth 57:264–270, 1985.

83. D'Athis F, Machebouef M, Thomas H, Robert C, Desch G, Galtier M, Mares P, Eledjam JJ: Epidural analgesia with a bupivacaine-fentanyl mixture in obstetrics: Comparison of repeated injections and continuous infusion. Can J Anaesth 35:116–122, 1988.

84. Bogod DG, Rosen M, Rees GAD: Extradural infusion of 0.125% bupivacaine at 10 ml·hr⁻¹ to women during labour. Br J Anaesth 59:325–330, 1987.

85. Celleno D, Capogna G: Epidural fentanyl plus bupivacaine 0.125 per cent for labour: Analgesic effects. Can J Anaesth 35:375–378, 1988.

86. Chestnut DH, Owen CL, Bates JN, Ostman LG, Choi WW, Geiger MW: Continuous infusion epidural analgesia during labor: A randomized double-blind comparison of 0.0625% bupivacaine/0.0002% fentanyl versus 0.125% bupivacaine. Anesthesiology 68:754–759, 1988.

87. Kavuri S, Janardhan Y, Fernando E, Shevde K, Eddi D: A comparative study of epidural alfentanil and fentanyl for labor pain relief. Anesthesiology 71:A846, 1989.

88. Van Steenberge A, Debroux HC, Noorduin H: Extradural bupivacaine with sufentanil for vaginal delivery—a double-blind trial. Br J Anaesth 59:1518–1522, 1987.

89. Gambling DR, Yu P, McMorland GH, Palmer L: A comparative study of patient controlled epidural analgesia (PCEA) and continuous infusion epidural analgesia (CIEA) during labour. Can J Anaesth 35:249–254, 1988.

90. Lysak SZ, Eisenach JC, Dobson CE: Patient-controlled epidural analgesia during labor: A comparison of three solutions with a continuous infusion control. Anesthesiology 72:44–49, 1990.

91. Crawford JS: The stages and phases of labour: An outworn nomenclature that invites hazard—The experts opine. Surv Anesthesiol 28:62–67, 1984.

92. Chestnut DH, Vandewalker GE, Owen CL, Bates JN, Choi WW: The influence of continuous epidural bupivacaine analgesia on the second stage of labor and method of delivery in nulliparous women. Anesthesiology 66:774–780, 1987.

93. Niv D, Ber A, Rudick W, Lujkin Y, David M, Geller E: Mode of vaginal delivery and epidural analgesia. Isr J Med Sci 24:80–83, 1988.

94. Chestnut DH, Laszewski LJ, Pollack KL, Bates JN, Manago NK, Choi WW: Continuous epidural infusion of 0.0625% bupivacaine-0.0002% fentanyl during the second stage of labor. Anesthesiology 72:613–618, 1990.

95. Chestnut DH, Bates JN, Choi WW: Continuous infusion epidural analgesia with lidocaine: Efficacy and influence during the second stage of labor. Obstet Gynecol 69:323–327, 1987.

96. Browne RA, Catton DV: The use of bupivacaine in labour. Can Anaesth Soc J 18:23–32, 1971.

97. Bailey PW, Howard FA: Epidural analgesia and forceps delivery: Laying a bogey. Anaesthesia 38:282–285, 1983.

98. Noble AD, deVere RD: Epidural analgesia in labour (letter). Br Med J 2:296, 1970.

99. Bakhoum S, Lewis BV, Tipton RH: Lumbar epidural analgesia in labour. Br Med J 1:641, 1977.

100. Naulty JS, Smith R, Ross R: Effect of changes in labor analgesic practice on labor outcome. Anesthesiology 69:A660, 1988.

101. Goodfellow CF, Hull MGR, Swaab DF, Dogterom J, Buijs RM: Oxytocin deficiency at delivery with epidural analgesia. Br J Obstet Gynaecol 90:214–219, 1983.

102. Amico JA, Seitchik J, Robinson AG: Studies of oxytocin in plasma of women during hypocontractile labor. J Clin Endocrinol Metab 58:274–279, 1984.

103. Saunders NJStG, Spily H, Gilbert L, Fraser RB, Hall JM, Mutton PM, Jackson A, Edmonds DK: Oxytocin infusion during second stage of labour in primiparous women using epidural analgesia: A randomised double blind placebo controlled trial. Br Med J 299:1423–1426, 1989.

104. Crawford JS: Lumbar epidural block in labour: A clinical analysis. Br J Anaesth 44:66–74, 1972.

105. Johnson WL, Winter WW, Eng M, Bonica JJ, Hunter CA: Effect of pudendal, spinal and peridural block anesthesia on the second stage of labor. Am J Gynecol 113:166–173, 1972.

106. Maltau JM, Anderson HT: Continuous epidural anaesthesia with a low frequency of instrumental deliveries. Acta Obstet Gynecol Scand 54:401–406, 1975.

107. Phillips KC, Thomas TA: Second stage of labour with or without extradural analgesia. Anaesthesia 38:972–976, 1983.

108. Belfrage P, Raabe N: Letter to the editor. Acta Obstet Gynecol Scand 55:469–470, 1976.

109. Hibbard B, Pearson JF, Walker SM, Weaver JB, Rees GAD, Rosen M: Lumbar epidural analgesia in labor (letter). Br Med J 1:286, 1977.

110. McQueen J, Mylrea L: Lumbar epidural analgesia in labor (letter). Br Med J 1:640–641, 1977.

111. Niswander KR, Gordon M: Safety of the low-forceps operation. Am J Obstet Gynecol 117:619–629, 1973.

112. Maresh M, Choong KH, Beard RW: Delayed pushing with lumbar epidural analgesia in labour. Br J Obstet Gynaecol 90:623–627, 1983.

113. Cohen WR: Influence of the duration of second stage labor on perinatal outcome and puerperal morbidity. Obstet Gynecol 49:266–269, 1977.

114. Committee on Obstetrics: Maternal and Fetal Medicine: Obstetric Forceps, ACOG Committee Opinion No. 59. 1988.

115. Goodfellow CF, Studd C: The reduction of forceps in primagravidae with epidural analgesia: Controlled trial. Br J Clin Pract 33:287–288, 1979.

116. Kaminski HM, Stafl A, Aiman J: The effect of epidural analgesia on the frequency of instrumental obstetric delivery. Obstet Gynecol 69:770–773, 1987.

117. Morgan BM, Rehar S, Lewis PJ: Epidural analgesia for uneventful labour. Anaesthesia 35:57–60, 1980.

118. Walton P, Reynolds F: Epidural analgesia and instrumental delivery. Anaesthesia 39:218–223, 1984.

119. James DK, Chiswick ML: Kielland's forceps: Role of antenatal factors in prediction of use. Br Med J 1:10–11, 1979.

120. Bleyaert A, Soetens M, Vaes L, Van Steenberge AL, Van der Donck A: Bupivacaine, 0.125 per cent, in obstetric epidural analgesia: Experience in three thousand cases. Anesthesiology 51, 435–438, 1979.

121. Doughty A: Selective epidural analgesia and the forceps rate. Br J Anaesth 41:1058–1062, 1969.

122. Hawkins JL, Skjonsby BS, Joyce TH III, Hess KR, Morrow DH: The association of epidural analgesia and forceps delivery. Anesth Analg 70:S150, 1990.

123. Youngstrom P, Sedensky M, Frankmann D, Spagnuolo S: Continuous epidural infusion of low-dose bupivacaine-fentanyl for labor analgesia. Anesthesiology 69:A686, 1988.

124. Johnsrud M-L, Dale PO, Lovland B: Benefits of continuous infusion epidural analgesia throughout vaginal delivery. Acta Obstet Gynecol Scand 67:355–358, 1988.

125. Feiss P, Collet D, Vincelot A: Peridural analgesia in labor: Comparison between bupivacaine and 2-chloroprocaine. Can Anesthesiol 34:95–98, 1986.

126. Smedstad KG, Morison DH: A comparative study of continuous and intermittent epidural analgesia for labour and delivery. Can J Anaesth 35:234–241, 1988.

127. Naulty JS, Barnes D, Becker R, Pate A, Griffith W: Epidural PCA vs. continuous infusion of sufentanil-bupivacaine for analgesia during labor and delivery. Anesthesiology 73:A963, 1990.

128. Ahn NN, Karambelkar D, Cannelli G, Rudy TE: Epidural alfentanil and bupivacaine for analgesia during labor. Anesthesiology 71:A845, 1989.

129. Naulty JS, Ross R, Bergen W: Epidural sufentanil-bupivacaine for analgesia during labor and delivery. Anesthesiology 71:A842, 1989.

130. Carp H, Johnson MD, Bader AM, Datta S, Ostheimer GW: Continuous epidural infusion of alfentanil and bupivacaine for labor and delivery. Anesthesiology 69:A687, 1988.

131. Hoyt M, Youngstrom P: Neonatal neurobehavioral effects of continuous epidural infusion of fentanyl/bupivacaine/epinephrine in labor. Anesthesiology 73:A984, 1990.

132. Vertommen JD, Vandermeulen E, Van Aken H, Vaes L, Soetens M, Van Steenberge A, Mourisse P, Willaert J, Noordvin H, Devlieger H, Van Assche AF: The effects of the addition of sufentanil to 0.125% bupivacaine on the quality of analgesia during labor and on the incidence of instrumental deliveries. Anesthesiology 74:809–814, 1991.

133. Thorp JA, Parisi VM, Boylan PC, Johnston DA: The effect of continuous epidural analgesia on cesarean section for dystocia in nulliparous women. Am J Obstet Gynecol 161:670–675, 1989.

133a. Gribble RK, Meier PR: Effect of epidural analgesia on the primary cesarean rate. Obstet Gynecol 78:231–234, 1991.

134. Neuhoff D, Burke MS, Porreco RP: Cesarean birth for failed progress in labor. Obstet Gynecol 73:915–920, 1989.

135. Belfrage P, Raabe N, Thalme B, Berlin A: Lumbar epidural analgesia with bupivacaine in labor. Determinations of drug concentration and pH in fetal scalp blood and continuous fetal heart rate monitoring. Am J Obstet Gynecol 121:360–365, 1975.

136. Pearson JF, Davies P: The effect of continuous lumbar epidural analgesia on the acid-base status of maternal arterial blood during the first stage of labour. J Obstet Gynaecol Br Commonw 80:218–224, 1973.

137. Thalme B, Belfrage P, Raabe N: Lumbar epidural analgesia in labour. I. Acid-base balance and clinical condition of mother, fetus, and newborn child. Acta Obstet Gynecol Scand 53:27–35, 1974.

138. Thalme B, Raabe N, Belfrage P: Lumbar epidural analgesia in labour. II. Effects on glucose, lactate, sodium, chloride, total protein, haematocrit and haemoglobin in maternal, fetal, and neonatal blood. Acta Obstet Gynecol Scand 53:113–119, 1974.

139. Livnat EJ, Fejgin M, Scommegna A, Bieniarz J, Burd L: Neonatal acid-base balance in spontaneous and instrumental vaginal deliveries. Obstet Gynecol 52:549–551, 1978.

140. Mc Bride WG, Black BP, Brown CJ, Dolby RM, Murray AD, Thomas DB: Method of delivery and developmental outcome at five years of age. Med J Aust 1:301–304, 1979.

141. Gilstrap LC, Hauth JC, Schiano S, Connor KD: Neonatal acidosis and method of delivery. Obstet Gynecol 63:681–685, 1984.

142. Friedman EA, Sachtleben-Murray MR, Dahrouge D, Neff RK: Long-term effects of labor and delivery on offspring. A matched-pair analysis. Am J Obstet Gynecol 150:941–945, 1984.

143. Chen S-Z, Aisaka K, Mori H, Kigawa T: Effects of sitting position on uterine activity during labor. Obstet Gynecol 69:67–73, 1987.

143a. Piper JM, Bolling DR, Newton ER: The second stage of labor: Factors influencing duration. Am J Obstet Gynecol 165:976–979, 1991.

143b. Walker MPR, Farine D, Rolbin SH, Ritchie JWK: Epidural anesthesia, episiotomy, and obstetric laceration. Obstet Gynecol 77:668–671, 1991.

144. Danforth DN, Ueland K: Physiology of uterine action. In Obstetrics and Gynecology. DN Danforth, JR Scott, eds. JB Lippincott, Philadelphia, 1986, pp 582–628.

145. Gunther RE, Bauman J: Obstetrical caudal anesthesia. I. A randomized study comparing 1 per cent mepivacaine with 1 per cent lidocaine plus epinephrine. Anesthesiology 31:5–19, 1969.

146. Gunther RE, Bellville JW: Obstetrical caudal anesthesia. II. A randomized study comparing 1 per cent mepivacaine with

1 per cent mepivacaine plus epinephrine. Anesthesiology 37:288–298, 1972.

147. Abboud TK, David S, Nagappala S, Costandi J, Yanagi T, Haroutanian S, Yeh S-U: Maternal, fetal, and neonatal effects of lidocaine with and without epinephrine for epidural anesthesia in obstetrics. Anesth Analg 63:973–979, 1984.

148. Abboud TK, Shiek-al-Eslam A, Yanagi T, Murakawa K, Costandi J, Zakarian M, Hoffman D, Haroutanian A: Safety and efficacy of epinephrine added to bupivacaine for lumbar epidural analgesia in obstetrics. Anesth Analg 64:585–591, 1985.

149. Abboud TK, Der Sakissian L, Terrasi J, Minekawa K, Zhu J, Longhitano M: Comparative maternal, fetal, and neonatal effects of chloroprocaine with and without epinephrine for epidural anesthesia in obstetrics. Anesth Analg 66:71–75, 1987.

150. Eisenach JC, Grice SC, Dewan DM: Epinephrine enhances analgesia produced by epidural bupivacaine during labor. Anesth Analg 66:447–451, 1987.

151. Grice SC, Eisenach JC, Dewan DM: Labor analgesia with epidural bupivacaine plus fentanyl: Enhancement with epinephrine and inhibition with 2-chloroprocaine. Anesthesiology 72:623–628, 1990.

152. Covino BC, Vassallo HG: Local Anesthetics: Mechanisms of Action and Clinical Use. Grune & Stratton, New York, 1976, p 104.

153. Lund PC, Cwik JC, Gannon RT: Extradural anesthesia: Choice of local anaesthetic agents. Br J Anaesth 47:313–321, 1975.

154. Mather LE, Tucker CT, Murphy TM, Stanton-Hicks Md'A, Bonica JJ: The effects of adding adrenaline to etidocaine and lignocaine in extradural anaesthesia. II. Pharmacokinetics. Br J Anaesth 48:989–993, 1976.

CHAPTER 5

Perinatal Pharmacology

Mieczyslaw Finster, M.D.
David H. Ralston, M.D.
Hilda Pedersen, M.B., Ch.B., F.F.A.R.C.S.

Perinatal pharmacology is concerned with the classic pharmacologic processes of drug absorption, distribution, biotransformation and excretion, not in one individual but in two—the mother and the fetus (1–4). The perinatal period begins with the preimplantation blastocyst and extends to the neonate at 28 days of age. The discovery of vaginal adenosis in young women whose mothers were exposed to diethylstilbesterol during pregnancy (5) demonstrates the long-term effect that drugs administered during the perinatal period are capable of producing. This chapter focuses on the period of parturition and the effect of anesthetic drugs on the fetus and neonate. The basic concepts of placental drug transfer (absorption) (6), fetal and neonatal disposition of anesthetic drugs (distribution, biotransformation, excretion) (7, 8), and the clinical implications of anesthetic drug effects on the newborn (9) are examined. Because local anesthetics are among the most commonly used group of drugs in obstetrics and are currently being studied extensively throughout the world, their pharmacology is used to illustrate principles of perinatal pharmacology.

DETERMINANTS OF PLACENTAL TRANSFER

To achieve a physiologic effect, a critical concentration of "free" drug (i.e., nonionized and nonprotein-bound) must arrive at and react with a given tissue receptor site (Fig. 5.1) (6–8, 10). To reach the fetus, a maternally administered drug must first traverse the placenta, a process determined by maternal, placental, and fetal factors (Fig. 5.2).

Maternal Factors

Drug delivery to the placental exchange site depends on the fraction of total uterine blood flow that perfuses the intervillous space. Total uterine blood flow in humans at term has been estimated at approximately 150 ml/min/kg of total weight of gravid uterus (11). In the sheep, total uterine blood flow is 250 to 350 ml/min/kg (12), and approximately 80% perfuses the intervillous space (Fig. 5.3) (13). A similar distribution probably exists in humans.

Little information is available on how changes in maternal hemodynamics alter delivery of a drug to the placenta. To illustrate the complexity of this process, assume that a drug is injected as a bolus into venous blood of a woman in active labor. During the peak of a uterine contraction, uterine arterial flow ceases; hence, the drug is unable to reach the placenta, at least during the first maternal circulation time. Indeed, lower concentrations of diazepam were demonstrated in infants born to mothers given the drug intravenously at the onset of uterine contraction, compared with the newborns whose mothers received diazepam during uterine diastole (14). However, if the drug arrived at the onset or decline of a uterine contraction when only uterine venous outflow was impeded, the drug could be sequestered in the intervillous space and potentially cross the placenta to a greater extent. The supine position with its attendant vena caval or aortic obstruction could also alter drug delivery to the placenta. Maternal hypotension or hypertension may also affect delivery of a drug to the placenta to an unknown extent. Studies of drug transfer across rabbit placenta, perfused in situ, showed that a decrease in maternal blood pressure by 35% reduced the placental clearance of meperidine, but not bupivacaine (15). Neither did the addition of adrenaline affect the placental clearance of bupivacaine (16). The uterine artery concentration of "free drug" (C_m) that arrives at the intervillous space is itself dependent on several factors (Table 5.1).

Increasing the total dose of drug, irrespective of the route of administration, increases the maternal arterial blood concentration (17). Fetal drug blood concentration increases as well.

Injection of local anesthetic into the highly vascular caudal epidural space results in higher peak maternal blood levels than occur after lumbar epidural administration (18), whereas maternal concentrations of local anesthetics are similar after injection into the lumbar epidural, pudendal, or paracervical areas (19).

Epinephrine reduces the peak maternal local anesthetic concentration by 30 to 50% with lidocaine or mepivacaine but has little effect on peak levels of bupivacaine or etidocaine (Fig. 5.4) (17, 20).

Maternal metabolism and elimination reduce drug

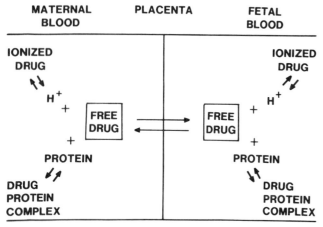

Figure 5.1. Drug in blood or tissue exists in several forms: ionized, protein bound, or as the nonionized, nonprotein-bound free form. It is this lipid-soluble, free form of the drug that readily passes biologic membranes such as the placenta.

concentrations at the intervillous space. In human volunteers, the elimination half-lives for the commonly administered local anesthetics range from 1.5 hr for lidocaine to 3.5 hr for bupivacaine (21). Detailed pharmacokinetic studies in pregnant females have not been possible, although available data suggest an elimination half-life of 60 to 90 min for lidocaine after intravenous bolus administration of 3 mg/kg (19). When bupivacaine is administered epidurally for cesarean section, the drug disappears from maternal blood in two phases, an initial rapid elimination with a half-life of 47 min and a slow elimination with a half-life of 9 hr (22). In another study, the times to maximum serum concentration (about 15 min) and terminal elimination half-life after epidural administration of bupivacaine were similar in pregnant and nonpregnant women (23).

Pretreatment with an H_2 receptor antagonist, cimetidine, to reduce the risk of acid pulmonary aspiration may alter maternal drug metabolism since cimetidine reduces hepatic blood flow and microsomal enzyme activity (24). Cimetidine has been shown to decrease the clearance of lidocaine but not of bupivacaine (25). Ranitidine, another H_2 blocker, is devoid of hepatic microsomal inhibition and has no effect on the metabolism of either local anesthetic (25).

Plasma protein binding of local anesthetic varies with the individual drug and its concentration (Fig. 5.5). At the usually encountered clinical concen-

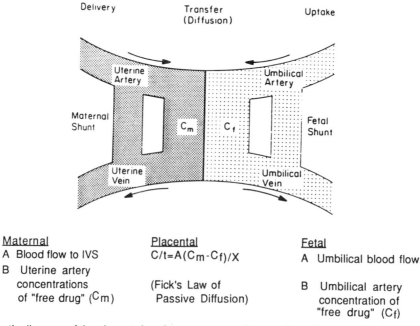

Maternal
A Blood flow to IVS
B Uterine artery concentrations of "free drug" (C_m)

Placental
$C/t = A(C_m - C_f)/X$

(Fick's Law of Passive Diffusion)

Fetal
A Umbilical blood flow
B Umbilical artery concentration of "free drug" (C_f)

Figure 5.2. A schematic diagram of the placental exchange site and the maternal, placental, and fetal factors that influence drug transfer and fetal drug uptake. *IVS*, intervillous space; *C/t*, rate of diffusion; *K*, diffusion constant of drug and membrane; *A*, surface available for transfer; C_m, drug concentration in maternal blood; C_f, drug concentration in fetal blood; *X*, thickness of membrane.

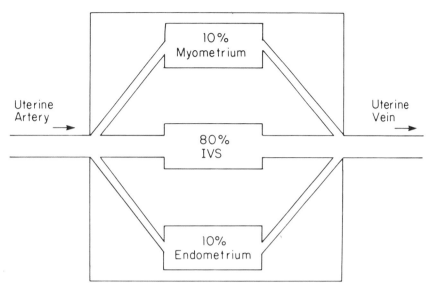

Figure 5.3. The distribution of uterine blood flow in the pregnant sheep. A similar distribution may occur in the human. (Modified from Makowski EL, Meschia G, Droegemueller W, Battaglia FC: Distribution of uterine blood flow in the pregnant sheep. Am J Obstet Gynecol 101:409–412, 1968.)

Table 5.1
Factors That Determine the Concentration of Free Drug in Uterine Arterial Blood (C$_m$)

Total dose
Route of administration
Presence of epinephrine in anesthetic solution
Maternal metabolism and excretion
Maternal protein binding
Maternal pH and pK$_a$ of drug

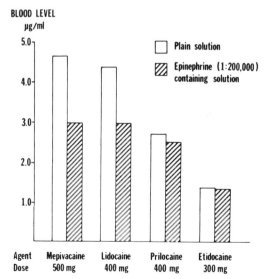

Figure 5.4. The peak concentration of various local anesthetics after epidural administration with and without epinephrine. (Reprinted by permission from Covino BG, Vassallo HG: *Local Anesthetics: Mechanisms of Action and Clinical Use*. Grune & Stratton, New York, 1976, p 104.)

trations, the percentage of binding for lidocaine or mepivacaine is 50 to 70% and for bupivacaine and etidocaine is 95% (21, 26). The higher degree of protein binding with bupivacaine and etidocaine may impede placental transfer by reducing the concentration of free drug available for diffusion (Fig. 5.1) (27–29). However, the lower umbilical vein/maternal vein concentration ratios of bupivacaine and etidocaine are due to the difference in fetal and maternal plasma protein binding (which is higher in the mother) rather than to maternal binding alone (27). Pregnancy reduces the protein binding of some drugs. For example, the binding of bupivacaine is lower in pregnant than nonpregnant ewes (30), whereas there is no effect on the binding of mepivacaine or ropivacaine (Fig. 5.6) (31). Plasma protein binding of bupivacaine is also reduced during human pregnancy (32). The rate of drug-protein dissociation is also important in assessing the significance of local anesthetic protein binding. Tucker (26) suggested that protein binding of local anesthetic does not significantly impede diffusion of drug across the placenta, because the dissociation of drug from protein is essentially instantaneous. This could not be substantiated for bupivacaine but was documented for fentanyl, an opioid bound to plasma albumin (33).

The pK$_a$ of a drug is the pH at which 50% of the drug is ionized and 50% is nonionized. Because most local anesthetics and narcotics are weak bases, with pK$_a$s above the maternal pH, a significant quantity of these drugs exist as the lipid-soluble, nonionized form in maternal blood.

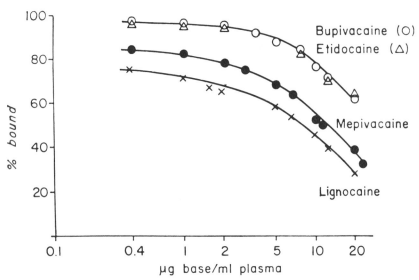

Figure 5.5. Plasma binding of four anilide local anesthetics at plasma concentrations of 0.4 to 20 µg/ml. (Reprinted by permission from Tucker GT, Mather LE: Pharmacokinetics of local anesthetic agents. Br J Anaesth 47:213–224, 1975.)

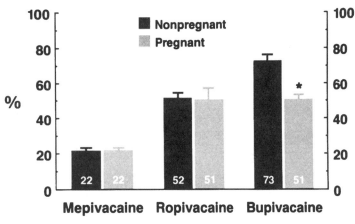

*Significantly different from nonpregnant; mean ± SEM

Figure 5.6. Serum protein binding of mepivacaine, ropivacaine, and bupivacaine in nonpregnant and pregnant ewes. (Adapted from Santos AC, Pedersen H, Harmon TW, Morishima HO, Finster M, Arthur GR, Covino BG: Does pregnancy alter the systemic toxicity of local anesthetics? Anesthesiology 70:991–995, 1989; and from Santos AC, Arthur GR, Pedersen H, Morishima HO, Finster M, Covino BG: Systemic toxicity of ropivacaine during ovine pregnancy. Anesthesiology 75:137–141, 1991.)

Placental Factors

Once a given drug has reached the intervillous space, the quantity transferred per unit time is described by Fick's equation of passive diffusion (34) (Fig. 5.2), expressed mathematically as

$$Q/t = K \cdot A \left(\frac{C_m - C_f}{X} \right)$$

where K is a diffusion constant determined by drug physicochemical properties such as molecular weight, lipid solubility, degree of ionization, and spatial configuration. This equation states that the amount of transfer is proportional to the free drug concentration difference between maternal and fetal blood and the surface area available for diffusion and is inversely related to the thickness of the membrane. At equilibrium the concentration of free drug on both sides of the membrane is equal. Therefore, placental drug transfer is facilitated by a high concentration of nonionized, lipid-soluble, nonprotein-bound drug. High molecular weight, poor lipid solubility, and a high degree of ionization will impede but not totally prevent the transfer of a drug across the placenta. Muscle relaxants such as succinylcholine, atracurium and vecuronium, which are highly ionized, do cross the placenta but only to a limited extent (35–37).

It has recently been proposed that, if the blood

flow to the fetal side of the placenta can be measured (such as in some animal studies), calculating the placental clearance is the more appropriate way of expressing drug transfer to the fetus (38). At steady state

$$Cl = \frac{Qu\,(Cuv - Cua)}{Cma}$$

where   Cl   =   clearance, in vol/time
       Qu   =   umbilical blood flow
       Cuv =   umbilical vein drug concentration
       Cua =   umbilical artery drug concentration
       Cma =   maternal arterial drug concentration

The capacity of the placenta to metabolize anesthetic drugs is too limited to be of significance in reducing their transfer to the fetus.

Fetal Factors

Fetal uptake, distribution, metabolism, and elimination determine drug disposition and physiologic effects once a drug has diffused across the placental exchange site.

FETAL UPTAKE OF DRUGS

Fetal uptake is determined by the solubility of the drug in fetal blood (which includes drug dissolved in plasma water, as well as drug bound to red blood cell and plasma protein components); the quantity and distribution of fetal blood flow to the intervillous space; and the concentration of drug in fetal blood returning to the placenta (Fig. 5.2). In addition, the pH gradient existing between maternal and fetal blood influences the concentration of drug at equilibrium. For example, local anesthetics are weak bases, with pK_as ranging from 7.6 for mepivacaine to 8.9 for procaine. At a higher hydrogen ion concentration (or lower pH) more local anesthetic exists in the ionized state. At pH 7.40 lidocaine is 24% nonionized, whereas at pH 7.0 11% exists in the nonionized form. Thus a 0.40 pH gradient would cause a 54% increase in the amount of ionized drug. Such a pH gradient may exist between a mother and an asphyxiated fetus. Because the ionized form of the drug does not pass through lipid membranes as readily as the lipid-soluble, nonionized form, a weakly basic drug may accumulate in the more acid fetal blood. Clinical and laboratory evidence suggests that this phenomenon of "ion trapping" may indeed occur. Brown et al. (39) found high umbilical vein (UV)/maternal vein (MV) concentration ratios of lidocaine and mepivacaine in neonates with umbilical artery pH values of 7.03 to 7.23. Biehl et al. (40) induced acidosis in fetal lambs during constant-rate lidocaine infusion into the mother. Higher fetal blood lidocaine concentrations were seen during fetal acidosis (pH 6.90 to 7.18)

than when fetal pH was normal (7.30 to 7.35). Correction of fetal acidosis with bicarbonate (fetal pH 7.22 to 7.40) resulted in a decrease in fetal blood lidocaine concentration (Fig. 5.7). Although ion trapping may account for the higher fetal blood levels of local anesthetics and narcotics, reduced fetal clearance of these drugs due to alterations in fetal cardiac output or umbilical or hepatic blood flow, or changes in the blood-to-tissue distribution of these drugs during metabolic acidosis, might also explain the observed findings. For example, the infusion of lidocaine into asphyxiated baboon fetuses resulted in increased drug uptake in the heart, brain, and liver, as compared with nonasphyxiated controls (41).

Fetal umbilical blood flow to the placental exchange site is obviously essential for fetal drug uptake (Fig. 5.8). Fetal-placental flow in the lamb is 200 to 250 ml/min/kg body weight, representing approximately 50% (Fig. 5.9) of the combined ventricular output (12, 42). The fraction of this output perfusing the placenta increases with fetal asphyxia (43) and may decrease with cord compression.

Local anesthetics transferred across the placenta may adversely affect fetal circulatory adaptation to asphyxia, including the increased placental blood flow. In the chronically instrumented pregnant ewe, lidocaine infusion resulting in clinically relevant maternal and fetal plasma levels of the drug is well tolerated by the partially asphyxiated mature fetal lamb (44). In contrast, the preterm fetus loses its cardiovascular adaptation to asphyxia and its condition deteriorates (45). Studies of drug transfer across rabbit placenta, perfused in situ, indicate that a reduction in umbilical blood flow may increase the fetal/maternal concentration ratio but reduce the rate of placental transfer of drugs such as bupivacaine, lidocaine, and meperidine (29). Further complicating the understanding of hemodynamic factors in fetal drug uptake is the nonhomogeneity of maternal and fetal blood flow in the placenta (46, 47). Inasmuch as most anesthetic drugs (similar to O_2 placental transfer) cross the placenta by a process of flow-dependent passive diffusion, changes in the maternal/fetal circulation ratios in various parts of the placenta undoubtedly modulate drug transfer. Little information is available in this area.

FETAL DISTRIBUTION OF DRUGS

The fetal circulation is unique in several ways and greatly modifies drug distribution (Fig. 5.10). Umbilical venous blood returning from the placenta either perfuses the liver or flows through the ductus venosus (48). Fetal hepatic perfusion may protect against attainment of high drug levels on the arterial side of the fetal circulation (49, 50). Dilution of um-

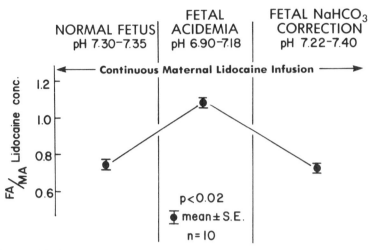

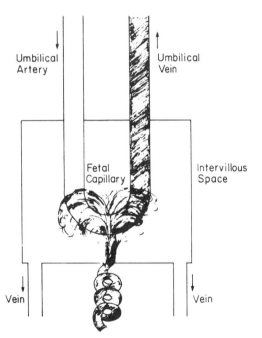

Figure 5.7. Fetal/maternal arterial (*FA/MA*) lidocaine ratios were significantly higher during fetal acidemia than during control or during pH correction with bicarbonate. (Reprinted by permission from Biehl D, Shnider SM, Levinson G, Callender K: Placental transfer of lidocaine: Effects of fetal acidosis. Anesthesiology 48:409–412, 1978.)

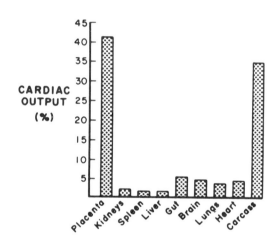

Figure 5.9. Percent distribution of combined ventricular output in fetal lamb near term (measured with radioactive microspheres). (Reprinted by permission from Pang LM, Mellins RB: Neonatal cardiorespiratory physiology. Anesthesiology 43:171–196, 1975.)

Figure 5.8. Circulatory pathways at the intervillous space. The fetal umbilical artery carries blood to the intervillous space, where exchange of oxygen, carbon dioxide, and drugs occurs. The maternal spinal artery enters at the base, and fountain-like spurts of blood bathe the branching villi, which contain fetal capillaries. Blood returns to the fetus via the umbilical vein, whereas uterine veins drain maternal blood from the intervillous space. Hemodynamic alterations may occur at several sites: umbilical artery or vein (cord compression); intervillous space (fetal capillary compression with increased intrauterine pressure); uterine vein (vena caval obstruction with a parturient in the supine position); or uterine artery (spinal hypotension or α-adrenergic stimulation). How hemodynamic changes influence placental transfer is poorly understood.

bilical venous blood in the fetal right atrium and shunting of blood across the foramen ovale and ductus arteriosus also modify fetal drug distribution.

The concentration of drug returning to the placenta in umbilical arterial blood (C_f) is determined by the quantity of drug entering the fetal circulation (the input), fetal tissue uptake, fetal pH, protein binding and, possibly, nonplacental routes of fetal drug elimination (Table 5.2). Rapid placental transfer of anesthetic drugs is paralleled by their rapid distribution to highly perfused fetal organs (49, 50). After inadvertent direct fetal administration of mepivacaine during caudal anesthesia, postmortem tissue drug concentrations in liver, brain, and kidney (51) were many times greater than blood concentrations.

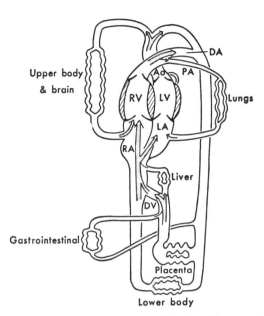

Figure 5.10. The fetal circulation. (Reprinted by permission from Rudolph AM: *Congenital Diseases of the Heart: Clinical-Physiologic Considerations in Diagnosis and Management.* Year Book Medical, Chicago, 1974, p 2.)

Table 5.2
Factors That Determine the Concentration of Free Drug in Fetal Umbilical Arterial Blood (C_f)

Umbilical venous blood concentration (input)
Fetal pH
Fetal protein binding
Fetal tissue uptake
Nonplacental routes of fetal drug elimination
    Fetal hepatic metabolism
    Fetal renal excretion

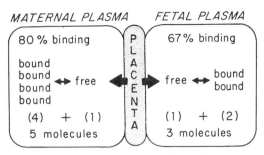

Figure 5.11. Differential protein binding of drug by maternal and fetal blood would account for differences in *total* drug concentrations on both sides of the placenta when free drug concentrations were, in fact, equal. (Reprinted by permission from DeJong RH: *Local Anesthetics.* Charles C Thomas, Springfield, IL, 1976, p 204.)

Table 5.3
Pharmacokinetics of Lidocaine in Adult Sheep and Newborn Lambs[a]

	Adult	Neonate
Vdβ (l/kg)	1.84	3.94
T½α (min)	5	5
T½β (min)	31	51
Cl (ml/min/kg)	41	54
Renal Cl (ml/min/kg)	1.0	9.2

[a]Adapted from Morishima HO, Finster M, Pedersen H, Fukunaga A, Ronfeld RA, Vassallo HG, Covino BG: Pharmacokinetics of lidocaine in fetal and neonatal lambs and adult sheep. Anesthesiology 50:431–436, 1979.

Fetal red blood cell and serum proteins bind local anesthetics to a lesser degree than do maternal red blood cells and proteins (52). This may be clinically significant because at a given total drug concentration more drug would be in the unbound free form, the fraction presumably responsible for physiologic effects (Fig. 5.11) (20).

FETAL METABOLISM AND EXCRETION OF DRUGS

Fetal hepatic enzyme activity is generally less than in adults. Oxidative and conjugative detoxification pathways, both of which are involved in the metabolism of many drugs, are deficient in the fetal or neonatal animal (53). In humans, although fetal metabolism of amide local anesthetics has not been studied, indirect evidence suggests that the human fetus can metabolize these drugs. Although hepatic cytochrome P-450 activity is absent in fetuses of several animal species either early or late in gestation, human fetal liver microsomes have significant cy-

tochrome P-450 levels and NADPH cytochrome C reductase as early as the 14th week of gestation (3, 54, 55). This suggests that even the premature human fetus can metabolize numerous drugs, including most local anesthetics.

A study comparing the pharmacokinetics of lidocaine among adult ewes and fetal and neonatal lambs showed that the metabolic clearance in the newborn was similar to, and renal clearance greater than, that in the adult (Table 5.3) (56). Nonetheless, the elimination half-life was more prolonged in the newborn. This was attributed to a greater volume of distribution and tissue uptake of the drug so that, at any given time, the neonate's liver and kidneys are exposed to a smaller fraction of lidocaine accumulated in the body. Similar results were obtained in another study involving administration of lidocaine to human infants in a neonatal intensive care unit (57). Prolonged elimination half-lives in the newborn compared with the adult have been noted for other amide local anesthetics (58).

References

1. Finnegan L: Clinical effects of pharmacologic agents on pregnancy, the fetus, and the neonate. Ann NY Acad Sci 281:74–89, 1976.
2. Mirkin BL: Research goals in developmental pharmacology. In *Perinatal Pharmacology: Problems and Priorities.* J Dancis, JC Hewang, eds. Raven Press, New York, 1974, p 221.
3. Yaffe SJ, Juchau MP: Perinatal pharmacology. Annu Rev Pharmacol 14:219–238, 1974.
4. Yaffe SJ, Stern L: Clinical implications of perinatal pharmacology. In *Perinatal Pharmacology and Therapeutics.* BL Mirkin, ed. Academic Press, New York, 1976.
5. Herbst AL, Ulfelder H, Poskanzer DC: Adenocarcinoma of the vagina: Association of maternal stilbesterol therapy with tumor appearance in young women. N Engl J Med 284:878–881, 1971.
6. Mirkin BL, Singh S: Placental transfer of pharmacologically active molecules. In *Perinatal Pharmacology and Therapeutics.* BL Mirkin, ed. Academic Press, New York, 1976, p 1.
7. Mirkin BL: Drug distribution in pregnancy. In *Fetal Pharmacology.* L Boreus, ed. Raven Press, New York, 1973, p 1.
8. Mirkin BL: Maternal and fetal distribution of drugs in pregnancy. Clin Pharmacol Ther 14:643–647, 1973.
9. Levinson G, Shnider SM: Placental transfer of local anesthetics: Clinical implications. In *Parturition and Perinatology.* GF Marx, ed. Davis, Philadelphia, 1973, p 173.
10. Mirkin BL: Perinatal pharmacology: Placental transfer, fetal localization, and neonatal disposition of drugs. Anesthesiology 43:156–170, 1975.
11. Assali NS, Douglass RA, Baird WM, Nicholson DB, Suyemoto R: Measurement of uterine metabolism. IV. Results in normal pregnancy. Am J Obstet Gynecol 66:248–253, 1953.
12. Comline RS, Silver M: Placental transfer of blood gases. Br Med Bull 31:25–31, 1975.
13. Makowski EL, Meschia G, Droegemueller W, Battaglia FC: Distribution of uterine blood flow in the pregnant sheep. Am J Obstet Gynecol 101:409–412, 1968.
14. Haram K, Bakke OM, Johanessen KH, Lund T: Transplacental passage of diazepam during labor: Influence of uterine contractions. Clin Pharmacol Ther 24:590–599, 1978.
15. Gaylard DG, Carson RJ, Reynolds F: Effect of umbilical perfusate pH and controlled maternal hypotension on placental drug transfer in the rabbit. Anesth Analg 71:42–48, 1990.
16. Laishley RS, Carson RJ, Reynolds F: Effect of adrenaline on placental transfer of bupivacaine in the perfused in situ rabbit placenta. Br J Anaesth 63:439–443, 1989.
17. Covino BG, Vassallo HG: *Local Anesthetics: Mechanisms of Action and Clinical Use.* Grune & Stratton, New York, 1976, p 100.
18. Lund PC, Bush DF, Covino BG: Determinants of etidocaine concentration in the blood. Anesthesiology 42:497–503, 1975.
19. Shnider SM, Way EL: The kinetics of transfer of lidocaine (Xylocaine^R) across the human placenta. Anesthesiology 29:944–950, 1968.
20. DeJong RH: *Local Anesthetics.* Charles C Thomas, Springfield, IL, 1977, p 197.
21. Tucker GT, Mather LE: Pharmacokinetics of local anesthetic agents. Br J Anaesth 47:213–224, 1975.
22. Magno R, Berlin A, Karlsson K, Kjellmer I: Anesthesia for cesarean section. IV. Placental transfer and neonatal elimination of bupivacaine following epidural analgesia for elective cesarean section. Acta Anaesth Scand 20:141–146, 1976.
23. Pihlajamäki K, Kanto J, Lindberg R, Karanko M, Kiilholma P: Extradural administration of bupivacaine: Pharmacokinetics and metabolism in pregnant and nonpregnant women. Br J Anaesth 64:556–562, 1990.
24. Feely J, Wilkinson GR, McAllister CB, Wood AJJ: Increased toxicity and reduced clearance of lidocaine by cimetidine. Ann Int Med 96:592–594, 1982.
25. O'Sullivan GM, Smith M, Morgan B, Brighouse D, Reynolds F: H$_2$ antagonists and bupivacaine clearance. Anaesthesia 43:93–95, 1988.
26. Tucker GT: Plasma binding and disposition of local anesthetics. Int Anesthesiol Clin 13:33–59, 1975.
27. Kennedy RL, Miller RP, Bell JU, Doshi D, deCousa H, Kennedy MJ, Heald D, David J: Uptake and distribution of bupivacaine in fetal lambs. Anesthesiology 65:247–253, 1986.
28. Kennedy RL, Bell JU, Miller RP, Doshi D, deSousa H, Kennedy MJ, Heald D, Bettinger R, David Y: Uptake and distribution of lidocaine in fetal lambs. Anesthesiology 72:483–489, 1990.
29. Hamshaw-Thomas A, Rogerson N, Reynolds F: Transfer of bupivacaine, lignocaine and pethidine across rabbit placenta: Influence of maternal protein binding and fetal flow. Placenta 5:61–70, 1984.
30. Santos AC, Pedersen H, Harmon TW, Morishima HO, Finster M, Arthur R, Covino BG: Does pregnancy alter the systemic toxicity of local anesthetics? Anesthesiology 70:991–995, 1989.
31. Santos AC, Arthur GR, Pedersen H, Morishima HO, Finster M, Covino BG: Systemic toxicity of ropivacaine during ovine pregnancy. Anesthesiology 75:137–141, 1991.
32. Wulf H, Münstedt P, Maier CH: Plasma protein binding of bupivacaine in pregnant women at term. Acta Anaesth Scand 35:129–133, 1991.
33. Vella LM, Knott C, Reynolds F: Transfer of fentanyl across the rabbit placenta. Br J Anaesth 58:49–54, 1986.
34. Gillette JR, Stripp B: Pre- and postnatal enzyme capacity for drug metabolite production. Fed Proc 34:172–178, 1975.
35. Drábková J, Crul JF, van der Kleijn E: Placental transfer of ^{14}C labelled succinylcholine in near-term Macaca mulatta monkeys. Br J Anaesth 45:1087–1095, 1973.
36. Flynn PJ, Frank M, Hughes R: Use of atracurium in caesarean section. Br J Anaesth 56:599–605, 1984.
37. Dailey PA, Fisher DM, Shnider SM, Baysinger CL, Shinohara Y, Miller RD, Abboud TK, Kim KC: Pharmacokinetics, placental transfer and neonatal effects of vecuronium and pancuronium administered during cesarean section. Anesthesiology 60:569–574, 1984.
38. Reynolds F, Knott C: Pharmacokinetics in pregnancy and placental drug transfer. In *Oxford Reviews of Reproductive Biology, Vol. 11.* SR Milligan, ed. Oxford University Press, New York, 1989, p 389.
39. Brown WU Jr, Bell GC, Alper MH: Acidosis, local anesthetics and the newborn. Obstet Gynecol 48:27–30, 1976.
40. Biehl D, Shnider SM, Levinson G, Callender K: Placental transfer of lidocaine: Effects of fetal acidosis. Anesthesiology 48:409–412, 1978.
41. Morishima HO, Covino BG: Toxicity and distribution of lidocaine in non-asphyxiated and asphyxiated baboon fetuses. Anesthesiology 54:182–186, 1981.
42. Rudolph AM, Heymann MA: The circulation of the fetus in utero. Circ Res 21:163–184, 1967.
43. Rudolph AM: *Congenital Diseases of the Heart: Clinical-Physiologic Considerations in Diagnosis and Management.* Year Book Medical Publishers, Chicago, 1974, p 1.
44. Morishima HO, Santos AC, Pedersen H, Finster M, Tsuji A, Hiraoka H, Arthur GR, Covino BG: Effect of lidocaine on the asphyxial responses in the mature fetal lamb. Anesthesiology 66:502–507, 1987.
45. Morishima HO, Pedersen H, Santos AC, Schapiro HM, Finster M, Arthur GR, Covino BG: Adverse effects of maternally administered lidocaine on the asphyxiated preterm fetal lamb. Anesthesiology 71:110–115, 1989.
46. Power GG, Hill EP, Longo LD: Analysis of uneven distribution of diffusing capacity and blood flow in placenta. Am J Physiol 222:740–746, 1972.
47. Power GG, Longo LD, Wagner NN, Kuhl DE, Forster RE II: Uneven distribution of maternal and fetal placental blood flow, as demonstrated using macroaggregates, and its response to hypoxia. J Clin Invest 46:2053–2063, 1967.
48. Pang LM, Mellins RB: Neonatal cardiorespiratory physiology. Anesthesiology 43:171–196, 1975.
49. Finster M, Morishima HO, Boyes RN, Covino BG: The placental transfer of lidocaine and its uptake by fetal tissues. Anesthesiology 36:159–163, 1972.

50. Finster M, Morishima HO, Mark LC, Perel JM, Dayton PG, James LS: Tissue thiopental concentrations in the fetus and newborn. Anesthesiology 36:155–158, 1972.

51. Sinclair JC, Fox HA, Lentz UF, Field GL, Murphy J: Intoxication of the fetus by a local anesthetic, a newly recognized complication of maternal caudal anesthesia. N Engl J Med 273:1173–1177, 1965.

52. Mather LE, Long G, Thomas J: The binding of bupivacaine to maternal and foetal plasma proteins. J Pharm Pharmacol 23:359–365, 1971.

53. Dawkins MJ: Biochemical aspects of developing function in newborn mammalian liver. Br Med Bull 22:27–33, 1966.

54. Waddell WJ, Marlowe GC: Disposition of drugs in the fetus. In *Perinatal Pharmacology and Therapeutics.* BL Mirkin, ed. Academic Press, New York, 1976, p 119.

55. Yaffe SJ: Developmental factors influencing interactions of drugs. Ann NY Acad Sci 281:90–97, 1976.

56. Morishima HO, Finster M, Pedersen H, Fukunaga A, Ronfeld RA, Vassallo HG, Covino BG: Pharmacokinetics of lidocaine in fetal and neonatal lambs and adult sheep. Anesthesiology 50:431–436, 1979.

57. Mihaly GW, Moore RG, Thomas J, Triggs EJ, Thomas D, Shanks CA: The pharmacokinetics and metabolism of the anilide local anaesthetics in neonates. Eur J Clin Pharmacol 13:143–152, 1978.

58. Brown WU Jr, Bell GC, Lurie AO, Scanlon JW, Alper MH: Newborn blood levels of lidocaine and mepivacaine in the first postnatal day following maternal epidural anesthesia. Anesthesiology 42:698–707, 1975.

ANESTHESIA FOR VAGINAL DELIVERY

CHAPTER 6

Choice of Local Anesthetics in Obstetrics

Philip R. Bromage, M.B., B.S., F.F.A.R.C., F.R.C.P. (C)

A broad range of local anesthetics are available for the relief of pain during labor. The selection often seems bewilderingly large, and frequently the anesthesiologist is left wondering whether a particular choice really matters, provided the selected drug works effectively and does no apparent harm. Opinions change as fresh data become available, and choices that seemed obvious a few years ago may not be as desirable in the light of new experience. This chapter attempts to set out guidelines to indicate the major advantages and disadvantages of agents currently available and to suggest those drugs and concentrations that are likely to be better than others under different circumstances and those that should be avoided.

DESIDERATA

As with any choice, the question must be asked: What do we really want? All too often this essential preliminary to the act of selection has not been thought through, but in the context of obstetric anesthesia most of the information that is needed to make a rational selection has been amassed by laborious investigation over the past 45 years. Five basic requirements must be met for relief of pain in labor and delivery, as set out in Table 6.1.

The drug must perform the intended clinical task. It must provide effective analgesia; and obviously, it must be safe to the mother. The fetus must not be jeopardized. In terms of the three Ps outlined in Table 6.1, this means that the expulsive forces of labor must be unaffected. In addition, tone should be preserved in the muscles of the birth canal so that rotation of the fetal head occurs in a normal fashion as the presenting part descends. Finally and very importantly, the fetus, or passenger, must not be intoxicated by placental transfer of potentially depressing drugs nor should the drugs jeopardize fetal gas exchange by reducing maternal blood flow to the uteroplacental unit. This implies that dosages should be kept to a minimum consistent with efficacy and that every means should be sought to minimize placental transfer. In addition, caution must be exercised when us-

ing vasoactive drugs that may diminish uterine blood flow.

The emphasis on each of these five requirements will shift, depending on whether delivery is by the vaginal route—when it is important to preserve normal tone in the *powers* and the *passages*—or by cesarean section, when it is not. Also, vaginal delivery requires less intense analgesia than abdominal section; therefore as a general rule one may expect that more dilute solutions of local anesthetics will be adequate for labor and vaginal delivery. In the defensive medicolegal climate of contemporary obstetric practice, cesarean section rates in the U.S. have climbed to 25 to 30%. Consequently, of all epidural catheters inserted for relief of pain in labor, one-fourth to one-third will end up providing surgical anesthesia for cesarean section. This change of purpose does not necessarily imply the need to change analgesic agents to one that will cause profound motor block of the abdominal muscles because these are already stretched and surgical conditions rarely require much additional relaxation.

LOCAL ANESTHETIC AGENTS: GENERAL CONSIDERATIONS

Two important new developments have narrowed the gap between the advantages of epidural and of subarachnoid anesthesia for cesarean section. First, the manufacture of fine narrow-gauge spinal needles such as the 26- to 29-gauge Quincke, 22- to 27-gauge Whitacre, the 22- to 24-gauge Sprotte, has reduced the incidence of spinal puncture headaches to a competitive level of 1 to 2% (the latter two types have noncutting needle tips) (1–5). Second, the efficacy and safety of modest doses of intrathecal morphine have brought spinal anesthesia into line with epidural analgesia and made it a simple and practical method for providing prolonged postoperative analgesia that is intense enough to alleviate the pain of a lower abdominal incision.

During labor and delivery very dilute epidural infusions of local anesthetics and opiates have approached closer to the goal of pain relief without motor block than has been possible in the past. In addition, there has been a decline in the incidence of delay in the second stage of labor and in the need for instrumental assistance. Thus, in this chapter it will be necessary to touch briefly on some technical aspects of local anesthetic-opiate mixtures, although the main treatment of spinal opiates will be presented in Chapter 10.

ESTER-LINKED AGENTS

Local anesthetics are divided into two main pharmacologic genera, depending on their molecular structure; those with an ester-type linkage in the molecule and those with an amide linkage (Fig. 6.1). The

esters, such as procaine, chloroprocaine and tetracaine, are broken down in the bloodstream by plasma pseudocholinesterase at different speeds, with chloroprocaine having the fastest rate of hydrolysis. Para-aminobenzoic acid, the end-product of ester cleavage, passes across the placenta freely, but it does not appear to cause appreciable fetal depression (6). Some esters, such as piperocaine (Metycaine) are broken down more readily by the liver than by plasma pseudocholinesterase (7).

Chloroprocaine (Nesacaine)

Chloroprocaine, an ester-type agent that is rapidly broken down in the bloodstream, is the least cardiotoxic and the fastest acting local anesthetic available in the U.S. For the infant, it is one of the safest agents for use in obstetrics (Figs. 6.2 and 6.3). Unfortunately, these major advantages have been offset by several practical disadvantages. However, the agent has a valuable if limited role to play in obstetric anesthesia.

In the recent past chloroprocaine was thought to be neurotoxic because of reports of arachnoiditis following its use for epidural analgesia (8–11). Subsequent investigations traced the cause of arachnoiditis

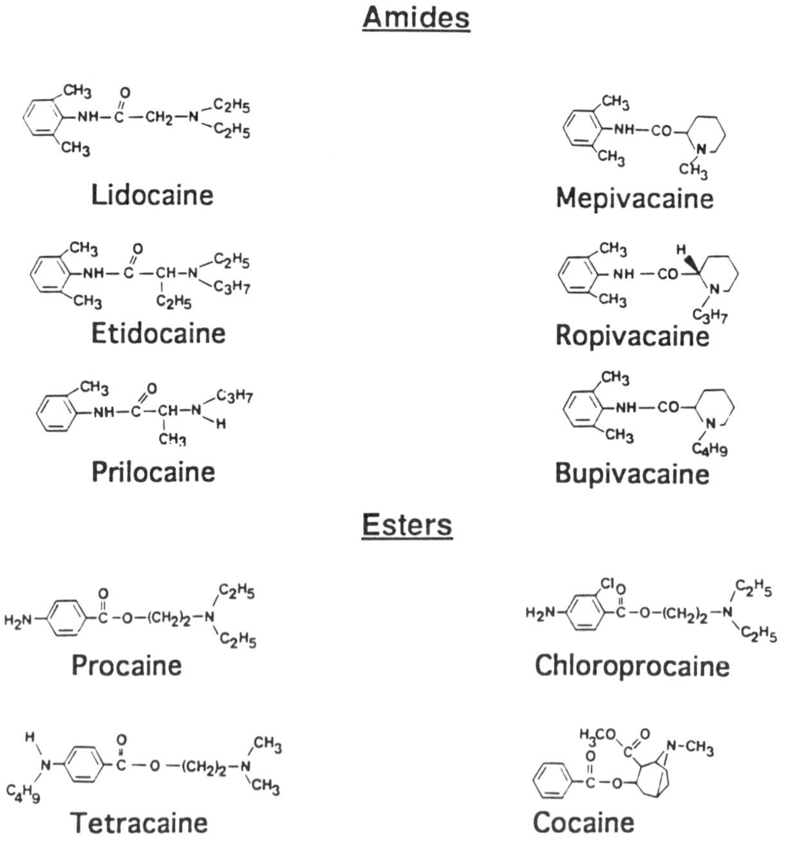

Table 6.1
Requirements of a Local Anesthetic Agent for Relief of Pain in Labor and Delivery

Effective and controllable analgesia
Maternal safety
No weakening of maternal powers
No alteration of maternal passages
No depression of the passenger (fetus)

Amides

Lidocaine

Mepivacaine

Etidocaine

Ropivacaine

Prilocaine

Bupivacaine

Esters

Procaine

Chloroprocaine

Tetracaine

Cocaine

Figure 6.1. Chemical structures of local anesthetics.

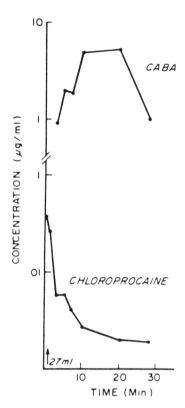

Figure 6.2. Plasma concentrations of chloroprocaine and chloroaminobenzoic acid (*CABA*) in a typical patient following epidural anesthesia (single injection of 27 ml of 3%) for cesarean section. (Reprinted by permission from Kuhnert BR, Kuhnert PM, Prochaska BS, Gross TL: Plasma levels of 2-chloroprocaine in obstetric patients and their neonates after epidural anesthesia. Anesthesiology 53:21–25, 1980.)

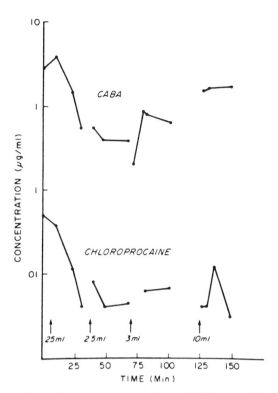

Figure 6.3. Plasma concentrations of chloroprocaine and chloroaminobenzoic acid (*CABA*) in a typical patient following epidural anesthesia (multiple injections) for vaginal delivery. (Reprinted by permission from Kuhnert BR, Kuhnert PM, Porochaska BS, Gross TL: Plasma levels of 2-chloroprocaine in obstetric patients and their neonates after epidural anesthesia. Anesthesiology 53:21–25, 1980.)

to sodium bisulfite that was added as an antioxidant to stabilize the formulation (Fig. 6.4 and Table 6.2). Replacement of metabisulfite by disodium ethylenediaminetetraacetic acid (EDTA) has removed the apparent associated danger of arachnoiditis and exchanged it for the less serious, but nonetheless distressing, side effect of backache that tends to accompany doses of the new formulation in excess of 23 to 25 ml. Volumes of less than 20 ml do not appear to cause trouble. The backache is severe, unrelenting, lasting for a period of several hours, and only relieved by a further dose of epidural local anesthetic or by 100 to 200 μg epidural fentanyl (13–16). In addition, chloroprocaine or one of its metabolites, 4-amino-2-chlorobenzoic acid, impairs the subsequent actions of epidural bupivacaine, fentanyl, and morphine if these agents are used together or sequentially (17–20).

In contrast, the analgesic actions of butorphanol, a mixed μ-receptor antagonist and κ-receptor agonist are not blocked by prior use of chloroprocaine, suggesting that chloroprocaine or its metabolites compete for nonagonist receptors within the spinal cord (21). The practical result of this competition is that the efficacy of the μ-receptor agonists, such as fentanyl and morphine, is impaired by chloroprocaine, and a choice of intraspinal narcotics is limited to κ-agonists such as butorphanol or nalbuphine, agents that are less desirable because of their short duration of action and their tendency to induce heavy sedation when given in effective analgesic doses.

These disadvantages tend to exclude chloroprocaine as an agent of first choice for cesarean section or as the local anesthetic component of opioid–local anesthetic epidural infusions for relief of pain in labor. Nevertheless, the low toxicity and rapid onset of chloroprocaine ensure that it has a limited but very useful role in specific circumstances, as discussed later in this chapter.

Chloroprocaine breaks down very rapidly in the presence of normal pseudocholinesterase. The in vitro plasma half-life is 21 sec for maternal blood and 43 sec for umbilical cord blood (Table 6.3). Thus it is unlikely to reach the fetus in appreciable amounts. If any of the drug did reach the fetus, it would prob-

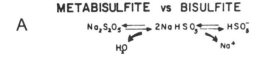

A

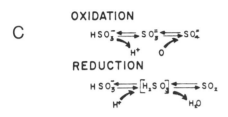

B S, SO_2, $SO_3^=$, $[H_2SO_3]$, HSO_3^-, $S_2O_5^=$, $[H_2SO_2]$, $SO_4^=$

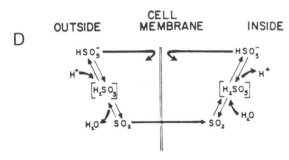

C   OXIDATION

REDUCTION

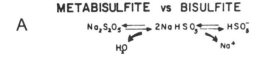

Figure 6.4. Diagram of sulfite chemistry. (*A*) Bisulfite ion appears whether metabisulfite salt or bisulfite salt is added to aqueous solution. (*B*) Ionic species of sulfur ion that appear in aqueous solution regardless of which ion is added to the solution. Relative concentrations determined by pH, ionic concentrations, and temperature. (*C*) Oxidation-reduction equations for bisulfite ion. Oxidation favored by high pH, reduction by low pH. (*D*) Effect of bisulfite ion (externally) in reducing intracellular pH by SO_2 migration through cell membrane. (Reprinted by permission from Gissen AJ, Datta S, Lambert D: The chloroprocaine controversy. II. Is chloroprocaine neurotoxic? Reg Anesth 9:135–145, 1985.)

Table 6.2
Effect of 3% Chloroprocaine Base, 3% Nesacaine, pH, and Bisulfite on Conduction in A and C Fibers of Rabbit Vagus Nerve[a]

Drug	pH	Bisulfite %	Recovery Time (min)	
			A fibers	C fibers
3% Chloroprocaine base	7.2	None	60	120
	3.2	None	60	120
	3.0	0.2	Irreversible block	
	7.3	0.2	60	120
3% Nesacaine	7.3	0.2	60	120
	3.0	0.2	Irreversible block	
Sodium bisulfite in Liley solution	7.0	0.2	No block	
	3.3	0.2	Irreversible block	

[a] Reprinted by permission from Gissen AJ, Datta S, Lambert D: The chloroprocaine controversy. II. Is chloroprocaine neurotoxic? Reg Anesth 9:135–145, 1984.

Table 6.3
Half-Life of Chloroprocaine (in sec)[a]

	Mean ± SD
Mothers (n = 7)	20.9 ± 5.8
Umbilical cords (n = 7)	42.6 ± 11.2
Male controls (n = 6)	20.6 ± 4.1
Female controls (n = 5)	25.2 ± 3.7
Homozygous atypical cholinesterase carriers	106.0 ± 45.0

[a] Reprinted by permission from O'Brien JE, Abbey V, Hinsvark O, Perel J, Finster M: Metabolism and measurement of 2-chloroprocaine, an ester-type anesthetic. J Pharmacol Sci 68:75–79, 1979.

ably be rapidly hydrolyzed in the fetal blood. Chloroprocaine has most of the attributes of a successful local anesthetic for obstetrics. It has a fast onset and good quality of sensory blockade and is safe due to its rapid rate of hydrolysis. However, it also has a very short duration of action, lasting only 35 to 50 min when epinephrine is added. Therefore frequent repeated injections are needed when prolonged analgesia is required. A concentration of 1.5 to 2% is adequate for relief of first-stage labor pain, but a 3% concentration is required for surgical anesthesia, for perineal analgesia and relaxation, or for cesarean section.

Piperocaine (Metycaine)

Piperocaine enjoyed a period of popularity in the 1940s and 1950s, but its slow hydrolysis rate gives it no advantage in terms of fetal toxicity, and it was discarded in favor of the more effective amide agents, such as lidocaine.

Tetracaine (Pontocaine)

Tetracaine has a long duration of action and might seem to be a desirable ester-linked agent for use in labor. Although tetracaine remained one of the most effective and popular drugs for subarachnoid block for many years, it is a poor choice for epidural analgesia. For reasons that are not altogether clear, epidural tetracaine produces a relatively profound motor block but inadequate analgesia (22). This pattern of dissociated blockade is particularly undesirable in obstetrics, in which sensory analgesia is needed, but motor block interferes with the active management of parturition.

AMIDE-LINKED AGENTS

The amide-linked agents include the most powerful and effective local anesthetics currently available. Unfortunately, these drugs are all broken down in the liver, and their half-lives are long. They have relatively low molecular weights (under 325) and high lipid solubilities, and they all pass the placenta in greater or lesser amounts. The ease of placental transfer is also determined by their degree of ionization at physiologic pH. Transfer is favored by a high proportion of nonionized drug, and this in turn is favored by a low dissociation constant, or pK_a and a high lipid solubility. For example, the five agents lidocaine, etidocaine, mepivacaine, ropivacaine, and bupivacaine can be ranked in order of pK_a and diffusibility. Thus:

mepivacaine (pK_a 7.65) > etidocaine (pK_a 7.76)
> lidocaine (pK_a 7.85) > ropivacaine (pK_a 8.1)
> bupivacaine (pK_a 8.16)

From this scale it can be seen that mepivacaine is likely to show the greatest degree of placental transfer and bupivacaine the least.

In the past it was thought that highly protein-bound local anesthetics such as bupivacaine and etidocaine (23, 24) would not traverse the placenta as easily as less highly protein-bound drugs such as lidocaine. However, Morishima et al. (25) demonstrated that low fetal *blood* levels do not imply limited placental transfer. Studies in the pregnant guinea pig indicated that the total amount of local anesthetic reaching the fetus was the same for lidocaine and etidocaine. Highly protein-bound and lipid-soluble drugs have greater tissue uptake, and therefore lower blood levels result. The influence of protein binding and lipid solubility on fetal uptake of local anesthetics is discussed more fully in Chapter 5.

Six of the more important amide drugs are briefly reviewed:

Mepivacaine (Carbocaine)

Mepivacaine is an effective agent with a slightly longer action than lidocaine. However, its long half-life in the neonate (9 hr versus less than 3 hr for lidocaine) has led to a decline in its use in obstetric practice (26, 27).

Prilocaine (Citanest)

Prilocaine was launched with high hopes that its rapid breakdown and low acute toxicity would make it a useful drug for obstetrics. Although prilocaine is probably the safest and most effective agent for such nonobstetric procedures as the Bier block for surgical anesthesia of limbs, its chemical properties make it unsuited for routine obstetric use. Unfortunately the phenolic breakdown product of prilocaine, α-ortho-toluidine, causes significant methemoglobinemia in doses above 600 mg (28, 29). Because the fetus is vulnerable to any reduction of oxygen supply, it is generally agreed that the risk for methemoglobinemia is a contraindication to the use of prilocaine for relief of pain in labor (30).

Lidocaine (Xylocaine)

For many years lidocaine hydrochloride was the standard agent for epidural analgesia in labor. Lidocaine provides dependable analgesia with a duration of action of about 60 min without epinephrine and 75 min when epinephrine 1:200,000 is added. Although placental transfer is appreciable, Apgar scores are usually high (31, 32) and the time to sustained respiration is short. However, neurobehavioral studies of the newborn after maternal lidocaine and mepivacaine epidurals indicated the possibility of subtle depression of some reflexes that was not seen after bupivacaine, chloroprocaine, or etidocaine (26, 33). More recent experience has questioned the practical significance of these neurobehavioral changes (34, 41), and the pendulum of opinion has swung back in favor of lidocaine with its long record of safety and reliability (Table 6.4). Carbonated lidocaine has been available in Canada and Europe since 1970, but not in the United States. Initial clinical studies with this agent showed great promise in terms of its faster onset and more intense analgesia, especially in the resistant segments of L5 and S1 (42–44). Later comparisons questioned the superiority of carbonated lidocaine over the orthodox hydrochloride salt (45–47). However, more recent double-blind evaluations have confirmed the significantly faster onset profiles of sensory and motor blockade with the carbonated salts (48, 49). In the absence of commercial carbonated lidocaine some shortening of latency still can be obtained by pH adjustment of the hydrochloride salt, as discussed under the section "Adjuvants" later in this chapter.

Bupivacaine (Marcaine, Sensorcaine)

Bupivacaine is a congener of mepivacaine, with three methyl groups added to the piperidine ring of the mepivacaine molecule. This important agent was introduced into clinical practice by Telivuo in 1963 (50).

Bupivacaine has two advantages in obstetric practice: (a) the quality of analgesia is high in relation to the degree of motor block; and (b) the duration is long, especially when epinephrine is added. The drug provides effective relief of first-stage labor pain in dilutions as low as 0.125% (51, 52) and at such low concentrations that every induction and top-up dose

Table 6.4
Effect of Lidocaine on Neonatal Neurobehavior

Delivery	Investigators	Comparative Drug Effects on Neonatal Neurobehavior
Vaginal	Scanlon et al., 1974 (26)	Lidocaine and mepivacaine worse than non-epidural
	Scanlon et al., 1976 (33)	Bupivacaine no different than original non-epidural
	Brown, 1977 (34)	Chloroprocaine no different than original non-epidural
	Higuchi and Takeuchi, 1982 (35)	Lidocaine and mepivacaine worse than chloroprocaine, bupivacaine epidural, or tetracaine spinal
	Abboud et al., 1982 (36)	Lidocaine no different than bupivacaine, chloroprocaine, or no medication
	Abboud et al., 1982 (37)	Relatively large doses of lidocaine no different than no medication
	Abboud et al., 1984 (39)	Continuous infusion lidocaine no different than infusions of bupivacaine or chloroprocaine
	Kuhnert et al., 1984 (41)	Trivial differences between lidocaine and chloroprocaine
Cesarean	Abboud et al., 1983 (38)	No difference among lidocaine, bupivacaine, or chloroprocaine
	Kileff et al., 1984 (40)	No difference between lidocaine and bupivacaine
	Kuhnert et al., 1984 (41)	Trivial difference between lidocaine and chloroprocaine

given in epidural analgesia for vaginal delivery can serve as a test dose (53). Ten milliliters of bupivacaine 0.125% plus epinephrine 1:800,000 contain 12.5 mg of bupivacaine and 12.5 μg of epinephrine. This qualifies as a reasonable test dose for both subarachnoid and intravascular injection. Weaker dilutions of bupivacaine (down to 0.0625%) are effective when used in conjunction with a suitable epidural opiate (54, 55). However, bupivacaine has the practical disadvantage of being very slow to produce surgical anesthesia, especially in the resistant segments L5–S1, and a 30-min wait may be needed to establish satisfactory epidural blockade for cesarean section when the 0.5% solution is used (56). The 0.75% solution provides faster onset and better surgical conditions, and for a while the 0.75% concentration enjoyed widespread popularity as a single-shot agent.

Unfortunately, a number of tragic cases of toxic reactions and refractory cardiac arrest have been associated with its use, and 0.75% bupivacaine is now proscribed from obstetric practice. Animal studies confirmed that bupivacaine appears to be potentially more cardiotoxic than lidocaine (Table 6.5 and Fig. 6.5), (57–72). The most likely mechanism for such cardiotoxicity relates to the action of bupivacaine on cardiac sodium channels (Fig. 6.6). Both lidocaine and bupivacaine block the sodium channels of nerve

and heart. These channels, which open briefly during the upstroke of the action potential, are responsible for fast conduction. Thus blockade of sodium channels slows or stops conduction. Such blockade at the level of the nerve membrane is considered the primary mechanism of action of local anesthetics. Blockade of cardiac sodium channels by lidocaine appears to be well tolerated by the heart; in fact, the drug is commonly used as an antiarrhythmic agent. In contrast, the action of bupivacaine on the heart appears toxic (71). When electrophysiologic differences between lidocaine and bupivacaine were compared using voltage clamp experiments with guinea pig papillary muscle, lidocaine was found to enter the sodium channel quickly and to leave quickly; bupivacaine was found to be a "fast-in, slow-out" agent (Fig. 6.7) (71). As a result, bupivacaine is a "potentially dangerous cardiac poison." Courtney (72) also has compared the effects of lidocaine and bupivacaine on contractility; bupivacaine is 16 times more potent than lidocaine in reducing isometric contractions by 33%.

Most of the reported cases of bupivacaine cardiotoxicity involved obstetric patients. The reason for the increased incidence of cardiotoxic reactions to bupivacaine in pregnancy is not clear. It may be due to the more frequent use of bupivacaine for obstetric

Table 6.5
Percentage of Significant Electrocardiographic Rhythm Abnormalities, Hemodynamic Changes, or Death in Acidotic Sheep after Injection of Lidocaine or Bupivacaine at Two Dose Levels[a]

	Lidocaine (%)		Bupivacaine (%)	
	5.7 mg/kg (n = 5)	11.4 mg/kg (n = 6)	2.1 mg/kg (n = 6)	4.2 mg/kg (n = 6)
Atrioventricular conduction block	0	0	0	50
Wide QRS complex rhythm	0	0	33	50
Wide QRS complex bradycardia	0	0	50	83
Wide QRS complex tachycardia	0	0	0	17
Electromechanical dissociation	0	0	17	66
Death	0	0	17	100

[a] Modified from data in Rosen MA, Thigpen JW, Shnider SM, Foutz SE, Levinson G, Koike M: Bupivacaine-induced cardiotoxicity in hypoxic and acidotic sheep. Anesth Analg 64:1089–1096, 1985.

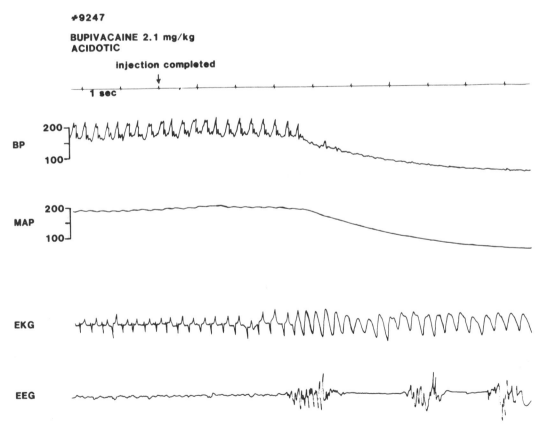

Figure 6.5. Hemodynamic effects of rapid intravenous injection (over 10 sec) of bupivacaine 2.1 mg/kg into a ewe with respiratory acidosis. Within seconds of completion of the injection, convulsant activity is noted on the electroencephalogram (*EEG*). The electrocardiogram (*EKG*) develops a wide QRS complex rhythm, and arterial blood pressure (*BP*) falls precipitously. (Reprinted by permission from Rosen MA, Thigpen JW, Shnider SM, Foutz SE, Levinson G, Koike M: Bupivacaine-induced cardiotoxicity in hypoxic and acidotic sheep. Anesth Analg 64:1089–1096, 1985.)

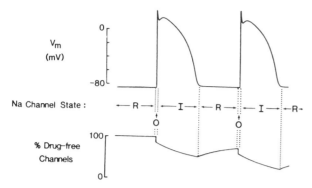

Figure 6.6. Schematic diagram illustrating time-dependent changes in sodium channel states (*middle*) and block of sodium channels (*bottom*) associated with the cardiac action potential (*top*) in the presence of a local anesthetic drug. The top trace shows two simulated ventricular muscular action potentials. V_m = transmembrane voltage. The drug binds to sodium channels in open (*O*) and inactivated (*I*) states but has a very low affinity for channels in the rested (*R*) state. Drug dissociation during diastole is time dependent and, with a drug such as bupivacaine, may be incomplete even at normal heart rates. This results in an accumulation of drug-associated (blocked) channels with successive beats. (Reprinted by permission from Clarkson CW, Hondeghem LM: Mechanism for bupivacaine depression of cardiac conduction: Fast block of sodium channels during the action potential with slow recovery from block during diastole. Anesthesiology 62:396–405, 1985.)

epidural blocks or because it is easier to accidentally puncture a dilated epidural vein during parturition. Also, physiologic changes during pregnancy may make the parturient patient more susceptible to such reactions or more difficult to resuscitate than the non-parturient patient. Animal studies on the possible increased sensitivity of pregnant patients to bupivacaine cardiotoxicity have yielded conflicting results. For example, Eisler et al. (73) found that the lethal dose for rapidly injected intravenous bupivacaine in rabbits did not change with pregnancy. However, Morishima et al. (Fig. 6.8) (74) and Crandell and Kotelko (75) found that pregnant sheep were more susceptible to the cardiotoxic effects of bupivacaine.

Despite its potential cardiotoxicity, bupivacaine is still a useful agent in obstetric anesthesia. When used for epidural blocks for labor, it produces high-quality analgesia with minimal motor blockade and has a relatively long duration of action. Moreover, it is effective as a sole agent in concentrations as low as 0.125%. Bupivacaine 0.5% has been found to be effective for cesarean sections. Although bupivacaine 0.75% may produce a more rapid onset and a denser block, the added hazard of the higher concentration justifies the recommendations of the Food and Drug Administration (FDA).

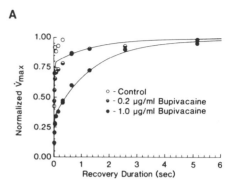

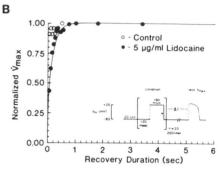

Figure 6.7. The time course of recovery from block under control conditions and in the presence of bupivacaine (*A*) or lidocaine (*B*). The pulse protocol is shown in the inset. (Reprinted by permission from Clarkson CW, Hondeghem LM: Mechanism for bupivacaine depression of cardiac conduction: Fast block of sodium channels during the action potential with slow recovery from block during diastole. Anesthesiology 62:396–405, 1985.)

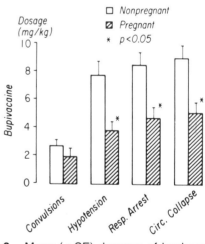

Figure 6.8. Mean ($\pm$SE) dosages of bupivacaine administered slowly (0.5 mg/kg/min) to nonpregnant and pregnant ewes up to the onset of each toxic manifestation. *Significantly different from nonpregnant ewes. (Reprinted by permission from Morishima HO, Pedersen H, Finster M, Hiraoka H, Tsuji A, Feldman HS, Arthur GR, Covino BG: Bupivacaine toxicity in pregnant and nonpregnant ewes. Anesthesiology 63:134–139, 1985.)

Etidocaine (Duranest)

The powerful lipophilicity of etidocaine attracts the drug out of the water phase in the cerebrospinal fluid and far into the lipid depths of the spinal cord to produce intense motor and sensory blockade (76). Unlike bupivacaine, etidocaine blocks A fibers before C fibers (77). These characteristics result in a more intense blockade of somatosensory-evoked potentials than any other local anesthetic in current clinical use (78, 79). Unfortunately, the propensity for large-fiber blockade causes a comparatively profound degree of motor blockade that tends to outlast sensory anesthesia. This is the reverse of what is required in an obstetric setting, where "de-afferentation" without "de-efferentation" is the stated goal (80). Hence, the drug is a poor choice both for relief of pain in labor and for cesarean delivery, in which abdominal muscles are already well stretched and further relaxation is not needed.

Ropivacaine

Preliminary data suggest that ropivacaine promises to become a popular agent in obstetric anesthetic practice. Ropivacaine is another homologue of the mepivacaine series, with one less methyl group than bupivacaine in the lipophilic amine–side chain of the anesthetic molecule. Based on predictions from structure-activity relationships the shorter side chain of ropivacaine should confer less toxicity than bupivacaine, but at the expense of less anesthetic potency (81). To date, animal and human studies in nonobstetric populations have borne out these theoretical predictions. Several important practical findings about ropivacaine have been reported. Cardiotoxicity in animals is reduced more than anesthetic potency, and during the early phases of resuscitation from supraconvulsive doses of ropivacaine, mean arterial pressure is maintained at a significantly higher level than after bupivacaine (82). The therapeutic index of potency/toxicity of ropivacaine appears to be more favorable than bupivacaine, with a comparative ratio of approximately 1.4 for ropivacaine to 1 for bupivacaine (83–85).

Currently, ropivacaine has not yet undergone critical evaluation in an obstetric population, and because crucially relevant data are missing from existing clinical studies, it is difficult to predict how the drug will perform in an obstetric setting. Specifically, no precise information exists on sensory onset profiles (after induction of subarachnoid or epidural anesthesia) as they relate to the salient of anesthetic delay in the resistant spinal segments L5 and S1. At present, all ropivacaine studies have either neglected to make sufficiently frequent observations to construct accurate onset profiles or have failed to record their findings on these spinal segments. This oversight will need to be corrected before a clear comparison can be made between the clinical merits of bupivacaine and ropivacaine. The importance of these segments, at least in North American obstetric practice, lies in their correlation with maternal pain or discomfort during eventration of the uterus for repair of the uterine incision at cesarean section. This is a nociceptive maneuver that has been widely adopted in North American, but less extensively in European obstetric practice (86). Interruption of the afferent pathway appears to be related to cutaneous analgesia in segments L5 and S1, which commonly escape effective blockade under epidural analgesia with 0.5% bupivacaine (author's unpublished data).

ADJUVANTS

Carbon Dioxide, Sodium Bicarbonate: pH Adjustment

Slow onset of epidural analgesia for cesarean section is a serious drawback in a busy obstetric unit. The onset of analgesia can be hastened by increasing the proportions of nonionized, lipid-soluble base in the anesthetic solution. Commercially prepared carbonated lidocaine, as a salt of carbonic acid, has an appreciably faster onset than the orthodox hydrochloride solution, especially in the resistant segments L5 and S1 (87, 88). Although the carbonated formulation of lidocaine has been available in Canada for the past 20 years, it is still not approved in the U.S., where pH adjustment with freshly added sodium bicarbonate is a workable but more primitive and less effective substitute (89, 90). One milliequivalent of sodium bicarbonate (i.e., 1 ml of 8.4% sodium bicarbonate solution) added to every 10 ml of lidocaine hydrochloride, or 3% chloroprocaine, increases the pH to between 7.08 and 7.51 (91). Bupivacaine is more troublesome because the margin between satisfactory alkalinization and complete precipitation of the base is very narrow and pH adjustment must be done carefully with one-tenth of the amount of bicarbonate used for lidocaine (91).

In spite of the handicap of having to add bicarbonate just before injection, the benefits are worthwhile in terms of the faster onset and more profound analgesia when chloroprocaine or lidocaine are chosen as the primary anesthetic agent. Bicarbonate does not appear to hasten onset when added to bupivacaine (66).

Epinephrine

Epinephrine has a long history as an important adjuvant for subarachnoid and epidural anesthesia. Recently, the use of epinephrine has become controversial, partly because of variables peculiar to the drug itself and partly because of physicochemical differences among the newer local anesthetics and opiate agents to which it is added in contemporary practice. The prime reason for using epinephrine is to slow vascular uptake of local anesthetics and opioids from the spinal canal and to favor their uptake into the lipids of the cord and canal, thereby increasing the intensity and duration of their neural blockade (93–97). At the same time, fetal uptake of local anesthetics and opioids is reduced through slowing of maternal vascular uptake and reduction of placental transfer (98).

In addition, epidural epinephrine alone at a concentration of 5 μg/ml has been shown to induce a mild degree of segmental analgesia in volunteers (99). Although this effect may add to the cumulative intensity of analgesia provided by local anesthetic–opioid mixtures, the intrinsic epinephrine contribution is too small to be distinguished from the more important vasoactive effects that determine competition for drug uptake between the aqueous and lipid phases within the spinal canal. The outcome of this competition between aqueous and lipid phases depends on the inherent lipid solubility of each local anesthetic or opiate under study; the more lipid-soluble the agent the less striking is the relatively smaller extra advantage from adding epinephrine. Thus the sensory and motor-blocking qualities of lidocaine, with a low lipid/water partition coefficient of 2.7, are markedly enhanced by adding epinephrine, whereas epidural bupivacaine with a lipid-solubility coefficient 10 times greater, is less affected, and it is difficult to demonstrate any enhancement of its sensory block from the addition of epinephrine, although intensification of motor block can be seen (100).

Similarly, epinephrine intensifies the sensory and side effects of epidural morphine to a greater degree than a more lipid-soluble agent such as sufentanil (97, 99). However, epinephrine does reduce the vascular uptake of the lipid-soluble narcotics, so that lower maternal blood levels and fetal drug transfer may be expected if epinephrine is added to a bolus injection of epidural fentanyl or sufentanil for cesarean section or to an epidural infusion for relief of pain in labor.

The practical role of epinephrine as an adjuvant may be summarized as:

1. In concentrations of 2 to 5 μg/ml (i.e., 1/500,000 to 1/200,000) as a logical adjuvant for bolus epidural doses of lidocaine or chloroprocaine, but not for bupivacaine or etidocaine.

2. In concentrations of 1.5 to 2 μg/ml as an adjuvant for epidural infusion of local anesthetics and opioids to discourage vascular uptake and fetal transfer of the opioid.

3. In subarachnoid anesthesia in amounts of 100 to 200 μg, as an adjuvant to lidocaine, tetracaine, and (probably) bupivacaine to intensify blockade and reduce the incidence of side effects (101, 102).

Finally, fears that intraspinal epinephrine may contribute to spinal cord ischemia have not been substantiated. Blood flow studies in animals with radioactive microspheres and with the hydrogen washout technique have failed to show any significant reduction of flow in the spinal cord after intrathecal or epidural injections of epinephrine, although a significant reduction of flow in the dura mater has been recorded (103–105).

OPIOIDS

Intraspinal opioids act on receptors in the small-cell networks of the dorsal horn of the spinal cord and modulate nociceptive impulses transmitted by C and delta-A fibers before they are relayed to the ascending spinothalamic tracts. Their analgesic action is complementary to the axonal blocking effects of local anesthetics. Thus their analgesic contribution is additive. No evidence of a true synergism between intraspinal opiates and local anesthetics has been uncovered.

Meperidine

Part opioid, part local anesthetic, this familiar narcotic is capable of producing corneal anesthesia in rabbits, sciatic nerve block in frogs (106), and subarachnoid block for surgical anesthesia in humans (107). Meperidine was among the first opioid agents to be tested as the sole epidural agent for relief of pain in labor. Initial reports were controversial, mainly as a result of the use of conservative doses of 25 mg (108), but later studies confirmed epidural analgesic efficacy when larger doses of meperidine were used alone or as an adjuvant to a dilute local anesthetic solution (109–111).

Because meperidine is part local anesthetic, it may reveal its true nature through the same sympathetic and motor side effects as does any other local anesthetic, with the potential for arterial hypotension and some degree of segmental motor impairment when high doses in excess of 100 mg are given. In addition, the opioid element of the drug carries the usual risk of respiratory depression. Thus local anesthetic mixtures with the less pharmacologically complicated opioids such as fentanyl or sufentanil are generally preferred for routine clinical use.

Opioids Without Local Qualitative Properties

The greatest success with intraspinal opiates for pain relief in obstetrics has been achieved with μ-receptor agonists such as morphine, fentanyl, and sufentanil. To date, comparatively little satisfaction has been obtained with κ-agonists or mixed agonist-antagonists such as nalbuphine or butorphanol (112, 113).

Successful use of μ-agonists depends on the practical application of three pharmacologic characteristics of these drugs. First, the intraspinal opiates have a ceiling effect beyond which further dosing increases the intensity of undesirable side effects without a comparable increase in analgesic efficacy. Second—and perhaps because of their site of action at complex relay networks with built-in time delays, the analgesia provided by the intraspinal opiates is more effective against steady ongoing pain than against the intermittent pain of labor in which stimulus-free periods alternate with intense crescendo pain involving sudden recruitment of large nociceptive neuronal pools. Third, undesirable maternal side effects are attributable to rostral spread in the neuraxis (114), whereas fetal side effects of respiratory depression are caused by excessive maternal vascular uptake and placental transfer.

The ceiling effect of intraspinal opiates is overcome by using mixtures of local anesthetics and opiates so that each class of drug complements the other. The precise anesthetic equivalence of opiate and local anesthetic remains to be determined. However, preliminary algesiometric observations with epidural bupivacaine and fentanyl suggest that a bolus dose of 100 μg of epidural fentanyl is approximately equivalent to the analgesic effect of 0.1% bupivacaine (115), and that an epidural infusion of 0.1% bupivacaine combined with 0.00015 to 0.0002% fentanyl provides a degree of analgesia that is approximately equivalent to 0.2% bupivacaine, without increasing the amount of motor block caused by 0.1% bupivacaine. The crescendo character of strong labor pain is effectively relieved by continuous epidural infusion of 0.065 to 0.1% bupivacaine when combined with 0.00015 to 0.0002% fentanyl at infusion rates of 7 to 15 ml/hr (54). Vascular uptake of both the opiate and local anesthetic is reduced by adding epinephrine in concentrations of 1/600,000 to 1/200,000 so that fetal transfer is discouraged and intraspinal blockade is prolonged (70, 17, 96, 20, 116).

During cesarean section, the intensity of analgesia and overall comfort are markedly improved by the addition of fentanyl or sufentanil to the subarachnoid or epidural anesthetic in the amounts shown in Table 6.6. Vascular absorption is reduced and duration is prolonged by using epinephrine in the mixture. As can be seen in Table 6.6, morphine is slow to produce satisfactory analgesia, but the prolonged duration provides approximately 75% pain relief for the moderate pain intensity of a lower abdominal incision. With this regimen most patients experience satisfactory analgesia for 18 to 24 hr and seldom require more supplementation than an oral nonsteroidal, anti-inflammatory agent, sometimes fortified with 30 to 60 mg of oral codeine. Respiratory competence is monitored by regular recording of the respiratory rate. In severely obese patients, pulse oximetry may be added as a further precaution against undetected delayed respiratory depression.

All adjuvants to sealed ampules or vials of local anesthetic imply some degree of added risk, because each time a substance is added to a local anesthetic there is a chance of error or bacterial contamination. Most adjuvants have more than one action, and obviously one of these must be clinically desirable for the substance to be considered at all. The other action may be neutral or even positively harmful and is to be avoided. For example, sodium bicarbonate may be required for pH adjustment to hasten the onset of blockade. With lidocaine the appropriate volume of 8.4% bicarbonate is 1 ml/10 ml 2% lidocaine, and this is a large enough amount to accommodate small volumetric errors. However, when added to bupivacaine, the volume is more critical and only 0.1 ml (10 times less) should be added to each 10 ml of 0.5% bupivacaine. A small excess of bicarbonate will lead to complete precipitation of the bupivacaine base, with possible adverse effects after injection (91).

Worse still, in a moment of stress or distraction, the anesthesiologist may pick up a look-alike ampule of some neurotoxic substance such as calcium chloride and inject that. Tragedies and near tragedies of this nature have included erroneous addition of hyperosmolar potassium chloride solutions, which in

Table 6.6
Intrathecal and Epidural Opiates as Adjuvants for Intraoperative and Postoperative Pain Relief in Cesarean Section

| Drug | Predelivery Dose | | Postdelivery Dose | | Onset (mins) | Duration with Epinephrine 1/200,000 (hr) |
	Subarachnoid (μg)	Epidural (μg)	Subarachnoid (μg)	Epidural (μg)		
Fentanyl	10–15	50–75	—	50–100	5–8	2–3
Sufentanil	5–10	20–30	—	30–50	5–8	5–7
Morphine	250–300	—	—	4000–5000	40–50	16–24

one case led to permanent paraplegia. In another infamous case, paraldehyde was injected, leading to permanent quadriplegia. The dismal list of such errors is long and should be viewed as a constant warning to label all adjuvants clearly and accurately and as a reminder of the fundamental medical injunction: "First do no harm."

SELECTION OF AGENTS AND CONCENTRATIONS FOR SPECIAL TASKS

Cesarean Section

Analgesic requirements for cesarean section are very different from those for vaginal delivery. First, active motor power is not required for expulsion of the fetus and profound muscle relaxation is also unnecessary since the abdominal muscles are well-stretched by the enlarged uterus. Second, analgesia must be profound in all lumbosacral segments including the resistant segments L5 and S1, which carry powerful nociceptive input during manipulation of the uterus and repair of the uterine incision. In contemporary North American obstetric practice this nociceptive input and the incidence of pain and nausea are heightened by the widely adopted maneuver of eventrating the uterus for uterine repair (86, 117, 118). In European practice, most uterine repairs are done less traumatically by the older technique of repair in situ, but even then, partial rotation of the uterus on its long axis may generate an appreciable incidence of pain if the L5 and S1 segments are not well anesthetized. Third, segmental analgesia must extend higher than the sixth thoracic dermatome which, on theoretic grounds, should be sufficient to interrupt all afferent impulses from the lower abdomen. Clinical experience shows that, contrary to theoretic expectations, analgesia is often inadequate unless blockade extends to include T4 or even to the apex of the axilla (i.e., T3) (119).

These clinical goals must be achieved by techniques and agents that provide profound and extensive segmental blockade without causing fetal depression. Subarachnoid and lumbar epidural blockade are the only two feasible techniques for the task. Caudal anesthesia requires excessively large amounts of local anesthetic, and it is not recommended for cesarean section.

SUBARACHNOID BLOCKADE

Subarachnoid block is favored by many as the technique of choice for cesarean section. It has great aesthetic appeal because intense and extensive analgesia is obtained from a tiny dose of local anesthetic and blood concentrations of local anesthetic never reach a level that could possibly have any depressant effect on the fetus. Moreover, the technique has the

virtue of speed. The block can be performed and an anesthetic level to T3 established in 5 to 10 min, whereas a carefully titrated epidural anesthetic will take 30 to 40 min to reach the same segmental level. Even then, proprioceptive sensation as measured by a tuning fork may still persist in segments L5 and S1. Weighed against the advantage of speed is the unpredictability of segmental analgesic spread. None of the traditional indices of anesthetic dose, such as height, spinal length, body weight, or ponderal index, exerts any degree of statistic power for predicting segmental analgesic spread in parturient patients (120). In one recent study of 52 cesarean sections, upper segmental levels of analgesia varied between T6 (in two patients) and C2 (in four patients) with a median at T2–T3 following a fixed dose of 15 mg of hyperbaric bupivacaine with 0.15 mg of morphine sulphate (120).

The great rapidity of sympathetic blockade is prone to cause precipitous changes of cardiovascular dynamics. As a result, the incidence of arterial hypotension is high and corrective vasopressor treatment is often needed, even when prophylactic measures of acute intravenous prehydration with 2 liters of crystalloid are taken, together with left uterine displacement (121).

Attempts to resolve the dilemma between hypotension and inadequate blockade, by the "two-needle technique" of combined subarachnoid puncture and epidural catheter placement has only partially solved the problem, since speed and technical simplicity are sacrificed to accuracy and risk factors are increased by combining the potential, although very remote, hazards of both methods. The two-needle technique is discussed more fully in Chapter 12. Here, discussion will be confined to the appropriate drugs for either subarachnoid or epidural block, but not when the two are combined together.

Subarachnoid and epidural blockade spreads further in obstetric patients than in the normal population, and most recommended dose schedules for subarachnoid anesthesia in cesarean section tend to err on the low side for safety's sake. The reader should be aware that, in following the dose schedules in this chapter, a small proportion of inadequate blocks may be encountered in which the upper level of spinal analgesia fails to reach as high as T6. For this reason, many anesthesiologists prefer to adopt a fixed volume routine for the majority of obstetric patients of average height and weight. For example, 60 to 75 mg of hyperbaric 5% lidocaine (i.e., 1.2 to 1.5 ml) administered in the sitting position at L3–4 will produce a reliable upper segmental level analgesia in the range of T4–C8. Similarly, 11.25 to 15 mg of hyperbaric 0.75% bupivacaine (i.e., 1.5 to 2 ml) will produce the same range of anesthesia in most patients. Table 6.7 outlines the generally accepted dose requirements for cesarean section under subarachnoid block.

Because spinal analgesia is of relatively short duration and segmental predictability is uncertain, intrathecal opiates have become almost routine additives in an effort to circumvent those shortcomings. Preservative-free morphine in a small dose of 0.1 to 0.25 mg is added to provide 16 to 24 hr of postoperative analgesia without respiratory depression (122). The quality of intraoperative analgesia is augmented by combining a short-acting lipophilic agent such as fentanyl (10 to 25 μg) or sufentanil (5 to 10 μg) with the intrathecal morphine. In doing so the total volume of the injectate is increased by a significant amount. For example, if 70 mg of hyperbaric 5% lidocaine (1.4 ml) with epinephrine 0.2 mg (0.2 ml) is chosen as the main anesthetic agent, the further addition of 0.3 mg of preservative-free morphine (Duramorph) and 15 μg of fentanyl will raise the total volume by 57% to 2.2 ml. To date, studies have not indicated whether such volume expansion causes more extensive segmental spread than usual. However, experience with other agents suggests that this is unlikely, since it is the mass of the intrathecal drug administered, rather than merely the volume, that determines segmental spread.

However, there have been anecdotal reports of delayed segmental spread with this type of polypharmacy (123, 124). Regression of cervical blockade was rapid in these few cases, and no adverse events arose. The pattern is dramatic enough to command close attention to the analgesia level, and to require that all appropriate resuscitative equipment and drugs are ready for immediate use. Provided these precautions are taken, the risks are no greater than in any routine spinal anesthetic and are more than justified by the superb quality of analgesia achieved. However, since the possibility of residual rostral spread of intrathecal fentanyl and morphine with extended respiratory depression cannot be excluded, these patients should be carefully monitored as described in Chapter 10.

EPIDURAL ANALGESIA

Unlike subarachnoid block, epidural analgesia requires dosages large enough to cause appreciable transfer of local anesthetic agents across the placenta, with the resulting possibility of fetal depression. Blockade, however, has a slower onset, and the maternal cardiovascular system is more readily controlled than in the precipitous onset of subarachnoid block. Moreover, when a continuous catheter technique is used, dosage can be titrated to achieve a more precise segmental level, and an inadequate initial level can be raised by injecting a small supplementary dose.

As with spinal anesthesia for cesarean section, narcotics have become standard adjuvants to improve the intraoperative quality of epidural analgesia and to prolong postoperative analgesia. However the narcotic doses required by the epidural route are five to ten times greater than when injected directly into the intrathecal space. Thus careful consideration must be given to minimizing maternal vascular uptake and placental transfer to the fetus. The following protocol is recommended:

1. Choose a rapid onset, short-acting lipophilic agent such as fentanyl in a small dose of 50 μg for intraoperative analgesia before birth of the baby.
2. Give the fentanyl time to work (i.e., 6 to 7 min before incision).
3. Give the fentanyl 5 to 10 minutes *after* the full dose of epidural local anesthetic has been administered with 1/300,000 to 1/200,000 epinephrine and after sufficient time has elapsed for epidural and dural vasoconstriction to occur to reduce maternal vascular uptake and obtain the maximum segmental analgesic effect (96). Under these circumstances, prior dilution of the fentanyl is unnecessary and it can be given as an undiluted bolus with full confidence that effective segmental analgesic augmentation will occur within 6½ to 7 min (115).
4. After the infant has been delivered and the cord clamped, administer a second bolus of 50 μg of epidural fentanyl to augment intraoperative comfort, followed by 4 mg of preservative-free morphine to provide prolonged postoperative pain relief.

Table 6.7
Subarachnoid Block for Cesarean Section, Dose Requirements

Drug	Dose (mg)	Predicted Spread[a]	Duration (hr)[b]
Tetracaine	7–10	T7–T5	2.5–3.0
Lidocaine	60–75	T7–C8	1.5–2.0
Bupivacaine	11.25–15	T5–C8	3.0–3.5

[a] Average and range.
[b] With 0.2 ml of 1:1000 epinephrine.

5. Write pain management nursing instructions for 24-hr postoperative respiratory surveillance of the mother.

At the present time, the choice of an anesthetic agent for epidural blockade is restricted to three or four drugs that stand out as superior for the special requirements of pain relief and safety in cesarean section. These are lidocaine, bupivacaine, and chloroprocaine. While etidocaine provides intense and prolonged motor and sensory blockade, it is not considered ideal for cesarean section for the reasons already discussed. Currently, ropivacaine awaits formal evaluation in an obstetric setting. Available evidence suggests that ropivacaine will prove ideal for obstetric use and that it will be high on the list of available choices for cesarean section. Regardless of which drug is chosen, the key to successful epidural analgesia is *time*. Enough time must be allowed for diffusion to occur from the epidural space, across the dura, and into the spinal roots and cord. Between 25 and 40 min is required for this to take place and to ensure solid analgesia, especially in segments L5 and S1. In a hurried milieu a high incidence of intraoperative pain or discomfort must be expected if the operating team does not appreciate and abide by this inherent constraint of epidural blockade.

CHLOROPROCAINE

In spite of the rapid potency and very low toxicity of chloroprocaine, the two major disadvantages of potential backache and interference with the analgesic efficacy of other adjuvants have relegated chloroprocaine to a relatively narrow role in obstetric analgesia (13–17, 21). However, there are two specific situations where chloroprocaine can prove valuable. First, the "chloroprocaine save" can salvage inadequate epidural anesthetics when it is believed that the catheter is lodged within the epidural space, but blockade fails to extend to an adequate segmental level after a maximum safe dose of amide local anesthetic has been administered. Supplementary doses of 11 to 24 ml of chloroprocaine may be sufficient to achieve a satisfactory surgical level of anesthesia (125). Second, the onset of analgesia with 3% chloroprocaine is fast enough to substitute for subarachnoid analgesia in many cases where fast low-spinal anesthesia is required for instrumental delivery, retained placenta, or extensive perineal repair. A low-lumbar epidural injection of 12 to 15 ml of 3% chloroprocaine will provide analgesia up to the umbilicus, or a caudal injection of 12 to 15 ml will provide sacral analgesia for perineal repair within 10 min or so. Obviously, a routine test dose must be used to exclude inadvertent massive subarachnoid injection, but the danger of systemic toxicity is extremely low because of the rapid breakdown of chloroprocaine by plasma pseudocholinsterase.

LIDOCAINE

For more than 45 years the most reliable agent for epidural anesthesia has been 2% lidocaine. For most cesarean sections, a total of 20 to 25 ml of 2% lidocaine in incremental doses will be needed to raise the upper segmental level of analgesia to the third or fourth thoracic segments. Epinephrine 1/200,000 should be added to reduce vascular absorption, since the large volume of lidocaine approaches the maximum recommended dose. Segmental analgesic efficacy and maternal comfort, without fetal depression, are increased by adding a small bolus of lipid-soluble opioid, such as fentanyl (50 μg) or sufentanil (30 μg) through the epidural catheter about 4 to 5 min *after* the lidocaine and epinephrine dose has been completed. In this way there is no need to add any diluent volume to the fentanyl, and the bolus of fentanyl takes effect within 5 to 7 min (115).

After delivery of the infant, epidural morphine (4 to 5 mg) may be given via the epidural catheter for prolonged postoperative analgesia.

BUPIVACAINE

Because low concentrations of bupivacaine (about 0.25%) do not give adequate surgical anesthesia, it is necessary to use a 0.5% solution in volumes of 17 to 25 ml (i.e., 85 to 125 mg of bupivacaine) to obtain satisfactory analgesia for cesarean section. However, as pointed out earlier, the onset of analgesia with 0.5% bupivacaine is very slow and 30 min may be required for adequate blockade to set in. Bupivacaine 0.75% became very popular as a single-shot agent for cesarean section because of its faster onset, greater intensity of blockade, and excellent neonatal outcome (126, 127). However, the high incidence of prolonged motor blockade of the legs and the subsequent risk of deep vein thrombosis was an undesirable feature. A more sinister objection arose from a number of cases of toxic reactions and recalcitrant cardiac arrest that occurred during induction of epidural blockade for cesarean section with the 0.75% solution. These have led to consensus that the 0.75% concentration is unsafe for obstetric anesthesia (57). In fairness, it must be pointed out that all of these cases of cardiac arrest occurred in women who were positioned on their backs for resuscitative purposes when toxic convulsions began, and it is probable that intractable cardiac arrest may have been due to the double and ironic iatrogenic insult of unrelieved aortic caval compression combined with the accidental intravenous injection of a potent and toxic local anesthetic. These cases highlight the essential need for constant vigilance to ensure safe maternal posture and uterine displacement at all times.

Motor block, but not sensory block from epidural bupivacaine, is enhanced by epinephrine (100). Nevertheless, if fentanyl or sufentanil are used as epidural adjuvants, the prior epidural injection of epinephrine will slow vascular absorption of the opiate and enhance analgesia as outlined above.

Bupivacaine is appreciably slower to establish an effective block than lidocaine, and 45 min or longer may be needed to achieve analgesia at S1, unless an epidural infusion has already been instituted for trial of labor. The duration of blockade is significantly longer than with lidocaine, and the patient may not be able to move her legs for 3 to 4 hr after returning to the recovery room—a contribution to venous stasis that may increase the hazard of deep vein thrombosis.

Vaginal Delivery

As set out at the beginning of this chapter, the analgesic requirements for vaginal delivery are quite clear-cut. Analgesia must be effective, controllable, and safe, and there should be no depression of the three Ps—that is, the powers of labor; the tone of the birth passage, or the infant, the passenger traveling through those passages. Effective analgesia must not be purchased at the expense of excessive dosage and consequent fetal depression. The art of choice lies in compromise and in choosing the least dose that will do the job. This implies rather close supervision of the patient to ensure that the delicate balance between effective analgesia and fetal depression does not tip one way or the other. The agents currently available are good, and failure to maintain the right balance is usually due to failure of supervision rather than to shortcomings of the drugs.

SUBARACHNOID BLOCKADE

Subarachnoid blockade has a very limited role to play in labor and vaginal delivery. It is usually a last-minute analgesic maneuver for delivery when circumstances have made continuous epidural blockade impossible or inappropriate. Subarachnoid analgesia produces intense motor block within the seg-

mental distribution of its influence. This property is desirable if forceps delivery is planned. However, if spontaneous delivery is desired, the block will violate two of the five desiderata for ideal analgesic conditions in labor set out at the beginning of this chapter. First, the muscular integrity of the birth passages is disturbed, because the pelvic floor is rendered atonic and patulous by blockade of the sacral segments. Second, the expulsive powers are diminished if blockade rises to affect the abdominal segments.

The choice of agents for spinal analgesia in labor and delivery depends to a great degree on when the block is induced. A long-lasting agent such as bupivacaine or tetracaine is indicated if spinal block is started before the cervix is fully dilated. A shorter acting agent such as lidocaine is indicated for a short period of perineal analgesia after the cervix is fully dilated and when delivery is imminent. Table 6.8 outlines the agents and doses that are suitable and their approximate duration of action.

CONTINUOUS EPIDURAL ANALGESIA

When properly administered, continuous epidural analgesia is the only technique that can offer quiet and gentle progress through all the painful stages of labor and delivery without undue risk and without the need for systemic analgesics. Introduction of intraspinal narcotics into clinical practice has added an enormously useful dimension to epidural analgesia for management of pain in labor.

LIDOCAINE

Before the introduction of bupivacaine for obstetrics, lidocaine was the standard agent for prolonged epidural analgesia in labor. At that time, the provision of effective pain relief was the principal aim, and in most units relatively little attention was paid to the maintenance of motor power and tone in the muscles of the birth canal. Moreover, infusion devices were primitive and imprecise (128); thus intermittent bolus doses of 1% lidocaine were customary. After the introduction of bupivacaine into obstetrics, it became clear that bupivacaine provided a more favorable ratio of sensory to motor block (129),

Table 6.8
Choice of Analgesic Agent for Subarachnoid Analgesia in Vaginal Delivery

Stage of Labor	Segments to be Anesthetized	Agent	Dose (mg)	Duration with Epinephrine Wash (hr)
Late first stage	T10–S5	Tetracaine	5–6	2.5
Second stage	T10–S5	Tetracaine	4–6	2.5
	T10–S5	Lidocaine	30–40	1.5
"Saddle block"	S1–S5	Tetracaine	3	2.5
	S1–S5	Lidocaine	25–30	1.5

and careful studies of maternal-to-fetal transfer showed that the fetal accumulation of the maternal dose was 2.8 times higher for lidocaine than for bupivacaine (130, 131).

Published studies of continuous lidocaine infusions for labor have not been uniformly enthusiastic. The few reports that exist used concentrations of 0.4 to 0.75% (128–135). The advantage claimed for lidocaine was less fetal heart disturbances than with bupivacaine (134), but this was achieved at the expense of less reliable perineal analgesia than with bupivacaine (135). Lidocaine-opioid mixtures for labor infusions have not been formally evaluated. Personal unpublished data using 0.3% lidocaine (32 to 45 mg) for an induction-test dose, followed by a 0.175% infusion with 0.000175% fentanyl and 0.000175% epinephrine has demonstrated good first-stage analgesia at infusion rates of 9 to 14 ml/hr and a mean consumption rate of 21 mg of lidocaine per hour (Table 6.9). Chestnut's findings of poor perineal spread with 0.75% lidocaine have been confirmed with the 0.175% lidocaine-fentanyl mixture, together with a greater tendency for the block to lateralize under the influence of gravity than bupivacaine, making it necessary to turn the patient every 20 to 30 min to ensure a bilaterally symmetric block.

In summary, current assessments of dilute lidocaine-opioid infusions for labor suggest:

1. In spite of a higher maternal-fetal transfer ratio, lidocaine appears to be less cardiotoxic to the fetus than bupivacaine, an advantage that is expected to be shared by ropivacaine (83–85).

2. Satisfactory analgesia is provided for first-stage labor and for second-stage spontaneous labor, but perineal analgesia is inadequate for forceps delivery.

3. There is a need for closer personal supervision of infusion rates and patient posture than with bupivacaine-opioid mixtures—a disadvantage that is likely to make the choice of lidocaine unpopular in those obstetric units where anesthesia coverage is marginally adequate.

These findings with dilute lidocaine-opioid mixtures may prove helpful in clarifying the hierarchic status of ropivacaine when its turn comes for evaluation as a preferred agent for pain relief in labor.

Bupivacaine in Labor

Bupivacaine has earned a place as the most reliable and least offensive amide local anesthetic for epidural analgesia in labor and delivery. Scanlon and his associates (33) used neurobehavior tests to assess the effect of absorbed bupivacaine on the newborn after 3 hr of maternal epidural analgesia with a rather high cumulative maternal dose of 112 mg of bupivacaine. They found that umbilical vein concentrations of 110 ± 20 ng/ml at delivery were apparently innocuous to the infant. Based on the evidence available, it seems extremely unlikely that these very low concentrations of local anesthetic can have any immediate or long-term adverse effects on the infant.

Early studies with bupivacaine for relief of pain in labor were marred by the use of excessive concentrations for the required task. Solutions of 0.5% and 0.25% bupivacaine provided excellent relief of pain, but at the cost of prolonged labors from excessive relaxation of the muscles of the pelvic floor. The pioneering clinical studies of Van Steenberge and his colleagues in 1974 were required to reevaluate the idea that a powerful induction dose was needed to establish an intense segmental blockade that could be allowed to continue throughout labor. A concentration of 0.125% bupivacaine with 1/800,000 epinephrine was shown to be adequate for an acceptable degree of comfort, while retaining sufficient tone in the pelvic muscles to steer the presenting fetal part along a smooth course through the birth passage (51–53).

Table 6.9
Lidocaine-Fentanyl Regimen for Epidural Analgesia in Labor

Induction	
Solution	5 ml of 1.5% lidocaine + 1/200,000 epinephrine diluted to 25 ml with normal saline (i.e., 0.3% lidocaine + 1/10^6 epinephrine)
Induction Dose	6 ml + 6 ml = 36 mg of lidocaine

Maintenance Infusion			
Normal saline 100 ml *plus*:		Final dilution	
2% lidocaine, 10 ml (200 mg)	=	1.75 mg/ml	
Fentanyl, 4 ml (200 μg)	=	1.75 mcg/ml	
Epinephrine, 0.2 (200 μg)	=	1.75 mcg/ml	
Epidural Infusion Rate			
8–14 ml/hr			

Turn patient every 30 min; check segmental levels (upper and lower) hourly

Since the advent of epidural narcotics for labor in the early 1980s, an empirical search has continued for the optimal mixture of bupivacaine and opioid to provide the best compromise of maternal comfort with the least depression of the fetus or the muscular powers of parturition. To date, 0.0625% bupivacaine with 0.0002% fentanyl appears to be one of the most popular epidural infusions, in terms of ease of management and good outcome (54). However, these concentrations of bupivacaine and fentanyl do carry a higher toxicity potential than the lidocaine-fentanyl mixture described above.

CONCLUSION

The agents available for obstetric regional anesthesia have undergone intense reevaluation in the past few years with significant improvements in the quality and safety of analgesia and the management of difficult labor. Part of this reevaluation stems from increased knowledge of the drugs themselves, but an important part of how we use these drugs today has arisen from technical developments in the way they can be delivered more safely and effectively to their target sites.

With the possible exception of chloroprocaine, coadministration of two or more analgesic agents with widely different target sites has superseded the traditional view that, in obstetric practice, local anesthetics are safest and best when given alone for major spinal blockade. Opiate adjuvants have played, and continue to play, a major role in this change of outlook. Currently, opiates of high and low lipophilicity are almost routine additives for intrathecal and epidural administration, although the practice still lacks official FDA approval. Fear of epinephrine as an appropriate adjuvant in both subarachnoid and epidural anesthesia has been put in a more correct perspective, and epinephrine's intrinsic contribution to the total analgesic picture as an α-agonist has been acknowledged.

α_2-adrenoreceptor agonists are under intense investigation as adjuvants for relief of pain. However, at present clonidine, the only α-2-agonist that has been widely studied in humans, remains unacceptable for obstetric use because of its side effects of vascular hypotension and sedation (136). But other α-2-agonists are being tested, and in due course we may expect to see some members of this class (with the side effects eliminated) that may prove appropriate as another factor in the choice of local anesthetic.

References

1. Ready LB, Cuplin S, Hascke RH, Nesly M: Spinal needle determinants of rate of transdural fluid leak. *Anesth Analg* 69:457–460, 1989.
2. Flaaten H: Postdural puncture headache: A comparison between 26- and 29-gauge needles in young patients. Anaesthesia 44:147–149, 1989.
3. Cesarini M, Torrielli R, Lahaye F, Mene JM, Cabiro C: Sprotte needle for intrathecal anaesthesia for caesarean section: Incidence of postdural puncture headache. Anaesthesia 45:656–658, 1990.
4. Sears DH, Leeman MI, O'Donnell RH, Kelleher JF, Santos GC: Incidence of postdural puncture headache in cesarean section patients using the 24-G Sprotte needle. Anesthesiology 73:A1003, 1990.
5. Ross BK, Chadwick HS, Mancusco JJ, Benedetti C: Incidence of postdural puncture headache in the obstetric patient: Sprotte vs Quincke tip needle. In *Abstracts of Scientific Papers.* Society for Obstetric Anesthesia and Perinatology, Madison, WS, 1990, p E-31.
6. Usubiaga JE, La Iuppa M, Moya F, Wikinski JA, Velazco R: Passage of procaine hydrochloride and para-aminobenzoic acid across the human placenta. Am J Obstet Gynecol 100:918–923, 1968.
7. de Jong RH: *Physiology and Pharmacology of Local Anesthesia,* 2nd ed. Charles C Thomas, Springfield, IL, 1977, pp 224–230.
8. Covino BG, Marx GF, Finster M, Zsigmond EK: Prolonged sensory/motor deficits following inadvertent spinal anesthesia. Anesth Analg 59:399–400, 1980.
9. Ravindran RS, Bond VK, Tasch MD, Gupta CD, Luerssen TG: Prolonged neural blockade following regional analgesia with 2-chloroprocaine. Anesth Analg 59:447–451, 1980.
10. Reisner LS, Hochman BN, Plumer MH: Persistent neurologic deficit and adhesive arachnoiditis following intrathecal 2-chloroprocaine injection. Anesth Analg 59:452–454, 1980.
11. Barsa J, Batra M, Fink BR, Sumi SM: A comparative in vivo study of local neurotoxicity of lidocaine, bupivacaine, 2-chloroprocaine and a mixture of 2-chloroprocaine and bupivacaine. Anesth Analg 61:561–567, 1982.
12. Gissen AJ, Datta S, Lambert D: The chloroprocaine controversy. II. Is chloroprocaine neurotoxic? Reg Anesth 9:135–145, 1984.
13. Fibuch EE, Opper SE: Back pain following epidurally administered nesacaine-MFP. Anesth Analg 69:113–115, 1989.
14. McLoughlin TM, DiFazio CA: More on back pain after nesacaine-MFP. Anesth Analg 71:562–563, 1990.
15. Hynson JM, Sessler DI, Glosten B: Back pain in volunteers after epidural anesthesia with chloroprocaine. Anesth Analg 72:253–256, 1991.
16. Stevens RA, Artuso JD, Kao TC, Bray JC, Spitzer L, Louwsma DL: Changes in human plasma catecholamine concentrations during epidural analgesia depend on the level of block. Anesthesiology 74:1029–1034, 1991.
17. Hodgkinson R, Husain FJ, Bluhm C: Reduced effectiveness of bupivacaine 0.5% to relieve labor pain after prior injection of chloroprocaine 2%. Anesthesiology 57:A201, 1982.
18. Kotelko DM, Thigpen JW, Shnider SM, Foutz SE, Rosen MA, Hughes SC: Postoperative epidural morphine analgesia after various local anesthetics. Anesthesiology 59:A413, 1983.
19. Corke BC, Carlson CG, Dettbarn WD: The influence of 2-chloroprocaine on the subsequent analgesic potency of bupivacaine. Anesthesiology 60:25–27, 1984.
20. Grice SC, Eisenach JC, Dewan DM: Labor analgesia with epidural bupivacaine plus fentanyl: Enhancement with epinephrine and inhibition with 2-chloroprocaine. Anesthesiology 72:623–628, 1990.
21. Camann WR, Hartigan PM, Gilbertson LI, Johnson M, Datta S: Chloroprocaine antagonism of epidural opioid analgesia: A receptor-specific phenomenon? Anesthesiology 73:860–863, 1990.
22. Bromage PR: A comparison of bupivacaine and tetracaine in epidural analgesia for surgery. Can Anaesth Soc J 16:37–45, 1969.
23. Tucker GT, Boyes RN, Bridenbaugh PO, Moore DC: Binding of anilide-type local anesthetics in human plasma. I. Relationships between binding, physicochemical properties, and anesthetic activity. Anesthesiology 33:287–303, 1970.

24. Tucker GT, Boyes RN, Bridenbaugh PO, Moore DC: Binding of anilide-type local anesthetics in human plasma. II. Implications in vivo, with special reference to transplacental distribution. Anesthesiology 33:304–314, 1970.

25. Morishima HO, Daniel SS, Finster M, Poppers PJ, James S: Transmission of mepivacaine hydrochloride (Carbocaine) across the human placenta. Anesthesiology 27:147–154, 1966.

26. Scanlon JW, Brown WU, Weiss JB, Alper MH: Neurobehavioral responses of newborn infants after maternal epidural anesthesia. Anesthesiology 40:121–128, 1974.

27. Brown WU Jr, Bell GC, Jurie AO, Weiss JB, Scanlon JW, Alper MH: Newborn blood levels of lidocaine and mepivacaine in the first postnatal day following maternal epidural anesthesia. Anesthesiology 42:698–707, 1975.

28. Fujimori M, Nishimura K: Methemoglobinemia due to local anesthetics (a preliminary report). Far East J Anaesth 4:4, 1964.

29. Lund PC, Cwik JC: Propitocaine (Citanest®) and methemoglobinemia. Anesthesiology 26:569–571, 1965.

30. Scott DB: Citanest® and methemoglobinemia: Discussion. In Citanest. S Wiedling, ed. Universitetsforlaget I Aarhus, Copenhagen, 1965, p 199.

31. Shnider SM, Way EL: Plasma levels of lidocaine (Xylocaine) in mother and newborn following obstetrical conduction anesthesia: Clinical applications. Anesthesiology 29:951–958, 1968.

32. Fox GS, Houle GL: Transmission of lidocaine hydrochloride across the placenta during cesarean section. Can Anaesth Soc J 16:135–143, 1969.

33. Scanlon JW, Ostheimer GW, Lurie AO, Brown WU, Weiss JB, Alper MH: Neurobehavioral responses and drug concentrations in newborns after maternal epidural anesthesia with bupivacaine. Anesthesiology 45:400–405, 1976.

34. Brown WU: Neonatal neurobehavioral tests following vaginal delivery under ketamine, thiopental, and extradural anesthesia: Guest discussion. Anesth Analg 56:548–553, 1977.

35. Higuchi M, Takeuchi S: Studies on the neurobehavioral response (Scanlon test) in newborns after epidural anesthesia with various anesthetic agents for cesarean section. Acta Obstet Gynecol Jpn 4:2143–2148, 1982.

36. Abboud TK, Khoo SS, Miller F, Doan T, Henriksen EH: Maternal, fetal and neonatal responses after epidural anesthesia with bupivacaine, 2-chloroprocaine or lidocaine, Anesth Analg 61:638–644, 1982.

37. Abboud TK, Sarkis F, Blikian A, Varakian L: Lack of adverse neurobehavioral effects of lidocaine. Anesthesiology 57:A404, 1982.

38. Abboud TK, Kyung CK, Noueihid R, Kuhnert BK, DerMardirossian N, Moumdijan J, Sarkis F, Nagappala S: Epidural bupivacaine, chloroprocaine or lidocaine for cesarean section: Maternal and neonatal effects. Anesth Analg 62:914–919, 1983.

39. Abboud TK, Afrasiabi A, Sarkis F, Daftarian F, Nagappala S, Noueihid R, Kuhnert BR, Miller F: Continuous infusion epidural analgesia in parturients receiving bupivacaine, chloroprocaine, or lidocaine: Maternal, fetal and neonatal effects. Anesth Analg 63:421–428, 1984.

40. Kileff ME, James FM III, Dewan DM, Floyd HM: Neonatal neurobehavioral responses after epidural anesthesia for cesarean section using lidocaine and bupivacaine. Anesth Analg 63:413–417, 1984.

41. Kuhnert BR, Harrison MJ, Linn PL, Kuhnert PM: Effect of maternal epidural anesthesia on neonatal behavior. Anesth Analg 63:301–308, 1984.

42. Bromage PR: A comparison of the hydrochloride salts of lidocaine and prilocaine for epidural analgesia. Br J Anaesth 37:753–761, 1965.

43. Bromage PR: Improved conduction blockade in surgery and obstetrics: Carbonated local anaesthetic solutions. Can Med Assoc J 97:1377–1384, 1967.

44. Bromage PR, Burfoot MF, Crowell DE, Truant AP: Quality of epidural blockade. III. Carbonated local anaesthetic solutions. Br J Anaesth 39:197–209, 1967.

45. Morison DH: A double-blind comparison of carbonated lidocaine and lidocaine hydrochloride in epidural anaesthesia. Can Anaesth Soc J 28:387–389, 1981.

46. Martin R, Lamarche Y, Tetreault L: Comparison of clinical effectiveness of lidocaine hydrocarbonate and lidocaine hydrochloride with and without epinephrine in epidural anaesthesia. Can Anaesth Soc J 28:224–227, 1981.

47. Cole CP, McMorland GH, Axelson JE: Evaluation of epidural blockade comparing lidocaine hydrocarbonate and lidocaine hydrochloride for caesarean section. Anesthesiology 59:A411, 1983.

48. Nickel PM, Bromage PR, Sherrill DR: Comparison of hydrochloride and carbonated salts of lidocaine for epidural analgesia. Reg Anesth 11:62–67, 1986.

49. Sukani R, Winnie AP: Clinical pharmacokinetics of carbonated local anesthetics. I. Subclavian perivascular brachial block model. Anesthesiology 66:739–745, 1987.

50. Telivus L: A new long-acting local anaesthetic for pain relief after thoracotomy. Ann Chir Gynaecol Fenn 52:513, 1963.

51. Geerinckx K, Vanderick G, Van Steenberge AL, Bouche R, De Muylder E: Bupivacaine 0.125% in epidural block analgesia during childbirth: Maternal and foetal plasma concentrations. Br J Anaesth 46:937–941, 1974.

52. Bleyaert A, Soetens M, Vaes L, Van Steenberge AL, Van Der Donck A: Bupivacaine 0.125% in obstetric epidural analgesia: Experience in three thousand cases. Anesthesiology 51:435–438, 1979.

53. Van Zundert A, Vaes L, Soetens M, De Vel M, Van Der AA, Van Der Donck A, Meeuwis H, De Wolf A: Every dose given in epidural analgesia for vaginal delivery can be a test dose. Anesthesiology 67:436–440, 1987.

54. Chestnut DH, Owen CL, Bates JN, Ostman LG, Choi WW, Geiger MW: Continuous infusion epidural analgesia during labor: A randomized, double-blind comparison of 0.0625% bupivacaine, 0.0002% fentanyl versus 0.125% bupivacaine. Anesthesiology 68:754–759, 1988.

55. Chestnut DH, Laszewski LJ, Pollack KL, Bates JN, Manago NK, Choi WW: Continuous epidural infusion of 0.0625% bupivacaine, 0.0002% fentanyl during the second stage of labor. Anesthesiology 72:613–618, 1990.

56. Bromage PR: A comparison of bupivacaine and tetracaine in epidural analgesia for surgery. Can Anaesth Soc J 16:37–45, 1969.

57. Albright GA: Cardiac arrest following regional anesthesia with etidocaine or bupivacaine. Anesthesiology 51:285–287, 1979.

58. Komai H, Rusy BF: Hyperkalemia and bupivacaine block of AV conduction. Anesthesiology 53:S210, 1980.

59. Loechning RW, Tanz RD: Bupivacaine is more cardiotoxic than lidocaine. Anesthesiology 55:A165, 1981.

60. Block A, Covino BG. Effect of local anesthetic agents on cardiac conduction and contractility. Reg Anesth 6:55–61, 1981.

61. Sage DJ, Feldman HS, Arthur GR, Datta S, Ferretti AM, Norway SB, Covino BG: Influence of lidocaine and bupivacaine on isolated guinea pig atria in the presence of acidosis and hypoxia. Anesth Analg 63:1–7, 1984.

62. de Jong RH, Bonin JD: Deaths from local anesthetic-induced convulsions in mice. Anesth Analg 59:401–405, 1980.

63. de Jong RH, Ronfeld RA, de Rosa RA: Cardiovascular effects of convulsant and supraconvulsant doses of amide local anesthetics. Anesth Analg 61:3–9, 1982.

64. Liu P, Feldman HS, Covino BM, Giasi R, Covino BG: Acute cardiovascular toxicity of intravenous amide local anesthetics in anesthetized ventilated dogs. Anesth Analg 61:317–322, 1982.

65. Kotelko DM, Shnider SM, Dailey PA, Brizgys RV, Levinson G, Shapiro WA, Koike M, Rosen MA: Bupivacaine-induced cardiac arrhythmias in sheep. Anesthesiology 60:10–18, 1984.

66. Rosen MA, Thigpen JW, Shnider SM, Foutz SE, Levinson G, Koike M: Bupivacaine-induced cardiotoxicity in hypoxic and acidotic sheep. Anesth Analg 64:1089–1096, 1985.

67. Liu PL, Feldman HS, Giasi R, Patterson MK, Covino BG:

Comparative CNS toxicity of lidocaine, etidocaine, bupivacaine, and tetracaine in awake dogs following rapid intravenous administration. Anesth Analg 62:375–379, 1983.

68. Sage DJ, Feldman HS, Arthur GR, Doucette AM, Norway SB, Covino BG: The cardiovascular effects of convulsant doses of lidocaine and bupivacaine in the conscious dog. Reg Anesth 10:175–183, 1985.

69. Munson ES, Tucker WK, Ausinsch B, Malagodi MH: Etidocaine, bupivacaine and lidocaine seizure thresholds in monkeys. Anesthesiology 42:471–478, 1975.

70. Eisler EA, Thigpen JW, Shnider SM, Halpern SH, Brookshire GL, Levinson G, Johnson J, Jones MJ: Bupivacaine cardiotoxicity in normal and acidotic rabbits. Anesthesiology 61:A233, 1984.

71. Clarkson CW, Hondeghem LM: Mechanism for bupivacaine depression of cardiac conduction: Fast block of sodium channels during the action potential with slow recovery from block during diastole. Anesthesiology 62:396–405, 1985.

72. Courtney KR: Relationship between excitability block and negative inotropic actions of antiarrhythmic drugs. Proc West Pharmacol Soc 27:181–184, 1984.

73. Eisler EA, Baker W, Shnider SM, Halpern SH, Levinson G, Dailey PA, Hughes SC, Rosen MA, Johnson J, Jones MJ: The lethal dose of intravenous bupivacaine in pregnant and nonpregnant rabbits. In *Abstracts of Scientific Papers*. Society for Obstetric Anesthesia and Perinatology, Washington, DC, 1985, p 92.

74. Morishima HO, Pedersen H, Finster M, Hiraoka H, Tsuji A, Feldman HS, Arthur GR, Covino BG: Bupivacaine toxicity in pregnant and nonpregnant ewes. Anesthesiology 63:134–139, 1985.

75. Crandell JT, Kotelko DM: Cardiotoxicity of local anesthetics during late pregnancy. Anesth Analg 64:S204, 1985.

76. Cusick JF, Myklebust JB, Abram SE: Differential neural effects of epidural anesthetics. Anesthesiology 53:299–306, 1980.

77. Gissen A, Covino BG, Gregus J: Differential sensitivity of fast and slow fibers in mammalian nerve. III. Effect of etidocaine and bupivacaine on fast/slow fibers. Anesth Analg 61:570–575, 1982.

78. Dahl JB, Rosenberg J, Lund C, Kehlet H: Effect of thoracic epidural bupivacaine 0.75% on somatosensory evoked potentials after dermatomal stimulation. Reg Anesth 15:73–75, 1990.

79. Lund C, Hansen OB, Kehlet H, Mogensen T, Qvitzau S: Effects of etidocaine administered epidurally on changes in somatosensory evoked potentials after dermatomal stimulation. Reg Anesth 16:38–42, 1991.

80. Bromage PR, Datta S, Dunford LA: Etidocaine: An evaluation in epidural analgesia for obstetrics. Can Anaesth Soc J 21:535–545, 1974.

81. Covino BG, Vassallo HG: Chemical aspects of local anesthetic agents. In *Local Anesthetics: Mechanisms of Action and Clinical Use*. Grune & Stratton, New York, 1976, pp 6–11.

82. Feldman HS, Arthur GR, Pitkanen M, Hurley R, Doucette AM, Covino BG: Treatment of acute systemic toxicity after the rapid intravenous injection of ropivacaine and bupivacaine in the conscious dog. Anesth Analg 73:373–384, 1991.

83. Reiz S, Häggmark G, Johansson G, Nath S: Cardiotoxocity of ropivacaine: A new amide local anaesthetic agent. Acta Anaesthesiol Scand 33:93–98, 1989.

84. Nancarrow C, Rutten AJ, Runciman WB, Mather LE, Carapetis RJ, McLean CF, Hipkins SF: Myocardial and cerebral drug concentrations and the mechanisms of death after fatal intravenous doses of lidocaine, bupivacaine and ropivacaine in sheep. Anesth Analg 69:276–283, 1989.

85. Brockway MS, Bannister J, McClure JH, McKeown D, Wildsmith JAW: Comparison of extradural ropivacaine and bupivacaine. Br J Anaesth 66:31–37, 1991.

86. Hershey DW, Quilligan EJ: Extraabdominal uterine exteriorization at cesarean section. Obstet Gynecol 52:189–192, 1978.

87. Bromage PR, Burfoot MF, Crowell DE, Trunant AP: Quality of epidural blockade. III. Carbonated local anaesthetic solutions. Br J Anaesth 39:197–209, 1967.

88. Nickel PM, Bromage PR, Sherrill DL: Comparison of hydrochloride and carbonated salts of lidocaine for epidural analgesia. Reg Anesth 11:62–67, 1986.

89. Galindo A: pH-adjusted local anesthetics: Clinical experience. Reg Anesth 8:35–36, 1983.

90. DiFazio CA, Carron H, Grosslight KR, Moscicki JC, Bolding WR, Johns RA: Comparison of pH-adjusted lidocaine solutions for epidural anesthesia. Anesth Analg 65:760–764, 1986.

91. Peterfreund RA, Datta S, Ostheimer GW: pH-adjustment of local anesthetic solutions with sodium bicarbonate: Laboratory evaluation of alkalinization and precipitation. Reg Anesth 14:265–270, 1989.

92. Stevens RA, Chester WL, Greutor JA, Schubert A, Brandon D, Clayton B, Spitzer L: The effect of pH-adjustment of 0.5% bupivacaine on the latency of epidural anesthesia. Reg Anesth 14:236–239, 1989.

93. Bromage PR, Robson JG: Concentrations of lignocaine in the blood after intravenous, intramuscular, epidural and endotracheal administration. Br J Anaesth 16:461–478, 1961.

94. Burfoot MF, Bromage PR: The effects of epinephrine on mepivacaine absorption from the spinal epidural space. Anesthesiology 35:488–492, 1971.

95. Burn AGL, Van Kleef JW, Gradines MP, Olthof G, Spierdijk J: Epidural anesthesia with lidocaine and bupivacaine: Effect of epinephrine on the plasma concentration profile. Anesth Analg 65:1281–1284, 1986.

96. Jamous MA, Hand CW, Moore RA, Teddy PJ, McQuay HJ: Epinephrine reduces systemic absorption of extradural diacetylmorphine. Anesth Analg 65:1290–1294, 1986.

97. Klepper ID, Sherrill DL, Boetger CL, Bromage PR: Analgesic and respiratory effects of extradural sufentanil in volunteers and the influence of adrenaline as an adjuvant. Br J Anaesth 59:1147–1156, 1987.

98. Abboud TK, David S, Nagappala S, Costandi J, Yanagi T, Haroutunian S, Yeh SU: Maternal, fetal and neonatal effects of lidocaine with and without epinephrine for epidural anesthesia in obstetrics. Anesth Analg 63:973–979, 1984.

99. Bromage PR, Camporesi EM, Durant PA, Nielsen CH: Influence of epinephrine as an adjuvant to epidural morphine. Anesthesiology 58:257–262, 1983.

100. Bromage PR, El-Faqih S, Husain I, Naguib M: Epinephrine and fentanyl as adjuvants to 0.5% bupivacaine for epidural analgesia. Reg Anesth 14:189–194, 1989.

101. Moore DC: Spinal anesthesia: Bupivacaine compared with tetracaine. Anesth Analg 59:743–750, 1980.

102. Malinow AM, Mokriski BLK, Nomara MK, Kaufman MA, Snell JA, Sharp GD, Howard RA: Effect of epinephrine on intrathecal fentanyl analgesia in patients undergoing postpartum tubal ligation. Anesthesiology 73:381–385, 1990.

103. Kozody R, Palahniuk RJ, Wade JG, Cumming M: The effect of subarachnoid epinephrine and phenylephrine on spinal cord blood flow. Can Anaesth Soc J 31:503–508, 1984.

104. Dohi S, Takeshima R, Naito H: Spinal cord blood flow in dogs: The effects of tetracaine, epinephrine, acute blood loss and hypercapnia. Anesth Analg 66:599–606, 1987.

105. Porter SS, Albin MS, Watson WA, Bunegin L, Pantoja G: Spinal cord and cerebral blood flow responses to subarachnoid injection of local anesthetics with and without epinephrine. Acta Anaesthesiol Scand 29:330–338, 1985.

106. Way EL: Studies on the local anesthetic properties of isonipecaine. J Am Pharmacol Assoc 35:44–47, 1946.

107. Framewo CE, Naguib M: Spinal anaesthesia with meperidine as the sole agent. Can Anaesth Soc J 32:553–557, 1985.

108. Perris BW: Epidural pethidine in labour: A study of dose requirements. Anaesthesia 35:380–382, 1980.

109. Husemeyer RP, Davenport HI, Cummings AJ: Comparison of epidural and intramuscular pethidine for analgesia in labour. Br J Obstet Gynaecol 88:711–717, 1981.

110. Baraka A, Maktabi M, Noueihid R: Epidural meperidine-bupivacaine for obstetric analgesia. Anesth Analg 61:652–656, 1982.

111. Brownridge P: Epidural bupivacaine-pethidine mixture chemical experience using a low-dose combination in labour. Aust N Z J Obstet Gynaecol 28:17–24, 1988.

112. Camann WR, Hurley RH, Gilbertson LI, Long ML, Datta S: Epidural nalbuphine for analgesia following caesarean delivery: Dose-response and effect of local anaesthetic choice. Can J Anaesth 38:728–732, 1991.

113. Marando R, Sinatra RS, Fu ES, Collins JG: Failure of intrathecally administered nalbuphine to suppress visceral pain in pregnant rats. Anesthesiology 67:A447, 1987.

114. Bromage PR, Camporsei EM, Durant PAC, Nielsen CH: Rostral spread of epidural morphine. Anesthesiology 56:431–436, 1982.

115. Bromage PR, Husain I, El-Faqih S, Bonsu AK, Kadiwal GH, Seraj P: Critique of the Dornier HM3 lithotripter as a clinical algesimeter. Pain 40:255–265, 1990.

116. Henry M, Graizon A, Seebacher J, Vauthier D, Levron JC, Viars P: Epidural fentanyl with and without epinephrine: Plasma levels and pain relief. Anesthesiology 69:A391, 1988.

117. Hibbard LT: Cesarean section and other surgical procedures. In *Obstetrics: Normal and Problem Pregnancies.* SG Gabbe, Niebyl JR, Simpson JL, eds: Churchill Livingstone, New York, 1986, pp 522–523.

118. Cunningham FG, MacDonald PC, Gant NF: Cesarean section and cesarean hysterectomy. In *Williams Obstetrics*, 18th ed. Appleton & Lange, Norwalk, CT, 1989, pp 441–459.

119. Crawford JS: Caesarean section. In *Principles and Practice of Obstetric Anaesthesia*, 5th ed. Blackwell Scientific Publications, Oxford, 1984, pp 284–343.

120. Norris MC: Patient variables and the subarachnoid spread of hyperbaric bupivacaine in the term patient. Anesthesiology 72:478–482, 1990.

121. Clark RB, Thompson DS, Thompson CH: Prevention of spinal hypotension associated with cesarean section. Anesthesiology 45:670–674, 1976.

122. Abboud TK, Dror A, Mosaad P, Zhu J, Mantila M, Swart F, Gangolly J, Silao P, Makar A, Moore J, Davis H, Lee J: Minidose intrathecal morphine for the relief of post-cesarean section pain. Anesth Analg 67:137–143, 1988.

123. Brockway MS, Noble DW, Sharwood-Smith GH, McClure JH: Profound respiratory depression after extradural fentanyl. Br J Anaesth 64:243–245, 1990.

124. Palmer CM: Early respiratory depression following intrathecal morphine combination. Anesthesiology 74:1153–1155, 1991.

125. Crosby E, Read D: Salvaging inadequate epidural anaesthetics: "The chloroprocaine save." Can J Anaesth 38:136–137, 1991.

126. McGuinness GA, Merkow AJ, Kennedy RL, Erenberg A: Epidural anesthesia with bupivacaine for cesarean section: Neonatal blood levels and neurobehavioral responses. Anesthesiology 49:270–273, 1978.

127. Magno R, Berlin A, Karlsson K, Kjellmer I: Anesthesia for cesarean section. IV. Placental transfer and neonatal elimination of bupivacaine following epidural analgesia for elective cesarean section. Acta Anaesthesiol Scand 20:141–146, 1976.

128. Spoerel WE, Thomas A, Gerula GR: Continuous epidural analgesia: Experience with mechanical injection devices. Can Anaesth Soc J 17:37–51, 1970.

129. Bromage PR: Epidural analgesia for obstetrics. In *Epidural Analgesia*. WB Saunders, Philadelphia, 1978, pp 547–550.

130. Kennedy RL, Miller RP, Bell JU, Doshi D, de Sousa H, Kennedy MJ, Heald DL, David Y: Uptake and distribution of bupivacaine in fetal lambs. Anesthesiology 65:247–253, 1986.

131. Kennedy RL, Bell JU, Miller RP, Doshi D, de Sousa H, Kennedy MJ, Heald DL, Bellinger R, David Y: Uptake and distribution of lidocaine in fetal lambs. Anesthesiology 72:483–489, 1990.

132. Zador G, Willdeck-Lund G, Nilsson BA: Continuous drip lumbar epidural anesthesia with lidocaine for vaginal delivery. I. Clinical efficacy and lidocaine concentrations in maternal, foetal and umbilical cord blood. Acta Obstet Gynecol Scand 34 (suppl):31–40, 1974.

133. Zador G, Nilsson BA: Continuous drip lumbar epidural anaesthesia with lidocaine for vaginal delivery. II. Influence on labour and foetal acid-base status. Acta Obstet Gynecol Scand 34 (suppl):41–49, 1974.

134. Abboud T, Abrasiabi A, Sarkis F, Daftarian F, Nagappala S, Noueihid R, Kuhnert BR, Miller F: Continuous infusion epidural analgesia in parturients receiving bupivacaine, chloroprocaine or lidocaine: Maternal, fetal and neonatal effects. Anesth Analg 63:421–428, 1984.

135. Chestnut DH, Bates JN, Choi WH: Continuous infusion epidural analgesia with lidocaine: Efficacy and influence during the second stage of labor. Obstet Gynecol 69:323–327, 1987.

136. Maze M, Tranquilli W: Alpha-2 adrenoceptor agonists: Defining the role in clinical anesthesia. Anesthesiology 74:581–605, 1991.

CHAPTER 7

Psychologic and Alternative Techniques for Obstetric Anesthesia

Samuel C. Hughes, M.D.
Jay S. DeVore, M.D.

The experience of childbirth ranges from agony to ecstasy. However, a comparison of pain scores revealed that the degree of pain accompanying labor ranged, on average, between that of cancer pain and amputation of a digit (Fig. 7.1) (1). There is a wide range in the pain experienced by parturients as judged by pain evaluation scores (Fig. 7.2). In some women, fear and anxiety may contribute to the pain generated by uterine contractions, cervical dilation, and perineal distension. Thus in recent years, the emphasis of both psychologic and physical preparation for childbirth has increased, and methods of anesthesia incorporating both approaches have been developed. It is possible that preparation for childbirth can decrease the amount of anesthetic and analgesic drugs used during labor and delivery. Furthermore, in the prepared mother, childbirth is more likely to be an enjoyable experience that may influence maternal feelings toward the child for years to come. Preparation of the father, so that both parents may participate in the birth of the child, may also be important.

A number of different methods of psychologic anesthesia have been used with varying degrees of success. These include (a) hypnosis; (b) "natural childbirth," as described by Dick-Read in his book, *Childbirth without Fear* (2); (c) "psychoprophylaxis," as described by Lamaze in his book *Painless Childbirth* (3); (d) acupuncture; (e) the LeBoyer technique, as described in his book *Birth without Violence* (4); and (f) transcutaneous electrical nerve stimulation (TENS) (5). These techniques have been used independently, in combination, and with modification, depending on the requirements of the mother and the situation.

HYPNOSIS

Hypnosis has been used as a method of pain relief in childbirth for many years (6). The hypnoidal trance achieves maternal analgesia with no obstruction of airway reflexes or hypotension and no drug depression of the neonate (7). Furthermore, several investigators have claimed that hypnosis shortens labor (8) and that the acid-base status of the neonate is better at birth and in the hour following than it is with general anesthesia (Fig. 7.3) (7).

Women who may be candidates for hypnosis—that is, those with extreme anxiety or in whom there might be contraindications to more conventional anesthetic techniques—can be evaluated for hypnotic suggestibility by any of several techniques. The eyeroll test of Spiegel (9) is simple and reliable. Those with high susceptibility can be conditioned for full hypnoanalgesia, whereas those with low susceptibility should be cautioned that supplemental chemical anesthesia may be necessary.

Preparation of the mother for hypnosis for childbirth consists of a series of conditioning sessions of approximately 30 min in length. With each session, greater degrees of trance are induced until a level of analgesia, generally of the hand, is achieved. The mother is then conditioned to transfer the analgesia from the hand to the abdomen and perineum to provide pain relief for labor and delivery. The well-conditioned parturient will be able to perform these maneuvers without the hypnotist's presence at the time of delivery.

The use of hypnoanalgesia for childbirth is not widespread. Aside from its time-consuming aspects, hypnosis occasionally produces undesirable side effects. Rosen (10) described the danger of hypnosis practiced by improperly trained physicians. Wahl (11) reported complications of hypnosis in obstetrics that ranged from states of acute anxiety to frank psychosis. He suggested that hypnoanalgesia for childbirth was strongly contraindicated by a documented history of psychosis or psychoneurotic hysterical conversion reactions; ambivalence regarding birth or motherhood; or prevalence of nightmares in the last

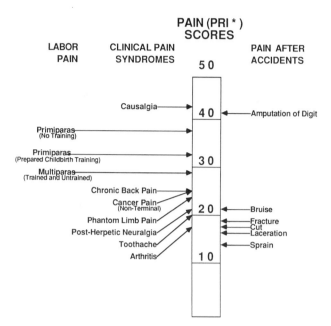

Figure 7.1. A comparison of pain scores using the McGill Pain Questionnaire, comparing labor pain and pain of other patients in a general hospital pain clinic. * McGill Pain Questionnaire Pain Rating Index. (Reprinted by permission from Melzack R: The myth of painless childbirth (The John J. Bonica Lecture). Pain 19:321–337, 1984.)

trimester. In sum, this technique is not always effective and is not without serious risk to some women.

NATURAL CHILDBIRTH

The "natural childbirth" method of Dick-Read (2) was widely used in the 1940s. It is now recognized as having some important limitations. The basis of his approach was that anxiety, fear, and pain were interlinked and that a simple and fearless approach to labor could render it painless. He believed that, during uncomplicated labor, uterine contractions should be painless because "there is no physiologic function in the body which gives rise to pain in the normal course of health" (2).

PSYCHOPROPHYLAXIS

The psychoprophylaxis method of Lamaze (3) is currently one of the most popular approaches. This technique combines positive conditioning of the mother with education on the process of childbirth. The basis of psychoprophylaxis is the belief that the pain of labor and delivery can be suppressed by reorganization of cerebral cortical activity. Conditioned pain reflexes associated with uterine contractions and perineal distension can be replaced by newly created "positive" conditioned reflexes. The mother is taught to respond to the beginning of a contraction by immediately taking a deep "cleansing breath," gently exhaling, then breathing in a specific shallow pattern until the con-

traction ends. She also focuses her eyes on a specific object or location away from herself, concentrates on release of muscle tension, and maintains the proper breathing rhythm with the help and "coaching" of a spouse or friend. The increased concentration required of her by these activities distracts from or inhibits the pain of uterine contraction. Lamaze preparation usually begins 6 weeks before delivery. Instruction includes the normal anatomy and physiology of pregnancy, labor, and delivery and provides the mother with knowledge and some "control" of the process she is undergoing.

Although there may appear to be some similarity between psychoprophylaxis and hypnosis, proponents of psychoprophylaxis point out that their technique freely engages the mother's conscious and cooperative efforts. When Samko and Schoenfeld (12) investigated the relationship between hypnotic susceptibility and successful Lamaze childbirth, they found no correlation.

A realistic approach to individual tolerance of pain is important to maternal self-esteem, satisfaction with the birth experience, and bonding with the newborn (13). Several women authors have noted, to their dismay, the tendency toward the dogmatic approach by many childbirth instructors (14, 15). A more flexible approach to pain management should result from good childbirth preparation so the patient can make informed choices. Psychoprophylaxis helps to reduce the amount of chemical anesthesia required by the mother (16). However, widespread experience indicates that a majority of women receiving Lamaze training will request pharmacologic analgesia or regional block during labor (Table 7.1) (1, 16). This is not surprising because, although childbirth preparation has been shown to decrease pain levels, it was not a dramatic reduction (1). Furthermore, childbirth training may be less effective with some types of labor pain (17). Thus it is important that Lamaze training include information about anesthetic aids and the awareness that labor is unlikely to be absolutely painless. Enduring excessive pain or anxiety over failure to control pain may result in more harm to the fetus than the judicious use of pharmacologic analgesia (18). It has been demonstrated that analgesic and anesthetic drugs administered to the mother cross the placenta and may sedate the fetus, depending on the drug and the amount administered. Therefore some authors have advocated not using chemical anesthesia for childbirth. However, Myers (18) and Morishima and co-workers (19) have demonstrated that, in the primate mother, psychologic stress during labor may cause hypoxia and acidosis in the fetus, probably due to decreased uterine blood flow (Figs. 7.4 and 7.5). Shnider and co-workers (20)

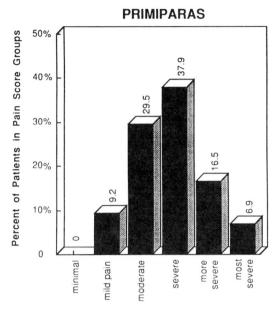

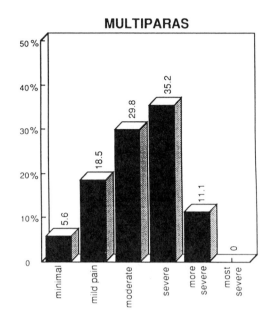

Figure 7.2. Distribution of Pain Rating Index (PRI) scores for primiparas and multiparas in six intervals of the PRI range. There is a wide range of pain scores in both primiparas and multiparas. (Adapted and reprinted with permission from Mel-

zack R, Taenzer P, Feldman P, Kinch RA: Labour is still painful after prepared childbirth training. Can Med Assoc J 125:357–363, 1981.)

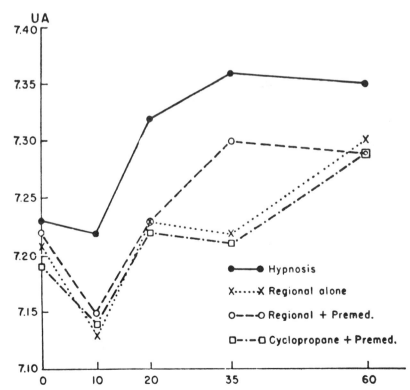

Figure 7.3. Mean serial arterial blood pH values in first hour after birth. Umbilical artery (UA) blood averages are plotted at zero time. Time in minutes is shown on *horizontal axis*;

pH is shown on *vertical axis*. (Reprinted by permission from Moya F, James LS: Medical hypnosis for obstetrics. JAMA 174:2026–2032, 1960.)

Table 7.1
Pharmacologic Methods of Pain Relief Used during Labor and Delivery[a]

| Analgesia and Anesthesia | Number of Mothers | | P Value |
	Lamaze Group (n = 129)	Control Group (n = 129)	
None during first stage of labor	36	9	<0.001
Sedatives or tranquilizers	28	39	NS[b]
Narcotics	84	109	<0.001
Paracervical	13	15	NS
Epidural or caudal	18	52	<0.001
Saddle	6	8	NS
General anesthesia	4	5	NS
Pudendal	83	59	<0.001
Local infiltration only	13	5	NS

[a] Reprinted by permission from Scott JR, Rose NB: Effect of psychoprophylaxis (Lamaze preparation) on labor and delivery in primiparas. N Engl J Med 294:1205–1207, 1976.
[b] NS = not significant.

have demonstrated that maternal stress results in increased plasma norepinephrine levels and reduced uterine blood flow in the pregnant ewe (Fig. 7.6). It has also been shown that catecholamine levels in the mother decrease during labor after administration of lumbar epidural anesthesia (21). Therefore avoidance of chemical analgesia must not be taken to an extreme that results in harm to the fetus or rejection of the newborn due to the unpleasantness of labor and delivery.

The use of regional anesthesia may be a reasonable compromise, minimizing stress but allowing participation of the mother and father. However, regional anesthesia may be inappropriate for women who want to fully experience childbirth. Some women have felt that the removal of pain deprives them of a major portion of the experience. Billewicz-Driemel and Milne (22) studied this feeling of deprivation to determine whether it has any long-term psychologic consequences. They found that a small percentage of women who gave birth using epidural analgesia felt deprived, but did not appear to experience long-term consequences. We believe that choices regarding pain management are best made by a well-informed pa-

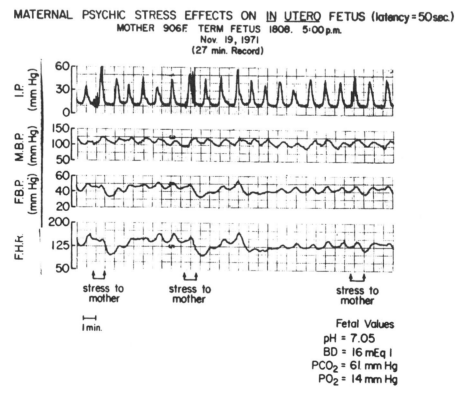

Figure 7.4. The effects of three 1-min episodes of "contrived" psychologic stress stimulation of a pregnant monkey timed with a stopwatch. In two instances, the fetus responded with clear-cut episodes of bradycardia. (Reprinted by permission from Myers RE: Maternal psychological stress and fetal asphyxia: A study in the monkey. Am J Obstet Gynecol 122:47–59, 1975.)

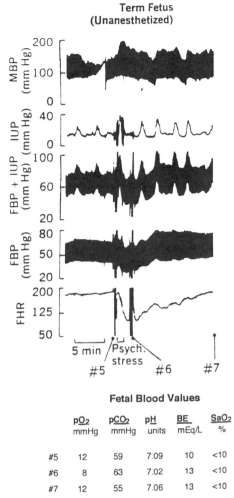

**Term Fetus
(Unanesthetized)**

Fetal Blood Values

	pO$_2$ mmHg	pCO$_2$ mmHg	pH units	BE mEq/L	SaO$_2$ %
#5	12	59	7.09	10	<10
#6	8	63	7.02	13	<10
#7	12	55	7.06	13	<10

Figure 7.5. Maternal blood pressure, intrauterine pressure, and fetal blood pressure and heart rate before, during, and after a pregnant monkey was exposed to a 1-min episode of psychologic stress. This produced marked fetal bradycardia and hypotension. These changes required 15 to 20 min for full recovery. Fetal blood samples taken immediately before, during, and following recovery demonstrated significant reductions in oxygen values during bradycardia. These data support the view that the fetal bradycardia and hypotension produced by stress of the mother are caused by enhanced asphyxia. (Reprinted by permission from Myers RE, Myers SE: Use of sedative, analgesic, and anesthetic drugs during labor and delivery: Bane or boon? Am J Obstet Gynecol 133:83–104, 1979.)

tient in consultation with the Lamaze coach, anesthesiologist, and obstetrician.

The question of whether or not Lamaze preparation results in healthier babies is unanswered. Scott and Rose (16) compared prepared and unprepared mothers and found that, although prepared mothers required less analgesia (Table 7.1), neonatal outcome was similar. There is no question, however, that preparation for the event of childbirth is of benefit to almost all women and, regardless of the type of anesthesia used, can make the experience more pleasant (23). The parturient who is well prepared and understands the birth process is often more able to participate in delivery and make intelligent choices on the use of anesthesia and the birth process, as clinically necessary.

ACUPUNCTURE

Acupuncture has been practiced in China for more than a thousand years for both its therapeutic and analgesic properties (24). Anecdotal reports have stimulated interest in the value of acupuncture as an alternative to conventional anesthesia (25, 26). It is only natural that acupuncture should receive attention as a possible obstetric anesthetic, inasmuch as it seems to be completely safe for mother and newborn. Because Chinese women traditionally have delivered their children without anesthesia, there are no traditional acupuncture points for vaginal delivery. In China, acupuncture anesthesia for surgery is reported to be successful in about 70% of patients. However, this success depends on careful patient selection, high patient motivation, and deeply embedded cultural conditioning (26).

Several American investigators have attempted to provide analgesia for labor and delivery using the acupuncture points for vaginal hysterectomy and dysmenorrhea (Fig. 7.7) (27, 28). Wallis et al. (27) studied manual and electrical acupuncture in 21 motivated volunteers. Nineteen of twenty-one mothers experienced inadequate analgesia (Fig. 7.8). The remaining women, both treated by manual acupuncture, reported significant relief of pain. Both had used a natural childbirth technique. Sixteen women requested an alternative method of analgesia. Among the five who did not, three had used natural childbirth methods. None of the 21 subjects were judged by the investigators to have obtained adequate analgesia from acupuncture. Obviously this technique seems less than ideal.

LEBOYER TECHNIQUE

The French obstetrician LeBoyer (4) has received much attention for promoting the concept of "childbirth without violence." He believed that the noise, bright lights, and other stimulation associated with the traditional delivery caused psychologic trauma to the newborn. His solution was to perform deliveries in near silence and semidarkness and to avoid stimulation of the newborn to prevent crying. Although there is no doubt that there is unnecessary noise in most delivery rooms, the authors believe good lighting is essential to evaluate the condition of the newborn and to care for the mother. Furthermore, LeBoyer's method of placing the newborn on

Figure 7.6. Effect of electrically induced stress (30 to 60 sec) on maternal arterial blood pressure, plasma norepinephrine levels, and uterine blood flow. All values subsequent to control are given as mean percentage change with standard error. (Reprinted by permission from Shnider SM, Wright RG, Levinson G, Roizen MF, Wallis KL, Rolbin SH, Craft JB: Uterine blood flow and plasma norepinephrine changes during maternal stress in the pregnant ewe. Anesthesiology 50:524–527, 1979.)

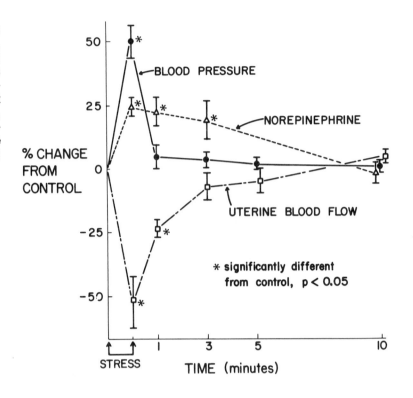

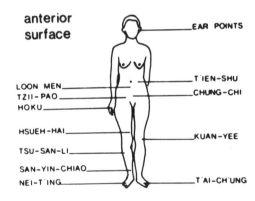

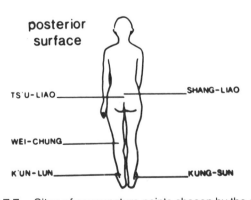

Figure 7.7. Sites of acupuncture points chosen by the acupuncturist to provide analgesia during labor. (Reprinted by permission from Wallis L, Shnider SM, Palahniuk RJ, Spivey HL: An evaluation of acupuncture analgesia in obstetrics. Anesthesiology 41:596–601, 1974.)

the mother's abdomen with the umbilical cord still intact and pulsating can result in a loss of blood from newborn to placenta that can be harmful. Furthermore, the authors believe there is a rather subtle suggestion in LeBoyer's technique that newborns who cannot survive without active resuscitation are already permanently damaged and that intervention should be avoided. This, of course, is not true (see Chapter 39).

TRANSCUTANEOUS ELECTRICAL NERVE STIMULATION

Transcutaneous electrical nerve stimulation (TENS) is a technique that was introduced as a screening procedure to predict which patients would respond well to indwelling dorsal column stimulators for analgesia (29, 30). Although TENS failed to predict implant outcome, it did produce local analgesia, suggesting other applications of the technique. The use of electricity for analgesia dates from the Greek and Roman use of the torpedo fish, which can emit 200 V (29). Although the use of electricity in modern medicine has been erratic and not always safe, developments in the field of electronics and publication of the gate theory of pain in 1965 revived interest in analgesia by electrical stimulation of the afferent nervous system (30).

The gate theory of pain hypothesizes that an area of central nervous system, the substantia gelatinosa in the dorsal horn, acts as a "gate" that, when acti-

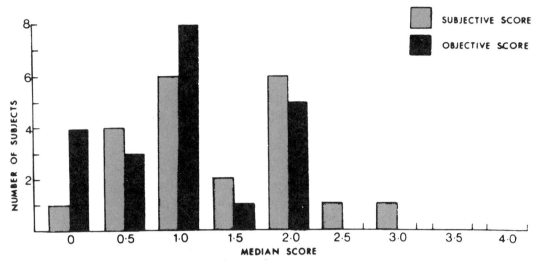

Figure 7.8. Histogram representing median analgesia scores during acupuncture treatment for all 21 subjects in the study. Subjective and observer scores are shown for each patient. Scores ≤2 were considered to indicate inadequate analgesia.

(Reprinted by permission from Wallis L, Shnider SM, Palahniuk RJ, Spivey HL: An evaluation of acupuncture analgesia in obstetrics. Anesthesiology 41:596–601, 1974.)

vated or "closed," inhibits pain sensations from reaching the conscious brain. Theoretically, it is stimulation of large, myelinated A-β nerve fibers that "close the gate," or increase the pain-modulating function of the substantia gelatinosa. Pain sensations or input transmitted by the A-Δ and C nerve fibers may thus be altered or blocked (31, 32). TENS is thought to affect the A-β fibers similarly, although this hypothesis is controversial (33, 34). Others have suggested that the endogenous opioid system is responsible for the effects of TENS (35, 36), although more recent work refutes this (38, 39). Regardless of its mechanism of action, TENS has proved effective in a variety of operative situations (40–42), although not all studies are supportive (42, 43). For obstetrics, TENS offers the possibility of analgesia for labor and delivery produced with minimal intervention and essentially no risk. The clinical results to date have been variable, however.

Technique

The use of this technique is fairly simple. The equipment can be set up in minutes, involving the parturient in the management of her analgesia by allowing her to adjust stimulation as required. Skin electrodes made of a conductive adhesive, 37 × 150 mm (Tenzcare), are applied symmetrically to either side of the T10–L1 region of the spine. Smaller electrode pads may be added to the sacral area for the second stage of labor to be used in combination with the T10–L1 stimulation (Fig. 7.9). The electrical current is a biphasic pulse from 30 to 250 μsec in duration, with an amplitude of 0 to 75 mA and a frequency of 40 to 150 Hz. Each manufacturer recommends slightly different limits, and there

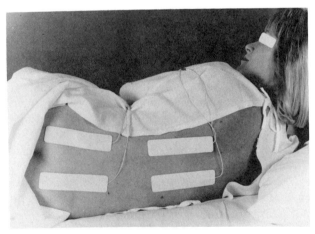

Figure 7.9. Placement of TENS electrodes on a patient's back. Electrodes are easily applied, much like an ECG pad, and have wires leading to a nerve stimulator. The apparatus is easily operated and can be placed at the bedside or clipped to a patient's gown if she is ambulatory.

is some disagreement on the shape of the stimulation waveform. The best results in obstetrics come from a continuous low level of stimulation during labor with a higher level instituted during contractions. The baseline level of stimulation is usually increased as labor progresses: otherwise, analgesia tends to fade. Some manufacturers offer hand-held devices that allow the mother to adjust (increase) the stimulation with contractions according to need. The mother experiences a tingling sensation in the areas around the electrodes, and the best analgesia is achieved when stimulation is increased until muscle activity around the area is stimulated. The degree of stimulation needed (and tolerated) varies from patient to patient.

The use of this technique seems to be completely safe; its greatest risk is unsatisfactory analgesia. In a European study, measurements of current density in urinary bladders of nonpregnant women using TENS have revealed a current that is below the proposed safety standard of 0.5 μA/mm (44). The stimulators used in the United States have an even lower output and should thus be within the safety limits.

Clinical Experience

To date, obstetric experience with TENS is generally limited and almost anecdotal. There are few well-controlled studies and thus little reliable information. Augustinsson and co-workers (45) used a two-channel stimulator with separate controls and a handswitch for rapid change between two different preset stimulation levels. Forty-four percent of their subjects ($n = 147$) experienced good to very good relief, and 44% obtained moderate relief. In a larger study, it was suggested that TENS was particularly good for pain localized to the back (34). In general, the results have been best for some relief of pain during the first stage of labor, with diminished relief during the second stage. It has also been reported that, with TENS, the use of narcotics during labor decreases (46). In a controlled study there was no significant decrease in the amount of narcotics or epidural anesthesia used when TENS was applied (47). However, TENS provides analgesia (as minimal as it might be) noninvasively, without risk to mother and newborn, and can be easily administered by nurse midwives or labor room nurses. It is also instantly "reversible" (48). The only complication thus far noted is signal artifact—that is, electrical interference with fetal heart rate tracing not unlike that encountered with Bovie equipment and ECG monitors in the operating room. With TENS, this happens rarely, has no effect on the true fetal ECG, and can be dealt with by turning off the TENS machine, if necessary, to read the monitor. A filter that can be applied to the nerve stimulators has been shown to block this interference, but this piece of equipment is not yet available in the United States (44).

Some authors have suggested that the effects of this technique beyond placebo are minimal (49). Other investigators have had somewhat positive results (47–51). It may prove particularly beneficial to the well-motivated patient who wishes minimal intervention.

FAMILY-CENTERED MATERNAL CARE

Currently, one of the most widely discussed concepts in the psychology of childbirth is that of family-centered maternity care. The belief is that the interaction between mother, father, and child in the first few minutes of the child's life can greatly influence the entire relationship of the child with its environment. Proponents of this philosophy believe that the traditional hospital maternity care is physician centered and sacrifices the individuality of the mother and psychologic well-being of the newborn to the convenience of the hospital staff. This has led to renewed interest in home deliveries. Advocates of home deliveries point out that most deliveries are perfectly normal and do not require the intervention of a physician. Unfortunately, it is impossible to predict accurately which patients will develop problems during labor, and, when problems do occur, immediate physician intervention is often necessary to preserve the lives of both mother and newborn. Data from 11 state health departments reported that out-of-hospital births posed two to five times greater risk to a newborn's life than hospital births (52). For example, in 1975 California had a perinatal mortality of 20 per 1000 births in the hospital compared with 42.3 per 1000 births for home deliveries. However, more recent data suggest that with *carefully selected* patients and rigorous standards, birth centers offer a "safe and acceptable alternative" (53).

In response to some of the objections to traditional hospital maternity care, the "birthing room" has been created. This is a room in which the mother both labors and delivers her baby. The room is in a hospital maternity suite that has been altered to provide a home-like atmosphere. Mothers are encouraged to bring their own personal belongings. The presence of the father is encouraged, no matter what mode of delivery is chosen. Latitude is allowed in the management of labor. All emergency facilities are immediately at hand. What is provided is, in effect, a home delivery in the hospital. A pleasant environment as well as continuous emotional support may have very positive effects on the outcome (54).

PRENATAL ANESTHESIA VISITS

Some anesthesiologists set up prenatal anesthesia clinics to provide mothers with the opportunity to discuss anesthesia for labor and delivery prior to the onset of labor. During the visit, a medical history is taken, choices of anesthesia are discussed, and the questions and concerns of the mother are addressed. If individual interviews are impractical, a session during which an anesthesiologist meets with a group of expectant parents to discuss anesthetic alternatives and address questions and concerns should be arranged. The prenatal anesthetic visit can avoid much of the mutual anxiety that often occurs on the labor floor when an anesthesiologist is called to see a parturient in pain about whom he or she knows nothing. Many anesthesia units distribute a brochure to prospective parents describing pain relief in childbirth. One such brochure is reprinted in the Appendix to this chapter.

References

1. Melzack R: The myth of painless childbirth (The John J. Bonica Lecture). Pain 19:321–327, 1984.
2. Dick-Read G: *Childbirth without Fear*, 2nd ed. Harper & Row, New York, 1959.
3. Lamaze F: *Painless Childbirth: Psychoprophylactic Method*. Burke, London, 1958.
4. LeBoyer F: *Birth without Violence*. Wildwood House, London, 1975.
5. Hughes SC: Approaches to pain relief in the obstetrical patient. In *ASA Refresher Course Lectures*, American Society of Anesthesiology, New Orleans, 1984, No 232.
6. August RV: *Hypnosis in Obstetrics*. McGraw-Hill, New York, 1961.
7. Moya F, James LS: Medical hypnosis for obstetrics. JAMA 174:2026–2032, 1960.
8. Flowers CE, Littlejohn TW, Wells HB: Pharmacologic and hypnoid analgesia. Obstet Gynecol 16:210–221, 1960.
9. Spiegel H: An eye-roll test for hypnotizability. Am J Clin Hypn 15:25–28, 1972.
10. Rosen H: Hypnosis: Applications and misapplications. JAMA 172:683–687, 1960.
11. Wahl CW: Contraindications and limitations of hypnosis in obstetric analgesia. Am J Obstet Gynecol 84:1869–1872, 1962.
12. Samko MR, Schoenfeld LS: Hypnotic susceptibility and the Lamaze childbirth experience. Am J Obstet Gynecol 121:631–636, 1975.
13. Hughes SC, Levinson G, Marut J, Shnider SM, Slavazza K, Rohdr JM, Dailey PA: Influence of epidural analgesia for labor on maternal self-esteem and perception of the newborn. Anesthesiology 57:A406, 1982.
14. Behan M: Childbirth machisma. Parenting April 1988.
15. Ephron N: Having a baby after 35. NY Times Mag, November 26, 1978.
16. Scott JR, Rose NB: Effect of psychoprophylaxis (Lamaze preparation) on labor and delivery in primiparas. N Engl J Med 294:1205–1207, 1978.
17. Melzack RM, Schaffelberg D: Low-back pain during labor. Am J Obstet Gynecol 156:901–905, 1987.
18. Myers RE: Maternal psychological stress and fetal asphyxia: A study in the monkey. Am J Obstet Gynecol 122:47–59, 1975.
19. Morishima HO, Pedersen H, Finster M: The influence of maternal psychological stress on the fetus. Am J Obstet Gynecol 131:286–290, 1978.
20. Shnider SM, Wright RG, Levinson G, Roizen MF, Wallis KL, Rolbin SH, Craft JB Jr: Uterine blood flow and plasma norepinephrine changes during maternal stress in the pregnant ewe. Anesthesiology 50:524–527, 1979.
21. Shnider SM, Abboud TK, Artal R, Henricksen EH, Stefani SJ, Levinson G: Maternal catecholamines decrease during labor after lumbar epidural anesthesia. Am J Obstet Gynecol 147:13–15, 1983.
22. Billewicz-Driemel AM, Milne MD: Long term assessment of extradural analgesia for the relief of pain in labour: Relevant or not? Br J Anaesth 48:139–144, 1976.
23. Doering SG, Entwisel DR: Preparation during pregnancy and ability to cope with labor and delivery. Am J Orthopsychiatry 45:825–837, 1975.
24. Vieth I: Acupuncture in traditional Chinese medicine: A historical review. Calif Med 118:70–79, 1973.
25. Reston J: Now, about my operation in Peking. In *The New York Times Report from Red China*. F Ching, ed. Quadrangle Books, New York, 1971, p 304.
26. Dimond EG: Acupuncture anesthesia: Western Medicine and Chinese traditional medicine. JAMA 218:1558–1563, 1971.
27. Wallis L, Shnider SM, Palahniuk RJ, Spivey HL: An evaluation of acupuncture analgesia in obstetrics. Anesthesiology 41:596–601, 1974.
28. Abouleish E, Depp R: Acupuncture in obstetrics. Anesth Analg 54:83–88, 1975.
29. Tyler E, Caldwell G, Ghia JN: Transcutaneous electrical nerve stimulation: An alternative approach to the management of postoperative pain. Anesth Analg 61:449–456, 1982.
30. Melzack R, Wall PD: Pain mechanisms: A new theory. Science 150:971–979, 1965.
31. Shealy CN, Mortiner JT, Reswick JB: Electrical inhibition of pain by stimulation of the dorsal columns. Anesth Analg (Curr Res) 46:489–491, 1967.
32. Long DM: External electrical stimulation as a treatment of chronic pain. Minn Med 57:195–198, 1974.
33. Melzack R, Taenzer P, Feldman P, Kinch RA: Labour is still painful after prepared childbirth training. Can Med Assoc J 125:357–363, 1981.
34. Bundsen P, Peterson L-E, Selstam U: Pain relief in labor by transcutaneous electrical nerve stimulation: A prospective matched study. Acta Obstet Gynecol Scand 60:459–468, 1981.
35. Woolf CJ, Mitchell D, Barrett GD: Antinociceptive effect of peripheral segmental electrical stimulation in the rat. Pain 8:237–252, 1980.
36. Solomon RA, Viernstein MC, Long DM: Reduction of postoperative pain and narcotic use by transcutaneous electrical nerve stimulation. Surgery 87:142–146, 1980.
37. Willer J-C, Roby A, Boulu P, Boureau F: Comparative effects of electracupuncture and transcutaneous nerve stimulation on the human blink reflex. Pain 14:267–278, 1982.
38. Abram SE, Reynolds AC, Cusick JF: Failure of naloxone to reverse analgesia from transcutaneous electrical stimulation in patients with chronic pain. Anesth Analg 60:81–84, 1984.
39. Stanley TH, Cazalaa JA, Atinault A, Coeytaux R, Limoge A, Louville Y: Transcutaneous cranial electrical stimulation decreases narcotic requirements during neurolept anesthesia and operation in man. Anesth Analg 61:863–866, 1982.
40. Rooney S-M, Jain S, Goldiner PL: Effect of transcutaneous nerve stimulation on postoperative pain after thoracotomy. Anesth Analg 62:1010–1012, 1983.
41. Bourke DL, Smith BAC, Erickson J, Gwartz B, Lessard L: TENS reduces halothane requirements during hand surgery. Anesthesiology 61:769–772, 1984.
42. McCallum MD, Glynn CJ, Moore RA, Lammer P, Phillips AM: Transcutaneous electrical nerve stimulation in the management of acute postoperative pain. Br J Anaesth 61:308–312, 1988.
43. Reynolds RA, Glandstone N, Ansari AM: Transcutaneous electrical nerve stimulation for reducing narcotic use after cesarean section. J Reprod Med 32:843–846, 1987.
44. Bundsen P, Ericson K: Pain relief in labor by transcutaneous electrical nerve stimulation: Safety aspects. Acta Obstet Gynecol Scand 61:1–5, 1982.
45. Augustinsson L-E, Bohlin P, Bundsen P, Carlsson C-A, Forssman L, Sjoberg P, Tyreman NO: Pain relief during delivery by transcutaneous electrical stimulation. Pain 4:59–65, 1977.
46. Miller Jones CMH: Transcutaneous nerve stimulation in labour (Forum). Anaesthesia 35:372–375, 1980.
47. Hughes SC, Dailey PA, Partridge C: Transcutaneous electrical nerve stimulation for labor analgesia. Anesth Analg 67:S99, 1988.
48. Stewart P: Transcutaneous nerve stimulation as a method of analgesia in labour. Anaesthesia 34:361–364, 1979.
49. Merry AF: Use of transcutaneous electrical stimulation in labour (letter). N Z Med J 96:635–636, 1983.
50. Harrison RF, Woods T, Shore M, Mathews G, Unwin A: Pain relief in labour using transcutaneous electrical nerve stimulation (TENS): A TENS/TENS placebo controlled study in two parity groups. Br J Obstet Gynaecol 93:739–746, 1986.
51. Harrison RF, Shore T, Woods T, Mathews G, Gardiner J, Unwin A: A comparative study of transcutaneous electrical nerve stimulation (TENS), entonox, pethidine + promazine and lumbar epidural for pain relief in labor. Acta Obstet Gynecol Scand 66:9–14, 1987.
52. American College of Obstetricians and Gynecologists: ACOG Newsletter 22:No 2, 1976.
53. Rooks JP, Weatherby NL, Ernst EK, Stapleton S, Rosen D, Rosenfield A: Outcomes of care in birth centers. N Engl J Med 321:1804–1811, 1989.
54. Kennell J, Klaus M, McGrath S, Robertson S, Hinkley C: Continuous emotional support during labor in a US hospital. JAMA 265:2197–2201, 1991.

Pain Relief During Childbirth

University of California, San Francisco

Doctors from the Department of Anesthesia at the University of California, San Francisco, are available 24 hr a day to assist women in the labor and delivery suite. These anesthesiologists are the members of the obstetric health care team skilled in the techniques for providing pain relief during labor, vaginal delivery, and cesarean section. The purpose of this pamphlet is to introduce you to these techniques. First, though, we want to stress that once hard labor has started, it is important that you do not eat any solid foods; restrict your intake to clear liquids only, such as tea or ginger ale.

On admission to the labor and delivery area, you will be examined and evaluated by an obstetrician or midwife, after which you will meet an anesthesiologist. The purpose of the anesthesiologist's visit is twofold: (a) to learn of any medical problems you may have which could influence the use and choice of anesthesia and (b) to advise you firsthand of the techniques available for relief from pain or discomfort during labor and delivery. You should discuss your choices with the anesthesiologist at this time. They are available to consult even if anesthesia is not necessary for the birth of your baby.

LABOR AND VAGINAL DELIVERY

During childbirth, you often must work hard (labor) to deliver your baby. Your uterus contracts repetitively, guiding the baby into and through the birth canal. These contractions can be painful, and additional pain or discomfort may result from pressure produced as the baby moves through the birth canal. However, the degree of discomfort during childbirth varies by person. For some women, the pain or discomfort is minimal and for others, significant. Many women attend childbirth classes and learn techniques that help to focus their concentration on lessening the experience of pain or discomfort. Often, these techniques succeed and babies are delivered without the use of anesthesia. Other options are available for women who do not find these techniques adequate or who have not learned them. The anesthesiologist's goal is to provide you the greatest comfort, while safeguarding the health of both you and the baby.

PAIN RELIEF DURING LABOR

Injection of Medication

During the early and middle part of labor, pain can be decreased by an injection of medication. Typically, narcotics (opiates) or tranquilizers are the medications used, but in very small doses. Larger doses cause drowsiness or sleep for you and, consequently, the baby. Because we want the baby to be vigorous at birth, not sleepy, we administer only very small doses which may not completely relieve the pain, but will "take the edge off" it. For some women, when combined with the techniques learned in childbirth classes, this is sufficient. Others may need greater pain relief.

Epidural Anesthetic

Once labor is "active," pain can be substantially relieved or eliminated by epidural administration of either an opiate, a local anesthetic, or a combination of both. An "epidural" works by introducing anesthetic into a space surrounding the spinal cord sac in the lower part of the back (the epidural space) and blocks the discomfort of uterine contractions. To introduce the anesthetic, we insert a needle between the vertebrae in the lower back and thread a small, flexible hollow tube (called a catheter) through the needle into the epidural space. Medication is injected into the catheter and partially or completely relieves the pain. You remain fully awake and aware that contractions are occurring by the sensation of pressure, but pain is abolished, or considerably reduced. The dose and concentration of medication can be varied to produce any level of analgesia from minimal to profound. The small, soft catheter is left in place to allow administration of additional anesthetic, throughout labor and even delivery usually by a constant slow infusion.

A properly administered "epidural" is a very effective pain relief technique. It is safe for both mother and baby and is a method used often at this and many other hospitals. As with all anesthetics or medications, complications are possible, though very uncommon, and most can be treated. An anesthesiologist will explain the epidural technique and the benefits, alternatives, and associated risks to help you evaluate your choices.

Inhalation Anesthetic

Relief from pain can also be obtained by inhaling a rapid-acting *analgesic gas* (nitrous oxide) from a hand-held device. This is called *inhalation analgesia*. You remain awake and experience a degree of pain relief that is likely to be satisfactory, although not comparable to that provided by the epidural method. Nitrous oxide is a safe gas for both mother and baby, the effects of which disappear rapidly when you stop inhaling it.

PAIN RELIEF DURING DELIVERY

An *epidural anesthetic* also may provide pain relief during delivery. The method of introducing anesthetic is the same as that for labor and is as effective and safe for both mother and baby. If you selected the epidural method for pain relief during labor, the same catheter will be used to administer local anesthetic for delivery.

A *spinal anesthetic* is another safe technique for relieving delivery pain. A "spinal" is similar to, but *not the same as*, an epidural, although the two are sometimes confused. Like an epidural, a spinal anesthetic, or "saddle block," is introduced through a needle inserted between the vertebrae in the lower back, and it numbs the nerves. However, a spinal anesthetic is given only once, as a single injection, and local anesthetic is introduced directly into the fluid-filled sac of the spinal cord, rather than into the epidural space around it. No catheter is inserted. Because the anesthetic is injected only once, the spinal technique is not useful for the type of long-term pain relief required for labor. However, it is very successful in relieving the immediate pain or discomfort of delivery or episiotomy. It is especially useful if the obstetrician needs to use forceps or other instruments to assist the delivery.

Injection of *local anesthetic* around the vagina will also relieve delivery pain. However, this technique can provide pain relief during *only* the very last part of delivery and the repair of an episiotomy. The local anesthetic is administered by an obstetrician or midwife; it does not require an anesthesiologist; and it does not affect the baby.

Inhaling *analgesic gas* (nitrous oxide) from a hand-held breathing device is another option. As during labor, this method will provide a degree of pain relief for delivery. Used alone, or in combination with the injection of local anesthetic around the vagina, the inhalation technique is safe for both mother and baby.

The most rapid onset of anesthesia is achieved with *general anesthesia*. In the rare emergency situations in which rapid, vaginal delivery of the baby is required, we therefore use general anesthesia—that is, you are completely asleep. The anesthesiologist will interview you quickly and administer a general anesthetic that is safe for both mother and baby. We do not use general anesthesia for routine vaginal delivery for several reasons: (a) with prolonged use the anesthetic may make the baby sleepy at birth; (b) the mother may vomit and inhale stomach contents as the anesthetic takes effect; (c) the pushing efforts important for delivery are absent because the mother is asleep, necessitating an instrument-assisted delivery; and (d) most women prefer to be awake for delivery of the baby.

ANESTHESIA FOR CESAREAN SECTION

If your obstetrician decides a cesarean section is necessary, an anesthesiologist will speak with you before surgery. If you chose an epidural to provide relief from labor pain, the epidural catheter is already in place and can be used to provide *epidural anesthesia* for the cesarean section. An epidural also can be administered at the time of the cesarean section. You remain awake, have no sensation of surgical pain, and can see the baby shortly after delivery.

When an epidural anesthetic is used for cesarean delivery, a *small* dose of morphine is usually administered through the epidural catheter just after delivery to provide good to excellent pain relief for up to 24 hr after surgery. Pain relief following epidural morphine is superior to that resulting from the more conventional technique of repetitive postoperative injection of morphine or other opiates. As with all medications, benefits are accompanied by risks of possible side effects. The anesthesiologist will discuss these with you.

A *spinal anesthetic* also can be used for a cesarean section. Spinal morphine can be administered for postoperative pain relief comparable to that provided by epidural morphine.

General anesthesia, unless necessary, is not recommended for cesarean section for reasons similar to those for routine vaginal delivery: (a) a sleepy baby at birth; (b) a mother at risk of vomiting and inhaling stomach contents; and (c) loss of the opportunity to be awake for the baby's birth. However, when general anesthesia is required for emergencies that restrict the time for proper administration of an epidural or spinal anesthetic, or when it is preferred by the mother, the anesthesiologist will confer with you and administer a general anesthetic that is safe for both mother and baby.

CONCLUSION

The degree of pain experienced over the course of childbirth varies by individual, and changes in each woman over the course of labor and delivery. The type of pain relief we provide, if requested, depends on the preferences of mother and physician and the health of mother and baby at the time of labor and delivery. Specific concerns you may have about the use of anesthesia because of medical, obstetric, or previous anesthesia-related problems can and should be addressed to both your obstetrician and anesthesiologist. The goal of your anesthesiologist is to provide you with the greatest comfort during childbirth, while safeguarding the health of you and your baby.

We hope this pamphlet has provided you with the basic information necessary to understand the options we offer at UCSF for pain relief during childbirth. We look forward to the opportunity to discuss the choices with you on an individual basis when you arrive in the labor and delivery suite at UCSF. We also can arrange for you to speak with an obstetric anesthesiologist well in advance of delivery.

CHAPTER 8

Systemic Medication for Labor and Delivery

Gershon Levinson, M.D.
Sol M. Shnider, M.D.

Despite the increasing use of regional analgesia during labor, systemic medications are still widely used to relieve pain and anxiety. There is no ideal, universally applicable analgesic agent for use during childbirth. All systemic medications used for pain relief in labor cross the placenta and may have a depressant effect on the fetus. The amount of depression will depend on the dose of the drug, the route and time of administration before delivery, and the presence of obstetric complications.

The systemic drugs administered during labor may be classified into five broad groups:

1. *Sedative-tranquilizers* are generally used during the first stage of labor, either alone or in combination with a narcotic.

2. *Narcotics* are used to relieve pain during the first and second stages of labor.

3. *Dissociative or amnestic drugs,* such as ketamine or scopolamine, are used infrequently. Ketamine in low subanesthetic doses may be used as an analgesic during the second stage of labor or as an adjunct to regional anesthesia for cesarean section. The use of ketamine as an induction agent for cesarean section is discussed in Chapter 12. Scopolamine has been used as an amnestic drug.

4. *Neuroleptanalgesia* with a drug preparation such as Innovar is not commonly used prior to birth.

5. *Antagonists* are drugs used to reverse possible adverse effects of the above medications.

SEDATIVE-TRANQUILIZERS

The amount of anxiety and fear a woman experiences during labor and delivery can be minimized by proper psychologic preparation and the continuous presence of supportive attendants and a sympathetic husband. In practice, however, many women still require some pharmacologic intervention to reduce their anxiety. Furthermore, these drugs promote sleep, and this hypnotic effect may be especially beneficial in early labor. In addition, all the phenothiazines, as well as drugs such as hydroxyzine and droperidol, are potent antiemetics and will reduce the nausea and vomiting commonly seen during labor.

Barbiturates

The use of short- or medium-acting barbiturates such as secobarbital (Seconal), pentobarbital (Nembutal), or amobarbital (Amytal) is no longer popular. These sedative-hypnotic drugs possess no analgesic action and, indeed, may produce an antianalgesic effect (1, 2). In the presence of severe pain, administration of these drugs may result in an excited, disoriented, and unmanageable parturient.

With low doses (secobarbital 50 to 200 mg intramuscularly) there is no significant maternal respiratory depression (3). In larger doses or with the addition of narcotics to smaller doses, barbiturates are associated with respiratory depression and obtundation of protective airway reflexes.

The principal objection to the use of barbiturates in obstetrics is their prolonged depressant effects on the neonate. All the barbiturates rapidly cross the placenta, and equilibrium between mother and fetus is achieved in minutes (Fig. 8.1) (4, 5). Shnider and Moya (6) showed that the addition of secobarbital (100 mg intramuscularly or 200 mg per os) to meperidine (50 to 100 mg intramuscularly) increased the incidence of depressed newborns. High doses of barbiturates alone (600 to 1000 mg) have been reported to produce neonatal somnolence, flaccidity, hypoventilation, and failure to feed for up to 2 days (7). Even with smaller doses, resulting in no apparent clinical depression as ascertained by the Apgar score, the newborn's attention span may be decreased for 2 to 4 days (8).

Currently, the primary indication for the use of barbiturates is as a sedative-hypnotic during the early latent phase of labor when delivery is not anticipated for 12 to 24 hr.

Phenothiazine Derivatives and Hydroxyzine

Promethazine (Phenergan) and propiomazine (Largon) are phenothiazine derivatives that may be useful during labor to relieve anxiety. Chlorpromazine (Thorazine), promazine (Sparine), and pro-

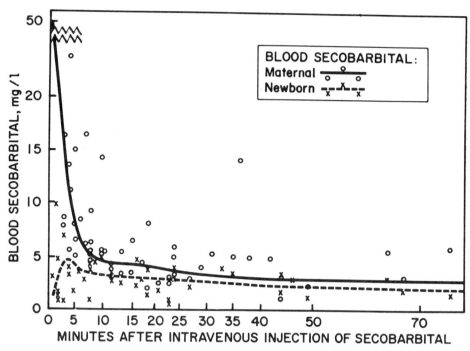

Figure 8.1. Scattergram of blood levels of secobarbital in maternal venous and umbilical cord blood after a single intravenous injection of 250 mg of sodium secobarbital from 1 to 75 min before delivery. Secobarbital crosses the placenta rapidly and the neonatal blood level at delivery is approximately 70% of that in the mother. (Reprinted by permission from Root B, Eichner E, Sunshine I: Blood secobarbital levels and their clinical correlation in mothers and newborn infants. Am J Obstet Gynecol 81:948–956, 1961.)

chlorperazine (Compazine)—also phenothiazine derivatives—are not as popular because they possess greater α-adrenergic blocking properties, resulting in hypotension. Hydroxyzine (Vistaril), although chemically unrelated to the phenothiazines, has similar ataractic properties.

Promethazine, propiomazine, and hydroxyzine seem to be equally effective in relieving anxiety, reducing narcotic requirements, and controlling emesis. Differences between these drugs are relatively minor. Propiomazine has a shorter onset time and duration than promethazine (9). Promethazine is a respiratory stimulant, whereas propiomazine is a mild respiratory depressant. Hydroxyzine has a slight disadvantage in that it cannot be used intravenously.

Despite the rapid placental transfer and decrease in beat-to-beat variability of the fetal heart rate, these drugs in the recommended doses do not seem to cause neonatal depression. For example, Powe et al. (9) compared three intramuscular analgesic regimens: meperidine 50 mg; meperidine 50 mg plus promethazine 50 mg; and meperidine 50 mg plus propiomazine 20 mg. Although increasing the sedation in the mother, the incidence of depressed newborns was not increased by the addition of either tranquilizer to the narcotic. Similarly, hydroxyzine 50 to 100 mg

combined with a narcotic or by itself produced increased tranquility without increased neonatal depression (10–12).

Benzodiazepines

In obstetrics, benzodiazepines may be used as sedatives, narcotic adjuvants, anticonvulsants, and premedicants prior to cesarean sections. These drugs possess anxiolytic, hypnotic, and anticonvulsant, muscle relaxant, and antegrade amnestic effects. Specific benzodiazepine receptors are found throughout the central nervous system. The pharmacologic effects of benzodiazepines have been attributed to an increase in the quantity or facilitation of the effectiveness of the inhibitory neurotransmitters gammaaminobenzoic acid (GABA) and glycine (Fig. 8.2). The glycine-mimetic actions in the spinal cord produce muscle relaxation. Enhanced inhibitory neurotransmitter effects of GABA result in sedation and anticonvulsant activity. The antianxiety effects are likely the result of both glycine- and GABA-mediated inhibition of neuronal pathways in the cortex and brain stem. Diazepam, lorazepam, and midazolam (Fig. 8.3) are the three benzodiazepines clinically used in obstetrics.

DIAZEPAM

Diazepam (Valium) has been most extensively used and studied in obstetrics. The drug rapidly crosses the placenta, and maternal and fetal blood levels are approximately equal within minutes of an intravenous dose (13). Some have reported that at birth fetal blood levels may actually exceed maternal levels (Fig. 8.4) (14–16). Diazepam is metabolized in the liver to a pharmacologically active metabolite, desmethyldiazepam, and to hydroxydiazepam. Diazepam has a half-life of 14 to 90 hr; desmethyldiazepam has a half-life of 30 to 100 hr and undergoes enterohepatic recirculation, which can cause a return of drowsiness 6 to 8 hr later. Although the neonate is capable of metabolizing small doses of diazepam, when the total maternal dosage during labor exceeds 30 mg the drug and its active metabolite persist in pharmacologically active concentrations for at least a week in the neonate (14). When diazepam 0.3 mg/kg intravenously was used for induction of general anesthesia for cesarean delivery, diazepam concentrations in neonates 2 hr after delivery were found to be in the lower range of plasma levels found in adults on daily therapy with diazepam 15 mg (17). The principal adverse effects of large doses of diazepam are hypotonia, lethargy, decreased feeding, and hypothermia (14, 17–20).

In small doses, the authors and other investigators (15) have found minimal fetal and neonatal effects. Although beat-to-beat variability of the fetal heart rate is markedly decreased even with small intravenous doses (5 to 10 mg) (21), there are no adverse effects on fetal or neonatal acid-base or clinical status (15, 22). Small doses (2.5 to 10 mg) of intravenous diazepam used as an antianxiety medication in patients undergoing cesarean section under regional anesthesia (23) did not sedate the newborn—as evidenced by total Apgar scores (Table 8.1)—and did not alter umbilical vein or artery oxygen or acid-base status, but did decrease newborn muscle tone. The Scanlon neurobehavioral examination also showed decreased tone at 4 hr but not at 24 hr of age (Table 8.2).

A theoretical objection to the use of diazepam in obstetrics has been raised by the work of Schiff et al. (24). These investigators found that sodium benzoate, which is used as a buffer in the injectable form of the drug, is a potent bilirubin-albumin uncoupler. The displacement of lipid-soluble bilirubin from its albumin-binding sites would increase the susceptibility of the infant to kernicterus. These workers therefore advised caution in using the drug as a relaxant for infants receiving mechanical intermittent positive pressure respiration or for the control of convulsions in the neonate when serum bilirubin levels are increased. In parturients, only small doses of diazepam are required and would seem very unlikely to cause subsequent problems with bilirubin binding in the neonate (25). Furthermore, the maternal liver should rapidly metabolize the sodium benzoate.

The authors believe that small intravenous doses of diazepam (2.5-mg doses up to a total of 10 mg) can help allay extreme apprehension and anxiety without producing significant adverse fetal or neonatal effects. When larger doses are used, as, for ex-

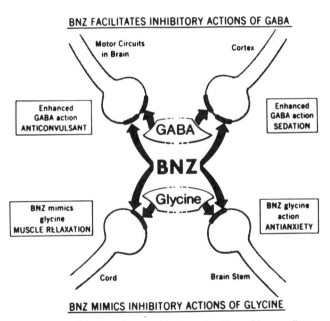

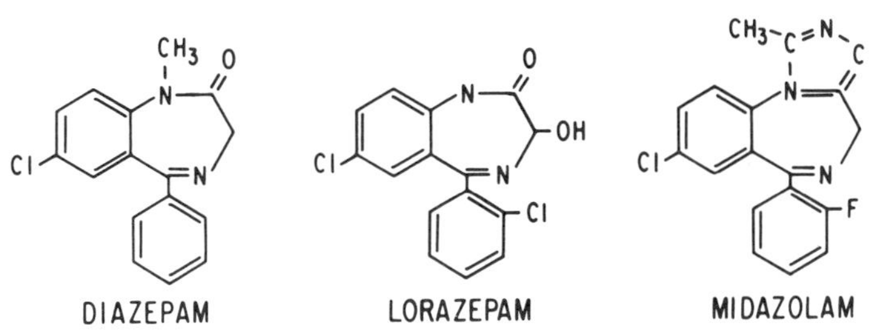

Figure 8.2. Mechanisms and sites of action of benzodiazepines (*BNZ*). (Reprinted by permission from Richter JJ: Current theories about the mechanisms of benzodiazepines and neuroleptic drugs. Anesthesiology 54:66–72, 1981.)

Figure 8.3. Structural formulas of midazolam and two commonly used benzodiazepines, diazepam and lorazepam. Note the fused imidazole ring that distinguishes midazolam from other benzodiazepines. (Reprinted by permission from Reves JG, Fragen RJ, Vinik HR, Greenblatt DJ: Midazolam: Pharmacology and uses. Anesthesiology 62:310–324, 1985.)

DIAZEPAM   LORAZEPAM   MIDAZOLAM

Figure 8.4. Mean plasma concentrations of diazepam and desmethyldiazepam showing cross-over in degradation curves. ○—○, diazepam; ●—●, desmethyldiazepam. (Reprinted by permission from Cree IE, Meyer J, Hailey DM: Diazepam in labour: Its metabolism and effect on the clinical condition and thermogenesis of the newborn. Br Med J 4:251–255, 1973.)

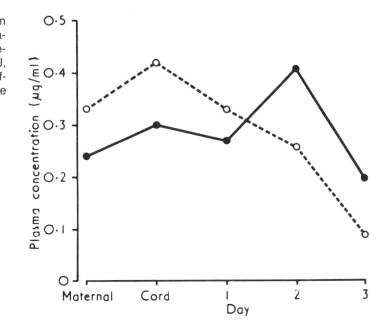

Table 8.1
Diazepam Effect on Newborns after Elective Cesarean Section Epidural Anesthesia[a]

Apgar Score	Without Diazepam (n = 179)	With Diazepam (n = 148)
1–4	1.6%	2.7%
5–7	26.2%	26.3%
8–10	72.2%	71.0%

[a]No significant differences.

ample, in the therapy of preeclampsia-eclampsia, particular care should be taken to maintain a warm environment for the newborn, and these infants should be observed carefully for at least 36 hr after delivery.

LORAZEPAM

Lorazepam is five times as potent as the same dose of diazepam (26). It differs from diazepam in that it has a much shorter half-life and less than 1% of the drug is transformed to other metabolites. Houghton (27) reported that lorazepam 0.05 mg/kg (approximately 3.5 mg) administered intramuscularly 90 min before elective cesarean section produced no measurable antianxiety or amnestic effects in the mother but did produce lower neurobehavioral scores on the Brazelton Neonatal Behavioral Assessment Scale in the neonate. In addition, the neonates had increased respiratory rates for up to 7 days. The drug did not have adverse effects on Apgar scores, neonatal blood gases at 8, 24, and 48 hr after birth, temperature, or feeding patterns. Other studies have demonstrated adverse effects on neonatal feeding after maternal premedication with lorazepam 1 mg per os (28) or

neonatal respiratory depression after lorazepam 2 mg per os (29). It would appear that, despite its short half-life and lack of pharmacologically active metabolites, lorazepam does not offer significant advantages over diazepam in obstetric anesthesia.

MIDAZOLAM

Midazolam differs from other commonly used benzodiazepines in that it is water soluble, has a rapid onset and short duration of action, and can be administered intravenously or intramuscularly without producing pain at the injection site. Similarly to other benzodiazepines, it has anxiolytic, sedative-hypnotic, amnestic, anticonvulsant, and muscle relaxant properties.

Midazolam is approximately 3 to 4 times as potent as diazepam. After intravenous administration first effects are seen immediately and maximum effects are seen by 3 min. Following intramuscular injection effects begin in 5 min and the maximum effects are seen in about 20 min. As with other benzodiazepines, clinically useful doses produce minimal cardiovascular or respiratory changes.

In the pregnant ewe the drug rapidly crosses the placenta but not to the same extent as diazepam (30, 31). Midazolam (5 mg) administered during labor or just prior to cesarean section was associated with lower Apgar scores (32).

One possible drawback to the use of the drug is the anterograde amnesia that is commonly produced. A 5-mg intravenous dose will produce approximately 30 min of amnesia (33). This is usually considered a desirable effect in the surgical patient. In the obstetric patient delivering under regional anesthesia,

Table 8.2
Percentage of Infants with High Scores on the Scanion Neurobehavioral Exam

	4 hr		24 hr	
	No Diazepam ($n = 19$)	Diazepam ($n = 10$)	No Diazepam ($n = 19$)	Diazepam ($n = 10$)
Muscle power and tone				
Pull-to-sitting	63	30	79	60
Arm recoil	58	50	74	50
Truncal tone	42[a]	0[a]	79	60
General tone	84	60	95	90
Reflex				
Rooting reflex	37	50	63	60
Sucking reflex	63	80	68	70
Moro reflex	100[a]	60[a]	79	80
Placing	95	80	84	90
Withdrawal	79	50	89	90
Response decrement				
Pinprick	95	100	100	90
Sound	89	90	95	100
Light	89	90	100	90
Moro	95	100	100	100
Alertness and general assessment				
Alertness	42	60	83	70
General assessment	79	80	94	70

[a]Significant difference between the "no diazepam" and the "diazepam" groups by chi-square test ($P < 0.05$).

full awareness and recall of the birth of the baby is usually highly desirable. Most women wish to recall the entire labor and delivery experience, especially if it is painless. Kanto et al. (33) administered midazolam 0.075 mg/kg (approximately 5 mg) intravenously following delivery of the baby in 11 patients having cesarean sections under epidural anesthesia. This dose of midazolam rapidly produced profound sedation. All the patients remembered the baby being delivered (no retrograde amnesia) but most remembered nothing further until moving to the recovery room.

NARCOTICS

Narcotics are the most effective systemic medication for the relief of pain. Although a wide variety of narcotics are available only a few are used currently in obstetrics. These include morphine, meperidine (Demerol), fentanyl (Sublimaze), butorphanol (Stadol), and nalbuphine (Nubain). Oxymorphone (Numorphan) and anileridine (Leritine) are not widely used in obstetrics because they have no advantages over meperidine and seem to be more depressant to the neonate than other narcotics. Alphaprodine (Nisentil) is no longer available (34, 35).

No narcotic currently available can produce effective analgesia without some respiratory depression. Complete analgesia for labor and delivery cannot be achieved in most parturients without also producing severe hypoventilation, obtundation of reflexes, and postural hypotension. Therefore narcotics are used to reduce pain rather than completely eliminate it. Because all narcotics in appropriate doses produce comparable pain relief, the choice of drug depends on potential maternal and neonatal side effects and the desired onset and duration of action.

Respiratory depression is the most significant side effect of narcotic administration. In equianalgesic doses most narcotics probably produce a comparable shift of the carbon dioxide response curve to the right. Some narcotics, such as fentanyl (36) and alphaprodine (37), may produce an extremely rapid, transient shift in the response curve. The peak respiratory depression of these narcotics may be of much greater magnitude than equianalgesic doses of other narcotics. Usually, serious problems do not occur with small doses of fentanyl and alphaprodine because of the short duration of the respiratory depression, but apnea may occasionally occur even with therapeutic doses (Fig. 8.5).

Another potentially serious side effect of all narcotics is orthostatic hypotension resulting from peripheral vasodilation (38). When the usual analgesic doses of narcotics are administered to parturients in the horizontal position, maternal blood pressure, heart rate, and rhythm are unaffected. However, if these patients are allowed to ambulate or sit up or are moved too vigorously, severe hypotension with maternal and

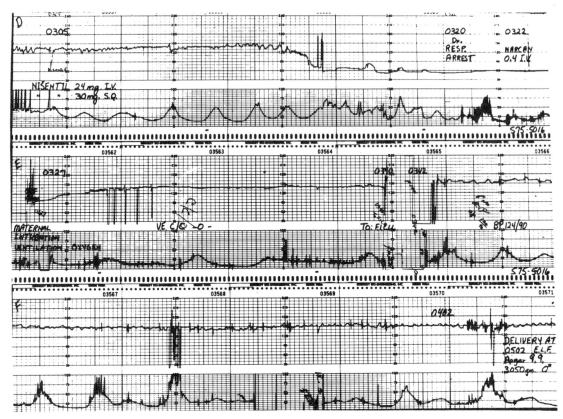

Figure 8.5. Continuous fetal heart rate monitor strip from a patient who received Nisentil intravenously and subcutaneously. Ten minutes after medication a sustained fetal bradycardia developed and maternal respiratory arrest was noted shortly thereafter. The mother was treated with Narcan, endotracheal intubation, and controlled ventilation with 100% oxygen. Fetal heart rate rapidly improved, and a vigorous neonate was delivered 2 hr later. (Labor record provided by RH Paul, MD, University of Southern California, Los Angeles.)

fetal distress may develop. Frequent monitoring of blood pressure is mandatory.

Narcotics produce nausea and vomiting probably by direct stimulation of the chemoreceptor trigger zone in the medulla. The emetic effects are dose related, and equianalgesic doses of the commonly used narcotics usually produce equal amounts of nausea and vomiting. However, some patients seem to be more sensitive to nausea with some narcotics than with others.

Although narcotics usually stimulate smooth muscle, gastric motility is decreased. During active labor, meperidine 100 mg and scopolamine 0.4 mg have been reported to produce retention of 20 to 43% of a test meal at 3 hr and 12 to 37% at 5 hr (39).

During the latent or early stages of labor, narcotics, like all analgesic agents, may decrease uterine activity, slow cervical dilation, and retard the progress of labor (40). Once labor is well established narcotics have been reported to shorten labor and correct incoordinate uterine contractions (41, 42). The mechanism of these effects seems to be related to relief of anxiety and pain rather than direct action on uterine

muscle. Low spinal anesthesia also exerts these actions.

All narcotics are rapidly transferred across the placenta (43–45) and are capable of producing neonatal respiratory depression and changes in neurobehavioral status. With most narcotics the maximum neonatal depression of Apgar scores occurs in newborns delivered 2 to 3 hr after maternal intramuscular administration (6, 46, 47). Drug absorption from traditional intramuscular injection sites may be altered during labor. Plasma levels after deltoid injection are higher than those after gluteus injection (Fig. 8.6) (48).

Meperidine (Demerol)

Meperidine is the most popular narcotic currently used in obstetrics. The usual dosage is 50 to 100 mg intramuscularly or 25 to 50 mg intravenously. The peak analgesic effect occurs 40 to 50 min after intramuscular and 5 to 10 min after intravenous administration. The duration of action is 3 to 4 hr.

The placental transfer and the fetal and neonatal effects of this drug have been studied extensively.

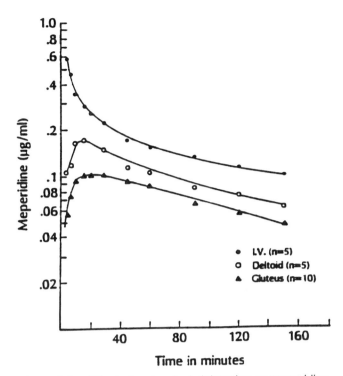

Figure 8.6.   Effect of route of administration on meperidine levels during labor. Gluteus versus intravenous curves are significantly different (F[1.8] = 10.53; P < 0.01). Gluteus versus deltoid curves are significantly different (F[1.8] = 9.7; P < 0.02). (Reprinted by permission from Lazebnik N, Kuhnert BR, Carr PC, Brashear WT, Syracuse CD, Mann LI: Intravenous, deltoid, or gluteus administration of meperidine during labor? Am J Obstet Gynecol 160:1184–1189, 1989.)

Meperidine reaches the fetal circulation within 90 sec of intravenous administration to the mother, and the fetal and maternal concentrations achieve equilibrium within 6 min (Fig. 8.7) (49). In most studies, at delivery maternal and umbilical cord blood levels are similar (50, 51).

The effects of meperidine on the fetus include altered electroencephalogram (52), decreased or arrested respiratory movements (53), and decreased beat-to-beat variability (54). The effect of meperidine on fetal blood pressure, heart rate, arterial oxygen, and acid-base status has been studied in pregnant ewes. Intravenous injections of small doses to the mother did not affect these variables (55).

Maternally administered meperidine may produce neonatal depression as evidenced by prolonged time to sustained respirations, decreased Apgar scores (6), lower oxygen saturation (56), decreased minute volume (47), respiratory acidosis (57), and abnormal neurobehavioral examinations (58, 59). These effects are related to the dose and to the time interval between maternal administration and delivery of the infant. Shnider and Moya (6) studied a group of parturients with no medical or obstetric complications. If meperidine was given within 1 hr of birth, there was no statistically significant difference in the incidence of depressed babies compared with a control, unmedicated group (Fig. 8.8). This was found even when the mother received up to 100 mg of drug.

Figure 8.7.   Plasma levels of meperidine at delivery after maternal intravenous administration of 50 mg at various intervals from 30 sec to 4 hr before delivery. (From data in Shnider SM, Way EL, Lord MJ: Rate of appearance and disappearance of meperidine in fetal blood after administration of narcotic to the mother. Anesthesiology 27:227–228, 1966.)

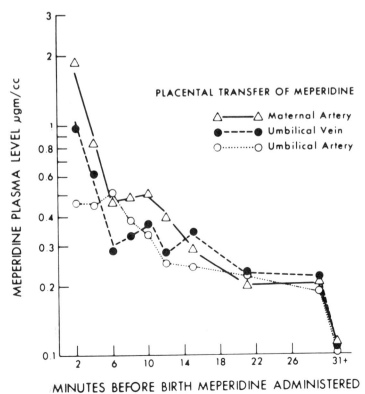

PLACENTAL TRANSFER OF MEPERIDINE

△——△ Maternal Artery
●----● Umbilical Vein
○·······○ Umbilical Artery

MINUTES BEFORE BIRTH MEPERIDINE ADMINISTERED

Figure 8.8. Correlation of the time of administration of meperidine and neonatal depression according to Apgar scores. (Reprinted by permission from Shnider SM, Moya F: Effects of meperidine on the newborn infant. Am J Obstet Gynecol 89:1009–1015, 1964.)

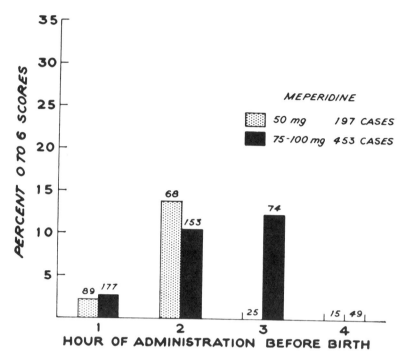

However, there was a significant increase in the percentage of depressed babies born during the second hour after drug administration. This was true even if mothers had received only 50 mg of meperidine. Increased doses tended to prolong the period in which significant neonatal depression was observed. The addition of a barbiturate not only prolonged the period but also increased the percentage of neonatal depression (Fig. 8.9).

The reason for the delay in the appearance of neonatal depression is unclear. One possibility is delayed uptake of drug after intramuscular administration. Another may be the presence of a pharmacologically active metabolite rather than the parent compound. Using a nonspecific colorimetric assay, Morrison et al. (60, 61) reported that, after intravenous administration of meperidine to pregnant women, there were three distinct types of metabolic patterns. Neonatal depression was associated with two of these patterns in which high and prolonged blood levels of unidentified metabolites were found. Of the known metabolites of meperidine only normeperidine is known to be a central nervous system depressant. Kuhnert et al. (62) reported that normeperidine levels in umbilical cord blood were highest 4 hr or more after administration of a single intravenous dose of meperidine to the mother. However, Freeman et al. (63) have shown that normeperidine levels in umbilical cord blood are unrelated to the time from maternal administration of meperidine to the delivery of the baby.

It is likely that the reason for the apparent safe period after a maternal administration of meperidine relates to the quantity of drug transferred across the placenta during the first hour after administration. Kuhnert et al. (62, 64, 65), using a very sensitive gas chromatography and mass spectrometry technique, measured the concentrations of meperidine and normeperidine in umbilical cord venous and arterial plasma at delivery and in the urine of the neonate for 3 days postpartum following administration of 50 mg intravenously to the mother. The amount of meperidine and normeperidine in the cord vein reflects the amount of drug that reaches the fetus following its dilution in the mother and transfer across the placenta. The difference between the umbilical cord vein drug level, at birth, and the umbilical cord artery level, at birth, reflects the amount of drug being taken up by fetal tissue. The urine drug level gives an indirect measure of the fetal tissue drug level and provides a rough estimate of the total amount of drug taken up by the fetus.

The investigators found that as the time from administration of the drug to delivery (drug-delivery interval [DDI]) increased, the level of meperidine in both cord vein and artery decreased. With a short DDI the cord vein levels were higher than cord artery levels, indicating fetal tissue uptake. With longer DDIs umbilical artery levels equaled or exceeded venous levels, indicating excretion of the drug across the placenta. Measurements of neonatal urine levels of meperidine indicated that fetal exposure to the drug

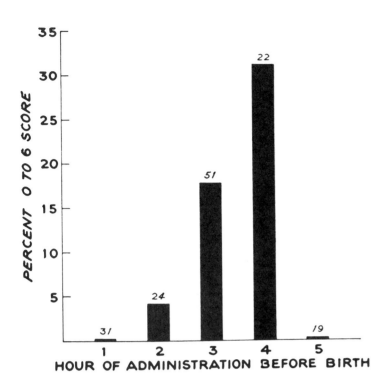

Figure 8.9. Correlation of the time of administration of meperidine-secobarbital and neonatal depression according to Apgar scores. (Reprinted by permission from Shnider SM, Moya F: Effects of meperidine on the newborn infant. Am J Obstet Gynecol 89:1009–1015, 1964.)

is highest 2 to 3 hr after administration of the narcotic to the mother. Neonates born to mothers who received meperidine 2 to 3 hr prior to delivery excreted the greatest amount of drug (Fig. 8.10). Those infants whose mothers had shorter or longer DDIs excreted significantly less drug, indicating that maximal fetal tissue uptake of meperidine occurs 2 to 3 hr following maternal administration. In contrast to meperidine, Kuhnert et al. found that cord blood levels of normeperidine increased with increases in the DDI and that the metabolite reached its highest level in fetal tissues with the longest DDIs (Fig. 8.11). Thus, meperidine reaches a peak in neonatal tissues at a 2 to 3 hr DDI and normeperidine reaches a peak much later.

Neonatal depression after meperidine may be prolonged. Oxygen saturation is significantly depressed for at least 30 min after birth in full-term babies of mothers who receive 100 mg of meperidine 2 to 4 hr before birth (56). Neonatal hypercapnea may persist for up to 5 hr (57). Depression of habituation to an auditory stimulus as well as other subtle neurobehavioral changes are directly proportional to the dose of meperidine (50 to 150 mg) given to the mother and have been found to be present 20 to 60 hr after birth (58, 59, 65). Kuhnert et al. showed that the longest DDIs resulted in the poorest scores on the Brazelton Neonatal Behavioral Assessment Scale (Fig.

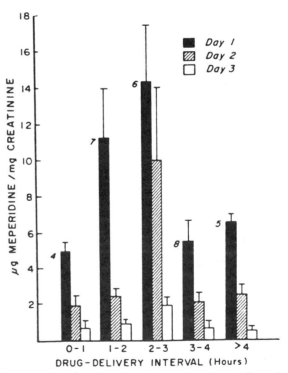

Figure 8.10. Relationship between the drug-delivery interval and the urinary excretion of meperidine by the neonate. (Reprinted by permission from Kuhnert BR, Kuhnert PM, Tu AL, Lin DCK: Meperidine and normeperidine levels following meperidine administration during labor. II. Fetus and neonate. Am J Obstet Gynecol 133:909–914, 1979.)

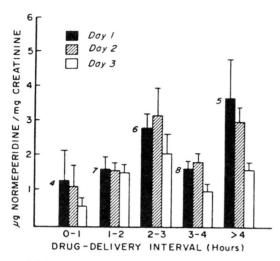

Figure 8.11.   Relationship between the drug-delivery interval and the urinary excretion of normeperidine by the neonate. (Reprinted by permission from Kuhnert BR, Kuhnert PM, Tu AL, Lin DCK: Meperidine and normeperidine levels following meperidine administration during labor. II. Fetus and neonate. Am J Obstet Gynecol 133:909–914, 1979.)

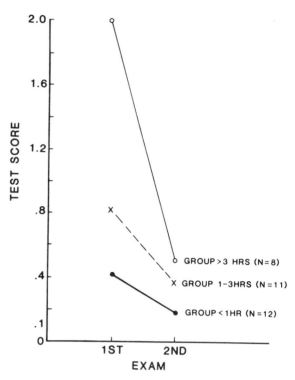

Figure 8.12.   The relationship between the drug-delivery interval and the mean number of abnormal reflexes in the meperidine group. (Reprinted by permission from Kuhnert BR, Linn PL, Kennard MJ, Kuhnert PM: Effects of low doses of meperidine on neonatal behavior. Anesth Analg 64:335–342, 1975.)

8.12) at both 12 hr and 3 days of age. Their results suggest that the poorer neonatal neurobehavioral test scores are due to normeperidine. **It would appear, therefore, that the acute neonatal effects of maternal administration of meperidine, as manifested by decreased Apgar scores, are due to high tissue levels of meperidine, whereas the more subtle and prolonged effects of neurobehavior are due to normeperidine.** It should be emphasized that the statistically significant differences in neurobehavioral examination scores were so slight as to be of doubtful clinical significance (66), although they are useful in elucidating pharmacologic mechanisms.

The elimination half-life of meperidine in the newborn has been reported to be between 13 (67) and 23 hr (68). The neonate will excrete meperidine for 3 to 6 days. The half-life of normeperidine is 62 hr, and doubtless it is present for even longer periods than meperidine (65). In a study in rhesus monkeys, administration of 2 mg/kg IV meperidine (or two such doses 4 hours apart) during labor produced respiratory depression (<60/min) in three out of eight newborns (69). The greatest respiratory depression occurred in newborns with the highest plasma levels of meperidine and normeperidine. In contrast to humans, in this monkey study plasma normeperidine concentrations were more closely associated with respiratory depression than were meperidine concentrations. They also found the normeperidine/meperidine ratios in the monkeys were considerably higher than in humans.

These same investigators performed neurobehavioral evaluations in neonatal monkeys exposed to narcotic analgesics during labor through their dams (70). Infants exposed to meperidine (2 mg/kg maternal dose) or alfentanil (0.1 mg/kg maternal dose) were compared with controls whose dams received no analgesic. Drug-exposed infants showed neurobehavioral effects over the first 3 days of life, including depressed respiration (at birth), depressed environmental response to aversive stimuli (days 0, 1, and 2), more overnight sleep (day 1), and more quiet behavior patterns while awake (day 30). In addition, drug exposure was associated with increased elicited muscle tone early in the neonatal period and earlier maturation of sitting, standing, and walking. Plots of daily weight over the first 2 weeks of life suggest more rapid growth in meperidine- or alfentanil-exposed infants than in controls from days 4 to 9 of life. Differences in activity and maturity were no longer apparent at the second-week test (day 10 of life).

Morphine

Morphine is no longer popular in obstetrics. When used it is usually administered in doses of 5 to 10 mg intramuscularly or 2 to 3 mg intravenously. The peak analgesic effect is 1 to 2 hr after intramuscular administration and 20 min after intravenous administration. The duration of action is 4 to 6 hr. In equianalgesic doses morphine produces more respiratory depression of the newborn than does meperidine (Fig. 8.13) (71).

Because of the delayed onset and prolonged duration of action in the mother, coupled with the greater sensitivity of the newborn's respiratory center to morphine, meperidine has replaced morphine as an obstetric analgesic.

Fentanyl (Sublimaze)

Fentanyl is a rapid-acting narcotic analgesic with properties similar to those of morphine. Fentanyl 100 μg is equianalgesic to morphine 10 mg. The usual doses are 50 to 100 μg intramuscularly and 25 to 50 μg intravenously. Intravenously administered fentanyl produces analgesia almost immediately; the peak effect follows within 3 to 5 min, and the duration of action is 30 to 60 min. After intramuscular administration analgesia begins in 7 to 8 min, peaks at about 30 min, and lasts 1 to 2 hr.

The placental transfer and fetal and neonatal effects of fentanyl have been studied (72–84). As would be expected, fentanyl is detectable in fetal blood as early as 1 min after maternal administration (Fig. 8.14; Table 8.3). There are no adverse effects on uterine tone or blood flow (74).

Eisele et al. administered fentanyl 1 μg/kg intravenously just prior to cesarean delivery (72). As shown in Table 8.3, there was a rapid peak and decline of fentanyl resembling that of thiopental. As compared

with a control group of babies, fentanyl did not produce adverse effects on Apgar scores, umbilical cord blood gases, or neurobehavioral scores (Fig. 8.15). If the babies with higher concentrations of fentanyl were compared with the babies with lower concentrations (Fig. 8.16), minimal differences were found at 4 hr but not 24 hr. The authors concluded that fentanyl might be a useful adjuvant for either regional or general anesthesia for cesarean delivery. Use of fentanyl for intrapartum labor analgesia has also been studied (75, 76). In a prospective study a total of 137 women with uncomplicated term pregnancies were offered a standard intravenous dose (50 μg or 100 μg hourly

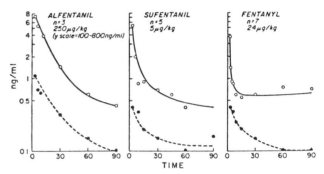

Figure 8.14. Washout curves from maternal (*solid line*) and fetal (*dashed line*) serum narcotic concentrations following an intravenous bolus of alfentanil 250 μg/kg (*left panel*), sufentanil 5 μg/kg (*center panel*), and fentanyl 24 μg/kg (*right panel*). Study was done on awake term pregnant sheep. (Reprinted by permission from Eisele JH: The use of short acting narcotics in obstetric anesthesia and the effects on the newborn. In *Opioids in Anesthesia.* FG Estafanous, ed. Butterworth, Boston, 1984, p 102.)

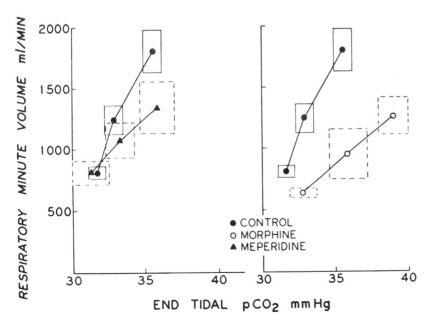

Figure 8.13. Effect of equianalgesic doses of morphine and meperidine on the CO_2 response curve in the newborn. The standard error of the means is indicated by the *rectangles* about each *point.* (Reprinted by permission from Way WL, Costley EC, Way EL: Respiratory sensitivity of the newborn infant to meperidine and morphine. Clin Pharmacol Ther 6:454–461, 1965.)

Table 8.3
Newborn and Maternal Concentration of Fentanyl[a]

Time (min)	Newborn (ng/ml)	Maternal (ng/ml)	Fetal-Maternal Ratio (ng/ml)
1	0.47	3.03	0.16
2	2.00	4.70	0.43
3	1.20	3.24	0.37
4	1.18	6.63	0.18
5	0.70	6.19	0.11
6	1.19	3.08	0.38
7	0.76	1.93	0.39
8	0.50	1.51	0.33
9	0.72	1.98	0.36
10	0.30	1.09	0.28
15	0.09	1.59	0.06

[a]Reprinted by permission from Eisele JH, Wright R, Rogge P: Newborn and maternal fentanyl levels at cesarean section. Anesth Analg 61:179–180, 1982.

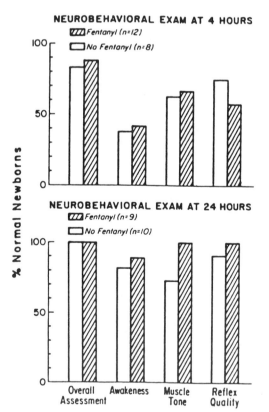

Figure 8.15. Neurobehavioral examination at 4 hr (*top*) and 24 hr (*bottom*) comparing newborns of mothers receiving fentanyl or no fentanyl at cesarean section. The percentage of newborns having normal scores is shown for each of four categories: overall assessment, awakeness, muscle tone, and reflex quality. (Reprinted by permission from Eisele JH: The use of short acting narcotics in obstetric anesthesia and the effects on the newborn. In *Opioids in Anesthesia*. FG Estafanous, ed. Butterworth, Boston, 1984, p 103.)

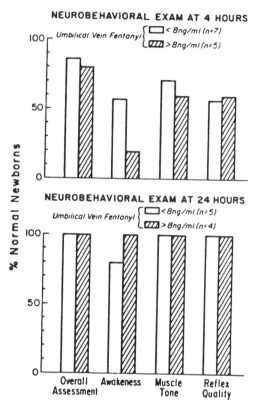

Figure 8.16. Neurobehavioral examination at 4 hr (*top*) and 24 hr (*bottom*) comparing newborns with umbilical cord fentanyl concentrations less than and more than 0.8 ng/ml at delivery. The percentage of newborns having normal scores is shown for each of four categories: overall assessment, awakeness, muscle tone, and reflex quality. (Reprinted by permission from Eisele JH: The use of short acting narcotics in obstetric anesthesia and the effects on the newborn. In *Opioids in Anesthesia*. FG Estafanous, ed. Butterworth, Boston, 1984, p 103.)

as needed) of fentanyl citrate during active labor (75). Temporary analgesia and mild sedation were apparent in each case. The cumulative dose varied in accordance with maternal needs (mean 140 ± 42 μg; range, 50 μg to 600 μg); but as seen in Figure 8.17, many women received multiple injections and relatively large cumulative doses. Regardless of the maternal dose, newborn drug levels were low and always less than maternal levels (Fig. 8.18).

Butorphanol (Stadol) and Nalbuphine (Nubain)

These drugs are two of the new synthetic agonist-antagonist narcotic analgesics. The major advantage reputed to these drugs is the ceiling effect for respiratory depression. In nonpregnant patients, analgesic doses of butorphanol (2 mg) and nalbuphine (10 mg) produce respiratory depression equivalent to 10 mg of morphine. However, whereas larger doses of mor-

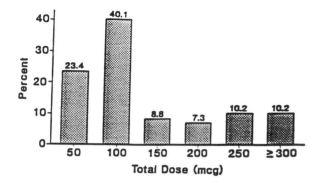

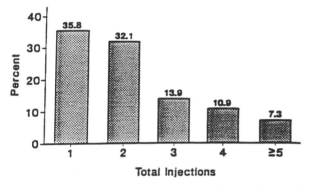

Figure 8.17. Fentanyl citrate use according to the number of injections and total cumulative dose. (Reprinted by permission from Rayburn W, Rathke A, Leuschen P, Chleborad J, Weidner W: Fentanyl citrate analgesia during labor. Am J Obstet Gynecol 161:202–206, 1989.)

phine produce more respiratory depression, increasing doses of butorphanol and nalbuphine do not (77) (Fig. 8.19). The proposed explanation for this ceiling effect is that they are primarily strong κ- and σ-agonists and weak μ-antagonists (see Chapter 10). The potential advantage of this ceiling effect on respiratory depression is usually not clinically significant in obstetric practice because of the comparable ceiling effect on analgesia.

Maduska and Hajghassemali (78) compared butorphanol 1 or 2 mg intramuscularly with meperidine (40 or 80 mg intramuscularly) as analgesics during labor and found them equally effective and safe for the neonate. Placental transfer of butorphanol was equivalent to meperidine, that is fetal-maternal serum drug concentration ratios were approximately the same. Hodgkinson et al. (79) studied the same doses of the drugs but administered them intravenously and also found them to be comparable, including having similar minimal neurobehavioral effects at 4 and 24 hr of age. Quilligan et al. (80) in a similar study reported that intravenous butorphanol (1 mg) produced greater analgesia at 30 min than meperidine 40 mg.

Nalbuphine is usually considered to be equipotent to morphine on a milligram-per-milligram basis. After intravenous administration to the mother in labor, measurement of umbilical cord blood nalbuphine concentrations demonstrated that nalbuphine crossed the placenta and entered the fetal circulation (81).

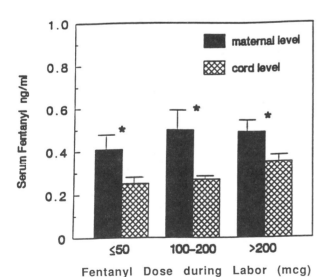

Figure 8.18. Maternal and cord serum fentanyl citrate concentrations at delivery according to maternal dose during labor (*P < 0.03; bars = SEM). (Reprinted by permission from Rayburn W, Rathke A, Leuschen P, Chleborad J, Weidner W: Fentanyl citrate analgesia during labor. Am J Obstet Gynecol 161:202–206, 1989.)

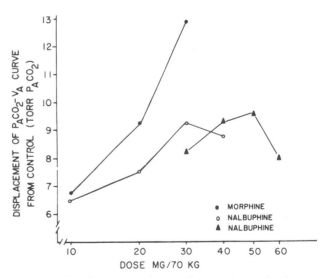

Figure 8.19. Dose-effect for respiratory depression by cumulative doses of morphine (●) and nalbuphine (○) in 8 subjects. Data of larger doses of nalbuphine (▲) were obtained from an additional 10 subjects who did not receive morphine. Abscissa is log scale. (Reprinted by permission from Romagnoli A, Keats AS: Ceiling effect for respiratory depression by nalbuphine. Clin Pharmacol Ther 27:478–485, 1980.)

Newborn concentrations varied substantially, ranging from one-third to six times the simultaneous maternal concentration. The effectiveness and safety of nalbuphine administered via the patient-controlled analgesia system were investigated in 82 parturients during labor (82). Comparison of nalbuphine via the patient-controlled system with 66 control patients receiving the same drug via intermittent intravenous bolus injection revealed it to be safe and effective in both cases. Complications from nalbuphine administration are rare, although a persistent sinusoidal heart pattern appearing after nalbuphine administration has been reported (83), as it has been for butorphanol (84).

The main side effects associated with both butorphanol and nalbuphine are drowsiness and dizziness. As with other narcotics, some patients complain of weakness, nausea, diaphoresis, and a sense of floating. They can cause psychotomimetic effects, but not as severe as with pentazocine. Butorphanol, but not nalbuphine, may increase mean pulmonary artery pressure, pulmonary capillary wedge pressure, mean aortic pressure, pulmonary vascular resistance, and myocardial work (85).

Pentazocine (Talwin)

Pentazocine is an older synthetic analgesic that, like nalbuphine and butorphanol, possesses both agonistic action and weak opioid antagonistic activity. Pentazocine is usually administered in doses of 20 to 30 mg intramuscularly or 10 to 20 mg intravenously. Analgesia occurs within 10 to 20 min after intramuscular administration or 2 to 3 min after intravenous administration. The duration of action is 3 to 4 hr.

The side effects of pentazocine, including respiratory depression and delayed gastric emptying, are similar to those of other narcotics. Possible advantages include less postural hypotension, nausea, and vomiting (45, 86). With doses above 60 mg, psychotomimetic effects—such as nightmares, hallucinations, and bizarre thoughts—have been reported (87). Pentazocine rapidly crosses the placenta. Within 10 min of intravenous administration fetal blood levels are approximately two-thirds of maternal levels. Compared to meperidine there do not seem to be any significant differences in neonatal depression with equianalgesic doses of pentazocine (45, 86–88).

DISSOCIATIVE OR AMNESTIC DRUGS

Ketamine (Ketalar, Ketaject)

Intramuscular or intravenous administration of ketamine produces a state referred to as "dissociative anesthesia," which is characterized by intense an-

algesia with only superficial sleep. In obstetrics the drug may be used in lieu of thiopental as an induction agent for general anesthesia (1 mg/kg) or in very small doses (0.25 mg/kg) in lieu of inhalation analgesia as a systemic analgesic in the awake parturient.

In both dose ranges the drug produces minimal respiratory depression and usually increases arterial blood pressure 10 to 25%. Undesirable hypertension may occur, and the drug should not be given to patients with high blood pressure. In low doses, maternal ketamine does not depress the neonate (Fig. 8.20).

Ketamine in intermittent intravenous doses of 10 to 15 mg can be titrated to produce intense maternal analgesia without loss of consciousness (89). Onset of action is less than 30 sec, and recovery is rapid (4 min), as evidenced by orientation to time, place, and person. Undesirable hallucinations are minimal, especially if the anesthesiologist provides pleasant verbal reassurance and encouragement.

Low-dose ketamine is particularly useful for parturients in whom imminent vaginal delivery of the fetus is expected or for parturients with spotty regional analgesia for either vaginal delivery or cesarean section. After the initial dose the patient should remain awake and responsive, and the dose may be repeated at intervals of 2 to 5 min. The total dose should not exceed 100 mg over a 30-min period. Amnesia for delivery is common and may be undesirable. A suggested technique is described in Table 8.4.

Scopolamine (Hyoscine)

Scopolamine, like atropine, is a belladonna derivative with vagolytic action. The drug, producing inhibition of acetylcholine at muscarinic and nicotinic receptor sites, results in decreased salivary secretions and gastric motility (94). Placental transfer is rapid; after intravenous administration (0.3 to 0.6 mg) fetal tachycardia and loss of beat-to-beat variability are produced within 10 to 25 min and last 60 to 90 min (95, 96). Unlike atropine, scopolamine crosses the blood-brain barrier and produces profound amnesia and mild sedation, presumably by its anticholinergic actions in the central nervous system (97). Amnesia does not occur until at least 20 min after intravenous administration. Scopolamine does not possess analgesic properties and, like most sedatives, will result in severe agitation, marked excitement, and loss of inhibitions in the presence of severe pain. Hallucinations and delirium are common if a parturient in active labor is given scopolamine without adequate narcotics. "Twilight sleep," once a popular analgesic-amnesic technique, consisted of the administration of a single dose of morphine and scopolamine during labor followed by later injections of scopol-

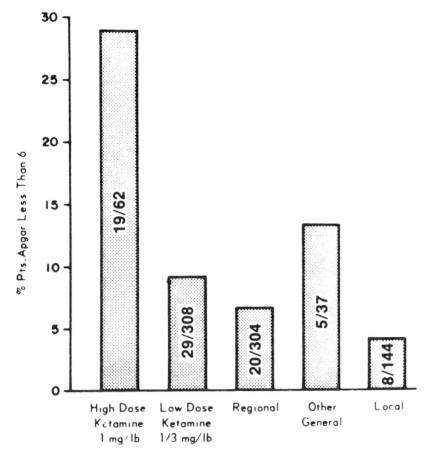

Figure 8.20. Comparison of high-dose and low-dose ketamine anesthesia with regional, local, and other general anesthetics. (Reprinted by permission from Janeczko GF, El-Etr AA, Younes S: Low-dose ketamine anesthesia for obstetrical delivery. Anesth Analg 53:828–831, 1974.)

Table 8.4
Low-Dose Ketamine Analgesia: A Suggested Technique

1. Administer 15 to 30 ml of antacid.
2. Check blood pressure.
3. Administer an initial dose of ketamine (10 to 15 mg), not to exceed 0.25 mg/kg.
4. Maintain continuous verbal contact with patient to provide reassurance and monitor her sensorium.
5. If necessary, give additional 10- to 15-mg doses of ketamine every 2 to 5 min, up to a maximum total dose of 100 mg.

amine only. Maternal amnesia for labor and delivery was intense, neonatal narcotic depression was common, and the parturient was difficult to manage. Scopolamine per se has no adverse effects on the progress of labor or significant respiratory depressant effects on the neonate (7).

The authors believe that scopolamine has little place as a sedative during labor, because maternal amnesia is no longer desired by most parturients. No good data exist to prove that scopolamine, when used as a premedicant prior to general anesthesia for cesarean section, decreases the incidence of maternal awareness for the operation.

NEUROLEPTANALGESIA

The state of psychic indifference to environmental stimuli produced by the combination of a major tranquilizer with a potent narcotic is known as neuroleptanalgesia. The most popular mixture of this type, Innovar, consists of droperidol (Inapsine) 2.5 mg/ml and fentanyl 0.05 mg/ml. Droperidol is a potent, long-acting tranquilizer with little or no direct effect on respiration, heart rate, myocardial contractile force, or cardiac output. It is an adrenergic blocking agent and can cause peripheral vasodilation and hypotention, particularly in hypovolemic patients. Droperidol, like other butyrophenones, may occasionally produce undesirable restlessness and extrapyramidal dyskinesia. Although most of the sedative-tranquilizer drugs possess antiemetic actions, droperidol seems to be vastly superior in this regard. Nausea and vomiting are common in parturients, especially in those receiving narcotics, and the antiemetic activity of droperidol is one of its most attractive properties. Santos and Datta (98) and Edelman et al. (99) have both demonstrated that small doses of droperidol (0.625 mg, 1.25 mg, and 2.5 mg) decrease the incidence of maternal nausea and vomiting during spinal anesthesia for cesarean section. The latter group also looked at neonatal neurobehavioral status at 4, 24, and 48 hr in babies whose mothers received those doses of droperidol and did not find any adverse effects. Fentanyl, the narcotic portion of Innovar, has been discussed previously.

Neuroleptanalgesia for childbirth is not a popular technique because of the potential for profound depressant effects on the newborn. The few studies available have indicated that Innovar probably does not cause more neonatal depression than other narcotic-tranquilizer combinations. For example, Ovadia and Halbrecht (100) administered Innovar for normal vaginal deliveries to 100 women. They gave 3 to 5 ml intramuscularly when the cervix was 4 cm dilated, followed by smaller doses at 30-min intervals if necessary. No medication was given after the cervix was fully dilated. They found that most of the women had considerably less discomfort, were able to sleep quietly between contractions, and were generally more cooperative than patients receiving a Demerol-Phenergan combination. Innovar decreased the duration and frequency of contractions, and almost all their patients received oxytocin or vacuum extraction. All the neonates had Apgar scores greater than 7, and none required any form of resuscitation. The lack of fetal depression was attributed to the short duration of action of fentanyl.

Although a few investigators have used Innovar for cesarean section without adverse maternal or fetal effects, most commonly the droperidol component has been administered during induction and the fentanyl withheld until after the umbilical cord is clamped (101) to avoid neonatal respiratory depression.

ANTAGONISTS

Physostigmine (Antilirium)

Physostigmine is an anticholinesterase agent that, unlike its analogue neostigmine, rapidly crosses the blood-brain barrier and increases central nervous system acetylcholine. It is extremely effective in reversing the delirium and sedation produced by scopolamine and other sedative drugs with anticholinergic activity (102, 103). It is most probably a nonspecific central nervous system stimulant, although some preliminary reports indicated that it may be specifically effective in reversing the sedative effects of diazepam (104), Innovar (105), and ketamine (102). The usual dose is 0.5 to 2 mg intravenously given in 0.5-mg increments. Total doses of 3 to 4 mg are occasionally necessary. The duration of action is 1 to 2 hr. Although bradycardia after physostigmine administration is uncommon, atropine should be readily available.

The drug has been used in obstetrics and found to be a safe and rapidly effective agent for reversing the delirium and somnolence produced by scopolamine. When used prior to delivery it is not associated with fetal bradycardia. The drug will reverse the decreased beat-to-beat variability produced by atropine and scopolamine (96). The clinical condition of newborns of mothers who have received physostigmine does not seen to be adversely affected (102, 103).

Naloxone (Narcan)

Naloxone is currently the preferred narcotic antagonist. Unlike nalorphine (Nalline) and levallorphan (Lorfan) it has no agonist activity and thus produces no cardiorespiratory or central nervous system depression. Narcotic antagonists have been administered in three ways: (a) to the mother with each dose of narcotic, (b) to the mother 10 to 15 min before delivery, and (c) to the neonate immediately after delivery.

The rationale for administering a narcotic and narcotic antagonist simultaneously is to provide maximum analgesia with minimal respiratory depression. Numerous studies have proved (107) that the antagonists will reverse the analgesia as well as the respiratory depression and therefore offer no advantage, except when used in conjunction with spinal opiates (see Chapter 10).

The rationale for administering naloxone just before delivery is to allow placental transfer and intrauterine reversal of narcotic depression in the fetus and neonate (108). Many consider this approach inadvisable, because removal of maternal analgesia immediately before delivery is unfair to the mother, may result in an uncontrollable and difficult delivery, and is usually unnecessary insofar as the neonate is concerned.

The rationale for administering naloxone routinely to all neonates whose mothers have received narcotics within 4 hr of delivery is that even apparently vigorous babies will have some central nervous system depression and alteration of neurobehavioral status (59, 109). The objection to this approach is based on the lack of documentation of long-term safety of naloxone. The short-term safety of naloxone is well documented. Even when administered in excessive doses no adverse effects are found.

However, it has become apparent that opiate receptors and endogenous opioid substances (enkephalins and endorphins) may have a normal physiologic function (110, 111). These compounds may be important neurotransmitters and be involved in hypothalamic-pituitary function and the integration of sensory stimuli. Naloxone acts by displacing narcotics from the receptor sites in the central nervous system and blocks the physiologic effects of enkephalins and endorphins; theoretically, it may adversely influence the neonate's response to stress. Indeed, several investigators, using animal models, have demonstrated that very large doses of naloxone administered directly to the fetus or neonate decreased their ability to respond to asphyxia (112–115). Until further studies are performed the routine administration of naloxone to all neonates is not recommended.

It should be emphasized that adverse neonatal effects of naloxone have never been demonstrated in humans and the drug should not be withheld when indicated. Parturients who receive an absolute or relative overdose of narcotics, as evidenced by obtundation or hypoventilation, should receive naloxone. Depressed infants who have a high probability of being narcotized and do not respond to routine resuscitation with oxygenation, ventilation, and tactile stimulation should also receive naloxone.

In adults the usual initial dose is 0.4 mg intravenously. The neonatal dose is 0.1 mg/kg either intravenously or, if perfusion is good, intramuscularly. Effects are seen within minutes and last 1 to 2 hr. Because of the relatively short duration of naloxone, the narcotically overdosed mother or neonate must be observed carefully and repeat doses of the antagonist administered if necessary. Naloxone should not be used in narcotic addicts or their neonates because acute withdrawal symptoms may be precipitated.

References

1. Clutton-Brock JC: Some pain threshold studies with particular reference to thiopentone. Anaesthesia 15:71–72, 1960.
2. Dundee JW: Alterations in response to somatic pain associated with anaesthesia. II. The effect of thiopentone and pentobarbitone. Br J Anaesth 32:407–414, 1960.
3. Keats AS, Kurosu Y: Increased ventilation after pentobarbital in man. Surv Anesthesiol 1:473–474, 1957.
4. Root B, Eichner E, Sunshine I: Blood secobarbital levels and their clinical correlation in mothers and newborn infants. Am J Obstet Gynecol 81:948–956, 1961.
5. Kosaka Y, Takahashi T, Mark LC: Intravenous thiobarbiturate anesthesia for cesarean section. Anesthesiology 31:489–506, 1969.
6. Shnider SM, Moya F: Effects of meperidine on the newborn infant. Am J Obstet Gynecol 89:1009–1015, 1964.
7. Snyder FF: Obstetric Analgesia and Anesthesia: Their Effects upon Labor and the Child. WB Saunders, Philadelphia, 1949.
8. Irving FC: Advantages and disadvantages of barbiturates in obstetrics. R I Med J 28:493, 1945.
9. Powe CE, Kiem IM, Fromhagen C, Cavanagh D: Propiomazine hydrochloride in obstetrical analgesia. JAMA 181:280–294, 1962.
10. Benson C, Benson RC: Hydroxyzine-meperidine analgesia and neonatal response. Am J Obstet Gynecol 84:37–43, 1962.
11. Brelje MC, Garcia-Bunuel R: Meperidine-hydroxyzine in obstetric analgesia. Obstet Gynecol 27:350–354, 1966.
12. Zsigmond EK, Patterson RL: Double blind evaluation of hydroxyzine hydrochloride in obstetric anesthesia. Anesth Analg 46:275–280, 1967.
13. Cavanagh D, Condo CS: Diazepam: A pilot study of drug concentrations in maternal blood, amniotic fluid and cord blood. Curr Ther Res 6:122–126, 1964.
14. Cree IE, Meyer J, Hailey DM: Diazepam in labour: Its metabolism and effect on the clinical condition and thermogenesis of the newborn. Br Med J 4:251–255, 1973.
15. Scher J, Hailey DM, Beard RW: The effects of diazepam on the fetus. J Obstet Gynaecol Br Commonw 79:635–638, 1972.
16. DeSilva JAF, D'Anconte L, Kaplan J: The determination of blood levels and the placental transfer of diazepam in humans. Curr Ther Res 6:115–121, 1964.
17. Bakkee OM, Haram K, Lygre T, Wallem G: Comparison of the placental transfer of thiopental and diazepam in caesarean section. Eur J Clin Pharmacol 21:221–227, 1981.
18. Flowers CE, Rudolph AJ, Desmond MM: Diazepam (Valium) as an adjunct in obstetric analgesia. Obstet Gynecol 34:68–81, 1969.
19. Shannon RW, Fraser GP, Aitken RG, Harper JR: Diazepam in preeclamptic toxaemia with special reference to its effect on the newborn infant. Br J Clin Pract 26:271–275, 1972.
20. Owen JR, Irani SF, Blair AW: Effect of diazepam administered to mothers during labour on temperature regulation of neonate. Arch Dis Child 47:107–110, 1972.
21. Hon E: An Atlas of Fetal Heart Rate Patterns. Harty Press, New Haven, CT, 1968, p 231.
22. Yeh SY, Paul RH, Cordero L, Hon EH: A study of diazepam during labor. Obstet Gynecol 43:363–373, 1974.
23. Rolbin SH, Wright RG, Shnider SM, Levinson G, Roizen MF, Johnson J, Jones M: Diazepam during cesarean section—Effects on neonatal Apgar scores, acid-base status, neurobehavioral assessment and maternal and fetal plasma norepinephrine levels. In Abstracts of Scientific Papers, American Society of Anesthesiologists, New Orleans, 1977, p 449.
24. Schiff D, Chan G, Stern L: Fixed drug combinations and the displacement of bilirubin from albumin. Pediatrics 48:139–141, 1971.
25. Nathenson G, Cohen MI, McNamara H: The effect of Na benzoate on serum bilirubin of the Gun rat. J Pediatr 86:799–803, 1975.
26. Comer WH, Elliot HW, Nomoff N, Navarro G, Ruelius HW, Knowles JA: Pharmacology of parenterally administered lorazepam in man. J Int Med Res 1:216–225, 1973.
27. Houghton DJ: Use of lorazepam as a premedicant for caesarean section: An evaluation of its effects on the mother and the neonate. Br J Anaesth 55:767–771, 1983.
28. Crawford JS: Premedication for elective caesarean section. Anaesthesia 34:892–897, 1979.
29. McAuley DM, O'Neill MP, Moore J, Dundee JWA: Lorazepam premedication for labour. Br J Obstet Gynaecol 89:149–154, 1982.
30. Conklin KA, Graham CW, Murad S, Randall FM, Katz RL, Cabalum R, Lieb SM, Brinkman CR III: Midazolam and diazepam: Maternal and fetal effects in the pregnant ewe. Obstet Gynecol 56:471–474, 1980.
31. Vree TB, Reekers-Ketting JJ, Fragen RJ, Arts THM: Placental transfer of midazolam and its metabolite 1-hydroxymethylmidazolam in the pregnant ewe. Anesth Analg 63:31–34, 1984.
32. Wilson CM, Dundee W, Moore J, Howard PJ, Collier PS: A comparison of the early pharmacokinetics of midazolam in pregnant and nonpregnant women. Anaesthesia 42:1057–1062, 1987.
33. Kanto J, Aaltonen L, Erkkola R, Aarimaa L: Pharmacokinetics and sedative effect of midazolam in connection with ceasarean section performed under epidural analgesia. Acta Anaesthesiol Scand 28:116–118, 1984.
34. Sentor MH, Solomon E, Kohl SG: An evaluation of oxymorphone in labor. Am J Obstet Gynecol 84:956–961, 1962.
35. Flowers CE: Systemic analgesia and amnesia. In Obstetrical Analgesia and Anesthesia. Harper & Row. New York, 1967, p 76.

36. Downes JJ, Kemp RA, Lambersen CJ: The magnitude and duration of respiratory depression due to fentanyl and meperidine in man. J Pharmacol Exp Therap 158:416–420, 1967.

37. Forrest WH, Bellville JW: Respiratory effects of alphaprodine in man. Obstet Gynecol 31:61–68, 1968.

38. Eckenhoff JE, Oech SR: The effects of narcotics and antagonists upon respiration and circulation in man. Clin Pharmacol Ther 1:483–524, 1960.

39. La Salvia LA, Steffen EA: Delayed gastric emptying time in labor. Am J Obstet Gynecol 59:1075–1081, 1950.

40. Friedman EA: The functional divisions of labor. Am J Obstet Gynecol 109:274–280, 1971.

41. DeVoe SJ, DeVoe K Jr, Rigsby WC, McDaniels BA: Effect of meperidine on uterine contractility. Am J Obstet Gynecol 105:1004–1007, 1969.

42. Filler WW Jr, Hall WC, Filler NW: Analgesia in obstetrics. Am J Obstet Gynecol 98:832–846, 1967.

43. Apgar V, Burns JJ, Brodie BB, Papper EM: Transmission of meperidine across human placenta. Am J Obstet Gynecol 64:1368–1370, 1952.

44. Moya F, Thorndike V: Passage of drugs across the placenta. Am J Obstet Gynecol 84:1778–1798, 1962.

45. Moore J, Carson RM, Hunter RJ: A comparison of the effects of pentazocine and pethidine administered during labour. J Obstet Gynaecol Br Commonw 77:830–836, 1970.

46. Shute E, Davis M: The effect on the infant of morphine administered in labor. Surg Gynecol Obstet 57:727, 1933.

47. Roberts H, Kane KM, Percival N, Snow P, Pease NW: Effects of some analgesic drugs used in childbirth. Lancet 1:128, 1957.

48. Lazebnik N, Kuhnert BR, Carr PC, Brashear WT, Syracuse CD, Mann LI: Intravenous, deltoid, or gluteus administration of meperidine during labor? Am J Obstet Gynecol 160:1184–1189, 1989.

49. Shnider SM, Way EL, Lord MJ: Rate of appearance and disappearance of meperidine in fetal blood after administration of narcotic to the mother. Anesthesiology 27:227–228, 1966.

50. Beckett AH, Taylor JF: Blood concentrations of pethidine and pentazocine in mother and infant at time of birth. J Pharm Pharmacol 19:50S–52S, 1967.

51. Moore J, McNabb TG, Glynn JP. The placental transfer of pentazocine and pethidine. Br J Anaesth 45(Suppl):798–801, 1973.

52. Rosen MG, Scibetta JJ, Hochberg CJ: Human fetal electroencephalogram. III. Pattern changes in presence of fetal heart rate alterations and after use of maternal medications. Obstet Gynecol 36:132–140, 1970.

53. Boddy K, Dawes GS: Fetal breathing. Br Med Bull 31:3–7, 1975.

54. Yeh SY, Forsythe A, Hon EH: Quantification of fetal heart beat-to-beat interval differences. Obstet Gynecol 41:355–363, 1973.

55. Jenkins VR II, Dilts PV Jr: Some effects of meperidine hydrochloride on maternal and fetal sheep. Am J Obstet Gynecol 109:1005–1010, 1971.

56. Taylor ES, vonFumetti HH, Essig LL, Goodman SN, Walker LC: The effects of Demerol and trichloroethylene on arterial oxygen saturation in the newborn. Am J Obstet Gynecol 69:348–351, 1955.

57. Koch G, Wandel H: Effect of pethidine on the postnatal adjustment of respiration and acid-base balance. Acta Obstet Gynecol Scand 47:27–37, 1968.

58. Brackbill Y, Kane J, Manniello RL, Abramson D: Obstetric meperidine usage and assessment of neonatal status. Anesthesiology 40:116–120, 1974.

59. Hodgkinson R, Bhatt M, Wang CN: Double blind comparison of the neurobehavior of neonates following administration of different doses of meperidine to the mother. Can Anaesth Soc J 25:405–411, 1978.

60. Morrison JC, Wiser WL, Rosser SI, Gayden JO, Bucovaz ET, Whybrew WD, Fish SA: Metabolites of meperidine related to fetal depression. Am J Obstet Gynecol 115:1132–1137, 1973.

61. Morrison JC, Whybrew WD, Rosser SI, Bucovaz ET, Wiser WL, Fish SA: Metabolites of meperidine in the fetal and maternal serum. Am J Obstet Gynecol 126:997–1002, 1976.

62. Kuhnert BR, Kuhnert PM, Tu AL, Lin DCK: Meperidine and normeperidine levels following meperidine administration during labor. II. Fetus and neonate. Am J Obstet Gynecol 133:909–914, 1979.

63. Freeman DS, Gjika HB, Van Vunakis H: Radioimmunoassay for normeperidine: Studies on the N-dealkylation of meperidine and anileridine. J Pharmacol Exp Therap 203:203–212, 1977.

64. Kuhnert BR, Kuhnert PM, Tu AL, Lin DCK, Foltz RL: Meperidine and normeperidine levels following meperidine administration during labor. I. Mother. Am J Obstet Gynecol 133:904–908, 1979.

65. Kuhnert BR, Kuhnert PM, Prochaska AL, Sokol RJ: Meperidine disposition in mothers, neonate, and nonpregnant females. Clin Pharmacol Ther 27:486–491, 1980.

66. Kuhnert BR, Linn PL, Kennard MJ, Kuhnert PM: Effects of low doses of meperidine on neonatal behavior. Anesth Analg 64:355–342, 1985.

67. Cooper LV, Stephen GW, Aggett PJA: Elimination of pethidine and bupivacaine in the newborn. Arch Dis Child 52:638–641, 1977.

68. Caldwell J, Wakile LA, Notarianni LJ, Smith RL, Correy GJ, Lieberman BA, Beard RW, Finnie MDA, Snedden W: Maternal and neonatal disposition of pethidine in childbirth: A study using quantitative gas chromatography-mass spectrometry. Life Sci 22:589–596, 1978.

69. Golub MS, Eisele JH Jr, Donald JM: Obstetric analgesia and infant outcome in monkeys: Neonatal measures after intrapartum exposure to meperidine of alfentanil. Am J Obstet Gynecol 158:1219–1225, 1988.

70. Golub MS, Eisele JH Jr, Kuhnert BR: Disposition of intrapartum narcotic analgesics in monkeys. Anesth Analg 67:637–643, 1988.

71. Way WL, Costley EC, Way EL: Respiratory sensitivity of the newborn infant to meperidine and morphine. Clin Pharmacol Ther 6:454–461, 1965.

72. Eisele JH Jr, Wright R, Rogge P: Newborn and maternal fentanyl levels at cesarean section. Anesth Analg 61:179–180, 1982.

73. Eisele JH Jr, Goetzman BW, Milstein JM, Bickers RG, Bennett SH, Martucci RW: Brain uptake of fentanyl in fetal lambs. Anesthesiology 57:A398, 1982.

74. Craft JB Jr, Coaldrake LA, Bolan JC, Mondino M, Mazel P, Gilman RM, Shokes LK, Woolf WA: Placental passage and uterine effects of fentanyl. Anesth Analg 62:894–898, 1983.

75. Rayburn W, Rathke A, Leuschen P, Chleborad J, Weidner W: Fentanyl citrate analgesia during labor. Am J Obstet Gynecol 161:202–206, 1989.

76. Rayburn WF, Smith CV, Parriott JE, Woods RE: Randomized comparison of meperidine and fentanyl during labor. Obstet Gynecol 74:604–606, 1989.

77. Gal TJ: Analgesic and respiratory depressant activity of nalbuphine: A comparison with morphine. Anesthesiology 55:367–374, 1982.

78. Maduska AL, Hajghassemali M: A double-blind comparison of butorphanol and meperidine in labour: Maternal pain relief and newborn outcome. Can Anaesth Soc J 25:398–404, 1978.

79. Hodgkinson R, Huff R, Hayashi R, Husain FJ: Double-blind comparison of maternal analgesia and neonatal neurobehaviour following intravenous butorphanol and meperidine. J Int Med Res 7:224–230, 1979.

80. Quilligan E, Keegan KA, Donahue MJ: Double-blind comparison of intravenously injected butorphanol and meperidine in parturients. Int J Gynaecol Obstet 18:363–367, 1980.

81. Wilson ST, Errick JK, Balkon J: Pharmacokinetics of nalbuphine during parturition. Am J Obstet Gynecol 155:340–344, 1986.

82. Podlas J, Breland BD: Patient-controlled analgesia with nalbuphine during labor. Obstet Gynecol 70:202–204, 1989.

83. Feinstein SJ, Lodeiro JG, Vintzileos AM, Campbell WA, Montgomery JT, Nochimson DJ: Sinusoidal fetal heart rate pattern after administration of nalbuphine hydrochloride: A case report. Am J Obstet Gynecol 154:159–160, 1986.
84. Hunt CO, Naulty JS, Malinow AM, Datta S, Ostheimer GW: Epidural butorphanol-bupivacaine for analgesia during labor and delivery. Anesth Analg 68:323–327, 1989.
85. Popio KA, Jackson DH, Ross AM, Schreiner BF, Yu PN: Hemodynamic and respiratory effects of morphine and butorphanol. Clin Pharmacol Ther 23:281–287, 1978.
86. Mowat J, Garrey MM: Comparison of pentazocine and pethidine in labour. Br Med J 2:757–759, 1970.
87. Paddock R, Beer EG, Bellville JW, Ciliberti BJ, Forrest WH Jr, Miller EV: Analgesic and side effects of pentazocine and morphine in a large population of postoperative patients. Clin Pharmacol Ther 10:355–365, 1969.
88. Duncan SLB, Ginsburg J, Morris NF: Comparison of pentazocine and pethidine in normal labor. Am J Obstet Gynecol 105:197–202, 1969.
89. Akamatsu TJ, Bonica JJ, Rehmet R, Eng M, Ueland K: Experiences with the use of ketamine for parturition. I. Primary anesthetic for vaginal delivery. Anesth Analg 53:284–287, 1974.
90. Meer FM, Downing JW, Coleman AJ: An intravenous method of anesthesia for caesarean section. II. Ketamine. Br J Anaesth 45:191–196, 1973.
91. Taylor PA, Towey RM: Depression of laryngeal reflexes during ketamine anaesthesia. Br Med J 2:688–689, 1971.
92. Bovill JG, Dundee JW, Coppell DL, Moore J: Current status of ketamine anaesthesia. Lancet 1:1285–1288, 1971.
93. Dich-Nielsen J, Holasek J: Ketamine as induction agent for caesarean section. Acta Anaesthesiol Scand 26:139–142, 1982.
94. Eger EI II: Atropine, scopolamine and related compounds. Anesthesiology 23:365–383, 1962.
95. Hellman LM, Morton GW, Wallach EE, Tolles WE, Fillisti LP: An analysis of the atropine test for placental transfer in 28 normal gravidas. Am J Obstet Gynecol 87:650–659, 1963.
96. Boehm FH, Smith BE, Egilmez A: Physostigmine's effect on diminished fetal heart rate variability caused by scopolamine. In *Abstracts of Scientific Papers*, Society for Obstetric Anesthesia and Perinatology, Philadelphia, 1975, p 18.
97. Safer DJ, Allen RP: The central effects of scopolamine in man. Biol Psychiatry 3:347–355, 1971.
98. Santos A, Datta S: Prophylactic use of droperidol for control of nausea and vomiting during spinal anesthesia for cesarean section. Anesth Analg 66:85–87, 1984.
99. Edelman C, Karambelkar D, Kennedy R, Vicinie A, McKenzie R: Neonatal effects after maternal prophylactic use of droperidol. In *Abstracts of Scientific Papers*, Society for Obstetric Anesthesia and Perinatology, Washington, DC, 1985, p 48.
100. Ovadia L, Halbrecht I: Neuroleptanalgesia: A new method of anesthesia for normal childbirth. Harefuah 72:143–145, 1967.
101. McGowan SW: Droperidol in obstetric practice. In *The Application of Neuroleptanalgesia in Anesthetic and Other Practice*. NW Shepard, ed. Pergamon Press, New York, 1965, p 69.
102. Smiler BG, Bartholomew EG, Sivak BV, Alexander GD, Brown EM: Physostigmine reversal of scopolamine delirium in obstetric patients. Am J Obstet Gynecol 116:326–329, 1973.
103. Smith DB, Clark RB, Stephens SR, Sherman RL, Hyde ML: Physostigmine reversal of sedation in parturients. Anesth Analg 55:478–480, 1976.
104. Larson GF, Hurlbert BJ, Wingard DW: Physostigmine reversal of diazepam induced depression. Anesth Analg 56:348–351, 1977.
105. Bidwai AV, Cornelius CR, Stanley TH: Reversal of Innovar-induced postanesthetic somnolence and disorientation with physostigmine. Anesthesiology 44:249–252, 1976.
106. Balmer HGR, Wyte SR: Antagonism of ketamine by physostigmine. Br J Anaesth 49:510, 1977.
107. Telford J, Keats AS: Narcotic-narcotic antagonist mixtures. Anesthesiology 22:465–484, 1961.
108. Clark RB: Transplacental reversal of meperidine depression in the fetus by naloxone. J Arkansas Med Soc 68:128–130, 1971.
109. Gerhardt T, Bancalari E, Cohen H, Rocha LF: Use of naloxone. J Pediatr 90:1009–1012, 1977.
110. Snyder SH: Opiate receptors in the brain. N Engl J Med 296:266–271, 1977.
111. Kosterlitz HW, Hughes J: Possible physiological significance of enkephalin: An endogenous ligand of opiate receptors. Adv Pain Res Therap 1:641, 1976.
112. Goodlin RC: Naloxone administration and newborn rabbit response to asphyxia. Am J Obstet Gynecol 140:340–341, 1981.
113. LaGamma EF, Itskovitz J, Rudolph AM: Effects of naloxone on fetal circulatory responses to hypoxemia. Am J Obstet Gynecol 143:933–940, 1982.
114. Young RSK, Hessert TR, Pritchard GA, Yagel SK: Naloxone exacerbates hypoxic-ischemic brain injury in the neonatal rat. Am J Obstet Gynecol 150:52–56, 1984.
115. Lou HC, Tweed WA, Davies JM: Naloxone reverses preferential brain stem perfusion in neonatal hypoxia. In *Abstracts of Scientific Papers*, Society for Obstetric Anesthesia and Perinatology, Washington, DC, 1985, p 75.

CHAPTER 9

Regional Anesthesia for Labor and Delivery

Sol M. Shnider, M.D.
Gershon Levinson, M.D.
David H. Ralston, M.D.

Regional anesthesia for labor and vaginal delivery has gained widespread use because of its effectiveness and, when properly conducted, its safety. Regional blocks provide analgesia while allowing the parturient to be awake and able to participate in labor and delivery. In contrast to parenteral or general inhalation anesthesia techniques, regional anesthesia decreases the likelihood of fetal drug depression and maternal aspiration pneumonitis. The most common forms of regional anesthesia are spinal, lumbar epidural, caudal, paracervical, pudendal, and local perineal infiltration. Each technique has a specific application and can be used to block some or all of the nerves carrying the pain impulses.

PAIN PATHWAYS

The pain of labor arises primarily from nociceptors in uterine and perineal structures. Nerve fibers transmitting pain sensation during the first stage of labor travel with sympathetic fibers and enter the neuraxis at the 10th, 11th, and 12th thoracic and first lumbar spinal segments (Fig. 9.1). These fibers synapse in, and make connections with, other ascending and descending fibers in the dorsal horn, particularly in lamina V (Figs. 9.2 and 9.3). In late first-stage and second-stage labor, pain impulses increasingly originate from pain-sensitive areas in the perineum and travel via the pudendal nerve to enter the neuraxis at the second, third, and fourth sacral segments. The afferent sensory component of pain can be largely relieved by blockade of the neural pathways at several anatomic sites. A list of regional obstetric anesthetic techniques, with examples of each and relevant anatomy, are given in Table 9.1 and Figures 9.4, 9.5.

MANAGEMENT OF COMPLICATIONS

Before performing any regional block in obstetrics, the physician must be prepared for the management of possible complications. Serious complications are unusual and if properly managed, rarely lead to permanent disability (1). Some of the more life-threatening complications—severe hypotension, local anesthetic convulsions and total spinal anesthesia—are discussed in Chapters 12 and 24.

Any room in which anesthesia is performed should have the following items immediately available before starting the block: apparatus for monitoring blood pressure, oxygen with positive pressure breathing apparatus and mask, suction with a wide-bore suction catheter, oral and nasal airways, a laryngoscope and endotracheal tubes, thiopental or diazepam to stop a convulsion, and ephedrine to treat hypotension. Prior to placing any block an intravenous route should be established. The bed should be capable of being placed in the Trendelenburg (head-down) position rapidly. The suggested contents of a mobile resuscitation cart are listed in Table 9.2. Resuscitation equipment should be checked prior to starting a block.

Hypotension

Hypotension remains the most common side effect of major conduction anesthesia for vaginal delivery (2); it is discussed fully in Chapter 22. The incidence and severity of hypotension depend on the height of the block, maternal position, the physical status of the parturient, and the prophylactic means taken to avoid hypotension. Measures to reduce the incidence of hypotension include administration of fluids prior to the block, left uterine displacement, and prophylactic administration of ephedrine (3–5). If hypotension occurs, more left uterine displacement should

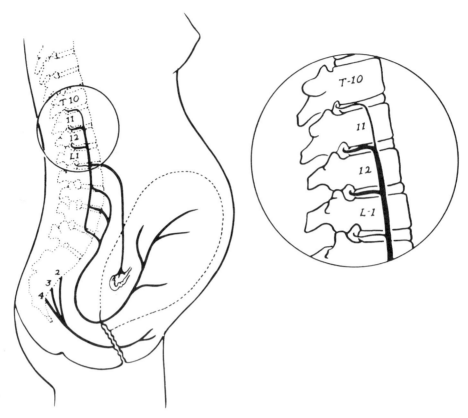

Figure 9.1. Parturition pain pathways. Afferent pain impulses from the cervix and uterus are carried by nerves that accompany sympathetic fibers and enter the neuraxis at T10, T11, T12, and L1 spinal level. Pain pathways from the perineum travel to S2, S3, and S4 via the pudendal nerve. (Reprinted by permission from Bonica JJ: The nature of pain of parturition. Clin Obstet Gynaecol 2:511, 1975.)

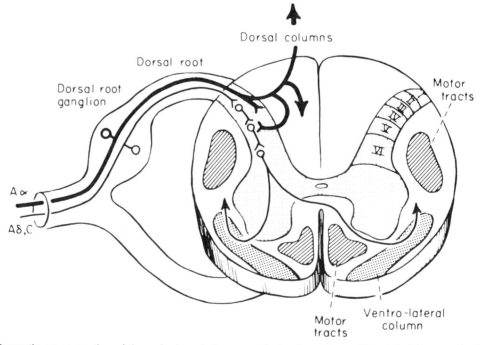

Figure 9.2. Schematic cross-section of the spinal cord. A-delta and C fibers make multiple synaptic connections in the dorsal horn. Cell bodies in lamina V send axons to the ipsilateral and contralateral ventral column to make up the spinothalamic system. (Reprinted by permission from Bonica JJ: The nature of pain of parturition. Clin Obstet Gynaecol 2:500, 1975.)

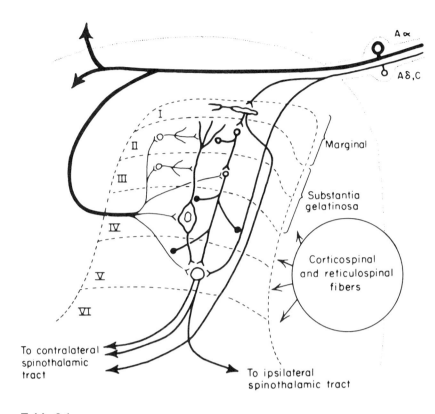

A∝

Aδ,C

I

II

III

Marginal

Substantia
gelatinosa

IV

V

Corticospinal
and reticulospinal
fibers

VI

To contralateral
spinothalamic
tract

To ipsilateral
spinothalamic tract

Figure 9.3. A simplified model of the synaptic connections within the six laminae of the dorsal horn. Pain impulses during parturition are transmitted via A-delta and C fibers to the dorsal horn, where multiple synaptic connections are made. Descending corticospinal and reticulospinal fibers carry impulses that may modulate pain information at the dorsal horn, a possible neurophysiologic mechanism for cortical modification of afferent pain stimuli. (Reprinted by permission from Bonica JJ: The nature of pain of parturition. Clin Obstet Gynaecol 2:501, 1975.)

Table 9.1
Regional Anesthetic Techniques in Obstetrics for Labor and Vaginal Delivery

Technique	Example	Area of Anesthesia
Infiltration	Local for episiotomy	Perineal skin and subcutaneous tissue
	Local for cesarean section	Skin, subcutaneous tissue fascia, peritoneum
Peripheral neural blockade		
Single nerve	Pudendal	S2–S4
Plexus	Lumbar sympathetic	T10–L1
	Paracervical	T10–L1
Central neural blockade		
Epidural	Lumbar	
	Standard	T10–S5
	Segmental	T10–L1
	Caudal	
	Standard	T10–S5
	High catheter	T10–S5
	Low catheter	S2–S5
	Combined	
	Segmental	T10–L1
	+	+
	Low caudal	S2–S5
Subarachnoid	Standard	T10–S5
	Low (saddle)	S1–S5

be applied, the patient placed in the Trendelenburg position, and intravenous fluids administered rapidly. If blood pressure is not restored within 1 to 2 min, ephedrine (5 to 15 mg) should be given intravenously. If blood pressure does not return to acceptable values promptly or if fetal heart abnormalities develop, additional vasopressor and oxygen should be administered. Transient maternal hypotension, if recognized and treated promptly, does not lead to maternal or neonatal morbidity.

The Test Dose

The function of a test dose is to allow recognition of either an accidental dural or intravascular punc-

Figure 9.4. Schematic diagram of lumbosacral anatomy showing needle placement for subarachnoid, lumbar epidural, and caudal blocks.

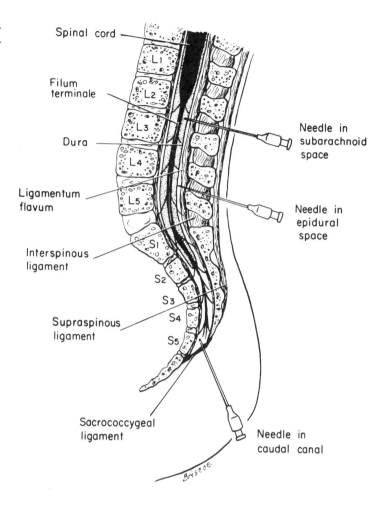

Spinal cord

Filum terminale

Dura

Ligamentum flavum

Interspinous ligament

Supraspinous ligament

Sacrococcygeal ligament

Needle in subarachnoid space

Needle in epidural space

Needle in caudal canal

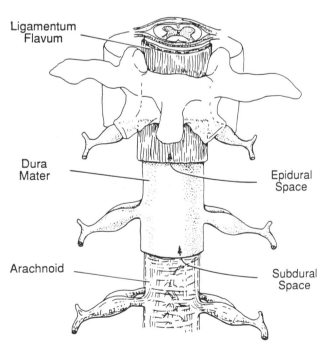

Ligamentum Flavum

Dura Mater

Arachnoid

Epidural Space

Subdural Space

Figure 9.5. Spinal cord and surrounding membranes.

Table 9.2
Resuscitation Cart

Positive pressure breathing apparatus
Oxygen supply
Laryngoscope: adult and infant blades
Endotracheal tubes: adult—6.5, 7, 7.5, 8
                    infant—2.5, 3, 3.5
Stylets: adult and infant
Oral airways: adult and infant
Nasal airways
Suction catheters: adult and infant
Board for closed-chest massage

Drugs: ephedrine	atropine, dopamine
CaCl₂	thiopental or diazepam
NaHCO₃	hydralazine, phentolamine
epinephrine	succinylcholine
naloxone	heparin

Nasogastric tubes
IV supplies, plasma expanders and electrolyte solution, syringes, needles, plastic indwelling catheters
Each labor room should contain an oxygen supply, suction, and bed capable of rapid Trendelenburg position. An ECG monitor and defibrillator should be readily available.

ture. A test dose should therefore contain an amount of local anesthetic sufficient to rapidly produce a low spinal block if injected into the subarachnoid space and also should provide a reliable indication of an accidental intravascular injection. An accidental subarachnoid block achieved with the test dose ideally should not exceed the upper thoracic dermatomes, and the response to an accidental intravascular injection should not produce serious toxicity to either the mother or fetus. Ideally, the test dose should use a readily available drug and should have a high degree of sensitivity and specificity—that is, few false positive or negative findings.

Fulfilling these criteria is difficult, and controversy exists on (a) the choice and dose of a local anesthetic, (b) the pros and cons of the addition of vasoactive drugs such as epinephrine, and (c) other methods such as air injection to detect intravascular injection.

Further complicating the selection is the lack of commercially available or easily preparable mixtures of the drugs one might consider preferable. For example, for detection of a subarachnoid injection, appropriate concentrations are available of hyperbaric lidocaine (3 ml of 1.5%) and bupivacaine (2 ml of 0.75%). However, these solutions are not available with an appropriate dose of epinephrine or isuprel in an ampule because catecholamines are not stable in dextrose containing solutions.

Currently, the most commonly used test dose is local anesthetic with 15 to 20 μgs of epinephrine—that is, 3 to 4 ml of a 1:200,000 solution. This dose, if injected into a blood vessel, should rapidly produce a transient increase in heart rate of 20 to 30 bpm and usually a slight increase in blood pressure. Although the original data by Moore and Batra (7) tested the intravenous dose of 15 μg of epinephrine in nonobstetric patients, similar changes occur in the parturient when an epidural vein is accidentally cannulated and epinephrine injected (Fig. 9.6) (8). The time of onset to tachycardia is approximately 30 sec and the duration is only approximately 30 sec. Thus the anesthesiologist must observe the tachometer during the first minute following the test dose to determine whether an accidental intravascular injection has occurred. Although tachycardia and perhaps a modest hypertension are the two most objective signs, occasionally epinephrine in this dosage may produce other obvious signs, such as acute perspiration and tachypnea or subjective signs such as patient complaints of apprehension or unease. She will often state that she feels "different," that she is

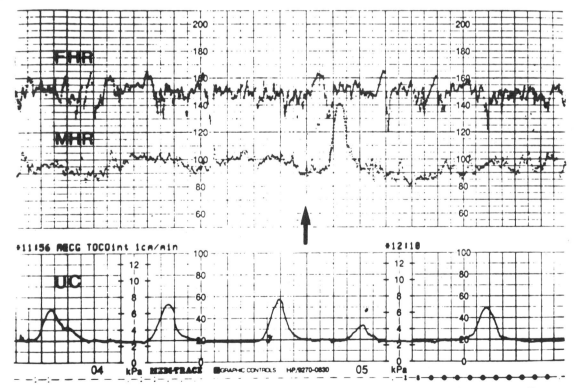

Figure 9.6. A peak increase in MHR lasting 40 sec in a laboring woman during intravenous injection of 12.5 mg of bupivacaine plus 12.5 μg of epinephrine in 10 ml of physiologic saline, recorded with the use of a direct ECG mode of fetal monitoring with dual heart rate capacity. *Arrow* shows start of injection. Thirty seconds is represented between each pair of vertical lines. (Reprinted by permission from Van Zundert AA, Vaes LE, De Wolf AM: ECG monitoring of mother and fetus during epidural anesthesia. Anesthesiology 66:584–585, 1987.)

apprehensive, possibly short of breath, or has palpitations or a "funny" feeling in her chest.

If uterine activity is being monitored with an intraamniotic catheter, it is not uncommon to find that the subsequent contraction is diminished in amplitude (Fig. 9.6) (8). This occurs because the small dose of epinephrine exerts a betamimetic effect on uterine activity. This change in uterine activity is not consistent and may be quite subtle, but when present, it is often dramatic.

Criticisms of using epinephrine as a test dose to determine accidental intravascular injection in the parturient include: (a) a high incidence of false-positive results both in laboring and nonlaboring patients (9); (b) the possibility of false-negative results in mothers with highly variable baseline heart rates (10); and possible adverse effects on uterine blood flow and fetal well-being (9, 11).

Epinephrine (10 to 20 µg) accidentally administered intravenously may produce a significant but very transient decrease in uterine blood flow (Fig. 9.7) (11). This decrease both in degree and duration, however, is similar to that which occurs with a uterine contraction during labor (Fig. 9.8). If a fetus can withstand a uterine contraction without developing severe distress, the fetus should be able to withstand the transient change in uterine blood flow that might occur with an intravascular injection of a small dose of epinephrine. It should be noted that the decrease in uterine blood flow following epinephrine only occurs in the instance when the drug is injected intravenously. It does not occur with epidural injection.

The incidence of false-positive results can be reduced by repeating the test dose in situations in which the response has been equivocal. The incidence of false-negative results should be reduced if one injects the test dose between contractions when the maternal heart rate is relatively slow and stable.

There are also potential problems with suggested alternatives to epinephrine. Subconvulsant doses of local anesthetics, such as 100 mg of lidocaine (12) or chloroprocaine (13), rely solely on the subjective responses of the mother, which may be unreliable in the anxious parturient. Furthermore, if injected subarachnoid, these doses may produce an unacceptably high block. Alternatives using doses of catecholamines that produce a greater increase in maternal heart rate, without adverse effects on uterine blood flow, such as isuprel 5 µg (14–17), involve the preparation of impractical dilutions of available drugs. The use of isoproterenol is also not recommended because, in an epidural anesthesia test dose, insufficient animal neurotoxicology data exist.

An injection of air (1 ml) and the use of the Doppler over the heart has also been suggested (18), but as yet has not achieved widespread popularity.

Precordial Doppler monitoring, utilizing standard external heart rate Doppler monitors, can detect air (microbubbles or a 1-ml bolus) injected through intravenously located epidural catheters (18, 19). The Doppler test has a low false-positive rate and a high positive predictive value. Thus far, no patients have developed complications from the air injection. Intrathecal injection of small amounts of air is safe; the

Figure 9.7. Changes in uterine blood flow (UBF) in the pregnant ewe following intravenous administration of various small amounts of epinephrine and bupivacaine. (Reprinted with permission of Hood DD, Dewan DM, Rose JC, James FM III: Maternal and fetal effects of intravenous epinephrine containing solutions in gravid ewes. Anesthesiology 59:A393, 1983.)

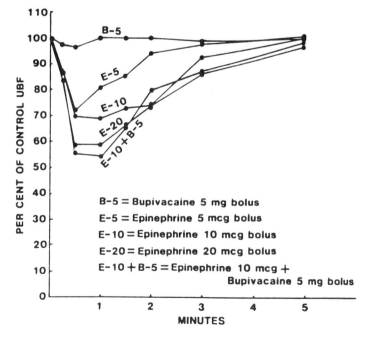

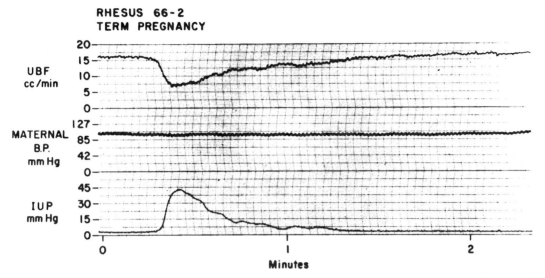

Figure 9.8. Uterine contraction in a pregnant monkey, showing the concomitant "mirror image" decrease in uterine blood flow. This phenomenon probably occurs with every contraction in every woman in labor. *UBF* = uterine blood flow (measured by electromagnetic flow meter); *IUP* = intrauterine pressure. (From Greiss F Jr: Uterine blood flow during labor. Clin Obstet Gynecol 11:96, 1968. Used with permission.)

radiographic technique of pneumoencephalography requires intrathecal injection of 20 to 30 ml of air. Intravenous injection of air (1 ml) is probably quite safe, for there are no reported cases of symptomatic air emboli following identification of the epidural space using the air loss-of-resistance technique, which is associated with a 43% incidence of precordial Doppler heart tone changes (20).

The Doppler test, however, requires a subjective interpretation of Doppler sound changes, requires additional personnel to position and hold the Doppler transducer, cannot be easily performed with the patient on her side, and precludes continuous monitoring of the fetus during injection unless a second external fetal heart rate monitor is available. The technique may be useful in selected patients in whom even small amounts of intravenous epinephrine are contraindicated.

In summary, using epinephrine in the test dose provides a reasonably, reliable indication of accidental intravascular placement of the epidural needle or catheter. The potential benefit outweighs the hazards of a brief decrease in uterine blood flow.

Despite confidence in the correct position of the epidural needle or catheter by a negative test dose response as well as negative aspiration, it is still prudent to administer the total dose in fractional amounts of perhaps 5 ml, then to wait and observe the patient for at least 30 sec between each injection.

Local Anesthetic Convulsions

Central nervous system toxicity occurs when a critical arterial blood (and brain tissue) concentration of local anesthetic is exceeded. High blood levels result from accidental intravascular injection, accumulation of local anesthetic during repeated injections over a prolonged period of time, and rapid systemic absorption of local anesthetic from a highly vascular area. The rate of administration, the total dose of drug, and the physical status of the patient affect tolerance to local anesthetics (21). Accidental intravascular injection may occur with any regional anesthetic technique, including paracervical and pudendal blocks (22). Therefore, when a needle or catheter is placed, aspiration should be performed before drug injection to determine whether a blood vessel has been entered. With epidural or caudal anesthesia a test dose should be injected.

The elimination half-life of amide local anesthetics is 2 to 3 hr. Therefore systemic accumulation of amide local anesthetics to near-toxic levels may occur with large doses repeated at frequent intervals. During properly conducted regional anesthesia, toxic concentrations of local anesthetics resulting from absorption are rarely seen (21, 23). The potential risk of systemic accumulation can be minimized by using the smallest quantity of drug necessary to achieve the desired anesthesia and by using agents that are rapidly metabolized.

The reported incidence of convulsions during obstetric regional anesthesia is low, varying from 0.03 to 0.5% (27–33). Of note is the lack of resultant maternal morbidity or mortality, suggesting that local anesthetic-induced toxic reactions, if properly treated, should not cause permanent sequelae. The intravascular injection of large doses of bupivacaine has been associated with cardiac toxicity. This subject has been discussed extensively in Chapter 6. A summary of the symptoms and signs of local anesthetic toxic reactions is shown in Table 9.3. Treatment involves:

1. Early recognition of the reaction. By constant observation of the patient and her vital signs and by talking to her, it is possible to become aware of the impending toxic reaction and to take steps to prevent it from becoming serious.

2. Prevention of progression of the reaction. Small doses of barbiturates given intravenously may prevent convulsions. The depressant effect of the barbiturate may intensify the depression that results from the local anesthetic, but small doses of thiopental (Pentothal, 50 to 100 mg) or diazepam (Valium, 5 mg), repeated as needed, are probably safe. At the same time, oxygen should be given by mask so that the patient is well oxygenated should a convulsion occur.

3. Maintenance of oxygenation despite convulsions and/or vomiting. Convulsions are not lethal, but the anoxia and acidosis that they produce may be. The airway should be cleared of foreign material and the patient ventilated with 100% oxygen with a positive pressure breathing apparatus. At times ventilating the unparalyzed convulsing patient may be difficult and it may be necessary to paralyze her with 60 to 80 mg of succinylcholine. Tracheal intubation with a cuffed endotracheal tube to facilitate ventilation and/or protect the airway from aspiration may also be necessary.

4. Support of the circulation. Elevation of the legs, displacement of the uterus to the left, and rapid administration of intravenous fluids and vasopressors may be needed to support the depressed circulation.

5. Treatment of cardiac arrest. Cardiac arrest should be treated in the usual way, with external cardiac massage, defibrillation if necessary, sodium bicarbonate, and appropriate cardiotonic drugs. Left uterine displacement should be maintained if possible. Delivery of the baby by relieving vena caval obstruction may facilitate cardiopulmonary resuscitation (34).

6. Consideration of the fetus. As soon as possible after the convulsion, the condition of the fetus should be assessed to enable the obstetrician to decide the subsequent course of delivery. Prompt maternal resuscitation usually will restore uterine blood flow and fetal oxygenation and will allow fetal excretion of local anesthetic to the mother via the placenta (35).

Total Spinal

Total spinal anesthesia may occur from an excessive spread of local anesthetic administered intrathecally, extradurally, or perhaps even subdurally. Dural perforation by an epidural catheter may occur when the catheter is initially inserted or during the course of a previously uneventful continuous epidural anesthetic (36). Although infrequent, the possibility of total spinal anesthesia necessitates the immediate presence of personnel who can promptly diagnose and treat this complication.

Treatment consists of establishing an airway and ventilating with oxygen. Endotracheal intubation should be performed as soon as possible to protect the airway from aspiration. A total spinal block will not produce relaxation of the jaw muscles, and succinylcholine may be required for intubation. The Trendelenburg position and left uterine displacement should be used to increase venous return to the heart. Fluids and ephedrine should be administered as necessary to maintain blood pressure. If a large dose of local anesthetic, intended for the epidural space, has accidentally been injected subarachnoid, then following stabilization of the patient's ventilation and circulation, consideration should be given to performing another lumbar puncture and draining the cerebrospinal fluid. This may be especially important if a local anesthetic solution containing bisulfite has been used.

Severe bradycardia progressing to cardiac asystole has been reported in young healthy subjects not premedicated with atropine (37–39). Decreases in heart rate to less than 60 bpm should be promptly treated by increasing venous return and, if necessary, by administering atropine and/or ephedrine. If conven-

---

Table 9.3
Signs and Symptoms of Local Anesthetic-Induced Systemic Toxicity

Central nervous system
  Cerebral cortex
    Stimulation—restlessness, nervousness, incoherent
      speech, metallic taste, dizziness, blurred vision,
      tremors, and convulsions
    Depression—unconsciousness
  Medulla
    Stimulation—increased blood pressure, heart and
      respiratory rate, nausea, and vomiting
    Depression—hypotension, apnea, and asystole
Cardiovascular
  Heart—bradycardia, ventricular tachycardia and
    fibrillation, decreased contractility
  Blood vessels—vasodilation and hypotension
Uterus
  Uterine vasoconstriction and uterine hypertonus resulting
    in fetal distress

tional doses of atropine or ephedrine are not effective, intravenous epinephrine should be administered.

In cases of cardiac arrest under high spinal anesthesia, comparatively poorer neurologic outcome has been reported with the usual cardiopulmonary resuscitation (CPR) techniques (39). It is believed that a high sympathetic blockade allows increased peripheral blood flow during CPR and prevents the usual preferential perfusion of the brain. It is therefore recommended that on recognition of cardiac arrest during a spinal or epidural anesthetic, a full-resuscitation dose of epinephrine, a potent α-agonist, be given immediately.

Vasopressor-Induced Hypertension

The interaction of vasoactive drugs and ergot derivatives may lead to severe maternal hypertension and possible cerebrovascular accidents (40). Particularly dangerous is the combination of a purely α-adrenergic agent, such as methoxamine, and the ergot derivatives ergonovine and methylergonovine. These ergot derivatives, when used alone, may also be associated with postpartum hypertension (23). Prophylactic vasopressors or ergot derivatives should be used with extreme caution in parturients with hypertension. If acute postpartum hypertension occurs, treatment includes: (a) labetalol, 10 to 20 mg intravenously, repeated every 5 min up to 1 mg/kg, (b) trimethaphan (Arfonad) drip (500 mg in 500 ml), (c) phentolamine (Regitine), 5 mg intravenously, or (d) nitroprusside (Nipride) drip (50 mg in 500 ml).

TECHNIQUES OF REGIONAL ANESTHESIA

Lumbar Epidural Anesthesia (Tables 9.4 and 9.5, and Figs. 9.9 to 9.15)

An enormous variety of techniques, variations on techniques, drug regimens with and without local

---

Table 9.4
Lumbar Epidural Anesthesia for Labor and Vaginal Delivery: Suggested Techniques

1. The patient should be examined by an individual qualified in obstetrics and the maternal and fetal status and progress of labor should be evaluated.
2. Check resuscitation equipment and oxygen-delivery system.
3. Start IV with 16- or 18-gauge plastic indwelling catheter.
4. Apply blood pressure cuff and check control pressure.
5. Administer 500 to 1000 ml balanced salt solution before starting block.
6. Position patient: Lateral decubitus is most commonly used, but sitting position may be useful in very obese patients. Have nurse available to reassure patient, to help with positioning, and to prevent movement during placement of the block.
7. Prepare with an appropriate antiseptic solution and drape the lumbar area.
8. Palpate lumbar spinous processes and choose widest interspace below L2.
9. A large-gauge epidural needle (16- to 18-gauge) is placed in the epidural space in the usual manner.

    a. Midline approach is most popular but lateral or paramedian approach is used by some.

    b. Loss-of-resistance technique with air- or saline-filled syringe most commonly used. Negative pressure method (e.g., hanging drop) is also used, but the incidence of dural puncture may be higher.
10. Aspirate for blood or cerebrospinal fluid.
11. Administer 5 ml of preservative-free saline to facilitate passage of catheter.
12. Insert catheter and remove needle. Catheter should be no more than 1 to 2 cm into the epidural space to prevent one-sided or single dermatome blocks. Aspirate catheter for blood or cerebrospinal fluid. If negative, inject test dose of local anesthetic.
13. Use 3-ml test dose of local anesthetic containing epinephrine 1:200,000 (15 μg). Observe for heart rate increase within 60 sec or evidence of spinal blockade within 3 to 5 min. If test dose is negative, administer additional drug as required to obtain desired pain relief.
14. Maintain patient in lateral position throughout labor to prevent aortocaval compression. If one-sided block occurs, place the patient on the unanesthetized side and give more local anesthetic. If the supine position is necessary for fetal scalp sampling or vaginal examination, duration of the procedure should be as short as possible.
15. Monitor blood pressure every 1 to 2 min for the first 10 min after injection of local anesthetic, then every 5 to 15 min until the block wears off.
16. During the first 20 min after the initial dose and after any top-up dose the patient must be observed continuously and not left unattended.
17. If hypotension occurs (fall in systolic blood pressure of 20 to 30% or to below 100 mm Hg), ensure left uterine displacement. Infuse intravenous fluids rapidly and place patient in 10- to 20 degree Trendelenburg position. If blood pressure is not restored within 1 to 2 min then administer ephedrine 5 to 15 mg IV. If hypotension persists, administer additional vasopressor and oxygen.
18. When possible, monitor fetal heart rate and uterine contractions continuously by electronic means before and after instituting an epidural block.
19. Aspirate catheter for blood or cerebrospinal fluid and administer test dose before each top-up dose if intermittent technique is used.
20. After delivery and episiotomy repair, remove catheter and check for hypotension when the patient's legs are taken out of stirrups.

anesthetics, opiates, and epinephrine have been described. Each has its advocates and rationale. Below are described techniques that are commonly used and that the authors have found to be satisfactory.

Once labor is well established with strong (50 to 70 mm Hg) contractions lasting 1 min and occurring 3 min apart, a continuous lumbar epidural block may be administered. After placement of a needle or plastic catheter in the epidural space, a test dose must be administered to rule out accidental subarachnoid or intravenous placement. Analgesia is then established by injecting the local anesthetic or opiate (Table 9.5). The mother is maintained on her side to prevent supine hypotension. If unilateral analgesia occurs, the patient is turned to the opposite side and more local anesthetic (5 to 10 ml) is injected. With con-

tinuous infusion techniques, sufficient perineal anesthesia is usually present and a perineal dose of local anesthetic not required. With intermittent injections segmental anesthesia is provided during labor with repeated injections until perineal anesthesia is required. With perineal distension by the fetal presenting part, the patient is placed in the sitting position, and 10 to 20 ml of drug are administered. The authors favor either lidocaine 1.5 to 2% or chloroprocaine 2% or 3% to produce rapid onset of profound analgesia and muscle relaxation.

Continuous Infusion Lumbar Epidural Anesthesia (Table 9.6)

Continuous infusion of low concentrations of local anesthetic with and without opiates into the epidural

---

Table 9.5
Drug Regimens for Lumbar Epidural Anesthesia for Labor and Vaginal Delivery

1. Epidural catheter is positioned and placement verified as described in Table 9.4.
2. Initial block—options:
   a. Bupivacaine 0.25% (10 ml)
   b. Sufentanil 10 to 15 μg in 10 ml of saline
   c. Bupivacaine 0.125% + fentanyl 1 μg/ml or sufentanil 10 to 15 μg in 10 ml of saline
3. Subsequent analgesia—options:
   a. Intermittent—repeat as above, as necessary, to maintain maternal comfort
   b. Continuous Infusions—10 to 15 ml/hr
      1. Bupivacaine 0.0625 to 0.125% + either fentanyl 1 to 2 μg/ml or sufentanil 0.1 to 0.2 μg/ml
      2. Bupivacaine 0.125 to 0.25% without opiate
4. If perineal anesthesia is required, place patient in semirecumbent or sitting position and administer 10 to 20 ml of local anesthetic. Suggest lidocaine 1.5 to 2% or chloroprocaine 2 to 3%.

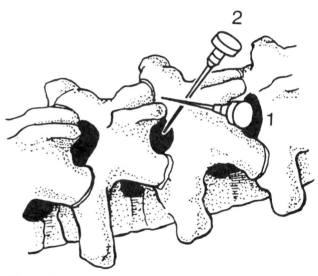

Figure 9.10. Vertebral position with patient in incorrect position. The vertebrae rotate forward, and if the needle is inserted in the usual way (*1*) the apophyseal joints are encountered. The direction the needle must follow is shown in *2*.

Figure 9.9. Incorrect position for placement of subarachnoid or epidural block. Shoulders have fallen forward, upper leg has rotated forward, and the patient is positioned too far on the bed so that there is no support from the edge and the back can curve.

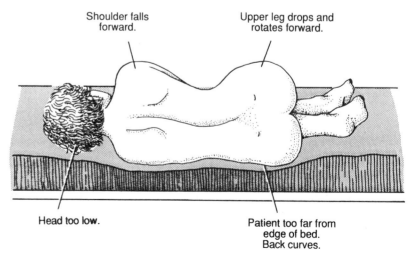

Shoulder falls forward.

Upper leg drops and rotates forward.

Head too low.

Patient too far from edge of bed. Back curves.

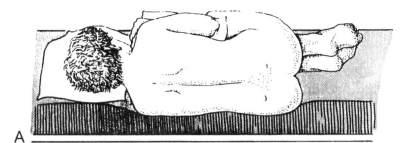

A

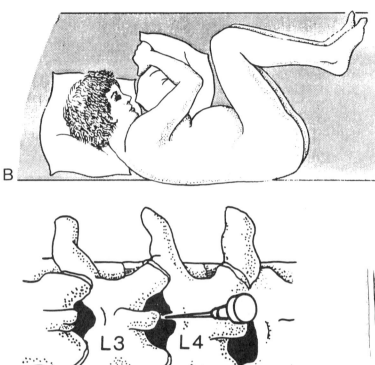

B

Figure 9.11. Correct position for placement of subarachnoid or epidural block. A, The back is straight and vertical, shoulders are square and the upper leg is prevented from rolling forward. B, Correct position viewed from above.

L3   L4

Figure 9.12. Vertebral position with patient correctly positioned.

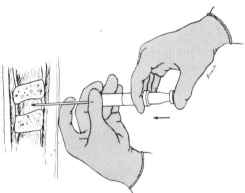

Figure 9.13. Loss-of-resistance technique for identifying epidural space. Needle is placed in interspinous ligament, and resistance to pressure on plunger of syringe is determined. Needle is stabilized with left hand while thumb of right hand applies intermittent pressure to plunger.

space is becoming increasingly popular. The technique provides a continuous stable anesthetic level, avoiding the fluctuations in pain relief often found with conventional intermittent epidural injections during labor. A number of studies have suggested significant advantages to this approach (41–55). Total amount of local anesthetic injected is usually less with this technique. Because of the dilute local anesthetic solutions used the amount of motor block is minimal. This allows the parturient greater mobility in bed. Pelvic muscle tone is maintained, possibly decreasing the incidence of malpositions, and the parturient is better able to make expulsive efforts during the second stage of labor.

There appear to be fewer hypotensive episodes during infusion epidurals (47, 50, 52), possibly due to fewer fluctuations in sympathetic block. The technique also offers advantages to the busy anesthesiologist. Without intermittent injections there is no need for the time-consuming repeat test doses or the necessary close monitoring of the patient for the first 20 min after a reinjection. This does not mean, however, that the anesthesiologist can ignore the patient following establishment of the block. To safely achieve optimum analgesia and patient satisfaction the anesthesiologist should examine and interview the patient at regular intervals. At this time he or she can make necessary adjustments in the rate of infusion

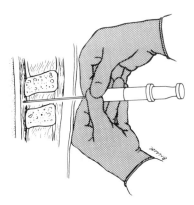

Figure 9.14. Needle is slowly advanced with both hands to prevent too rapid progression and inadvertent dural puncture. Following each incremental advance, intermittent pressure is applied to plunger.

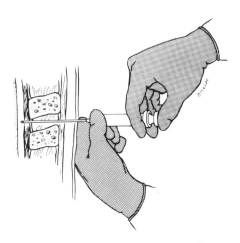

Figure 9.15. When needle passes through ligamentum flavum and enters the epidural space, there will be a sudden loss of resistance.

Table 9.6
Continuous Infusion Lumbar Epidural for Labor and Vaginal Delivery: Suggested Technique

1. Place epidural catheter in usual manner.
2. Use appropriate test dose of local anesthetic, containing epinephrine 15 μg, to rule out accidental intravascular or subarachnoid injection.
3. At the appropriate time (depending on agent used for initial block), start infusion.
4. Check sensory level and adequacy of anesthesia hourly. Adjust infusion rate up or down depending on dermatome level. Increase concentration of local anesthetic or add opiate if block is not dense enough.
5. Maintain patient in lateral position throughout labor to prevent aortocaval compression. Patient should turn from side-to-side every hour to avoid a one-sided block.
6. Monitor blood pressure every 1 to 2 min for the first 10 min after initial injection of local anesthetic, then every 5 to 15 min during the infusion and until the block wears off.
7. Ability of the patient to lift legs should be checked every half hour to monitor motor block.
8. Careful nursing supervision is mandatory.
9. Diminishing analgesia may indicate intravascular migration. A repeat test should be administered before any bolus injections.
10. Development of motor block may indicate subarachnoid migration. Catheter location should be verified by aspiration, careful sensory motor examination and, if necessary, cautious administration of test dose.

or concentration of local anesthetic and note any signs of intravascular or subarachnoid migration of the catheter. Between visits the patient must be closely supervised by trained nurses. Staff experienced in managing possible complications of epidural analgesia must be immediately available.

A variety of infusion devices may be used. However, it is important that the device used should have a number of safety features. Flow rate should be adjustable and accurate, with adjustment controls that cannot be changed by accident. The solution reservoir and tubing should be clearly and prominently labeled, and precautions must be taken to eliminate the possibility of injection of other drugs by mistake.

The potential complications of this technique are intravascular or subarachnoid migration of the catheter during the infusion or the development of progressively higher levels of anesthesia with resulting hypotension and ventilatory difficulties. In reality it

is unlikely that serious complications would occur with the technique as outlined above. Should the epidural catheter migrate into a blood vessel, the only side effect would probably be loss of pain relief. Significant systemic toxicity is avoided because of the very low rate of infusion of local anesthetic. For example, bupivacaine 0.125% infused at 10 ml/hr would only inject 12.5 mg of drug/hr—an amount that would not cause systemic toxicity.

Should the epidural catheter accidently puncture the dura mater the onset of motor block would be slow and easily diagnosed. During a 30-min period, 6.25 mg of bupivacaine would be infused, an amount that would prevent the patient from raising her legs, thereby alerting the staff to an intrathecal injection. If the infusion rate is too high, the slowly ascending sensory level will be easily recognized. Despite the inherent safety of continuous infusion epidurals for obstetric anesthesia, mishaps may occur if a properly trained and vigilant medical and nursing staff are not in attendance.

Caudal Anesthesia (Table 9.7)

A caudal block is also administered after labor is well established. Caudal blocks are performed with patients positioned either on their side (Fig. 9.16) or prone with a bolster placed under the thighs. Using the coccyx as a landmark for the midline, the sacral cornu and sacrococcygeal ligament are palpated (Fig. 9.17). Once the needle is placed in the canal (Figs. 9.18 and 9.19), the drapes are removed and a rectal examination is performed to exclude the possibility of accidental puncture of the fetal presenting part and subsequent anesthetic intoxication of the fetus (Fig. 9.20) (56). After replacing drapes and gloves the caudal catheter is introduced through the needle. After aspiration a test dose of local anesthetic is given through the needle and/or catheter, because it is possible to puncture the dural sac that ends at the second vertebra or a dural sleeve of a sacral nerve root and produce spinal anesthesia. The volume necessary to provide a T10 block usually varies between 15 and 20 ml, with subsequent doses of 15 ml to maintain

analgesia. Placing the patient in a head-down position may be necessary to achieve a T10 block with smaller volumes of drug.

Lumbar epidural may be preferable to caudal anesthesia for the following reasons: (a) segmental T10 to T12 levels can be achieved in early labor when sacral anesthesia is not required; (b) less drug is needed during labor; (c) pelvic muscles retain their tone, and rotation of the fetal head is more easily accomplished; and (d) even though there is an increased risk of dural puncture, often a lumbar epidural is technically easier for the anesthesiologist to administer and less painful for the patient during the placement of the needle than a caudal anesthetic. Caudal anesthesia administered just before delivery has advantages over lumbar epidural anesthesia in that the onset of perineal anesthesia and muscle relaxation is more rapid.

Double-Catheter Technique

This technique consists of inserting two catheters, a lumbar epidural catheter for pain relief during stage one labor and a caudal catheter for delivery. Usually the caudal catheter is inserted immediately after the epidural catheter, because this is more convenient for both the physician and the patient. Also, labor pains can be diminished during performance of the caudal block.

The double-catheter technique has several advantages. It allows the use of a smaller total dose of local anesthetic. It also permits one to achieve a segmental block (T10 to L1) early in labor. Then at the time of delivery, by not injecting the lumbar epidural catheter but instead activating the caudal catheter, it allows the mother to feel contractions, have maximum ability to push, and still have profound perineal anesthesia.

The technique is not currently popular because of the added hazards and discomfort of two needle and catheter insertions. In addition, either lumbar epidural or caudal alone may be used satisfactorily to achieve analgesia for a normal labor and delivery.

Table 9.7
Caudal Block for Labor and Vaginal Delivery

1. Prepare as for epidural block (Table 9.4, steps 1 to 4).
2. Position patient: Lateral decubitus is most commonly used, but prone position with bolster under hips is also popular. Have nurse available to reassure patient, to help with positioning, and to prevent movement during placement of the block.
3. Prepare and drape the caudal area.
4. Using the coccyx as a landmark for the midline, palpate the sacral hiatus and the sacrococcygeal ligament.
5. Place a 16- to 18-gauge epidural needle in the caudal canal in the usual manner.
   a. After positioning the needle, remove drapes and perform rectal examination to exclude the possibility of inadvertent puncture of the rectum, cervix, and fetal presenting part and subsequent anesthetic intoxication of the fetus.
   b. Change gloves, replace drape, and pass catheter through needle.
6. Aspirate for blood or cerebrospinal fluid.
7. Administer local anesthetic as for epidural anesthetic. For a T10 level, a total volume of 15 to 20 ml of local anesthetic is often necessary.

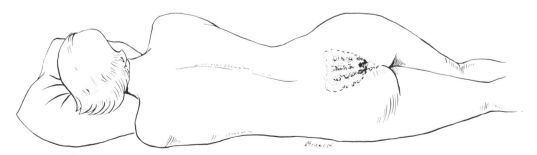

Figure 9.16. Lateral position for caudal block. Note forward tilt of upper hip. For the right-handed physician, the patient should lie on her left side.

Figure 9.17. Sacrum, showing bony landmarks for identifying sacral cornua and sacral hiatus. Sacral hiatus is usually located 2.5 inches above the tip of coccyx or at the apex of an equilateral triangle formed by posterior superior iliac spines and sacrococcygeal ligament.

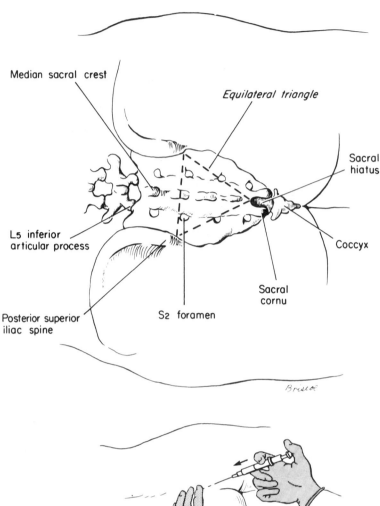

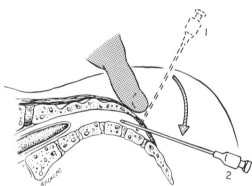

Figure 9.18. Technique of caudal anesthesia. Thumb is placed between sacral cornua at apex of sacral hiatus. Needle is inserted through sacrococcygeal ligament at an angle of approximately 45 degrees (needle position 1). Once ligament is penetrated, needle is repositioned as shown and advanced 1 to 2 cm into caudal canal (needle position 2).

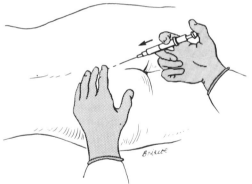

Figure 9.19. Position of needle in caudal canal verified by rapidly injecting a 2- to 3-ml bolus of saline and not palpating an impulse under the fingertips.

larger doses of tetracaine (4 mg), lidocaine (30 mg), or bupivacaine (7.5 mg). Small-bore needles will decrease the incidence of postdural puncture headache (57). Care must be taken not to administer the drug just before or during a uterine contraction lest the accompanying Valsalva maneuver result in an excessively high anesthetic level.

CONTINUOUS SPINAL ANESTHESIA (TABLE 9.9)

Passing a catheter into the subarachnoid space has several advantages. Intermittent doses of small amounts of local anesthetic or opiate can be administered until the appropriate level of anesthesia is

Spinal Anesthesia (Table 9.8)

Spinal, often called saddle block, anesthesia is administered immediately before delivery. For a true saddle block, a small dose of hyperbaric local anesthetic (e.g., tetracaine 3 mg or lidocaine 15 to 20 mg), injected into the subarachnoid space with the patient in the sitting position, is needed to accomplish only sacral anesthesia. More commonly, however, a T10 to S5 dermatome anesthetic distribution is desired and can be accomplished with slightly

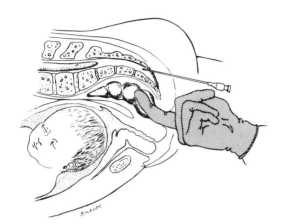

Figure 9.20. Prior to injection of medication or placement of catheter, a rectal examination is performed to rule out inadvertent misplacement of needle with rectal or fetal puncture.

Table 9.8
Spinal Anesthesia for Vaginal Delivery:
A Suggested Technique

1. Check resuscitation equipment and anesthesia machine prior to block.
2. Start IV with plastic indwelling catheter and infuse 500 to 1000 ml of dextrose-free solution rapidly.
3. Apply blood pressure cuff and check control pressure.
4. Position patient: The sitting position is most common. Lateral decubitus with reverse Trendelenburg may be used, especially if there is a preterm infant or a multigravida in whom fetal descent may be very rapid.
5. Prepare and drape lumbar area.
6. Palpate lumbar spinous processes and choose widest interspace below L2.
7. Place needle in subarachnoid space in the usual manner. Use small gauge (22 to 27), noncutting (Sprotte or Whitacre) needle. If cutting tip (Quincke) is used, bevel should be inserted parallel to longitudinal dural fibers.
8. Inject hyperbaric solution of tetracaine, 4 mg, lidocaine, 30 mg, or bupivacaine, 7.5 mg; immediately after a uterine contraction when the patient is relaxed and not straining.
9. Maintain patient in sitting or reverse Trendelenburg position for 30 sec, then place supine with legs in stirrups.
10. Monitor blood pressure every 1 to 2 min for the first 10 min after injection of local anesthetic, then every 5 to 10 min.
11. If hypotension occurs (fall in systolic blood pressure of 20 to 30% or below 100 mm Hg), ensure left uterine displacement, infuse intravenous fluids rapidly, and place patient in 10- to 20-degree Trendelenburg position. If blood pressure is not restored within 1 to 2 min, then administer ephedrine 5 to 15 mg IV. If hypotension persists, administer additional vasopressor and oxygen.
12. Following delivery and episiotomy repair, check for hypotension when the patient's legs are taken out of stirrups.

achieved. This is particularly useful for high risk patients in whom an unplanned high block may produce serious cardiovascular or respiratory problems. It is also useful in very obese patients in whom placement of an epidural is technically difficult or impossible. Occasionally, following an accidental dural puncture during a planned epidural ("wet tap"), the anesthesiologist may choose to proceed with continuous spinal anesthesia.

Disadvantages of the technique include an increased risk for infection and nerve trauma, although this has not proved to be a significant problem. Concern that the large-bore needle commonly used for continuous techniques would produce an unacceptably high incidence of postdural puncture headaches has also not been supported by clinical studies (58–60). It has been postulated that the catheter produces an inflammatory reaction, which helps seal the hole in the dura and prevent CSF leakage, thereby reducing the incidence of headache.

Table 9.9
Continuous Spinal Anesthesia

1. Lumbar puncture is performed in the usual manner. Any approach to the subarachnoid space may be used, although the paramedian approach provides the best angle for catheter insertion. A standard Touhy epidural needle with a Huber point is usually used. If use of microcatheter is planned, a standard 25- or 26-gauge spinal needle or a specially designed Sprotte needle may be used.
2. The bevel of the needle should be positioned laterally (i.e., parallel to the longitudinal dural fibers) until the dura is pierced, then directed cephalad.
3. The catheter is passed only 2 to 3 cm beyond the tip of the needle. This distance is sufficient to prevent accidental dislodgement but short enough to prevent curling or passage of the catheter into a dural sleeve. If the catheter cannot be threaded into the subarachnoid space, the needle and catheter should be withdrawn together and the procedure repeated. A catheter should never be withdrawn through a needle because a portion of it may be sheared off.
4. After the catheter has been inserted, the needle is slowly withdrawn over the catheter, taking care not to simultaneously remove the catheter.
5. Aspiration of CSF indicates proper placement of the catheter. With a 32-gauge microcatheter, aspiration of CSF may not be possible.
6. Any spinal local anesthetic solution or opiate may be used, but if precise titration is desired, drugs with a rapid onset are preferred. Drugs are usually administered in a volume of at least 1.0 ml.
7. Suggested drugs are hyperbaric lidocaine 1.5% or 5% (15 to 30 mg increments); bupivacaine 0.75% (3.25 to 7.5 mg increments); meperidine, 10 to 20 mg; sufentanil, 5 to 10 μg; fentanyl, 10 to 25 μg; morphine, 125 to 250 μg.

Recently a microcatheter that will pass through a standard 25 or 26 gauge spinal needle has become available. Experience with microcatheters is still limited. Serious questions of safety in regard to neurologic injury have been raised (61, 62), and as of June 1992 the U.S. Food and Drug Administration has recalled these catheters. If technical difficulties with insertion and maintenance of these microcatheters prove surmountable and the question of safety is resolved, the continuous technique may become much more popular.

Contraindications to Epidural, Caudal, and Spinal Anesthesia

There are relatively few absolute contraindications to major conduction anesthesia. These include: (a) patient refusal, (b) infection at site of needle injection, (c) hypovolemic shock, and (d) coagulopathies. The use of epidural anesthesia in patients receiving minidose heparin or aspirin and having a normal coagulation profile is controversial, although the authors believe it to be safe.

Preexisting neurologic disease of the spinal cord or peripheral nerves is a relative contraindication, but at times regional anesthesia may be in the best interest of the mother and neonate. Each case should be evaluated individually.

Paracervical Block Anesthesia

Paracervical block is a relatively simple method used by obstetricians to provide analgesia during labor. Local anesthesia is injected submucosally into the fornix of the vagina lateral to the cervix. Frankenhauser's ganglion, containing all the visceral sensory nerve fibers from the uterus, cervix, and upper vagina, is anesthetized. The somatic sensory fibers from the perineum are not blocked; thus the technique is only effective during the first stage of labor. The major disadvantage of paracervical block anesthesia is the relatively high frequency of fetal bradycardia following the block. This bradycardia is associated with decreased fetal oxygenation (Fig. 9.21), fetal acidosis, and an increased likelihood of neonatal depression. Bradycardia usually develops within 2 to 10 min and lasts from 3 to 30 min (Fig. 9.22).

The etiology of bradycardia is still unclear, but evidence suggests that it is related to a combination of decreased uterine blood flow from uterine vasoconstriction from the local anesthetic applied in close proximity to the artery (Fig. 9.23) and from high fetal blood levels of local anesthetics (63). Fetal drug levels in infants with bradycardia are occasionally higher than simultaneously drawn maternal levels, suggesting that local anesthetics may reach the fetus by a more direct route than maternal systemic absorption. Some investigators have postulated that high concentrations of local anesthetics reach the fetus by diffusion across the uterine arteries.

Although the precise cause of fetal bradycardia may be controversial, the significance is not. Paracervical block bradycardia indicates fetal distress. Increased neonatal morbidity and, indeed, mortality occur when bradycardia follows paracervical block. Currently, American and European medical journals contain reports of more than 50 perinatal deaths associated with paracervical block. Because of the potential fetal and neonatal hazards, the authors believe that this technique should not be used in cases of uteroplacental insufficiency or where there is pre-

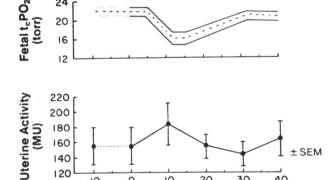

Figure 9.21. Decreased fetal oxygenation in association with fetal bradycardia following paracervical block anesthesia. (Reprinted by permission from Baxi LV, Petrie RH, James LS: Human fetal oxygenation following paracervical block. Am J Obstet Gynecol 135:1109–1112, 1979.)

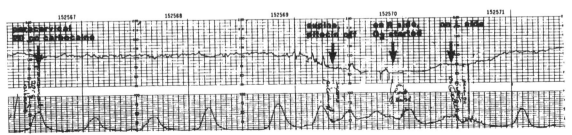

Figure 9.22. Course of fetal bradycardia induced by paracervical block. (Reprinted by permission from Parer JT: *Handbook of Fetal Heart Monitoring*, Saunders, Philadelphia, 1983, p 87.)

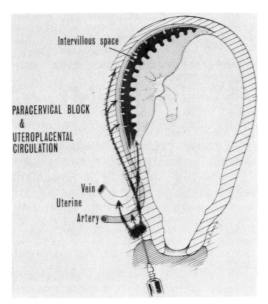

Figure 9.23. Diagram of paracervical area in relation to uteroplacental circulation. (Reprinted by permission from Asling JH, Shnider SM, Margolis AJ, Wilkinson GL, Way EL: Paracervical block anesthesia in obstetrics. II. Etiology of fetal bradycardia following paracervical block anesthesia. Am J Obstet Gynecol 107:626–634, 1970.)

existing fetal distress. There may be exceptions if other anesthetic techniques are contraindicated or pose a greater hazard to the mother or fetus.

When the technique is used the drug dosage must be kept to a minimum. Safe use of this technique requires that injections be superficial (i.e., just below the mucosa), aspiration be done before injection, and the fetal heart rate monitored closely after the injection. The block is performed with the patient in the lithotomy position. A needle is placed through the vaginal mucosa just lateral to the cervix at the three-o'clock position. After aspiration for blood, 5 to 10 ml of a low-concentration local anesthetic are injected. The fetal heart rate is monitored continuously during the next 5 min. If there is no bradycardia, the block is repeated on the other side just lateral to the cervix at the nine-o'clock position with the same volume of drug. The fetal heart rate and maternal blood pressure and pulse are monitored closely during the next 10 min. The duration of pain relief will vary from 40 min with 1.5% chloroprocaine to 90 min with 1% mepivacaine. Bupivacaine is contraindicated for paracervical block anesthesia in obstetrics. The block may be repeated at intervals depending on the duration of action of the local anesthetic. If the cervix has reached 8 cm of dilation, the block should be used with caution lest an injection into the fetal scalp occur.

Lumbar Sympathetic Block

Bilateral lumbar sympathetic block interrupts the pain impulses from the uterus, cervix, and upper third of the vagina and may be used to provide analgesia during the first stage of labor. For relief of perineal pain during the second stage, pudendal nerve blocks or a subarachnoid block must be added.

The lumbar sympathetic block is usually performed at the level of the second lumbar vertebra. Using a 22-gauge, 10-cm needle, the transverse process is located; the needle is then redirected and advanced an additional 5 cm so that the tip is at the anterolateral surface of the vertebral column just anterior to the medial attachment of the psoas muscle (64). The needle is aspirated in two planes to detect blood or cerebrospinal fluid, and then following a test dose a total of 10 ml of local anesthetic is injected in fractionated amounts. This volume will allow the anesthetic to spread along the length of the sympathetic chain. The procedure must be performed on both sides. Bupivacaine 0.5% will provide 2 to 3 hr of anesthesia.

Following the block the patient must be monitored as closely as with a lumbar epidural or caudal anesthetic. Maternal hypotension may occur and is especially common with larger volumes of local anesthetic that spread to and anesthetize the celiac plexus and splanchnic nerves. Systemic toxic reactions from accidental intravascular injection or accidental spinal or epidural injections may also occur. Consequently, prior to performing the block, preparations for those complications must be made. There is some evidence that lumbar sympathetic block accelerates the first stage of labor (65), and it should be used cautiously in the presence of rapidly progressive labor lest tumultuous contractions result (66).

Compared to continuous lumbar epidural analgesia, lumbar sympathetic block is a technically more difficult block to perform, involves more painful needle placement, and does not provide second-stage analgesia. Consequently, it is seldom performed in obstetrics.

Pudendal Block and Local Perineal Infiltration Anesthesia

The blocks are usually administered by the obstetrician just before delivery. Pudendal block is most commonly performed transvaginally. With the patient in the lithotomy position the physician palpates the ischial spine, places a needle guide (Iowa trumpet) under the spine, and introduces a 20-gauge needle through the guide until the point rests on the vaginal mucosa. The needle is advanced, approximately ½ inch, piercing the sarcospinous ligament; after aspirating for blood, 10 ml of local anesthetic (lidocaine or mepivacaine 1% or chloroprocaine 2%) are injected. The technique is then repeated on the opposite side.

Guidelines for Regional Anesthesia

The current **American Society of Anesthesiologists' guidelines for regional anesthesia in obstetrics** is included as an Appendix to this chapter.

References

1. Scott DB, Hibbard BM: Serious non-fatal complications associated with extradural block in obstetric practice. Br J Anaesth 64:537–541, 1990.
2. Shnider SM: Experience with regional anesthesia for vaginal delivery. In *The Anesthesiologist, Mother and Newborn.* SM Shnider, F Moya, eds. Williams & Wilkins, Baltimore, 1974, p 38.
3. Clark RB, Thompson DS, Thompson CH: Prevention of spinal hypotension associated with cesarean section. Anesthesiology 45:670–674, 1976.
4. Gutsche BB: Prophylactic ephedrine preceding spinal analgesia for cesarean section. Anesthesiology 45:462–465, 1976.
5. Wollman SB, Marx GF: Acute hydration for prevention of hypotension of spinal anesthesia in parturients. Anesthesiology 29:374–379, 1968.
6. Brizgyz RV, Dailey PA, Shnider SM, Kotelko DM, Levinson G: The incidence and neonatal effects of maternal hypotension during epidural anesthesia for cesarean section. Anesthesiology 67:782–786, 1987.
7. Moore DC, Batra MS: The components of an effective test dose prior to epidural block. Anesthesiology 55:693–696, 1981.
8. Van Zundert AA, Vaes LE, De Wolf AM: ECG monitoring of mother and fetus during epidural anesthesia. Anesthesiology 66:584–585, 1987.
9. Cartwright PD, McCarroll SM, Antzaka C: Maternal heart rate changes with a plain epidural test dose. Anesthesiology 65:226–228, 1986.
10. Leighton BL, Norris MC, Sosis M, Epstein R, Chayen B, Larijant GE: Limitations of epinephrine as a marker of intravascular injection in laboring women. Anesthesiology 66:688–691, 1987.
11. Hood DD, Dewan DM, James FM: Maternal and fetal effects of epinephrine in gravid ewes. Anesthesiology 64:610–613, 1986.
12. Roetman KJ, Eisenach JC: Evaluation of lidocaine as an intravenous test dose for epidural anesthesia. Anesthesiology 69:A669, 1988.
13. Grice SC, Eisenach JC, Dewan DM: Effect of 2-chloroprocaine test dosing on the subsequent duration of labor analgesia with epidural bupivacaine-fentanyl-epinephrine. Anesthesiology 69:A668, 1988.
14. Baker BW, Longmire S, Jones M, Gallen J, Palacios Q, Joyce TH III, Morrow D: The epidural test dose in obstetrics reconsidered. In *Abstracts of Scientific Papers,* Annual Meeting, Society for Obstetric Anesthesia and Perinatology, Halifax, Nova Scotia, 1987, p 69.
15. DeSimone CA, Leighton BL, Norris MC, Chayen B, Menduke H: The chronotropic effect of isoproterenol is reduced in term pregnant women. Anesthesiology 69:626–628, 1988.
16. Cleaveland CR, Rango RE, Shand DG: A standardized isoproterenol sensitivity test. Arch Intern Med 130:47–52, 1972.
17. Leighton BL, DeSimone CA, Norris MC, Chayen B: Isoproterenol is an effective marker of intravenous injection in laboring women. Anesthesiology 71:206–209, 1989.
18. Leighton BL, Gross JB: Air: An effective indicator of intravenously located epidural catheters. Anesthesiology 71:848–851, 1989.
19. Leighton BL, Norris MC, DeSimone CA, Rosko T, Gross JB: The air test as a clinically useful indicator of intravenously placed epidural catheters. Anesthesiology 73:610–613, 1990.
20. Naulty JS, Ostheimer GW, Datta S, Knapp R, Weiss JB: Incidence of venous air embolism during epidural catheter insertion. Anesthesiology 57:410–412, 1982.
21. Moore DC, Bridenbaugh LD, Thompson GE, Balfour RI, Horton WG: Factors determining dosages of amide-type local anesthetic drugs. Anesthesiology 47:263–268, 1977.
22. Grimes DA, Cates W Jr: Deaths from paracervical anesthesia used for first-trimester abortion. N Engl J Med 295:1397–1399, 1976.
23. Poppers PJ: Evaluation of local anesthetic agents for regional anaesthesia in obstetrics. Br J Anaesth 47:322–327, 1975.
24. Zsigmond EK: Obstetric use of 2-chloroprocaine. N Engl J Med 289:868, 1973.
25. Kuhnert BR, Kuhnert PM, Prochaska BS, Gross TL: Plasma levels of 2-chloroprocaine in obstetric patients and their neonates after epidural anesthesia. Anesthesiology 53:21–25, 1980.
26. Gross TL, Kuhnert PM, Kuhnert BR, Pimental R: Plasma levels of 2-chloroprocaine and lack of sequelae following an apparent inadvertent intravenous injection. Anesthesiology 54:173–174, 1981.
27. Adamson DH: Continuous epidural anesthesia in the community hospital. Can Anaesth Soc J 20:687–692, 1973.
28. Crawford JS: The second thousand epidural blocks in an obstetric hospital practice. Br J Anaesth 44:1277–1287, 1972.
29. Kandel PF, Spoerel WE, Kinch RAH: Continuous epidural analgesia for labour and delivery: Review of 1000 cases. Can Med Assoc J 95:947–953, 1966.
30. Bush RC: Caudal analgesia for vaginal delivery. II. Analysis of complications. Anesthesiology 20:186–191, 1959.
31. Dogu TS: Continuous caudal analgesia and anesthesia for labor and vaginal delivery. Obstet Gynecol 33:92–97, 1969.
32. Epstein HM, Sherline DM: Single-injection caudal anesthesia in obstetrics. Obstet Gynecol 33:496–500, 1969.
33. Gunther RE, Bellville JW: Obstetrical caudal anesthesia. II. A randomized study comparing 1 per cent mepivacaine with 1 per cent mepivacaine plus epinephrine. Anesthesiology 37:288–298, 1972.
34. Marx GF: Cardiopulmonary resuscitation of late-pregnant women. Anesthesiology 56:156, 1982.
35. Morishima HO, Adamsons K: Placental clearance of mepivacaine following administration to the guinea pig fetus. Anesthesiology 28:343–348, 1967.
36. Philip JH, Brown WU Jr: Total spinal anesthesia late in the course of obstetric bupivacaine epidural block. Anesthesiology 44:340–341, 1976.
37. Akamatsu TJ: Cardiovascular response to spinal anesthesia. In *Regional Anesthesia: Recent Advances and Current Status.* JJ Bonica, ed. FA Davis, Philadelphia, 1969.
38. Wetstone DL, Wong KC: Sinus bradycardia and asystole during spinal anesthesia. Anesthesiology 41:87–89, 1974.
39. Caplan RA, Ward RJ, Posner K, Cheney FW: Unexpected cardiac arrest during spinal anesthesia: A closed claims analysis of predisposing factors. Anesthesiology 68:5–11, 1988.
40. Casady GN, Moore CD, Bridenbaugh LD: Postpartum hypertension after use of vasoconstrictor and oxytocic drugs. JAMA 172:1011–1015, 1960.
41. Morrison DH, Smedstad KG: Continuous infusion epidurals for obstetric analgesia. Can Anaesth Soc J 32:101–104, 1985.
42. Scott DB, Walker LR: Administration of continuous epidural analgesia. Anaesthesia 18:82–83, 1963.
43. Spoerel WE, Thomas A, Gerula GR: Continuous epidural analgesia: Experience with mechanical injection devices. Can Anaesth Soc J 17:37–51, 1970.
44. Zador G, Willdeck-Lund C, Nilsson BA: Continuous drip lumbar epidural anesthesia with lidocaine for vaginal delivery. 1. Clinical efficacy and lidocaine concentrations in maternal, fetal and umbilical cord blood. Acta Obstet Gynecol Scand 34(Suppl):31–40, 1974.
45. Glover DJ: Continuous epidural analgesia in the obstetric patient: A feasibility study using a mechanical infusion pump. Anaesthesia 32:499–503, 1977.
46. Evans KRL, Carrie LES: Continuous epidural infusion of bu-

pivacaine in labour: A simple method. Anaesthesia 34:310–315, 1979.

47. Matouskova A, Hanson B, Elmen H: Continuous mini-infusion of bupivacaine into the epidural space during labor. III. A clinical study of 225 parturients. Acta Obstet Gynecol Scand 83(Suppl):43–52, 1979.

48. Davies AO, Fettes IW: A simple safe method for continuous infusion epidural analgesia in obstetrics. Can Anaesth Soc J 28:484–487, 1981.

49. Taylor HJC: Clinical experience with continuous epidural infusion of bupivacaine at 6 ml per hour in obstetrics. Can Anaesth Soc J 30:277–285, 1983.

50. Rosenblatt R, Wright R, Denson D, Raj P: Continuous epidural infusions for obstetric analgesia. Reg Anesth 8:10–15, 1983.

51. Abboud TK, Afrasiabi A, Sarkis F, Daftarian F, Nagappala S, Noueihid R, Kuhnert B, Miller F: Continuous infusion epidural analgesia in parturients receiving bupivacaine, chloroprocaine, or lidocaine—maternal, fetal, and neonatal effects. Anesth Analg 63:421–428, 1984.

52. Chestnut DH, Bates JN, Choi WW: Continuous infusion epidural analgesia with lidocaine: Efficacy and influence during the second stage of labor. Obstet Gynecol 69:323–327, 1987.

53. Chestnut DH, Owen Bates JN, Ostman LG, Choi WW, Geiger MW: Continuous infusion epidural analgesia during labor: A randomized, double-blind comparison of 0.0625% bupivacaine/0.0002% fentanyl versus 0.125% bupivacaine. Anesthesiology 68:754–759, 1988.

54. Phillips G: Continuous epidural analgesia in labor: The effect of adding sufentanil to 0.125% bupivacaine. Anesth Analg 67:462–465, 1988.

55. Chestnut DH, Vandewalker GE, Owen CL, Bates JN, Choi WW: The influence of continuous epidural bupivacaine analgesia on the second stage of labor and method of delivery in nulliparous women. Anesthesiology 66:774–780, 1987.

56. Sinclair JC, Fox HA, Lentz JF, Fuld GL, Murphy J: Intoxication of fetus by a local anesthetic: A newly recognized complication of maternal caudal anesthesia. N Engl J Med 273:1173–1177, 1965.

57. Greene BA: A 26-gauge lumbar puncture needle: Its value in the prophylaxis of headache following spinal analgesia for vaginal delivery. Anesthesiology 11:464–469, 1950.

58. Peterson DO, Borup JL, Chestnut JS: Continuous spinal anesthesia: Case review and discussion. Reg Anesth 8:109–113, 1983.

59. Kallos T, Smith TC. Continuous spinal anesthesia with hypobaric tetracaine for hip surgery in lateral decubitus. Anesth Analg 51:766–773, 1972.

60. Denny N, Masters R, Pearson D, Read J, Sihota M, Selander D: Postdural puncture headache after continuous spinal anesthesia. Anesth Analg 66:791–794, 1987.

61. Rigler M, Drasner K, Krejcie T, Yelich S, Scholnick F, DeFontes J, Bohner D: Cauda equina syndrome after continuous spinal anesthesia. Anesth Analg 72:275–281, 1991.

62. Rigler M, Drasner K: Distribution of catheter-injected local anesthetic in a model of the subarachnoid space. Anesthesiology 75:684–692, 1991.

63. Ralston DH, Shnider SM: The fetal and neonatal effects of regional anesthesia in obstetrics. Anesthesiology 48:34–64, 1978.

64. Bonica JJ: *Principles and Practice of Obstetric Analgesia and Anesthesia, Vol 1.* Davis, Philadelphia, 1967, p 253.

65. Hunter CA Jr: Uterine motility studies during labor: Observations on bilateral sympathetic nerve block in the normal and abnormal first stage of labor. Am J Obstet Gynecol 85:681–686, 1983.

66. James FM III: Clinical obstetrical anesthesia: Labor and delivery. In *Annual Refresher Course Lectures.* American Society of Anesthesiologists, Chicago, 1978, 126A.

Guidelines for Regional Anesthesia in Obstetrics

(Approved by the House of Delegates on October 12, 1988 and last amended on October 30, 1991)

These guidelines apply to the use of regional anesthesia or analgesia in which local anesthetics are administered to the parturient during labor and delivery. They are intended to encourage quality patient care but cannot guarantee any specific patient outcome. Because the availability of anesthesia resources may vary, members are responsible for interpreting and establishing the guidelines for their own institutions and practices. These guidelines are subject to revision from time to time as warranted by the evolution of technology and practice.

GUIDELINE I

REGIONAL ANESTHESIA SHOULD BE INITIATED AND MAINTAINED ONLY IN LOCATIONS IN WHICH APPROPRIATE RESUSCITATION EQUIPMENT AND DRUGS ARE IMMEDIATELY AVAILABLE TO MANAGE PROCEDURALLY RELATED PROBLEMS.

Resuscitation equipment should include, but is not limited to: sources of oxygen and suction, equipment to maintain an airway and perform endotracheal intubation, a means to provide positive pressure ventilation, and drugs and equipment for cardiopulmonary resuscitation.

GUIDELINE II

REGIONAL ANESTHESIA SHOULD BE INITIATED BY A PHYSICIAN WITH APPROPRIATE PRIVILEGES AND MAINTAINED BY OR UNDER THE MEDICAL DIRECTION (1) OF SUCH AN INDIVIDUAL.

Physicians should be approved through the institutional credentialing process to initiate and direct the maintenance of obstetric anesthesia and to manage procedurally related complications.

GUIDELINE III

REGIONAL ANESTHESIA SHOULD NOT BE ADMINISTERED UNTIL: (*a*) THE PATIENT HAS BEEN EXAMINED BY A QUALIFIED INDIVIDUAL (2); and (*b*) THE MATERNAL AND FETAL STATUS AND PROGRESS OF LABOR HAVE BEEN EVALUATED BY A PHYSICIAN WITH PRIVILEGES IN OBSTETRICS WHO IS READILY AVAILABLE TO SUPERVISE THE LABOR AND MANAGE ANY OBSTETRIC COMPLICATIONS THAT MAY ARISE.

Under circumstances defined by department protocol, qualified personnel may perform the initial pelvic examination. The physician responsible for the patient's obstetrical care should be informed of her status so that a decision can be made regarding present risk and further management (2).

GUIDELINE IV

AN INTRAVENOUS INFUSION SHOULD BE ESTABLISHED BEFORE THE INITIATION OF REGIONAL ANESTHESIA AND MAINTAINED THROUGHOUT THE DURATION OF THE REGIONAL ANESTHETIC.

GUIDELINE V

REGIONAL ANESTHESIA FOR LABOR AND/OR VAGINAL DELIVERY REQUIRES THAT THE PARTURIENT'S VITAL SIGNS AND THE FETAL HEART RATE BE MONITORED AND DOCUMENTED BY A QUALIFIED INDIVIDUAL. ADDITIONAL MONITORING APPROPRIATE TO THE CLINICAL CONDITION OF THE PARTURIENT AND THE FETUS SHOULD BE EMPLOYED WHEN INDICATED. WHEN EXTENSIVE REGIONAL BLOCKADE IS ADMINISTERED FOR COMPLICATED VAGINAL DELIVERY, THE STANDARDS FOR BASIC INTRAOPERATIVE MONITORING (3) SHOULD BE APPLIED.

GUIDELINE VI

REGIONAL ANESTHESIA FOR CESAREAN DELIVERY REQUIRES THAT THE STANDARDS FOR BASIC INTRA-OPERATIVE MONITORING (3) BE APPLIED AND THAT A PHYSICIAN WITH PRIVILEGES IN OBSTETRICS BE IMMEDIATELY AVAILABLE.

GUIDELINE VII

QUALIFIED PERSONNEL, OTHER THAN THE ANESTHESIOLOGIST ATTENDING THE MOTHER, SHOULD BE IMMEDIATELY AVAILABLE TO AS-

SUME RESPONSIBILITY FOR RESUSCITATION OF THE NEWBORN (2).

The primary responsibility of the anesthesiologist is to provide care to the mother. If the anesthesiologist is also requested to provide brief assistance in the care of the newborn, the benefit to the child must be compared to the risk to the mother.

GUIDELINE VIII

A PHYSICIAN WITH APPROPRIATE PRIVILEGES SHOULD REMAIN READILY AVAILABLE DURING THE REGIONAL ANESTHETIC TO MANAGE ANESTHETIC COMPLICATIONS UNTIL THE PATIENT'S POSTANESTHESIA CONDITION IS SATISFACTORY AND STABLE.

GUIDELINE IX

ALL PATIENTS RECOVERING FROM REGIONAL ANESTHESIA SHOULD RECEIVE APPROPRIATE POSTANESTHESIA CARE. FOLLOWING CESAREAN DELIVERY AND/OR EXTENSIVE REGIONAL BLOCKADE, THE STANDARDS FOR POSTANESTHESIA CARE (4) SHOULD BE APPLIED.

1. A Postanesthesia Care Unit (PACU) should be available to receive patients. The design, equipment and staffing should meet requirements of the facility's accrediting and licensing bodies.

2. When a site other than the PACU is used, equivalent postanesthesia care should be provided.

GUIDELINE X

THERE SHOULD BE A POLICY TO ASSURE THE AVAILABILITY IN THE FACILITY OF A PHYSICIAN TO MANAGE COMPLICATIONS AND TO PROVIDE CARDIOPULMONARY RESUSCITATION FOR PATIENTS RECEIVING POSTANESTHESIA CARE.

References

1. Anesthesia care team (approved by ASA House of Delegates October 14, 1987).
2. American Academy of Pediatrics and American College of Obstetricians and Gynecologists: Guidelines for Perinatal Care. The Academy, 1988.
3. Standards for basic intra-operative monitoring (approved by ASA House of Delegates October 21, 1986; last amended October 23, 1990).
4. Standards for postanesthesia care (approved by ASA House of Delegates October 12, 1988; last amended October 23, 1990).

CHAPTER 10

Intraspinal Opiates in Obstetrics

Samuel C. Hughes, M.D.

Since their introduction in 1979, the intraspinal (epidural and spinal) opiates rapidly have become an exciting addition to the field of obstetric anesthesia (1, 2). This chapter reviews the physiologic and pharmacologic bases of intraspinal opiate action, the benefits of using the intraspinal technique to treat labor, delivery, and postoperative pain, and the side effects produced by the use of this method. Although there are distinct advantages to the intraspinal technique, their use is not without a price (3). No other area in obstetric anesthesia has drawn as much attention in the last 8 to 10 years.

ENDOGENOUS OPIATES AND OPIATE RECEPTORS

The opiates have a long history of therapeutic relevance and still are among the most widely used drugs in medicine (4). Narcotics have been used as anesthetics, analgesics, sedatives, antitussives, and antidiarrheals, typically administered as intravenous, intramuscular or oral agents. (Their use in obstetrics is described in Chapter 8.) The discovery of opiate receptors, the sites on cell membranes that interact with opiate drugs, combined with the discovery of endogenous opiate-like substances (Table 10.1) implied that exogenous opiates could be administered to specific sites (5, 6). The additional finding that opiate receptors were concentrated in discrete areas in the central nervous system (CNS) helped to explain the multiple actions of the opiates (Table 10.2). When morphine was administered to the chief site of action for intraspinal narcotics—the substantia gelatinosa of the dorsal horn of the spinal column—it was shown to produce a highly selective depressant action on nociceptive pathways in the Rexed laminae of the dorsal horn, without affecting motor, sympathetic, or proprioceptive pathways (7–10). Opiates administered in minute doses to other receptor-laden areas in animals (e.g., the cortex) had no significant effect on nociceptive pathway action. Taken together, these outcomes indicated that opiate effects on a specific brain or other region dense with opiate receptors depended on the function routinely served by that region. We can therefore attempt to apply an opiate to a specific receptor site to obtain a specific and limited outcome, rather than administer systemic narcotics that activate multiple and peripheral receptors throughout the CNS.

A wide variety of chemical compounds with opiate activity produce effects via recognition by a receptor (11). The biochemical profile of this receptor is debated and recently was reviewed (Fig. 10.1) (12). Opiates may function by activating receptors presynaptically, thereby blocking the release of a primary afferent neurotransmitter responsible for depolarizing neurons, substance P (13). In the dorsal horn, opiates may function by modulating transmission to interneurons. Supraspinal (descending) pathways mediated by enkephalins may inhibit primary afferent transmission by activating serotonin or noradrenalin pathways. Regardless of the mechanism, it is clear that the use of intraspinal opiates engages an endogenous system composed of opiate receptors and opiate-like substances that function as neurotransmitters or neuromodulators. Systemic narcotics probably combine the effects of the supraspinal and direct spinal actions of the drugs administered (14, 15). Intraspinal narcotics may just be the beginning of our use of the expanding knowledge of pain transmission (Fig. 10.2).

Opiate-like Peptides

A number of researchers are involved in determining the structure and genesis of the opiate-like substances. In 1965 Li discovered β-lipotropin, a pituitary peptide chain composed of 91 amino acids (16). β-lipotropin was later shown to be composed of several biologically active peptides, including the pentapeptides, methionine-enkephalin, leucine-enkephalin, and β-endorphin (Fig. 10.3) (17). The exact function of such long-chain peptides in pituitary and brain function is unclear, as is the relationship between the enkephalins and β-lipotropin; the latter may serve as a precursor from which the active peptides are cleaved (4). The subunit β-endorphin, which exhibits potent opiate agonist activity, has been synthetized and administered intrathecally in humans, producing profound analgesia (18).

Opiate Receptors and Subpopulations

Soon after the initial recognition of the opiate receptors in the CNS, the likelihood of there being multiple types or subpopulations of receptors became clear. Comparing several agents, researchers demonstrated that both morphine and ethylketocyclazocine (EKC) blocked spinal nociceptive reflexes in

animal models. However, it required a much higher dose of the antagonist naloxone to reverse the effects of EKC than to reverse those of morphine. Furthermore, animals tolerant to EKC were not cross-tolerant to morphine (19). These results suggested the presence of different receptors for these drugs, called μ and κ receptors. Subsequent research indicated that there are at least five different receptors (with perhaps multiple subunits), each paired with endogenous or exogenous opiate substances or peptides having a corresponding affinity, and each triggering or controlling different functions (Table 10.3) (20–24). However, individual receptors may serve more than one function, and an opiate may target more than one specific receptor. The result is a great deal of crossover in receptor binding. In spite of the crossover, there is great interest in identifying receptor-specific drugs—that is, drugs that will affect only a specific receptor or receptor subunit. Research continues in this direction (25, 26). However, research and clinical trials using so-called "κ-specific" drugs have not been rewarding.

THE PHARMACOKINETICS OF INTRASPINAL NARCOTICS

The effects of opiate substances are determined not only by their relative affinity for particular receptors, but also by their ability to reach those receptors. For intraspinal receptors, the action depends on narcotics reaching the receptor site by penetrating the superficial laminae of the dorsal horn. The drug may be administered directly into the cerebrospinal fluid (CSF) or into the epidural space. The onset of the effects of epidural and intrathecal narcotics is very similar, indicating that penetration of neural tissue (not the dura) is the rate-limiting step.

The effects of intraspinal narcotics, like local anesthetics, are modulated by a number of factors, in-

Table 10.1
Endogenous Opiates and Opiate Receptors: An Outline of Terms

Opiate receptor	Specific sites on cell membranes, primarily in the CNS, that interact with opiate drugs or endogenous opiate-like substances. There are five or more different types of opiate receptors and probably a subpopulation of those five types.
Endogenous opiates	Naturally occurring substances (opioid peptides) isolated in humans and having opiate-like properties. The term *endorphin* is often used generically to describe any endogenous opiate, but is perhaps best applied to those isolated from the pituitary gland.
Enkephalins	Two short-chain peptides isolated from the CNS that have opiate activity (methionine– and leucine–enkephalin). They interact with opiate receptors and function as neurotransmitters.
β-Lipotropin	A pituitary peptide containing 91 amino acids. It may break down to form active subunits.
β-Endorphin	A fragment of β-lipotropin (amino acids 61–91) having potent opiate activity. It has been synthesized and manufactured for intraspinal application on an experimental basis.

Table 10.2
Opiate Receptor and Response[a]

Opiate Receptor Site	Physiologic and Pharmacologic Response
Medullary and pontine respiratory centers	Respiratory depression
Thalamus	
Lateral thalamus	Discrete, localized pain
Medial thalamus	Poorly localized, deep pain
(receptor density greater in medial thalamus)	
Substantia gelatinosa (dorsal horn of spinal cord)	First site in CNS for integration of sensory information (analgesia achieved)
Solitary nuclei	Depression of cough reflex; orthostatic hypotension
Area postrema (chemoreceptor trigger area)	Nausea and vomiting
Amygdala	Emotional behavior; euphoria
Gastrointestinal tract	Decreased motility (constipation)

[a] Adapted from Snyder SH: Opiate receptors in the brain. N Engl J Med 296:266–271, 1977.

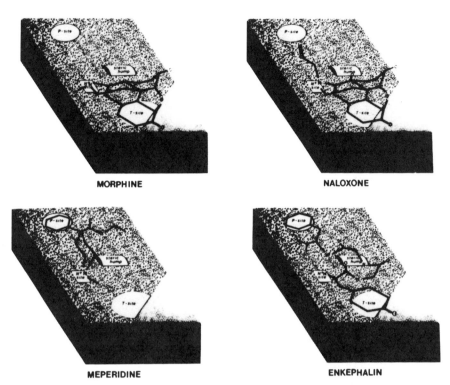

MORPHINE

NALOXONE

MEPERIDINE

ENKEPHALIN

Figure 10.1. Morphine, naloxone, meperidine, and enkephalin as they are envisioned to interact with the model of an opiate receptor. The receptor consists of two aromatic binding sites (*T-site* and *P-site*) and one anionic site (N^+-*site*) responsible for binding a nitrogen ion. The receptor is probably a complex site that does not interact with all narcotics, antagonists, and endogenous opiate peptides in the same "lock and key" fashion. (Reprinted by permission from Thorpe DH: Opiate structure and activity—a guide to understanding the receptor. Anesth Analg 63:143–151, 1984.)

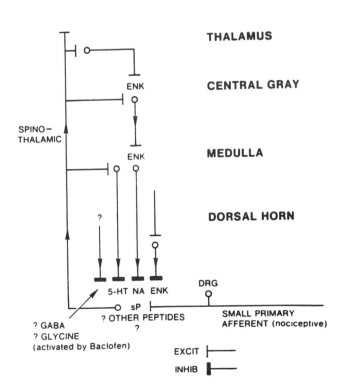

Figure 10.2. Model of pain transmission. Proposed excitatory (*excit*) and inhibitory (*inhib*) pathways and transmitters are shown. *DRG* = dorsal root ganglion; *DP* = substance P; *5-HT* = serotonin; *NA* = noradrenaline (norepinephrine); *ENK* = enkephalin; *GABA* = gamma-amino butyric acid. Primary afferent nociceptive impulses are conducted by way of DRG to spinothalamic and spinoreticular neurons in the dorsal horn with substance P as transmitter. Collaterals supply medulla and central gray matter. Enkephalin activates descending pathways (GABA, 5HT, NA), which inhibit primary afferent transmission. Within dorsal horn, there are local enkephalin (opioid) inhibitory systems. (Reprinted by permission from Cousins MJ, Cherry DA, Gourlay GK: Acute and chronic pain: Use of spinal opioids. In *Neural Blockade in Clinical Anesthesia and Management of Pain*, 2nd ed. MJ Cousins, PO Bridenbaugh, eds. JB Lippincott, Philadelphia, 1988, p 961.)

PEPTIDE	AMINO ACID SEQUENCE
β Lipotropin	¹ NH₂-GLU-LEU-ALA-GLY-ALA-PRO-PRO-GLU-PRO-ALA-ARG-ASP-PRO-GLU-ALA-PRO-ALA-GLU-GLY-ALA-ALA-ALA- ²⁰ -ARG-ALA-
β Lipotropin (continued)	³⁷ GLU-LEU-GLU-TYR-GLY-LEU-VAL-ALA-GLU-ALA-GLN-ALA-ALA-GLU-LYS-LYS-ASP-GLU-GLY-PRO-TYR-LYS
β-MSH	ALA-GLU-LYS-LYS-ASP-GLU-GLY-PRO-TYR-ARG-
β Lipotropin (continued)	⁴⁷ MET-GLU-HIS-PHE-ARG-TRY-GLY-SER-PRO-PRO-LYS-ASP-LYS-ARG-TYR-GLY-GLY-PHE-MET-THR-SER-GLU-LYS-SER- ⁶¹
β-MSH (continued)	MET-GLU-HIS-PHE-ARG-TRY-GLY-SER-PRO-PRO-LYS-ASP
ACTH 4-10	MET-GLU-HIS-PHE-ARG-TRY-GLY
α Endorphin	TYR-GLY-GLY-PHE-MET-THR-SER-GLU-LYS-SER
β Endorphin	TYR-GLY-GLY-PHE-MET-THR-SER-GLU-LYS-SER
Methionine enkephalin	TYR-GLY-GLY-PHE-MET
β Lipotropin (continued)	⁷⁶ GLN-THR-PRO-LEU-VAL-THR-LEU-PHE-LYS-ASN-ALA-ILE-VAL-LYS-ASN-ALA-HIS-LYS-LYS-GLY-GLN-OH ⁹¹
α Endorphin (continued)	GLN-THR-PRO-LEU-VAL-THR
β Endorphin (continued)	GLN-THR-PRO-LEU-VAL-THR-LEU-PHE-LYS-ASN-ALA-ILE-VAL-LYS-ASN-ALA-HIS-LYS-LYS-GLY-GLN-OH

Figure 10.3. Amino acid sequence of β-lipotropin, isolated from the pituitary, which may serve as a precursor for several active peptides. The amino acid residue 61–91, β-endorphin, accounts for the greater part of the pituitary's opioid activity. The pituitary also possesses opiate receptors, which may explain why opiates cause release of antidiuretic hormone. (Reprinted by permission from Snyder SH: Opiate receptors in the brain. N Engl J Med 296:266–271, 1977.)

Table 10.3
Receptors, Subpopulation, and Postulated Types

Type	Physiologic Response	Activators	
		Endogenous	Exogenous
μ	Miosis, analgesia; bradycardia; respiratory depression	Met-Leu-enkephalin β-endorphin	Morphine
κ	Sedation; no respiratory depression	Dynorphin	Ethylketocyclazocine; bremazocine
σ	Excitatory symptoms; tachycardia; hypertonia; tachypnea	?	Phencyclidine; SKF10047
δ	Analgesia?	Met-Leu-enkephalin β-endorphin	DADL[a]; Dezocine? (μ and δ)
ε	?		

[a] α-leu₅-enkephalin.

cluding pK$_a$. The greater the percentage of the drug that is in the anionic (base) form at a pH of 7.4, the more rapid the penetration of membranes such as the dura mater and dorsal horn, and consequently, the more rapid the onset of narcotic effect. For example, alfentanil, with a lower pK$_a$ of 6.5, would be expected to have a more rapid onset than morphine, which has a pK$_a$ of 7.9 (Table 10.4).

Lipid solubility also plays a key role. Fentanyl has a lipid solubility 800 times greater than that of morphine and more rapid onset clinically when administered epidurally (27–30).

Molecular weight undoubtedly is also a factor in membrane transport of intraspinal narcotics (31). For example, the molecular weights of the two narcotics commonly used as intraspinal agents, morphine (285) and fentanyl (336), are similar to the molecular weights of the two local anesthetics used intraspinally, lidocaine (271) and bupivacaine (324), suggesting comparable influence.

Movement of Narcotics within Cerebrospinal Fluid: Rostral Spread

Because of factors such as lipid solubility and pK$_a$, different types of narcotics have different rates of absorption and movement in the CSF that produce different actions and side effects. For example, the rapid tissue penetration and receptor uptake of fentanyl and meperidine limit the amount of narcotic moving centrally through the CSF. When ¹⁴C-mor-

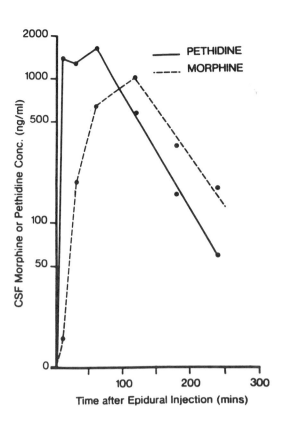

Figure 10.4. Cervical CSF concentrations of morphine and pethidine (meperidine) as a function of time following lumbar epidural administration. Morphine (10 mg) and pethidine (50 mg) in 10 ml of normal saline were administered simultaneously by means of a lumbar epidural catheter at L2–L3 interspace, and CSF samples were collected from the C7–T1 interspace at the times shown on the graph. Peak cervical CSF concentrations of pethidine were achieved earlier and declined sooner in comparison to those of morphine. Also, the peak concentrations of pethidine were lower than those of morphine, considering the doses of the two drugs injected. The rapid appearance of pethidine in CSF is in keeping with rapid diffusion through the dura. (Reprinted by permission from Gourlay GK, Cherry DA, Plummer JL, Armstrong PJ, Cousins MJ: The influence of drug polarity on the absorption of opioid drugs into CSF and subsequent cephalad migration following lumbar epidural administration: Application to morphine and pethidine. Pain 31:297–305, 1987.)

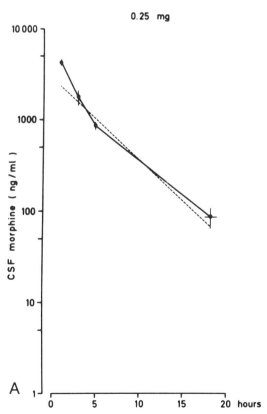

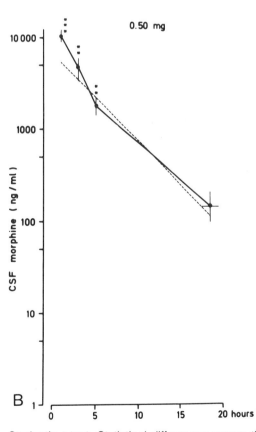

Figure 10.5. CSF morphine concentration contrasted with time plots following a single intrathecal dose of either 0.25 (*A*) or 0.50 (*B*) mg of morphine in five and six patients, respectively. Values shown are mean ± SEM. The *dotted line* represents the regression line obtained by a monoexponential fit to the individual data points. Statistical evaluation by Student's *t* test. Statistical differences versus the 0.25 mg group: $**P < 0.01$; $***P < 0.001$. (Reprinted by permission from Nordberg G, Hedner T, Mellstrand T, Dahlström B: Pharmacokinetic aspects of intrathecal morphine analgesia. Anesthesiology 60:448–454, 1984.)

Table 10.4
Molecular Weight, pK$_a$, Lipid Solubility, and Relative Potential for CNS Entry for Various Narcotic Agents[a]

Narcotic	Molecular Weight	pK$_a$[b]	Octanol Water Partition Coefficient	Relative Potential for CNS Entry[c]
Morphine	285	7.9	1.4	1
Meperidine	247	8.5	39	12
Fentanyl	336	8.4	816	133
Sufentanil	386	8.0	1757	133
Alfentanil	417	6.5	129	10
Methadone	309	9.3	116	—
Lidocaine	271	7.9	2.9[d]	
Bupivacaine	324	8.1	27.5[d]	

[a] Adapted from Hug CC Jr: Pharmacokinetics of new synthetic narcotic analgesics. In *Opioids in Anesthesia*. FG Estafanous, ed. Butterworth, Boston, 1984, p 52.
[b] At 37°C.
[c] Apparent partition coefficient at pH 7.4 multiplied by the free fraction of drug in plasma and divided by the value for morphine.
[d] n-Heptane/pH 7.4 buffer, partition coefficient.

phine and ^{3}H-fentanyl were injected intrathecally in animal models, the more hydrophilic morphine could be traced in the CSF over time, whereas the lipophilic fentanyl was quickly cleared (32). The movement of hydrophilic metrizamide has been studied with computerized tomographic (CT) scanning (33). With the patient in the supine position, metrizamide, which is slightly hyperbaric, spread upward from the lumbar subarachnoid space to the medulla within 30 min, suggesting that hydrophilic narcotics such as morphine may travel relatively rapidly and freely in the CSF to higher CNS centers. The risk of such movement is that narcotics might reach the ventral surface of the medulla where the central reflex control of respiratory function resides and induce respiratory depression. The potentially harmful effects of intraspinal narcotics are thus dose-related to the rates of narcotic absorption and movement in the CSF. Clinical work has now demonstrated that, although there is rapid central movement of morphine and the lipid-soluble narcotics, the onset of side effects is graded (Fig. 10.4) (34–36).

Although the rapid absorption of lipophilic narcotics into the CNS and other tissues results in fewer side effects, it also produces a much shorter duration of action than hydrophilic narcotics—that is, the rapid onset and tissue uptake that may decrease central CSF movement of lipophilic drug means that the elimination of such drugs also is rapid. For example, meperidine and fentanyl have been shown to provide 2 to 6 hr of analgesia, whereas morphine can provide 15 to 30 hr. The lipid soluble narcotics are "fast in" and "fast out." In many cases their clinical epidural action is very close in duration to an intramuscular application.

Concentration of Narcotics in Cerebrospinal Fluid and Duration of Narcotic Action

It appears that the concentration of narcotics in the CSF determines the duration and effectiveness of analgesia obtained. The concentration achieved depends on both the dose administered and the route selected. Results from a study by Nordberg and co-workers (37) demonstrated that as little as 0.25 to 0.5 mg of intrathecal morphine produced very high CSF morphine levels 16 to 19 hr later (Fig. 10.5). These authors also found that the clearance of intrathecal morphine from the CSF (terminal elimination half-life) was similar to that from plasma following various forms of administration. They concluded that the significant "pharmacokinetics parameter related to the long duration of analgesia after intrathecal morphine administration probably is the high CSF concentration" (37). This suggests that analgesia is dose related and opiate CSF concentration depends on the route of administration (Figs. 10.5 and 10.6) (38).

The results of the Nordberg et al. study are of particular interest when comparing analgesia provided for labor using epidural morphine with that provided by intrathecal morphine. Small intrathecal doses of morphine (0.25 to 0.5 mg) yield a relatively high concentration of narcotic in the CSF and good analgesia; epidurally administered morphine requires much higher doses (3 to 5 mg) to achieve an adequate CSF concentration and analgesia. However, the analgesia achieved epidurally can be nearly as effective as that obtained intrathecally, but may result in significant side effects. Further research in this area may help to define the parameters for effective application of intraspinal narcotics.

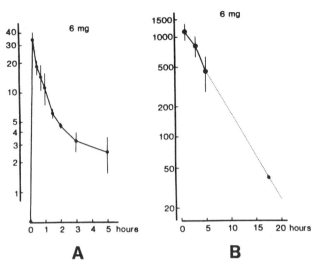

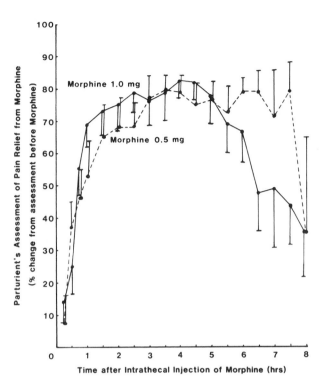

Figure 10.6. The plasma concentration of morphine (*A*) over time following the epidural administration of 6 mg of morphine compared with the CSF concentration of morphine (*B*). The elimination half-lives from plasma and CSF were similar, but the amount in the CSF far exceeded the plasma concentration after epidural administration. Not shown are peak CSF morphine levels after 2 and 4 mg of epidural morphine of approximately 350 ng/ml and 425 ng/ml, respectively. (Reprinted by permission from Nordberg G, Hedner T, Mellstrand T, Dahlström B: Pharmacokinetic aspects of epidural morphine analgesia. Anesthesiology 58:545–551, 1983.)

Figure 10.7. The parturient's assessment of pain relief from morphine during labor. Pain relief was achieved with 0.5 mg (*n* = 12) and 1 mg (*n* = 18) of intrathecal morphine in 7.5% dextrose administered when the cervix was 4 to 8 cm dilated. Both doses provided excellent pain relief during the first stage of labor. (Reprinted by permission from Abboud TK, Shnider SM, Dailey PA, Raya JA, Sarkis F, Grobler NM, Sadri S, Khoo SS, DeSousa B, Baysinger CL, Miller F: Intrathecal administration of hyperbaric morphine for the relief of pain in labor. Br J Anaesth 56:1351–1360, 1984.)

CLINICAL APPLICATION

The concept of intraspinal narcotics is simple: long-lasting analgesia produced with minimal doses of narcotics. This is achieved by the limited and almost direct application of narcotics (epidural or spinal) to the dorsal horn of the spinal column, resulting in analgesia without the systemic effects of narcotics. The remainder of this chapter examines the use of intraspinal narcotic analgesia for labor, delivery, and intra- and postoperative cesarean section pain and the side effects accompanying the use of this technique.

Labor and Delivery

When Wang and co-workers (1) demonstrated the successful and safe use of 0.5 to 1 mg of intrathecal morphine for patients with chronic pain, the implications for obstetrics were clear. They had achieved 10 to 24 hr of pain relief with no sympathetic or motor blockade using very low doses of narcotics. In general, the use of systemic narcotics in obstetrics is limited by the possibility of maternal respiratory depression; orthostatic hypotension; nausea, vomiting, and delayed gastric motility; decreased uterine activity when administered during early labor; and placental transfer of narcotic resulting in neonatal respiratory depression. However, all these problems

are dose related, and some may be avoided or ameliorated with the use of lower intraspinal doses.

INTRATHECAL OPIATES

The intrathecal application of as little as 0.5 mg of morphine has been successful in relieving the pain of the first stage of labor (Fig. 10.7) (39). In contrast, for nonobstetric patients as much as 20 mg of morphine has been used to relieve some forms of pain (40, 41). The ideal dose for analgesia during labor has not been determined, but 0.5 to 1.5 mg of morphine appears to be the appropriate range. High CSF levels of narcotic can be achieved with as little as 0.25 mg of intrathecal morphine, suggesting that the lower dose range is useful (Fig. 10.5).

Scott and co-workers were the first to use 1.5 mg of intrathecal morphine to provide pain relief during labor (42). Although the study was small (n = 12), they made several important observations. First, patients obtained pain relief but "felt contractions," implying that opiate blockade of pain is not as complete as that achieved using local anesthetics. This effect potentially benefits patients who want pain relief but also fuller participation in the delivery experience. Second, they observed that 1.5 mg of intrathecal morphine did not provide adequate pain relief for the second stage of labor. Intraspinal narcotics achieve analgesia, not surgical anesthesia! If surgical manipulation during labor or delivery were necessary (e.g., the use of forceps or an episiotomy), local anesthetic would have to be administered via the epidural or spinal route (or other technique) to provide further analgesia or anesthesia. Compared with the flexibility offered by initially using a continuous epidural route, single-injection intrathecal administration has a distinct disadvantage. One early investigator overcame this problem by following single-bolus injection of intrathecal morphine with placement of an epidural catheter to permit administration of local anesthetic if needed for delivery (43). The use of the "combined technique" or passing a long spinal needle through an epidural needle has made this approach easier. This allows for the easy spinal application of narcotics, followed by the placement of an epidural catheter for later use as needed.

One limitation of the intrathecal technique is the slow onset of analgesia. Although early reports suggested a rapid onset, 30 to 45 min usually is required with morphine alone (Fig. 10.8). This may be an unacceptable delay when the patient is in extreme pain. One possible approach to the problem is to combine a local anesthetic with morphine. Local anesthetics clearly have a potentiating effect on spinal morphine antinociception (44). In patients undergoing transurethral resection of the prostate, tetracaine (12 to 14 mg) has been used successfully with morphine (1 mg) for anesthesia and postoperative pain (45). This approach also may be effective in obstetric patients who may require immediate and long-lasting pain relief.

Another approach might be to apply intrathecal narcotics during early labor, perhaps when the cervix is 3 to 4 cm dilated and the patient is in good labor with only mild to moderate pain; this would allow for the onset of morphine's effects in early labor. One approach is to give 0.25 mg intrathecal morphine and 25 μg of fentanyl through a long spinal needle placed through an epidural needle. The epidural catheter is then placed to allow for the addition of a local anesthetic, which is generally needed in the second stage of labor (if not before) and which also can be used if a surgical delivery is required. Bupivacaine 0.125% is definitely more effective if the patient has previously received intrathecal morphine (46). The combination of intrathecal morphine and fentanyl was described by Leighton et al., but it is not anesthetic *nirvana* (Fig. 10.9) (47).

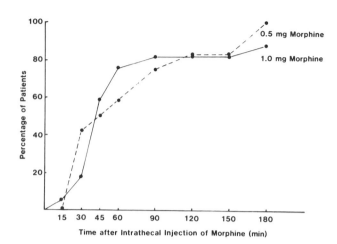

Figure 10.8. Onset of pain relief with intrathecal morphine. (Reprinted by permission from Abboud TK, Shnider SM, Dailey PA, Raja JA, Sarkis F, Grobler NM, Sadri S, Khoo SS, DeSousa B, Baysinger CL, Miller F: Intrathecal administration of hyperbaric morphine for the relief of pain in labor. Br J Anaesth 56:1351–1360, 1984.)

Intrathecal morphine has significant side effects, specifically the potential for delayed respiratory depression, the risk of which must be carefully considered if this technique is to be used. Patients must be appropriately monitored for 12 to 24 hr for late respiratory depression, and equipment for emergency resuscitation must be immediately available.

Other side effects include nausea, vomiting, urinary retention, and pruritus (Table 10.5) (39). Pruritus is the most common of these effects and may range from a mild facial itching to a generalized, highly irritating itch that requires immediate treatment. Aggressive treatment with naloxone (0.04 to 0.1 mg IV, repeated as necessary), including the possible use of naloxone infusion (0.2 to 0.4 mg/hr), may provide a positive pain relief experience resulting in good patient satisfaction, particularly during labor. A postdural puncture headache may also occur in the obstetric patient; the incidence ranges from 3.3 to 16% or higher (39, 48). This may be an unacceptable risk for routine analgesia during labor. However, the lower incidence of spinal headaches with the pencil-point spinal needles may help to make spinal narcotics a reasonable approach, particularly when an epidural catheter is placed at the same time.

Although the use of fentanyl, newer spinal needles, microspinal catheters and the combined technique (spinal and epidural) have solved many of the problems associated with the intrathecal approach, one has to ask if it's worth the effort in routine cases. Moreover, at this point, the routine use of the new microspinal catheters is not recommended despite the anecdotal reports in the literature (49). This is discussed in some detail in Chapter 9. With the mi-

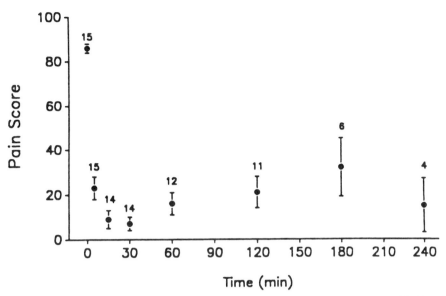

Figure 10.9. Mean ± SEM pain scores (*0* = no pain, *100* = worst imaginable pain) after intrathecal injection of fentanyl (25 µg) and morphine (0.25 mg) for pain relief during labor. The number of patients still laboring under intrathecal narcotic analgesia appears above each value. (Redrawn from Leigh-ton BL, DeSimone CA, Norris MC, Ben-David B: Intrathecal narcotics for labor revisited: The combination of fentanyl and morphine intrathecally provides rapid onset of profound, prolonged analgesia. Anesth Analg 69:122–125, 1989.)

Table 10.5
Percentages of Patients Having Adverse Side Effects after Intrathecal Injection of 0.5 mg or 1 mg Morphine[a]

| Side Effects | Morphine | | Combined Data |
	0.5 mg (n = 12) (%)	1 mg (n = 18) (%)	(n = 30) (%)
Pruritus[b]	58	94	80
Nausea/vomiting	50	56	53
Urinary retention	42	44	43
Drowsiness/dizziness	33	50	43
Respiratory depression	0	6	3
Headache	0	5	3

[a]This table demonstrates the incidence of side effects demonstrated by one study, but is representative of what might be expected. Pruritus is the most common side effect. Incidence of urinary retention is very high and probably related to labor and delivery. (Adapted from Abboud TK, Shnider SM, Dailey PA, Raya JA, Sarkis F, Grobler NM, Sadri S, Khoo SS, DeSousa B, Baysinger CL, Miller F: Intrathecal administration of hyperbaric morphine for the relief of pain in labor. Br J Anaesth 56:1351–1360, 1984.)
[b]$P = 0.02$: 0.5 mg vs. 1 mg.

crocatheters there is a potential risk of neurotoxicity, purportedly from high-dose local anesthetic administration and maldistribution (51, 52), an ever-present risk of infection and concern for neurotoxicity of intrathecal agents such as butorphanol and possibly sufentanil (50). As of June 1992 these catheters have been recalled by the United States Food and Drug Administration.

Progress of Labor

The effect of intrathecal morphine on the progress of labor has been questioned recently (47). Baraka and co-workers (43) demonstrated that neither 1 mg nor 2 mg of intrathecal morphine affected the rate of cervical dilation (Fig. 10.10). When epidural meperidine (100 mg) was compared with bupivacaine 0.25%, the results were the same—that is, no difference was found in the progress of labor (53) (although there was no control group in this study). Two other studies (39, 54) have reported normal progress for the first stage of labor in 74 and 88% (respectively) of parturients given intrathecal morphine for labor. All but one patient delivered vaginally. In the first study (n = 30), the incidence of midforceps delivery was 23%, and in the second (n = 40), approximately 15%. In the first study 41% of the patients had a prolonged second stage of labor, and in the second study, 28%. The relatively high incidence of midforceps deliveries and prolonged second-stage labor is probably attributable to the decrease in the patient's urge to bear down and push during the second stage. However, Abouleish et al. noted a prolonged first, but not second, stage labor after intrathecal morphine administration (0.2 mg) (47). Various hypotheses were proposed, including: (a) hypothalamic-pituitary level action of morphine; (b) a spinal cord site of action resulting in an effect similar to that of morphine upon micturition; and (c) direct uterine opioid receptor effects (47, 55, 56). In contrast, Cohen et al. observed that epidural sufentanil actually shortened labor (57).

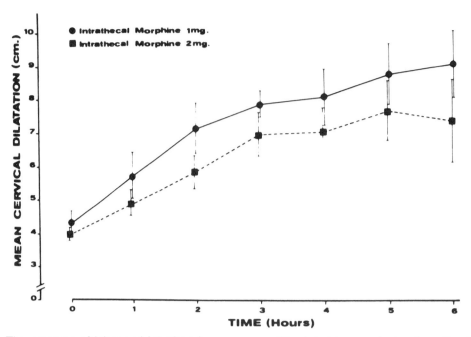

Figure 10.10. The progress of labor and intrathecal morphine: cervical dilation versus time. Mean cervical dilation versus time is represented for seven patients who were given 1 mg of intrathecal morphine and thirteen patients given 2 mg. (Reprinted by permission from Baraka A, Noueihid R, Hajj S: Intrathecal injection of morphine for obstetric analgesia. Anesthesiology 54:136–140, 1981.)

The answer is clouded and further studies are necessary. This potential problem must be considered if intrathecal morphine is to become a routine approach to analgesia for labor and delivery.

Although intrathecal administration is not recommended for routine use at this time, it may confer special benefits to parturients in whom the cardiovascular effects of routine regional anesthesia are undesirable. For certain cardiac patients, complications arise when there is a decrease in systemic vascular resistance during regional anesthesia. This can be avoided with the use of intraspinal narcotics. Studies in animal models (58, 59) document that few if any cardiovascular effects accompany the use of epidural morphine (Fig. 10.11) (60, 61). Several case reports of patients with complex cardiac problems demonstrate that intrathecal morphine has also been used successfully (62–64). The use of intrathecal opiates (combined with an epidural catheter) might benefit women with preeclampsia, although more investigation of this technique in these patients is necessary before the intrathecal approach can become routine. In general, obstetric patients with aortic stenosis, tetralogy of Fallot, Eisenmenger's syndrome, coarctation of the aorta, or pulmonary hypertension should be considered candidates for the intraspinal technique, with or without an epidural catheter placed at the same time.

EPIDURAL OPIATES

The use of continuous epidural infusion is a standard part of pain relief in labor. When Behar et al.

(2) reported good pain relief achieved with 2 mg of epidural morphine, their finding appeared to have particular relevance for labor and delivery. The possibility of providing good obstetric analgesia with such a small amount of narcotic and no resultant sympathectomy or motor blockade was intriguing. The continuous epidural technique, if effective, would have a distinct advantage over intrathecal administration because it is readily adaptable to changing clinical situations—for example, a sudden decision to perform a cesarean section.

Although one of the first reports following that of Behar et al. sounded optimistic (65), subsequent reports have not been as encouraging. Most investigators have reported generally unsatisfactory results using low-dose epidural morphine for analgesia during labor. Husemeyer and co-workers (62) tried to repeat the work of Behar et al. using 2 mg of preservative-free epidural morphine for women in labor and found that it provided no appreciable pain relief. Overall, investigators using 2 to 5 mg of epidural morphine or equivalent doses of meperidine have demonstrated that these doses are inadequate (66–71). These findings contrast sharply with the effectiveness of as little as 0.5 mg of intrathecal morphine for analgesia for labor or 2 to 5 mg of epidural morphine for postoperative analgesia. Studies performed by Hughes and co-workers (72) suggest a dose response. At similar doses, intrathecal injection introduces more morphine into the CSF than does epidural administration (Table 10.6), indicating that epidural morphine doses must be much higher than intrathecal doses to achieve similarly effective analgesia.

Hughes and co-workers (72) compared the effectiveness of preservative-free epidural morphine, at doses of 2 (n = 7), 5 (n = 10), and 7.5 mg (n = 11), with that of bupivacaine (n = 10) at 0.5% concentration. At 2 and 5 mg, morphine was ineffective, but at 7.5 mg it produced satisfactory analgesia in seven

of the eleven patients (Fig. 10.12) (72). The analgesia produced by 0.5% bupivacaine (no longer commonly used for labor) was superior, although repeated doses were necessary and resulted in the expected motor and sympathetic blockade.

Administering higher doses of epidural morphine has produced mixed results. Initial reports from Germany indicated that eight of ten parturients given 10 mg of epidural morphine experienced "fair" analgesia (73). Dick and co-workers (74) reported that six parturients given 10 mg of epidural morphine experienced inadequate pain relief accompanied by nausea, vomiting, and increased drowsiness. Although the results suggest a dose response, the incidence of side effects is unacceptable. Thus epidural morphine alone is a poor choice. Of particular concern during epidural administration of high-dose morphine (or other narcotic) to obstetric patients is that the high level of narcotic produced in the mother may lead to significant narcotic levels in the newborn via placental transfer (Fig. 10.13) (75).

Epidural meperidine (53), fentanyl (76), sufentanil (77), alfentanil (78), and lofentanil also have been used for analgesia for labor and delivery. These more lipophilic agents have a rapid onset but shorter duration of action than morphine. According to one study 100 mg of epidural meperidine provided satisfactory analgesia for obstetric patients for only 160.8 ± 90.3 min (53). Epidural fentanyl also is effective but of short duration. Analgesia of such short duration may be significantly related to systemic absorption. Epidural sufentanil has been reported to provide significant dose-related analgesia for labor at doses as low as 5 to 10 μg (Fig. 10.17) (77) with no neonatal complications. All patients received a lidocaine-epinephrine test dose. Thus, for short labors, several doses of perhaps 10 μg each of sufentanil with 10 ml of saline might provide good analgesia for the first and most of the second stages of labor (see Chapter 9). Epidural alfentanil in large doses (30 μg/kg), in contrast to smaller doses (96, 99), has led to neonatal hypotonia and the high doses should be avoided (78). Thus the current interest focuses on the combination of a local anesthetic with a narcotic, given as a continuous infusion. The most common local

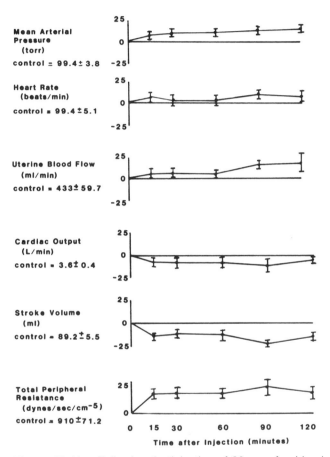

Figure 10.11. Following the injection of 20 mg of epidural morphine in the pregnant ewe, there were no significant changes in maternal cardiovascular parameters or uterine blood flow. Not shown are fetal data that demonstrated no change in blood pressure, heart rate, or acid-base status. (Data from Rosen MA, Hughes SC, Curtis JD, Norton M, Levinson G, Shnider SM: Effects of epidural morphine on uterine blood flow and acid-base status in the pregnant ewe. Anesthesiology 57:A383, 1982.)

Table 10.6
Intraspinal Morphine and CSF Concentration[a]

Site of Administration and Dose	Concentration (Time after Administration)	
	1 hr	18 hr
Epidural, 2–6 mg	200–1000 ng/ml	25–40 ng/ml
Spinal, 0.25–0.50 mg	4000–10,000 ng/ml	180–200 ng/ml

[a] Adapted from Nordberger G, Hedner T, Mellstrand T, Dahlström B: Pharmacokinetic aspects of intrathecal morphine analgesia. Anesthesiology 60:448–454, 1984.

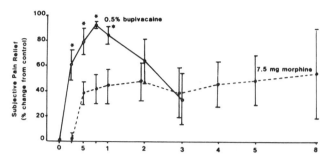

Figure 10.12. Subjective pain relief calculated from the visual linear analogue scale (mean ± SEM) contrasting 0.5% epidural bupivacaine with 7.5 mg of epidural morphine over time. *Asterisk* indicates a significant difference ($P < 0.01$). (Reprinted by permission from Hughes SC, Rosen MA, Shnider SM, Abboud TK, Stefani SJ, Norton M: Maternal and neonatal effects of epidural morphine for labor and delivery. Anesth Analg 63:319–324, 1984.)

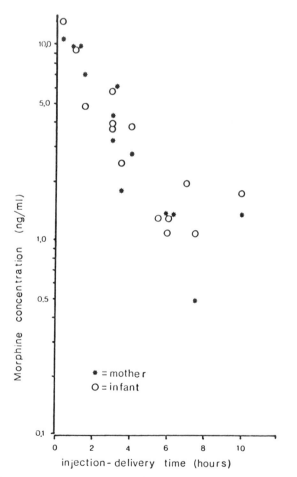

Figure 10.13. Epidural narcotics and newborn drug levels. (Reprinted by permission from Nybell-Lindahl G, Carlsson C, Ingemarsson I, Westgren M, Paalzow L: Maternal and fetal concentrations of morphine after epidural administration during labor. Am J Obstet Gynecol 139:20–21, 1981.)

anesthetic is bupivacaine (0.0625 to 0.25%) with fentanyl or sufentanil added.

LOCAL ANESTHETICS AND LIPID-SOLUBLE NARCOTICS

Justins et al. suggested that 80 μg of fentanyl added to 3 ml of 0.5% bupivacaine provided a faster onset and longer duration of analgesia than did a similar volume and concentration of bupivacaine and saline (79). This landmark paper and one that followed (Fig. 10.14) (80) have led to scores of recipes or variations on this basic theme—that is, bupivacaine (variable concentrations and volumes) plus some narcotic (most popularly fentanyl or sufentanil). Careful examination of this work and the many papers that followed is necessary to make firm judgments as to its appropriateness.

The use of a very low volume of local anesthetic (3 ml of 0.5%), is an unusual approach that has been repeated by others (81, 82). It is not surprising that a narcotic might "improve" such blocks. Additionally, the claim of rapid onset of pain relief was not well documented and a later report seemed to refute this suggestion (Fig. 10.15) (57). With a technique in which a block is first established with bupivacaine 0.2 to 0.25% and then followed by 12.5 ml/hr of 0.125% bupivacaine, the addition of fentanyl did not improve the mean pain scores or the patients' assessment of the quality of analgesia during the first or second stage of labor (Fig. 10.16) (83). The dilute solutions with fentanyl may have some appeal during the second stage of labor (84). The only proven

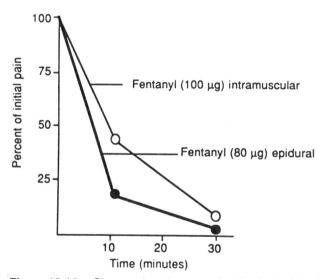

Figure 10.14. Changes in pain score after the first epidural injection of 0.5% bupivacaine in the intramuscular fentanyl group (-O-) and in the epidural fentanyl group (-●-). (Reprinted by permission from Justins DM, Knott C, Luthman J, Reynolds F: Epidural versus intramuscular fentanyl analgesia and pharmacokinetics in labour. Anaesthesia 38:937–942, 1983.)

Onset of Analgesia

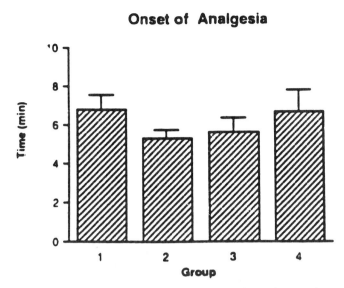

Figure 10.15. Epidural fentanyl/bupivacaine mixtures for obstetric analgesia: Whether patients received bupivacaine alone, group I (9 cc, 0.25%); bupivacaine (9 cc, 0.25%) and fentanyl (50 or 100 μg), groups 2 and 3; or bupivacaine (0.068%) and fentanyl (100 μg), the onset time of analgesia was the same. Thus even high dose fentanyl (100 μg, group 3) with a concentrated local anesthetic (bupivacaine 0.25%) did not have a faster onset when compared to plain bupivacaine 0.25% (group 1). (Reprinted by permission from Cohen SE, Tan S, Albright GA, Halpern J: Epidural fentanyl/bupivacaine mixtures for obstetric analgesia. Anesthesiology 67:403–407, 1987.)

benefits in this (83, 84) or any of the many similar studies is the finding of less motor blockade—that is, epidural fentanyl or sufentanil will allow a more dilute solution of bupivacaine to be used (0.0625 to 0.125%) and spare motor loss. This has not been shown to lead to any change in outcome, such as the incidence of forceps delivery, length of second stage, or rate of cesarean section, in a controlled study. A large review of an obstetric service that switched to the use of local anesthetics plus narcotics has purported such benefits, but they also "switched" from using 0.5% bupivacaine for labor to using the more routine dilute local anesthetics (85). On the other hand patients may clearly prefer less motor blockade, and this technique may increase patient and nursing satisfaction in some cases. However, in some patients bupivacaine 0.0625% or even 0.125% plus fentanyl (1 μg/ml) does not relieve labor pain. Thus, bupivacaine 0.25% is used as a "top-up" or as a continuous infusion. Although the dilute solutions of local anesthetics add a useful tool, they are not always ideal and the benefits may be marginal (86).

Does sufentanil improve 0.25% bupivacaine an-

algesia in any tangible way? Phillips (87) studied sufentanil in a manner similar to that of Justins et al. (79, 80). He and subsequent investigators hoped that sufentanil's higher lipid solubility (1727 vs. 816) and greater receptor affinity relative to that of fentanyl would confer an advantage (88–90). This does not seem to be the case when one examines the effects of comparable doses of these two agents. When given epidurally for labor, a bolus of sufentanil (30 μg) plus bupivacaine 0.25% was required to achieve a significant difference in analgesia compared with bupivacaine 0.25% alone. The addition of 10 or 20 μg of sufentanil to bupivacaine demonstrated no significant difference. Surely, doses as high as 30 μg sufentanil for labor analgesia routinely is questionable. Even the suggested dose of sufentanil, 1 μg/ml, plus bupivacaine 0.125% at the rate of 10 ml/hr may be excessive. Some clinicians have even suggested sufentanil, 2 μg/ml (91), in which case a labor lasting 20 hr would result in administration of a total sufentanil dose of at least 400 μg. This could prove excessive in some cases, particularly if the neonate is already compromised by meconium aspiration or is otherwise less than vigorous. Various dose regimens have been suggested, but there is no clear consensus (91–95). The doses used by clinicians range from 0.1 μg/ml of sufentanil to 2 μg/ml added to the local anesthetic solution (bupivacaine 0.0312 to 0.25%). There are essentially no comparative controlled data suggesting an appropriate dose when using sufentanil or even fentanyl. Is 0.1 μg/ml as good as 1 μg/ml of either drug? Widespread clinical experience suggests that fentanyl, 1 to 2 μg/ml, added to a local anesthetic infused at 10 to 12 ml/hr is a reasonable approach. No more than 1 μg/ml of sufentanil in a local anesthetic solution is necessary, and as suggested in Chapter 9, 0.1 to 0.2 μg/ml may be adequate.

Other agents have been suggested. Alfentanil does not appear to offer any substantial benefits over other agents (78, 96–99). Epidural butorphanol (100–102) at doses of 2 to 3 mg has resulted in maternal somnolence and a sinusoidal fetal heart rate pattern in 100% of fetuses whose mothers received the 3-mg dose (101). Butorphanol appears to offer no real advantage over epidural fentanyl or morphine.

Finally, morphine should not be forgotten as a possible additive to epidural local anesthetic. Administration of 2 mg of epidural morphine in early labor (cervical dilation of 3 cm) followed by bupivacaine when contractions were painful, significantly prolonged the duration of analgesia (Fig. 10.18) (103). Intrathecal morphine, 0.2 mg, has similar positive results (104) and deserves more widespread consideration.

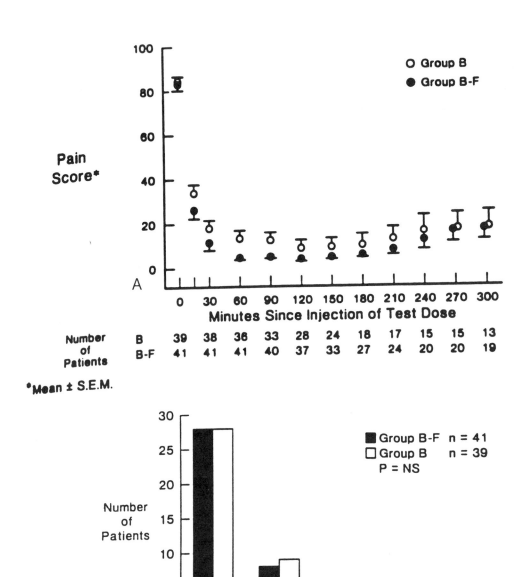

Figure 10.16. Continuous infusion epidural analgesia during labor. A, Mean ± SEM pain scores over time during the first stage of labor. B, Patient assessment of analgesia quality during first stage of labor. Patients received either bupivacaine (0.125%, group B) or bupivacaine and fentanyl (0.0625% bupivacaine + 2 μg/ml fentanyl, groups B to F). Both groups had similar onset and good quality analgesia, as judged by a visual analogue pain scale and the patients' verbal response. While group B to F had less motor loss (more dilute local anesthetic), this was achieved by giving 25 μg/hr of fentanyl. (Reprinted by permission from Chestnut DH, Owen CL, Bates JN, Ostman LG, Choi WW, Geiger MW: Continuous infusion epidural analgesia during labor: A randomized, double-blind comparison of 0.0625% bupivacaine/0.0002% fentanyl versus 0.125% bupivacaine. Anesthesiology 68:754–759, 1988.)

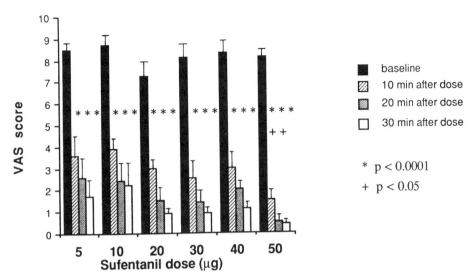

Figure 10.17. Effect of various dosages of epidural sufentanil alone for labor analgesia. All patients received a lidocaine with epinephrine test dose prior to injection of epidural sufentanil. There was a highly significant reduction in VAS scores at 10, 20, and 30 min at all doses ($P < 0.0001$). (Modified from Steinberg R, Powell G, Hu X, Dunn S: Epidural sufentanil for analgesia for labor and delivery. Reg Anesth 14:225–228, 1989.)

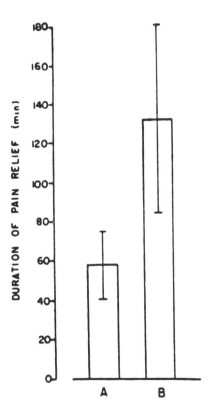

Figure 10.18. The duration in minutes (mean ± SD) of pain relief in groups A and B. Group A was treated with 8 ml of epidural bupivacaine, 0.25%. Group B was treated with epidural morphine HCL (2 mg in 10 ml of saline) in early labor followed by 8 ml of 0.25% bupivacaine when the patient was in active labor. Pain relief until the next epidural injection was significantly longer in group B than in group A. (Reprinted by permission from Niv D, Valery R, Golan A, Chayan MS: Augmentation of bupivacaine analgesia in labor by epidural morphine. Obstet Gynecol 67:206–209, 1986.)

Table 10.7
Epidural Narcotics and Local Anesthetics for Labor: A Suggested Regimen[a]

1. Establish a solid block to T10 with bupivacaine 0.125 to 0.25% or lidocaine 1.5% (usually 10 cc in divided doses, with or without epinephrine). A bolus of fentanyl (50 μgs?) or sufentanil (10 to 30 μgs?) is added to the local anesthetic.
2. Continuous infusion of bupivacaine 0.125%[b] plus fentanyl 1 μg/cc or sufentanil 0.1 to 1 μg/cc at a rate of 10 to 12 cc/hr. Adjust level by changing volume.
3. Top-up doses PRN for pain of 5 cc of bupivacaine 0.25% plain, lidocaine 1.5% plain, or bupivacaine 0.125% 10 cc.

[a] An alternative regimen is described in Chapter 9, Table 9.5.
[b] More dilute solutions may be effective in some patients (e.g., bupivacaine 0.03125 or 0.0625%).

Thus, although the benefits of the combination of various narcotics and dilute local anesthetics may be limited to better maternal motor tone, this method nonetheless has been adopted by many clinicians and is widely used. (An acceptable protocol is suggested in Table 10.7.) The clinician is urged, however, to consider the benefits carefully and limit the total dose of narcotics administered. The condition of the infant always must be considered, as well as the risk of possible neurotoxicity of various agents, particularly when administered in high doses or intrathecally in error. Epidural fentanyl has been used widely and does appear safe when dose limits are considered.

THE LIPID-SOLUBLE AGENTS— POSSIBLE USES

There may be specific indications for combining a lipid-soluble agent with a local anesthetic for analgesia during labor or delivery. Fentanyl, 50 μg, added to a top-up dose for low back pain unrelieved by plain bupivacaine 0.125% may produce adequate analgesia without the further motor blockade that would result from increasing the concentration of the local anesthetic. This might have implications for the second stage of labor (84). However, although the single dose of 50 to 100 μg of epidural fentanyl may be helpful at the start of labor, it would be inappropriate for repeated top-up doses. Ultimately, narcotics must not be used to make up for a bad epidural block, and clinicians must accept that some patients will need a more concentrated local anesthetic instead of large doses of epidural narcotics. Finally, during cesarean delivery the use of epidural fentanyl, 1 μg/kg, may be beneficial to alleviate the pain often experienced with exteriorization of the uterus or closing of the

peritoneum (105). This application remains controversial and the benefits are probably subtle, compared with those of a solid epidural block (106). At best, the use of epidural narcotics for labor analgesia is another tool in the anesthesiologist's armamentarium. There may be real benefits in specific situations, but pure local anesthetics continue to be the benchmark by which alternatives must be judged.

POSTOPERATIVE PAIN MANAGEMENT
Epidural Opiates

The use of epidural opiates to relieve the postoperative pain of cesarean delivery has been very successful. The approval by the Federal Drug Administration of a preservative-free morphine (Duramorph) in late 1984 has led to its widespread use and changed postoperative pain management for our nonobstetric anesthesia colleagues and patients as well (107).

In 1979 Wolfe and Nicholas (108) reported that fentanyl, 100 μg, diluted with 8 ml of 0.9% sodium chloride administered via an epidural catheter successfully relieved postoperative pain in 20 patients who had undergone elective cesarean section. Although time has shown epidural fentanyl to be less than ideal, this work led to real changes in early pain management (107, 109, 110). In one study it was suggested that, morphine, 10.3 mg ($\pm$ 2.5 SD) was required following upper abdominal surgery and 7.5 mg ($\pm$ 2.1 SD) following lower abdominal surgery (111). Several authors found 2 mg of epidural morphine effective for chronic pain and some postoperative and traumatic pain, but inadequate for postcesarean pain (112–114). Rosen and co-workers (115) found 2 mg of epidural morphine inadequate for postcesarean pain, but 5 and 7.5 mg were equally effective (Fig. 10.19).

Although epidural morphine, 4 to 5 mg, has become the routine approach in many institutions, a wide variety of drugs have been examined. Epidural fentanyl is probably the other most common approach to pain management in postcesarean section patients and has been widely investigated (108, 116). However, many believe that the systemic effects achieved by absorption from the epidural space (not unlike an intramuscular injection) explain much of fentanyl's effects (Fig. 10.20). The analgesic effects of epidural lidocaine 2% with 1/200,000 epinephrine or epidural bupivacaine 0.5%, alone, generally outlast the effects of epidural fentanyl. Epidural fentanyl still has its adherents (116, 117), despite the work by Malinow et al. (118) who demonstrated that "analgesia . . . after a single epidural dose of fentanyl is of

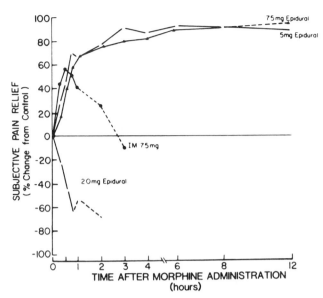

Figure 10.19. Epidural morphine relief of postoperative pain of cesarean delivery. (Reprinted by permission from Rosen MA, Hughs SC, Shnider SM, Abboud TK, Norton M, Dailey PA, Curtis JD: Epidural morphine for relief of postoperative pain after cesarean delivery. Anesth Analg 62:666–672, 1983.)

clinically insignificant duration after the use of lidocaine or bupivacaine anesthesia for cesarean section." Later work indicates that a single dose of fentanyl added to 2% lidocaine and epinephrine (probably the most common epidural agent for cesarean section) has no effect on postoperative pain (119, 120). The use of patient-controlled analgesia (PCA) by Sevarino et al. (120) for postoperative pain management after epidural lidocaine and fentanyl (vs. lidocaine and saline) further demonstrated the minimal contribution of epidural fentanyl to postoperative pain relief. What has been suggested by several authors is some contribution to better intraoperative conditions when epidural fentanyl (1 μg/kg) is added to 2% lidocaine for cesarean section (105). The potential intraoperative benefits of epidural fentanyl when added to bupivacaine was first noted in 1983 by Milon et al. (121). However, these investigators used approximately 1.7 μg/kg of epidural fentanyl and, in this as in many similar studies, one wonders if the same dose of fentanyl given intramuscularly before surgery would not have a similar effect (116, 122). Indeed, an epidural dose of 1.7 μg/kg of fentanyl

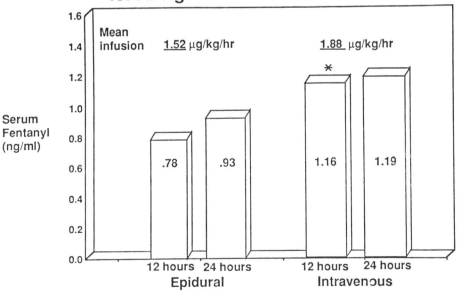

Figure 10.20. In a randomized double-blind comparison of epidural versus intravenous fentanyl infusions for analgesia for cesarean section, no clinical advantage to the epidural infusion over IV infusion could be demonstrated. While the serum fentanyl levels were significantly higher in the IV group at 12 hr, there was no difference by 24 hr. The infusion rates

were obviously quite similar. (Reprinted by permission from Ellis DJ, Millar WI, Reisner LS: A randomized double-blind comparison of epidural versus intravenous fentanyl infusion for analgesia after cesarean section. Anesthesiology 72:981–986, 1990.)

resulted in umbilical arterial plasma concentrations as high as 0.8 ng/ml (121). The effects on the newborn always must be considered, and many prefer to administer epidural narcotics after the umbilical cord is clamped. (This is discussed later in the section on fetal effects of epidural narcotics.) However, if the epidural block is not fully effective and intravenous narcotics are considered necessary it seems a reasonable alternative to administer 1 μg/kg of fentanyl through the epidural catheter, diluted to a volume of 10 ml (with more local anesthetic or saline) (123).

Finally, when considering the combination of a lipid-soluble agent and morphine, it is suggested that there is an interaction or potentiating effect of alfentanil, fentanyl, or sufentanil on morphine such that a more rapid onset is achieved, resulting in the use of a lower dose of morphine, fewer side effects, and a duration of analgesia equivalent to that obtained with larger doses of morphine alone (124). This alternative is appealing, but remains to be documented in a large series of patients. The application of significant amounts of a lipid-soluble narcotic should produce a rapid onset of analgesia. However, Sinatra et al. (125) could not demonstrate a potentiating effect of sufentanil, 30 μg, added to 3 mg of morphine epidurally; the duration of analgesia was longer with 5 mg of epidural morphine. The mean time before use of PCA in the morphine-only group was 13 hours, compared with 2.8 hours in the sufentanil and morphine group (i.e., sufentanil did not potentiate the morphine). The use of PCA is a valuable tool when evaluating the effectiveness of agents used to control pain, because the patient determines when and how much drug to administer. The lack of potentiation demonstrated by Sinatra et al. is confirmed by others, but larger studies are needed to elucidate the issue further.

Epidural sufentanil also has been widely investigated in obstetrics, as well as other postoperative pain management situations (126–130). The chief benefit of epidural sufentanil is its rapid onset and profound analgesia. Whether the analgesia is "better" than that achieved with fentanyl is uncertain, and sufentanil has many limitations (as previously discussed), including a brief duration of action in the epidural space (2 to 4 hr) (127). However, it is a reasonable agent to initiate a block in an acute pain situation, to top-up a patchy epidural block, or perhaps to administer after delivery (after verifying epidural placement intraoperatively) to help blunt the pain of uterine exteriorization. Profound respiratory depression has occurred with epidural sufentanil and patients must be monitored carefully in the acute period after administration. No caregiver should administer this drug, unless he or she is capable of

managing acute respiratory depression. Also of some concern is the effect of higher doses of sufentanil (50 to 100 μg) on central temperature control. While the patient's central temperature drops, there is no shivering. The risk of asymptomatic hypothermia has been raised by several authors, but appears not to be a concern when reasonable epidural doses are used (25 to 30 μg) (131, 132). Smaller doses of epidural narcotics may decrease the shivering that does occur with epidural anesthesia. The dose of epidural sufentanil for postoperative pain is probably 30 μg, diluted to a volume of approximately 10 to 15 ml. Sufentanil can be given as a continuous infusion, but 15 μg/hr may be needed (133).

Meperidine is another agent that is widely used epidurally (134–137). A dose of 50 mg in 10-ml saline provides analgesia lasting approximately 3 to 4 hr, a duration similar to that with intramuscular meperidine (135). However, epidural onset is rapid and analgesia may be better. Its short duration of action is a limiting factor, especially when compared to the success and longer duration of epidural morphine.

Many other epidural narcotic agents, including diamorphine, phenoperidine, butorphanol, alfentanil, hydromorphone, and buprenorphine, have been used in patients undergoing cesarean section (138–151). None of these agents has any particular advantage and, in fact, may have significant disadvantages. Lofentanil and buprenorphine are resistant to naloxone and may lead to catastrophic respiratory depression. Even epidural ketamine and droperidol have been combined with morphine for postoperative pain management (152–157), but neurotoxicity studies for many of these new epidural agents are few and results are questionable.

In conclusion, while there may well be a place for epidural fentanyl, sufentanil, or meperidine, the clear success with epidural morphine has made it the epidural agent of choice in the obstetric population for postoperative pain management (158–160).

Experience with Epidural Morphine

When Kotelko et al. (160) and Leicht et al. (200) reviewed the experience at UCSF of using 5 mg of epidural morphine for analgesia in healthy women undergoing cesarean delivery, they found that good to excellent analgesia had been achieved, lasting 24 to 36 hr for 83% of the patients (Table 10.8). Satisfactory postcesarean analgesia using the low-dose epidural technique has been reported at other centers as well (161–164). As a result, the administration of 5 mg of epidural morphine is now standard practice for many anesthesiologists. Preservative-free morphine sulfate, 5 mg (Duramorph 0.5 mg/ml), is added through the epidural catheter once the neonate is

Table 10.8
Epidural Morphine after Cesarean Section—
1000 Patients

Good to excellent pain relief (none or poor = 5.9%)	84.6%
Duration of analgesia	22.9 hrs. S.D. 13.8
Patients requiring only oral analgesics	44%
Patients requiring NO subsequent analgesics	16%

a Data from experience at University of California San Francisco; and from Leicht CH, Hughes SC, Dailey PA, Shnider SM, Rosen MA: Epidural morphine sulfate for analgesia after cesarean section: A prospective study of 1,000 patients. Anesthesiology 65:A366, 1986.

Table 10.9
Epidural Morphine after Cesarean Section—
1000 Patients

Pruritus			
None	38.8%		
Mild	20.3%	*treated*	28.6%
Moderate	35.5%		
Severe	3.9%		
Nausea	20.4%	*treated*	10.5%
Vomiting	14.8%		
Respiratory depression	0.4%	"obviously real"	0.1%

a Data from experience at University of California San Francisco; and from Leicht CH, Hughes SC, Dailey PA, Shnider SM, Rosen MA: Epidural morphine sulfate for analgesia after cesarean section: A prospective study of 1,000 patients. Anesthesiology 65:A366, 1986.

delivered. This is done in the operating room at the time of delivery to allow the analgesic to take effect before the local anesthetic has diminished, because epidural onset may take as long as 60 min and is still improving at 90 min. The experience of 1000 consecutive patients who received epidural morphine after cesarean section is shown in Table 10.8.

The most common side effect encountered is pruritus, which occurs in approximately 50% of patients. The most significant side effect is delayed respiratory depression (Table 10.9). To avoid this risk, a precise monitoring schedule is established during which respiratory rate is monitored and the adequacy of ventilation is evaluated (Table 10.10). Although some authors suggest that precise monitoring might include continuous measurement of end-tidal CO_2 or the use of an impedance apnea monitor, pulse oximetry or intensive care units, attentive nursing on the postpartum unit has proven to be satisfactory and adequate in this patient population. Experience over the last 13 years substantiates this approach.

The product labeling package insert for epidural morphine stresses that facilities using this drug must be equipped with resuscitative equipment, oxygen, naloxone, and appropriate resuscitative drugs. Moreover, patients must be carefully monitored for 12 to 24 hr following administration of the drug. Chronically ill or debilitated patients may be at particular risk for delayed respiratory depression. In addition, the depressant effects of morphine may be potentiated by the presence of other CNS depressants. Generalized sedation is a serious sign (rare) and such patients should be watched very closely.

A thoughtful approach combined with thorough knowledge of the subject is necessary when using any new drug or technique. Clearly, good monitoring is the key to the safe use of epidural morphine or any narcotic, by any route of administration.

INTRATHECAL NARCOTICS

The use of intraspinal narcotics initially was limited to the epidural route of administration. This followed from: (a) the initial success of epidural morphine in parturients; (b) the extensive investigation of various epidural dosing regimens and drugs; and (c) the initial reports of severe side effects with intrathecal narcotics. The latter, no doubt, was related to the very high doses of intrathecal morphine given to patients (2.0 to 20.0 mg of morphine). Not surprisingly, the side effects were significant and clinicians shied away from the use of intrathecal narcotics. Clearly, these problems were related to misunderstanding the dose requirements.

Intrathecal morphine now has been investigated more thoroughly and has proven to be a very reasonable choice for postcesarean section analgesia (165–167). Intrathecal fentanyl (168), sufentanil (169), and methadone (170), among other narcotics, also have been studied, but intrathecal morphine clearly has become the preferred agent. Some authors even propose that intrathecal morphine is superior to epidural morphine for postoperative pain management (171), although this is highly debatable (172). Certainly, in the obstetric population, intrathecal morphine is effective and provides another solid option for pain management. However, there is much greater experience with epidural morphine and more flexibility with a continuous epidural technique.

The ideal dose-response study for intrathecal morphine has not been performed, but a review of several papers suggests morphine, 0.25 mg, is a satisfactory dose in the cesarean section patient. While higher doses (0.3 to 1.0 mg) probably are not harmful, 0.25 mg provides 20 to 25 hr of pain relief in most patients, and the side effects can be easily managed with na-

Table 10.10
Suggested Postpartum Epidural or Intrathecal Narcotic Nursing Orders

1. The patient has received the following:
   Morphine _____ mg or _____
   Route: Epidural/Intrathecal (circle)
   Date _____ Time _____
2. Bed and kardex and chart to be labeled "Intraspinal narcotic patient."
3. Naloxone (Narcan) ampule (0.4 mg/1 ml) and syringe must be readily available at the nursing station.
4. Oxygen flow meter with nipple adapter and self-inflating bag with mask must be immediately accessible, either at nursing station or at patient's bedside.
5. No PO, IM, IV or SQ narcotics are to be given for 24 hr, except by order of an anesthesiologist: beeper # _____ or extension # _____ or as listed below.
6. Check and record respiratory rate q̄ 30 min for 12 hr, than q 1 hr until 24 hr after intraspinal narcotic administration.
7. Call anesthesiologist (beeper # _____) and house officer for *any* of the following:
   a. Respiratory rate is below 11
   b. Evidence of airway obstruction
   c. Change in respiratory pattern
   d. Decreased respiratory effort
   e. Pin-point pupils
   f. Patient is very drowsy or sedated or appears unexpectedly somnolent.
   g. Patient complains of severe itching, urinary retention, excessive nausea, vomiting
8. If respiratory rate <8/min or patient in respiratory distress, nurse may administer naloxone 0.2 mg IV (0.5 ml) and repeat if necessary.
9. Maintain IV access for 24 hr after last epidural injection.
10. For continued pain administer one of the following:
    Morphine sulfate, 1 to 2 mg IV q̄ 1 to 2 hr prn pain (hold if RR≤10.)
    Nalbuphine 5 to 10 mg IM q̄ 2 to 3 hr or
    Nalbuphine 1 to 2 mg IV q̄ 1 to 2 hr
11. For mild or moderate nausea or vomiting:
    Metoclopramide 10 mg I V q 2 hr *or*
    Droperidol 0.625 mg IV or IM q 4 hr PRN for nausea.
12. For mild or moderate pruritus:
    a. Diphenhydramine 25 mg IV or IM q 2 hr prn itching *or*
    b. Naloxone 0.1 mg (0.25 ml) q̄ 15 min PRN × 3. If symptoms relieved by IV bolus may repeat q 1 hr PRN
    c. If no relief by 45 min, start naloxone infusion at 0.2 mg/hr. This is prepared as follows:
       1.6 mg (4 ml) naloxone in 1000 ml at 125 ml/hr *or*
       0.8 mg (2 ml) naloxone in 500 ml at 125/hr *or*
       0.4 mg (1 ml) naloxone in 250 ml at 125 ml/hr
    d. If symptoms are not improved by 60 min of infusion, increase rate to 0.4 mg/hr by adding more naloxone to IV fluids.
    e. Pitocin and naloxone are compatible and can be mixed together.
    f. Discontinue naloxone infusion after 3 hr. If pruritus returns, restart naloxone infusion for an additional 3 hr.
    g. If surgical pain returns, stop infusion and call anesthesia resident.

FLAG CHART TO INDICATE NEW ORDER	Signature _____ M.D.	Beeper # _____ M.D. # _____
	Checked by _____ R.N.	Time _____ Date _____

loxone. Higher doses (1.0 mg or more?) result in some degree of respiratory depression (increasing end-tidal CO_2). Thus, using more than 0.5 mg would seem unnecessary and likely unreasonable in the routine management of postoperative pain in cesarean section patients. Of note is that the studies by both Abouleish et al. (intrathecal) and Brose and Cohen (epidural) found as much or more respiratory depression with parenteral narcotics as with intraspinal narcotics (166, 173). Morphine, 0.25 mg, is commonly added to bupivacaine or other local anes-

thetics for management of postoperative pain following cesarean section.

Intrathecal fentanyl has been shown to provide some analgesia, but of very brief duration. It is suggested that as little as 6.25 μg is an appropriate dose for postoperative pain management (168). Fentanyl may improve intraoperative conditions (less pain with uterine exteriorization), may decrease the need for intraoperative narcotics, and may provide a smoother transition to postoperative pain relief. Intrathecal morphine is slow in onset (30 to 45 min) and still improving at 90 min. Thus, the addition of a small dose of fentanyl (6.25 to 25.0 μg) to local anesthetics may be helpful, although this is controversial (174).

In conclusion, intrathecal morphine is now a well-established choice for pain management (165). Monitoring and treatment of side effects should be no different than those described for epidural morphine. Intrathecal morphine is an effective and safe choice for postoperative pain management in the obstetric patient.

Does the Addition of Local Anesthetic Affect the Efficacy of Epidural Morphine?

A review of the use of epidural morphine by Kotelko and co-workers (175) revealed that the intraoperative use of chloroprocaine for anesthesia adversely affected the successful use of epidural morphine for postoperative analgesia. They speculated that the chloroprocaine solution (pH 2.7) lowers pH in the epidural space to such an extent that morphine remains highly ionized, which delays its onset and reduces its potency. However, their results contrast with those of Youngstrom et al. (161) who found that cesarean delivery patients anesthetized with chloroprocaine and given 4 mg of epidural morphine for postoperative pain experienced pain relief lasting 20 hr. Multiple studies have debated the possibility of chloroprocaine antagonism of epidural morphine or fentanyl (118, 176–182). Of the numerous case studies and comments reporting adverse effects of the use of chloroprocaine, the work by Schlalret et al. (177) is most intriguing. They demonstrated that a small test dose of 2% chloroprocaine vs. 2% lidocaine, followed by anesthesia with 0.5% bupivacaine, reduced the efficacy of postoperative analgesia with epidural morphine (5.0 mg). Chloroprocaine may, in fact, have an antagonistic effect, but the mechanism of action is uncertain.

Epinephrine and Epidural Opiates

The addition of epinephrine to a local anesthetic solution offers the advantages of increasing the duration of action, lowering the peak serum local anesthetic level, and increasing the intensity of neural blockade, all of which might be beneficial for the patient given epidural opiates. As early as 1904, it was demonstrated that analgesia could be achieved with epinephrine alone and, by 1950, in parturients (183). The latter study by Priddle and Andros involved several experiments, including administration of 1.0 mg of epinephrine (1 ml of 1:1000) mixed with 1 ml of 5% dextrose to parturients for labor analgesia. The result was complete pain relief. This approach is not recommended. The potential of neural damage from profound and prolonged vasoconstriction is very real. However, when combined with ep-

idural agents, epinephrine clearly potentiates analgesia. We now know this potentiation to be mediated through α₂-adrenoreceptors and the inhibition of substance P and dorsal horn neuron firing (184–187).

It has been demonstrated in cats that spinally administered epinephrine suppresses noxiously evoked activity in the dorsal horn (188) (Fig. 10.21). These investigators suggested that adrenergic agonists "may act in a multiplicative fashion with spinally administered opiates to produce a profound suppression of noxiously evoked activity" (188). The use of epinephrine, norepinephrine, and now clonidine and its analogs, makes further use of our increasing knowledge of intraspinal mechanisms of pain transmission. Investigations by Eisenach (186, 189–192) and others (193–197) may lead to the routine clinical use of clonidine or similar drugs. The use of intraspinal narcotics may be just the beginning of very specific modulation of pain pathways, but our initial application of new drugs must be cautious (198).

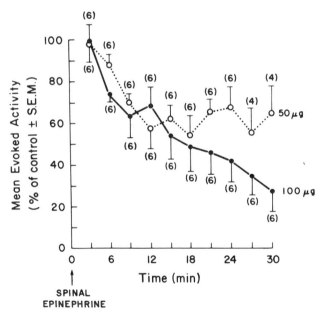

Figure 10.21. Spinally administered epinephrine suppresses noxiously evoked activity of WDR neurons in the dorsal horn of the spinal cord. "Effects of 50 μg and 100 μg of spinally administered epinephrine on the mean evoked activity of all the neurons included in this study. Abscissa: time in minutes after spinal epinephrine administration. Ordinate: mean evoked activity expressed as a percent of control. The numbers in parentheses indicate the number of cells studied at each point. The flats represent ± SEM." (Reprinted by permission from Collins JG, Kitahata LM, Matsumoto N, Homma E, Suzukawa M: Spinally administered epinephrine suppresses noxiously evoked activity of WDR neurons in the dorsal horn of the spinal cord. Anesthesiology 60:269–275, 1984.)

COMPLICATIONS OF INTRASPINAL NARCOTICS

The chief side effects of intraspinal narcotics are pruritus, nausea, vomiting, somnolence, urinary retention, and late respiratory depression. The reported incidence of side effects varies greatly, possibly because of the small number of patients and absence of controls in many studies.

The most extensive early study of the side effects of epidural morphine was conducted by Reiz and Westberg (199). They clearly outlined the potential problems with the use of the technique, but reported a significantly lower incidence of side effects than previously encountered. In a study of 1200 patients, they found a 17% incidence of nausea and vomiting. Following use of a standard morphine solution, the incidence of pruritus was 15% but decreased to 1% with preservative-free morphine. A large review (n = 1002) revealed a 60% incidence of pruritus, a finding consistent with many others (Table 10.9) (200).

Bromage and co-workers (201) reported a significantly higher incidence of side effects when 1:200,000 epinephrine was added to 10 mg of epidural morphine than with administration of the same dose of morphine alone. While this finding represented only three volunteer patients without surgical pain, this finding generally has been supported by others (202). Bromage et al. (201) also reported a decrease in peak plasma morphine level from 44 ± 12.9 ng/ml to 13.7 ± 6.7 ng/ml with epidural morphine solutions containing epinephrine. Vasoconstriction of epidural veins by epinephrine leads to increased CSF levels of narcotic, i.e., a slower systemic uptake of narcotic. This may produce greater analgesia but also will increase side effects. Clearly, side effects are dose-related.

Delayed Respiratory Depression

The most serious side effect, delayed respiratory depression, has occurred with the use of both epidural and spinal opiates since the first use of this technique (16), and has occurred with both morphine and the lipid-soluble agents (203–214). All narcotics, whether administered as intravenous, intramuscular, intrathecal, or epidural agents, can and have caused respiratory depression. All patients who receive narcotics should be monitored closely (173). Respiratory depression may occur when epidurally administered narcotic reaches its peak plasma level or, more seriously, 6 or more hours after the initial administration of narcotic.

Respiratory depression can and does occur in obstetric patients (200). In a retrospective study of delayed respiratory depression, the Swedish Society of Anesthesiologists estimated that, in 6000 to 9000 pa-

tients, the incidence of respiratory depression was 0.25 to 0.40% with epidural opiates and 4 to 7% with intrathecal opiates (215). Respiratory depression appeared to be related to the age of the patient (with increased incidence in those 70 years of age or older), the presence of pulmonary disease, the addition of systemic narcotics, or the thoracic administration of epidural morphine. The dose of narcotic also has been shown to be important; as little as 1.0 mg of intrathecal morphine (or less!) may cause respiratory depression (205). Therefore, all patients given epidural or intrathecal morphine must be monitored for respiratory depression (Table 10.10) (200).

Reports of respiratory depression are numerous and no longer unusual (Table 10.11) (107, 200, 203–214, 216). The body of work concerning the respiratory response to narcotics administered by various routes is growing (217, 218). Should anyone be surprised that 400 mg of epidural morphine (given inadvertently) causes respiratory depression (219)? Profound respiratory depression with as little as 100 μg of epidural fentanyl has been reported (213). Respiratory depression may occur at a rate of approximately 0.1 to 0.25% in cesarean section patients given epidural morphine. A nursing staff that is capable of and allowed to administer intramuscular narcotics has the necessary skills and general knowledge to monitor patients who have received epidural narcotics. After appropriate education concerning the specific side effects of epidural or intrathecal narcotics, monitoring these patients in the routine obstetric-postpartum wards is appropriate.

Table 10.11
Respiratory Depression—How Much of a Problem?

	Patients (n)[a]	Respiratory Depression
Cesarean section—UCSF experience (prospective study)		
Leicht C et al. (200)	1000	4 (0.4%)[b]
General surgery		
Stenseth R et al. (216)	1085	10 (0.9%)
National survey—all patients		
Rawal N et al. (275)	15,100	13 (0.9%)
General surgery		
Ready B et al. (107)	623	4 (0.6%)
Cesarean section		
Fuller J et al. (276)	4880	12 (0.25%)

[a] In these papers the patients with respiratory depression (both simple decreased respiratory rate or clear depression [see Fig. 10.22]) all recovered with no adverse sequelae. Many were simply observed, whereas some required naloxone and oxygen therapy.
[b] In the study at UCSF only one of the four patients, or 0.1%, had true respiratory depression (Fig. 10.22).

TIME SEQUENCE OF RESPIRATORY
DEPRESSION IN ONE PATIENT

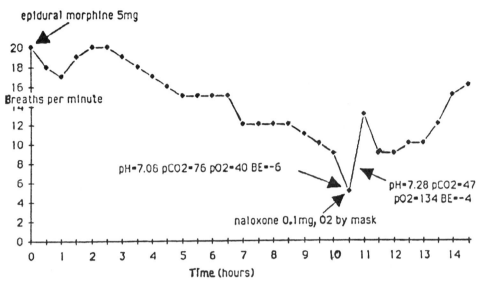

Figure 10.22. This represents the respiratory rate (*RR*) of an obstetric patient who received 5 mg of epidural morphine after a cesarean section. The patient became progressively sedate and had a decreasing RR. She was given naloxone and recovered uneventfully. (Reprinted by permission from Leicht CH, Hughes SC, Dailey PA, Shnider SM, Rosen MA: Epidural morphine sulfate for analgesia after cesarean section: A prospective report of 1000 patients. Anesthesiology 65:A366, 1986.)

Clinical experience suggests that the period when the patient is at greatest risk for delayed respiratory depression is 4 to 8 hr after the epidural administration of narcotic. A biphasic ventilatory response to epidural morphine has been suggested, with initial respiratory depression caused by the serum level, and depression occurring at 8 hr by movement in the CSF (220). This also was suggested by Camporesi and co-workers (221), who demonstrated that CO_2 response curves in volunteers were maximally depressed at 0.5 hr following intravenous administration of morphine and at 6 to 10 hr following epidural administration. Although it is probably still prudent to monitor for 24 hr after epidural morphine, the risk period probably does not extend beyond 12 hr, assuming the patient is alert and free of other side effects at that time (Fig. 10.22).

Providing pain relief always invites risk, and perhaps no medical intervention is without risk. However, the potential for respiratory depression must be a key caveat to the use of narcotics, whether the route is intraspinal, intramuscular, or intravenous.

PRURITUS

The most common side effect of intraspinal narcotics is pruritus (Table 10.9), which is nonsegmental and highly variable in nature. Onset occurs shortly after analgesia develops. Although many patients do not complain of this condition and thus appear asymptomatic, when asked, they respond affirmatively. The cause of pruritus is unknown and does not appear to be related to histamine release (222). Treatment may include intravenous administration of naloxone (0.1 to 0.2 mg) or diphenhydramine (25 to 50 mg), although the latter regimen seems best suited to inducing sleep so the patient no longer "cares" about the itching. It also has been suggested that nalbuphine (10 mg subcutaneously) will decrease pruritus (223, 224). Some prefer the use of small intravenous doses of naloxone or, potentially, a continuous infusion (see order sheet, Table 10.10).

Figure 10.23 illustrates the incidence of pruritus and the number treated in patients given 5 mg of epidural morphine for postcesarean delivery pain (175). In patients given 1 mg of morphine for labor and delivery pain, Baraka and co-workers found a 100% incidence of pruritus (43). Since side effects are dose-related and thus intensify with increasing levels of narcotic in CSF, the onset of pruritus probably is related to the central migration of morphine in the CSF. The treatment of pruritus must be prompt and aggressive if the patient is to achieve satisfactory analgesia without complaint.

It has been suggested that there is a relationship

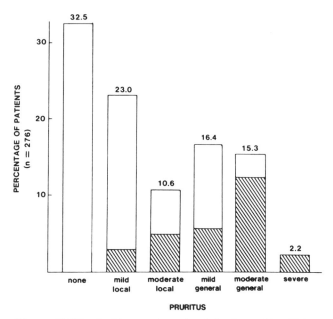

Figure 10.23. Incidence of pruritus following epidural injection of 5 mg of morphine for cesarean delivery. *Shaded areas* represent the percentage of patients in each group who were given treatment. *Open areas* represent the total percentage of patients having pruritus. (Reprinted by permission from Kotelko DM, Dailey PA, Shnider SM, Rosen MA, Hughes SC, Brizgys RV: Epidural morphine analgesia after cesarean delivery. Obstet Gynecol 63:409–413, 1984.)

between epidural morphine, facial pruritus, and herpes labialis (cold sores) that may combine to reactivate oral herpes simplex virus. This was first noted by Carden (225) after spinal morphine administered to children for enuresis, and again in two interesting studies in patients undergoing cesarean section (226, 227). Several studies provide support for a central or "ganglion trigger" mechanism (228–231). Some suggest that patients with a history of herpes labialis should be warned of a possible reactivation of their infection, although this is not universally followed.

URINARY RETENTION

Urinary retention is a minor but annoying side effect. Although not always apparent and difficult to judge in the obstetric population, the reported incidence among nonobstetric patients is 15 to 90% and may be highest in males (199, 232). There is evidence that the cause of urinary retention is the rapid onset of detrusor muscle relaxation produced by the local sacral spinal action of narcotics (Fig. 10.24) (233). There is now a series of interesting studies investigating this mechanism (234–237). Onset occurs with analgesia and thus appears earlier than pruritus, nausea, and vomiting, which are centrally mediated. If necessary, urinary retention can be treated with naloxone, but ambulating the patient or performing a

single straight urinary catheterization often succeeds in relieving the problem. Since a Foley catheter commonly is placed in the cesarean section patient and often patients in labor, urinary retention is less of a problem in obstetric anesthesia.

NAUSEA AND VOMITING

Nausea and vomiting are side effects whose causes are difficult to separate from surgical events or pregnancy itself. Nausea also may result from an earlier oral intake of food stimulated by the patient's general sense of well-being following significant pain relief. Although the incidence of these effects is variable, the onset is predictable. Small doses of an antiemetic or naloxone can be used to treat them while maintaining analgesia. Metaclopromide (10 mg intravenously) is recommended by some, whereas others administer droperidol (0.625 mg IV). Several investigators have found moderate success with transdermal scopolamine patches (1.5 mg scopolamine) placed behind the patient's ear (238–240). Common side effects of this method include dry mouth (67%), drowsiness (18%), and occasionally blurred vision. However, all side effects can be bothersome, and the use of scopolamine patches may be a reasonable choice.

Side Effects and Use of Naloxone

Almost all side effects of intraspinal morphine can be decreased or relieved completely by administering naloxone intravenously. Analgesia can be maintained if the dosage of naloxone is titrated carefully. Because central opiate receptors in the brain appear to be responsible for most of the side effects of intraspinal narcotics (urinary retention excluded), high blood flow to the brain delivers enough naloxone to reverse side effects. The relatively low blood flow to the dorsal horn, which is dense with morphine-laden opiate receptors, allows analgesia to continue. Dailey and co-workers found a significantly decreased incidence of pruritus in obstetric patients given a continuous infusion (Table 10.12) of 0.4 to 0.6 mg/hr naloxone following 1 mg of intrathecal morphine during labor (54). Analgesia was maintained despite the naloxone infusion (Fig. 10.25). Similar work with human volunteers and surgical patients demonstrated that a naloxone infusion of 5 to 10 μg/kg/hr increased minute ventilation and respiratory frequency to preepidural morphine levels and decreased end-tidal CO_2, which had increased in response to the epidural narcotic (241). The routine addition of 0.4 mg of naloxone to each liter of intravenous fluids (usually administered at 125 ml/hr) to prevent respiratory depression obviously is a homeopathic dose and probably ineffective. If naloxone is required to treat side effects, 0.1 to 0.6 mg/hr is

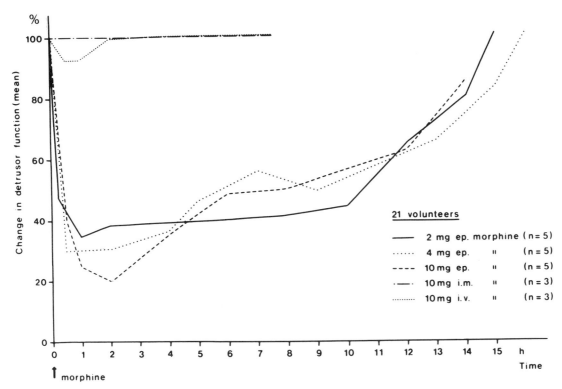

Figure 10.24. The urodynamic effects of epidural and intravenous morphine in male volunteers. Detrussor muscle function depression persisted for many hours following even 2 mg of epidural morphine. This does not occur with systemic narcotics, and a local spinal cause (i.e., opiate receptors) is probable. (Reprinted by permission from Rawal N, Möllefors K, Axelsson K, Lingardh G, Widman B: An experimental study of urodynamic effects of epidural morphine and of naloxone reversal. Anesth Analg 62:641–647, 1983.)

Table 10.12
Intravenous Naloxone Decreases Side Effects after Intrathecal Morphine (1 mg)[a]

Side Effect	Saline Infusion (%) (n = 17)	Naloxone Infusion (%) (n = 23)	Statistical Significance
Pruritus	35	9	$P < 0.05$
Vomiting	53	26	NS
Drowsiness/ dizziness	65	35	NS

[a] Adapted from Dailey PA, Brookshire GL, Shnider SM, Abboud TK, Kotelko DM, Noueihid R, Thigpen JW, Khoo SS, Raya JA, Foutz SE, Brizgys RV, Goebelsman U, Lo MW: Naloxone decreases side effects after intrathecal morphine for labor. Anesth Analg 64:658–666, 1985.

the appropriate dose range. However, if the dose of naloxone reaches 10 μg/kg/hr, the duration of analgesia may be shortened by about 25% (242).

Although intravenous infusion of naloxone may help to reduce the side effects of intraspinal narcotics and may even prevent respiratory depression if given in higher doses, the routine use of this technique cannot be recommended for obstetrics, if only because of the inconvenience and expense. Intravenous

naloxone also may cause serious maternal problems. Furthermore, although the effects on the newborn of clinical doses of naloxone appear to be benign, there is evidence in animal models that very high levels of naloxone may reduce the resistance of the fetus to hypoxic stress (243). There is no evidence of this vulnerability in humans: Parenteral doses as high as 200 μg/kg have been given to neonates without detectable adverse effects (244). However, naloxone does cross the placenta (245) and may increase the number and amplitude of fetal heart rate accelerations and affect fetal behavior (240). Intravenous naloxone also may cause serious maternal problems and is to be used cautiously.

In the nonobstetric literature, there are multiple case reports of pulmonary edema and cardiac arrest after naloxone administration (247–252). While this problem seems unlikely in the obstetric setting, the use of narcotic antagonists should not be undertaken without some consideration. Oral naltrexone (6 mg) has been suggested as a possible prophylactic drug to treat pruritus (253, 254), and an intravenous antagonist, nalmefene, may prove useful (255). The latter may be effective in reversing respiratory depression for 4 hr or more. Further investigation is needed

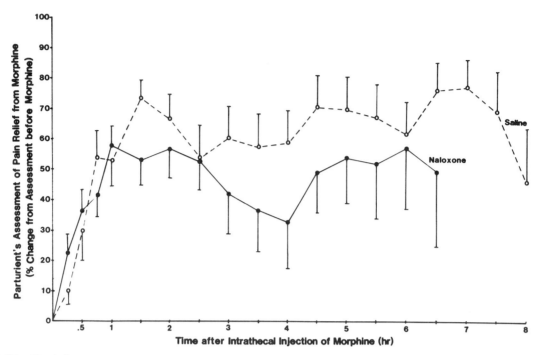

Figure 10.25. Predelivery maternal pain relief following the intrathecal administration of 1 mg of morphine. One hour later, an intravenous bolus of naloxone 0.4 mg was given, followed by a naloxone infusion of 0.4 to 0.6 mg/hr. (Reprinted by permission from Dailey PA, Brookshire GL, Shnider SM, Ab- boud TK, Kotelko DM, Noueihid R, Thigpen JW, Khoo SS, Raya JA, Foutz SE, Brizgys RV, Goebelsman U, Lo MW: Naloxone decreases side effects after intrathecal morphine for labor. Anesth Analg 64:658–666, 1985.)

in this area before these drugs can be recommended for routine use.

Antagonism of side effects by the agonist-antagonist nalbuphine also might be considered; however, there are conflicting results and it is not without risks (223, 224, 256–258).

NEONATAL EFFECTS OF INTRASPINAL OPIATES

The effects of narcotics on the newborn are well known. Concern for the newborn, in part, stimulated the initial interest in the use of the intraspinal narcotics: Low-dose effective analgesia would pose less risk to the newborn while providing adequate pain relief to the mother. The safe and effective use of intrathecal morphine has been demonstrated in the gravid rat and rabbit and supported by early clinical reports (42, 43, 259). Newborns delivered of mothers given 2, 5, and 7.5 mg of epidural morphine had high Apgar and Neurologic and Adaptive Capacity Scores and normal values for umbilical arterial and venous blood-gas tensions (72). Nevertheless, the rapid placental transfer of epidural narcotics is to be expected and should limit the dose given during labor (Fig. 10.12). Whether it is morphine, fentanyl, sufentanil, or some other narcotic, placental transfer occurs and thus limits the amount which can be given safely.

Others have documented the safe use of intrathe-

cal morphine (39, 42, 43). When a low dose of intrathecal morphine is used (0.5 to 1 mg), this finding is not surprising (39). Dailey and co-workers (54) also found that a continuous infusion of naloxone in the mother did not adversely affect the infant. During labor, there was no change in fetal heart rate or variability resulting from either intrathecal morphine injection or continuous naloxone infusion in the mother. At the time of delivery, the mean plasma concentration of naloxone was 1.92 ± 0.28 ng/ml in the umbilical venous blood. This is a relatively low concentration, especially when considering the typically high dose of naloxone used in pediatric resuscitation.

Dailey and co-workers (54) also determined that the β-endorphin concentrations in the umbilical venous blood were not significantly different when saline rather than naloxone was infused. The β-endorphin levels were 78.7 ± 15.9 fmol/ml in newborns of mothers given saline, and 57.0 ± 8.2 fmol/ml in newborns of mothers given naloxone. These levels decreased as analgesia developed, but increased at delivery to preintrathecal morphine levels. The physiologic significance of plasma β-endorphin levels during labor and delivery is unknown; increased plasma β-endorphin levels resulting from stress are not associated with increased β-endorphin levels in the brain or CSF (260).

The increasing use of epidural fentanyl and sufentanil for labor analgesia has increased the concerns regarding fetal effects. If 10 to 20 μg/hr of sufentanil is to be used (as some authors have suggested) or 10 to 30 μg/hr of fentanyl plus potential bolus injections (50 to 100 μg) to treat incomplete pain relief (as some clinicians now practice), then the effects on the newborn must be carefully considered. All narcotics cross the placenta, including the lipid-soluble narcotics. Neurobehavioral changes (short term) can be seen with all narcotics. A recent investigation of intravenous alfentanil and meperidine in monkeys (*Macaca mulatta*) in labor found behavioral differences for up to 72 hr and possibly longer (261, 262). This is discussed fully in Chapter 8. There also is concern that the umbilical plasma narcotic levels measured and so often quoted as "low" may not be as important as brain tissue narcotic levels. In dogs, the high lipid content of the brain and the significant lipid solubility of fentanyl result in higher narcotic concentrations in brain (nanograms per gram of brain tissue) than in plasma (nanograms/milliliter serum) (Fig. 10.26) (261). Hypocarbia (hyperventilation with incomplete pain relief) also leads to higher brain fentanyl levels in dogs. Furthermore, there is accumulation of fentanyl in the sheep fetus when the ewe receives fentanyl (262) and a similar accumulation of meperidine in the fetal rabbit brain (Reynolds, personal communication).

When considering the practical aspects of the addition of lipid-soluble narcotics to local anesthetics, higher doses of narcotics may lead to changes in fetal heart rate, whereas low-dose, single-injection narcotics appear to be safe (263). The question of where and how long to monitor these patients after the epidural narcotic analgesia also arises. Certainly, they should be monitored for 4 to 6 hr after receiving lipid-soluble narcotics, with immediate treatment of side effects as they occur. The possibility of profound respiratory depression with 100 μg of epidural fentanyl as late as 100 min after injection should be kept in mind (213). As we mix more and more drugs, such as epinephrine, sodium bicarbonate, clonidine, local anesthetics, and, perhaps, several narcotics, there may be a potential for catastrophic neurotoxicity. Already reported are cases involving administration of gross amounts of narcotics (400 mg of epidural morphine or 100 μg of intrathecal sufentanil). Obviously, high-dose intrathecal narcotic may be neurotoxic, as has already been demonstrated in an animal study using butorphanol (50). Clinicians must therefore consider carefully the mixing and addition of multiple epidural and spinal agents. Issues of potential neurotoxicity of epidural or intrathecal narcotics and various combinations cannot be ignored.

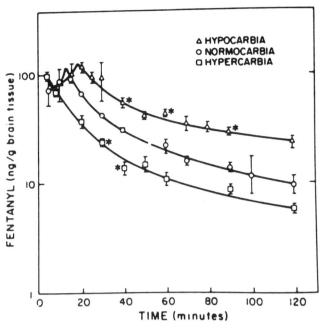

Figure 10.26. Fentanyl levels in brain measured over 2 hr in three groups of dogs during normocarbia, and hypercarbia. *indicates significant difference ($P < 0.05$) when compared with normocarbia by the Student's *t* test. (Reprinted by permission from Ainslie FG, Eisele JH, Corkhill B: Fentanyl concentrations in brain and the serum during respiratory acid base changes in the dog. Anesthesiology 80:295–297, 1979.)

In summary, the routine use of epidural or intrathecal narcotics for labor analgesia should be considered thoughtfully and investigated further. Clinicians must carefully consider the risks and benefits and analyze new reports closely. Questions to ask include: How many patients were studied? Were there satisfactory study controls? Was the statistical difference a *clinical difference*? Are the results from a small study of healthy parturients generalizable? Several authors have appropriately suggested that a stressed fetus might not tolerate what the healthy fetus does in experimental protocols (264, 265).

Other Side Effects of Intraspinal Opiates

When using narcotics, the potential for narcotic irritation of neural tissue always must be considered. There is ample evidence that morphine has no deleterious effect on neural tissue, and research is now underway to determine the effects of fentanyl, sufentanil, alfentanil, and other drugs (50, 266–268). However, clinicians are urged to be cautious when considering any new agent for intraspinal use: Many agents are being suggested without adequate study of possible neurotoxicity (198). Even low doses of intrathecal butorphanol may cause neurotoxicity (Fig. 10.27) (50).

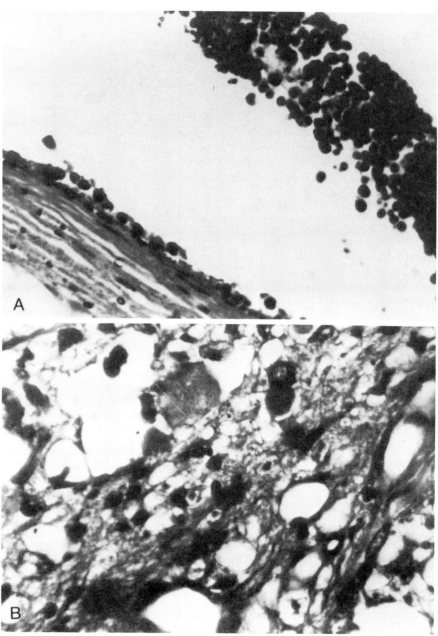

Figure 10.27. *A*, Section at level of catheter up. Inflammatory changes suggestive of suppurative meningitis due to irritating effect of small dose (0.075 mg/kg) of intrathecal butorphanol (electron microscopy ×400). *B*, Axonal and neuronal degeneration following small dose intrathecal butorphanol. Hemorrhages near catheter insertion: Section at level of catheter insertion (electron microscopy ×400). (Reprinted by permission from Rawal N, Nuutinen L, Raj PP, Lovering SL, Gobuty AH, Hargardine J, Lehmkuhl L, Herva R, Abouleish E: Behavioral and histopathologic effects following intrathecal administration of butorphanol, sufentanil, and nalbuphine in sheep. Anesthesiology 75:1025–1034, 1991.)

In addition, unusual complications have been associated with the use of intraspinal narcotics. In one case a cancer patient in whom chronic administration of very large doses of narcotic was discontinued when analgesia was provided with 1 mg of intrathecal morphine manifested opiate withdrawal (269). Although this is not likely to be a problem in the obstetric population, it might well occur in chronic pain patients treated by long-term narcotic therapy before the use of intraspinal narcotics. Epidural butorphanol has caused withdrawal in an obstetric patient with a "silent" narcotic abuse history. Another report suggested the synergistic action of droperidol and epidural narcotics (270), but this was not substantiated in a large review (200). However, when additional narcotics, sedatives, or tranquilizers are given to a patient who has received intraspinal narcotics, increased monitoring of the patient is required. Another rare but potential problem is suggested by a fascinating case report of an anaphylactic reaction to epidural fentanyl (271).

Although the analgesia achieved with intraspinal narcotics is very real, so are the side effects. In most cases these can be treated quite easily, but must be acknowledged as part of the price for analgesia. When undertaking the use of intraspinal narcotics, the anesthesiologist must be prepared to consider and treat the side effects.

WHY USE INTRASPINAL NARCOTICS?

The best results with this technique have been in providing good postoperative analgesia for cesarean delivery patients. The pain relief obtained is superior to that provided by traditional methods. Patients can ambulate, care for their newborn, and interact with family members immediately postpartum. Although one might expect greater maternal-infant bonding as a result, this has not been the case. One study suggests that the chief benefits of using epidural morphine in postcesarean patients are improved analgesia and early ambulation without improvement in maternal-infant bonding (272).

Some patients might benefit from the improved pulmonary function produced by analgesia without motor blockade. Bromage and co-workers (7) demonstrated that an increased forced expiratory volume (FEV_1) (determined by percentage of preoperative FEV_1) resulted after upper abdominal surgery when an epidural, but not intravenous, narcotic was used for postoperative pain relief. Another study demonstrated that earlier ambulation, improved pulmonary function, and fewer days of hospitalization followed gastric surgery in the grossly obese patient when epidural rather than intramuscular morphine was used for postoperative pain relief (273). Epidural fentanyl reportedly produces a decrease in stress-induced elevation of plasma vasopressin that may be beneficial to the patient (274). Clearly, the potential benefits of the intraspinal technique go beyond better pain relief but remain to be fully defined.

For the patient in labor, intraspinal narcotics are a promising technique that requires more investigation. This approach provides an alternative for both anesthesiologist and patient. Particular patients in labor may benefit from this approach. For the patient in postoperative pain following cesarean delivery, the benefits appear to be great and the risks minimal.

References

1. Wang JK, Nauss LA, Thomas JE: Pain relief by intrathecally applied morphine in man. Anesthesiology 50:149–151, 1979.
2. Behar M, Magora F, Olshwang D, Davidson JT: Epidural morphine in treatment of pain. Lancet 1:527–528, 1979.
3. Bromage PR: The price of intraspinal narcotic analgesia: Basic constraints. Anesth Analg 60:461–463, 1981.
4. Snyder SH: Opiate receptors in the brain. N Engl J Med 296:266–271, 1977.
5. Pert CB, Kuhar J, Snyder SH: Opiate receptor: Autoradiographic localization in rat brain. Proc Natl Acad Sci 73:3729–3733, 1976.
6. Atweh SF, Kuhar MJ: Autoradiographic localization of opiate receptors in rat brain. I. Spinal cord and lower medulla. Brain Res 124:53–67, 1977.
7. Bromage PR, Camporesi E, Chestnut D: Epidural narcotics for postoperative analgesia. Anesth Analg 59:473–480, 1980.
8. Calvillo O, Henry JL, Neuman RS: Effects of morphine and naloxone on dorsal horn neurones in the cat. Can J Physiol Pharmacol 52:1207–1211, 1974.
9. Kitahata LM, Kosaka Y, Taub A: Lamina-specific suppression of dorsal-horn unit activity by morphine sulfate. Anesthesiology 41:39–48, 1974.
10. Le Bars D, Menetrey D, Conseiller C, Bessen J-M: Comparaison chez le chat spinal et le chat decerebre, des effets de la morphine sur les activities des interneurones de type V de la corne dorsale de la moelle. CR Seances Acad Sci (III) 279:1369–1371, 1974.
11. Beckett AH, Casy AF: Synthetic analgesics: Stereochemical considerations. J Pharm Pharmacol 6:986–1001, 1954.
12. Thorpe DH: Opiate structure and activity: A guide to understanding the receptor. Anesth Analg 63:143–151, 1984.
13. Yaksh TL, Jessle TM, Gamse R, Mudge AW, Leeman SE: Intrathecal morphine inhibits substance P release from mammalian spinal cord in vivo. Nature 287:155–157, 1980.
14. Yaksh TL, Rudy TA: Studies on the direct spinal action of narcotics in the production of analgesia in the rat. J Pharmacol Exp Ther 202:411–428, 1977.
15. Yaksh TL, Rudy TA: Narcotic analgesics: CNS sites and mechanisms of action as revealed by intracerebral injection techniques. Pain 4:299–359, 1978.
16. Li CH, Barnafi I, Chretien M, Chung D: Isolation and amino-acid sequence of β-LPH from sheep pituitary glands. Nature 208:1093–1094, 1965.
17. Hughes J, Smith TW, Kosterlitz HW, Fothergill LA, Morgan BA, Morris HR: Identification of two related pentapeptides from the brain with potent opiate agonist activity. Nature 258:577–579, 1975.
18. Oyama T, Matsuki A, Taneichi T, Ling N, Guillemin R: β-endorphin in obstetric analgesia. Am J Obstet Gynecol 137:613–616, 1980.
19. Martin WR, Eades CG, Thompson JA, Huppler RE, Gilbert PE: The effects of morphine- and nalorphine-like drugs in the nondependent and morphine-dependent chronic spinal dog. J Pharmacol Exp Ther 197:517–532, 1976.
20. Martin WR: Mini-symposium. II. Multiple opioid receptors. Life Sci 28:495–499, 1977.
21. Lord JAH, Waterfield AA, Hughes J, Kosteritz HW: Endogenous opioid peptides: Multiple agonists and receptors. Nature 267:495–499, 1977.
22. Wuster M, Schulz R, Herz A: The direction of opioid agonists towards μ-, d- and e-receptors in the vas deferens of the mouse and the rat. Life Sci 27:163–170, 1980.
23. Audigier Y, Mazarguil H, Gout R, Cros J: Structure-activity relationships of enkephalin analogs at opiate and enkephalin receptors: Correlation with analgesia. Eur J Pharmacol 63:35–46, 1980.
24. Goodman RR, Snyder SH, Kuhar MJ, Young WS III: Differentiation of delta and mu opiate receptor localizations by light microscopic autoradiography. Proc Natl Acad Sci 77:6239–6243, 1980.
25. Freye E, Hartung E, Shenk GK: Bremazocine: An opiate that induces sedation and analgesia without respiratory depression. Anesth Analg 62:483–488, 1983.
26. Rowlingson JC, Moscicki JC, DiFazio CA: Anesthetic potency of dezocine and its interaction with morphine in rats. Anesth Analg 62:899–902, 1983.
27. Bailey PW, Smith BE: Continuous epidural infusion of fentanyl for postoperative analgesia. Anaesthesia 35:1002–1006, 1980.

28. Torda TA, Pybus DA: Comparison of four narcotic analgesics for extradural analgesia. Br J Anaesth 54:291–295, 1981.

29. Carrie LES, O'Sullivan GM, Seegobin R: Epidural fentanyl in labour. Anaesthesia 36:965–969, 1981.

30. Justins DM, Francis D, Houlton PG, Reynolds F: A controlled trial of extradural fentanyl in labour. Br J Anaesth 54:409–414, 1982.

31. Bromage PR: Extradural and intrathecal opiates. In 33rd Annual Refresher Course Lectures, American Society of Anesthesiologists, Las Vegas, 1982, p 138.

32. Schubert P, Teschemacher H, Kreutzberg GW, Herz A: Intracerebral distribution pattern of radioactive morphine and morphine-like drugs after intraventricular and intrathecal injection. Histochemie 22:277–288, 1970.

33. Drayer BP, Rosenbaum AE: Studies of the third circulation: Amipaque CT cisternography and ventriculography. J Neurosurg 48:946–956, 1978.

34. Gourlay GK, Cherry DA, Plummer JL, Armstrong PJ, Cousins MJ: The influence of drug polarity on the absorption of opioid drugs into CSF and subsequent cephalad migration following lumbar epidural administration: Application to morphine and pethidine. Pain 31:297–305, 1987.

35. Bromage PR, Camporesi EM, Durant PAC, Nielsen CH: Rostral spread of epidural morphine. Anesthesiology 56:431–436, 1982.

36. Hansdottir V, Hedner T, Woestenborghs R, Nordberg G: The CSF and plasma pharmacokinetics of sufentanil after intrathecal administration. Anesthesiology 74:264–269, 1991.

37. Nordberg G, Hedner T, Mellstrand T, Dahlstrom B: Pharmacokinetic aspects of intrathecal morphine analgesia. Anesthesiology 60:448–454, 1984.

38. Nordberg G, Hedner T, Mellstrand T, Dahlstrom B: Pharmacokinetic aspects of epidural morphine analgesia. Anesthesiology 58:545–551, 1983.

39. Abboud TK, Shnider SM, Dailey PA, Raya JA, Sarkis F, Grobler NM, Sadri S, Khoo SS, DeSousa B, Baysinger CL, Miller F: Intrathecal administration of hyperbaric morphine for the relief of pain in labor. Br J Anaesth 56:1351–1360, 1984.

40. Samii K, Chauvin M, Viars P: Postoperative spinal analgesia with morphine. Br J Anaesth 53:817–820, 1981.

41. Cousins MJ, Mather LE, Glynn CJ, Wilson PR, Graham JR: Selective spinal analgesia (letter). Lancet 1:1141–1142, 1979.

42. Scott PV, Bowen FE, Cartwright P, Rao BCM, Deeley D, Wotherspoon HG, Sumrein IMA: Intrathecal morphine as sole analgesic during labour. Br Med J 281:351–353, 1980.

43. Baraka A, Noueihid R, Hajj S: Intrathecal injection of morphine for obstetric analgesia. Anesthesiology 54:136–140, 1981.

44. Åkerman B, Arweström E, Post C: Local anesthetics potentiate spinal morphine antinociception. Anesth Analg 67:943–938, 1988.

45. Cunningham AJ, McKenna JA, Skene DS: Single injection spinal anesthesia with tetracaine and morphine for transurethral prostatectomy. Anesth Analg 62:255, 1983.

46. Abouleish E, Rawal N, Shaw J, Lorenz T, Rashad N: Intrathecal morphine 0.2 mg versus epidural bupivacaine 0.125% or their combination: Effects on parturients. Anesthesiology 74:711–716, 1991.

47. Leighton BL, DeSimone CA, Norris MC, Ben-David B: Intrathecal narcotics for labor revisited: The combination of fentanyl and morphine intrathecally provides rapid onset of profound, prolonged analgesia. Anesth Analg 69:122–125, 1989.

48. Bonnardot JP, Maillet M, Colau JC, Millot F, Deligne P: Maternal and fetal concentrations of morphine after intrathecal administration during labour. Br J Anaesth 54:487–489, 1982.

49. Johnson MD, Hurley RJ, Gilbertson LL, Datta S: Continuous microcatheter spinal anesthesia with subarachnoid meperidine for labor and delivery. Anesth Analg 70:658–661, 1990.

50. Rawal N, Nuutinen L, Raj PP, Lovering SL, Gobuty AH, Hargardine J, Lehmkuhl L, Herva R, Abouleish E: Behavioral and histopathologic effects following intrathecal administration of butorphanol, sufentanil, and nalbuphine in sheep. Anesthesiology 75:1025–1034, 1991.

51. Rigler ML, Drasner K, Krejcie TC, Yelich SJ, Scholnick FT, DeFontes J, Bohner D: Cauda equina syndrome after continuous spinal anesthesia. Anesth Analg 72:275–281, 1991.

52. Rigler ML, Drasner KD: Distribution of catheter injected local anesthetic in a model of the subarachnoid space. Anesthesiology 75:684–692, 1991.

53. Baraka A, Maktabi M, Noueihid R: Epidural meperidine-bupivacaine for obstetric anesthesia. Anesth Analg 61:652–656, 1982.

54. Dailey PA, Brookshire GL, Shnider SM, Abboud TK, Kotelko DM, Noueihid R, Thigpen JW, Khoo SS, Raya JA, Foutz SE, Brizgys RV, Goebelsman U, Lo MW: Naloxone decreases side effects after intrathecal morphine for labor. Anesth Analg 64:658–666, 1984.

55. Bicknell RJ, Leng G, Russell JA, Dyer RG, Mansfield S, Zhao BG: Hypothalmic opioid mechanisms controlling oxytocin neurones during parturition. Brain Res Bull 20:743–749, 1988.

56. Sivalingam T, Pleuvry BJ: Actions of morphine pethidine and pentazocine on the oestrus and pregnant rat uterus in vitro. Br J Anaesth 57:430–433, 1985.

57. Cohen SE, Tan S, Albright GA, Halpern J: Epidural fentanyl/bupivacaine mixtures for obstetric analgesia. Anesthesiology 67:403–407, 1987.

58. Rosen MA, Hughes SC, Curtis JD, Norton M, Levinson G, Shnider SM: Effects of epidural morphine on uterine blood flow and acid-base status in the pregnant ewe. Anesthesiology 57:A383, 1982.

59. Craft JB Jr, Bolan JC, Coaldrake LA, Mondino M, Mazel P, Gilman RM, Shokes IK, Woolf WA: The maternal and fetal cardiovascular effects of epidural morphine in the sheep model. Am J Obstet Gynecol 142:835–839, 1982.

60. Power KJ, Avery AF: Extradural analgesia in the intrapartum management of a patient with pulmonary hypertension. Br J Anaesth 63:116–120, 1989.

61. Robinson DE, Leicht CH: Epidural analgesia with low-dose bupivacaine and fentanyl for labor and delivery in a parturient with severe pulmonary hypertension. Anesthesiology 68:285–288, 1988.

62. Ahmad S, Hawes D, Dooley S, Faure E, Brunner E: Intrathecal morphine in a parturient with a single ventricle. Anesthesiology 54:515–517, 1981.

63. Abboud TK, Raya I, Noueihid R, Daniel J: Intrathecal morphine for relief of labor pain in a parturient with severe pulmonary hypertension. Anesthesiology 59:477–479, 1983.

64. Copel JA, Harrison D, Whittemore R, Hobbins JC: Intrathecal morphine analgesia for vaginal delivery in a woman with a single ventricle: A case report. J Reprod Med 31:274–276, 1986.

65. Booker PD, Wilkes RG, Bryson TH, Beddard J: Obstetric pain relief using epidural morphine. Anaesthesia 35:377–379, 1980.

66. Husemeyer RP, O'Connor MC, Davenport HT: Failure of epidural morphine to relieve pain in labour. Anaesthesia 35:161–163, 1980.

67. Writer WDR, James FM III, Wheeler AS: Double-blind comparison of morphine and bupivacaine for continuous epidural analgesia in labor. Anesthesiology 54:215–219, 1981.

68. Magora F, Olshwang D, Eimerl D, Shorr J, Katzenenson R, Cotev S, Davidson JT: Observations on extradural morphine analgesia in various pain conditions. Br J Anaesth 52:247–252, 1980.

69. Crawford JS: Forum: Experiences with epidural morphine in obstetrics. Anaesthesia 36:207–209, 1981.

70. Perriss BW: Epidural pethidine in labour. Anaesthesia 35:380–382, 1980.

71. Perriss BW: Epidural opiates in labour. Lancet 2:422, 1979.

72. Hughes SC, Rosen MA, Shnider SM, Abboud TK, Stefani SJ, Norton M: Maternal and neonatal effects of epidural morphine for labor and delivery. Anesth Analg 63:319–324, 1984.

73. Von Hartung H-J, Wiest W, Klose R, Bauknect H, Hettenbach A: Epidurale morphin-injektion zur schmerzbekampfung in der geburtshilfe. Fortschr Med 98:500, 1980.

74. Dick W, Traub E, Moller RM: Epidural morphine in obstetric anesthesia. Obstet Anesth Digest 2:29–31, 1982.

75. Nybell-Lindahl G, Carlsson C, Ingemarsson I, Westgren M,

Paalzow L: Maternal and fetal concentrations of morphine after epidural administration during labor. Am J Obstet Gynecol 139:20–21, 1981.

76. Carrie LES, O'Sullivan GM, Seegobin R: Epidural fentanyl in labour. Anaesthesia 36:965–969, 1981.

77. Steinberg RB, Powell G, Hu X, Dunn SM: Epidural sufentanil for analgesia for labor and delivery. Reg Anesth 14:225–228, 1989.

78. Heytens L, Cammu H, Camu F: Extradural analgesia during labour using alfentanil. Br J Anaesth 59:331–337, 1987.

79. Justins DM, Francis D, Houlton PG, Reynolds F: A controlled trial of extradural fentanyl in labor. Br J Anaesth 54:409–414, 1982.

80. Justins DM, Knott C, Luthman J, Reynolds F: Epidural versus intramuscular fentanyl analgesia and pharmacokinetics in labour. Anaesthesia 38:937–942, 1983.

81. Vella LM, Willats DG, Knott C, Lintin DJ, Justins DM, Reynolds F: Epidural fentanyl in labour. Anaesthesia 40:741–747, 1985.

82. Deprats R, Mandry J, Grandjean H, Amar B, Pontonnier G, Lareng L: Analgesie peridurale au cours du travail: Etude comparative de l'association fentanyl-marcaïne et de la marcaïne seule. J Gynecol Obstet Biol Reprod (Paris) 12:901–905, 1983.

83. Chestnut DH, Owen CL, Bates JN, Ostman LG, Choi WW, Geiger MW: Continuous infusion epidural analgesia during labor: A randomized, double-blind comparison of 0.0625% bupivacaine/0.0002% fentanyl versus 0.125% bupivacaine. Anesthesiology 68:754–759, 1988.

84. Chestnut DH, Laszewski LJ, Pollack KL, Bates JN, Manago NK, Choi WW: Continuous epidural infusion of 0.0625% bupivacaine-0.0002% fentanyl during the second stage of labor. Anesthesiology 72:613–618, 1990.

85. Naulty JS, Smith R, Ross R: Effect of changes in labor analgesia practice on labor outcome. Anesthesiology 69:A660, 1989.

86. Reynolds F: Extradural opioids in labour. Br J Anaesth 63:251–253, 1989.

87. Phillips G: Epidural sufentanil/bupivacaine combinations for analgesia during labor: Effect of varying sufentanil doses. Anesthesiology 67:835–838, 1987.

88. Donadoni R, Rolly G, Noorden H, Vanden Bussche G: Epidural sufentanil for postoperative pain relief. Anaesthesia 40:634–638, 1985.

89. Niemegeers CJ, Schellenkens KHL, Van Bever WFM, Janssen PAJ: Sufentanil, a very potent and extremely safe intravenous morphine-like compound in mice, rats, and dogs. Arzneimittelforschung 26:1551–1556, 1976.

90. Leysen JE, Gommeren W, Niemegeers CJE: (^{3}H) sufentanil, a superior ligand for μ-opiate receptors: Binding properties and regional distribution in rat brain and spinal cord. Eur J Pharmacol 87:209–225, 1983.

91. Phillips G: Combined epidural sufentanil and bupivacaine for labor analgesia. Reg Anesth 12:165–168, 1987.

92. Naulty JS, Ross R, Bergen W: Epidural sufentanil-bupivacaine for analgesia during labor and delivery. Anesthesiology 71:A842, 1989.

93. Phillips G: Continuous infusion epidural analgesia in labor: The effect of adding sufentanil to 0.125% bupivacaine. Anesth Analg 67:462–465, 1988.

94. Van Steenberge A, Debroux HC, Noorduin H: Extradural bupivacaine with sufentanil for vaginal delivery. Br J Anaesth 59:1518–1522, 1987.

95. Vertommen JD, Vandermeulen E, Van Aken H, Vaes L, Soetens M, Van Steenberge A, Mourisse P, Willaert J, Noorduin H, Devlieger H, Van Assche AF: The effects of the addition of sufentanil to 0.125% bupivacaine on the quality of analgesia during labor and on the incidence of instrumental deliveries. Anesthesiology 74:809–814, 1991.

96. Huckaby T, Gerard K, Scheidlinger J, Johnson MD, Datta S: Continuous epidural infusion of alfentanil-bupivacaine for labor and delivery. Anesthesiology 71:A846, 1989.

97. Fernando E, Shevde K, Eddi D: A comparative study of epidural alfentanil and fentanyl for labor pain relief. Anesthesiology 71:A846, 1989.

98. Carp H, Johnson MD, Datta S, Ostheimer GW: Continuous epidural infusion of alfentanil and bupivacaine for labor and delivery. Anesthesiology 69:A687, 1988.

99. Ahn NN, Karambelkar D, Cannelli G, Rudy TE: Epidural alfentanil and bupivacaine analgesia during labor. Anesthesiology 71:A845, 1989.

100. Abboud TK, Reyes A, Steffens Z, Afrasiabi A, D'Onofrio L, Davidson J, Zhu J, Khoo N, Paul R, Mantilla, Mosaad P: Bupivacaine/butorphanol/epinephrine for epidural anesthesia in obstetrics: Maternal and neonatal effects. Reg Anesth 14:219–224, 1989.

101. Hunt CO, Naulty JS, Malinow AM, Datta S, Ostheimer GW: Epidural butorphanol-bupivacaine for analgesia during labor and delivery. Anesth Analg 68:323–327, 1989.

102. Rodriguez J, Abboud TK, Reyes A, Payne M, Zhu J, Steffens Z, Afrasiabi A: Continuous infusion epidural analgesia during labor: A randomized, double-blind comparison of 0.0625 bupivacaine/0.002% butorphanol versus 0.125% bupivacaine. Anesthesiology 71:A840, 1989.

103. Niv D, Rudick V, Golan A, Chayen MS: Augmentation of bupivacaine analgesia in labor by epidural morphine. Obstet Gynecol 67:206–209, 1986.

104. Abouleish E, Rawal N, Shaw J, Lorenz T, Rashad N: Intrathecal morphine, 0.2 mg versus epidural bupivacaine 0.125% or their combination: Effects on parturients. Anesthesiology 74:711–716, 1991.

105. Preston PG, Rosen MA, Hughes SC, Glosten B, Ross BK, Daniels D, Shnider SM, Dailey PA: Epidural anesthesia with fentanyl and lidocaine for cesarean section: Maternal effects and neonatal outcome. Anesthesiology 68:938–943, 1988.

106. Breen TW, Janzen JA: Epidural fentanyl and lidocaine for cesarean section: When should fentanyl be given? In Abstracts of Scientific Papers, Society for Obstetric Anesthesia and Perinatology, Boston, 1991.

107. Ready LB, Oden R, Rooke BA, Caplan R, Chadwick HS, Wild LM: Development of an anesthesiology-based postoperative pain management service. Anesthesiology 68:100–106, 1988.

108. Wolfe MJ, Nicholas ADG: Selective epidural analgesia. Lancet 1:150–151, 1979.

109. Ellis DJ, Millar WI: Reisner LS: A randomized double-blind comparison of epidural versus intravenous fentanyl infusion for analgesia after cesarean section. Anesthesiology 72:981–986, 1990.

110. Loper KA, Ready LB, Downey M, Sandler AN, Nessly M, Rapp S, Badner N: Epidural and intravenous fentanyl infusions are clinically equivalent after knee surgery. Anesth Analg 70:72–75, 1990.

111. Bromage PR, Camporesi E, Chestnut D: Epidural narcotics for postoperative analgesia. Anesth Analg 59:473–480, 1980.

112. Chayen MS, Rudick V, Borvine A: Pain control with epidural injection of morphine. Anesthesiology 53:338–339, 1980.

113. Rawal N, Sjöstrand U, Dahlström B: Postoperative pain relief by epidural morphine. Anesth Analg 60:726–731, 1981.

114. Yu CM, Youngstrom PC, Cowan RI, Spagnuolo SET: Postcesarean epidural morphine: Double-blind study. Anesthesiology 53:A216, 1980.

115. Rosen MA, Hughes SC, Shnider SM, Abboud TK, Norton M, Dailey PA, Curtis JD: Epidural morphine for pain relief of postoperative pain after cesarean delivery. Anesth Analg 62:666–672, 1983.

116. Naulty JS, Datta S, Ostheimer GW, Johnson MD, Burger G: Epidural fentanyl for postcesarean delivery pain management. Anesthesiology 63:694–698, 1985.

117. King MJ, Bowden MI, Cooper GM: Epidural fentanyl and 0.5% bupivacaine for elective cesarean section. Anaesthesia 45:285–288, 1990.

118. Malinow AM, Mokriski BLK, Wakefield ML, McGuinn WJ, Martz DG, Desverreaux JN, Matjasko MJ: Choice of local anesthetic affects post-cesarean epidural fentanyl analgesia. Reg Anesth 13:141–145, 1988.

119. Mahesh KT, Heavner JE: Post cesarean section analgesia requests are independent of when epidural fentanyl is given. Anesth Analg 70:S255, 1990.

120. Sevarino FB, McFarlane C, Sinatra RS: Epidural fentanyl

does not influence intravenous PCA requirements in the post-caesarean patient. Can J Anaesth 38:450–453, 1991.

121. Milon D, Bentue-Ferrer D, Noury D, Reymann JM, Sauvage J, Allain H, Saint-Marc C, van den Driessche J: Anésthesie péridurale pour césarienne par association bupivacaïne-fentanyl. Ann Fr Anesth Reanim 2:273–279, 1983.

122. Gaffud MP, Bansal P, Lawton C, Velasquez N, Watson WA: Surgical analgesia for cesarean delivery with epidural bupivacaine and fentanyl. Anesthesiology 65:331–334, 1986.

123. Birnbach DJ, Johnson MD, Arcario T, Datta S, Naulty JS, Ostheimer GW: Effect of diluent volume on analgesia produced by epidural fentanyl. Anesth Analg 68:808–810, 1989.

124. Naulty JS, Parmet J, Pate A, Becker R, Loeffler C, Barnes D: Epidural sufentanil and morphine for post-cesarean delivery analgesia. Anesthesiology 73:A965, 1990.

125. Sinatra RS, Savarino FB, Chung JH, Graf G, Paige D, Takla V, Silverman DG: Comparison of epidurally administered sufentanil, morphine, and sufentanil-morphine combination for postoperative analgesia. Anesth Analg 72:522–527, 1991.

126. Rosen MA, Dailey PA, Hughes SC, Leicht CH, Shnider SM, Jackson CE, Baker BW, Cheek DB, O'Connor DE: Epidural sufentanil for postoperative analgesia after cesarean section. Anesthesiology 68:448–454, 1988.

127. Donaldoni R, Rolly G, Noaduin H, Banden Bussche G: Epidural sufentanel for postoperative pain. Anaesthesia 40:634–638, 1985.

128. Cohen SE, Tan S, White PF: Sufentanil analgesia following cesarean section: Epidural vs. intravenous administration. Anesthesiology 68:129–134, 1988.

129. Whiting WC, Sandler AN, Lau LC, Chovaz PM, Slavchenko P, Daley D, Koren G: Analgesic and respiratory effects of epidural sufentanil in patients following thoracotomy. Anesthesiology 69:36–43, 1988.

130. Vertommen JD, Van Aken H, Vandermeulen E, Vangerven M, Devlieger H, Van Assche AF, Shnider SM: Maternal and neonatal effects of adding epidural sufentanil to 0.5% bupivacaine for cesarean delivery. J Clin Anesth 3:371–376, 1991.

131. Johnson MD, Sevarino FB, Lema MJ: Cessation of shivering and hypothermia associated with epidural sufentanil. Anesth Analg 68:70–71, 1989.

132. Sevarino FB, Johnson MD, Lema MJ, Datta S, Ostheimer GW, Naulty JS: The effect of epidural sufentanil on shivering and body temperature in the parturient. Anesth Analg 68:530–533, 1989.

133. Rosen MA, Hughes SC, Shnider SM, Curry GR, Glaze GM, Thirion AV, Vertommen JD: Continuous epidural sufentanil for postoperative analgesia. Anesth Analg 70:S331, 1990.

134. Brownridge P, Frewin DB: A comparison study of techniques of postoperative analgesia caesarean section and lower abdominal surgery. Anaesth Intensive Care 13:123–130, 1985.

135. Perriss BW, Latham BV, Wilson IH: Analgesia following extradural and IM pethidine in post-caesarean section patients. Br J Anaesth 64:355–357, 1990.

136. Sjöström S, Hartvig P, Persson P, Tamsen A: Pharmacokinetics of epidural morphine and meperidine in humans. Anesthesiology 67:877–888, 1987.

137. Glynn CJ, Mather LE, Cousins MJ, Graham JR, Wilson PR: Peridural meperidine in humans: Analgetic response, pharmacokinetics and transmission into CSF. Anesthesiology 55:520–526, 1981.

138. Macrae DJ, Munishankrappa S, Burrow LM, Milne MK, Grant IS: Double-blind comparison of the efficacy of extradural diamorphine, extradural phenoperidine and IM diamorphine following caesarean section. Br J Anaesth 59:354–359, 1987.

139. Abboud TK, Moore M, Zhu J, Murakawa K, Minehart M, Longhitano M, Terrasi J, Klepper ID, Choi Y, Kimball S, Chu G: Epidural butorphanol or morphine for the relief of postcesarean section pain: Ventilatory responses to carbon dioxide. Anesth Analg 66:887–893, 1987.

140. Chrubasik J, Wüst H, Schulte-Mönting J, Thon K, Zindler M: Relative analgesic potency of epidural fentanyl, alfentanil, and morphine in treatment of postoperative pain. Anesthesiology 68:929–933, 1988.

141. Penon C, Negre I, Ecoffey CF, Gross JB, Levron J, Samii K: Analgesia and ventilatory response to carbon dioxide after intramuscular and epidural alfentanil. Anesth Analg 67:313–317, 1988.

142. Dann WL, Hutchinson A, Cartwright DP: Maternal and neonatal responses to alfentanil administered before induction of general anaesthesia for caesarean section. Br J Anaesth 59:1392–1396, 1987.

143. Chestnut DH, Choi WW, Isbell TJ: Epidural hydromorphone for postcesarean analgesia. Obstet Gynecol 68:65–69, 1986.

144. Dougherty TB, Baysinger CL, Gooding DJ: Epidural hydromorphone for postoperative analgesia after delivery by cesarean section. Reg Anesth 11:118–122, 1986.

145. Dougherty TB, Baysinger CL, Henenberger JC, Gooding DJ: Epidural hydromorphone with and without epinephrine for postoperative analgesia after cesarean delivery. Anesth Analg 68:318–322, 1989.

146. Henderson SK, Matthew EB, Cohen H, Avram MJ: Epidural hydromorphone: A double-blind comparison with intramuscular hydromorphone for postcesarean section analgesia. Anesthesiology 66:825–830, 1987.

147. Wüst HJ, Bromage PR: Delayed respiratory arrest after epidural hydromorphone. Anaesthesia 42:404–406, 1987.

148. Bilsback P, Rolly G, Tampubolon O: Efficacy of the extradural administration of lofentanil, buprenorphine or saline in the management of postoperative pain: A double-blind study. Br J Anaesth 57:943–948, 1985.

149. Lanz E, Simko G, Theiss D, Glocke MH: Epidural buprenorphine: A double blind study of postoperative analgesia and side effects. Anesth Analg 63:593–598, 1984.

150. Jensen FM, Jensen NH, Holk IK, Ravnborg M: Prolonged and biphasic respiratory depression following epidural buprenorphine. Anaesthesia 42:470–475, 1987.

151. Knape JT: Early respiratory depression resistant to naloxone following epidural buprenorphine. Anesthesiology 64:382–384, 1986.

152. Ravat F, Dorne R, Baechle JP, Beaulaton A, Lenoir B, Leroy P, Palmier B: Epidural ketamine or morphine for postoperative analgesia. Anesthesiology 66:819–822, 1987.

153. Naji P, Farschtschian M, Wilder-Smith O, Wilder-Smith C: Epidural droperidol and morphine for postoperative pain. Anesth Analg 70:583–588, 1990.

154. Kawana Y: Epidural ketamine for postoperative pain relief after gynecologic operations: A double-blind study and comparison with epidural morphine. Anesth Analg 67:798–802, 1988.

155. Van der Auwera D, Verborgh C, Camu F: Epidural ketamine for postoperative analgesia. Anesth Analg 66:1340, 1987.

156. Kawana Y, Sato H, Shimada H, Fujita N, Ueda Y, Hayashi A, Araki Y: Epidural ketamine for postoperative pain relief after gynecologic operations: A double-blind study and comparison with epidural morphine. Anesth Analg 66:735–738, 1987.

157. Brock-Utne JG, Rubin J, Mankowitz RJ: Epidural ketamine for control of postoperative pain (letter). Anesth Analg 65:990, 1986.

158. Hughes SC: Intraspinal narcotics for analgesia after cesarean section. Curr Opin Anaesth 2:295–302, 1989.

159. Loper KA, Ready LB, Nessly MN, Wild BS: Epidural morphine provides safe and effective analgesia on hospital wards. Anesth Analg 70:S248, 1990.

160. Kotelko DM, Dailey PA, Shnider SM, Rosen MA, Hughes SC, Brizgys RV: Epidural morphine analgesia after cesarean delivery. Obstet Gynecol 63:409–413, 1984.

161. Youngstrom PC, Cowan RI, Suttheimer C, Eastwood DW, Yu JCM: Pain relief and plasma concentrations from epidural and intramuscular morphine in post-cesarean patients. Anesthesiology 57:404–409, 1982.

162. Coombs DW, Danielson DR, Pageau MG, Rippe E: Epidurally administered morphine for postcesarean analgesia. Surg Gynecol Obstet 153:385–388, 1982.

163. Carmichael FJ, Rolbin SH, Hew EM: Epidural morphine for analgesia after cesarean section. Can Anaesth Soc J 29:359–363, 1982.
164. Binsted RJ: Epidural morphine after cesarean section. Anaesth Intensive Care 11:130–134, 1983.
165. Chadwick HS, Ready LB: Intrathecal and epidural morphine sulfate for postcesarean analgesia: A clinical comparison. Anesthesiology 68:925–929, 1988.
166. Abouleish E, Rawal N, Fallon K, Hernandez D: Combined intrathecal morphine and bupivacaine for cesarean section. Anesth Analg 67:370–374, 1988.
167. Abboud TK, Dror A, Mosaad P, Zhu J, Mantilla M, Swart F, Gangolly J, Silao P, Makar A, Moore J, Davis H, Lee J: Minidose intrathecal morphine for the relief of post-cesarean section pain: Safety, efficacy, and ventilatory responses to carbon dioxide. Anesth Analg 67:137–143, 1988.
168. Hunt CO, Naulty JS, Bader AM, Hauch MA, Vartikar JV, Datta S, Hertwig LM, Ostheimer GW: Perioperative analgesia with subarachnoid fentanyl-bupivacaine for cesarean delivery. Anesthesiology 71:535–540, 1989.
169. Donaldoni R, Vermeulen H, Noorduin, Rolly G: Intrathecal sufentanil as a supplement to subarachnoid anaesthesia with lignocaine. Br J Anaesth 59:1523–1527, 1987.
170. Jacobson L, Chabal D, Brody MC, Ward RJ, Ireton RC: Intrathecal methadone and morphine for postoperative analgesia: A comparison of the efficacy, duration and side effects. Anesthesiology 70:742–746, 1989.
171. Stoelting RK: Intrathecal morphine: An underused combination for postoperative pain management. Anesth Analg 68:707–709, 1989.
172. Campbell C: Epidural opioids: The preferred route of administration. Anesth Analg. 68:710–711, 1989.
173. Brose WG, Cohen SE: Oxyhemoglobin saturation following cesarean section in patients receiving epidural morphine, PCA, or IM meperidine analgesia. Anesthesiology 70:948–953, 1989.
174. Boerner TF, Norris MC, Leighton BL, Arkoosh VA, Witkowski TA, Torjman M: Intrathecal fentanyl does not improve intrathecal morphine analgesia after cesarean section. In Abstracts of Scientific Papers, Society for Obstetric Anesthesia and Perinatology, Boston, 1991.
175. Kotelko DM, Thigpen JW, Shnider SM, Foutz SE, Rosen MA, Hughes SC: Postoperative epidural morphine analgesia after various local anesthetics. Anesthesiology 59:A413, 1983.
176. Hughes SC, Wright RG, Murphy D, Preston P, Hughes W, Rosen M, Shnider S: The effect of pH adjusting 3% 2-chloroprocaine on the quality of post-cesarean section analgesia with epidural morphine. Anesthesiology 69:A689, 1988.
177. Schlairet TJ, Eisenach JC, Dobson CE: Effect of catheter testing with 2-chloroprocaine on the duration of epidural morphine analgesia following cesarean section. Anesthesiology 71:A917, 1989.
178. Phan CQ, Machernis EA, Lobo WD, Azar I, Lear E: The effect of alkalinization of 2-chloroprocaine on the onset and the quality of epidural morphine analgesia. Anesthesiology 71:A891, 1989.
179. Phan CQ, Machernis EA, Zung N, Azar I, Lear E: The quality of epidural morphine-fentanyl analgesia following epidural anesthesia with 2-chloroprocaine. Anesthesiology 71:A835, 1989.
180. Ackerman WE, Juneja MM: 2-chloroprocaine decreases the duration of analgesia of epidural fentanyl. Anesth Analg 68:S2, 1989.
181. Naulty JS, Hertwig L, Hunt CO, Hartwell B, Datta S, Ostheimer GW, Covino BG: Duration of analgesia of epidural fentanyl following cesarean delivery: Effects of local anesthesia drug selection. Anesthesiology 65:A180, 1986.
182. Durkan WJ, Baker LT, Leicht CH: Postoperative epidural morphine analgesia after 3% 2-chloroprocaine (nesacaine-MPF) or lidocaine epidural anesthesia. Anesthesiology 71:A834, 1989.
183. Priddle HD, Andros GJ: Primary spinal anesthetic effects of epinephrine. Anesth Analg (Curr Res) 29:156–162, 1950.
184. Kuraishi Y, Hirota N, Sato Y, Kaneko S, Satoh M, Takagi H: Noradrenergic inhibition of the release of substance P from the primary afferents in the rabbit spinal dorsal horn. Brain Res 359:177–182, 1985.
185. Fleetwood-Walker SM, Mitchell R, Hope PH, Molony V, Iggo A: An alpha-2 receptor mediates the selective inhibition by noradrenaline of nociceptive responses of identified dorsal horn neurones. Brain Res 334:243–254, 1985.
186. Eisenach JC, Lysak SZ, Vicsomi CM: Epidural clonidine analgesia following surgery: Phase I. Anesthesiology 71:640–646, 1989.
186. Kitahata LM: Spinal analgesia with morphine and clonidine. Anesth Analg 68:191–193, 1989.
188. Collins JG, Kitahata LM, Matsumoto M, Homma E, Suzukawa M: Spinally administered epinephrine suppresses noxiously evoked activity of WDR neurons in the dorsal horn of the spinal cord. Anesthesiology 60:269–275, 1984.
189. Eisenach JC, Dewan DM, Rose JC, Angelo JM: Epidural clonidine produces antinociception, but not hypotension, in sheep. Anesthesiology 66:496–501, 1987.
190. Eisenach JC, Castro MI, Dewan DM, Rose JC, Grice SC: Intravenous clonidine hydrochloride toxicity in pregnant ewes. Am J Obstet Gynecol 160:471–476, 1988.
191. Eisenach JC, Castro MI, Dewan DM, Rose JC: Epidural clonidine analgesia in obstetrics. Sheep studies. Anesthesiology 70:51–56, 1989.
192. Eisenach JC, Rauck RL, Buzzanell C, Lysak SZ: Epidural clonidine analgesia for intractable cancer pain: Phase I. Anesthesiology 71:647–652, 1989.
193. Post C, Gordh T, Minor B, Archer T, Freedman J: Antinociceptive effects and spinal cord tissue concentrations after intrathecal injection of guanfacine or clonidine into rats. Anesth Analg 66:317–324, 1987.
194. Leimdorfer A, Metzner WRT: Analgesia and anesthesia induced by epinephrine. Am J Physiol 157:116–121, 1949.
195. Reddy SVR, Maderdrut JL, Yaksh TL: Spinal cord pharmacology of adrenergic agonist-mediated antinociception. J Pharmacol Exp Ther 213:525–533, 1980.
196. Yaksh TL, Reddy SVR: Studies in the primate on the analgetic effects associated with intrathecal actions of opiates, a-adrenergic agonists and baclofen. Anesthesiology 54:451–467, 1981.
197. Huntoon M, Eisenach JC, Boese P: Epidural clonidine after cesarean section: Appropriate dose and effect of prior local anesthetic. Anesthesiology 76:187–193, 1992.
198. Yaksh T, Collins JG: Studies in animals should precede human use of spinally administered drugs. Anesthesiology 70:4–6, 1989.
199. Reiz S, Westberg M: Side-effects of epidural morphine. Lancet 2:203–204, 1980.
200. Leicht CH, Hughes SC, Dailey PA, Shnider SM, Rosen MA: Epidural morphine sulfate for analgesia after cesarean section: A prospective report of 1000 patients. Anesthesiology 65:A366, 1986.
201. Bromage PR, Camporesi EM, Durant PA, Nielsen CH: Influence of epinephrine as an adjuvant to epidural morphine. Anesthesiology 58:257–262, 1983.
202. Boas RA: Hazards of epidural morphine. Anaesth Intensive Care 8:377–378, 1980.
203. Christensen V: Respiratory depression after extradural morphine. Br J Anaesth 52:841, 1980.
204. Davies GK, Tolhurst-Cleaver CL, James TL: CNS depression from intrathecal morphine. Anesthesiology 52:280, 1980.
205. Glynn CJ, Mather LE, Cousins MJ, Wilson PR, Graham JR: Spinal narcotics and respiratory depression. Lancet 2:356–357, 1979.
206. Jones RDM, Jones JG: Intrathecal morphine: Naloxone reversed respiratory depression but not analgesia. Br Med J 281:645, 1980.
207. Liolios A, Anderson FH: Selective spinal analgesia. Lancet 2:357, 1979.
208. Scott DB, McClure J: Selective epidural analgesia. Lancet 1:1410–1411, 1979.

209. Wüst HJ, Bromage PR: Delayed respiratory arrest after epidural hydromorphone. Anaesthesia 42:404–406, 1987.

210. London SW: Respiratory depression after single epidural injection of local anesthetic and morphine. Anesth Analg 66:797–799, 1987.

211. Streinstra R, Van Poorten F: Immediate respiratory arrest after caudal epidural sufentanil. Anesthesiology 71:993–994, 1989.

212. Brockway MS, Noble DW, Sharwood-Smith GH, McClure JH: Profound respiratory depression after extradural fentanyl. Br J Anaesth 64:243–245, 1990.

213. Krane BD, Kreutz JM, Johnson DL, Mathson JE: Alfentanil and delayed respiratory depression: Case studies and review. Anesthesiology 70:557–561, 1990.

214. Palmer DM: Early respiratory depression following intrathecal fentanyl-morphine combination. Anesthesiology 174:1153–1155, 1991.

215. Gustafsson LL, Schildt B, Jacobsen K: Adverse effects of extradural and intrathecal opiates: Report of a nationwide survey in Sweden. Br J Anaesth 54:479–486, 1982.

216. Stenseth R, Sellevold O, Breivik H: Epidural morphine for postoperative pain: Experience with 1085 patients. Acta Anaesthesiol Scand 29:148–156, 1985.

217. Daley MD, Sandler AN, Turner KE, Vosu H, Slavchenko P: A comparison of epidural and intramuscular morphine in patients following cesarean section. Anesthesiology 72:289–294, 1990.

218. Wheatly RG, Somerville ID, Sapsford DJ, Jones JG: Postoperative hypoxaemia: Comparison of extradural, IM and patient-controlled opioid analgesia. Br J Anaesth 64:267–275, 1990.

219. Dahl JB, Jacobson JB: Accidental epidural narcotic overdose. Anesth Analg 70:321–322, 1990.

220. Kafer ER, Brown JT, Scott D, Findlay JWA, Butz RF, Teeple E, Ghia JN: Biphasic depression of ventilatory responses to CO_2 following epidural morphine. Anesthesiology 58:418–427, 1983.

221. Camporesi EM, Nielsen CH, Bromage PR, Durant PAC: Ventilatory CO_2 sensitivity after intravenous and epidural morphine in volunteers. Anesth Analg 62:633–640, 1983.

222. Korsh J, Ramanathan S, Parker F, Turndorf H: Systemic histamine release by epidural morphine. Anesthesiology 67:A445, 1987.

223. Davies G, From R: A blinded study using nalbuphine for prevention of pruritus induced by epidural fentanyl. Anesthesiology 69:763–765, 1988.

224. Morgan PJ, Mehta S: Prophylactic nalbuphine in cesarean section patients treated with epidural morphine. Anesth Analg 68:S203, 1989.

225. Cardan E: Herpes simplex after spinal morphine. Anaesthesia 39:1031, 1984.

226. Gieraerts R, Navalgund A, Vaes L, Soetens M, Chang J, Jahr J: Increased incidence of itching and herpes simplex in patients given epidural morphine after cesarean section. Anesth Analg 66:1321–1324, 1987.

227. Crone LA, Conly JM, Clark KM, Crichlow AC, Wardell GC, Zbitnew A, Rea LM, Cronk SL, Anderson CM, Tan LK, Albritton WL: Recurrent herpes simplex virus labialis and the use of epidural morphine in obstetric patients. Anesth Analg 67:318–323, 1988.

228. Crone LA, Conly JM, Storgard C, Zbitnew A, Cronk SL, Rea LM, Greer K, Berenbaum E, Tan LK, To T: Herpes labialis in parturients receiving epidural morphine following cesarean section. Anesthesiology 73:208–213, 1990.

229. Ugolani G, Kuypers HG, Simmons A: Retrograde transneuronal transfer of herpes simplex virus type 1 (HSV 1) from motoneurones. Brain Res 422:242–256, 1987.

230. Ugolani, Kuypers HG, Strick PL: Transneuronal transfer of herpes virus from peripheral nerves to cortex and brainstem. Science 243:89–91, 1989.

231. Scott PV, Fischer HBJ: Spinal opiate analgesia and facial pruritus: A neural theory. Postgrad Med J 58:531–535, 1986.

232. Weddel SJ, Ritter RR: Epidural morphine: Serum levels and pain relief. Anesthesiology 53:A419, 1980.

233. Rawal N, Mollefors K, Axelsson K, Lingardh G, Widman B: An experimental study of urodynamic effects of epidural morphine and of naloxone reversal. Anesth Analg 62:641–647, 1983.

234. Durant P, Yaksh T: Micurition in the unanesthetized rat: Effects of intrathecal capsaicin, N-vanillylnonanamide, 6-hydoxydopamine and 5,6-dihydroxytryptamine. Brain Res 451:301–308, 1988.

235. Durant P, Lucas P, Yaksh T: Micturition in the unanesthetized rat: Spinal vs. peripheral pharmacology of the adrenergic system. J Pharm Exper Ther 245:426–435, 1988.

236. Durant P, Yaksh T: Drug effects on urinary bladder tone during spinal morphine-induced inhibition of the micturition reflex in unanesthetized rats. Anesthesiology 68:325–334, 1988.

237. Dray A: Epidural opiates and urinary retention: New models provide new insights. Anesthesiology 68:323–324, 1988.

238. Loper KA, Ready LB, Dorman BH: Prophylactic transdermal scopolamine patches reduce nausea in postoperative patients receiving epidural morphine. Anesth Analg 68:144–146, 1989.

239. Bailey PL, Streisand JB, Pace NL, Bubbers SJM, East KA, Mulder S, Stanley TH: Transdermal scopolamine reduces nausea and vomiting after outpatient laparoscopy. Anesthesiology 72:977–980, 1990.

240. Kotelko DM, Rottman RL, Wright WC, Stone JJ, Yamashiro AY, Rosenblatt RM: Transdermal scopolamine decreases nausea and vomiting following cesarean section in patients receiving epidural morphine. Anesthesiology 71:675–678, 1989.

241. Rawal N, Wattwil M: Respiratory depression after epidural morphine: An experimental and clinical study. Anesth Analg 63:8–14, 1984.

242. Rawal N, Schött U, Dahlström B, Inturrisi CE, Tandon B, Sjöstrand U, Wennhager M: Influence of naloxone infusion on analgesia and respiratory depression following epidural morphine. Anesthesiology 64:194–201, 1986.

243. Young RSK, Hessert TR, Pritchard GA, Yagel SK: Naloxone exacerbates hypoxic-ischemic brain injury in the neonatal rat. Am J Obstet Gynecol 50:52–56, 1984.

244. Wiener PC, Hogg MIJ, Rosen M: Effects of naloxone on pethidine-induced neonatal depression. Br Med J 2:228–231, 1977.

245. Hibbard BM, Rosen M, Davies D: Placental transfer of naloxone. Br J Anaesth 58:45–48, 1986.

246. Arduini D, Rizzo G, Dell'Acqua S, Mancuso S, Romanini C: Effect of naloxone on fetal behavior near term. Am J Obstet Gynecol 156:474–478, 1987.

247. Flacke JW, Flacke WE, Williams GD: Acute pulmonary edema following naloxone reversal of high-dose morphine anesthesia. Anesthesiology 47:376–378, 1977.

248. Andree RA: Sudden death following naloxone administration. Anesth Analg 59:782–784, 1980.

249. Taff RH: Pulmonary edema following naloxone administration. Anesth Analg 59:576–577, 1983.

250. Prough DS, Raymond R, Baumgarner J, Shannon G: Acute pulmonary edema in healthy teenagers following conservative doses of intravenous naloxone. Anesthesiology 60:485–486, 1984.

251. Partridge BL, Ward CF: Pulmonary edema following low-dose naloxone administration. Anesthesiology 65:709–710, 1986.

252. Wride SRN, Smith RER, Courtney PG: A fatal case of pulmonary edema in a healthy young male following naloxone administration. Anaesth Intensive Care 17:374–377, 1989.

253. Mok MS, Shuai SP, Lee C, Lee TY, Lippmann M: Naltrexone pretreatment attenuates side effects of epidural morphine. Anesthesiology 65:A200, 1986.

254. Abboud TK, Afrasiabi A, Davison J, Zhu J, Reyes A, Khoo N, Steffens Z: Prophlactic oral naltrexone with epidural morphine: Effect on adverse reactions and ventilatory responses to carbon dioxide. Anesthesiology 72:233–237, 1990.

255. Knoieczko KM, Jones JG, Barrowcliffe MP, Jordan C, Altman DG: Antagonism of morphine-induced respiratory depression with nalmefene. Br J Anaesth 61:318–323, 1988.

256. Des Marteau JK, Cassot AL: Acute pulmonary edema resulting from nalbuphine reversal of fentanyl-induced respiratory depression. Anesthesiology 65:237, 1986.

257. Blaise GA, McMichan JC, Nugent M, Hollier LH: Nalbuphine produces side-effects while reversing narcotic-induced respiratory depression. Anesth Analg 65:S19, 1986.

258. Penning JP, Samson B, Baxter A: Nalbuphine reversal epidural morphine induced respiratory depression. Anesth Analg 65:S119, 1986.

259. Yaksh TL, Wilson PR, Kaiko RF, Inturrisi CE: Analgesia produced by a spinal action of morphine and effects upon parturition in the rat. Anesthesiology 51:386–392, 1979.

260. Steinbrook RA, Carr DB, Datta S, Naulty SJ, Lee C, Fisher J: Dissociation of plasma and cerebrospinal fluid beta-endorphin-like immunoactivity levels during pregnancy and parturition. Anesth Analg 61:893–897, 1982.

261. Golub MS, Eisele JH, Donald JM: Obstetric analgesia and infant outcome in monkeys: Infant development after intrapartum exposure to meperidine or alfentanil. Am J Obstet Gynecol 159:1280–1286, 1988.

262. Golub MS, Eisele JH, Donald JM: Obstetric analgesia and infant outcome in monkeys: Neonatal measures after intrapartum exposure to meperidine or alfentanil. Am J Obstet Gynecol 158:1219–1225, 1988.

263. Mokriski B, Malinow AM, St. Amant MC, Kaufman MA, Snell JA, Nagey DA: Epidural narcotic analgesia for labor and fetal heart rate variability. Anesthesiology 71:A856, 1989.

264. Copogna G, Celleno D, Costantino P, Sebastiani M, Muratori F, Emanuelli M: Epidural morphine and buprenorphine for analgesia during and after cesarean section: Maternal effects and neonatal outcome. Reg Anesth 15:S26, 1990.

265. Banlabed M, Midgel M, Dreizzen E, Escourou P, Ecoffey C, Gaultier C: Neonatal pattern of breathing after cesarean section with or without epidural fentanyl. Anesthesiology 69:A651, 1988.

266. Noueihid R. Durant P, Yaksh TL: Studies on the effect of intrathecal sufentanil, fentanyl, and alfentanil in rats and cats. Anesthesiology 61:A218, 1984.

267. Abouleish E, Barmada MA, Nemoto EM, Tung A, Winter P: Acute and chronic effects of intrathecal morphine in monkeys. Br J Anaesth 53:1027–1032, 1981.

268. Yaksh TL, Rudy TA: Chronic catheterization of the spinal subarachnoid space. Physiol Behav 17:1031–1036, 1976.

269. Tung AS, Tenicela R, Winter PM: Opiate withdrawal syndrome following intrathecal administration of morphine. Anesthesiology 53:340, 1980.

270. Cohen SE, Rothblatt AJ, Albright GA: Early respiratory depression with epidural narcotic and intravenous droperidol. Anesthesiology 59:559–560, 1983.

271. Zucker-Pinchoff B, Ramanathan S: Anaphylactic reaction to epidural fentanyl. Anesthesiology 71:599–601, 1989.

272. Cohen SE, Woods WA: The role of epidural morphine in the postcesarean patient: Efficacy and effects on bonding. Anesthesiology 58:500–504, 1983.

273. Rawal N, Sjostrand U, Christoffersson E, Dahlstrom B, Arvill A, Rydman H: Comparison of intramuscular and epidural morphine for postoperative analgesia in the grossly obese: Influence on postoperative ambulation and pulmonary function. Anesth Analg 63:583–592, 1984.

274. Bormann BV, Weidler B, Dennhardt R, Sturm G, Scheld HH, Hempelmann G: Influence of epidural fentanyl on stress-induced elevation of plasma vasopressin (ADH) after surgery. Anesth Analg 62:727–732, 1983.

275. Rawal N, Arner S, Gustafsson LL, Allvin R: Present state of extradural and intrathecal opioid analgesia in Sweden. Br J Anaesth 59:791–799, 1987.

276. Fuller JG, McMorland GH, Douglas MJ, Palmer L: Epidural morphine for analgesia after caesarean section: A report of 4880 patients. Can J Anaesth 37:636–640, 1990.

CHAPTER 11

Inhalation Analgesia and Anesthesia for Vaginal Delivery

Sheila E. Cohen, M.B., Ch.B., F.F.A.R.C.S.

Since 1847 when James Simpson first administered ether to a woman in labor, almost every new inhalation anesthetic has been used for this purpose. However, for a variety of reasons, few agents have retained their place in the obstetric anesthesiologist's armamentarium. In a 1986 survey of obstetric anesthesia practice in the United States performed by the American Society of Anesthesiologists and the American College of Obstetricians and Gynecologists, none of the responding hospitals reported the use of inhalation agents to provide analgesia during labor [1]. However, 6% of women received inhalation analgesia for vaginal delivery, whereas 3% received general anesthesia for this purpose. If these statistics still hold true, it means that each year in the United States approximately 350,000 women receive inhalation agents during their deliveries. Inhalation techniques are used with even greater frequency in obstetric practice in the United Kingdom and elsewhere. This chapter discusses the role of inhalation agents in modern obstetric practice and their effects, both beneficial and adverse, on the mother, the fetus, and the process of labor. Detailed consideration of individual anesthetic agents is restricted to those of most relevance to current anesthetic practice.

It is important to define the terms inhalation analgesia and inhalation anesthesia. *Inhalation analgesia* describes the administration of subanesthetic concentrations of inhalation agents to provide analgesia for the first and second stages of labor, either alone or as a supplement to regional or local anesthesia. The object of this technique is for the mother to remain awake throughout, to be able to cooperate, and to maintain protective laryngeal reflexes while achieving analgesic levels of the agent. The anesthetic is usually administered via a mask or mouthpiece, either by an anesthesiologist or other qualified individual or by the patient herself. The term *inhalation anesthesia* describes the practice of administering inhalation agents with the intention of producing unconsciousness for the purpose of performing cesarean section, vaginal delivery with forceps, or vacuum extraction or in cases in which uterine relaxation is required.

INDICATIONS FOR INHALATION ANALGESIA

Inhalation analgesia provides a degree of pain relief that, although not comparable with that obtained with regional anesthesia, is rated as "satisfactory" by more than 80% of parturient patients [2]. Many women elect not to have regional anesthesia because of a fear of needles and spinal headaches or because they believe regional anesthesia will render them unable to participate in the delivery. In such cases the choice of analgesic techniques for the first stage of labor falls among inhalation agents, opioids, or other systemic drugs and paracervical block. Although opioids are easily administered, they have the potential for causing neonatal respiratory and neurobehavioral depression. The high incidence of fetal bradycardia after paracervical block has led to the infrequent use of this technique. Thus inhalation techniques may provide an acceptable alternative, particularly when labor is progressing rapidly.

When a brief period of analgesia is required during the second stage of labor in the absence of, or to supplement, regional or local anesthesia, inhalation agents again may be used. Ketamine in low doses also may be used in this circumstance [3]. Although effective and without adverse fetal effects, ketamine is associated with a high incidence of amnesia for delivery, which many patients consider unsatisfactory. The use of ketamine in obstetrics is discussed in Chapter 8.

Historically, the majority of obstetric anesthetics in this country, and perhaps in the world, have been administered by personnel who have had no formal anesthesia training. The 1986 survey of obstetric anesthesia practice mentioned previously revealed that an anesthesiologist administered or supervised care in only 53% of the cases in which inhalation analgesia was used for vaginal delivery and in 66% of cases in which general anesthesia was used (1). Nurse anesthetists directed by an obstetrician, the delivery room nurse, the obstetrician, and the house officer administered the remainder of anesthetics. This survey further reported that only 21% of hospitals in the United States had 24-hr coverage provided by anesthesiologists, and only 15% had 24-hr coverage by nurse anesthetists. Although attempts have been made to improve this situation, it is likely that a major problem still exists, and the reality of present limitations in personnel must be faced. Thus there is a need for an analgesic method that is simple to administer and that has a high degree of safety for both mother and fetus. Inhalation analgesia in some respects fulfills these requirements; it has been widely used by nurse anesthetists and obstetric nurses in the United States and by midwives in the United Kingdom (4). However, in view of the absence of trained anesthesia personnel in many situations in which inhalation analgesia is used, it is critical that those administering it are specifically educated in the technique and its potential hazards.

INDICATIONS FOR INHALATION ANESTHESIA

Because the risk of aspiration of vomitus is significantly lower with regional anesthesia or inhalation analgesia, the author does not recommend the use of general anesthesia for vaginal delivery unless there is a specific indication. If acute fetal distress occurs during the second stage of labor and operative vaginal delivery is indicated, general anesthesia may be the most satisfactory technique because of the rapidity with which it can be instituted. If regional techniques are contraindicated (see Chapter 9) and inhalation analgesia or low-dose ketamine is inadequate to allow for a safe, controlled delivery, general anesthesia may be necessary. Probably the most common indication for general anesthesia for vaginal delivery is the necessity for uterine relaxation. Intrauterine manipulations for internal podalic version, complete breech extraction, manual removal of the placenta, and replacement of an inverted uterus usually are performed under general anesthesia with a volatile inhalation agent. In addition, uterine relaxation might be necessary for relief of a tetanic uterine contraction or during a breech delivery when the uterus has clamped down before delivery of the head. Recent reports (5, 6) of the use of low doses (i.e., 50 μg bolus) of intravenous nitroglycerin to produce uterine relaxation for removal of a retained placenta suggest that volatile anesthetics may not always be necessary in these circumstances. If, after wider testing, nitroglycerin proves safe and effective as a myometrial relaxant, it may be used for this purpose, with regional anesthesia, inhalation analgesia or intravenous agents administered for patient comfort.

INHALATION ANALGESIA AND ANESTHESIA: GENERAL CONSIDERATIONS

Maternal Safety

Perhaps the greatest pitfall of inhalation techniques is their apparent simplicity. The ease of administration using devices that the patient holds herself may lead busy attendants to neglect her, which can produce disastrous results. This is particularly hazardous because anesthesia is induced rapidly in the parturient patient for a variety of reasons. Physiologic changes in pregnancy, including a reduction in functional residual capacity and an increase in alveolar ventilation, lead to a more rapid equilibration of alveolar and inspired anesthetic concentrations. This results in more rapid induction of anesthesia and fluctuations of anesthetic level in response to changes in inspired concentration. Pregnancy also is associated with reduced anesthetic requirements, perhaps as a result of elevated β-endorphin and progesterone levels. In one study the minimum alveolar concentration (MAC) was decreased 32% for methoxyflurane, 25% for halothane, and 40% for isoflurane (7). Opioids given in labor will further reduce MAC and thus contribute to the risk of unexpected loss of consciousness.

Therefore the major risk from inhalation analgesia is accidental anesthetic overdose with loss of protective reflexes. Vomiting or silent regurgitation may then occur, resulting in immediate respiratory obstruction and asphyxia or delayed development of aspiration pneumonitis. In the past, maternal deaths caused by anesthesia have made up 5 to 15% of all maternal deaths in the United States, with approximately half of these due to aspiration (8, 9). In the state of Indiana during a 7-year period (1967 to 1974), 14 of 154 maternal deaths were directly related to anesthesia, and of those, 10 women died of pulmonary failure resulting from aspiration of gastric fluid (10). In these reports it is often unclear whether inhalation agents had been administered with the intention of producing general anesthesia or only analgesia, and in many instances there is no mention of endotracheal intubation.

More recent data suggest that both anesthesia-related maternal mortality and deaths resulting from aspiration are decreasing. Two reports of maternal mortality in the United States (11, 12), which together cover the period from 1974 to 1986, found that 4 to 5% of deaths were associated with anesthesia, with aspiration responsible for 25 to 29% of cases. However, the true number of anesthetic deaths may be considerably higher than this, because widespread underreporting of maternal mortality has been demonstrated in the United States (11, 12). Anesthetic mishaps in which medicolegal issues are involved may be particularly likely to be misreported. In a 1991 analysis of closed malpractice claims performed by the American Society of Anesthesiologists, pulmonary aspiration was cited in 8% of obstetric claims (16 of 190), compared with only 2% of nonobstetric claims (13). In seven of the obstetric cases in which aspiration occurred, anesthesia was administered by mask, whereas in six others it occurred during difficult esophageal intubation. Because claims for maternal death and respiratory events were significantly more common in cases involving general anesthesia, the report concluded that regional anesthesia was markedly safer than general anesthesia in pregnant women.

The most accurate statistics on maternal mortality come from the United Kingdom, where a triennial report, *The Report on Confidential Enquiries into Maternal Deaths*, examines the cause and circumstances of every maternal death in that country. Between 1976 and 1978, approximately 50% of maternal anesthetic deaths were related to aspiration of gastric contents, with the majority occurring during either induction of or recovery from anesthesia (14). In the most recent report covering mortality between 1985 and 1987, aspiration was responsible for only 12.5% of the total number of anesthetic deaths, which also had decreased compared with previous years (15). Substandard care administered by inexperienced personnel was a factor in all the deaths directly attributed to anesthesia.

The pregnant woman must always be regarded as being at risk for acid aspiration syndrome whenever analgesia or anesthesia is undertaken (see Chapter 23). The presence of a large volume of gastric juice or a dangerously low gastric pH cannot be excluded in any parturient patient, regardless of the time of last food intake or the onset of labor (16). Routine administration of oral antacids to every pregnant patient before induction of general anesthesia has therefore been recommended. (Prophylaxis of aspiration is dealt with more fully in Chapter 23.)

Because the risk of aspiration can never be completely avoided, routine endotracheal intubation is indicated whenever general anesthesia is induced in the pregnant patient (17). This includes those situations in which inhalation analgesia is converted to anesthesia, for whatever reason. Rarely, face mask-administered general anesthesia may be appropriately undertaken as part of a difficult intubation drill.

This should only be undertaken if the anesthesiologist can maintain a satisfactory airway. Cricoid pressure should be continued during the entire anesthetic procedure.

In addition to the physiologic changes of pregnancy described above, there is a higher metabolic rate and increased oxygen consumption, which further increases during labor. These factors predispose the pregnant patient to the rapid development of hypoxia in the event of respiratory depression or airway obstruction. Hypercapnia and acidosis also develop extremely quickly in such circumstances. In the obese woman who has additional derangement of pulmonary function and in whom airway management frequently is difficult, these changes are exaggerated.

The advent of noninvasive methods of continuously monitoring oxygen saturation has clarified the respiratory effects of inhalation agents administered during labor, which formerly were thought to be minimal. An early study in which arterial blood was intermittently sampled during inhalation of nitrous oxide or methoxyflurane during labor found increases in mean arterial oxygen tension at the end of periods of inhalation. Although episodes of mild hypoxemia occurred in individual patients, severe hypoxemia was rarely detected (18). In a more recent study in which oxygen saturation was continuously monitored during nitrous oxide analgesia in labor, Reed et al. demonstrated frequent transient episodes of moderate desaturation (to <90%) and occasional episodes of profound desaturation (to <70%) (19). During the first stage of labor, hypoxemia occurred most frequently between contractions, whereas in the second stage it occurred in association with breath-holding during contractions. It is well known that, even in nonmedicated pregnant women, relative hypoventilation can follow the hyperventilation and resultant hypocapnia induced by painful contractions. It appears that nitrous oxide may exacerbate this phenomenon, a theory supported by a study in nonpregnant volunteers, which found more severe desaturation after hyperventilation with 50% nitrous oxide than after hyperventilation with a mixture of 79% nitrogen and oxygen (20). Possible mechanisms to explain these findings include an effect of nitrous oxide on ventilatory drive, diffusion hypoxia, or ventilation/perfusion mismatch. Another study in nonpregnant volunteers suggests that modification of ventilatory control by subanesthetic concentrations of nitrous oxide is the most likely explanation (21). In the laboring patient, the respiratory depressant effect of concurrently administered opioids further exacerbates the hypoxemia associated with nitrous oxide analgesia (18, 19, 22). Therefore routine monitoring of maternal oxygenation using pulse oximetry is recommended whenever inhalation techniques are used. In addition, supplemental oxygen should be administered during and between periods of inhalation.

Effects on the Fetus and Neonate

Placental transfer of all inhalation agents occurs rapidly, because these agents are highly lipid soluble, un-ionized, and of fairly low molecular weight. Anesthetic levels rise rapidly in the fetal brain, and in general the degree of fetal and neonatal depression is directly proportional to the depth and duration of maternal anesthesia (23). Neonatal depression may be a result of drug effect or of physiologic changes, such as hypoventilation or hypotension, induced in the mother.

Deep halothane or isoflurane anesthesia has been shown to be associated with fetal hypoxia and acidosis (24, 25), probably as a result of maternal hypotension, which occurs in such cases (Fig. 11.1). Because these agents are rapidly transmitted across the placenta, they also can exert direct effects on the fetus. Studies in animals have found that MAC for halothane and isoflurane are significantly less for the fetus than for the mother (26, 27). This finding also has been reported for isoflurane in preterm infants (28). The cause for this is speculative but has been attributed both to the elevated levels of progesterone and endorphins present during pregnancy and to structural changes in the developing nervous system of the neonate. Another unexplained finding is the decreased solubility coefficient for inhalation agents in fetal, as compared with maternal, blood (29). Despite this decrease in anesthetic requirement, the healthy fetus does not appear to be unduly sensitive to the cardiovascular depressant effects of the halogenated agents. Using the pregnant sheep model, Biehl et al. studied the cardiovascular responses of the mother and fetus to the administration of anesthetic concentrations of halothane (30). Following maternal administration of 1.5% halothane for 8 min, a significant decrease in fetal blood pressure occurred, which was maintained throughout the 90-min experiment. However, fetal cardiac output and regional blood flow to vital organs (including the brain) were not significantly altered, and fetal acid-base status remained stable. Thus it can be deduced that fetal hypotension was a consequence of a decrease in peripheral vascular resistance rather than of myocardial depression. In similar studies by the same group using isoflurane, prolonged exposure to 2% isoflurane resulted in progressive fetal acidosis after 48 min and in a decrease in fetal cardiac index after 60 min (31). However, in a subsequent study in which isoflurane was administered for only 30 min, fetal acidosis and myocardial depression did not develop (27).

Studies of the effects of inhalation agents in the stressed sheep fetus have yielded controversial results, suggesting that fetal condition, drug concentration, and duration of exposure, all can influence outcome. Palahniuk et al. investigated the effects of halothane administration in the presence of an acidotic fetus (32). In this circumstance, halothane caused marked fetal hypotension, hypoxia, and worsening of the acidosis. Whereas fetal acidosis before halothane exposure had been associated with increased cerebral blood flow, following halothane administration cerebral autoregulation was lost and cerebral blood flow decreased. Other investigators have demonstrated that with more moderate asphyxia (33) or a shorter exposure to halothane (34), fetal hypotension occurred, but the protective reflexes of increased cerebral and coronary blood flow and decreased cerebral metabolic rate of oxygen (CMR_{O_2}) were not abolished. Baker et al. found similar results following 15 min of 1% isoflurane administration to the mother of the asphyxiated fetal lamb; fetal acidosis deteriorated further, but redistribution of cerebral and cardiac blood flow was maintained and the balance of oxygen supply/demand remained favorable (35).

The clinical implications of the above data are that brief exposure of either the healthy or the stressed fetus to moderate doses of volatile agents is unlikely to be detrimental. When uterine relaxation is needed to facilitate delivery of a second twin or in breech presentation when the fetal head is entrapped by an incompletely dilated cervix, several minutes of inhalation of a volatile agent is usually all that is required. If the fetus is severely depressed, the volatile agent should be discontinued as soon as the desired degree of myometrial relaxation has been obtained.

Prolonged general anesthesia with nitrous oxide also has been associated with an increased number of depressed infants (36, 37). Infants born after a drug-delivery interval of 15 to 17 min had higher Apgar scores than those born after an interval of 23 to 36 min. This seems to correlate with the finding of a nitrous oxide concentration ratio for umbilical artery/umbilical vein of 89% at 36 min by Stenger et al. (37) and with similar findings by Marx et al. (38), who recorded 87% equilibration in the fetal tissues after 15 to 19 min (Fig. 11.2). Stenger et al. found a very wide maternal artery/uterine vein (umbilical vein) gradient for nitrous oxide early in the course of anesthesia. Fetal concentrations apparently approach maternal levels as the anesthetic is continued (Fig. 11.3). In addition to the time factor, placental transfer of the anesthetic agent also may relate to the adequacy of placental blood flow. Hay demonstrated a higher umbilical vein/maternal artery nitrous oxide concentration ratio in infants with higher Apgar scores and

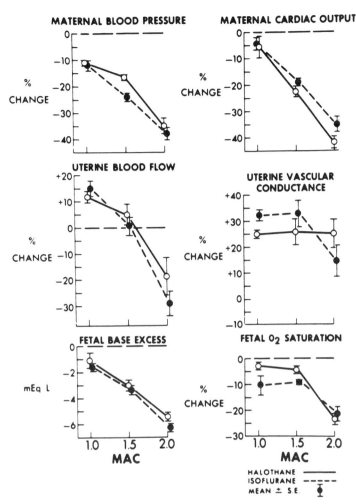

Figure 11.1. Changes from control values in mean maternal blood pressure, cardiac output, uterine blood flow, uterine vascular conductance, fetal arterial base excess, and fetal arterial O_2 saturation at 1, 1.5, and 2 MAC halothane and isoflurane. Values represent means of results obtained at 15, 30, 60, and 90 min. (Reprinted by permission from Palahniuk RJ, Shnider SM: Maternal and fetal cardiovascular and acid-base changes during halothane and isoflurane anesthesia in the pregnant ewe. Anesthesiology 41:462–472, 1974.)

birth weights, and suggested that all these factors were indicators of better uteroplacental perfusion (39). Furthermore, newborn status following administration of inhalation agents, particularly nitrous oxide, depends on maternal oxygenation. Marx and Mateo found that newborns were more vigorous when "high" (i.e., 67%), rather than "medium" (33%) concentrations of maternal oxygen were inhaled, despite the addition of a volatile agent to deepen nitrous oxide anesthesia to a level at which awareness was abolished (40). Piggot et al. similarly demonstrated higher umbilical venous Po_2 and decreased need for neonatal resuscitation following emergency cesarean section when 100% oxygen with 1.5 MAC of isoflurane, rather than 50% nitrous oxide, was administered (41).

Analgesic concentrations of inhalation agents, in contrast to the deeper levels required to produce complete anesthesia, do not appear to cause neonatal depression even when administration is prolonged (42, 43). However, Clark and associates demonstrated that, when prolonged methoxyflurane analgesia was followed by anesthesia with the same agent and nitrous oxide for delivery, the incidence of neonatal depression was increased (44). This was associated with higher umbilical vein levels of methoxyflurane, as measured at delivery. Recent studies in which neurobehavioral assessment of the newborn have been performed following cesarean or vaginal delivery have not demonstrated any adverse effects resulting from analgesic concentrations of halothane, enflurane, isoflurane, or nitrous oxide (2, 43, 45, 46).

When used in low concentrations, inhalation agents provide a considerable advantage for the fetus over systemic narcotics, because termination of the hypnotic effect is not dependent on metabolism and ex-

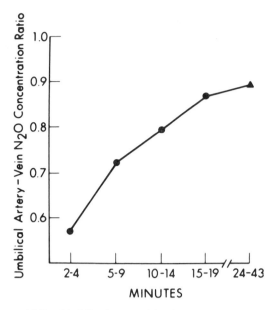

Figure 11.2. Umbilical artery blood nitrous oxide concentration, expressed as the ratio of umbilical vein blood N_2O concentration in relation to duration of N_2O administration. (Reprinted by permission from Marx GF: Newer aspects of general anesthesia for cesarean section. NY State J Med 71:1084, 1971. Drawn from data in Marx GF, Joshi CW, Orkin LR: Placental transmission of nitrous oxide. Anesthesiology 32:429–432, 1970.)

cretion is effected by the lungs. As long as the infant is breathing and circulation is adequate, depression from inhalation agents should progressively diminish in the period immediately after birth. Even if neonatal depression does occur, artificial ventilation can be instituted with the expectation of rapid improvement.

Effects on Labor and Uterine Tone

Most of the inhalation agents used in obstetric anesthesia cause dose-related depression of uterine contractility and tone (this is discussed fully in Chapter 4). Uterine relaxation may prolong labor and, of more importance, may result in increased blood loss following delivery. Early experiences with ether, chloroform, and halothane confirmed that these agents were profound myometrial depressants, particularly in the pregnant individual (47). Naftalin et al. noted a dose-related decrease in resting tension in both pregnant and nonpregnant animal and human myometrium exposed in vitro to halothane (48, 49). At low concentrations, the depressant effect was more profound on gravid myometrium. Studies by Munson and Embro of isolated human uterine muscle demonstrated that halothane, enflurane, and isoflurane are equally depressant when used in equipotent concentrations (50). Uterine contractility was significantly inhibited at 0.5 MAC, with further depression

proportional to dosage; resting myometrial tension at this anesthetic level was not affected with any of these agents. Intrauterine pressure measurements performed during labor or postpartum confirm that methoxyflurane (51), halothane, and enflurane (52) significantly depress the myometrium, whereas cyclopropane in low concentrations seems to have little effect on uterine contractility (53). Clinical experience and reported trials demonstrate the safety in this respect of analgesic concentrations of nitrous oxide, isoflurane, and enflurane, the agents currently used to provide analgesia during labor and vaginal delivery (2, 43). Marx et al. demonstrated, in vivo, that oxytocics counteracted the depression of uterine contractility caused by low concentrations of halothane or enflurane, but were unable to do so when concentrations greater than 0.8 to 0.9 MAC were present. An in vitro study similarly demonstrated that the depressant effect of up to 1.5% isoflurane could be reversed by oxytocin (54). Because isoflurane is excreted more rapidly than halothane, it may be preferable if a volatile anesthetic is administered specifically to produce uterine relaxation. The greater cardiovascular stability associated with isoflurane is an additional benefit in this circumstance.

Environmental Pollution

Epidemiologic evidence suggests that the operating room may be an environmentally hazardous location (55). The abnormality most consistently reported has been an increased incidence of spontaneous abortion among female anesthetists (56). Some studies also have suggested that, in these women, there is a slightly higher incidence of certain malignancies and a larger number of congenital abnormalities among their offspring. Exposure to trace concentrations of inhalation agents may be the cause of these problems, although this is controversial (56). Other factors related to working in the operating room, such as stress or radiation exposure, may be responsible. Although many scavenging systems have been designed to reduce pollution in the operating room, all self-administration analgesic devices in use in this country result in pollution of the environment from expired air containing inhalation agents. In the United Kingdom, Munley et al. found that midwives were potentially at risk from excessive occupational exposure when working in delivery suites in which self-administered nitrous oxide was used (57). In three of the hospitals studied, the average exposure was 100 ppm; in a fourth, a poorly ventilated unit, exposure was 360 ppm. A trial scavenging system introduced into the latter reduced levels to only 100 ppm. Although it is not known what level of exposure if any is harmful, the National Institute of Oc-

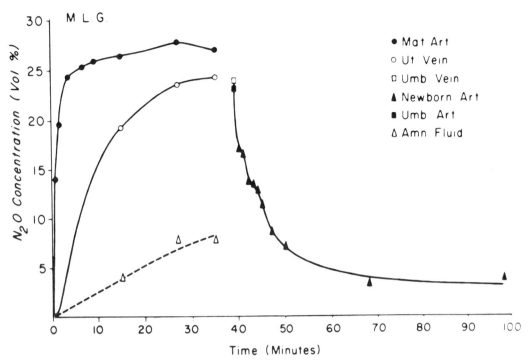

Figure 11.3. Serial concentrations of nitrous oxide during a prolonged anesthetic for a cesarean section. Note very wide maternal artery-uterine vein (umbilical vein) gradient for nitrous oxide early in the anesthesia. Fetal concentrations apparently approach maternal levels as the anesthetic is continued. (Reprinted by permission from Stenger VG, Blechner JN, Prystowsky H: A study of prolongation of obstetric anesthesia. Am J Obstet Gynecol 103:901–907, 1969.)

cupational Safety and Health in the United States has set a maximum permitted limit of 25 ppm, while the Swedish legal limit is 100 ppm. Currently, in most institutions in the United States inhalation analgesia is only administered in a delivery or operating room via an anesthetic machine equipped with a scavenging device.

Apparatus

Inhalation analgesics may be administered either from a standard anesthetic machine or a flow-over vaporizer. When nitrous oxide is used for self-administered analgesia, it usually is combined with oxygen by a blender apparatus, producing varying concentrations, dependent on the requirements of the patient. Volatile anesthetics are administered via several types of vaporizers, most of which are now of only historical interest. Examples of handheld vaporizers include the Cyprane (Fig. 11.4) and Duke inhalers. Currently, precision vaporizers that are attached to the anesthetic machine and that allow for the concomitant use of oxygen and nitrous oxide are most often employed. A vaporizer used for inhalation analgesia must be capable of delivering a reliable concentration, or range of concentrations, or anesthetic vapor. These concentrations should be safe and should not be significantly altered by the patient's minute ventilation, peak flow, or variations in

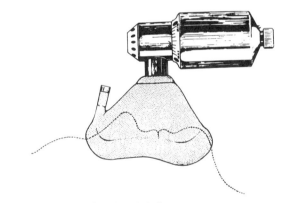

Figure 11.4. A Cyprane inhaler.

room temperature. These considerations are especially important because of the wide variations in minute ventilation that occur during labor. Some devices incorporate a fail-safe device, requiring the patient to generate a negative pressure to initiate gas flow. These mechanisms assume that the patient will be unable to operate them if excessively anesthetized and that deepening of anesthesia will cause the mouthpiece or mask to fall from the face. However, patients may learn to circumvent these intended safety mechanisms by such ingenious maneuvers as holding on to the mouthpiece with their teeth or by propping the inhaler against the pillow.

Studies of various inhalers have found that patients prefer a mask to a mouthpiece, as it enables them to breathe through either their mouth or their nose (58, 59).

Problems with older handheld vaporizers included the possibility of position changes causing flooding of the system and consequent delivery of high concentrations of anesthetic vapor; the inability to administer supplemental oxygen; and the lack of temperature compensation so that increasing temperature with use resulted in an excessive anesthetic concentration.

Nitrous oxide may be administered by an anesthesiologist, using a conventional anesthetic machine or by the patient herself on demand. Several favorable reports evaluating apparatus designed to deliver a premixed concentration of nitrous oxide and oxygen have appeared in the literature in the United States (60, 61). However, these units have not gained wide acceptance, perhaps because they are unwieldy. In the United Kingdom, a premixed container of 50% nitrous oxide and 50% oxygen, marketed under the name of Entonox, is widely used. It is delivered from a single cylinder fitted with a reducing valve. This connects to a face mask, which operates only when a negative pressure opens the valve. A possible danger of this mixture is that, if the cylinder is allowed to reach $-7°C$, separation of the two gases occurs, allowing pure oxygen and then pure nitrous oxide to be delivered as the cylinder is progressively emptied. This can be avoided by adequate mixing and warming of the cylinder. Recommendations for the use of nitrous oxide-oxygen apparatus in obstetric analgesia, including specifications as to desired limits of accuracy, flow resistance, and safety features, are included in a report by the subcommittee of the Medical Research Council in England (62).

TECHNIQUES OF INHALATION ANALGESIA

Inhalation analgesics are administered either *intermittently* (only during contractions) or *continuously* (during and between uterine contractions). With either technique the anesthesiologist should first instruct the patient in the proper use of the equipment. The anesthesiologist must maintain verbal contact with the patient and provide continuous reassurance and encouragement. Rather than using a fixed concentration of anesthetic, the concentration must be regulated according to the patient's response. If the patient becomes confused, drowsy, excited, or uncooperative, the inspired concentration should be lowered quickly. Otherwise she may lose her laryngeal reflexes, vomit or passively regurgitate, and

Table 11.1
Intermittent Inhalation Analgesia: A Suggested Technique

1. Administer 30 ml of a nonparticulate antacid.
2. Check blood pressure.
3. Start intravenous infusion with indwelling catheter.
4. Apply pulse oximeter.
5. If the contractions are regular, initiate the inhalation analgesic 30 sec before the onset of a contraction.
6. If the contractions are irregular, initiate the inhalation analgesic with the onset of the contraction.
7. Begin with $N_2O:O_2$ 70:30%, enflurane 0.5%, isoflurane 0.4–0.7%, or a combination of nitrous oxide and the volatile agent. Decrease nitrous oxide to 50% after the first few breaths.
8. During the first stage of labor apply the face mask and have the patient take three deep breaths and then take three to four normal breaths.
9. During the second stage of labor, the technique is modified by the patient bearing down forcefully after the third deep breath and maintaining her expulsive effort as long as she is able. After another deep breath, the patient should bear down again. This sequence should be continued until the contraction ends or she becomes drowsy.
10. Maintain verbal contact with the patient and be reassuring. If the patient becomes confused, drowsy, excited, or uncooperative, the inspired concentration should be lowered and 100% oxygen administered.
11. Remove the mask between contractions and instruct the patient to relax in a comfortable position and breathe normally. Administer 100% oxygen via the anesthetic face mask or via a plastic oxygen mask or nasal cannulae between contractions if oxygen saturation decreases.
12. Because this technique does not provide complete analgesia, the obstetrician should infiltrate the perineum with local anesthetic or perform a pudendal block for delivery.

aspirate. Close monitoring of maternal oxygenation using pulse oximetry is recommended.

Intermittent Analgesia (Table 11.1)

There is a time lag between the initiation of inhalation analgesia and the maximum analgesic effect, called the *latency of analgesia*. The latency of analgesia is shortened by a high inspired concentration, increased alveolar ventilation, and low lipid solubility of the agent. Unfortunately, there is only a brief interval between the onset of a uterine contraction and the perception of pain. If possible, the patient or anesthesiologist should time the uterine contractions so that administration of the analgesic agent is started about 30 sec *before* the onset of the contraction. An adequate gas tension then will be achieved in the brain by the time the contraction becomes painful. If this is not possible, the latency of the analgesia

Table 11.2
Continuous Inhalation Analgesia:
A Suggested Technique

1. Administer 30 ml of a nonparticulate antacid.
2. Check blood pressure.
3. Start intravenous infusion with indwelling catheter.
4. Apply pulse oximeter.
5. Initiate inhalation analgesia when the patient becomes uncomfortable during either the late first stage or, more commonly, the second stage of labor.
6. Begin with N_2O 40%, or isoflurane, or enflurane 0.3% or a mixture of N_2O 30% and isoflurane or enflurane 0.2 to 0.3% and oxygen.
7. Use these low concentrations initially and gradually increase them until the maximum concentration is reached at which the patient is cooperative, oriented, and comfortable.
8. With each expulsive effort instruct the patient to take three deep breaths and then bear down.
9. Maintain verbal contact with the patient and be reassuring. If the patient becomes confused, drowsy, excited, or uncooperative or if oxygen saturation decreases, immediately lower the inspired concentration and administer 100% oxygen.
10. The obstetrician should infiltrate the perineum with a local anesthetic or perform a pudendal block for added analgesia.

may be shortened by using a higher concentration for a brief period of time (30 to 60 sec) and by starting the administration at the onset of the contraction. When this is done, careful attention must be paid to the patient's level of consciousness and signs of excitement. If the patient takes three to six deep breaths at the onset of administration, the increased alveolar ventilation will also shorten the latency of analgesia.

The inhalation analgesics may also be self-administered. The technique is the same as when intermittent analgesia is administered by an anesthesiologist. An experienced attendant should instruct the patient early in labor in the proper use of the equipment, should ascertain later that she is bearing down effectively, and most importantly, should monitor any change in the level of consciousness.

Continuous Technique (Table 11.2)

This technique offers the advantage of a more stable and more effective level of analgesia. Although the continuous technique may be used in a labor room during the first stage of labor, it is most commonly used in the delivery room shortly before birth. During the expulsive stage of labor, contractions are usually very frequent and the interval between the onset of a contraction and the perception of pain is only 5 to 10 sec. Because the parturient must push with each contraction, precluding inhalation of an-

esthetic, the intermittent technique is less effective (Fig. 11.5). When using the continuous technique, a low concentration of the inhalation analgesic is administered initially, then the concentration is gradually increased until the maximum concentration is reached at which the patient has achieved an analgetic state and remains oriented and cooperative. The anesthetist must maintain continuous verbal contact with the patient and lower the concentration of the agent if the patient becomes confused, drowsy, or uncooperative. Analgesia is improved if the patient takes two to three deep breaths before each expulsive effort and during crowning of the fetal head. To ensure more effective pain relief during delivery and repair of the episiotomy, inhalation analgesia can be supplemented with a pudendal block or local infiltration of the perineum.

TECHNIQUES OF GENERAL ANESTHESIA

A "standard" obstetric general anesthetic technique has gained enormous popularity because of its maternal safety and relatively low depressant effects on the newborn. This technique, outlined in Table 11.3, is similar to that used for general anesthesia for cesarean section. When uterine relaxation is necessary, isoflurane and halothane are presently the most popular agents. Here again, induction of anesthesia should be effected with oxygen inhalation, thiopental and succinylcholine administration, endotracheal intubation, and then (solely for the purpose of uterine relaxation) administration of oxygen with isoflurane, enflurane, or halothane. Currently, isoflurane is favored by many practitioners because it maintains cardiovascular stability better than do the other agents and is excreted rapidly. Up to 50% nitrous oxide can be added if needed to prevent light anesthesia. Because the patient is paralyzed, great caution must be exercised not to overdose the patient with the volatile agent. Immediately after the intrauterine manipulation and delivery, the volatile agent can be discontinued and an intravenous opioid substituted if necessary; the patient is hyperventilated with nitrous oxide and oxygen or oxygen alone; the uterus is massaged and an intravenous infusion of oxytocin is administered. Excessive uterine bleeding is unusual.

INDIVIDUAL AGENTS

The ideal inhalation agent for use in obstetrics should have excellent analgetic and little hypnotic effects, thus minimizing the risk of aspiration at analgesic concentrations. It also should be nonflammable, nontoxic, excreted wholly by the lungs, and have no effect on uterine contractility. Of course, no single agent exists with all these properties. A num-

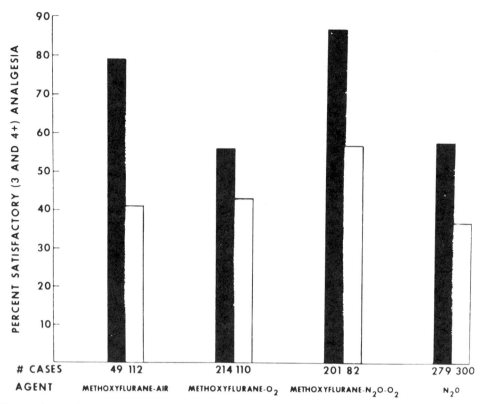

Figure 11.5. Comparison of continuous and intermittent techniques of inhalation analgesia. (Reprinted by permission from Steffenson J: Inhalation analgesia—nitrous oxide, methoxyflurane. In *Obstetrical Anesthesia: Current Concepts and Practice*. SM Shnider, ed. Williams & Wilkins, Baltimore, 1970, p 85.)

ber of agents, which for a variety of reasons are no longer used, exhibited considerable favorable properties for obstetric analgesia. Cyclopropane achieved great popularity in obstetrics because it enabled the rapid induction of anesthesia, caused little uterine relaxation, and (in analgesic concentrations) did not adversely affect the fetus. It was not usually associated with hypotension, perhaps because its administration resulted in a high level of circulating catecholamines. Cyclopropane's flammability and arrhythmogenic potential led to its removal from modern anesthetic practice.

Trichloroethylene and methoxyflurane, both of which are potent and extremely soluble in blood and fat, also were widely used in obstetrics. The constant level of analgesia obtained with continuous inhalation of low concentrations of these agents made them almost ideal for this purpose. Unfortunately, trichloroethylene interacts with soda-lime to form toxic products, and methoxyflurane, because of its biotransformation to inorganic fluoride and oxalic acid, is a potential nephrotoxin (63, 64). Although levels of inorganic fluoride associated with polyuric renal failure (i.e., those greater than 80 μmol/liter) seldom resulted from the use of methoxyflurane during labor

(65–67), individual variations in metabolism make this a potential hazard. Similarly, although neonatal serum inorganic fluoride levels ranged only from 5 to 15 μmol/liter after maternal inhalation of methoxyflurane (65–67), little is known about the renal effects of this ion in the neonate. Trichloroethylene and methoxyflurane are rarely used in the United States. Only those agents used in modern obstetric practice are considered here.

Nitrous Oxide

Various concentrations of nitrous oxide have been administered either by continuous or intermittent inhalation to provide pain relief in labor. A report of a large clinical trial in Great Britain (4) showed little difference in the analgesic effect between intermittent inhalation of 50% and 70% nitrous oxide, except in abnormal labors in which the higher concentration was slightly superior. Approximately 70% of women considered their relief in the first and second stages of labor to be complete or good, and 90% said that use of the agent "helped them." Although both concentrations in this study proved safe for the mother and neonate, 3% of women receiving 70% nitrous oxide lost consciousness, as compared with only 0.4%

Table 11.3
General Anesthesia for Vaginal Delivery:
A Suggested Technique[a]

1. Premedicate the patient with 30 ml of a nonparticulate oral antacid within 30 min of induction.
2. Start intravenous infusion with a large-bore plastic cannula.
3. Apply pulse oximeter, blood pressure cuff and electrocardiograph leads.
4. Preoxygenate the patient for 3 min if possible. Use high flow rates (greater than 6 liters/min).
5. When delivery is imminent and forceps are to be applied, administer thiopental 4 mg/kg and succinylcholine 1.5 mg/kg at the start of uterine contraction. An assistant should apply cricoid pressure until the trachea is sealed by the cuff of the endotracheal tube.
6. Verify correct tracheal placement of tube by identification of CO_2 in expired air (via capnograph or chemical detector).
7. If uterine relaxation is not necessary, administer N_2O 5 liters/min + O_2 5 liters/min. Use muscle relaxant as necessary.
8. If uterine relaxation is necessary, administer isoflurane or halothane with oxygen 99% (or N_2O, 50%) commencing with 1% and increasing concentration up to 3% until desired conditions are obtained. Controlled ventilation with high concentrations of volatile agents, particularly halothane, should be used with extreme caution, with careful and constant monitoring of maternal heart sounds and blood pressure and only if uterine hypertonus is resulting in fetal jeopardy. The volatile agent should be discontinued after delivery of the infant and uterine tone restored with intravenous infusion of oxytocin drip and uterine massage. An IV opioid can be substituted to maintain adequate anesthetic depth during repair of episiotomy.
9. Extubate the patient when she is fully awake.

[a]General anesthesia is not the preferred technique for routine vaginal delivery. Its use should be reserved for situations in which anesthesia is necessary but regional techniques are either contraindicated or inadequate. Some examples are acute fetal distress during the second stage of labor, intrauterine manipulations requiring uterine relaxation, or an uncontrollable patient whose physical activity may damage the newborn during delivery.

of those receiving 50% nitrous oxide. Because there was considerable variability in the mother's response to nitrous oxide, the authors emphasized the need for careful supervision.

Because nitrous oxide has a very low blood solubility, concentrations in the brain rise and fall rapidly. Theoretic calculations of the kinetics of nitrous oxide distribution during intermittent administration for labor suggest that the optimal method of delivery is achieved by administration of a 50% mixture for 50 sec *before* the start of each contraction, continuing for a period equal to half the time between contractions (68). In this way, the highest nitrous oxide brain levels will coincide with the maximum intensity of pain, but the patient will be awake between contractions. Intermittent inhalation of 50% nitrous oxide is equivalent to breathing a 26.8% concentration of nitrous oxide continuously until equilibrium occurs (69). If nitrous oxide is inhaled continuously, a mean concentration of 41.2% is necessary to provide adequate analgesia while maintaining consciousness (70). Because the onset of contractions is often unpredictable, intermittent administration seldom is begun before the uterine contraction starts and maximum analgesic effectiveness is not achieved. Consequently, continuous analgesia is more reliable.

Nitrous oxide administered in analgesic concentrations appears to cause minimal maternal cardiovascular or respiratory depression and does not affect uterine contractility. The potential for hypoxemia during nitrous oxide analgesia, particularly when administered following opioids, has been discussed earlier in this chapter. Occasionally, restlessness may occur during nitrous oxide administration, resulting in an uncooperative patient. This complication was less common with methoxyflurane or trichloroethylene (71) and may be less frequent with isoflurane or enflurane. Although accepted as safe for the fetus when used for obstetric analgesia, nitrous oxide has been implicated as a contributing factor in fetal deterioration when anesthesia was prolonged during cesarean section (37). In studies of pregnant ewes, Palahniuk and Cumming (72) found a significant decrease in fetal pH after only a brief period of anesthesia when a thiopental induction was followed by 70% nitrous oxide. There was a fall in fetal PaO_2 after induction of anesthesia, and uterine blood flow was reduced by 18 to 30%. Although the fetus seemed to be most susceptible to the changes following induction of anesthesia, further deterioration occurred and was thought to be caused by reduced uterine perfusion related to light anesthesia and increased endogenous maternal catecholamines. Indeed, Shnider et al. showed that noxious stimulation of a pregnant ewe during nitrous oxide-oxygen anesthesia was associated with an increase in maternal blood pressure, a decrease in uterine blood flow, and an increase in plasma norepinephrine of 71% from the awake control state (Fig. 11.6) (73). In contrast, noxious stimulation during nitrous oxide-oxygen anesthesia that was supplemented with either 0.5% halothane or 1% enflurane did not increase plasma catecholamines or adversely affect uterine blood flow. In fact, uterine blood flow rose 20% from control levels during nitrous oxide-oxygen halothane anesthesia. High con-

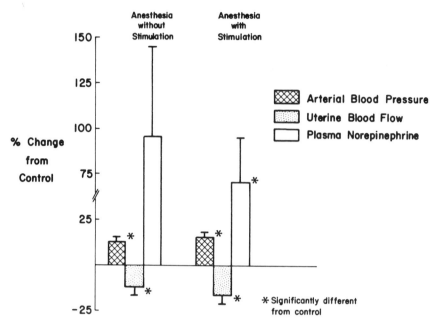

Figure 11.6. Effects of nitrous oxide (50%) anesthesia, with and without noxious stimulation, on maternal plasma norepinephrine, blood pressure, and uterine blood flow in the pregnant ewe. (Reprinted by permission from Shnider SM, Wright RG, Levinson G, Roizen MF, Rolbin SH, Biehl D, Johnson J, Jones M: Plasma norepinephrine and uterine blood flow changes during endotracheal intubation and general anesthesia in the pregnant ewe. In *Abstracts of Scientific Papers*, Annual Meeting, American Society of Anesthesiologists, Chicago, 1978, p 115.)

centrations of nitrous oxide also may be deleterious to the fetus by limiting the availability of oxygen. Multiple reports now have confirmed the benefit to the fetus of high maternal oxygen concentrations (40, 41, 74).

Diffusion hypoxia in the neonate after maternal administration of nitrous oxide is a theoretic cause of neonatal depression if a high concentration of the agent is administered over a prolonged period. Although investigators have been unable to demonstrate this when alveolar nitrous oxide levels have been measured in the newborn (75, 76), it seems prudent to administer oxygen to the newborn until it is clear that hypoxemia is absent.

Halothane

The use of halothane in obstetric anesthesia has been controversial in the past as a result of fears that it would cause excessive myometrial depression. Although the uterine relaxant effect of this agent, even at low concentrations, is well established, its use in concentrations of less than 0.8% for cesarean section (74) or vaginal delivery (77) has not been associated with increased blood loss. When used for cesarean section, it has proved superior to 70% nitrous oxide, particularly when the effects on the fetus are considered (74). This probably results from the ability to use a higher percentage of inspired oxygen and from improved uterine blood flow caused by the in-

hibition of endogenous catecholamine secretion by halothane (73). However, 0.5% halothane is considered preferable to 0.8% because the incidence of hypotension with the higher concentration is unacceptable (74). Halothane is not used to provide analgesia during labor, because the patient is likely to become unconscious before satisfactory analgesic levels have been obtained. There are other specific indications for its use, such as when rapid, profound uterine relaxation is needed. However, it is doubtful whether halothane is a better myometrial relaxant than the other inhalation agents. Furthermore, its slower elimination and potential for causing cardiac arrhythmias may prove relatively disadvantageous in this circumstance.

Enflurane

Several reports detail the use of enflurane in obstetric practice. Coleman and Downing administered low doses to supplement anesthesia with 50% nitrous oxide and a muscle relaxant for cesarean section (78). No adverse effects were noted in the neonate, nor was blood loss excessive. When used for vaginal delivery some investigators found that enflurane, like halothane, produced little analgesic effect unless administered in concentrations that resulted in unconsciousness (79, 80). In contrast, Abboud et al. reported that enflurane (0.25 to 1.25%) was an effective analgesic for delivery (43). In a study comparing continuous analgesia with either nitrous oxide or enflurane, obstetricians rated enflurane superior to nitrous oxide. In a similar study McGuinness and Rosen also found lower pain scores with 1% enflurane, as compared to 50% nitrous oxide, although drowsiness was greater with enflurane (81). Neonatal condition appears unaffected by brief maternal inhalation of low concentrations of enflurane (46). Like halothane, enflurane causes a dose-related depression of uterine contractility, and in high doses (e.g., 3%), it may produce increased postpartum uterine blood loss (52). Thus enflurane and halothane share many characteristics, and indications for their use in obstetric anesthesia are similar. An advantage of enflurane, as compared to halothane, is that its effects are more rapidly reversible because of its lower blood solubility. Enflurane is metabolized to inorganic fluoride, although to a much lesser extent than is methoxyflurane. Despite this, its use in patients with renal impairment should be avoided and other agents chosen in preference. In morbidly obese patients increased biotransformation of enflurane occurs (82) and has resulted in potentially nephrotoxic inorganic fluoride levels after surgical anesthesia (83, 84). Its use, therefore, should be avoided in such individuals, as well as in patients receiving drugs, such as isoniazid, which are known to induce its metabolism.

Isoflurane

This agent has gained wide acceptance in the United States because of its favorable properties of low blood solubility, low arrhythmogenic potential, apparent freedom from hepatic and renal toxicity, and maintenance of cardiovascular stability. At equipotent concentrations, its effect on uterine contractility is similar to that of halothane and enflurane (50). McLeod and co-workers administered 0.75% isoflurane in oxygen over the course of five contractions during the first stage of labor, comparing it to 50% nitrous oxide (Entonox) with each patient acting as her own control (85). Although linear analog pain scores were lower with isoflurane (Fig. 11.7), more drowsiness occurred with this agent. In a study comparing 0.2 to 0.7% isoflurane with 30 to 60% nitrous oxide administered during the second stage of labor, Abboud et al. reported similar analgesia with both agents (2). Using average concentrations of 0.4% isoflurane and 33% nitrous oxide, analgesia was rated as satisfactory by more than 83% of patients, obstetricians, and anesthesiologists. Maternal acceptance of isoflurane was high and amnesia was rare. Although blood loss was not measured precisely, it was estimated to be normal and similar in both groups. Neonatal outcome, assessed by Apgar scores, cord blood gases, and neuro-

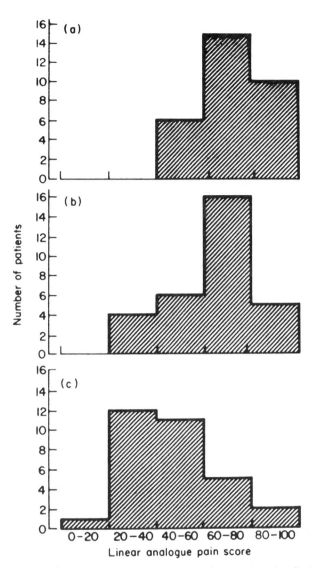

Figure 11.7. Linear analogue pain scores during the first stage of labor during (a) control period, (b) inhalation of 50% nitrous oxide, or (c) inhalation of 0.75% isoflurane in oxygen. Pain scores were significantly lower with isoflurane than with nitrous oxide ($p < 0.001$). (Reprinted with permission from McLeod DD, Ramayya GP, and Tunstall ME: Self-administered isoflurane in labour. Anaesthesia 40:424–426, 1985.)

behavioral examinations, was equally good in both groups. Renal toxicity was absent, as evidenced by unchanged maternal serum and urine inorganic fluoride levels and low neonatal urinary fluoride levels. The authors concluded that subanesthetic concentrations of isoflurane in oxygen provide safe and effective analgesia for normal vaginal delivery and have an advantage over nitrous oxide of permitting delivery of a high inspired oxygen concentration.

Isoflurane also appears appropriate for use in general anesthesia performed for operative vaginal or cesarean delivery. Warren et al. studied the maternal and neonatal effects of 50% oxygen and 50% nitrous oxide alone and combined with 0.5% halothane, 1.0% enflurane, or 0.75% isoflurane in healthy women undergoing general anesthesia for elective cesarean section (45). Endotracheal intubation was performed following thiopental and succinylcholine for induction. Two of twelve (17%) patients given nitrous oxide-oxygen alone had recall; none who received a potent inhalation agent had any recall. Blood loss was similar in all four groups. There were no significant differences among the groups in the incidence of Apgar scores of less than 7 at 1 and 5 min, in maternal and fetal blood gas tensions, in acid-base balances, in lactate values, and in early neonatal neurobehavioral scores at 2 to 4 hr. Warren et al. concluded that analgesic concentrations of halothane, enflurane, or isoflurane can be added safely to nitrous oxide-oxygen (50:50) to prevent maternal awareness during general anesthesia for cesarean delivery, while maintaining normal maternal and neonatal conditions. More recently, Ghaly et al. found 0.75% isoflurane preferable to 0.5% halothane in this circumstance because of the more rapid recovery from anesthesia, the decreased need for muscle relaxant, and the surgeon's assessment that uterine relaxation and bleeding were less with isoflurane (86). Neonatal condition was similar with both agents.

New Agents

Although isoflurane appears to have some advantages over the other volatile anesthetic agents, it is recommended for use in low concentrations and for relatively brief periods only as are the other agents. The ideal inhalation agent with excellent analgesic properties, low blood and gas solubility, freedom from toxicity, and lack of myometrial and newborn depressant effects is yet to be discovered. Two new agents, sevoflurane and desflurane, are undergoing investigation for possible introduction into clinical practice. Sevoflurane, an agent with a low blood-gas coefficient (0.6), promises rapid recovery from anesthesia but appears to cause myometrial depression similar to that of the other volatile agents when administered for cesarean section (87). Preliminary results of studies in the pregnant sheep model suggest that sevoflurane preserves maternal hemodynamic stability, while causing greater increases in uterine blood flow than does isoflurane (88). The major problem with this agent is that, when administered with soda-lime, a number of potentially toxic metabolites are formed (89). Therefore sevoflurane should not be administered in a closed or semiclosed anesthetic circuit, a problem which might hinder its usefulness in the United States. Sevoflurane also undergoes bio-

transformation resulting in inorganic fluoride levels comparable with those associated with enflurane administration.

Desflurane also has a low blood-gas solubility coefficient (0.4) but, in contrast to sevoflurane, is extremely stable and does not interact with soda-lime. It is metabolized to a significantly lesser degree than are other volatile anesthetics and thus has a minimal potential for causing organ toxicity. The disadvantage with desflurane is that its vapor pressure is close to 1 atm at room temperature; thus it requires a special vaporizer to permit its administration.

The properties of sevoflurane and desflurane and their possible role in anesthetic practice are discussed in an excellent review by Jones (90). No judgment can be made on their potential usefulness in obstetric practice until more extensive studies have been performed, both in pregnant and nonpregnant patients.

References

1. Gibbs CP, Krischer J, Peckham BM, Sharp H, Kirschbaum TH: Obstetric anesthesia: A national survey. Anesthesiology 65:298–306, 1986.
2. Abboud TK, Gangolly J, Mosaad P, Crowell D: Isoflurane in obstetrics. Anesth Analg 68:388–391, 1989.
3. Akamatsu TJ, Bonica JJ, Rehmet R, Eng M, Ueland K: Experiences with the use of ketamine for parturition. I. Primary anesthetic for vaginal delivery. Anesth Analg 53:284–287, 1974.
4. Committee on Nitrous Oxide Analgesia in Midwifery, Sir Dugald Baird, Chairman. Clinical trials of different concentrations of oxygen and nitrous oxide for obstetric analgesia. Br Med J 1:709–713, 1970.
5. Peng ATC, Gorman RS, Shulman SM, Demarchis E, Nyunt KM, Blancato L: Intravenous nitroglycerin for uterine relaxation in patients with retained placenta. Anesthesiology 71:172–173, 1989.
6. De Simone CA, Norris MC, Leighton BL: Intravenous nitroglycerin aids manual extraction of a retained placenta. Anesthesiology 73:787, 1990.
7. Palahniuk RJ, Shnider SM, Eger EI II: Pregnancy decreases the requirement for inhaled anesthetic agents. Anesthesiology 41:82–83, 1974.
8. Bonica JJ: Anesthetic deaths. In *Principles and Practice of Obstetric Analgesia and Anesthesia*. FA Davis, Philadelphia, 1972, pp 751–760.
9. Merrill RB, Hingson RA: Study of incidence of maternal mortality from aspiration of vomitus during anesthesia occurring in major obstetrical hospitals in the United States. Anesth Analg 30:121–135, 1951.
10. Bond VK, Ragan WD: Anesthetic-related mortality in Indiana. J IN State Med Assoc 72:266–267, 1979.
11. Kaunitz AM, Hughes JM, Grimes DA, Smith JC, Rochat RW, Kafrissen ME: Causes of maternal mortality in the United States. Obstet Gynecol 65:605–612, 1985.
12. Atrash HK, Koonin LM, Lawson HW, Franks AL, Smith JC: Maternal mortality in the United States, 1979–1986. Obstet Gynecol 76:1055–1060, 1990.
13. Chadwick HS, Posner K, Caplan RA, Ward RJ, Cheney FW: A comparison of obstetric and nonobstetric anesthesia malpractice claims. Anesthesiology 74:242–249, 1991.
14. Tomkins J, Turnbull A, Robson G, Dawson I, Cloake E, Adelstein AM, Ashley J: *Report on Confidential Enquiries into Maternal Deaths in England and Wales, 1976–1978*. Depart-

ment of Health and Social Security, Her Majesty's Stationery Office, London, 1982, No 26.

15. Turnbull A, Tindall VR, Beard RW, Robson G, Dawson IMP, Cloake EP, Ashley JSA, Botting B: Report on Confidential Enquiries into Maternal Deaths in England and Wales, 1982–1984. Department of Health and Social Security, Her Majesty's Stationery Office, London, 1989, No 34.

16. Roberts RB, Shirley MA: Reducing the risk of acid aspiration during cesarean section. Anesth Analg 53:859–868, 1974.

17. Smiler BG, Goldberger R, Sivak BJ, Brown EM: Routine endotracheal intubation in obstetrics. Am J Obstet Gynecol 103:947–949, 1969.

18. Davies JM, Hogg M, Rosen M: Maternal arterial oxygen tension during intermittent inhalation analgesia. Br J Anaesth 47:370–377, 1975.

19. Reed PN, Colquhoun AD, Hanning CD: Maternal oxygenation during normal labour. Br J Anaesth 62:316–318, 1989.

20. Wilkins CJ, Reed PN, Aitkenhead AR: Hypoxaemia after inhalation of 50% nitrous oxide and oxygen. Br J Anaesth 63:346–347, 1989.

21. Northwood D, Sapsford DJ, Jones JG, Griffiths D, Wilkins: Nitrous oxide sedation causes post-hyperventilation apnoea. Br J Anaesth 67:7–12, 1991.

22. Zelcer J, Owers H, Paull JD: A controlled oximetric evaluation of inhalational, opioid and epidural analgesia in labour. Anaesth Intensive Care 17:418–421, 1989.

23. Moya F: Volatile inhalation agents and muscle relaxants in obstetrics. Acta Anesth Scand 25(suppl):368–375, 1966.

24. Palahniuk RJ, Shnider SM: Maternal and fetal cardiovascular and acid-base changes during halothane and isoflurane anesthesia in the pregnant ewe. Anesthesiology 41:462–472, 1974.

25. Cosmi EV, Marx GF: The effect of anesthesia on the acid-base status of the fetus. Anesthesiology 30:238–242, 1969.

26. Gregory GA, Wade JG, Biehl DR, Ong BY, Sitar DS: Fetal anesthetic requirement (MAC) for halothane. Anesth Analg 62:9–14, 1983.

27. Bachman CR, Biehl DR, Sitar D, Cumming M, Pucci W: Isoflurane potency and cardiovascular effects during short exposures in the foetal lamb. Can Anaesth Soc J 33:41–47, 1986.

28. LeDez KM, Lerman J: The minimum alveolar concentration (MAC) of isoflurane in preterm neonates. Anesthesiology 67:301–307, 1987.

29. Gibbs CP, Munson ES, Tham MK: Anesthetic solubility coefficients for maternal and fetal blood. Anesthesiology 43:100–103, 1975.

30. Biehl DR, Tweed WA, Cote J, Wade JG, Sitar D: Effect of halothane on cardiac output and regional flow in the fetal lamb in utero. Anesth Analg 62:489–492, 1983.

31. Biehl DR, Yarnell R, Wade JG, Sitar D: The uptake of isoflurane by the foetal lamb in utero: Effect on regional blood flow. Can Anaesth Soc J 30:581–586, 1983.

32. Palahniuk RJ, Doig GA, Johnson GN, Pash MP: Maternal halothane anesthesia reduces cerebral blood flow in the acidotic sheep fetus. Anesth Analg 59:35–39, 1980.

33. Cheek DBC, Hughes SC, Dailey PA, Field DR, Pytka S, Rosen MA, Parer JT, Shnider SM: Effect of halothane on regional cerebral blood flow and cerebral metabolic oxygen consumption in the fetal lamb in utero. Anesthesiology 67:361–366, 1987.

34. Yarnell R, Biehl DR, Tweed WA, Gregory GA, Sitar D: The effect of halothane anaesthesia on the asphyxiated foetal lamb in utero. Can Anaesth Soc J 30:474–479, 1983.

35. Baker BW, Hughes SC, Shnider SM, Field DR, Rosen MA: Maternal anesthesia and the stressed fetus: Effects of isoflurane on the asphyxiated fetal lamb. Anesthesiology 72:65–70, 1990.

36. Finster M, Poppers PJ: Safety of thiopental used for induction of general anesthesia in elective cesarean section. Anesthesiology 29:190–191, 1968.

37. Stenger VG, Blechner JN, Prystowsky H: A study of prolongation of obstetric anesthesia. Am J Obstet Gynecol 103:901–907, 1969.

38. Marx GF, Joshi CW, Orkin LR: Placental transmission of nitrous oxide. Anesthesiology 32:429–432, 1970.

39. Hay DM: Nitrous oxide transfer across the placenta and condition of the newborn at delivery. Br J Obstet Gynaecol 85:299–302, 1978.

40. Marx GF, Mateo CV: Effects of different oxygen concentrations during general anaesthesia for elective caesarean section. Can Anaesth Soc J 18:587–593, 1971.

41. Piggott SE, Bogod G, Rosen M, Rees AD, Harmer M: Isoflurane with either 100% oxygen or 50% nitrous oxide in oxygen for caesarean section. Br J Anaesth 65:325–329, 1990.

42. Shnider SM, Steffenson JL, Margolis AJ: Methoxyflurane analgesia in obstetrics. Obstet Gynecol 33:594–595, 1969.

43. Abboud TK, Shnider SM, Wright RG, Rolbin SH, Craft JB, Henriksen EH, Johnson J, Jones MJ, Hughes SC, Levinson G: Enflurane analgesia in obstetrics. Anesthesiology 60:133–137, 1981.

44. Clark RB, Cooper JO, Brown WE, Greifenstein FE: The effect of methoxyflurane on the foetus. Br J Anaesth 42:286–294, 1970.

45. Warren TW, Datta S, Ostheimer GW, Naulty JS, Weiss JB, Morrison JA: Comparison of the maternal and neonatal effects of halothane, enflurane and isoflurane for cesarean delivery. Anesth Analg 62:516–520, 1983.

46. Stefani SJ, Hughes SC, Shnider SM, Abboud TK, Henriksen EH, Williams V, Johnson J: Neonatal neurobehavioral effects of inhalation analgesia for vaginal delivery. Anesthesiology 56:351–355, 1982.

47. Munson ES: Uterine activity and anesthesia. In Obstetrical Anesthesia: Current Concepts and Practice. SM Shnider, ed. Williams & Wilkins, Baltimore, 1969, pp 29–36.

48. Naftalin NJ, Phear WPC, Goldberg AH: Halothane and isometric contractions of isolated pregnant rat myometrium. Anesthesiology 42:458–463, 1975.

49. Naftalin NJ, McKay DM, Phear WPC, Goldberg AH: The effects of halothane on pregnant and nonpregnant human myometrium. Anesthesiology 46:15–19, 1977.

50. Munson ES, Embro WJ: Enflurane, isoflurane and halothane and isolated human uterine muscle. Anesthesiology 46:11–14, 1977.

51. Ishikawa M, Shimizu T, Matsuda S: The effects of obstetric anesthetic agents on the uterine contractility with special reference to intrauterine pressure. Acta Obstet Gynaecol 20:67–71, 1973.

52. Marx GF, Kim YO, Lin CC, Halevy S, Schulman H: Postpartum uterine pressures under halothane or enflurane anesthesia. Obstet Gynecol 51:695–698, 1978.

53. Munson ES, Maier WR, Caton D: Effects of halothane cyclopropane and nitrous oxide on isolated human uterine muscle. J Obstet Gynaecol Br Commonw 76:27–33, 1969.

54. Abadir AR, Humayun SG, Calvello D, Gintautas J: Effects of isoflurane and oxytocin on gravid human uterus in vitro. Anesth Analg 66:S1, 1987.

55. Ad Hoc Committee: The effect of trace anesthetics on the health of operating room personnel: A national study. Anesthesiology 41:321–340, 1974.

56. Buring JE, Hennekens CH, Mayrent SL, Rosner B, Greenberg ER, Colton T: Health experience of operating room personnel. Anesthesiology 62:325–330, 1985.

57. Munley AJ, Railton R, Gray WM, Carter KB: Exposure of midwives to nitrous oxide in four hospitals. Br Med J 293:1063–1064, 1986.

58. Marx GF, Chen LK, Tabora JA: Experiences with a disposable inhaler for methoxyflurane analgesia during labour. Clinical and biochemical results. Can Anaesth Soc J 16:66–71, 1969.

59. Enrile LL, Roux JF, Wilson R, Lebherz TB: Methoxyflurane (Penthrane) inhalation in labor. Obstet Gynecol 41:860–864, 1973.

60. Hanisch EC, Sankawa H, Gauert WB, Overman JW: Clinical and mechanical evaluation of an A.E. gas machine for obstetric analgesia and anesthesia. Anesth Analg 50:190–194, 1971.

61. Wilson RD, Priano LL, Allen CR, Phillips MT, Bryant TF:

Demand analgesia and anesthesia in obstetrics. South Med J 65:556–562, 1972.

62. Cole PV, Crawford JS, Doughty AG, Epstein HG, Hill ID, Rollason WN, Tunstall ME: Specifications and recommendations for nitrous oxide/oxygen apparatus to be used in obstetric analgesia. Anaesthesia 25:317–327, 1970.

63. Mazze RI, Trudell JR, Cousins MJ: Methoxyflurane metabolism and renal dysfunction: Clinical correlation in man. Anesthesiology 35:247–252, 1971.

64. Cousins MJ, Mazze RI: Methoxyflurane nephrotoxicity: A study of dose response in man. JAMA 225:1611–1616, 1973.

65. Creasser CW, Stoelting RK, Krishna G, Peterson C: Methoxyflurane metabolism and renal function after methoxyflurane analgesia during labor and delivery. Anesthesiology 41:62–66, 1974.

66. Young SR, Stoelting RK, Bond VK, Peterson C: Methoxyflurane biotransformation and renal function following methoxyflurane administration for vaginal delivery or cesarean section. Anesth Analg 55:415–419, 1976.

67. Clark RB, Beard AG, Thompson DS, Barclay DL: Maternal and neonatal plasma inorganic fluoride levels after methoxyflurane analgesia for labor and delivery. Anesthesiology 45:88–91, 1976.

68. Waud BE, Waud DR: Calculated kinetics of distribution of nitrous oxide and methoxyflurane during intermittent administration in obstetrics. Anesthesiology 32:306–316, 1970.

69. Latto IP, Molloy MJ, Rosen M: Arterial concentrations of nitrous oxide during intermittent patinet-controlled inhalation of 50% nitrous oxide in oxygen (Entonox) during the first stage of labour. Br J Anaesth 45:1029–1034, 1973.

70. Jones PL, Rosen M, Mushin WW, Jones EV: Methoxyflurane and nitrous oxide as obstetric analgesics. I. A comparison by continuous administration. Br Med J 3:255–259, 1969.

71. Rosen M, Mushin WW, Jones PL, Jones EV: Field trial of methoxyflurane, nitrous oxide, and trichloroethylene as obstetric analgesia. Br Med J 3:263–267, 1969.

72. Palahniuk RJ, Cumming M: Foetal deterioration following thipentone-nitrous oxide anaesthesiain the pregnant ewe. Can Anaesth Soc J 24:361–370, 1977.

73. Shnider SM, Wright RG, Levinson G, Roizen MF, Wallis KL, Rolbin SH, Craft JB: Uterine blood flow and plasma norepinephrine changes during maternal stress in the pregnant ewe. Anesthesiology 50:524–527, 1979.

74. Moir DD: Anaesthesia for caesarean section: An evaluation of a method using low concentrations of halothane and 50 percent of oxygen. Br J Anaesth 42:136–142, 1970.

75. Reid DHS: Diffusion anoxia at birth. Lancet 1:757–758, 1958.

76. Mankowitz E, Brock-Utne JG, Downing JW: Nitrous oxide elimination by the newborn. Anaesthesia 36:1014–1016, 1981.

77. Stallabras P: Halothane and blood loss at delivery. Acta Anaesth Scand 25(suppl):376, 1966.

78. Coleman AJ, Downing JW: Enflurane anesthesia for cesarean section. Anesthesiology 43:354–357, 1975.

79. Westmoreland RT, Evans JA, Chastain GM: Obstetric use of enflurane (Ethrane). South Med J 67:527–530, 1974.

80. Devoghel JC: Enflurane (Ethrane) in obstetrics. Acta Anaesthesiol Belg 2:283–288, 1974.

81. McGuinness C, Rosen M: Enflurane as an analgesic in labour. Anaesthesia 39:24–26, 1984.

82. Strube PJ, Hulands GH, Halsey MJ: Serum fluoride levels in morbidly obese patients: enflurane compared with isoflurane anesthesia. Anaesthesia 42:685–689, 1987.

83. Mazze RI, Calverly RK, Smith NT: Inorganic fluoride nephrotoxicity: prolonged enflurane and halothane anesthesia in volunteers. Anesthesiology 46:265–271, 1977.

84. Maduska AL: Serum inorganic fluoride levels in patients receiving enflurane anesthesia. Anesth Analg 53:351–353, 1974.

85. McLeod DD, Ramayya GP, Tunstall ME: Self-administered isoflurane in labour. Anaesthesia 40:424–426, 1985.

86. Ghaly RG, Flynn RJ, Moore J: Isoflurane as an alternative to halothane for caesarean section. Anaesthesia 43:5–7, 1988.

87. Asada A, Fujimori M, Tomada S, Hikada A: Sevoflurane anesthesia for elective cesarean section. J Anesth 1:66–72, 1990.

88. Stein D, Masaoka T, Wlody D, Santos A, Pederson H, Morishima HO, Finster M: The effects of sevoflurane on uterine blood flow and fetal well being in sheep. In Abstracts of Scientific Papers, Society for Obstetric Anesthesia and Perinatology, Boston, 1991.

89. Strum DP, Johnson BH, Eger EI II: Stability of sevoflurane in soda lime. Anesthesiology 67:779–781, 1987.

90. Jones RM: Desflurane and sevoflurane: Inhalation anaesthetics for this decade? Br J Anaesth 65:527–536, 1990.

OBSTETRIC COMPLICATIONS

CHAPTER 12

Anesthesia for Cesarean Section

Sol M. Shnider, M.D.
Gershon Levinson, M.D.

Delivery of a baby by cesarean section has become increasingly common. In the past, 4 to 6% of deliveries were via the abdominal route. The most common indications were cephalopelvic disproportion, uterine dystocia, hemorrhage, and acute fetal distress. Currently cesarean section rates of 25% are common; in high-risk centers with disproportionately increased incidences of preeclampsia-eclampsia, diabetes, Rh isoimmunization, prematurity, and other high-risk problems the rates are even higher. Despite wide differences in cesarean section rates between different countries (Fig. 12.1) (1), the annual rate of increase for all countries appears to be similar (Fig. 12.2) (2).

A number of factors account for the increased section rate. It has become commonly accepted that serious trauma to the baby can be eliminated by avoiding potentially difficult midforceps or vaginal breech deliveries and performing a cesarean section instead. The widespread use of electronic and biochemical fetal monitoring prior to and during labor (see Chapters 36 and 37) has made it easier to identify a fetus in jeopardy and promptly deliver the baby by the abdominal route. The clinical impression that cesarean section is less traumatic for the tiny fetus and some cases of multiple gestations, and concerns over potential lawsuits in cases of poor neonatal outcome, have also encouraged obstetricians to perform cesarean sections with less positive indications than in the past.

Although several reports indicate that maternal mortality is higher with cesarean birth versus vaginal delivery, it is still a very rare occurrence. Reported rates are between 0 and 105 cases per 100,000 operations (Table 12.1) (3–6). In comparison, the mortality from automobile accidents in women of childbearing age is approximately 20 per 100,000 women. Despite the marked increase in cesarean births, there has been a continuing decline in overall maternal mortality (Fig. 12.3). Similarly, perinatal mortality has also continued to decline, despite the rising ce-

sarean birth rate (Fig. 12.4). Thus, in borderline cases, obstetricians often opt for the cesarean delivery. Indications for cesarean section are listed in Table 12.2.

CHOICE OF ANESTHESIA

The choice of anesthesia for cesarean section depends on the reason for the operation, the degree of urgency, the desires of the patient, and the judgment of the anesthesiologist. There is no one ideal method of anesthesia for cesarean section; the advantages and disadvantages of spinal, epidural, and general anesthesia are discussed in this chapter and suggested methods for these techniques are outlined. The anesthesiologist must choose the method that he or she believes (a) is safest and most comfortable for the mother; (b) is least depressant to the newborn; and (c) provides the optimal working conditions for the obstetrician.

Surveys indicate that conduction anesthesia is the most commonly used anesthetic for cesarean section (Table 12.3) (4, 5). Spinal anesthesia appears to be the preferred technique nationwide. However, in residency training programs, spinal anesthesia is less popular, and this preference for epidural over spinal anesthesia has been reflected in the increasing popularity of epidural anesthesia nationwide. In part, the increased usage of epidural anesthesia for cesarean section reflects the fact that many of the patients already had functioning epidural anesthetics in place for labor. The most recent survey by the American College of Obstetricians and Gynecologists and American Society of Anesthesiologists has shown that 21% of all cesarean sections are performed under epidural anesthesia. The experience of two major obstetric anesthesia teaching centers has shown even higher rates (Fig. 12.5 and Table 12.4). At both of these institutions during the last 10 years, more than 50% of all cesarean deliveries were done under epidural anesthesia. In contrast, in the 1970s only 3 to 10% were performed using this technique.

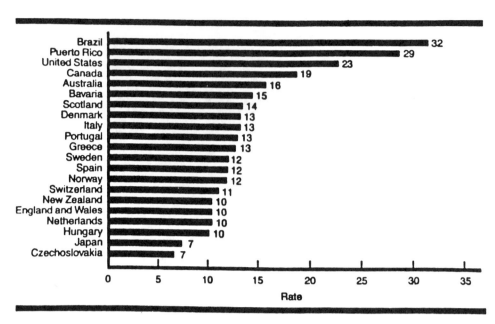

Figure 12.1. Cesarean section rates per 100 hospital deliveries in selected countries for 1985 or most recent year for which data were available (1981 through 1986 for Brazil; 1984 and 1985 for Puerto Rico and Canada; 1982 for Italy; 1987 for Portugal; 1983 for Greece; 1983 through 1986 for Switzerland; and 1986 for Czechoslovakia). There was incomplete coverage of cesarean section rates for Australia, Bavaria, Portugal, Spain, and Switzerland. (Reprinted by permission from Notzon FC: International differences in the use of obstetric interventions. JAMA 263:3286-3291, 1990.)

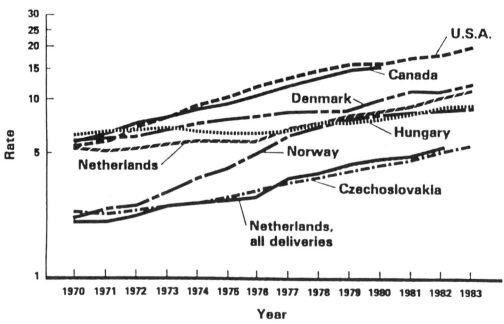

Figure 12.2. Rates of cesarean sections. (Reprinted by permission from Notzon FC, Placek PJ, Taffel SM: Comparisons of national cesarean section rates. N Engl J Med 316:386–389, 1987.)

Table 12.1
Maternal Mortality for Cesarean Section

Population	Years	Number of Cesarean Sections	Rate (Per 100,000 C-Sections)
Rhode Island (3)	1965–76	12,941	69.5
Georgia	1975–76	15,188	105.3
Survey of Hospitals by Commission on Professional and Hospital Activities (5)	1970, 1974, 1978	350,892	60.7
Boston Women's Hospital (6)	1968–78	10,231	0.0

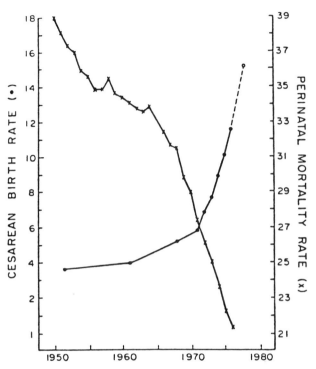

Figure 12.4. Cesarean birth rates and perinatal mortality in the United States from 1950 to 1976. The cesarean birth rate is per 100 deliveries, and the perinatal mortality is per 1000 deliveries. (Reprinted by permission from Bottoms SF, Rosen MG, Sokol RJ: Current concepts—The increase in the cesarean birth rate. N Engl J Med 302:559–563, 1980.)

Table 12.2
Common Indications for Cesarean Section

Previous section
Cephalopelvic disproportion
Failure to progress
Failure of induction
Malpresentation
Breech presentation
Failed forceps delivery
Hemorrhage
Placenta previa
Toxemia
Chorioamnionitis
Herpes genitalia
Fetal distress
Chronic uteroplacental insufficiency
Rh isoimmunization
Prolapsed cord
Hypertonic uterus

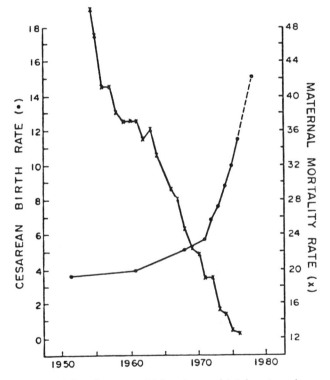

Figure 12.3. Cesarean birth rates and total maternal mortality in the United States from 1950 to 1976. The cesarean birth rate is per 100 deliveries, and the maternal mortality is per 100,000 deliveries. (Reprinted by permission from Bottoms SF, Rosen MG, Sokol RJ: Current concepts—The increase in the cesarean birth rate. N Engl J Med 302:559–563, 1980.)

Table 12.3
Cesarean Sections Classified by Type of Anesthesia Used

Type of Anesthesia	ACOG 1970[a] (%)	CPHA 1974[b] (%)	Obstetric Anesthesia Centers[c]	ACOG/ASA 1981[d] (%)
General anesthesia	32	55	43	41
Regional anesthesia				
Spinal	53	35	24	35
Epidural	3	4	32	21
TOTAL	56	39	56	56
Local	1	0	0	0
Combination	10	6	0	0

[a] Data from American College of Obstetricians and Gynecologists: *A Report of the Committee on Maternal Health: National Study of Maternity Care. Survey of Obstetric Practice and Associated Services in the Hospitals in the United States.* American College of Obstetricians and Gynecologists, Chicago, 1970.
[b] Data from Lowe JA, Klassen DF, Loop RJ: Commission on Professional and Hospital Activities. PAS Reporter 14:29, 1976.
[c] Data from Hicks JS, Levinson G, Shnider SM: Obstetric anesthesia training centers in the U.S.A.—1975. Anesth Analg 55:839–845, 1976.
[d] Data from Gibbs CP, Krischer J, Peckham BM, Sharp H, Kirschbaum TH: Obstetric anesthesia: A national survey. Anesthesiology 65:298–306, 1986.

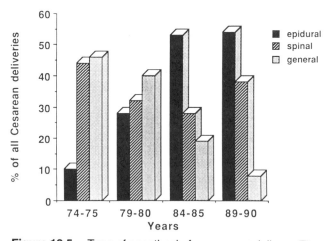

Figure 12.5. Type of anesthesia for cesarean delivery: The Brigham and Women's Hospital experience. Note the decreased use of general and increased used of epidural anesthesia. The popularity of spinal anesthesia gradually decreased, but recently its usage has been increasing. (Modified from Ostheimer GW: *Manual of Obstetric Anesthesia*, 2nd ed. GW Ostheimer, ed. Churchill Livingstone, London, 1992.)

Table 12.4
Type of Anesthesia Used for Cesarean Section at UCSF[a]

Year	Percentage of Total			Total Number of Cases
	Epidural (%)	Spinal (%)	General (%)	
1985	83	1	16	363
1986	84	2	14	351
1987	84	1	15	383
1988	86	1	13	350
1989	82	4	14	353
1990	85	14	11	405
1991	75	17	8	411

[a] During the 6-year period, the use of general anesthesia decreased and the use of spinal anesthesia dramatically increased.

REGIONAL ANESTHESIA

Epidural or spinal anesthesia for cesarean section allows the mother to be awake, minimizes or completely avoids the problems of maternal aspiration, and avoids neonatal drug depression from general anesthetics.

Choice of Regional Technique

A subarachnoid block is easily administered and rapidly and reliably produces profound analgesia. Nevertheless, many anesthesiologists prefer the continuous epidural technique. It is their belief that, with epidural anesthesia, hypotension occurs less precipitously and, consequently, is easier to prevent or treat. The anesthetic level is also more controllable with epidural anesthesia because, if the initial dose does not produce a satisfactory sensory block, more drug can be injected through the epidural catheter. A suggested technique for regional anesthesia for cesarean section is outlined in Tables 12.5, 12.6, and 12.7. The rationale for these recommendations is discussed below.

Antacid Administration

The hazards of aspiration pneumonitis and the use of oral antacids are discussed fully in Chapter 23. Approximately 30% of women undergoing elective scheduled cesarean section will have significant amounts of acidic contents in their stomach unless they have received antacid within 1 hr before surgery (9). Because a small proportion of patients receiving a block will require a general anesthetic, we believe it is prudent to give *all* patients an oral antacid prior to cesarean section.

Maternal Hypotension: Prevention and Therapy

Pregnant women are particularly prone to arterial hypotension following sympathetic blockade. When

Table 12.5
Preparation for Regional Anesthesia for Cesarean Section

1. Administer a nonparticulate oral antacid within 1 hr of induction of anesthesia.
2. Transport the patient to the operating room in the lateral position.
3. Measure vital signs. Supine hypotension unresponsive to left uterine displacement may make regional anesthesia inadvisable.
4. Administer rapidly 1000 to 2000 ml of dextrose-free balanced salt solution IV.
5. Before starting the block, check resuscitation equipment and drugs: (a) oxygen delivery system and the anesthesia machine; (b) airways; (c) laryngoscope; (d) endotracheal tubes; (e) thiopental or diazepam for possible convulsion; (f) ephedrine for hypotension; and (g) suction apparatus.
6. If subarachnoid anesthesia is planned, administer ephedrine (10 to 15 mg IV) or (25 to 50 mg IM). Avoid in hypertensive or preeclamptic patients.
7. Administer oxygen by plastic face mask or nasal prongs.

the parturient lies in the supine position, her gravid uterus compresses the inferior vena cava and decreases venous return to the heart. With sympathetic blockade she may not be able to compensate adequately for the venous obstruction. A fall in blood pressure is associated with a comparable fall in uterine blood flow and placental perfusion and may lead to fetal hypoxia and acidosis. Therefore the patient should not be permitted to lie in the supine position either in transit to the operating room or after the block is performed. After regional blockade the patient should be positioned with left uterine displacement to prevent aortocaval compression and in a slight Trendelenburg position to increase venous return.

The authors have reviewed their experience with 583 consecutive cesarean sections performed under epidural anesthesia (10). All patients received a rapid intravenous infusion of at least 1 liter of lactated Ringer's solution prior to the block. About half the patients received ephedrine (25 to 50 mg) intramuscularly to prevent hypotension. All patients were positioned with left uterine displacement after the block. The overall incidence of hypotension was 29%. Hypotension occurred more frequently in women not in labor (36%) than in those who were in labor (24%) (Table 12.8). With prehydration and uterine displacement, intramuscular prophylactic ephedrine, administered 15 min before the block, did not appear to provide additional protection against hypotension. In all cases maternal hypotension was promptly recognized and promptly treated. Neither Apgar scores nor time to sustained respiration was affected by ma-

Table 12.6
Regional Anesthesia for Cesarean Section: A Suggested Technique

Spinal anesthesia
Use smallest needle possible and/or needle with noncutting point (Sprotte or Whitacre).

Local anesthetic options:
1. 7 to 10 mg of hyperbaric tetracaine (tetracaine 1% and equal volumes of 10% dextrose in water) or
2. 60 to 75 mg of lidocaine (1.2 to 1.5 ml of lidocaine 5% with 7.5% glucose) or
3. 12 to 15 mg of bupivacaine (1.6 to 2 ml of bupivacaine 0.75% with 8.25% dextrose)

Intrathecal narcotic options—added to above local anesthetics
1. Fentanyl, 10 to 25 μg (0.2 to 0.5 ml of fentanyl 50 μg/ml solution)
2. Morphine, 0.1 to 0.25 mg (0.2 to 0.5 ml of preservative-free morphine 5 mg/10 ml)
3. Both fentanyl and morphine in above doses

Epinephrine option—if unusually prolonged surgery is anticipated, 0.1 to 0.2 mg of epinephrine may be added

Epidural anesthesia
Local anesthetic options:
1. 1.5 to 2.0% lidocaine
2. 0.5% bupivacaine
3. 3.0% chloroprocaine
Epinephrine may be added to a maximum concentration of 1:200,000.
Test Dose: Use 3-ml test dose of local anesthetic containing epinephrine 1:200,000 (15 μg). Observe for heart rate increase within 60 sec or evidence of spinal blockade within 3 to 5 min. If test dose produces negative results, administer up to 20 ml of local anesthetic in fractional increments of no more than 5 ml per 30 sec. Insert epidural catheter. Inject additional drug as required through catheter (after another test dose) to obtain sensory blockade up to fourth thoracic dermatome. Alternatively, the catheter may be passed initially and test dose and local anesthetic injected through the catheter.

pH adjustment option:
1. Add 1 ml (1 mEq) sodium bicarbonate (8.4%) to 10 ml of lidocaine or chloroprocaine or
2. 0.1 ml (0.1 mEq) sodium bicarbonate to 20 ml of bupivacaine

Epidural narcotic options:
1. Fentanyl, 50 to 100 μg, or sufentanil, 10 to 20 μg, may be added to above local anesthetics to potentiate intraoperative analgesia
2. Morphine 5 mg may be administered through the epidural catheter following delivery
Position patient with left uterine displacement, slight (10-degree) Trendelenburg tilt and head on pillow.
Monitor arterial blood pressure every minute until birth of the baby, then every 5 min for duration of block.
Monitor ECG and oxygen saturation (pulse oximeter).

Table 12.7
Management of Complications of Regional Anesthesia for Cesarean Section

1. If systolic blood pressure falls by 30% or below 100 torr, ensure left uterine displacement and increase IV infusion rate. If blood pressure is still not restored, administer 5 to 15 mg of ephedrine IV; repeat if necessary.
2. Treat anxiety and incomplete or "spotty" anesthesia with one or more of the following agents prior to delivery of the infant: (a) 2.5 mg of diazepam in increments up to 10 mg IV; (b) fentanyl up to 1 μg/kg IV; (c) 40% nitrous oxide (by mask); (d) 0.25 mg/kg of ketamine IV; (e) 10–20 ml 0.5% lidocaine intraperitoneally.
3. If analgesia is inadequate, proceed to general anesthesia with endotracheal intubation.
4. If supplementation to spinal or epidural blockade is necessary after delivery, administer small doses of narcotic.
5. Metoclopramide (10 mg IV) or droperidol (0.5 mg IV) may be administered to reduce the likelihood of nausea and vomiting.

Table 12.8
Effects of Ephedrine on the Incidence of Hypotension[a,b]

	No Ephedrine Prophylaxis (%)	Ephedrine Prophylaxis (%)
Repeat cesarean section (no labor, $n = 183$)	43	35
Primary cesarean section (no labor, $n = 39$)	35	21
Repeat cesarean section (in labor, $n = 88$)	26	26
Emergency cesarean section (in labor, $n = 273$)	27	17
TOTAL ($n = 583$)	32	26

[a] Adapted from Brizgys RV, Shnider SM, Kotelko DM, Dailey PA, Levinson G: The incidence and neonatal effects of maternal hypotension during epidural anesthesia for cesarean section. Anesthesiology 57:A395, 1982.
[b] No significant differences were found.

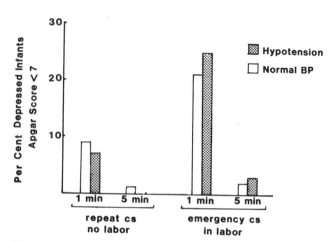

Figure 12.6. Lack of significant effect of rapidly treated maternal hypotension, produced by epidural anesthesia, on neonatal Apgar scores following cesarean delivery. (Reprinted by permission from Brizgys RV, Dailey PA, Shnider SM, Kotelko DM, Levinson G: The incidence and neonatal effects of maternal hypotension during epidural anesthesia for cesarean section. Anesthesiology 67:782–786, 1987.)

ternal hypotension (Fig. 12.6) nor were umbilical venous (UV) and umbilical arterial (UA) P_{O_2} and P_{CO_2} values. There were some small statistically significant differences in UV and UA pH and base excess values between hypotensive and normotensive patients, especially in women not in labor (maximum pH difference 0.04 units, maximum base excess difference 2 mEq/liter). While the use of prophylactic ephedrine to prevent hypotension has not been demonstrated to be useful in epidural anesthesia, this may not be true for spinal anesthesia where the onset of the sympathetic block is far more rapid (11, 12). The authors have found that, following either epidural or spinal anesthesia, the incidence of hypoten-

sion is more than 80% if no prophylactic measures are instituted. With intravenous hydration and left uterine displacement this can be markedly reduced. While prehydration with 1000 ml of crystalloid decreases the incidence of hypotension, with high regional block (13) increasing the crystalloid prehydration to 2000 ml is more effective (14).

Following institution of the block the patient's blood pressure should be monitored every minute for the first 20 min and then every 5 min for the duration of surgery. Some anesthesiologists monitor blood pressure every minute until the baby is born. If hypotension occurs (either a systolic pressure of less than 100 torr or a fall of 30% from preanesthetic levels), left uterine displacement should be increased and fluids rapidly infused. If hypotension is not corrected within 30 to 60 sec, a dose of ephedrine (5 to 15 mg intravenously) should be administered.

In the past, the use of vasopressors in the pregnant patient has been criticized on the basis of uterine vasoconstriction that could lead to fetal hypoxia and acidosis. This problem can be avoided by using vasopressors such as ephedrine, mephentermine (Wyamine), or metaraminol (Aramine). These drugs, in contrast to methoxamine (Vasoxyl) and phenylephrine (Neo-Synephrine), have slight α-adrenergic activity and do not cause uterine vasoconstriction (15, 16) (see Fig. 3.14). In the experimental animal, ephedrine, mephentermine, and metaraminol restore uterine blood flow toward normal when used to treat spinal hypotension. A prophylactic dose of ephedrine has no adverse effect on uterine blood flow (17) (see Fig. 3.16). Recent clinical data in normal parturients not in labor indicate that phenylephrine in small (20 to 100 μg) increments can be safely used to treat spinal (12) or epidural (18) hypotension.

Toxic Reactions and Total Spinals

With administration of spinal or epidural block, a total spinal with hypotension and respiratory insufficiency or a toxic reaction with convulsions, hypoxia, and cardiovascular collapse may occur. Therefore, before starting any block the anesthesia machine, laryngoscope, airways, endotracheal tubes, suction apparatus, and monitoring equipment should be checked, and thiopental and ephedrine should be immediately available. Treatment of these complications is outlined in Chapters 6 and 9.

Supplementary Oxygen

Parturients receiving a spinal or epidural block should be given supplementary oxygen. The use of nasal prongs or a clear plastic face mask is more acceptable to most parturients than an anesthesia face mask. The added maternal oxygen may increase fetal oxygenation. In healthy women undergoing elective cesarean sections under lumbar epidural anesthesia, increasing inspired maternal oxygen concentrations from 21 to 100% resulted in an increase in umbilical venous PO_2 from 28 to 47 torr and umbilical artery PO_2 from 15 to 25 torr, respectively (Fig. 12.7) (19).

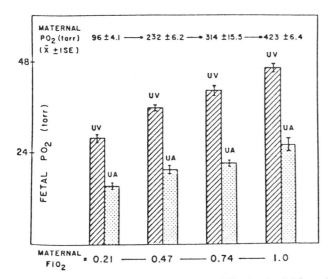

Figure 12.7. Histograms showing umbilical vein (*UV*) and umbilical artery (*UA*) PO_2 levels at different maternal levels of FIO_2. Maternal PaO_2 levels at four levels of FIO_2 are shown at top. Values are means ± 1 SE (*n* = 10). (Reprinted by permission from Ramanathan S, Gandhi S, Arismendy J, Chalon J, Turndorf H: Oxygen transfer from mother to fetus during cesarean section under epidural anesthesia. Anesth Analg 61:576–581, 1982.)

The increased maternal oxygenation may also provide additional maternal safety should hypoventilation or hypotension not be recognized immediately.

Subarachnoid Block: Anesthetic Solutions

The most popular drugs for spinal anesthesia for cesarean section are **bupivacaine** 0.75% in dextrose 8.25%, **lidocaine** 5% in glucose 7.5%, and **tetracaine** 1% mixed with dextrose. Lidocaine rapidly produces a profound sensory and motor block usually lasting 45 to 75 min. For cesarean section with speedy surgeons this agent is ideal. For most cesarean sections either bupivacaine or tetracaine is appropriate. For unusually long cesarean sections tetracaine with epinephrine may be necessary. The effect of the addition of epinephrine to bupivacaine or lidocaine solutions is controversial with some investigators claiming no clinically useful purpose (20), and others finding improved and prolonged sensory and motor block (21, 22).

A number of reports have indicated that bupivacaine is superior to tetracaine in that it has a faster onset, lesser motor block (23), produces fewer failed blocks (22), and results in greater patient satisfaction (21). These findings, however, are debated by others (24, 25). Nonetheless, bupivacaine is becoming the spinal local anesthetic of choice, especially the hyperbaric solution of 0.75%.

Several studies have evaluated the subarachnoid spread of hyperbaric bupivacaine in the term parturient (26–28). In his first study Norris et al. chose a uniform dose of 12 mg to administer to 50 parturients (26), and in a subsequent study, 15 mg were used (27). In these studies it was apparent that it was *not* necessary to vary the dose of injected hyperbaric bupivacaine according to the patient's age, height, weight, body mass, or vertebral column length. For either dose, these variables did not affect the level of anesthesia. For very reliable blocks, many anesthesiologists are using the larger dose of 15 mg. This dose will produce a high level of sensory block (up to T2), with occasional patients showing analgesic levels of C2 (Fig. 12.8). The Trendelenburg position (10 degrees) is important to ensure adequate venous return, but care must be taken that the drug does not spread cephalad to the medullary respiratory center. We recommend that a pillow be placed under the head *immediately* following spinal anesthesia for cesarean section.

Fentanyl, sufentanil, and morphine have been administered into the subarachnoid space immediately before, after, or combined with local anesthetic administration of either hyperbaric tetracaine 1% or hyperbaric bupivacaine 0.75%. Subarachnoid fen-

Figure 12.8. Maximum cephalad extent of analgesia to pin prick and anesthesia to light touch in 52 term parturients following subarachnoid injection of 15 mg hyperbaric bupivacaine and 0.15 mg morphine. (Adapted from Norris MC: Patient variables and the subarachnoid spread of hyperbaric bupivacaine in the term patient. Anesthesiology 72:478–482, 1990.)

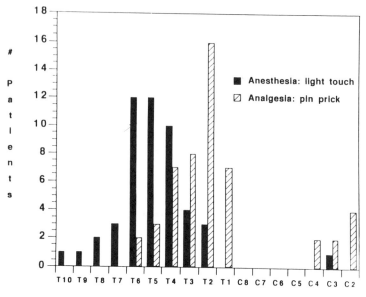

Maximum Level of Sensory Blockade

tanyl in doses of 6.25 μg or greater (29) significantly increases the duration and intensity of analgesia and provides postoperative pain relief lasting 5 to 6 hr. High doses (37.5 to 50 μg) do not appear to prolong analgesia, but do increase the incidence of side effects, notably pruritus. However, no respiratory depression was reported, even with 50 μg. Good improvement of intraoperative analgesia with a low incidence of side effects are achieved with doses of 10 to 25 μg.

Subarachnoid sufentanil 10 μg mixed with 15 mg of hyperbaric bupivacaine 0.75% also improves intraoperative analgesia and prolongs postoperative analgesia (4 hr) with few side effects (30).

Subarachnoid morphine in doses of 0.1 to 0.5 mg combined with 0.75% hyperbaric bupivacaine improves intraoperative analgesia and prolongs postoperative pain relief (18 to 27 hr) with minor side effects such as pruritus and nausea and vomiting (31–34). Although respiratory depression has not been reported, even "minidoses" of morphine (0.1 mg) administered into the subarachnoid space achieve significant CSF concentrations and have the potential for rostral spread, resulting in late respiratory depression. Close monitoring to avoid respiratory depression and related side effects is necessary.

Epidural Anesthesia: Anesthetic Solutions

In contrast to spinal blockade, epidural anesthesia requires large amounts of local anesthetic, and the fetus and neonate may be affected adversely by placental transfer of these drugs. This subject is discussed extensively in Chapters 5 and 6. The preferred

local anesthetic for epidural anesthesia for cesarean section is controversial. The ones most commonly used are **lidocaine, bupivacaine,** and **2-chloroprocaine.** Each has advantages and potential disadvantages.

Bupivacaine 0.5% is effective for cesarean section anesthesia, but its onset is very slow and some authors find the block not dense enough. The 0.75% concentration has a faster onset and provides better surgical conditions, but because of the cardiac arrests associated with its accidental intravascular injection, this concentration is no longer recommended for use in obstetrics. Chloroprocaine 3% rapidly produces profound anesthesia and, in doses of 25 to 30 ml, is an excellent choice for cesarean section anesthesia. Chloroprocaine is useful for cesarean section because of its rapid onset of surgical anesthesia. This characteristic, in addition to its short half-life in both maternal and fetal serum, make this an attractive local anesthetic for situations of fetal distress and the need for urgent cesarean section.

However, in 1979 four cases of prolonged neurologic deficit were reported following unintentional subarachnoid injection of a large dose of chloroprocaine. Studies have suggested that sodium bisulfite, the antioxidant present in chloroprocaine in high concentrations may be neurotoxic (35, 36), and this may explain some of the reported complications that have occurred. The preparation of Nesacaine (as marketed by Astra) does not contain sodium metabisulfite but does contain disodium EDTA (Table 12.9). This preparation has been reported to cause severe paralumbar muscle pain, usually when larger vol-

Table 12.9
Contents (mg/ml) of Various Solutions of Chloroprocaine 3%[a]

	Pennwalt Nesacaine[b]	Astra Nesacaine-MPF	Abbott Chloro-procaine
Chloroprocaine	30	30	30
Na-Metabisulfite	—	—	1.8
Na-Bisulfite	2.0	—	—
Disodium EDTA	—	0.11	—
pH	2.7–4.0	2.7–4.0	2.7–4.0

[a]Modified from Stevens RA, Chester WL, Artuso JD, Bray JG, Nellestein JA: Back pain after epidural anesthesia with chloroprocaine in volunteers: Preliminary report. Reg Anesth 16:199–203, 1991.
[b]Pennwalt Nesacaine is no longer manufactured.

umes (20 to 25 ml) of the anesthetic is administered (37–39). It is postulated that, because the sodium salts of EDTA are active chelating agents of heavy metals, they cause an acute lowering of tissue calcium and thus muscle spasm. Which preparation of chloroprocaine is chosen depends on the judgement of the anesthesiologist.

There are other potential problems with chloroprocaine. The rapid onset of the block may be associated with a higher incidence of hypotension (40). Chloroprocaine may interfere with the efficacy of subsequent epidural narcotics or bupivacaine (41–44). This does not appear to be an effect of pH (41, 45), but may be due to a metabolite of chloroprocaine. Initial evaluations of efficacy of epidural morphine after different local anesthetic drugs suggested that the morphine was less effective after chloroprocaine. However, follow-up studies revealed that, since chloroprocaine is short acting, it may wear off before the epidural morphine has begun to provide analgesia. Supplemental analgesia (either continued use of epidural local anesthetics or systemic narcotics) may be necessary in patients who have received chloroprocaine for surgical anesthesia.

Epinephrine

Epinephrine is frequently added to local anesthetics to decrease systemic absorption and peak blood levels, intensify the motor block, and prolong the duration of the anesthetic (46–48). Some have avoided epinephrine in obstetrics because of concern that the α-adrenergic effects of epinephrine may decrease uterine blood flow and its betamimetic effects may decrease uterine activity and prolong labor (49–55). Absorbed epinephrine from the epidural space probably does not have significant effects on uterine blood flow (56–58). In pregnant ewes epidural epinephrine (100 μg) did not decrease uterine blood flow (57).

Epidural anesthesia with epinephrine 1:200,000 did not alter human intervillous blood flow (58).

The betamimetic effects of systemically absorbed epinephrine have been shown to decrease uterine contractility and prolong labor (51–55). Because, in epidural anesthesia for vaginal delivery, the addition of epinephrine (except for the test dose) is unnecessary due to the small amounts of drug used and the lack of need for an intense motor block, it should probably be avoided. For cesarean delivery, since larger doses of local anesthetic are used and more intense motor block desired, the addition of epinephrine 1:200,000 may be advantageous.

Test Dose

Aspiration that does not produce CSF or blood does not preclude intravascular or subarachnoid injection. Therefore the anesthesiologist must administer an effective test dose and monitor results before giving the full dose of local anesthetic. The test dose should contain an amount of local anesthetic sufficient to produce a T10 spinal block if injected subarachnoid. This dose is usually too small to allow recognition of an intravascular injection; thus either a second larger test dose is administered or 15 to 20 μg of epinephrine are added to the local anesthetic. This dose of epinephrine will usually produce a rapid increase in heart rate of 20 to 30 bpm. Some authors object to the use of epinephrine in a test dose because of unreliability in the obstetric patient and possible adverse effects on uterine blood flow. The controversy regarding the preferred test dose has been discussed fully in Chapter 9. When using a continuous catheter technique, test doses should be given prior to the original dose and all reinforcing doses because plastic tubing in the epidural space can migrate. Finally, the local anesthetic should be administered slowly in fractional doses rather than by rapid bolus injections.

Alkalinization of Local Anesthetics

Alkalinization of local anesthetic solutions has been advocated to speed the onset of and prolong and intensify epidural blocks. As pH increases the proportion of the nonionized lipid-soluble form of the local anesthetic increases; therefore the drug should be more quickly available at the site of action. Clinical studies have shown that alkalinization of lidocaine is effective (59, 60), but studies of chloroprocaine and bupivacaine have been contradictory (61–66). DiFazio et al. (59) studied the onset of anesthesia (loss of sensation of tetanic stimulation at L2) in patients undergoing cesarean section or orthopedic procedures with pH-adjusted epidural lidocaine (1.5%). Three pH values of lidocaine were studied: 4.55, 6.35, and 7.20. The onset of anesthesia was significantly more rapid in the higher pH groups (Fig. 12.9). A potential side effect of pH-adjusting local anesthetics is a higher incidence of hypotension subsequent to the more rapid onset of epidural anesthesia. Parnass et al. (67) found a greater fall in blood pressure in patients who received pH-adjusted 2% lidocaine for epidural anesthesia for cesarean section when compared with those who received the commercial preparation (Fig. 12.10). Hypotension also developed more quickly in these patients. Possible adverse effects of hypotension on uteroplacental blood flow suggest that caution be used in the use of alkalinized lidocaine in high risk obstetrical patients. The usual recommended recipes are to add 2 ml of an 8.4% bicarbonate solution to the 20 ml of lidocaine or chloroprocaine and 0.1 ml to 20 ml of bupivacaine (68). If excess bicarbonate is added, precipitation may occur. This is especially true with bupivacaine for which the margin of error is very small. Visible precipitation has been noted after only 0.2 ml of 7.5% bicarbonate (0.18 mEq) added to 30 ml of 0.5% bupivacaine (69).

Epidural Opiates

Epidural **fentanyl** (50 to 100 μg) has been found to potentiate intraoperative analgesia (70–73), decrease nausea and vomiting during uterine manipulation (71), and decrease requirements for supple-

mental opiate medication (72, 73) with no adverse maternal (70–73) or neonatal effects (73). Several studies have evaluated the neonatal pattern of breathing, neonatal respiratory rates, and neurobehavioral status following epidural fentanyl (100 μg) used before the infant has been delivered at cesarean section and have found no adverse effects (74–76). The volume of diluent used with epidural fentanyl can affect its efficacy. Volumes greater than 10 ml appear to be necessary to provide complete analgesia (74).

The addition of **sufentanil** (20 to 30 μg) to 0.5% bupivacaine with epinephrine 1:200,000 produced significantly better intraoperative anesthesia, longer postoperative analgesia than bupivacaine alone, minimal maternal side effects, and no adverse neonatal effects (78). Epidural sufentanil (20 to 30 μg) appears to be equivalent to fentanyl (100 μg) (79). Both opiates provide rapid onset but short duration of postoperative analgesia.

Epidural **morphine** is widely used to provide postoperative cesarean section pain relief. Five milligrams of epidural morphine provides effective, safe, and prolonged (24 hr) analgesia after cesarean delivery with only mild and easily treatable side effects (80). In a prospective study of 1000 patients given 5 mg of epidural morphine (81), it was found that 85% obtained good to excellent postoperative analgesia lasting 23 hr. Sixteen percent required no additional

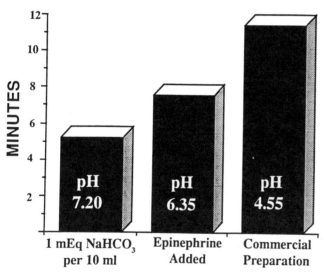

Figure 12.9. Times for onset of surgical anesthesia as measured with a nerve stimulator and the pH of the lidocaine epidural solution used. The patients received either a commercial preparation of lidocaine with epinephrine 1:200,000 (pH 4.55), plain lidocaine to which epinephrine was added to a final concentration of 1:200,000 (pH 6.35), or a commercially prepared solution of lidocaine with epinephrine 1:200,000 plus 1 mEq of NaHCO$_3$ added per 10 ml of solution (pH 7.20). (Modified with permission from DiFazio CA: Comparison of pH-adjusted lidocaine solutions for epidural anesthesia. Anesth Analg 65:760–764, 1986.)

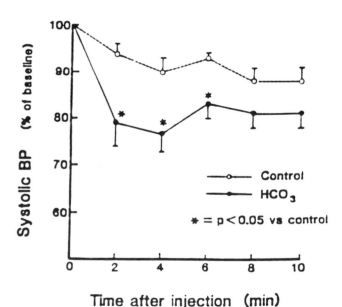

Time after injection (min)

Figure 12.10. Time course of average systolic blood pressure (*BP*) readings (mean ± SEM) expressed as a percentage of the baseline value. (Reprinted by permission from Parnass SM, Curran MJA, Becker GL: Incidence of hypotension associated with epidural anesthesia using alkalinized and nonalkalinized lidocaine for cesarean section. Anesth Analg 66:1148–1150, 1987.)

analgesia before discharge, and 44% required only oral analgesics. Side effects included 29% moderate to severe pruritus, 20% nausea or vomiting, and 0.1% (one patient) severe respiratory depression, which responded promptly to oxygen and intravenous naloxone. A later Canadian retrospective study of approximately 5000 patients confirmed these results (82). Studies of potential respiratory depression following the use of epidural morphine compared to IM morphine or patient-controlled analgesia (PCA) following cesarean section have been performed by a number of investigators (83–87). Although mild decreases in oxygen saturation have been seen, no maternal morbidity has been reported. Thus these reports confirm the efficacy of epidural morphine for analgesia after cesarean section and suggest that its use is safe when basic monitoring criteria are rigidly followed and treatment is expeditiously instituted.

Epidural morphine has been compared to PCA for postoperative pain relief. Both provide excellent analgesia (87–89), epidural morphine more so than PCA (Fig. 12.11) (87, 88). PCA produces more sedation (Fig. 12.12), and epidural morphine more pruritus (Fig. 12.13) (89). Finally, the use of epidural morphine for post-cesarean section pain relief appears to be safe for the neonate who breastfeeds (90).

Supplementary Drugs for Anxiety and Analgesia

Treatment of maternal anxiety may often facilitate performance of the regional block and, with attainment of an adequate sensory level, provide the mother with a more pleasant delivery. Low doses of intravenous diazepam (2.5 mg increments, up to 10 mg)

may be used with minimal neonatal effects (91). If the sensory block is not completely satisfactory, then 30 to 40% nitrous oxide and oxygen or a low dose of ketamine (0.25 mg/kg) intravenously (92) may be used safely, as long as the mother remains awake and maintains her laryngeal reflexes. Fentanyl (1 μg/kg intravenously) has also been used as an adjuvant for regional anesthesia for cesarean section without adverse effects on the neonate (93). If the sensory level is clearly inadequate, general anesthesia with endotracheal intubation should be performed.

Dosage

In the pregnant woman, the dose of local anesthetic required to achieve a given level with spinal anesthesia is approximately 50 to 70% of the dose required for nonpregnant women (94). With epidural anesthesia, some authors have reported that dose re-

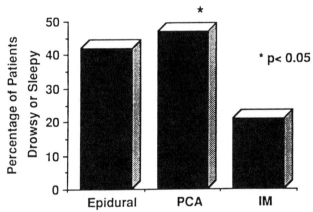

Figure 12.12. Postcesarean section pain relief. Incidence of sedation. (Modified with permission from Harrison DM, Sinatra R, Morgese L, Chung JH: Epidural narcotic and patient-controlled analgesia for post-cesarean section pain relief. Anesthesiology 68:454–457, 1988.)

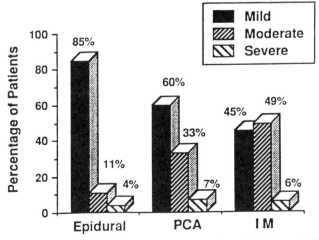

Figure 12.11. Post-cesarean section pain relief: Amount of pain. (Modified from Harrison DM, Sinatra R, Morgese L, Chung JH: Epidural narcotic and patient-controlled analgesia for post-cesarean section pain relief. Anesthesiology 68:454–457, 1988.)

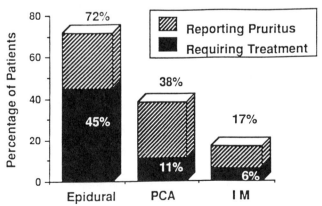

Figure 12.13. Post-cesarean section pain relief: Incidence of pruritus. (Modified with permission from Harrison DM, Sinatra R, Morgese L, Epidural narcotic and patient-controlled analgesia for post-cesarean section pain relief. Anesthesiology 68:454–457, 1988.)

quirements are also reduced (Fig. 12.14) (95). On the other hand, other studies suggest that with equal amounts of local anesthetic, there is no significant difference in sensory levels in pregnant and non-pregnant patients (Table 12.10) (96).

Postdural Puncture Headache (PDPH)

One of the most troublesome and annoying complications of spinal anesthesia is postdural puncture headache. This subject is discussed in Chapter 24 and is briefly reviewed below.

PREVENTION

A variety of approaches have been taken to minimize the incidence of PDPH.

1. Needle Size. The incidence can be minimized by using the smallest needle possible (97–112). There is, however, a wide variation in the reported incidence of headache between different investigators using the same size needle, although all agree the smaller the needle the less likely is a PDPH.

2. Direction of Needle Bevel. Insertion of the needle with the bevel parallel to the longitudinal fibers of the dura appears to produce a smaller rent and a lower incidence of headache. The microscopic arrangement of dural fibers probably minimizes the size of the dural hole if the needle bevel is directed parallel to the longitudinal axis of the vertebral col-

umn (Fig. 12.15) (113). Mihic (114) randomly assigned patients to either parallel or perpendicular insertion of the spinal needle bevel and found a high significant reduction in the incidence of headache if parallel insertion was employed. Similarly, with epidural needles, the incidence of headache after accidental dural puncture was significantly lower with parallel insertion of the needle (115).

Table 12.10
Comparison of Spread of Epidural Anesthesia in Pregnant and Nonpregnant Women[a]

	Volume of Bupivacaine 0.75% (ml)	Most Cephalad Thoracic Dermatome Anesthetized to Pinprick
Nonpregnant (n = 32)	15	5.7 ± 1.7
Pregnant (n = 60)	15	5.5 ± 1.2
Nonpregnant (n = 29)	20	4.7 ± 1.7
Pregnant (n = 29)	20	4.2 ± 1.5

[a] Adapted from Grundy EM, Zamora AM, Winnie AP: Comparison of spread of epidural anesthesia in pregnant and nonpregnant women. Anesth Analg 57:544–546, 1978. (Note that, although bupivacaine 0.75% is no longer recommended for use in obstetrics, the findings in this study are still significant.)

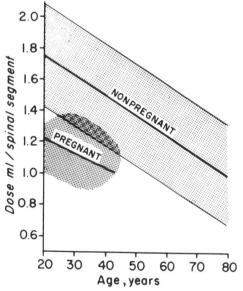

Figure 12.14. Regression lines for dose of epidural solution and age in nonpregnant women and in pregnant women at term. The gravida obviously requires much less drug. (Reprinted by permission from Bonica JJ: *Principles and Practice of Obstetric Analgesia and Anesthesia, vol 1.* Davis, Philadelphia, 1967, p 624; modification by Bonica from Bromage PR: Continuous lumbar epidural analgesia for obstetrics. Can Med Assoc J 85:1136–1140, 1961.)

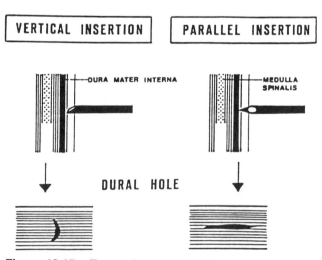

Figure 12.15. Types of needle insertion by lumbar punctures. In vertical versus parallel insertion, the bevel of the spinal needle is inserted through the dura mater interna perpendicular to (versus parallel to) the longitudinal dural fibers. The number of severed dural fibers is greater by vertical insertion. (Reproduced with permission from Mihic DN: Postdural headache and relationship of needle bevel to longitudinal dural fibers. Reg Anesth 10:76–81, 1985.)

3. Type of Needle. "Pencil" point needles (Fig. 12.16) that spread rather than cut dural fibers have a lower incidence of spinal headache (106, 110, 116–119). The Whitacre needle has a conical shaped solid tip with a lateral eye. The Sprotte needle has a ogival shaped solid tip and a lateral opening, which is larger than the Whitacre. Both needles come in various sizes, ranging from 22 to 27 gauge. The 22-gauge needles are firmer and easier to insert than the smaller ones, which usually require an introducer. However, as with the cutting needle, larger sizes produce more headaches. Currently, the 24-gauge Sprotte needle is very popular because of the combination of reasonable ease of placement, excellent flow characteristics allowing for easy identification of the subarachnoid space, and a minimal incidence of headache.

4. Angle of Insertion. Based on an in vitro study, it has been postulated that, if the dura mater is punctured at an acute angle, the resulting holes in the dura and arachnoid would not be opposed, creating a flap valve that would reduce fluid leak (120). However, two randomized prospective trials that compared the incidence of spinal headache between the midline and paramedian approach failed to validate this hypothesis (121, 122).

5. Prophylactic Bed Rest. While many clinicians routinely keep the patients on bed rest following either a subarachnoid block or accidental dural puncture, there is little evidence that this reduces the likelihood of developing a spinal headache. In a study of 100 neurology patients having diagnostic lumbar punctures with an 18-gauge needle, half were allowed to ambulate immediately after the puncture and half were kept in bed for 24 hr (123). The incidence and duration of the spinal headache was similar in both groups (Fig. 12.17).

6. Increased Hydration. Increased hydration after dural puncture has little or no effect on the incidence of subsequent headache. Animal studies have shown that relatively large increases in fluid intake do not increase CSF production (124). In humans the incidence of PDPH is independent of fluid intake (125).

7. Management of Accidental Dural Puncture. The occurrence of accidental dural puncture associated with epidural anesthesia will, of course, vary with the experience of the anesthesiologist. In training centers the incidence reported is usually between 1 and 2%. If a dural puncture occurs after the use of a 16-gauge needle and the epidural technique is abandoned, almost 80% of patients develop a headache. However, if an epidural anesthetic is administered using another interspace (directing the catheter away from the dural hole), approximately 55% of patients develop a headache. The local anesthetic solution in

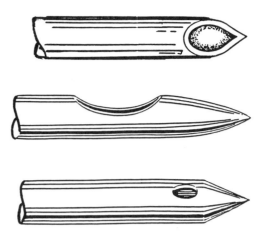

Figure 12.16. Comparison of Quincke point (*top*), Sprotte (*center*), and Whitacre (*bottom*) needles.

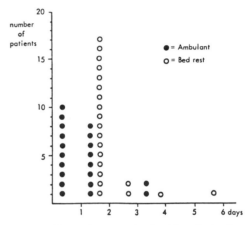

Figure 12.17. Time of onset of spinal headache in neurology patients following diagnostic lumbar puncture (18-gauge needle) who were either allowed to ambulate at will immediately following the block or were kept on bed rest for a 24-hr period. Duration of the headache was also similar in both groups. (Reprinted by permission from Carbaat PAT, van Crevel H: Lumbar puncture headache: Controlled study on the preventive effect of 24 hours' bed rest. Lancet 2:1133–1135, 1981.)

the epidural space likely reduces the pressure gradient between the subarachnoid and epidural space, decreasing CSF leak and promoting dural healing. Local anesthetic injected into the epidural space following an accidental dural puncture may rarely result in a high spinal block (126, 127). Slow injection of fractionated doses and frequent monitoring of anesthetic dermatome levels and vital signs are recommended.

Several investigators have suggested that instillation of preservative-free salt solution through the epidural catheter decreases the incidence of spinal headache (128–130). In all cases the epidural anesthetic was allowed to wear off. Protocols range from a single 60-ml injection to multiple injections of 30 to 60 ml every 6 hr for 24 hr, or a continuous infusion of a liter over a 24-hr period. Effectiveness with all protocols has been good. For example, Craft et al. (129) reported that, after accidental dural puncture with a 16-gauge needle, one 60-ml injection of saline following delivery reduced the incidence of spinal headache from 76 to 12%. Administration of a **prophylactic epidural blood patch** via either the epidural catheter or spinal needle has been suggested (131, 132).

Uncontrolled retrospective studies were not able to demonstrate any prophylactic effect of blood patch instituted within 24 hr of a dural tap (133, 134). Randomized prospective trials of immediate blood patch, given through an epidural catheter, have found this to be of value (135–138). Possibly, the use of larger volumes of autologous blood (15 to 20 ml), rather than the smaller amount (10 ml) used in earlier reports, may account for the difference (139). The very high incidence of headache after dural puncture with an epidural needle would make the prophylactic use of an epidural blood patch attractive. The potential for infection may be higher if blood is injected through an epidural catheter that has been in position for many hours, and some authors argue that, since spinal headache is not an inevitable consequence of dural puncture, prophylactic blood patch is not justifiable. The occurrence of an epidural abscess after epidural blood patch, either as a de novo procedure or through an existing catheter, has not been reported.

TREATMENT
1. **Bed rest** in the prone, lateral, or supine position will relieve the headache. In many mild cases this is all the therapy that is necessary.
2. **Oral analgesics** may be required and should be used to allow the patient more mobility.
3. **Intravenous caffeine sodium benzoate** has been reported to be effective (140). The mechanism is believed to be related to cerebral vasoconstriction. Abboud et al. (141) confirmed that intravenous caffeine sodium benzoate (500 mg) relieved headaches in the majority of patients, but there was a 42% recurrence rate. Camann et al. (142) demonstrated a beneficial effect of oral caffeine (300 mg) on headache, although again there was a significant recurrence rate of 30%. Seizures have been reported in a postpartum patient with elevated blood pressure after treatment of spinal headache with blood patch and caffeine sodium benzoate (143). Caffeine is a central nervous system stimulant and may have been an etiologic factor. Oral theophylline, 300 mg in a sustained release tablet, has also been reported to ameliorate spinal headache (144, 145).
4. **A blood patch epidural** using autologous blood may be performed in patients suffering from severe refractory postdural puncture headaches. Using a rig-

idly aseptic technique, 15 to 20 ml of blood are withdrawn via a venipuncture and immediately placed into the epidural space at the site of the dural rent. The success rate reported has ranged between 94 and 100% (Table 12.11). A long-term follow-up of 118 patients for 2 years has indicated that epidural blood patch is without serious complication. No cases of infection, adhesive arachnoiditis, or cauda equina syndrome have been reported (155). Backache is the most common complication. It is seldom severe or incapacitating and usually disappears within 48 hr, although it may occasionally last up to 3 months.

Successful epidural anesthesia following prior epidural blood patch has been reported (158). Although a high incidence of poor analgesia in patients with previous accidental dural punctures has been reported, it does not appear to be related to whether or not the patient was originally treated with a blood patch epidural (159). Preliminary experience of blood patch in HIV-positive patients has been encouraging (160, 161).

5. The use of **epidural dextran 40**, in a volume of 20 to 30 ml, has been suggested as an alternative to autologous blood. Complete relief has been reported to occur within 2 hours with no major complications (162). This may be useful in patients in whom autologous blood is contraindicated or unacceptable.

COMBINED SPINAL-EPIDURAL ANESTHESIA

The use of both spinal and epidural anesthesia in the same patient has been suggested (8, 9, 11, 12, 14, 20, 40, 62, 163–170). To obtain the benefits of each technique, an epidural needle is placed in the usual

Table 12.11
Blood Patch Epidural for Dural Puncture Headache

Investigator	Number of Patients	Success Rate (%)
Gormley (146)	7	100
DiGiovanni and Dunbar (147)	45	91.1
DiGiovanni et al. (148)	63	96.8
Glass and Dupont[a]	43	93
Glass and Kennedy (149)	50	94
Dupont and Shire (150)	41	97.5
Vondrell and Bernards (151)	60	96.5
Blok (152)	22	91
Balagot et al. (153)	7	100
Ostheimer et al. (154)	185	98.5
Abouleish et al. (155)	118	97.5
Loeser et al. (156)	31	96
Abouleish (157)	3	100
TOTAL	675	AVERAGE 96

[a]Personal communication cited in DiGiovanni AJ, Galbert MW, Wahle WM: Epidural injection of autologous blood for post-lumbar-puncture headache. II. Additional clinical experiences and laboratory investigation. Anesth Analg 51:226–232, 1972.

way, then a long spinal needle is inserted through the epidural needle into the CSF. The alleged advantages are the rapid onset and reliability of spinal block with the flexibility to reinforce or raise the anesthetic level of a continuous epidural without the hazards of a spinal catheter. The technique described for cesarean section limited the spinal anesthetic to the lower segments and extended anesthesia by epidural injection (171). Other investigators have advocated using spinal anesthesia intraoperatively and the epidural catheter for postoperative analgesia with local anesthetic, opioids, or both (172).

GENERAL ANESTHESIA

In contrast to regional anesthesia, general anesthesia has the advantages of a more rapid induction, less hypotension and cardiovascular instability, and better control of the airway and ventilation. Some patients are terrified of "needles in the back" or the prospect of being awake during major abdominal surgery. In addition, general anesthesia may be preferable in patients with preexisting neurologic or lumbar disc disease, coagulopathies, or infections.

If general anesthesia is used, important considerations include: (a) prevention of aspiration pneumonitis; (b) having a plan of action for failed intubation; (c) prevention of supine hypotension; (d) maintenance of normal maternal ventilation and oxygenation; and (e) minimizing the duration of general anesthesia. Management of general anesthesia for cesarean section is outlined in Table 12.12.

Table 12.12
General Anesthesia for Cesarean Section: A Suggested Technique

1. Administer a nonparticulate oral antacid within 1 hr of induction.
2. Utilize left uterine displacement.
3. Start IV infusion with a large-bore plastic cannula.
4. Preoxygenate with high flow rates (greater than 6 liters/min).
5. When the surgeon is ready to begin, an assistant should apply cricoid pressure (and maintain until position of endotracheal tube is verified and trachea is sealed by inflated cuff).
6. Administer 4 mg/kg of thiopental and 1.5 mg/kg of succinylcholine, wait 30 to 60 sec, then intubate trachea.
7. Administer N_2O (5 liters/min) + O_2 (5 liters/min) plus either halothane 0.5%, isoflurane 0.75% or enflurane 1%. Use muscle relaxant as necessary.
8. Avoid maternal hyperventilation.
9. After the umbilical cord is clamped, deepen anesthesia with nitrous oxide, narcotic, or barbiturate; the halogenated hydrocarbon may be continued.
10. Extubate when the patient is awake.

Prevention of Aspiration

Aspiration of gastric contents during general anesthesia is a major cause of maternal morbidity and mortality. Routine administration of antacid prior to induction significantly raises gastric pH (173). However, use of antacids will not diminish the risk of aspiration of particulate matter.

The risk of regurgitation and aspiration is decreased by (a) rapid endotracheal intubation; (b) avoiding positive pressure ventilation prior to intubation, which could inflate the stomach and make the patient more prone to regurgitate; (c) use of cricoid pressure (Sellick maneuver) to occlude the esophagus and prevent passive regurgitation during endotracheal intubation (174); and (d) extubating the patient only after she is fully awake and able to protect her airway.

We do not routinely administer a nondepolarizing muscle relaxant prior to succinylcholine to prevent fasciculations. A nondepolarizing muscle relaxant will make intubation more difficult since it prolongs the onset time of succinylcholine paralysis and reduces the duration and intensity of the block. Furthermore, pregnant women have less abdominal muscle tone and presumably will have less rise in intragastric pressure with fasciculations. It has also been noted that pregnant women do not have intense fasciculations or postsuccinylcholine muscle pain (175), possibly due to increased progesterone levels. Finally, and most significantly, it has been demonstrated in *nonpregnant* patients that, with fasciculations, the rise in the pressure in the lower esophageal junction is *greater* than the rise in intragastric pressure. Thus the barrier pressure, which prevents passive regurgitation, actually increases with fasciculations (176). However, it is unclear whether this latter study can be applied to pregnant women.

Since morbidity and mortality is markedly increased when the volume of aspirate exceeds 0.4 ml/kg and the pH is less than 2.5 (177), an effort is made to routinely increase maternal gastric pH and decrease gastric volume. Routine administration of an antacid prior to induction significantly raises gastric pH. Particulate or colloidal antacids are avoided since they themselves may cause severe physiologic insult and pulmonary damage if aspirated (178, 179). Sodium citrate (0.3 molar), a clear nonparticulate antacid, is effective and relatively benign if aspirated (180, 181). Bicitra and Alka-Seltzer Gold are commercially available preparations consisting primarily of sodium citrate and appear to be safe and effective (182, 183). Sodium citrate, 15 to 30 ml, is effective if administered in one dose 10 to 15 min before anesthesia.

Preanesthetic administration of a histamine H_2-

receptor antagonist, such as cimetidine or ranitidine, has been suggested to decrease gastric acidity and volume (184–186). Both these drugs require an interval of at least 1 to 2 hr after oral administration and 45 to 60 min after IV or IM administration to be effective. The drugs are probably not indicated routinely, with the possible exceptions of *elective* cesarean sections under general anesthesia or when the parturient has an unusual problem such as peptic ulcer disease or morbid obesity. Metoclopramide is an antiemetic that increases stomach emptying and raises gastroesophageal sphincter tone (187–192). Its efficacy and safety for aspiration prophylaxis in obstetrics has not been fully elucidated. Because of its possible beneficial effects on gastroesophageal sphincter tone and gastric volume, its use might be considered in parturients with unusual problems predisposing to gastric regurgitation.

Failed Intubation

Failed or difficult intubation is the leading cause of anesthetic related maternal mortality. The incidence of failed intubation in obstetrics is much greater than in the surgical patient (193–196). Postulated reasons are the presence of full dentition, increased incidence of laryngeal and pharyngeal edema, obstruction to laryngoscope placement by large pendulous breasts, and failure to allow adequate time for succinylcholine to be effective. Physical characteristics associated with difficulty in airway management and intubation are short muscular necks, receding lower jaws (micrognathia) with obtuse mandibular angles, protruding upper incisors, poor mobility of the mandible, long high-arched palate with a long narrow mouth, and increased alveolar mental distance (anterior depth of the mandible).

Carefully performed preoperative evaluation of the patient will frequently alert the anesthesiologist to a potentially difficult intubation (197, 198).

1. Viewing the patient from the lateral and anterolateral positions should identify patients with maxillary overgrowth (protruding upper incisors) or receding mandible (micrognathia).

2. Viewing and palpating the neck anteriorly allows the anesthesiologist to estimate the mandibular space. The space anterior to the larynx determines how easily the laryngeal axis will line up with the pharyngeal axis during laryngoscopy. Also, when there is a large mandibular space, the tongue does not have to be pulled maximally forward to reveal the larynx and visualization is much easier. The mandibular space is most easily evaluated by measuring the thyromental distance with either a ruler or number of finger breadths (Fig. 12.18). The normal measurement is 6.5 cm or greater. If the distance is 6 to 6.5 cm without other anatomic problems, laryngoscopy and intubation are difficult, but usually possible. A

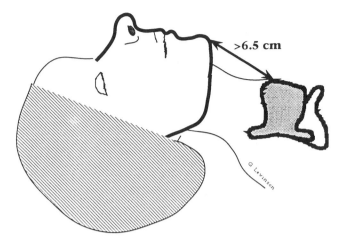

Figure 12.18. The distance from the thyroid notch to the tip of the chin is measured with the neck fully extended. If the distance is less than 6.5 cm, visualization of the vocal cords by direct laryngoscopy may be difficult or impossible.

distance of less than 6 cm suggests that laryngoscopy may be impossible (199). Other reports have confirmed the value of this measurement in predicting difficult intubation (200).

3. Flexing and extending the neck maximally will identify limitations that might prevent optimal alignment of the oral, pharyngeal, and laryngeal axes. The normal atlanto-occipital joint allows 35 degrees of extension (201).

4. The relation of the size of the tongue to that of the oral cavity is estimated by visual examination of the oral pharynx. The patient sits upright with the head in the neutral position. She is asked to open her mouth as widely as possible (normal maximum mandibular opening is 5 to 6 cm) (202) and to protrude her tongue to a maximum. The observer sits opposite at eye level and inspects the pharyngeal structures. The airway is then classified according to the structures seen. If the soft palate, faucial pillars, and uvula are fully visualized, exposure of the glottis on direct laryngoscopy is usually easy. If the uvula is masked by the base of the tongue, some difficulty in exposing the glottis can be anticipated. If only the soft palate is visible or, indeed, if the soft palate is also masked by the base of the tongue, visualization of the glottis may not be possible using the conventional laryngoscope (Fig. 12.19) (203–205). If possible difficulty in intubating the parturient is suspected, an alternative to the usual rapid-sequence intubation should be used. This may include regional anesthesia, awake nasal intubation, or awake fiberoptic intubation. A vasoconstrictor should be applied to the nasal mucosa prior to nasal intubation. Cocaine 4% or a mixture of lidocaine 4% and neosynephrine 0.25% are both effective.

Despite careful preoperative evaluation, there still may be times when, following rapid-sequence induction, the anesthesiologist is unable to intubate the patient. A plan to manage a failed intubation is shown in Figure 12.20. Persistent attempts at intubation and repeated doses of succinylcholine should be avoided. Maternal hypoxia and chances of aspiration are more likely during prolonged attempts at intubation when tracheal intubation is unsuccessful. A call for help should be initiated, cricoid pressure maintained, and the patient ventilated by mask with 100% oxygen. The surgical team should be apprised of the problem and alerted to prepare for transtracheal jet ventilation and/or cricothyroidotomy.

If the indications for cesarean section are not immediately life threatening to the mother or fetus, the mother should be allowed to awaken and anesthesia continued with either an awake intubation or a regional block. If there is an immediate life-threatening maternal or fetal problem, a judgment must be made concerning the relative risks of proceeding. If mask ventilation is relatively easy, general anesthesia without intubation may be an acceptable alternative. The preferred anesthetic agent for this approach, the method of ventilation, and decisions about subsequent attempts at intubation after delivery of the baby are controversial. Under any circumstance, adequate maternal oxygen and ventilation should be maintained, adequate depth of anesthesia provided, and cricoid pressure continuously applied. Halothane is frequently chosen because it is the least irritating of the halogenated agents. An anesthetic dose of halothane may prevent adequate postpartum uterine contraction, and consideration should be given to the use of methergine or other potent oxytocics and/or

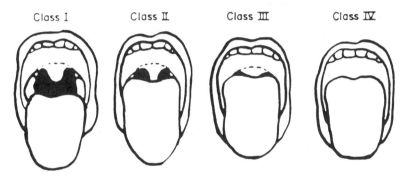

Figure 12.19. Pictorial classification of the pharyngeal structures as seen during examination of the oral pharynx. Class III and IV have been associated with difficulty in visualizing the larynx. (Modified by permission from Samsoon GLT, Young JRB: Difficult tracheal intubation: A retrospective study. Anaesthesia 42:487–490, 1987.)

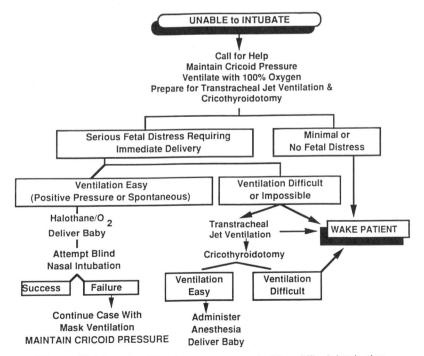

Figure 12.20. Algorithm for management of the difficult intubation.

reducing the concentration of the halogen by supplementing with nitrous oxide, low-dose ketamine, or narcotic.

If ventilation is difficult or impossible, the mother should be allowed to awaken or the airway established surgically. To immediately provide oxygen to the mother, either an appropriately sized laryngeal mask airway (206) is inserted or transtracheal jet ventilation through a percutaneous IV catheter (207) should be instituted. After adequate oxygenation is established, a cricothyroidotomy or tracheostomy may be performed, a cuffed tracheal tube inserted, and anesthesia and surgery should proceed. Under extreme circumstances, some anesthesiologists may choose to proceed with cesarean section under local anesthesia while maternal airway management is in progress. A minimal system for transtracheal jet ventilation is shown in Figure 12.21. The laryngeal mask airway is shown in Chapter 23 (see Fig. 23.8).

There is little clinical experience concerning the safety of either of these two techniques in the obstetric patient with a full stomach. The laryngeal mask is not designed for use in either apneic patients or patients with full stomachs (208–212). Both of these techniques are designed to briefly provide oxygen to the mother while she is awakening or an airway is being established surgically.

Preoxygenation

Oxygen consumption at term is 20% higher than in the nonpregnant state (213). In addition, in pregnant women functional residual capacity is reduced 20% because of upward displacement of the diaphragm (214). Because of the reduced functional residual capacity, the mother is more likely to become hypoxic during induction of anesthesia than is the nonpregnant patient. During a 1-min period of apnea (due to paralysis after preoxygenation), a parturient will sustain a 150-torr reduction in PaO_2, in contrast to a 50-torr reduction in a nonpregnant woman (215). Occasionally, difficult laryngoscopy and several attempts at intubation are encountered. Thus maternal hypoxia is less likely with preoxygenation before induction. The usual method of preoxygenating before induction of general anesthesia is to have the patient breathe 100% oxygen for 3 to 5 min using a tight-fitting face mask. It has been demonstrated that having parturients take four maximally deep inspirations of 100% oxygen within 30 sec of induction of anesthesia is as effective in raising maternal PaO_2 as the standard 3-min preoxygenation (Table 12.13) (216). However, the duration of apnea in these patients was relatively brief ($PaCO_2$ rose only 8 to 9 torr). In a similar study using nonpregnant patients, oxygen saturation decreased more rapidly in subjects preoxygenated with four breaths compared to those preoxygenated for 3 min (Table 12.14) (217).

Table 12.13
Maternal Blood Gas Values with Preoxygenation for Cesarean Section[a]

	Blood Gas	100% Oxygen	
		3 Min ($n = 8$)	4 Deep Breaths ($n = 9$)
Baseline	PaO_2	101	103
	$PaCO_2$	31	32
After preoxygenation	PaO_2	376	408
	$PaCO_2$	32	31
After intubation	PaO_2	264	313
	$PaCO_2$	40	40

[a] Modified from Norris MC, Dewan DM: Preoxygenation for cesarean section: A comparison of two techniques. Anesthesiology 62:827–829, 1985.

Table 12.14
Time to Arterial Desaturation for Subjects Preoxygenated with Two Different Techniques[a,b]

Saturation (%)	3 Min ($n = 6$)	4 Breaths ($n = 6$)
97	7.9	5.6
95	8.4	6.0
93	8.6	6.3
90	8.9	6.8

[a] Modified from Gambee AM, Hertzka RE, Fisher DM: Preoxygenation techniques: Comparison of three minutes and four breaths. Anesth Analg 66:468–470, 1987.
[b] Subjects were not pregnant. Pregnant patients would be expected to desaturate more quickly because of their decreased Functional Residual Capacity (FRC) and increased oxygen consumption.

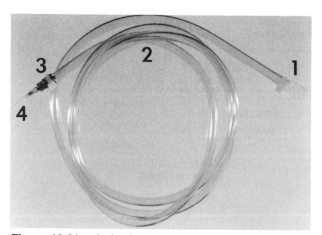

Figure 12.21. A simple transtracheal jet ventilation system designed to use the anesthesia machine fresh-gas outlet and flush valve. The components are (1) 15-mm ETT tube adapter, (2) oxygen-supply tubing, (3) hose barb male luer lock, and (4) intravenous catheter with standard hub.

Reduced Anesthetic Requirements

Anesthetic requirements are decreased during pregnancy. In the experimental animal, minimum alveolar concentration (MAC) for halothane, isoflurane, or methoxyflurane is 25 to 40% less in pregnant animals than in nonpregnant animals (Table 12.15) (218). Also, the reduced maternal functional residual capacity results in a faster rate of equilibration between inspired and alveolar (brain) gas tension. Therefore the rate of induction of anesthesia is much more rapid in the pregnant patient, and overdose may easily occur.

Table 12.15
MAC Presented as Percent End-Tidal Anesthetic Concentration (Means ± SE)[a]

	Nonpregnant Ewes ($n = 6$)	Pregnant Ewes ($n = 6$)	Change (%)
Halothane	0.97 ± .04	0.73[b] ± .07	−25
Isoflurane	1.58 ± .07	1.01[c] ± .06	−40
Methoxyflurane	0.26 ± .02	0.18[d] ± .01	−32

[a] Reprinted by permission from Palahniuk RJ, Shnider SM, Eger EI II: Pregnancy decreases the requirements for inhaled anesthetic agents. Anesthesiology 41:82–83, 1974.
[b] $P < .001$.
[c] $P < .010$.
[d] $P < .025$.

Maternal Ventilation

Under anesthesia, excessive positive pressure ventilation (maternal $PaCO_2$ less than 20 torr) may result in fetal hypoxemia and acidosis (219). The etiologic factors include reduced uterine and umbilical blood flow and increased affinity of maternal hemoglobin for oxygen (Bohr effect), resulting in less placental transfer of oxygen (Figs. 12.22, 12.23, and 12.24). The anesthesiologist should try to maintain a normal $PaCO_2$, which at term ranges between 30 and 33 torr.

Maternal and Fetal Effects of Anesthetic Agents

THIOPENTAL

Thiopental rapidly crosses the placenta, and it is not possible to deliver the baby before the drug is transferred to the fetus. After a single maternal intravenous dose, the drug can be detected in umbilical venous blood within 30 sec (Fig. 12.25) (220). Thiopental reaches its peak concentration in umbilical venous blood in 1 min and in umbilical arterial blood in 2 to 3 min. At delivery, the umbilical vein/maternal vein ratio is close to 1 (221). Why, then, is the neonate not affected? The fetal brain will not be exposed to high concentrations of barbiturate if the induction dose is less than 4 mg/kg. With this dose, umbilical arterial levels of thiopental are much lower than the umbilical venous levels (Fig. 12.26) (222).

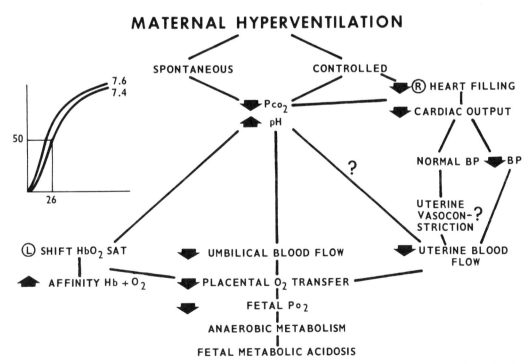

Figure 12.22. Pathophysiology of maternal hyperventilation. (Reprinted by permission from Shnider SM, Moya F: *The Anesthesiologist, Mother and Newborn*. Williams & Wilkins, Baltimore, 1973, p 98.)

Figure 12.23. Changes from control values in mean maternal and fetal arterial oxygen content during five periods of positive pressure ventilation. Mean maternal $PaCO_2$ during each period is indicated at the top of the figure. (Reprinted by permission from Levinson G, Shnider SM, deLorimier AA, Steffenson JL: Effects of maternal hyperventilation on uterine blood flow and fetal oxygenation and acid-base status. Anesthesiology 40:340–347, 1974.)

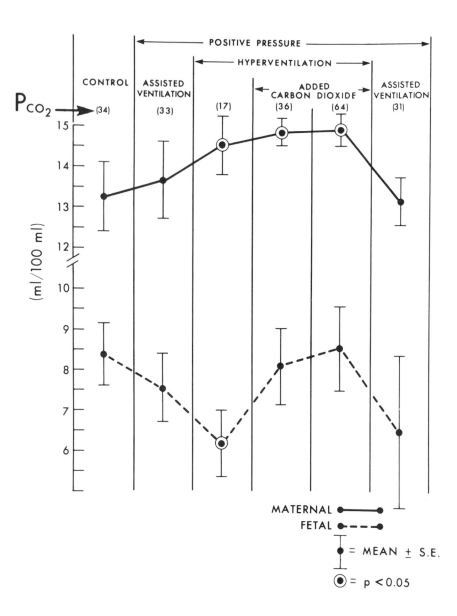

Figure 12.24. The relationship of umbilical vein PO_2 (mm Hg) plotted against maternal end-tidal PCO_2 (mm Hg). The *horizontal broken line* indicates the normal value of fetal umbilical vein PO_2 (28 mm Hg) in 27 healthy patients undergoing cesarean section under general anesthesia. (Reprinted by permission from Cook PT: The influence on foetal outcome of maternal carbon dioxide tension at caesarean section under general anaesthesia. Anesth Intensive Care 12:296–302, 1984.)

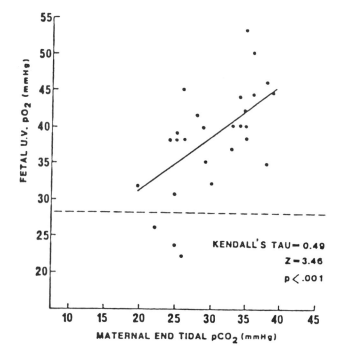

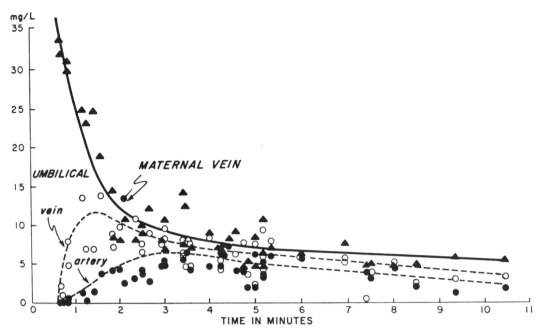

Figure 12.25. The level of thiopental in maternal vein, umbilical vein, and umbilical artery after injection of a single dose of 4 mg/kg for induction of anesthesia. Note the rapid decay of the maternal venous blood level and the rapid transfer to the fetus. (Reprinted by permission from Kosaka Y, Takahashi T, Mark LC: Intravenous thiobarbiturate anesthesia for cesarean section. Anesthesiology 31:489–506, 1969.)

Figure 12.26. Relationship between the concentration of thiopental in umbilical artery and umbilical vein at birth. (Reprinted by permission from Finster M, Mark LC, Morishima HO, Moya F, Perel JM, James LS, Dayton PG: Plasma thiopental concentrations in the newborn following delivery under thiopental-nitrous oxide anesthesia. Am J Obstet Gynecol 95:621–629, 1966.)

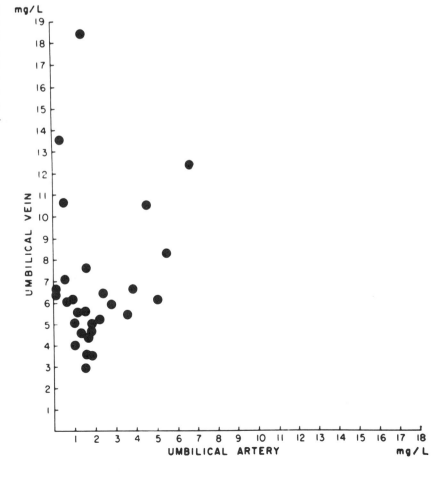

Blood from the placenta either passes through the liver or traverses the ductus venosus into the inferior vena cava. Therefore most of the thiopental is either cleared by the liver or diluted by blood from the lower extremities and viscera. Uptake of thiopental by fetal liver is probably not a significant factor in the observed resistance of the fetal brain to maternally administered barbiturate following a single intravenous injection. Other reasons for lack of neonatal depression after a sleep dose of thiopental are swift decline of the drug concentration in maternal blood due to redistribution, nonhomogeneity of blood in the intervillous space, and progressive dilution in the circulation due to shunting. There is no advantage to delaying delivery until the thiopental has redistributed in the mother or fetus. It should be stressed that, after large doses of thiobarbiturate (8 mg/kg), babies are depressed (220).

KETAMINE

Ketamine is used for induction of anesthesia in patients with possible hypovolemia or with acute asthma. The drug produces minimal respiratory depression and usually increases arterial blood pressure 10 to 25%. Undesirable hypertension may occur, and the drug should not be given to patients with high blood pressure. In the bleeding hypotensive patient, cardiovascular stimulation is desirable, and ketamine may be the preferred induction agent for general anesthesia. Emergence delirium and hallucinations are common with high doses in unpremedicated patients (223). Premedication with, or coadministration of, diazepam decreases the incidence of psychotomimetic side effects (224).

Because ketamine has vasopressor effects and many vasoactive compounds decrease uterine blood flow, several investigators have examined the effects of ketamine on uterine perfusion. In both pregnant ewes and monkeys, the increase in maternal blood pressure was not associated with a reduction in uterine blood flow (225–227). Ketamine produces a dose-related oxytocic effect on uterine tone when administered during the second trimester of pregnancy (228, 229) (see Fig. 14.20). However, when ketamine (2 mg/kg) is administered at term for cesarean section, no increase in intrauterine pressure is noted (see Fig. 14.21).

Ketamine crosses the placenta rapidly but does not produce neonatal depression unless used in doses above 1 mg/kg (see Fig. 8.20) (230, 231). At higher doses, low Apgar scores and neonatal muscular hypertonicity have been reported. In several instances, even with endotracheal intubation, ventilation of the infant has been difficult because of excessive muscle tone.

When ketamine is used in a single intravenous dose of 1 mg/kg for induction of general anesthesia for cesarean section, neonatal neurobehavioral test scores are slightly higher than after thiopental (4 mg/kg) (232). The Apgar scores and fetal acid-base status at birth are similar after ketamine or thiopental anesthesia (233, 234). However, it is unlikely that ketamine will replace thiopental as the routine induction agent of choice because of ketamine's psychotomimetic properties. On the other hand, ketamine offers distinct advantages over thiopental in the severely hypotensive, hypovolemic parturient or the patient with severe asthma (235). Ketamine should not be administered to the obstetric patient in doses greater than 1 mg/kg because an unacceptably high incidence of neonatal depression is found.

Some authors have suggested that anesthesia be induced with ketamine (0.5 to 0.7 mg/kg) combined with a smaller dose of thiopental (2 mg/kg). Reputed advantages of this approach are: less hemodynamic effects, ability to use 100% oxygen, less maternal recall, and better neonatal neurobehavioral scores. However, a study comparing the induction of anesthesia with either thiopental (4 mg/kg) to induction with a combination of thiopental (2 mg/kg) and ketamine (0.5 mg/kg) did not demonstrate any advantage in regard to maternal recall, hemodynamic responses, or neonatal neurobehavioral scores (236).

PROPOFOL

Propofol is a new intravenous anesthetic agent that is becoming increasingly popular in nonobstetric patients for induction of anesthesia and, using an infusion technique, for maintenance of anesthesia. Desirable properties of the drug include rapid induction followed by rapid recovery with a low incidence of postoperative side effects. The drug has not yet been approved for obstetric anesthesia and clinical experiences are still limited.

Studies in pregnant sheep indicate that anesthetic induction and maintenance with propofol has no direct adverse effects on ovine uterine blood flow or fetal well-being (237). The adverse effects of laryngoscopy and intubation on uterine blood flow were not accentuated by propofol but were exacerbated significantly with thiopental. A number of clinical studies have compared propofol (2 to 2.8 mg/kg) to thiopental (4 to 5 mg/kg) for induction of cesarean section anesthesia (238–247). Propofol induction did not produce more hypotension than thiopental. With both drugs, arterial blood pressure rose significantly with endotracheal intubation but the rise was less with propofol. Increases in heart rate accompanying intubation were similar for both drugs, although in one small study 2 of 6 patients developed severe bradycardia following administration of propofol and succinylcholine (248). Similarly, in pregnant sheep, propofol exaggerated the effects of succinylcholine on maternal heart rate, causing severe bradycardia during induction (237). This effect suggests that combining propofol with succinylcholine conveys potential maternal risk, which may limit the usefulness of propofol. Placental transfer of propofol appears to be similar to thiopental. The neonatal condition as appraised by Apgar scores, umbilical cord acid-base status, and NACS has been reported to be comparable to thiopental induction in most studies, but there have been some reports of lower Apgar scores, muscular hypotonus, and transient somnolence after propofol administration (238).

ETOMIDATE

Etomidate, a carboxylated imidazole, has minimal effects on cardiorespiratory function when used for the induction of anesthesia in a dose of 0.3 mg/kg. It is not a popular induction agent for cesarean section despite a favorable report (249). This is probably due to the high incidence of pain on injection and the involuntary muscle movements in unpremedicated patients (250). It also suppresses cortisol production in the neonate (251).

MUSCLE RELAXANTS

Muscle relaxants are commonly used prior to delivery to facilitate rapid endotracheal intubation and provide optimum operating conditions in a lightly anesthetized patient. Muscle relaxants have low lipid solubility and are highly ionized at physiologic pH. When conventional doses are administered clinically, insignificant placental transfer occurs (252–256).

Succinylcholine administered to the mother in high doses (2 to 3 mg/kg) is detectable in fetal blood and may cause alterations in the electromyograph (257), but it has no depressant effects on neonatal respiration. Only with maternal administration of massive doses (10 mg/kg) does enough placental transfer occur to cause neonatal depression (258). Despite reduced plasma pseudocholinesterase in parturients (259, 260), metabolism of moderate doses of succi-

nylcholine is usually not prolonged (Table 12.16) (261). In some patients, however, pseudocholinesterase levels are so low they result in a prolonged block (259). Also, in patients with atypical cholinesterase, prolonged maternal and neonatal respiratory depression have been reported (262). After injection of an intubating dose of succinylcholine, return of neuromuscular function should be ensured before additional relaxant is administered.

Nondepolarizing muscle relaxants may be administered in small doses to prevent fasciculations from succinylcholine and in larger doses to maintain muscle relaxation during surgery. Because these nondepolarizing relaxants are easily reversible, the authors prefer them to a continuous infusion of succinylcholine. Pancuronium and curare had been the more commonly used relaxants, but atracurium and vecuronium, because of their shorter duration of action, have become the preferred agents (254–256, 263). As with curare (264) and pancuronium (265), placental transfer does occur (with similar umbilical venous/maternal venous ratios of approximately 0.1 to 0.2) (254–256). With clinical doses (curare, 0.2 mg/kg; pancuronium or vecuronium, 0.05 mg/kg; or atracurium, 0.5 mg/kg), there are no adverse neonatal effects of these drugs as measured by Apgar scores, umbilical cord acid-base status, or neonatal neurobehavioral scores.

NITROUS OXIDE

Nitrous oxide is the most popular inhalation agent in obstetric anesthesia. It produces no significant uterine relaxation. It is rapidly transferred across the placenta, but fetal tissue uptake during the first 20 min reduces the fetal arterial concentration and subsequent neonatal depression (266, 267) (see Figs. 11.2 and 11.3). It is well documented that, the longer the duration of anesthesia with nitrous oxide, the more anesthetized the newborn may be (268, 269). These studies were done using 70%, rather than the currently more common 50%, nitrous oxide, and the effect of the time from induction to delivery was more exaggerated. With current techniques, time may not be as critical. Nevertheless, the duration of anesthesia prior to delivery should be as brief as possible.

Table 12.16
Time to Twitch Recovery after Succinylcholine[a]

	Succinylcholine (mg)	Twitch Recovery (min)		
		10%	50%	90%
Nonpregnant women (n = 15)	144	10.2	11.9	13.3
Cesarean sections (n = 10)	148	9.9	11.5	12.9

[a] Adapted from Blitt CD, Petty WC, Alberternst EE, Wright BJ: Correlation of plasma cholinesterase activity and duration of action of succinylcholine during pregnancy. Anesth Analg 56:78–81, 1977.

This can be accomplished by delaying induction of anesthesia until the patient is prepped and draped and the obstetrician is ready to begin the operation.

HALOGENATED AGENTS

The use of low-dose halothane (0.5%), isoflurane (0.75%) or enflurane (1.0%) as supplements to nitrous oxide anesthesia is very common. The nitrous oxide concentration is usually reduced from 70 to 50%. The halogenated agents (a) decreased the likelihood of maternal postoperative recall and awareness of intraoperative events; (b) permit higher maternal inspired oxygen tension; (c) may improve uterine blood flow; (d) do not result in increased uterine bleeding; and (e) do not depress the newborn.

Maternal Awareness

Several surveys have reported a high incidence of maternal awareness of surgery and birth with subsequent unpleasant experiences such as nightmares following nitrous oxide-oxygen relaxant technique for vaginal delivery or cesarean section (Table 12.17) (270–278). The incidence of awareness appears to vary inversely with the concentration of nitrous oxide. For example, in one study approximately 9% of parturients who received 67% nitrous oxide in oxygen were aware of the delivery, whereas 26% were aware if 50% nitrous oxide was used (270). No maternal awareness of pain has been reported if halothane 0.1 to 0.65%, enflurane 0.5 to 1.5%, methoxyflurane 0.1%, or isoflurane 0.75% is added to 50% nitrous oxide before delivery (272–280).

Higher Maternal Oxygen

Maternal hyperoxia should improve fetal oxygenation and neonatal clinical condition at birth. In a study of 75 healthy women undergoing elective cesarean section under general anesthesia, oxygen tension, saturation, and content of fetal blood increased significantly with increases in maternal inspired oxygen concentration until maternal PaO_2 reached approximately 300 torr (Table 12.18) (281). The clinical condition of the newborn was also better in the higher oxygen groups. It was noted that there was no additional fetal or neonatal benefit if the maternal oxygen tension was above 300 torr.

Other investigators (282, 283) compared anesthesia with either 50% oxygen (balance nitrous oxide and halogenated agent) to anesthesia with 100% ox-

Table 12.17
Maternal Awareness of Surgery and Birth after Barbiturate-Relaxant Induction

Anesthetic and Investigator	Incidence of Awareness (%)
Nitrous oxide 50%	
Crawford (246)	26
Wilson and Turner (247)	19
Warren et al. (255)	17
Abboud et al. (256)	12
Nitrous oxide 67–75%	
Crawford (246)	9
Wilson and Turner (247)	10
Moir (248)	4
Palahniuk et al. (249)	5
Nitrous oxide 25–40% + halothane 0.3–0.5% (Galbert and Gardner [250])	0
Nitrous oxide 50% + halothane 0.1–0.65%	
Moir (248)	0
Wilson (251)	0
Latto and Waldron (252)	0
Warren et al. (255)	0
Abboud et al. (256)	0
Nitrous oxide 50% + enflurane 0.5–1.5%	
Coleman and Downing (253)	0
Warren et al. (255)	0
Abboud et al. (256)	0
Nitrous oxide 33% + methoxyflurane 0.1% (Crawford et al. [254])	3.5
Nitrous oxide 50% + isoflurane 0.75% (Warren et al. [255])	0

Table 12.18
Improvement in Umbilical Venous and Umbilical Arterial Blood Oxygen Tensions and Neonatal Condition at Birth with Increasing Maternal Oxygen Tension[a]

	61–100	101–160	181–240	241–300	301–360	361–420	421–520
Maternal arterial PO_2 (torr)							
Number	13	12	3	10	19	11	7
Umbilical venous PO_2 (torr)	29	31	29	35	38	41	41
Umbilical artery PO_2 (torr)	16	20	21	23	25	26	25
Time necessary for infant to establish sustained respiration (sec)	62	54	33	27	11	13	14
Number of infants with Apgar score of 6 or less	4	2	1	0[b]	0	0	0

[a]Modified from Marx GF, Mateo CV: Effects of different oxygen concentrations during general anaesthesia for elective caesarean section. Can Anaesth Soc J 18:587–593, 1971.
[b]There was no further change as maternal arterial PO_2 rose above 300 torr.

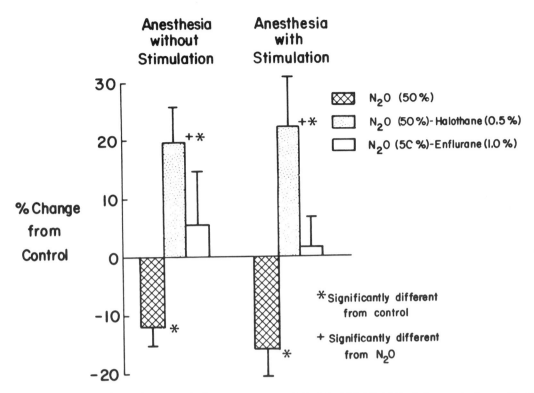

Figure 12.27. Uterine blood flow changes during anesthesia in the pregnant ewe with and without noxious stimulation. The three anesthetics administered for 1 hr each were nitrous oxide 50%, nitrous oxide 50% plus halothane 0.5%, and nitrous oxide 50% plus enflurane 1.0%. (Reprinted by permission from Shnider SM, Wright RG, Levinson G, Roizen MF, Rolbin SH, Biehl D, Johnson J, Jones M: Plasma norepinephrine and uterine blood flow changes during endotracheal intubation and general anesthesia in the pregnant ewe. In *Abstracts of Scientific Papers*, American Society of Anesthesiologists, Chicago, 1978, p 115.)

ygen and halogenated agent. The use of 100% oxygen significantly improved fetal oxygenation with particular benefit in emergency cases. Babies born to mothers who received 100% oxygen required less resuscitation than those whose mothers received 50% oxygen.

Improved Uterine Blood Flow

Anesthetic agents modify sympathetic activity. The authors have shown that, in pregnant sheep, noxious stimulation during nitrous oxide-oxygen anesthesia was associated with an increase in maternal blood pressure, a decrease in uterine blood flow, and an increase in plasma norepinephrine compared to the awake control state (284). By contrast, noxious stimulation during nitrous oxide-oxygen anesthesia supplemented with either 0.5% halothane or 1% enflurane did not increase plasma catecholamines. Blood pressure remained unchanged in both groups, and uterine blood flow increased with halothane but did not change with enflurane (Fig. 12.27).

Uterine Bleeding

The main concerns associated with the administration of halogenated agents are that they may decrease uterine muscle tone and that postpartum blood loss will increase. The halogenated agents produce a dose-related decrease in uterine contractility and tone (285–289). However, several studies have failed to reveal any increased blood loss with low-dose halothane 0.1 to 0.8% (Tables 12.19 and 12.20) (272, 274–276, 280, 290), enflurane 0.5 to 1.5% (277), or isoflurane 0.75% during cesarean section. At these low concentrations, the uterus in the immediate postpartum period is responsive to oxytocin stimulation (289). One study (291) did show that the addition of halogenated agents was associated with a greater fall in postpartum hematocrit and an increased requirement for blood transfusion. However, it is apparent that, in this retrospective analysis, the group receiving halogenated agent was not comparable to the other groups. When higher concentrations of halogenated agents are used (282, 283), blood loss is still not clinically significantly increased and their regimens, as described in Table 12.21, may be useful when

Table 12.19
Influence of Anesthesia on Blood Loss of 145 Cesarean Sections[a]

	Anesthetic			
	N_2O-O_2 (70:30) (50 Cases)	N_2O-O_2 (50:50) + 0.5% Halothane (50 Cases)	N_2O-O_2 (50:50) + 0.8% Halothane (25 Cases)	Epidural Analgesia (20 Cases)
Loss (mean ± SD) (ml)	792 ± 388	688 ± 206	702 ± 294	378 ± 146

[a] Reprinted by permission from Moir DD: Anaesthesia for caesarean section: An evaluation of a method using low concentrations of halothane and 50 percent of oxygen. Br J Anaesth 42:136–142, 1970.

Table 12.20
Hematocrit Values before and after Cesarean Section[a]

Anesthetic Technique[b]	Hematocrit (Preoperative)	Hematocrit Postoperative Day 1	Postoperative Day 2
Halothane predelivery (n = 22)	37.7 ± 9.1	31.8 ± 4.3	31.4 ± 4.4
Halothane pre- and postdelivery (n = 20)	36.9 ± 3.9	30.8 ± 4.6	29.6 ± 4.3
Epidural (n = 23)	37.9 ± 9.1	33.1 ± 4.6	31.7 ± 4.1

[a] Reprinted by permission from Thirion A-V, Wright RG, Messer CP, Rosen MA, Shnider SM. Maternal blood loss associated with low dose halothane administration for cesarean section. Anesthesiology 69:A693, 1988.
[b] Effect of low-dose halothane during cesarean section on intraoperative blood loss as estimated by postpartum hematocrit changes. Patients received (a) nitrous oxide and halothane 0.5% predelivery and nitrous oxide and narcotic postdelivery; (b) nitrous oxide with halothane 0.5% throughout the operation; (c) epidural anesthesia.

Table 12.21
Effect of Various Anesthetic Regimens on Blood Loss and Change in Hemoglobin over 48 Hours Following Cesarean Section[a]

	N_2O/O_2–50:50, Halothane 0.5%		100% O_2, Halothane 1.1% × 5 min, then Halothane 0.75%		100% O_2, Enflurane 2.5% × 5 min, then Enflurane 1.7%		100% O_2, Isoflurane 1.8% × 5 min, then Isoflurane 1.2%	
	Elective	Emergent	Elective	Emergent	Elective	Emergent	Elective	Emergent
Mean blood loss	619	896	689	740	874[b]	610	613	641
SD	87	559	197	191	317	270	205	145
Mean maximum decrease in Hb (%)	5.5	13.1	7.4	21.4	8.3	12.8	11.4*	15.6
SD	2.8	5.3	5.3	10.3	5.6	7.5	4.8	7.2

[a] Modified with permission from Piggott SE, Bogod DG, Rosen M, Rees GAD, Harmer M. Isoflurane with either 100% oxygen or 50% nitrous oxide in oxygen for caesarean section. Br J Anaesth 65:325–329, 1990.
[b] $p < 0.05$

high inspired maternal oxygen concentrations are indicated.

Neonatal Depression

A potential hazard of the use of these potent inhalational agents is neonatal depression. However, clinical experience indicates that the slight increase in maternal anesthetic depth is not reflected in the neonate at birth (272–280, 282, 283).

REGIONAL VERSUS GENERAL ANESTHESIA: CONDITION OF THE NEWBORN

A neonate is conventionally evaluated by Apgar score, acid-base status, and neurobehavioral exami-

nation. Although it is widely believed that regional anesthesia is safer for the newborn, many studies indicate that either technique can result in vigorous, well-oxygenated babies.

Apgar Score

Virginia Apgar was the first to point out that babies were more vigorous following cesarean section under conduction (spinal) than general (cyclopropane) anesthesia (292). Since then numerous studies have confirmed these findings. For example, the Collaborative Project (a research study involving 15 medical centers) found that, in 405 normal gravidas undergoing elective repeat cesarean section, more than five times as many neonates were depressed at 1 min (Apgar 0 to 3) when delivery occurred under general anesthesia as compared to regional anesthesia (293). Moreover, in this study, three times as many newborns had depressed Apgar scores at 5 min after general anesthesia in contrast to regional anesthesia. This prolonged depression, the authors believe, probably represents inadequate management of the newborn. The authors have found that, after general anesthesia with a thiopental induction followed by 70% nitrous oxide, despite a high incidence of depressed newborns at 1 min, by 5 min of age (after stimulation and assisted ventilation) babies are as vigorous as those after regional anesthesia (Table 12.22). The low initial Apgar score in these babies is clearly due to transient sedation rather than asphyxia. This transient sedation can be markedly reduced with anesthetic techniques that include higher concentrations of oxygen and only 50% nitrous oxide, combined with low-dose halogenated agents, continuous lateral tilt, and reasonably expeditious delivery times (less than 10 to 15 min from induction to delivery).

In the largest study to date (294), a review of 3940 cesarean deliveries between 1975 and 1983, a multivariate analysis showed the risk of poor neonatal outcome was greater after general than regional anesthesia. They found that general anesthesia, whether for elective or emergency cesarean section, was an independent risk factor for low Apgar scores after controlling for numerous other variables. Furthermore, the analysis of the elective cesarean group also found significantly better Apgar scores after regional anesthesia.

Although the infants born of mothers given general anesthesia had lower 1-min Apgar scores and required more active respiratory resuscitation after birth, there was marked improvement in the 5-min Apgar scores and no significant difference in the neonatal death rates between the infants delivered by cesarean section under regional anesthesia and those under general anesthesia. With any technique, babies delivered shortly after the induction of general anesthesia are as vigorous as those born with regional anesthesia (Tables 12.23 and 12.24). The authors found

that neonatal depression after general anesthesia is related to the duration of anesthesia, which is in agreement with numerous other studies (267, 268, 295, 296). For example, Stenger et al. (267) reported a 15% incidence of depressed neonates when the mean duration of nitrous oxide anesthesia was 15 min and a 54% incidence when the duration was 36 min. Finster and Poppers (268) found that, when duration of anesthesia was less than 10 min, the mean Apgar score was 7.7; it decreased to 6.8 in the group delivered after 11 to 20 min and to 6.3 when the duration of anesthesia before delivery exceeded 21 min.

Thus, when general anesthesia is chosen, expeditious delivery of the newborn is necessary to minimize neonatal depression. If a prolonged operating time is anticipated, regional anesthesia may be preferable. In contrast to general anesthesia, the authors have found that a prolonged duration of epidural anesthesia does not result in depressed neonates (Table 12.24). In addition, the hypotension so common with regional anesthesia, when properly and promptly treated, does not result in low Apgar scores (Table 12.25 and Fig. 12.6).

Table 12.23
Elective Cesarean Section: Duration of (General Anesthesia (N₂O–o₂) Antepartum and Apgar Scores[a]

Minutes of Anesthesia	Apgar Score: 7 to 10	
	Number	Percent
<5	16	88
6–10	47	74
11–20	36	69
21–30	20	50
31–60	11	36

[a] Reprinted by permission from Rolbin SH, Levinson G, Shnider SM: Current status of anesthesia for cesarean section. *Weekly Anesthesiology Update, Volume 1, Lesson 7*. Weekly Anesthesiology Update, Inc., Princeton, NJ, 1977.

Table 12.24
Elective Cesarean Section: Duration of Epidural Anesthesia Antepartum and Apgar Scores

Minutes of Anesthesia	Apgar Score: 7 to 10	
	Number	Percent
<20	20	85
21–30	44	93
31–60	214	92
61–120	40	90
>120	5	100

[a] Reprinted by permission from Rolbin SH, Levinson G, Shnider SM: Current status of anesthesia for cesarean section. *Weekly Anesthesiology Update, Volume 1, Lesson 7*. Weekly Anesthesiology Update, Inc., Princeton, NJ, 1977.

Table 12.22
Elective Cesarean Section: Clinical Condition of Newborn

	Apgar Score: 7 to 10 (%)	
	1 Min	5 Min
Spinal (n = 151)	92	97
Epidural (n = 327)	91	99
General (n = 163)	69	97

Table 12.25
Elective Cesarean Section: Hypotension and Condition of Infant

		Number	Apgar Scores 7 to 10 (%)	
Spinal	Hypotension	104	91	
	No hypotension	47	100	NS[a]
Epidural	Hypotension	102	88	
	No hypotension	227	93	NS

[a]NS = No statistically significant difference between hypotension and no hypotension.

Acid-Base Status

Numerous investigators have compared fetal acid-base status in umbilical cord blood sampled from a doubly clamped segment immediately after elective cesarean section delivery (269, 273, 297–300). As seen in Table 12.26, the differences between the techniques are minimal and not clinically significant. With any technique the acid-base status of the neonate should be in the normal range. Even with prolonged general anesthesia and depressed Apgar scores (i.e., sleepy babies), fetal acid-base status is normal.

If fetal hypoxia and acidosis are found with elective cesarean section, a number of etiologic factors may exist. With general anesthesia, maternal hypoxia, excessive hyperventilation, aortocaval compression, or anesthetic overdose may all cause fetal asphyxia. With regional anesthesia, unrecognized or improperly treated hypotension is the most likely cause of fetal acidosis. ***With either technique a prolonged uterine incision-to-delivery time has been found to be directly related to fetal hypoxia and acidosis.***

Crawford and Davies (301) found that, with cesarean section under general anesthesia, the condition of the infant, both clinical and biochemical, was directly related to the time that elapsed from the initial uterine incision to completion of delivery. This was confirmed by Datta et al. (302), who found that, with both general and spinal anesthesia, uterine incision-to-delivery intervals exceeding 3 min were associated with a significantly lower pH in the baby and a higher incidence of depressed Apgar scores. Prolonged uterine incision-delivery intervals during regional anesthesia results in elevated fetal umbilical artery norepinephrine concentrations and associated fetal acidosis (303).

Neurobehavioral Examination

Even when neonates are not depressed at birth as ascertained by low Apgar scores, more subtle neurobehavioral changes in the subsequent neonatal period may occur. This is discussed fully in Chapter

Table 12.26
Fetal Acid-Base Status with General Versus Regional Anesthesia

	MA		UV		UA	
	pH	BD	pH	BD	pH	BD
Marx et al. (274)						
General (n = 14)	7.42	3.5	7.30	4.9	7.23	6.5
Spinal (n = 10)	7.40	4.6	7.30	5.1	7.24	6.0
Datta and Brown (275)						
General (n = 15)	7.46	0.6	7.38	—	7.30	1.9
Spinal (n = 15)	7.43	0.7	7.34	—	7.28	1.4
Shnider (245)						
General (n = 39)	7.46	3.6	7.36	2.3	7.29	2.9
Spinal (n = 26)	7.42	3.9	7.33	3.3	7.23	4.7
James et al. (277)						
General (n = 20)	7.47	3.0	7.38	1.9	7.32	1.8
Epidural (n = 15)	7.44	3.0	7.35	1.6	7.30	1.3
Palahniuk et al. (249)						
General (n = 11)	7.42	2.8	7.37	4.2	7.31	4.2
Epidural (n = 14)	—	—	7.34	4.5	7.30	6.3
Shnider[b]						
General (n = 41)	7.46	3.6	7.36	2.3	7.29	2.9
Epidural (n = 30)	7.45	3.8	7.32	5.1	7.23	5.7
Fox et al. (276)						
General (n = 20)	7.39	4.6	7.35	3.4	7.31	3.9
Epidural (n = 20)	7.44	4.4	7.36	3.5	7.29	5.0

[a]MA = maternal arterial blood; UV = umbilical venous blood; UA = umbilical arterial blood; BD = base deficit.
[b]Data from a review of UCSF data on elective cesarean sections.

38. Using the early neonatal behavioral scale on infants delivered by cesarean section, Scanlon et al. (304) reported that infants born after general anesthesia with nitrous oxide were more depressed 6 to 8 hr later than those born after regional anesthesia. Palahnuik et al. (273), Hodgkinson et al. (305), and Abboud et al. (306) reported similar results. In all studies, the neurobehavioral effects were subtle and essentially disappeared by 24 hr of age. Hollmén et al. (307) found that neurobehavioral scores were lower in infants born after epidural rather than general anesthesia, but several of the mothers had hypotension that was not promptly treated. Abboud et al. (308) found that hypotension, when promptly treated, did not result in babies with depressed neurobehavioral scores.

EMERGENCY CESAREAN SECTION

Sudden, unexpected complications during late pregnancy or labor that adversely affect the mother or fetus may necessitate an immediate emergency cesarean section. Examples include massive third-trimester bleeding, prolapsed umbilical cord, or severe fetal distress. When the mother or fetus is in immediate jeopardy, cesarean section should not be

239

delayed to establish an adequate sensory level with either a spinal or epidural block. For some emergency cesarean sections in which neither the mother nor fetus is in imminent danger, immediate delivery is not crucial. Examples include repeat section in early labor, failure of induction, failure to progress, failed forceps delivery, chorioamnionitis, malpresentation, and mild to moderate fetal distress. In these situations either regional or general anesthesia may be administered (309, 310).

Anesthesia for cesarean section in the presence of some of the more common and significant obstetric and medical complications is discussed in the chapters on preeclampsia-eclampsia (Chapter 17) and placenta previa, abruptio placentae, and ruptured uterus (Chapter 21); parturients with cardiac disease (Chapter 27); and the diabetic parturient (Chapter 29).

References

1. Notzon FC: International differences in the use of obstetric interventions. JAMA 263:3286–3291, 1990.
2. Notzon FC, Placek PJ, Taffel SM: Comparisons of national cesarean-section rates. N Engl J Med 316:386–389, 1987.
3. Evrard J, Gold EM: Cesarean section and maternal mortality in Rhode Island: Incidence and risk factors, 1965–1975. Obstet Gynecol 50:594–597, 1977.
4. Rubin GL, Peterson HB, Rochat RW, McCarthy BJ, Terry JS: Maternal death after cesarean section in Georgia. Am J Obstet Gynecol 139:681–685, 1981.
5. Petitti DB, Cefalo RC, Shapiro S, Whalley P: In-hospital maternal mortality in the United States: Time trends and relation to method of delivery. Obstet Gynecol 59:6–12, 1982.
6. Frigoletto RD Jr, Ryan KJ, Phillippe M: Maternal mortality rate associated with cesarean section: An appraisal. Am J Obstet Gynecol 136:969–970, 1980.
7. Hicks JS, Levinson G, Shnider SM: Obstetric anesthesia training centers in the U.S.A.—1975. Anesth Analg 55:839–845, 1976.
8. Gibbs CP, Krischer J, Peckham BM, Sharp H, Kirschbaum TH: Obstetric anesthesia: A national survey. Anesthesiology 65:298–306, 1986.
9. Roberts RB, Shirley MA: The obstetrician's role in reducing the risk of aspiration pneumonitis with particular reference to the use of oral antacids. Am J Obstet Gynecol 124:611–617, 1976.
10. Brizgys RV, Dailey PA, Shnider SM, Kotelko DM, Levinson G: The incidence and neonatal effects of maternal hypotension during epidural anesthesia for cesarean section. Anesthesiology 67:782–786, 1987.
11. Gutsche BB: Prophylactic ephedrine preceding spinal analgesia for cesarean section. Anesthesiology 45:462–465, 1976.
12. Moran D, Perillo M, LaPorta R, Bader A, Datta S: Phenylephrine in the prevention of hypotension following spinal anesthesia for cesarean delivery. J Clin Anesth 3:301–305, 1991.
13. Wollman SB, Marx GF: Acute hydration for prevention of hypotension of spinal anesthesia in parturients. Anesthesiology 29:374–380, 1968.
14. Lewis M, Thomas P, Wilkes RG: Hypotension during epidural analgesia for caesarean section. Anaesthesia 38:250–253, 1983.
15. James FM III, Greiss FC Jr, Kemp RA: An evaluation of vasopressor therapy for maternal hypotension during spinal anesthesia. Anesthesiology 33:25–34, 1970.
16. Shnider SM, deLorimier AA, Holl JW, Chapler FK, Morishima HO: Vasopressors in obstetrics. I. Correction of fetal acidosis with ephedrine during spinal anesthesia. Am J Obstet Gynecol 102:911–919, 1968.
17. Ralston DH, Shnider SM, deLorimier AA: Effects of equipotent ephedrine, metaraminol, mephentermine, and methoxamine on uterine blood flow in the pregnant ewe. Anesthesiology 40:354–370, 1974.
18. Ramanathan S, Grant GJ: Vasopressor therapy for hypotension due to epidural anesthesia for cesarean section. Acta Anaesthesiol Scand 32:559–565, 1988.
19. Ramanathan S, Gandhi S, Arismendy J, Chanon J, Turndorf H: Oxygen transfer from mother to fetus during cesarean section under epidural anesthesia. Anesth Analg 61:576–581, 1982.
20. Chambers WA, Littlewood DG, Scott DB: Spinal anesthesia with hyperbaric bupivacaine: Effect of added vasoconstrictors. Anesth Analg 61:49–52, 1982.
21. Abouleish EI: Epinephrine improves the quality of spinal hyperbaric bupivacaine for cesarean section. Anesth Analg 66:395–400, 1987.
22. Moore DC: Spinal anesthesia: Bupivacaine compared with tetracaine. Anesth Analg 59:743–750, 1980.
23. Santos A, Pedersen H, Finster M, Edström H: Hyperbaric bupivacaine for spinal anesthesia in cesarean section. Anesth Analg 63:1009–1013, 1984.
24. Logan MR, McClure JH, Wildsmith JAW: Plain bupivacaine: An unpredictable spinal anesthetic agent. Br J Anaesth 58:292–296, 1986.
25. Russell IF: Spinal anesthesia for cesarean section. Br J Anaesth 55:309–313, 1983.
26. Norris MC: Height, weight and the spread of hyperbaric bupivacaine in the term parturient. Anesth Analg 67:555–558, 1988.
27. Norris MC: Patient variables and the subarachnoid spread of hyperbaric bupivacaine in the term parturient. Anesthesiology 72:478–482, 1990.
28. Hartwell BL, Aglio LS, Hauch MA, Datta S: Vertebral column length and the spread of hyperbaric subarachnoid bupivacaine in the term parturient. Reg Anesth 16:17–19, 1991.
29. Hunt CO, Naulty JS, Bader AM, Hauch MA, Vartikan JV, Datta S, Hertwig LM, Ostheimer GW: Perioperative analgesia with subarachnoid fentanyl-bupivacaine for cesarean delivery. Anesthesiology 71:535–540, 1989.
30. de Sousa H, de la Vega S: Spinal sufentanil. Reg Anesth 13:S23, 1988.
31. Abboud TK, Dror A, Mosaad P, Zhu J, Mantilla M, Swart F, Gangolly J, Silao P, Makar A, Moore J: Mini-dose intrathecal morphine for the relief of post-cesarean section pain: Safety, efficacy, and ventilatory responses to carbon dioxide. Anesth Analg 67:137–143, 1988.
32. Abouleish E, Rawal N, Fallon K, Hernandez D: Combined intrathecal morphine and bupivacaine for cesarean section. Anesth Analg 67:370–374, 1988.
33. Chadwick SH, Ready LB: Intrathecal and epidural morphine sufate for post-ceasrean analgesia: A clinical comparison. Anesthesiology 68:925–929, 1988.
34. Stenkamp SJ, Easterling TR, Chadwick HS: Effect of epidural and intrathecal morphine on the length of hospital stay after cesarean section. Anesth Analg 68:66–69, 1989.
35. Wang BC, Hillman DE, Spielholz NI, Turndorf H: Chronic neurological deficits and Nesacaine-CE: An effect of the anesthetic, 2-chloroprocaine, or the antioxidant, sodium bisulfite? Anesth Analg 63:445–447, 1984.
36. Gissen AJ, Datta S, Lambert D: The chloroprocaine controversy: Is chloroprocaine neurotoxic? Reg Anesth 9:135–145, 1984.
37. Fibuch EE, Opper SE: Back pain following epidurally administered Nesacaine-MPF. Anesth Analg 69:113–115, 1989.
38. McLoughlin TM, DiFazio CA: More on back pain after Nesacaine-MPF. Anesth Analg 71:562–563, 1990.
39. Stevens RA, Chester WL, Artuso JD, Bray JG, Nellestein JA: Back pain after epidural anesthesia with chloroprocaine in volunteers: Preliminary report. Reg Anesth 16:199–203, 1991.
40. James FM III: Chloroprocaine vs. bupivacaine for lumbar

epidural analgesia for elective cesarean section. Anesthesiology 52:488–491, 1980.

41. Chestnut DH: The influence of pH-adjusted 2-chloroprocaine on the quality and duration of subsequent epidural bupivacaine analgesia during labor: A randomized, double-blind study. Anesthesiology 70:437–441, 1989.

42. Naulty JS, Hertwig L, Hunt CO: Duration of analgesia of epidural fentanyl following cesarean delivery: Effects of local anesthetic drug selection. Anesthesiology 65:A180, 1986.

43. Malinow AM, Mokriski BLK, Wakefield ML, McGuin WJ, Martz DG, Desverreaux JN, Matjesko MJ: Anesthetic choice affects postcesarean epidural fentanyl analgesia. Anesth Analg 67:S138, 1988.

44. Ackerman WE, Juneja MM: 2-chloroprocaine decreases the duration of analgesia of epidural fentanyl. Anesth Analg 68:S2, 1989.

45. Hughes SC, Wright RG, Murphy D, Preston P, Hughes W, Rosen M, Shnider S: The effect of pH adjusting 3% 2-chloroprocaine on the quality of post-cesarean section analgesia with epidural morphine. Anesthesiology 69:A689, 1988.

46. Bromage PR, Robson JG: Concentrations of lignocaine in the blood after intravenous, intramuscular epidural and endotracheal administration. Anaesthesia 16:461, 1961.

47. Mather LE, Tucker GT, Murphy TM, Stanton-Hicks D'A, Bonica JJ: The effects of adding adrenaline to etidocaine and lignocaine in extradural anaesthesia. II. Pharmacokinetics. Br J Anaesth 48:989–994, 1976.

48. Scott DB, Jebson PJR, Braid DP, Örtengren B, Frisch P: Factors affecting plasma levels of lignocaine and prilocaine. Br J Anaesth 44:1040–1049, 1972.

49. Rosenfeld CR, Barton MD, Meschia G: Effects of epinephrine on distribution of blood flow in the pregnant ewe. Am J Obstet Gynecol 124:156–163, 1976.

50. Wallis KL, Shnider SM, Hicks JS, Spivey HT: Epidural anesthesia in the normotensive pregnant ewe: Effects on uterine blood flow and fetal acid-base status. Anesthesiology 44:481–487, 1976.

51. Rucker MP: The action of adrenalin on the pregnant uterus. South Med J 18:412–418, 1925.

52. Gunther RE, Bauman J: Obstetrical caudal anesthesia. I. A randomized study comparing 1% mepivacaine with 1% lidocaine plus epinephrine. Anesthesiology 31:5–19, 1969.

53. Gunther RE, Bellville JW: Obstetrical caudal anesthesia. II. A randomized study comparing 1 per cent mepivacaine with 1 per cent mepivacaine plus epinephrine. Anesthesiology 37:288–298, 1972.

54. Matadial L, Cibils LA: The effect of epidural anesthesia on uterine activity and blood pressure. Am J Obstet Gynecol 125:846–854, 1976.

55. Zador G, Englesson S, Nilsson BA: Continuous drip epidural anesthesia in labour. II. Influence on labour and foetal acid-base status. Acta Obstet Gynecol 34(Suppl):41–49, 1974.

56. Levinson G, Shnider SM, Krames E, Ring G: Epidural anesthesia for cesarean section: Effects of epinephrine in the local anesthetic solution. In Abstracts of Scientific Papers, American Society of Anesthesiologists, Chicago, 1975, p 285.

57. deRosayro AM, Hahrwold ML, Hill AB: Cardiovascular effects of epidural epinephrine in the pregnant sheep. Reg Anesth 6:4–7, 1981.

58. Albright GA, Jouppila R, Hollmén AI, Joupila P, Vierola H, Kiovula A: Epinephrine does not alter human intervillous blood flow during epidural anesthesia. Anesthesiology 54:131–135, 1981.

59. DiFazio CA, Carron H, Grosslight KR, Moscicki JC, Bolding WR, Johns RA: Comparison of pH-adjusted lidocaine solutions for epidural anesthesia. Anesth Analg 65:760–764, 1986.

60. Galindo A: pH-adjusted local anesthetics: Clinical experience. Reg Anesth 8:35–36, 1983.

61. Douglas MJ: The effect of pH adjustment of bupivacaine on epidural anesthesia for cesarean section. Anesthesiology 65:A380, 1986.

62. McMorland GH, Douglas MJ, Jeffrey WK, Ross PLE, Axelson JE, Kim JHK, Gambling DR, Robertson K: Effect of pH-adjustment of bupivacaine on onset and duration of epidural analgesia in parturients. Can Anaesth Soc J 33:537–541, 1986.

63. Tackley RM: Alkalinized bupivacaine and adrenaline for epidural caesarean section. Anaesthesia 43:1019–1021, 1988.

64. Benhamou D, Labaille T, Bonhomme L, Perrachon N: Alkalinization of epidural 0.5% bupivacaine for cesarean section. Reg Anesth 14:240–243, 1989.

65. Glosten B, Dailey PA, Preston PG, Shnider SM, Ross BK, Rosen MA, Hughes SC: pH-adjusted 2-chloroprocaine for epidural anesthesia in patients undergoing postpartum tubal ligation. Anesthesiology 68:948–950, 1988.

66. Ross BK: Evaluation of epidural pH-adjusted 2% 2-chloroprocaine for labor analgesia. Anesthesiology 67:A629, 1987.

67. Parnass SM, Curran MJA, Becker GL: Incidence of hypotension associated with epidural anesthesia using alkalinized and nonalkalinized lidocaine for cesarean section. Anesth Analg 66:1148–1150, 1987.

68. Peterfreund RA, Datta S, Ostheimer GW: pH adjustment of local anesthetic solutions with sodium bicarbonate: Laboratory evaluation of alkalinization and precipitation. Reg Anesth 14:265–270, 1989.

69. Ikuta PT: pH adjustment schedule for the amide local anesthetics. Reg Anesth 14:229–235, 1989.

70. Naulty JS, Datta S, Ostheimer GW, Johnson MD, Burger GA: Epidural fentanyl for postcesarean delivery pain management. Anesthesiology 63:694–698, 1985.

71. Ackerman WE, Juneja MM, Colclough GW, Kaczorowski DM: Epidural fentanyl significantly decreases nausea and vomiting during uterine manipulation in awake patients undergoing cesarean section. Anesthesiology 69:A679, 1988.

72. Gaffud MP, Bansal P, Lawton C, Velasquez N, Watson WA: Surgical analgesia for cesarean delivery with epidural bupivacaine and fentanyl. Anesthesiology 65:331–334, 1986.

73. Preston PG, Rosen MA, Hughes SC, Glosten B, Ross BK, Daniels D, Shnider SM, Dailey P: Epidural anesthesia with fentanyl and lidocaine for cesarean section: Maternal effects and neonatal outcome. Anesthesiology 68:938–943, 1988.

74. Benlabed M, Midgal M, Dreizzen E, Escourrou P, Ecoffey C, Gaultier C: Neonatal pattern of breathing after cesarean section with or without epidural fentanyl. Anesthesiology 69:A651, 1988.

75. Schlesinger TS, Miletich DJ: Epidural fentanyl and lidocaine during cesarean section: Maternal efficacy and neonatal safety using impedance monitoring. Anesthesiology 69:A649, 1988.

76. Capogna G, Celleno D, Tomassetti M, Castantino P, Feo GD, Nisini R: Epidural versus intravenous fentanyl for cesarean section delivery: Neonatal neurobehavioral effects. Reg Anesth 13:S17, 1988.

77. Arcario T, Vartikar J, Johnson MD, Lema MJ, Datta S, Ostheimer GW, Naulty JS: Effect of diluent volume on analgesia produced by epidural fentanyl. Anesthesiology 67:A441, 1987.

78. Vertommen JD, Van Aken H, Vandermeulen E, Vanderven M, Devlieger H, Van Assche AF, Shnider SM: Maternal and neonatal effects of adding sufentanil to 0.5% bupivacaine for cesarean delivery. J Clin Anesth 3:371–376, 1991.

79. Madej TH, Stunin L: Comparison of epidural fentanyl with sufentanil. Anaesthesia 42:1156–1161, 1987.

80. Rosen MA, Hughes SC, Shnider SM, Abboud TK, Norton M, Dailey PA, Curtis JD: Epidural morphine for relief of postoperative pain after cesarean delivery. Anesth Analg 62:666–672, 1983.

81. Leicht CH, Hughes SC, Dailey PA, Shnider SM, Rosen MA: Epidural morphine sulfate for analgesia after cesarean section: A prospective report of 1000 patients. Anesthesiology 65:A366, 1986.

82. Fuller JG, McMorland GH, Douglas J, Palmer L, Constantine LV: Epidural morphine for postoperative pain after caesarean section: A review. In Abstracts of Scientific Papers, Society for Obstetric Anesthesia and Perinatology, 1988, San Francisco, p 94.

83. Turner K, Sandler AN, Vosu H, Daley D, Slavchenko P, Lau L: Respiratory pattern in post-cesarean section patients after

epidural or intramuscular morphine. Anesth Analg 68:S296, 1989.

84. Brose WG, Cohen SE: Oxyhemoglobin saturation following cesarean section in patients receiving epidural morphine, PCA or im meperidine analgesia. Anesthesiology 70:948–953, 1989.

85. Choi HJ, Little MS, Fujita RA, Garber SZ, Tremper KK: Pulse oximetry for monitoring during ward analgesia: Epidural morphine versus parenteral narcotics. Anesthesiology 65:A371, 1986.

86. Östman LP, Owen CL, Bates JM, Scamman FL, Davis K: Oxygen saturation in patients the night prior to and the night after cesarean section during epidural morphine analgesia. Anesthesiology 69:A691, 1988.

87. Cohen SE, Subak LL, Brose WG, Halpern J: Analgesia after cesarean delivery: Patient evaluations and cost of five opioid techniques. Reg Anesth 16:141–149, 1991.

88. Harrison DM, Sinatra R, Morgese L, Chung JH: Epidural narcotic and patient-controlled analgesia for post-cesarean section pain relief. Anesthesiology 68:454–457, 1988.

89. Eisenach JC, Grice SC, Dewan DM: Patient-controlled analgesia following cesarean section: A comparison with epidural and intramuscular narcotics. Anesthesiology 68:444–448, 1988.

90. Bernstein J, Patel N, Moszczynski Z, Parker F, Ramanathan S, Turndorf H: Colostrum morphine following epidural administration. Anesth Analg 68:S23, 1989.

91. Rolbin SH, Wright RG, Shnider SM, Levinson G, Roizen MF, Johnson J, Jones M: Diazepam during cesarean section: Effects of neonatal Apgar scores, acid-base status, neurobehavioral assessment and maternal and fetal plasma norepinephrine levels. In *Abstracts of Scientific Papers*, American Society of Anesthesiologists, New Orleans, 1977, p 449.

92. Akamatsu TJ, Bonica JJ, Rehmet R, Eng M, Ueland K: Experiences with the use of ketamine for parturition. I. Primary anesthetic for vaginal delivery. Anesth Analg 53:284–287, 1974.

93. Eisele JH, Wright R, Rogge P: Newborn and maternal fentanyl levels at cesarean section. Anesth Analg 61:179–180, 1982.

94. Assali NS, Prystowsky H: Studies on autonomic blockade. II. Observations on the nature of blood pressure fall with high selective spinal anesthesia in pregnant women. J Clin Invest 29:1367–1375, 1950.

95. Bromage PR: Continuous lumbar epidural analgesia for obstetrics. Can Med Assoc J 85:1136–1140, 1961.

96. Grundy EM, Zamora AM, Winnie AP: Comparison of spread of epidural anesthesia in pregnant and nonpregnant women. Anesth Analg 57:544–546, 1978.

97. Arner O: Complications following spinal anesthesia: Their significance and technique to reduce their incidence. Acta Chir Scand 167(Suppl):7, 1952.

98. Greene BA: A 26-gauge lumbar puncture needle: Its value in the prophylaxis of headache following spinal analgesia for vaginal delivery. Anesthesiology 11:464–469, 1950.

99. Harris LM, Harmel MH: The comparative incidence of post-lumbar puncture headache following spinal anesthesia administered through 20 and 24 gauge needles. Anesthesiology 14:390–397, 1953.

100. Krueger JE: Etiology and treatment of postspinal headaches. Anesth Analg 32:190–198, 1953.

101. Hart JR, Whitacre RJ: Pencil-point needle in prevention of postspinal headache. JAMA 147:657–658, 1951.

102. Ebner H: An evaluation of spinal anesthesia in obstetrics. Anesth Analg 38:378–387, 1959.

103. Phillips OC, Nelson AT, Lyons WB, Graff TD, Harris LC, Frazier TM: Spinal anesthesia for vaginal delivery: A review of 2016 cases using Xylocaine. Obstet Gynecol 13:437–441, 1959.

104. Myers L, Rosenberg M: The use of the 26-gauge spinal needle: A survey. Anesth Analg 41:509–515, 1962.

105. Tarrow AB: Solution to spinal headaches. Int Anesth Clin 1:877–887, 1963.

106. Cesarini M, Torrielli R, Lahaye F, Meme JM, Cabiro C: Sprotte needle for intrathecal anaesthesia for caesarean section: Incidence of post-dural puncture headache. Anaesthesia 45:656–658, 1990.

107. Flaatten H, Rodt SA, Vamnes J, Rosland J, Wisborg T, Koller ME: Postdural puncture headache—A comparison between 26 and 29 gauge needles in young patients. Anaesthesia 44:147–149, 1989.

108. Lesser P, Bembridge M, Lyons G, MacDonald R: An evaluation of a 30-gauge needle for spinal anaesthesia for caesarean section. Anaesthesia 45:767–768, 1990.

109. Barker P: Are obstetrical headaches avoidable? Anaesth Intensive Care 18:553–554, 1990.

110. Snyder GE, Person DL, Flor CE, Wilden RT: Headache in obstetric patients; Comparison of Whitacre needle versus Quincke needle. Anesthesiology 71:A860, 1989.

111. Ready LB, Cuplin S, Haschke R, Nessley M: Spinal needle determinants of rate of transdural fluid leak. Anesth Analg 69:457–460, 1989.

112. Cruickshank RH, Hopkinson JM: Fluid leak through dural puncture sites. Anaesthesia 44:415–418, 1989.

113. Fink BR, Walker S: Orientation of fibers in human dorsal lumbar dura mater in relation to lumbar puncture. Anesth Analg 69:768–772, 1989.

114. Mihic D: Postspinal headache and relationship of needle bevel to longitudinal dural fibers. Reg Anesth 10:76–81, 1985.

115. Norris MC, Leighton BL, DeSimone CA: Needle bevel direction and headache after inadvertent dural puncture. Anesthesiology 70:729–731, 1989.

116. Hart JR, Whitacre RJ: Pencil-point needle in prevention of spinal headache. JAMA 147:657–658, 1981.

117. Cappe BE: Prevention of post spinal headache with a 22-gauge pencil-point needle and adequate hydration. Anesth Analg 39:463–465, 1960.

118. Sprotte G, Schedel R, Pajunk H: An atraumatic needle for single shot regional anaesthesia. Reg Anesth 10:104–108, 1987.

119. Kreuscher HP, Sandmann G: Prevention of postspinal headache by using Whitacre's pencil-point needle. Reg Anesth 11:5, 1988.

120. Ready LB, Cuplin S, Haschke RH, Nessly M: Spinal needle determinants of rate of transdural fluid leak. Anesth Analg 69:457–460, 1989.

121. Stasiuk R, Jenkins L: Post-spinal headache; A comparison of midline and laminar approaches. Can J Anaesth 37:S58, 1990.

122. Jorgensen N: Post-dural puncture headache is more common with the paramedian approach. Anesth Analg 72:S131, 1991.

123. Carbaat PAT, van Crevel H: Lumbar puncture headache: Controlled study on the preventive effect of 24 hours' bed rest. Lancet 2:1133–1135, 1981.

124. McLeskey CH, Hornbein TF, Pavlin EG: Hydration and post-spinal headache. In *Abstracts of Scientific Papers*, American Society of Anesthesiologists, San Francisco, 1976, p 455–456.

125. Dieterich M, Brandt T: Incidence of post-lumbar puncture headache is independent of fluid intake. Eur Arch Psychiatr Neurol Sci 237:194–196, 1988.

126. Hodgkinson R: Total spinal block after epidural injection into an interspace adjacent to an inadvertent dural perforation. Anesthesiology 55:593–594, 1981.

127. Leach A, Smith GB: Subarachnoid spread of epidural local anaesthetic following dural puncture. Anaesthesia 43:671, 1988.

128. Crawford JS: The prevention of headache consequent upon dural puncture. Br J Anaesth 44:598–599, 1972.

129. Craft JB Jr, Epstein BS, Coakley CS: Prophylaxis of dural-puncture headache with epidural saline. Anesth Analg 52:228–231, 1973.

130. Smith BE: Prophylaxis of epidural wet tap headache. In *Abstracts of Scientific Papers*, American Society of Anesthesiologists, San Francisco, 1979, p 119.

131. Ozdil T, Powell WF: Postlumbar puncture headache: An effective method of prevention. Anesth Analg 44:542–545, 1965.

132. Gutterman P, Bezier H: Prophylaxis of post myelogram headache. J Neurol 49:869–871, 1978.
133. Loeser EA, Hill GE, Bennett GM, Sedeberg JH: Time vs success rate for epidural blood patch. Anesthesiology 49:147–148, 1978.
134. Palahnuik RJ, Cumming M: Prophylactic blood patch does not prevent post-lumbar puncture headache. Can Anaesth Soc J 26:132–133, 1979.
135. Quaynor H, Corbey M: Extradural blood patch—why delay? Br J Anaesth 57:538–540, 1985.
136. Cheek TG, Banner R, Sauter J, Gutsche B: Prophylactic extradural blood patch is effective. Br J Anaesth 61:340–342, 1988.
137. Ackerman W, Juneja M, Kaczorowski D: The attenuation of a postdural puncture headache with a prophylactic blood patch in labor patients. Anesth Analg 68:S1, 1989.
138. Colonna-Romano P, Shapiro BE: Unintentional dural puncture and prophylactic epidural blood patch in obstetrics. Anesth Analg 69:522–523, 1989.
139. Szeinfeld M, Ihmeidan IH, Moser M, Machado R, Klose J, Serafini AN: Epidural blood patch: Evaluation of the volume and spread of blood injected into the epidural space. Anesthesiology 64:820–822, 1986.
140. Sechzer P, Abel L: Post-spinal analgesia headache treated with caffeine: Evaluation with the demand method. I. Curr Therap Res 24:307–312, 1978.
141. Abboud T, Zhu J, Reyes A, Steffens Z, Afrasiabi A, Gendein D: Efficacy of intravenous caffeine for post-dural puncture headache. Anesthesiology 73:A936, 1990.
142. Camann W, Murray R, Mushlin PS, Lambert DH: Effects of oral caffeine on post-dural puncture headache: A double-blind placebo controlled trial. Anesth Analg 70:181–184, 1990.
143. Bolton VE, Leicht CH, Scanlon TS: Postpartum seizure after epidural blood patch and intravenous caffeine sodium benzoate. Anesthesiology 70:146–149, 1989.
144. Fuerstein T, Zeides A: Theophylline relieves headache following lumbar puncture. Klin Wochenschr 64:216–218, 1986.
145. Schwalbe S, Schiffmiller M, Marx G: Theophylline for postdural puncture headache. Anesthesiology 75:A1082, 1991.
146. Gormley JB: Treatment of postspinal headache. Anesthesiology 21:565–566, 1960.
147. DiGiovanni AJ, Dunbar BS: Epidural injections of autologous blood for postlumbar puncture headache. Anesth Analg 49:268–271, 1970.
148. DiGiovanni AJ, Galbert MW, Wahle WM: Epidural injection of autologous blood for postlumbar-puncture headache. II. Additional clinical experiences and laboratory investigation. Anesth Analg 51:226–232, 1972.
149. Glass PM, Kennedy WF Jr: Headache following subarachnoid puncutre: Treatment with epidural blood patch. JAMA 219:203–204., 1972.
150. DuPont FS, Shire RD: Epidural blood patch: An unusual approach to the problem of post-spinal anesthetic headache. Mich Med 71:105–107, 1972.
151. Vondrell JJ, Bernards WC: Epidural "blood patch" for the treatment of postspinal headaches. Wis Med J 72:132–134, 1973.
152. Blok RJ: Headache following spinal anesthesia: Treatment by epidural blood patch. J Am Osteopath Assoc 73:128–130, 1973.
153. Balagot RC, Lee T, Liu C, Kwan BK, Ecanow B: The prophylactic epidural blood patch (letter). JAMA 228:1369–1370, 1974.
154. Ostheimer GW, Palahnuik RJ, Shnider SM: Epidural blood patch for postlumbar-puncture headache (letter). Anesthesiology 41:307–308, 1974.
155. Abouleish E, de la Vega S, Blendinger J, Tiong-Oen T: Long-term follow-up of epidural blood patch. Anesth Analg 54:459–463, 1975.
156. Loeser EA, Hill GE, Bennett GM, Sederberg JH: Time vs. success rate for epidural blood patch. Anesthesiology 49:147–148, 1978.
157. Abouleish E: Epidural blood patch for the treatment of chronic postlumbar-puncture cephalgia. Anesthesiology 49:291–292, 1978.
158. Naulty JS, Herold R: Successful epidural anesthesia following epidural blood patch. Anesth Analg 57:272–273, 1978.
159. Ong BY, Graham CR, Ringaert KR, Cohen MM, Palahniuk RJ: Impaired epidural analgesia after dural puncture with and without subsequent blood patch. Anesth Analg 70:76–79, 1990.
160. Bevacqua B, Slucky A: Epidural blood patch in a patient with HIV infection (letter). Anestheiology 74:952–953, 1991.
161. Frame W, Lichtmann M: Blood patch in the HIV-positive patient (letter). Anesthesiology 73:1297, 1990.
162. Barrios-Alarcon J, Aldrete JA, Paragas-Tapia D: Relief of postlumbar puncture headache with epidural dextran 40: A preliminary report. Reg Anesth 14:78–80, 1989.
163. Brownridge P: Epidural and subarachnoid analgesia for elective caesarean section. Anaesthesia 36:70, 1981.
164. Carrie LES: Epidural versus combined spinal epidural block for caesaeran section. Acta Anaesthesiol Scand 32:595–596, 1988.
165. Carrie LES: Spinal and/or epidural blockade for caesarean section. In Epidural and Spinal Analgesia In Obstetrics. F Reynolds, ed, Bailliére Tindall, London, 1990, pp 139–150.
166. Carrie LES, O'Sullivan GM: Subarachnoid bupivacaine 0.5% for caesarean section. Eur J Anaesth 1:275–283, 1984.
167. Coates MB: Combined subarachnoid and epidural techniques. Anaesthesia 37:89–90, 1982.
168. Dennison B: Combined subarachnoid and epidural block for caesarean section. Can Anaesth Soc J 34:105–106, 1987.
169. Kumar CM: Combined subarachnoid and epidural block for caesarean section. Can Anaesth Soc J 34:329–330, 1987.
170. Rawal N: Single segment combined subarachnoid and epidural block for caesarean section. Acta Anaesthesiol Scand 32:61–66, 1988.
171. Rawal N, Schollin J, Wesstrom G: Epidural versus combined spinal epidural block for caesarean section. Acta Anaesthesiol Scand 32:61–66, 1988.
172. Randalls B, Broadway JW, Browne DA, Morgan BM: Comparison of four subarachnoid solutions in a needle-through-needle technique for elective caesarean section. Br J Anaesth 66:314–318, 1991.
173. Roberts RB, Shirley MA: Reducing the risk of acid aspiration during cesarean section. Anesth Analg 53:859–868, 1974.
174. Sellick BA: Cricoid pressure to control regurgitation of stomach contents during induction of anesthesia. Lancet 2:404–406, 106.
175. Thind GS, Bryson THL: Single dose suxamethonium and muscle pain in pregnancy. Br J Anaesth 55:743–745, 1983.
176. Smith G, Dalling R, Williams TIR: Gastro-esophageal pressure gradient changes produced by induction of anaesthesia and suxamethonium. Br J Anaesth 50:1137–1143, 1978.
177. Roberts RB, Shirley MA: Reducing the risk of acid aspiration during cesarean section. Anesth Analg 53:859–868, 1974.
178. Gibbs CP, Hempling RE, Wynne JW, Hood CI: Antacid pulmonary aspiration. Anesthesiology 51:A290, 1979.
179. Eyler SW, Cullen BF, Murphy ME, Welch WD: Antacid aspiration in rabbits: A comparison of Mylanta and Bicitra. Anesth Analg 61:288–292, 1982.
180. Gibbs CP, Spohr L, Schmidt D: The effectiveness of sodium citrate as an antacid. Anesthesiology 57:44–46, 1982.
181. Abboud TK, Curtis JP, Shnider SM, Earl S, Henriksen EH: Comparison of the effects of sodium citrate and Gelusil on gastric acidity and volume. Anesth Analg 61:167, 1982.
182. Gibbs CP, Banner TC: Effectiveness of Bicitra as a preoperative antacid. Anesthesiology 61:97–99, 1984.
183. Chen CT, Toung TJR, Haupt HM, Hutchins GM, Cameron JL: Evaluation of Alka-Seltzer Effervescent in gastric acid neutralization. Anesth Analg 63:325–329, 1984.
184. Pickering BG, Palahniuk RJ, Cumming M: Cimetidine premedication in elective cesarean section. Can Anaesth Soc J 27:33–35, 1980.

185. Williams JG: H₂ receptor antagonists and anaesthesia. Can Anaesth Soc J 30:264–269, 1983.

186. Manchikanti L, Kraus JW, Edds SP: Cimetidine and related drugs in anesthesia. Anesth Anaig 61:595–608, 1982.

187. Brock-Utne JG, Rubin J, Downing JW, Dimopoulos CE, Moshal MG, Naicker M: The administration of metoclopramide with atropine: A drug interaction effect on the gastrooesphageal spincter in man. Anaesthesia 31:1186–1190, 1976.

188. McNeill MJ, Ho ET, Kenny GNC: Effect of I.V. metoclopramide on gastric emptying after opioid premedication. Br J Anaesth 64:450–452, 1990.

189. Brock-Utne JG, Dow TGB, Welman S, Dimopoulos GE, Moshal MG: The effect of metoclopramide on lower oesophageal sphincter tone. Anaesth Intens Care 6:26–29, 1978.

190. Chestnut DH, Vandewalker GE, Owen CL, Bates JN, Choi WW: Administration of metoclopramide for prevention of nausea and vomiting during epidural anesthesia for elective cesarean section. Anesthesiology 66:563–566, 1987.

191. Murphy DF, Nally B, Gardiner J, Unwin A: Effect of metoclopramide on gastric emptying before elective and emergency caesarean section. Br J Anaesth 56:1113–1116, 1984.

192. Wyner MB, Cohen S: Gastric volume in early pregnancy. Anesthesiology 57:209–212, 1982.

193. Lyons G: Failed intubation. Anaesthesia 40:759–762, 1985.

194. Lyons G, MacDonald R: Difficult intubation in obstetrics. Anaesthesia 40:1016, 1985.

195. Cormack RS, Lehane J: Difficult tracheal intubation in obstetrics. Anaesthesia 39:1105–1111, 1984.

196. Samsoon GLT, Young JRB: Difficult tracheal intubation: A retrospective study. Anaesthesia 42:487–490, 1987.

197. McIntyre JR: The difficult tracheal intubation. Can J Anaesth 34:204–213, 1987.

198. Wilson ME, Spigekhalter D, Robertson JA, Lesser P: Predicting difficult intubation. Br J Anaesth 61:211–216, 1988.

199. Patil VU, Stehling LC, Zauder HL: *Fiberoptic Endoscopy in Anesthesia.* Year Book Medical Publishers, Chicago, 1983.

200. Mathew M, Hanna LS, Aldrete JA: Pre-operative indices to anticipate difficult tracheal intubation. Anesth Analg 68:S187, 1989.

201. Brechner VL: Unusual problems in the management of airways. I. Flexion-extension mobility of the cervical spine. Anesth Analg 47:362–373, 1968.

202. Finucane BT, Santora AH: Evaluation of the airway prior to intubation. In *Principles of Airway Management.* Davis, Philadelphia, 1988, pp 69–83.

203. Mallampati SR: Clinical signs to predict difficult tracheal intubation (hypothesis). Can Anaesth Soc J 30:316–317, 1983.

204. Mallampati SR, Gatt SP, Gugino LD, Desai SP, Waraksa B, Freiberger D, Liu PL: A clinical sign to predict difficult tracheal intubation: A prospective study. Can Anaesth Soc J 32:429–434, 1985.

205. Samsoon GLT, Young JRB: Difficult tracheal intubation: A retrospective study. Anaesthesia 42:487–490, 1987.

206. Brain AIJ: Three cases of difficult intubation overcome by laryngeal mask airway. Anaesthesia 40:353–355, 1985.

207. Benumof JL, Scheller MS: The importance of transtracheal jet ventilation in the management of the difficult airway. Anesthesiology 71:769–778, 1989.

208. Tunstall ME, Sheikh A: Failed intubation protocol: Oxygenation without aspiration. In Clinics in Anaesthesiology, Obstetric Analgesia, and Anaesthesthia, Vol 4. GW Ostheimer, ed. WB Saunders, Philadelphia, 1986, pp 171–187.

209. McClune S, Regan M, Moore J: Laryngeal mask airway for caesarean section. Anaesthesia 45:227–228, 1990.

210. O'Sullivan G, Stoddart PA: Failed tracheal intubation. Br J Anaesth 67:225, 1991.

211. King TA, Adams AP: Failed tracheal intubation. Br J Anaesth 67:225, 1991.

212. Ansermino JM, Blogg CE, Carrie LES: Failed tracheal intubation at caesarean section and the laryngeal mask. Br J Anaesth 68:54–59, 1992.

213. Widlund G: Cardio-pulmonary function during pregnancy: A clinical-experimental study with particular respect to ventilation and oxygen consumption among normal cases in rest and after work tests. Acta Obstet Gynecol Scand 25(Suppl):1–125, 1945.

214. Cugell DW, Frank NR, Gaensler ER, Badger TL: Pulmonary function in pregnancy. I. Serial observations in normal women. Am Rev Tuberc 67:568–597, 1953.

215. Archer GW Jr, Marx GF: Arterial oxygen tension during apnoea in parturient women. Br J Anaesth 46:358–360, 1974.

216. Norris MC, Dewan DM: Preoxygenation for cesarean section: A comparison of two techniques. Anesthesiology 62:827–829, 1985.

217. Gambee AM, Hertzka RE, Fisher DM: Preoxygenation techniques: Comparison of three minutes and four breaths. Anesth Analg 66:468–470, 1987.

218. Palahniuk RJ, Shnider SM, Eger EI II: Pregnancy decreases the requirements for inhaled anesthetic agents. Anesthesiology 41:82–83, 1974.

219. Levinson G, Shnider SM, deLorimier AA, Steffenson JL: Effects of maternal hyperventilation on uterine blood flow and fetal oxygenation and acid-base status. Anesthesiology 40:340–347, 1974.

220. Kosaka Y, Takahashi T, Mark LC: Intravenous thiobarbiturate anesthesia for cesarean section. Anesthesiology 31:489–506, 1969.

221. Bach V, Carl P, Ravio O, Crawford ME, Jensen AG, Mikkelsen BO, Crevoisier C, Heizmann P, Fattinger K: A randomized comparison between midazolam and thiopental for elective cesarean section anesthesia. III. Placental transfer and elimination in neonates. Anesth Analg 68:238–247, 1989.

222. Finster M, Mark LC, Morishima HO, Moya F, Perel JM, James LS, Dayton PG: Plasma thiopental concentrations in the newborn following delivery under thiopental-nitrous oxide anesthesia. Am J Obstet Gynecol 95:621–629, 1966.

223. Bovill JG, Dundee JW, Coppell DL, Moore J: Current status of ketamine anaesthesia. Lancet 1:1285–1288, 1971.

224. Dich-Nielsen J, Holasek J: Ketamine as induction agent for caesarean section. Acta Anaesthesiol Scand 26:139–142, 1982.

225. Levinson G, Shnider SM, Gildea J, deLorimier AA: Maternal and foetal cardiovascular and acid base changes during ketamine anaesthesia. Br J Anaesth 45:1111–1115, 1973.

226. Eng M, Berges PU, Bonica JJ: The effects of ketamine on uterine blood flow in the monkey. In *Abstracts of Scientific Papers,* Society for Gynecological Investigation, Atlanta, 1973, p 48.

227. Craft JB Jr, Coaldrake LA, Yonekura ML, Dao SD, Co EG, Roizen MF, Mazel P, Gilman R, Shokes L, Trevor AJ: Ketamine, catecholamines, and uterine tone in pregnant ewes. Am J Obstet Gynecol 146:429–434, 1983.

228. Galloon S: Ketamine for obstetric delivery. Anesthesiology 44:522–524, 1976.

229. Oats JN, Vasey DP, Waldron BA: Effects of ketamine on the pregnant uterus. Br J Anaesth 51:1163–1166, 1979.

230. Little B, Chang T, Chucot L, Dill WA, Emile LL, Glazko AJ, Jassani M, Kretchmer H, Sweet AY; Study of ketamine as an obstetric agent. Am J Obstet Gynecol 113:247–260, 1972.

231. Janeczko GF, El-Etr AA, Younes S: Low-dose ketamine anesthesia for obstetrical delivery. Anesth Analg 53:828–831, 1974.

232. Hodgkinson R, Marx GF, Kim SS, Miclat NM: Neonatal neurobehavioral tests following vaginal delivery under ketamine, thiopental and extradural anesthesia. Anesth Analg 56:548–553, 1977.

233. Pelz B, Sinclair DM: Induction agents for caesarean section: A comparison of thiopentone and ketamine. Anaesthesia 28:37–42, 1973.

234. Downing JW, Mahomedy MC, Jeal DE, Allen PJ: Anaesthesia for caesarean section with ketamine. Anaesthesia 31:883–892, 1976.

235. Corssen G, Gutierrez J, Reves JG, Huber FC: Ketamine in the anesthetic management of asthmatic patients. Anesth Analg 51:588–596, 1972.

236. Schultetus RR, Hill CR, Dharamraj CM, Banner TE, Berman LS: Wakefulness during cesarean section after anesthetic in-

duction with ketamine, thiopental, or ketamine and thiopental combined. Anesth Analg 65:723–728, 1986.

237. Alon E, Rosen MA, Shnider SM, Ball RH, Parer JT: Maternal and fetal effects of propofol anesthesia in the ewe. Anesthesiology 75:A1077, 1991.

238. Celleno D, Capogna G, Tomassetti M, Costantino P, DiFeo G, Nisini R: Neurobehavioral effects of propofol on the neonate following elective caesarean section. Br J Anaesth 62:649–654, 1989.

239. Dailland P, Jaquinot P, Lirzin JD, Jorrot JC, Harmey JL, Conseiller C: Neonatal effects of propofol administered maternally for anesthesia for cesarean section. Cahiers d'Anesthesiologie 37:429–433, 1989.

240. Dailland P, Cockshott ID, Lirzin JD, Jacquinot P, Jorrot JC, Devery J, Harmey JL, Conseiller C: Intravenous propofol during cesarean section: Placental transfer, concentrations in breast milk, and neonatal effects—A preliminary study. Anesthesiology 71:827–834, 1989.

241. Flynn RJ, Moore J, Sharpe TDE: A comparative study of propofol and thiopental as induction agents for cesarean section. Anesth Analg 68:S321, 1989.

242. Valtonen M, Kanto J, Rosenberg P: Comparison of propofol and thiopentone for induction of anaesthesia for elective caesarean section. Anaesthesia 44:758–762, 1989.

243. Moore J, Bill KM, Flynn RJ, McKeating KT, Howard PJ: A comparison between propofol and thiopentone as induction agents in obstetric anaesthesia. Anesthesiology 44:753–757, 1989.

244. Gin T, Gregory MA, Oh TE: The hemodynamic effects of propofol and thiopental for induction of caesarean section. Anaesth Intensive Care 18:175–179, 1990.

245. Gin T, Gregory MA, Chan K, Oh TE: Maternal and fetal levels of propofol at caesarean section. Anaesth Intensive Care 18:180—184, 1990.

246. Yau G, Gin T, Ewart MC, Kotur CF, Leung RK, Oh TE: Propofol for induction and maintenance of anaesthesia at caesarean section. A comparison with thiopentone/enflurane. Anaesthesia 46:20–23, 1991.

247. Gin T, Yau G, Chan K, Gergory MA, Oh TE: Disposition of propofol infusions for caesarean section. Can J Anaesth 38:31–36, 1991.

248. Baraka A: Severe bradycardia following propofol-suxamethonium squence. Br J Anaesth 61:482–483, 1988.

249. Dowing JW, Buley RJR, Brock-Utne JG, Houlton PC: Etomidate for induction of anaesthesia at caesarean section: Comparison with thiopentone. Br J Anaesth 51:135–139, 1979.

250. Suresh MS, Solanki DR, Andrews JJ, Hedges P, Nguyen S: Comparison of etomidate with thiopental for induction of anesthesia at cesarean section. Anesthesiology 65:A400, 1985.

251. Reddy BK, Pizer B, Bull PT: Neonatal serum cortisol suppression by etomidate compared with thiopentone for elective caesarean section. Eur J Anaesth 5:171–176, 1988.

252. Cohen EN, Paulson WJ, Wall J, Elert B: Thiopental, curare, and nitrous oxide anesthesia for cesarean section with studies on placental transmission. Surg Gynecol Obstet 97:456-462, 1953.

253. Moya F, Kvisselgaard N: The placental transmission of succinylcholine. Anesthesiology 22:1–6, 1961.

254. Dailey PA, Fisher DM, Shnider SM, Baysinger CL, Shinohara Y, Miller RD, Abboud TK, Kim KC: Pharmacokinetics, placental transfer, and neonatal effects of vecuronium and pancuronium administered during cesarean section. Anesthesiology 60:569–574, 1984.

255. Demetriou M, Depoix JP, Diakite B, Fromentin M, Duvaldestin P: Placental transfer of Org NC45 in women undergoing cesarean section. Br J Anaesth 54:643–645, 1982.

256. Flynn PJ, Frank M, Hughes R: Use of atracurium in caesarean section. Br J Anaesth 56:599–605, 1984.

257. Drabkova J, Crul JF, Van Der Kleijn E: Plaental transfer of ^{14}C-labelled succinylcholine in near-term Macaca mulatta monkeys. Br J Anaesth 45:1087–1095, 1973.

258. Kvisselgaard N, Mya F: Investigation of placental thresholds to succinylcholine. Anesthesiology 22:7–10, 1961.

259. Shnider SM: Serum cholinesterase activity during pregnancy, labor and puerperium. Anesthesiology 26:335–339, 1965.

260. Leighton BL, Cheek TG, Gross JB, Apfelbaum JL, Shantz BB, Gutsche BB, Rosenberg H: Succinylcholine pharmacodynamics in peripartum patients. Anesthesiology 64:202–205, 1986.

261. Blitt CD, Petty WC, Alberternst EE, Wright BJ: Correlations of plasma cholinesterase activity and duration of action of succinylcholine during pregnancy. Anesth Analg 56:78–81, 1977.

262. Baraka A, Haroun S, Bassili M, Abu-Haider G: Response of the newborn to succinylcholine injection in homozygote atypical mothers. Anesthesiology 43:115–116, 1975.

263. Baraka A, Noueihid R, Sinno H, Wakid N, Agoston S: Succinylcholine vecuronium (Org NC45) sequence for cesarean section. Anesth Analg 62:909–913, 1983.

264. Kivalo I, Saarikoski S: Placental transmission and foetal uptake of ^{14}C-dimethyltubocurarine. Br J Anaesth 44:557–561, 1972.

265. Abouleish E, Wingard LB Jr, de la Vega S, Uy N: Pancuronium in caesarean section and its placental transfer. Br J Anaesth 52:531–536, 1980.

266. Marx GF, Joshi CW, Orkin LR: Placental transmission of nitrous oxide. Anesthesiology 32:429–432, 1970.

267. Stenger VG, Blechner JN, Prystowsky H: A study of prolongation of obstetric anesthesia. Am J Obstet Gynecol 103:901–907, 1969.

268. Finster M, Poppers PJ: Safety of thiopental used for induction of general anesthesia in elective cesarean section. Anesthesiology 29:190–191, 1968.

269. Shnider SM: Anesthesia for elective cesarean section. In *Obstetrical Anesthesia: Current Concepts and Practice.* SM Shnider, ed. Williams & Wilkins, Baltimore, 1970, p 94.

270. Crawford JS: Awareness during operative obstetrics under general anesthesia. Br J Anaesth 43:179–182, 1971.

271. Wilson J, Turner DJ: Awareness during caesarean section under general anaesthesia. Br Med J 1:280–283, 1969.

272. Moir DD: Anaesthesia for caesarean section: An evaluation of a method using low concentrations of halothane and 50 percent of oxygen. Br J Anaesth 42:136–142, 1970.

273. Palahniuk RJ, Scatliff J, Biehl D, Wieve H, Sankaran K: Maternal and neonatal effects of methoxyflurane, nitrous oxide and lumbar epidural anaesthesia for caesarean section. Can Anaesth Soc J 24:586–596, 1977.

274. Galbert MW, Gardner AE: Use of halothane in a balanced technique for cesarean section. Anesth Analg 51:701–704, 1972.

275. Wilson J: Methoxyflurane in caesarean section. Br J Anaesth 45:233, 1973.

276. Latto IP, Waldron BA: Anaesthesia for caesarean section. Br J Anaesth 49:371–378, 1977.

277. Coleman AJ, Downing JW: Enflurane anesthesia for cesarean section. Anesthesiology 43:354–357, 1975.

278. Crawford JS, Burton OM, Davies P: Anaesthesia for section: Further refinement of a technique. Br J Anaesth 45:726–731, 1973.

279. Warren TM, Datta S, Ostheimer GW, Naulty JJ, Weiss JB, Morrison JA: Comparison of the maternal and neonatal effects of halothane, enflurane and isoflurane for cesarean delivery. Anesth Analg 62:516–520, 1983.

280. Abboud TK, Kim SH, Henriksen EH, Chen T, Eisenman R, Levinson G, Shnider SM: Comparative maternal and neonatal effects of halothane and enflurane for cesarean section. Acta Anaesthesiol Scand 29:663–668, 1985.

281. Marx GF, Mateo CV: Effects of different oxygen concentrations during general anesthesia for elective caesarean section. Can Anaesth Soc J 18:587–593, 1971.

282. Bogod DG, Rosen M, Rees GAD: Maximum F$_{IO_2}$ during caesarean section. Br J Anaesth 61:255–262, 1988.

283. Piggott SE, Bogod DG, Rosen M, Rees GAD, Harmer M: Isoflurane with either 100% oxygen or 50% nitrous oxide in oxygen for caesarean section. Br J Anaesth 65:325–329, 1990.

284. Shnider SM, Wright RG, Levinson G, Roizen MF, Rolbin SH, Biehi D, Johnson J, Jones M: Plasma norepinephrine and uterine blood flow changes during endotracheal intubation and general anesthesia in the pregnant ewe. In *Abstracts of Scientific Papers*, American Society of Anesthesiologists, Chicago, 1978, p 115.

285. Naftalin NJ, Phear WPC, Goldberg AH: Halothane and isometric contractions of isolated pregnant rat myometrium. Anesthesiology 42:458–463, 1975.

286. Naftalin NJ, McKay DM, Phear WPC, Goldberg AH: The effects of halothane on pregnant and nonpregnant human myometrium. Anesthesiology 40:15–19, 1977.

287. Munson ES, Maier WR, Caton D: Effects of halothane, cyclopropane and nitrous oxide on isolated human uterine muscle. J Obstet Gynaecol Br Commonw 76:27–33, 1969.

288. Munson ES, Embro WJ: Enflurane, isoflurane, and halothane and isolated human uterine muscle. Ansthesiology 46:11–14, 1977.

289. Marx GF, Kim YI, Lin CC, Halevy S, Schulman H: Postpartum uterine pressures under halothane or enflurane anesthesia. Obstet Gynecol 51:695–698, 1978.

290. Thirion A-V, Wright RG, Messer CP, Rosen MA, Shnider SM: Maternal blood loss associated with low dose halothane administration for cesarean section. Anesthesiology 69:A693, 1988.

291. Gilstrap LC, Hauth JC, Hankins GDV, Patterson AR: Effect of type of anesthesia on blood loss at cesarean section. Obstet Gynecol 69:328–332, 1987.

292. Apgar V, Holaday DA, James LS, Prince CE, Weisbrot IM: Comparison of regional and general anesthesia in obstetrics. JAMA 105:2155–2161, 1957.

293. Benson RC, Shubeck F, Clarke WM, Berendes H, Weiss W, Deutschberger J: Fetal compromise during elective cesarean section. Am J Obstet Gynecol 91:645–651, 1965.

294. Ong BY, Cohen MM, Palahniuk RJ: Anesthesia for cesarean section: Effects on neonates. Anesth Analg 68:270–275, 1989.

295. Kalappa R, Ueland K, Hansen JM, Eng M, Parer JT: Maternal acid-base status during cesarean section under thiopental, N$_2$O and succinylcholine anesthesia. Am J Obstet Gynecol 109:411–420, 1971.

296. Hodges RJ, Tunstall ME: The choice of anaesthesia and its influence on perinatal mortality in caesarean section. Br J Anaesth 33:572–588, 1961.

297. Marx GF, Cosmi EV, Wollman SB: Biochemical status and clinical condition of mother and infant at cesarean section. Anesth Analg 48:986-993, 1969.

298. Datta S, Brown WU Jr: Acid-base status in diabetic mothers and their infants following general or spinal anesthesia for cesarean section. Anesthesiology 47:272–276, 1977.

299. Fox GS, Smith JB, Namba Y, Johnson RC: Anesthesia for cesarean section: Further studies. Am J Obstet Gynecol 133:15–19, 1979.

300. James FM, Crawford JS, Hodgkinson R, Davies P, Naiem H: A comparison of general anesthesia and lumbar epidural analgesia for elective cesarean section. Anesth Analg 56:228–235, 1977.

301. Crawford JS, Davies P: A return to trichloroethylene for obstetric anaesthesia. Br J Anaesth 47:482–489, 1975.

302. Datta S, Ostheimer GW, Weiss JB, Brown WU, Jr, Alper MH: Neonatal effect of prolonged anesthetic induction for cesarean section. Obstet Gynecol 58:331–335, 1981.

303. Bader AM, Datta S, Arthur GR, Benvenuti E, Courtney M, Hauch M: Maternal and fetal catecholamines and uterine incision-to-delivery interval during elective cesarean section. Obstet Gynecol 75:600–603, 1990.

304. Scanlon JW, Shea E, Alper MH: Neurobehavioral responses of newborn infants following general or spinal anesthesia for cesarean section. In *Abstracts of Scientific Papers*, American Society of Anesthesiologists, Chicago, 1975, p 91.

305. Hodgkinson R, Bhatt M, Kim SS, Grewal G, Marx GP: Neonatal neurobehavioral tests following cesaeran section under general and spinal anesthesia. Am J Obstet Gynecol 132:670–674, 1978.

306. Abboud TK, Nagapppala S, Murakawa K, David S, Haroutunian S, Zakarian M, Yanagi T, Sheik-Ol-Eslam A: Comparison of the effects of general and regional anesthesia for cesarean section on neonatal neurologic and adaptive capacity scores. Anesth Analg 64:996–1000, 1985.

307. Hollmén Al, Jouppila R, Koivisto M, Maatta L, Pihlajaniemi R, Puukka M, Rantakyla P: Neurologic activity of infants following anesthesia for cesarean section. Anesthesiology 48:350–356, 1978.

308. Abboud TK, Blikian A, Noueihid R, Nagappala S, Afrasiabi A, Henriksen EH: Neonatal effects of maternal hypotension during spinal anesthesia as evaluated by a new test. Anesthesiology 59:A421, 1983.

309. Marx GF, Luykx WM, Cohen S: Fetal-neonatal status following caesarean section for fetal distress. Br J Anaesth 56:1009–1013, 1984.

310. Ramanathan J, Ricca DM, Sibai BM, Angel JJ: Epidural vs general anesthesia in fetal distress with various abnormal fetal heart rate patterns. Anesth Analg 67:S180, 1988.

CHAPTER 13

Anesthesia for Postpartum Sterilization Surgery

Stephen H. Rolbin, M.D.C.M., F.R.C.P.(C)

Pregnancy, labor, and delivery are associated with major physiologic changes. These changes have been known for some time and their understanding has resulted in improved anesthetic care of the mother, fetus, and newborn. However, these changes do not revert immediately with delivery of the newborn but continue into the puerperium, which is the period from termination of labor to complete involution of the uterus during which the body returns to a normal nonpregnant state. This period usually lasts about 6 weeks but may vary from 4 to 12 weeks (1). The term *postpartum* is defined as after childbirth or following or occurring as a sequel of childbirth (2). There is no precise definition as to when the "postpartum period" ends. Common usage of the term *postpartum tubal ligation* seems to refer to the fact that the procedure occurs during the same admission as the delivery and not any particular time period.

This chapter discusses the physiologic changes that occur in the puerperium. The implications of these changes for the anesthetic management of these patients is discussed from the perspective of providing the safest possible anesthetic.

PUERPERAL ANATOMIC AND PHYSIOLOGIC CHANGES

Immediately after expulsion of the placenta, the fundus of the contracted body of the uterus is about midway between the umbilicus and symphysis (1, 3). The uterus remains approximately the same size during the next 2 days and then atrophies so that, within 2 weeks, it has descended into the true pelvis and can no longer be felt above the symphysis. It usually regains its nonpregnant size in 5 to 6 weeks. The abdominal wall remains soft and flabby as a result of the prolonged distension by the pregnant uterus. This returns to normal over a period of several weeks.

A bradycardia of 40 to 50 beats/min lasting 24 to 48 hr occasionally occurs. The increase in blood volume during pregnancy returns to normal over a period of 2 to 3 weeks.

In the first 2 to 3 days postpartum, there is a 15 to 30% increase in circulatory blood volume resulting from elimination of the placental circulation, an increase in venous return, and a shift of fluid from the interstitial compartment into the circulation (1, 3). The usual result is a 35% increase in cardiac output (1), which is potentially hazardous in patients with a limited cardiac reserve. However, in a study that measured blood volume changes with ^{131}I-albumin, Ueland failed to find any rise in blood volume in the early puerperium (4). Instead, the blood volume showed a steady decline to the third postpartum day in the vaginal delivery group and remained fairly stable until the fifth postpartum day in the cesarean delivery group. The physiologic changes of pregnancy, such as increased cardiac output, increased blood volume, and hemodilution result in better perfusion of the alveoli. These changes result in a reduced arterial to end-tidal carbon dioxide tension difference during anesthesia for tubal ligation, which persists for 8 days following delivery (5).

The leukocytosis found during pregnancy and labor continues for several days. Values of 20,000 to 30,000/mm^3 are common, and the increase is mainly neutrophilic. Any rise in the patient's temperature during puerperium is likely to be an infection, often in the urinary tract (3). Bladder infections are common because the bladder is often injured to some extent during labor and delivery. Dilation of the ureters and the renal pelvis is also common (1). All these factors favor the development of urinary tract infections.

The glomerular filtration rate remains high for the first week. This, coupled with the increase in circulatory blood volume, accounts for a marked diuresis for 4 or 5 days postpartum. Glycosuria is found in 20% of patients; proteinuria lasts for 1 or 2 days in 50% of patients (1).

The respiratory changes that occur during pregnancy have been reviewed in Chapter 1 and elsewhere (6). Changes in ventilation and some lung volumes take weeks to return to normal (6).

Acid production is increased in the first trimester of pregnancy (7), and gastric emptying is delayed in pregnancy and labor and by certain drugs, such as narcotics. It is not known how long after delivery it takes for these changes to revert to normal, and therefore the anesthesiologist must be aware that the patient may be at increased risk for aspiration.

POSTPARTUM TUBAL STERILIZATION

Surgical sterilization has become an increasingly common method of birth control. By 1982 it was used by 6,783,000 U.S. women (8). Not only is the total number of procedures increasing but the incidence relative to the population and live births also is increasing. This trend has developed from a broadening of the general indications for carrying out such procedures (9, 10). Close to one million female sterilizations are performed each year in North America. Most of those are done by laparoscopy (11).

Currently, criteria for performing postpartum tubal ligation are based on the wishes and consent of the wife and husband. The advantage of postpartum sterilization is that the fallopian tubes are more easily accessible because of the altered anatomy produced by the enlarged uterus, resulting in a simpler surgical procedure than when complete involution of the uterus has taken place. Puerperal sterilization usually does not lengthen the hospital stay, and obviously it eliminates the need for rehospitalization for this procedure. This should reduce the patient's stress and total medical bills.

In recent years there has been a tendency to consider postpartum tubal ligation as a semiurgent operation (i.e., immediately postpartum). The hope was that infection would be reduced with immediate postpartum tubal ligation. It is believed that performing postpartum tubal ligations more than 48 hr after delivery is not prudent because bacteria are present in the uterus, and thus the risk of infection is increased. A survey conducted among obstetric anesthesiologists expressed concern about aspiration of gastric contents should general anesthesia be given (12). Indeed, 4 out of 30 anesthesiologists encountered aspiration of gastric contents in patients with general anesthesia in the postpartum period. The consensus from this survey was that immediate postpartum tubal ligation could be performed safely under a continuous epidural anesthetic that had been effective for labor and delivery, but that the risk of aspiration should limit the induction of general anesthesia in the immediate postpartum period. The com-

mon practice is to wait at least 8 hr before performing surgery.

Often, patients with complications of pregnancy or medical conditions are advised to have sterilization performed when a complete involution of the uterus has taken place (i.e., 6 months after delivery). Even after such a delay, several patient factors increase the risk of complications twofold or more: diabetes mellitus, previous abdominal or pelvic surgery, lung disease, a history of pelvic inflammatory disease, and obesity (13).

RISK OF MATERNAL ASPIRATION

The risk of aspiration in pregnant patients has been well recognized since Mendelson first described a syndrome associated with aspiration of gastric acid (14). Clearly the postpartum patient is also at risk for aspiration and must be treated as such, but it is not yet known for how long this risk is present.

Several factors predispose pregnant patients to gastric retention and regurgitation. The large uterus at term mechanically obstructs the duodenum; progesterone decreases intestinal motility and relaxes the gastroesophageal sphincter; and pain and analgesic drugs may delay gastric emptying. The important question, however, is when does gastric emptying return to normal in the postpartum period? The answer is not known. General anesthesia itself puts the patient at risk. Berson and Adriani; conducted a study on the incidence of silent aspiration in 926 surgical patients using a dye to identify gastric contents in the respiratory tract (15). Gastric contents refluxed in 14% and were aspirated in 7% of patients. The incidence of reflux of gastric contents or endotracheal aspiration was greater with difficult inductions. Of these patients, 30% were intubated, and this also resulted in a greater incidence of aspiration. None of these patients developed any of clinical or radiologic changes of pneumonitis.

A widely quoted study of gastric volume and pH in postpartum patients was conducted by Blouw and co-workers (Table 13.1) (14). They assessed 21 patients between 9 and 42 hr postpartum and compared them to a group of 11 patients who had not recently been pregnant and were undergoing elective tubal ligations. An indicator dilution method was used to assess the amount of gastric contents. The authors concluded that if an 8-hr interval is allowed between delivery and anesthesia, the postpartum patient is no more at risk than the elective surgical patient. However, they found that, in both groups, a significant number of patients (33 to 64%) had greater than 25 ml of fluid at a pH of less than 2.5. This is considered to be the criterion for being at risk for aspiration

Table 13.1
Gastric Volume and pH in Postpartum Versus Elective Tubal Ligation[a,b]

	Postpartum Group (n = 21)	Control Group (n = 11)
Average (± SE) hours postpartum	19.5 ± 1.3	—
Range	9–42	—
Average gastric volume (ml)	30	28
Range	8–88	12–50
Average gastric pH	2.65	2.37
Range	1.33–6.90	1.51–5.10

[a] Adapted from Blouw R, Scatliff J, Craig DB, Palahniuk RJ: Gastric volume and pH in postpartum patients. Anesthesiology 45:456–457, 1976.

[b] Elective tubal ligation patients had not recently been pregnant.

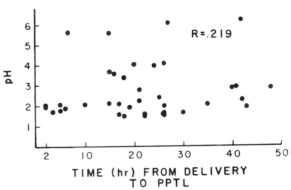

Figure 13.2. Scattergram showing the relationship of pH of gastric contents to the number of hours from a parturient's delivery to the induction of general anesthesia for postpartum tubal ligation (PPTL). (Data reprinted by permission from Uram M, Abouleish E, McKenzie R, Phityakorn P, Tantisira B, Uy N: The risk of aspiration pneumonitis with postpartum tubal ligation. In *Abstracts of Scientific Papers*, Society for Obstetric Anesthesia and Perinatology, Annual Meeting, Jackson Hole, WY, 1982, p 2.)

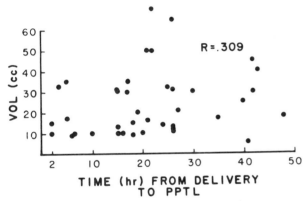

Figure 13.1. Scattergram showing the relationship of gastric volume to the number of hours from a parturient's delivery to the induction of general anesthesia for postpartum tubal ligation (PPTL). (Data reprinted by permission from Uram M, Abouleish E, McKenzie R, Phityakorn P, Tantisira B, Uy N: The risk of aspiration pneumonitis with postpartum tubal ligation. In *Abstracts of Scientific Papers*, Society for Obstetric Anesthesia and Perinatology, Annual Meeting, Jackson Hole, WY, 1982, p 2.)

pneumonitis (16). Furthermore, in the postpartum patients they found no significant correlation between gastric fluid volume and number of hours of fasting after the 9-hr period. They did not study any patients less than 9 hr postpartum.

A study of Uram and co-workers found a similar incidence of high-risk patients (Figs. 13.1 and 13.2) (17). They concluded that the patient's safety is not improved by delaying a general anesthesia for postpartum tubal ligation beyond 2 hr. A study by James and co-workers looked at three postpartum time intervals: 1–8 hr, 9–23 hr, and 24–45 hr (18). No postpartum group differed significantly from the control group. Moreover, the incidence of risk was high in all groups (Table 13.2).

Should one conclude that the patient is safe after 2 hr or that she is at risk for a period of greater than 36 hr?

The effects of pregnancy and labor on gastric motility have recently been assessed by a paracetamol absorption technique (19). Healthy nonpregnant females of reproductive age were used as control groups. With pregnancy the gastric emptying time was unchanged during the third trimester and also was normal in the first 24 to 48 hr postpartum. A second report using noninvasive measurements of gastric emptying (by impedance technique) showed no difference between pregnant and nonpregnant females. However, labor caused a significant delay in gastric emptying (20). The data presented did not include those patients who had undergone epidural anesthesia without prior intramuscular narcotics nor did it assess how long after delivery the delay in gastric emptying persisted.

The conflicting results of these studies emphasize that the postpartum patient is at high risk. In this author's opinion, the studies to date do not conclusively prove a safe delivery-to-surgery interval. Therefore preventative measures should be taken for postpartum surgery (18, 21). No one time interval will absolutely guarantee that a specific patient is free of risk (21). Attention to all details of induction of general anesthesia is mandatory; this is described in the section on general anesthesia in this chapter. Furthermore, the use of regional anesthesia whenever possible will greatly reduce the incidence of maternal aspiration syndrome.

Table 13.2
pH and Volume of Gastric Contents of Postpartum Patients Studied by the Delivery-to-Surgery Interval (DSI)[a]

	Average (± SD) DSI	Mean Volume (ml) (Range)	Mean pH (Range)	% Patients with pH < 2.5	% Patients with pH < 1.4	% Patients with Gastric Contents pH < 2.5 & Volume >25 ml
Control	—	38 (10–82)	1.56 (1.08–6.47)	100	26	60
1–8 hr	4.8 ± 2.1	39 (7–73)	1.53 (1.27–2.24)	100	33	73
9–23 hr	17.3 ± 4.7	24 (6–56)	1.48 (1.14–2.07)	80	40	40
24–45 hr	32.6 ± 6.9	41 (8–73)	1.40 (0.98–2.80)	80	46	67

[a] Adapted from James CF, Gibbs CP, Banner TE: Postpartum perioperative risk of pulmonary aspiration pneumonia. Anesthesiology 61:756–759, 1984.

TUBAL LIGATION VERSUS LAPAROSCOPIC STERILIZATION

Tubal ligation and laparoscopic coagulation are the two commonly used methods for postpartum sterilization. Postpartum tubal ligation is more common than laparoscopic procedures (10, 22). There are over 100 variations of this technique for accomplishing interruption of the continuity of the fallopian tubes. Of these, only a few are in common use today (23). Tubal ligation is easily accomplished in the immediate puerperal period. It requires less experience than laparoscopic coagulation and does not depend on expensive equipment (24).

Postpartum laparoscopy has also been used and has been found to be safe, practical, and acceptable by many authorities (25–29). However, follow-up of these patients has shown a higher complication rate, and laparoscopic sterilization is no longer performed in the immediate puerperium (28), even though convalescence is said to be more rapid and comfortable (21).

Selection of an optimal postpartum day for laparoscopic surgery is not possible. Some authorities believe that the fundal height is optimal on the second to fourth postpartum day (29); others wait at least 5 days (27). Other potential problems during the puerperium include pelvic bleeding, difficulty in mobilizing the bulky uterus, increased infection, and the breakdown of an episiotomy as the result of increased abdominal pressure. Although postpartum laparoscopic tubal coagulation has its advocates, most obstetricians favor the use of postpartum tubal ligation.

PHYSIOLOGIC CHANGES INDUCED BY LAPAROSCOPY

Carbon dioxide or nitrous oxide can be used for inducing pneumoperitoneum. Carbon dioxide is usually chosen as the gas for peritoneal insufflation. Its high solubility results in a rapid absorption of any remaining postoperative gas and gives some safety if the gas is accidentally injected intravenously (30). Nitrous oxide is associated with less diaphragmatic and peritoneal irritation, and use of nitrous oxide also diminishes shoulder pain in the postoperative period (31). This advantage has resulted in nitrous oxide commonly being used when the surgery is being performed with the patient receiving local anesthesia or regional blockade.

Anesthesia for a patient undergoing laparoscopy with CO_2 insufflation involves several important considerations. Rising intraabdominal pressure by gas insufflation may result in cardiovascular depression; reflux of gastric contents may be encouraged; and cardiac arrhythmias may occur from hypercarbia.

Artificial ventilation is considered safer than spontaneous ventilation because high arterial Pa_{CO_2} can be prevented with mechanical ventilation (32, 33). Several factors contribute to rising Pa_{CO_2} during laparoscopy when the patient is given a general anesthetic with spontaneous ventilation. Respiratory depression could occur from premedicant or anesthetic drugs, absorption of carbon dioxide from the peritoneal cavity, and impairment of ventilation by mechanical factors such as abdominal distension and the Trendelenburg position. Theoretically, mechanical ventilation decreases the risk of hypercarbia, but it has occurred in some studies (34–37). It has been suggested that adequate clearance of CO_2 can be ensured by increasing ventilation to one and one-half times the normal ventilation required (31). When nitrous oxide is used to insufflate the abdomen, no significant elevation in arterial Pa_{CO_2} or decrease in Pa_{O_2} is seen (34, 36), and presumably the tendency to develop arrhythmias is less.

Laparoscopy with intraperitoneal insufflation up to 20 mm Hg is accompanied by circulatory stimulation with elevated arterial and central venous pressures, tachycardia, hypercarbia, and a decrease in pH (35–38). Further increases in intraabdominal pressure to 30 mm Hg cause decreases in central venous pressure, systolic pressure, pulse pressure, and cardiac output (35, 39). This suggests that impairment of venous return is a primary cause of the changes observed. High peripheral resistance, elevated peak respiratory pressure, and high arterial halothane concentrations might also contribute to circulatory depression. However, animal studies indicate that these hemodynamic changes occur during nitrous oxide anesthesia alone; therefore it is not the volatile agent that is causing the depression of the cardiovascular system. With release of the intraabdominal pressure, all values return to normal (35, 36). The clinical relevance of these findings is that, during laparoscopy, elevation of intraperitoneal pressure above 20 mm Hg may be potentially dangerous and that, should it occur, the release of intraabdominal pressure results in a rapid return of cardiovascular indices to normal.

Reduced blood volume in the postpartum period also contributes to the occurrence of hypotension (28, 29, 31). Keith and coworkers have found a 10% incidence of hypotension and recommend that the blood volume be acutely increased by 750 ml of Ringer's lactate solution (28, 29, 31).

Cardiac arrhythmias occur frequently during laparoscopy in patients receiving halothane anesthesia with spontaneous ventilation. Ventricular extrasystoles occurred in 17 of 100 patients receiving CO_2 insufflation compared to 2 of 45 patients receiving nitrous oxide insufflation (40). The authors believed that the arrhythmias were related to the high $PaCO_2$ in conjunction with carbon dioxide insufflation and spontaneous ventilation. The occurrence of cardiac arrhythmias is greatly reduced by control of ventilation (33, 34).

Cardiac arrhythmias have been frequently noted during anesthesia. Aside from hypercarbia and hypoxia, vasovagal reflexes also have been implicated in the production of arrhythmias. This may be related to CO_2 insufflation, manipulation of the pelvic organs, or the rise in central venous pressure (31). Atropine and glycopyrrolate have been recommended as premedicants because of their vagal-blocking effects (31).

Pneumothorax or pneumomediastinum are other potentially serious complications. The gas may pass retroperitoneally through congenital foraminae, through defects in the diaphragm, or weak points of the aortic or esophageal hiatus. Gas embolism also may occur. These infrequent but potentially fatal complications of laparoscopy must be ruled out whenever a patient becomes hypoxic, difficult to ventilate, or hypotensive (41).

As can be seen, a rather complex situation arises from peritoneal insufflation. The hemodynamic changes are a result of the interaction of many factors. If the intraabdominal pressure is not allowed to rise above 20 cm, it is unlikely that these changes will be of clinical significance. Finally, it should be emphasized that the patient must be adequately ventilated to prevent hypercarbia.

GENERAL ANESTHESIA FOR POSTPARTUM STERILIZATION SURGERY

If general anesthesia is selected for postpartum tubal ligation or laparoscopic coagulation, the physiologic changes related to the pregnancy and the specific requirements of the surgery must be considered. Even young, healthy patients (ASA status I) may have a significant mortality related to general anesthesia (42, 43).

Sterilization procedures are associated with a very low mortality. An international collaborative study reported that the mortality (adjusted for individuals lost to follow-up) is 13 per 100,000 sterilizations for interval procedures, 53.3 per 100,000 for postabortion procedures, and 43.4 per 100,000 after vaginal delivery (44). Multiple factors contribute to such deaths, but infection, anesthesia, and hemorrhage are the most common causes.

It has been estimated that the mortality for tubal sterilization in the United States is between approximately 1 and 5 per 100,000 procedures (45). Data collected by the Centers for Disease Control suggest that general anesthesia is the leading cause of mortality (45, 46). Hypoventilation appears to be a major cause of these anesthesia-related deaths. These estimates are based on sterilization-attributable mortality statistics from the years 1977 to 1980 (45). At this time endotracheal intubation was not routinely performed for this procedure, and it is worth noting that, in none of the deaths attributed to general anesthesia, had the patient been intubated (45–47). Although no deaths caused by local and regional anesthesia were reported in the United States, further study is required to determine whether the risk of death is less than that with general anesthesia.

A substantial amount of time is required to obtain useful information. Indeed, the information referred to in the paragraph above was all that was published as late as 1989 (45). Techniques have changed markedly since the last available data has been assessed. Until more recent information is available, we can only be aware that death attributable to tubal sterilization is rare and that anesthesia-related complications were among the leading cause of such deaths.

The patient must be assessed before surgery. If there are any medical or obstetric problems (such as preeclampsia), it is best to postpone surgery until the disease states can be treated and optimal physiologic conditions prevail.

Laboratory investigations should be the same as for any patient undergoing surgery. Postpartum hemoglobin and hematocrit analyses are essential because blood loss at delivery is difficult to estimate. Premedication is optional and is determined by the wishes of the mother or anesthesiologist. As described earlier in this chapter, it is not known when the postpartum stomach has returned to normal. One could speculate on the benefit of using a combination of an H_2 blocker and a nonparticulate antacid. This has been shown to be effective in reducing the risk of acid aspiration in pregnancy and should have a similar effect as a premedicant before postpartum surgery. Thus it might be prudent to routinely prophylactically administer antacid with or without other drugs (e.g., ranitidine and metoclopramide) to neutralize acid present in the stomach, encourage gastric emptying, and prevent reflux of gastric contents. However, proof that such protocols will reduce morbidity or mortality is lacking (48, 49).

Intraoperative monitoring by the anesthesiologist should include electrocardiography, blood pressure measurements, precordial stethoscopy, and temperature measurements. Intraabdominal pressure is monitored by the gynecologist to observe any marked increases during insufflation. The question of the induction is controversial. As discussed earlier, studies to date have not clearly documented when the risk of aspiration pneumonitis is reduced to normal levels. Individual variation and ongoing medical therapy might influence the return of normal function. The author believes that a period of at least 8 hr should elapse between the birth of the infant and the scheduled surgery (14). Obviously, no food should be consumed by the patient during this interval. However, no one time interval will guarantee that the patient is free of risk.

The routine use of endotracheal intubation, cricoid pressure, and a rapid-sequence induction should further reduce the risk of pulmonary aspiration and is also recommended. Others do not recommend the routine use of intubation for postpartum tubal ligation surgery (30). However, endotracheal intubation is a must for laparoscopic surgery (45–47). The author believes that the risk of relatively minor complications of laryngoscopy and intubation are more than justified in light of the major morbidity and mortality associated with pulmonary aspiration of gastric contents. Similarly, extubation of these patients should be done when they are awake and the neuromuscular blockade is fully reversed. Patients should recover in the lateral position.

Thiopental remains the intravenous induction agent of choice until further investigations show a clear advantage over other agents. Nitrous oxide is the standard inhalational anesthetic drug used for maintenance. Volatile agents or narcotics can be used for maintenance. Overall the best volatile agent is probably the one with the least amount of biodegradation. Isoflurane appears to be a good choice based on this criterion. Enflurane is not recommended in patients with seizure disorders (50) and impaired renal function (51, 52). Thus its use in toxemic patients has been questioned, although no studies have been done concerning its safety in previously toxemic patients. The minimum alveolar concentration of anesthetic agents decreases in pregnancy (53). It is not known how long after delivery it takes for values to return to normal. This should not provide a problem for the anesthesiologist, who would normally adjust the concentration of the volatile agent used to meet a given patient's needs. Regardless of which halogenated hydrocarbon is chosen, high inspired concentrations should be avoided lest uterine atony and postpartum bleeding occur. Oxytocin should be added to the intravenous infusion (20 U/1000 ml) and the inspired concentration of halothane maintained below 1.5 vol/100 ml and isoflurane and enflurane below 2 to 3 vol/100 ml.

Narcotic anesthesia is a suitable alternative to volatile agents. Fentanyl with nitrous oxide is a popular combination because of their short durations of action (30). Muscle relaxants may be necessary. Succinylcholine infusion or gallamine have been used so that the duration of action does not exceed that of the surgery. Both drugs are highly ionized and minimal quantities reach the mother's breast milk. Newer short-acting muscle relaxants such as vecuronium or atracurium may be useful because of their short duration and ease of reversibility. It is not known whether these drugs are excreted in human breast milk and, as a result, their use in nursing women has not yet been approved.

The use of cimetidine and ranitidine has not prolonged the effects of succinylcholine (54, 55) or altered the duration of action of vecuronium (56). However, metoclopramide can inhibit plasma cholinesterase activity, and this results in a doubling of the duration of action of succinylcholine (57). In addition, vecuronium-induced neuromuscular blockade is prolonged in postpartum patients, as compared with nonpregnant controls (58).

Anesthesia for laparoscopy poses the added problems of hypotension and cardiac arrhythmias. The incidence of hypotension is greatly reduced when the intraabdominal pressure is kept below 20 mm Hg (35, 39). Blood pressure should be measured every 5 min and every minute during insufflation of CO_2 to detect hypotension. Since halothane is known to have a lower arrhythmia threshold than isoflurane (59), isoflurane would be a better choice. Enflurane has an arrhythmia threshold between those of halothane and isoflurane. Narcotics have the highest arrhythmia thresholds and reduce the amount of volatile anesthetic agent needed. As discussed earlier, it is safer to control the patient's ventilation than to allow spontaneous ventilation in patients undergoing anesthesia for laparoscopy. In comparing halothane, enflurane, and isoflurane for a short anesthetic, no agent is superior to the others in terms of quick discharge from the recovery room (41).

The author routinely passes a suction catheter into the stomach to ensure deflation of the stomach in the hope of preventing the occurrence of gastric perforation, which has been reported (31). Finally, the anesthesiologist must prevent patient movement caused by light anesthesia or inadequate muscle relaxation during the moment of coagulation of the fallopian tubes.

REGIONAL ANESTHESIA FOR POSTPARTUM STERILIZATION SURGERY

Many anesthesiologists use regional anesthesia for postpartum tubal ligation. A block up to T4 would result in excellent surgical conditions and patient satisfaction (60). A block to T10 might be adequate, but patients might be uncomfortable if more than the usual stimulation is necessary to locate the tubes.

Pregnancy is associated with certain physiologic changes that necessitate the modification of the doses of anesthetic drugs administered for spinal or epidural anesthesia. It is accepted that the dose of local anesthetic required to obtain any level of block is reduced by one-third in the last trimester of pregnancy (61–63).

Assali and Prystowsky used a continuous spinal technique with 0.2% procaine in 10 women both before and after delivery and noted that, 36 to 48 hr postpartum, there was an increase of three or four times in the amount of anesthetic required to produce the same sensory level and a marked decrease in the cardiovascular effects (Table 13.3) (63). When the effects of equal doses of spinal anesthesia (tetracaine 5 mg, dextrose 50 mg) were compared in full-term pregnant and healthy young gynecologic patients, there was a faster onset, higher level, and longer duration of blockade in the parturients (64). Also, when Marx studied spinal anesthesia in postpartum women undergoing tubal ligation, she found a progressive decline in the duration of blockade over the first 3 days postpartum (64). More recently Abouleish and co-workers found that postpartum tubal ligation pa-

Table 13.3
Blood Pressure Fall in Normotensive Patients Following High Spinal Anesthesia (Dermatome Levels T2–C3)[a]

	Systolic	Diastolic
Nonpregnant ($n = 5$)	7%	4%
Term pregnant ($n = 12$)	43%	53%
36–48 hr postpartum ($n = 10$)	12%	12%

[a] Adapted from Assali NS, Prystowsky H: Studies on autonomic blockade: Comparison between the effects of tetraethylammonium chloride (TEAC) and high selective spinal anesthesia on blood pressure of normal and toxemic pregnancy. J Clin Invest 29:1354–1366, 1950.

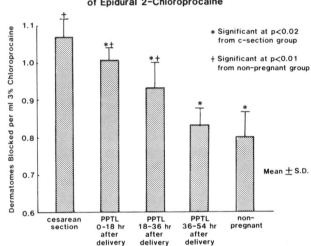

Figure 13.3. Comparison of the number of dermatomes blocked per milliliter of 3% chloroprocaine with epidural anesthesia in pregnant patients having cesarean deliveries, postpartum patients having postpartum tubal ligations (PPTL) at various intervals after delivery, and nonpregnant patients undergoing gynecologic procedures. (Reprinted with permission from Brooks GZ, Mandel ALZ: The early postpartum dermatomal spread of epidural 2-chloroprocaine. In *Abstracts of Scientific Papers*, Society for Obstetric Anesthesia and Perinatology, Annual Meeting, San Antonio, TX, 1984, p 25.)

tients require 30% or more (bupivacaine 0.75% in 8.25% dextrose) per segment than do elective repeat cesarean section patients (65).

Similarly, Brooks and Mandel found that there was a progressive decrease in the dermatomal spread of epidural anesthesia beginning during the first 18 hr postpartum compared to antepartum cesarean section patients (66). After 36 postpartum hr, epidural dose requirements were not significantly different from those in nonpregnant patients (Fig. 13.3).

The mechanisms for increased spread of epidural or spinal anesthesia in pregnant women at term have not been proven. Increased blood flow to the highly vascular pia mater may result in increased penetration of nerve roots by the local anesthetic agents. This would result in a more rapid onset of blockade. Distension of epidural veins has been implicated in the increased spread of anesthetic solution. Elevated intraabdominal pressure and inferior vena cava compression from the pregnant uterus have been suggested as likely causes during labor. In addition, the exaggerated lumbar lordosis of pregnancy may contribute to the increased cephalad spread of anesthetic solutions. Spread of intrathecally or epidurally injected contrast media shows a greater spread of contrast material in epidural rather than in the subarachnoid space (67).

The reduced dose requirement and reduced capacity of the intrathecal space do not appear to be directly related to uterine obstruction of the inferior vena cava. The reduced dose requirements persist even with adequate left uterine displacement and in the full-lateral position.

In fact, there is an increased spread of epidural anesthesia during the first trimester of pregnancy (68). This occurs at a time when mechanical factors are unlikely to play a significant role (68). A more likely explanation would be that these findings are attributable to hormonal changes. Dose requirements for volatile agents decrease in both the early and late phases of pregnancy (53, 69). However, it would appear that uptake of epidural anesthetic agents occurs by similar mechanisms in both pregnant and nonpregnant patients (68), and therefore it would be unlikely that hormones would have a significant additive effect on local anesthetics during pregnancy.

Another mechanism has been proposed by Fagraeus and co-workers (68). They postulate that hyperventilation associated with pregnancy results in an alkalosis that is compensated for by lowered bicarbonate levels. This would result in decreased buffering capacity and allow the local anesthetic agent to remain as a salt for a longer time. Therefore the agent would remain in the epidural space for a longer period of time. This would result in an increase in the time needed to reach complete analgesia; also, the drug would have time to spread further within the epidural space. The decreased buffering capacity during pregnancy might account for both the increased spread of local anesthetics and the increased time needed to achieve analgesia (68).

There is no clear recommendation about the dosage requirements of spinal or epidural anesthesia in the first day or two postpartum. Marx used a dose of 6 mg of hyperbaric tetracaine with satisfactory results (64). McKenzie recommended at least 75 mg of 5% lidocaine to obtain anesthesia at the T10 level in the average patient, with a dosage range of 60 to 90 mg depending on the patient's height (30). Tetracaine of 6 to 9 mg with 10% glucose achieves similar blockade heights (30). However, the author recommends a block to at least the T4 level to ensure patient comfort and ideal operating conditions. To obtain this, other authorities have previously recommended administering 8 to 12 mg of tetracaine or the equivalent dose of lidocaine, which might be preferred because of its shorter duration of action (31). The doses of 0.75% bupivacaine in 8.25% dextrose that have been successfully used are 12 mg or 10.6 mg for a 150-cm patient with an increase or decrease of 0.25 mg of bupivacaine for each 2.5 cm above or below this height (65, 70).

It is also worth noting that the incidence of postspinal headache following postpartum tubal ligation with a 25-gauge needle is the same (high level of 24%) as that found in parturients (71). This is significantly higher than in nonpregnant patients (72).

The precise doses of epidural anesthetics are not known. Ghosh and Tipton reported on 51 patients who achieved satisfactory epidural anesthesia for tubal ligation surgery within 10 hr (mean 2 hr) of delivery (73). They used 10 to 15 ml of 0.5% bupivacaine. Since dosage requirements are variable, some recommend using an epidural catheter and starting with doses similar to that used in pregnancy. If further anesthetic is needed, it can be added easily.

LOCAL ANESTHETIC FOR POSTPARTUM STERILIZATION SURGERY

Laparoscopic sterilization is usually an outpatient procedure. Local anesthesia is reported to have the advantage of rapid onset, ease of administration, rapid recovery time, and less nausea, vomiting, and other postoperative side effects. A prospective, randomized study that compared local analgesia (20 ml of bupivacaine 0.5% onto the peritoneal surface of the fallopian tubes) with general anesthesia concluded that it is a safe technique (74). It should be emphasized that nitrous oxide must be used for insufflation because carbon dioxide causes diaphragmatic irritation. Other studies have used 80 ml of intraperitoneal lidocaine 0.5% (75) or 20 ml of bupivacaine 0.5% (76) with satisfactory results. Postpartum tubal ligation can even be done under local infiltration of the periumbilic area plus neurolept anesthesia (77).

Although this author has had no experience with this technique, it may be an acceptable alternative. The extent to which local anesthetic techniques affect the fatality rate is unknown. Rochat and co-workers have speculated that perhaps the use of local anesthetic techniques in developing countries has reduced the higher risk of death that might otherwise have been expected (44). Anesthesia-related deaths are among the leading causes of such deaths (44, 46,

78, 79). Further assessment may help define the usefulness of this technique.

IMMEDIATE TIMING OF POSTPARTUM TUBAL LIGATION AFTER VAGINAL DELIVERY

In February 1987 the American College of Obstetricians and Gynecologists, Committee on Obstetrics, Maternal and Fetal Medicine issued a *Committee Opinion* on the appropriate timing of surgery after vaginal delivery.

If a woman has had a major anesthetic for her delivery and the anesthetic can be continued safely, there is no contraindication to proceeding with a tubal sterilization in the immediate postpartum period if the mother's condition is satisfactory and no maternal complication suggests that deferral is necessary.

If, in order to accomplish the tubal sterilization, it is necessary to induce a major anesthetic (regional or general), the patient should be carefully evaluated by the responsible anesthesiologist. It should be recognized that a postpartum sterilization is an elective procedure, and one should not proceed unless the patient is in near-optimal condition. In patients who have had significant medical or obstetric complications during their pregnancy or who have cardiovascular, respiratory, or metabolic derangements during the peripartum period (including significant anemia, hypovolemia, upper respiratory infections, or hypertension), the procedure probably should be deferred unless there are overriding medical considerations to proceed. Major physiologic changes occur at delivery in all parturients, and the cardiovascular stability of the patient should be ensured before proceeding. Neonatal condition and survivability may also be a consideration. In addition, because the parturient may have an increased risk of regurgitation and aspiration of acidic gastric contents, many anesthesiologists prefer to wait a period of time following delivery in order to allow for increased gastric emptying.

The decision as to when to proceed with anesthesia and surgery should be based on the anesthesiolgist's assessment of the patient and judgment of the relative risks and benefits for that patient (79a).

The author agrees with the above statement but wishes to emphasize that manpower considerations and the availability of personnel to provide emergency obstetric anesthesia frequently require that tubal sterilizations are performed during normal working hours.

BREAST-FEEDING AND ANESTHETIC DRUGS

Breast-feeding is considered the optimal method of infant feeding (80, 81). However, drugs do appear in breast milk. Factors involved in the transfer from plasma to milk include those of lipid solubility, ionization, concentration, degree of protein binding, and special transport mechanisms. In general, water-soluble drugs are excreted in higher concentration into colostrum, whereas lipid-soluble drugs are excreted in greater concentration into breast milk. However, there is a lack of detailed information on the excretion of maternally administered drugs in milk.

General neurobehavior responses of infants are normal whether a general or an epidural anesthetic is given (82). It is interesting to note that a significantly higher breast-feeding frequency and longer periods of breast-feeding are found up to 6 months postpartum after epidural anesthesia rather than after general anesthesia (83). One can only speculate as to whether patients who choose epidural anesthesia were more motivated to continue breast-feeding, whether epidural anesthesia facilitates mother-child bonding, or whether some drugs present in the breast milk interfere with early mother-child bonding.

It is safe to assume that most drugs given to the mother will be excreted in her milk. Recent investigations of the relationship between maternal labor analgesia and delay in the initiation of breast-feeding in healthy neonates in the early neonatal periods have suggested that even small doses of narcotics, when administered 1 to 3 hr before delivery, can delay effective breast-feeding for hours or even days (84). For most drugs, however, the quantity excreted in the milk is insufficient to have any clinical effects (85–89, 92).

Narcotics such as codeine, meperidine, and morphine result in insignificant levels with therapeutic doses (86–88, 90, 91). There would be no effects from acetaminophen, codeine, and morphine in recommended doses (92). This may not be the case when excessive doses of salicylates, acetaminophen or caffeine are taken (92). Fentanyl has also been assessed. Total doses of 50 to 400 µg were given to 10 mothers in labor. There was a lack of fentanyl excretion in breast milk. All infants had normal Apgar scores at birth and normal neurobehavior assessment scores (93).

On the other hand, it has been suggested that prescribed opioids in breast milk can cause or contribute to unexplained episodes of apnea, bradycardia, and cyanosis occurring during the first week of life in full-term infants (94). Although much more investigation needs to be done to confirm this suggestion, it may be prudent that neonates who experience such episodes avoid further exposure to the breast milk of women taking opioid analgesia (94).

Thiopental is found in breast milk but probably has insignificant effects on the newborn (85–87, 89). Intravenous propofol, one of the newer intravenous anesthetic agents, has been assessed for cesarean section anesthesia. The concentration of propofol is very low in milk or colostrum. In addition, propofol is rapidly cleared from the neonatal circulation so that exposure through breast milk is negligible and should have minimal effect on healthy newborns (95). Other authorities have found the opposite results following elective cesarean section (96, 97). Propofol (2.8 mg/kg) results in neonates with lower Apgar scores, some degree of hypotonia, and evidence of cortical depression, as compared to thiopental (5 mg/kg). Until further investigations clarify these contradictory findings, thiopental remains the induction agent of choice.

All benzodiazepines appear in human milk. Only high or repeated clinical doses might be expected to exert a possible effect on the newborn (98, 99). Diazepam, in particular, should be avoided in the neonatal period (85, 87–90). It has been reported that appreciable plasma levels of active substances are found in the neonate for up to 10 days after a single maternal dose of diazepam (99, 100). The concentration in the infant, however, is very low (98). Nevertheless, most authorities strongly advise against its use (85, 87, 88, 90, 91, 98, 100, 101).

Atropine and antihistamines cause decreased lactation with large doses, even though they may not be appreciably excreted (81, 87, 90, 91). Atropine may also cause anticholinergic side effects in infants (81, 85, 87).

In addition, many aspects of drug pharmacokinetics are impaired in the premature infant. Possible pharmacokinetic mechanisms include differences in absorption, metabolism, distribution, and elimination. Although evidence is lacking, it is commonly believed that the blood-brain barrier is more permeable in the premature infant. These factors might or might not be clinically relevant when a premature infant is given breast milk (102).

References

1. Frisoli G: Physiology and pathology of the puerperium. In *Principles and Practice of Obstetrics and Perinatology, Vol 2.* L Iffy, HA Kaminetzky, eds. John Wiley & Sons, New York, 1981, p 1657.
2. Taylor NB: *Stedman's Medical Dictionary,* 24th ed. Williams & Wilkins, Baltimore, 1982, p 1128.
3. Pritchard JA, MacDonald PC, eds: The puerperium. In *Williams Obstetrics.* Appleton-Century-Crofts, New York, 1980.
4. Ueland K: Maternal cardiovascular dynamics. VII. Intrapartum blood volume changes. Am J Obstet Gynecol 126:671–677, 1976.
5. Shankar KB, Moseley H, Kumar Y, Vemula V, Krishnan A: Arterial to end-tidal carbon dioxide tension difference during anaesthesia for tubal ligation. Anaesthesia 42:482–486, 1987.
6. Cohen SE: Why is the pregnant patient different? Semin Anesth 1:73, 1982.
7. Attia RR, Ebeid AM, Fischer JE, Goudsouzian NG: Maternal, foetal and placental gastrin concentrations. Anaesthesia 37:18–21, 1982.
8. Ory HW, Forrest JD, Lincoln R, eds: Making choices. In *Evaluating the Health Risks and Benefits of Birth Control Methods.* The Alan Guttmacher Institute, New York, 1983, p 11.
9. Moore JG, Russell KP: Maternal medical indications for female sterilization. Clin Obstet Gynecol 7:54–56, 1964.
10. Little WA: Current aspects of sterilization: The selections

and applications of various surgical methods of sterilization. Am J Obstet Gynecol 123:12–18, 1975.
11. Taylor PJ, Gomel V: Introduction. In *Laparoscopy and Hysteroscopy in Gynecologic Practice.* V Gomel, PJ Taylor, AA Yuzpe, JE Rious, eds. Year Book Medical Publishers, Chicago, 1986, pp 1–6.
12. Bilateral tubal ligation—An emergency? (Newsletter) Society for Obstetric Anesthesia and Perinatology July 1, 1973.
13. Destefano F. Greenspan JR, Dicker RC, Peterson HB, Strauss LT, Rubin GL: Complications of internal laparoscopic tubal sterilization. Obstet Gynecol 61:153–158, 1983.
14. Blouw R, Scatliff J, Craig DB, Palahnuik RJ: Gastric volume and pH in postpartum patients. Anesthesiology 45:456–457, 1976.
15. Berson W, Adriani J: Silent regurgitation and aspiration during anesthesia. Anesthesiology 15:644–649, 1954.
16. Roberts RB, Shirley MA: Reducing the risk of acid aspiration during cesarean section. Anesth Analg 53:859–868, 1974.
17. Uram M, Abouleish E, McKenzie R, Phityakorn P, Tantisira B, Uy N: The risk of aspiration pneumonitiis with postpartum tubal ligation. In *Abstracts of Scientific Papers,* Society for Obstetric Anesthesia and Perinatology, Annual Meeting, Jackson Hole, WY, 1982. p 2.
18. James CF, Gibbs CP, Banner TE: Postpartum perioperative risk of pulmonary aspiration pneumonia. Anesthesiology 61:756–759, 1984.
19. Whitehead EM, Smith M, O'Sullivan G: An evaluation of gastric emptying times in pregnancy and the puerperium. In *Abstracts of Scientific Papers,* Society of Obstetric Anesthesia and Perinatology, Annual Meeting, Madison, WI, 1990, p F-1.
20. O'Sullivan GA, Sutton AJ, Thompson SA, Cornie LE, Bullingham RE: Noninvasive measurement of gastric emptying in obstetric patients. Anesth Analg 66:505–511, 1987.
21. Rennie AL, Richard JA, Milne MK, Dalrymple DG: Postpartum sterilizaiton: An anaesthetic hazard? Anaesthesia 34:267–287, 1979.
22. Campbell AA: The incidence of operations that prevent conception. Am J Obstet Gynecol 89:694–700, 1964.
23. Overstreet EW: Techniques of sterilization. Clin Obstet Gynecol 7:109–125, 1964.
24. Devanesan M: Postpartum contraception. In *Principles and Practice of Obstetrics and Perinatology, Vol 2.* L Iffy, HA Kaminetzky, eds. John Wiley & Sons, New York, 1981, p 1677.
25. Clark DH, Schneider GT, McManus S: Tubal sterilization: Comparison of outpatient laparoscopy and postpartum ligation. J Reprod Med 13:69–70, 1974.
26. Paterson PJ, Grimwade JC: Laparoscopic sterilization during the puerperium. Med J Aust 2:312–313, 1972.
27. Neely MR, Elkady AA: Modified technique of puerperal laparoscopic sterilization. J Obstet Gynaecol Br Commonw 79:1025–1027, 1972.
28. Keith L, Webster A, Houser K, Procknicki L, Lash A, Barton J: Laparoscopy for puerperal sterilization. Obstet Gynecol 39:616–621, 1972.
29. Keith L, Webster A, Lash A: A comparison between puerperal and nonpuerperal laparoscopic sterilization. Int Surg 56:325–330, 1971.
30. McKenzie R: Postpartum tubal ligation. In *Pain Control in Obstetrics.* E Abouleish, ed. Lippincott, Philadelphia, 1977, pp 411–425.
31. Fishburne JI, Keith L: Anesthesia. In *Laparoscopy.* JM Phillips, ed. Williams & Wilkins, Baltimore, 1977, pp 69–85.
32. Desmond J, Gordon RA: Ventilation in patients anaesthetized for laparoscopy. Can Anaesth Soc J 17:378–387, 1970.
33. Hodgson C, McClellan RMA, Newton JR: Some effects of the peritoneal insufflation of carbon dioxide and laparoscopy. Anaesthesia 25:382–392, 1970.
34. Alexander GD, Brown EM: Physiologic alterations during pelvic laparoscopy. Am J Obstet Gynecol 105-1078-1081, 1969.
35. Motew M, Ivankovich AD, Bieniarz J, Albrecht RF, Zahed B, Scommegna A: Cardiovascular effects and acid-base and blood

gas changes during laparoscopy. Am J Obstet Gynecol 115:1002–1012, 1973.

36. Ivankovich AD, Miletich DK, Albrecht RF, Heyman HJ, Bonnet RF: Cardiovascular effects of peritoneal insufflation of carbon dioxide and nitrous oxide in the dog. Anesthesiology 42:281–287, 1975.

37. Pillalamarri ED, Bhangdia P, Rudin RS, Chadry RM, Tadoon PR, Abadir AR: Effects of CO_2 pneumoperitoneum during laparoscopy on A.B.G.'s, end-tidal CO_2 and cardiovascular dynamics. Anesthesiology 59:A424, 1983.

38. Smith I, Benzie RJ, Gordon NLM, Kelman GR: Cardiovascular effects of peritoneal insufflation of carbon dioxide for laparoscopy. Br Med J 3:410–411, 1971.

39. Lenz RJ, Thomas TA, Wilkins DG: Cardiovascular changes during laparoscopy: Studies of stroke volume and cardiac output using impedance cardiography. Anaesthesia 31:4–12, 1976.

40. Scott DB, Julian DG: Observations on cardiac arrhythmias during laparoscopy. Br Med J 1:411–413, 1976.

41. Spielman FJ: Laparoscopic surgery. Prob Anesth 3:151–159, 1989.

42. Vacanti CJ, Van Houten RJ, Hill RC: A statistical analysis of the relationship of physical status to postoperative mortality in 68,388 cases. Anesth Analg 49:564–566, 1970.

43. Goldstein A, Keats AS: The risk of anesthesia. Anesthesiology 33:130–143, 1970.

44. Rochat RW, Bhiwandiwala PP, Feldblum PJ, Peterson HB: Mortality associated with sterilization: Preliminary results of an international collaborative study. Int J Gynaecol Obstet 24:274–284, 1986.

45. Escobedo LG, Peterson HB, Grubb GS, Franks AL: Case-fatality rates for tubal sterilization in U.S. hospitals, 1979–80. Am J Obstet Gynecol 160:147–150, 1989.

46. Peterson HB, De Stefano F, Rubin GL, Greenspan JR, Lee NC, Ory HW: Deaths attributable to tubal sterilization in the United States, 1977 to 1981. Am J Obstet Gynecol 146:131–136, 1983.

47. Leads from the MMWR: Tubal sterilization-related deaths in the US, 1977–1981. JAMA 249:3011, 1983.

48. Cohen SE: Aspiration syndromes in pregnancy. Anesthesiology 51:375–377, 1979.

49. Moir DD: Cimetidine, antacids and pulmonary aspiration. Anesthesiology 59:81–83, 1983.

50. Shapiro HM: Anesthesia effects upon cerebral blood flow, cerebral metabolism, and the electroencephalogram. In *Anesthesia, Vol 2*. RD Miller, ed. Churchill-Livingstone, New York, 1982, p 811.

51. Eichhorn JH, Hedley-Whyte J, Steinman TI, Kaufmann JM, Laasberg H: Renal failure following enflurane anesthesia. Anesthesiology 45:557–560, 1976.

52. Mazze RI, Calverly RK, Smith NT: Inorganic fluoride nephrotoxicity: Prolonged enflurane and halothane anesthesia in volunteers. Anesthesiology 46:265–271, 1977.

53. Palahniuk RJ, Shnider SM, Eger EI II: Pregnancy decreases the requirements for inhaled anesthetic agents. Anesthesiology 41:82–83, 1974.

54. Bogod D: The effects of H_2 antagonists on duration of action of suxamethonium in the parturient. Anaesthesia 44:591–593, 1989.

55. Woodworth GE, Sears DH, Grove T, Ruff RH, Kosek PS, Katz RL: The effects of cimetidine and ranitidine on the duration of action of succinylcholine. Anesth Analg 68:295–297, 1989.

56. Hawkins JL, Adenwala J, Camp C, Joyce TH III: The effect of H_2-receptor antagonist premedication on the duration of vecuronium-induced neuromuscular blockade in postpartum patients. Anesthesiology 71:175–177, 1989.

57. Kao YJ, Turner DR: Prolongation of succinylcholine block by metoclopramide. Anesthesiology 70:905–908, 1989.

58. Camp CE, Tessem J, Adenwala J, Joyce TH III: Vecuronium and prolonged neuromuscular blockade in postpartum patients. Anesthesiology 67:1006–1008, 1987.

59. Johnson RR, Eger EI II, Wilson C: A comparative interaction of epinephrine with enflurane, isoflurane and halothane in man. Anesth Analg 55:709–712, 1976.

60. Moore DC: *Regional Block*, 4th ed. Charles C Thomas, Springfield, IL, 1973, p 381.

61. Bromage PR: Spread of analgesia solutions in the epidural space and their site of action: A statistical study. Br J Anaesth 34:161–178, 1962.

62. Sharrock NE, Greenidge J: Epidural dose responses in pregnant and nonpregnant patients. Anesthesiology 51:S298, 1979.

63. Assali NS, Prystowsky H: Studies on autonomic blockade: Comparison between the effects of tetraethylammonium chloride (TEAC) and high selective spinal anesthesia on blood pressure of normal and toxemic pregnancy. J Clin Invest 29:1354–1366, 1950.

64. Marx GF: Regional analgesia in obstetrics. Der Anaesth 21:84–91, 1972.

65. Abouleish EI: Postpartum tubal ligation requires more bupivacaine for spinal anesthesia than does cesarean section. Anesth Analg 65:897–900, 1986.

66. Brooks GZ, Mandel ALZ: The early postpartum dermatomal spread of epidural 2-chloroprocaine. In *Abstracts of Scientific Papers*, Society for Obstetric Anesthesia and Perinatology, Annual Meeting, San Antonio, TX, 1984, p 25.

67. Hipona FA, Yules R, Hehre FW: Venous encroachment on the spinal peridural space due to experimental IVC occlusion. Invest Radiol 1:157–161, 1966.

68. Fagraeus L, Urban BJ, Bromage PR: Spread of epidural analgesia in early pregnancy. Anesthesiology 58:184–187, 1983.

69. Strout CD, Nahrwold ML: Halothane requirement during pregnancy and lactation in rats. Anesthesiology 55:322–323, 1981.

70. De Simone CA, Norris MC, Leighton BL, Epstein RH, Palmer C: Spinal anesthesia for cesarean section and postpartum tubal ligation. Anesthesiology 71:A836, 1989.

71. Williams R, Silverstein PI, Levin KR. Incidence of postspinal headache following tubal ligation 24–48 hours post partum. Reg Anesth 13:21S, 1988.

72. Vandam LD, Dripps RD: Long-term follow-up of patients who received 10,098 spinal anesthetics. JAMA 161:586–591, 1956.

73. Ghosh AK, Tipton RH: Early postpartum tubal ligation under epidural analgesia. Br J Obstet Gynaecol 83:731–732, 1976.

74. Peterson HB, Hulka JF, Spielman FJ, Lee S, Marchbanks PA: Local versus general anesthesia for laparoscopic sterilization: A randomized study. Obstet Gynecol 70:903–908, 1987.

75. Cruikshank DP, Laube DW, De Bacher LJ: Intraperitoneal lidocaine anesthesia for postpartum tubal ligation. Obstet Gynecol 39:127–130, 1973.

76. Speilman FJ, Hulka JF, Ostheimer GW: Pharmacokinetics and pharmacodynamics of local analgesia for laparoscopic tubal ligations. Am J Obstet Gynecol 146:821–824, 1983.

77. Munson AK, Scott JR: Postpartum ligation under local anesthesia. Obstet Gynecol 39:756–758, 1972.

78. Mintz M: Risks and prophylaxis in laparoscopy: A survey of 100,000 cases. J Reprod Med 18:269–272, 1977.

79. Grimes DA, Satterthwaite AP, Rochat RW, Akhter N: Deaths from contraceptive sterilization in Bangladesh: Rates, causes and prevention. Obstet Gynecol 60:635–639, 1982.

79a. American College of Obstetricians and Gynecologists, Committee on Obstetrics, Maternal and Fetal Medicine: *Committee Opinion*, February 1987.

80. American Academy of Pediatrics, Committee on Nutrition: Breast feeding. Pediatrics 62:591–601, 1978.

81. *Breastfeeding: A Guide for the Medical Profession*, 3rd ed. RA Lawrence, ed. CV Mosby, St. Louis, 1989, pp 198–199.

82. Kangas-Saarela T, Koivisto M, Jouppila R, Jouppila P, Hollmén A: Comparison of the effects of general and epidural anaesthesia for caesarean section on the neurobehavioral responses of newborn infants. Acta Anaesthesiol Scand 33:313–319, 1989.

83. Lie B, Jual J: Effects of epidural vs. general anesthesia on breastfeeding. Acta Obstet Gynecol Scand 67:207–209, 1988.

84. Matthews MK: The relationship between maternal labour

analgesia and delay in the initiation of breastfeeding in healthy neonates in the early neonatal period. Midwifery 5:3–10, 1989.

85. Drugs in breast milk. Med Lett 16:25–27, 1974.
86. Kwit NT, Hatcher RA: Excretion of drugs in milk. Am J Dis Child 49:900–904, 1935.
87. O'Brien TE: Excretion of drugs in human milk. Am J Hosp Pharm 31:844–854, 1974.
88. Feilberg VL, Rosenborg D, Christensen CB, Morgensen JV: Excretion of morphine in human breast milk. Acta Anaesthesiol Scand 33:426–428, 1989.
89. Anderson LW, Quist T, Hertz J, Mogensen F: Concentrations of thiopentone in mature breast milk and colostrum following an induction dose. Acta Anaesthesiol Scand 31:30–32, 1987.
90. Knowles JA: Excretion of drugs in milk: A review. Pediatr Pharmacol Therap 66:1068–1082, 1965.
91. Anderson PO: Drugs and breast feeding. Semin Perinatol 3:271–278, 1979.
92. Findlay JWA, De Angelis RL, Kearney MF, Welch RM, Findlay JM: Analgesic drugs in breast milk and plasma. Clin Pharmacol Ther 29:625–633, 1981.
93. Leuschen MP, Wolf LJ, Rayburn WF: Fentanyl excretion in breast milk. Clin Pharm 9:336–337, 1990.
94. Naumburg EG, Meny RG: Breast milk opioids and neonatal apnea. Am J Dis Child 142:11–12, 1988.
95. Dailland P, Cockshott ID, Lirzin JD, Jacquinot P, Jorrott JC, Devery J, Harmey JL, Conseiller C: Intravenous propofol during cesarean section: Placental transfer, concentrations in breast milk and neonatal effects—A preliminary study. Anesthesiology 71:827–834, 1989.
96. Celleno D, Capogna G, Tomassetti M, Costantino P, Di Feo G, Nisini R: Neurobehavioral effects of propofol on the neonate following elective caesarean section induction. Br J Anaesth 62:649–654, 1989.
97. Gin T, Yau G, Gregory MA: Propofol during cesarean section. Anesthesiology 73:789, 1990.
98. Kanto JH: Use of benzodiazepines during pregnancy, labour and lactation, with particular reference to pharmacokinetic considerations. Drugs 23:354–380, 1982.
99. Summerfield RJ, Nielsen MS: Excretion of lorazepam into breast milk. Br J Anaesth 57:1042–1043, 1985.
100. Cole AP, Hailey DM: Diazepam and active metabolite in breast milk and their transfer to the neonate. Arch Dis Child 50:741–742, 1975.
101. Erkkola R, Kanto J: Diazepam and breastfeeding. Lancet 1:1235–1236, 1972.
102. Atkinson HC, Begg EJ, Darlow BA: Drugs in human milk: Clinical pharmacokinetic considerations. Clin Pharmacokinet 14:217–240, 1988.

CHAPTER 14

Anesthesia for Surgery during Pregnancy

Gershon Levinson, M.D.
Sol M. Shnider, M.D.

The incidence of surgery during pregnancy reportedly ranges from 0.3 to 22.2% (1–5). Shnider and Webster (1) reported that 1 in every 116 pregnant women has a major surgical anesthetic. Others have reported that as many as 2% of all operations carried out in women are performed during pregnancy (3). Based on these reports it has been estimated that each year in the United States up to 50,000 pregnant women may receive an anesthetic for surgery during pregnancy. These women require special attention in their anesthetic management if maternal morbidity and fetal wastage are to be avoided. The basic objectives in the anesthetic management of pregnant women undergoing surgery are: *(a) maternal safety; (b) avoidance of teratogenic drugs; (c) avoidance of intrauterine fetal asphyxia; and (d) prevention of preterm labor.*

MATERNAL SAFETY

The physiologic changes that occur during pregnancy are discussed in Chapter 1. Many of these changes are due to hormonal factors, as well as to the mechanical effects of the enlarging uterus, and occur during the first and second trimesters. The changes of greatest relevance to the anesthesiologist are summarized below.

Alveolar ventilation is increased about 25% by the fourth month of pregnancy and rises progressively to 70% at term (Fig. 14.1) (6). End-tidal P_{CO_2} falls to 33 torr by the third month of pregnancy (Fig. 14.2) (6). Functional residual capacity is decreased 10% at 6 months and 20% at term (Fig. 14.3) (7). Oxygen consumption increases significantly during mid-pregnancy (Fig. 14.4) due to the developing placenta, fetus, and uterine muscle. Anesthetic requirement for halogenated agents is decreased up to 40% by the second trimester (8, 9).

Induction of and emergence from anesthesia is more rapid because of the increased ventilation and decreased functional residual capacity. The likelihood of anesthetic overdose is increased. The increased oxygen consumption and decreased functional re-

sidual capacity make the pregnant patient more likely to become hypoxic with respiratory obstruction or difficult endotracheal intubation. Even during rapid endotracheal intubation (30 sec of apnea) arterial P_{O_2} can fall to 50 to 60 mm Hg in mothers who are not preoxygenated.

Cardiac output and stroke volume are increased 35 to 40% (10–12) (see Fig. 27.2), and blood volume is increased 20 to 30% by 20 to 24 weeks gestation (13, 14). Cardiac output increases 1000 ml/min by 8 weeks gestation (Fig. 14.5) primarily because of stroke volume rather than heart rate (Fig. 14.6) (15). Inferior vena caval occlusion, although most pronounced in women near term, is also significant during the second trimester (Fig. 14.7) despite the apparently small size of the uterus. Lateral tilt to prevent supine hypotension and uterine hypoperfusion should be used for all surgical procedures if possible.

The increase in femoral venous pressure shown in Figure 14.7 is likely also reflected in the epidural veins and may be relevant in explaining the reduced dosage of local anesthetic necessary to achieve a given level of spinal or epidural anesthesia during pregnancy. Because of epidural venous engorgement the size of the subarachnoid and epidural spaces may be decreased, and less local anesthetic is required to produce a given level of anesthesia.

However, this explanation of reduced local anesthetic requirement does not account for the interesting findings of Fagraeus et al. (16). They showed that, in women having epidural anesthesia during early pregnancy (8 to 12 weeks gestation), a given dose of local anesthetic produced a significantly higher anesthetic level than in nonpregnant women (Fig. 14.8). In fact, the dose requirement was similar to that found in pregnant women at term. This early in pregnancy, because of the small uterine size, venous engorgement is not prominent.

In rats there is a progressive increase in the pain threshold throughout pregnancy (Fig. 14.9) (17), likely due to a progressive increase in endogenous endorphins in the substantia gelatinosa, which can be

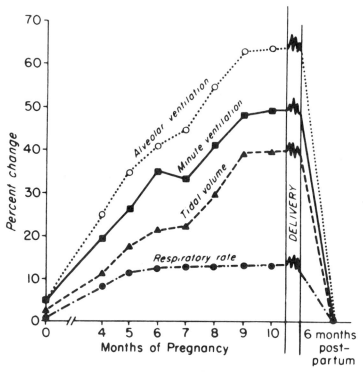
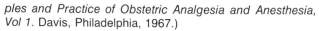

Figure 14.1. Changes in respiratory parameters during pregnancy. (Reprinted by permission from Bonica JJ: *Principles and Practice of Obstetric Analgesia and Anesthesia, Vol 1.* Davis, Philadelphia, 1967.)

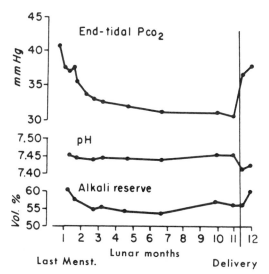

Figure 14.2. Progressive changes of alveolar carbon dioxide tensions, pH, and alkali reserve throughout pregnancy. (Reprinted by permission from Bonica JJ: *Principles and Practice of Obstetric Analgesia and Anesthesia, Vol 1.* Davis, Philadelphia, 1967.)

blocked by naltrexone administration (Fig. 14.10). Datta et al. (18) compared the effects of bupivacaine on nerve conduction in the isolated vagus nerve from pregnant and nonpregnant rabbits. The onset of block was significantly faster in nerves from pregnant an-

imals. These studies indicate that during pregnancy either nerve fibers have increased sensitivity to local anesthetics or there is enhanced diffusion of the local anesthetic to the membrane receptor site. Therefore the amount of local anesthetic should be reduced by 25 to 30% during any stage of pregnancy lest an excessively high level of anesthesia occur.

It is unclear precisely at which point in gestation a pregnant woman becomes more susceptible to regurgitation and aspiration under anesthesia. Plasma gastrin levels, believed to be of placental origin, are elevated throughout gestation but are especially high in the second half (19).

Wyner and Cohen (20) have shown that women under 20 weeks gestation do not have increased gastric volumes or decreased pH compared to nonpregnant women. Nonetheless, in both groups more than a third of the women have a gastric volume greater than 25 ml with a pH less than 2.5. Other studies have indicated that *during pregnancy* lower esophageal sphincter tone is decreased, predisposing the pregnant woman to passive regurgitation. This reduced sphincter tone is especially apparent in women with symptoms of heartburn, and has been documented to be present as early as 15 weeks gestation (20). Some suggest that all pregnant patients undergoing anesthesia should be premedicated with an oral antacid. Certainly, the authors believe, any preg-

Figure 14.3. Serial measurements of lung compartments, pulmonary mixing index, and maximum breathing capacity during normal pregnancy. *RV* = residual volume; *TLC* = total lung capacity. (Reprinted by permission from Bonica JJ: *Principles and Practice of Obstetric Analgesia and Anesthesia, Vol 1.* Davis, Philadelphia, 1967.)

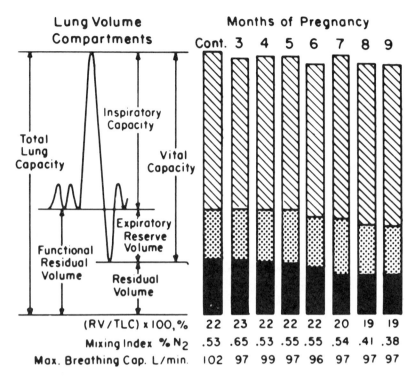

	Cont.	3	4	5	6	7	8	9
(RV/TLC) x 100,%	22	23	22	22	22	20	19	19
Mixing Index % N$_2$	.53	.65	.53	.55	.55	.54	.41	.38
Max. Breathing Cap. L/min.	102	97	99	97	96	97	97	97

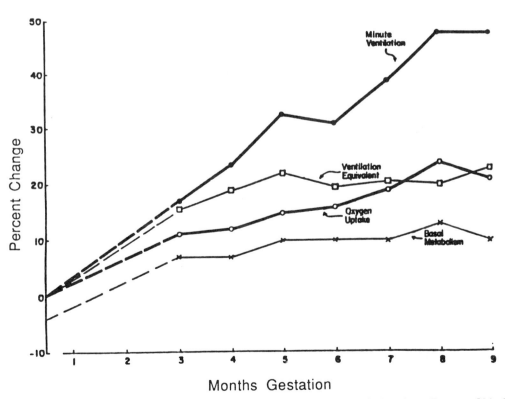

Months Gestation

Figure 14.4. Percentage of changes in minute ventilation, oxygen uptake, basal metabolism, and the ventilation equivalent for oxygen at monthly intervals throughout pregnancy.

(Reprinted by permission from Prowse CM, Gaensler EA: Respiratory and acid-base changes during pregnancy. Anesthesiology 26:381–392, 1965.)

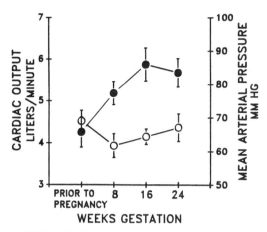

Figure 14.5. Cardiac output (*filled circles*) and mean arterial pressure (*open circles*) components of systemic vascular resistance are presented for four study periods. (Reprinted by permission from Capeless EL, Clapp JF: Cardiovascular changes in early phase of pregnancy. Am J Obstet Gynecol 161:1449–1453, 1989.)

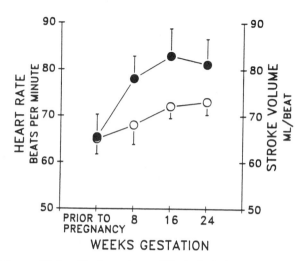

Figure 14.6. Stroke volume (*filled circles*) and heart rate (*open circles*) components of cardiac output are presented for four study periods. (Reprinted by permission from Capeless EL, Clapp JF: Cardiovascular changes in early phase of pregnancy. Am J Obstet Gynecol 161:1449–1453, 1989.)

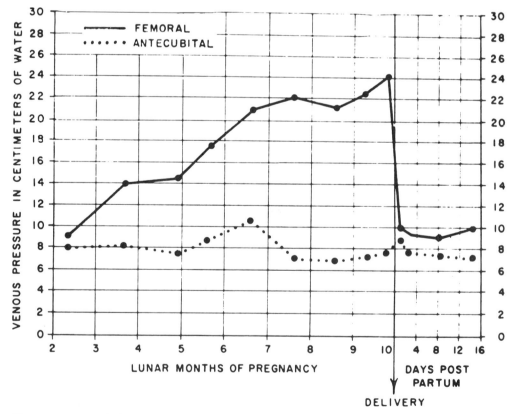

Figure 14.7. Venous pressure during pregnancy in the femoral and antecubital veins. (Reprinted by permission from Bonica JJ: *Principles and Practice of Obstetric Analgesia and Anesthesia, Vol 1.* Davis, Philadelphia, 1967.)

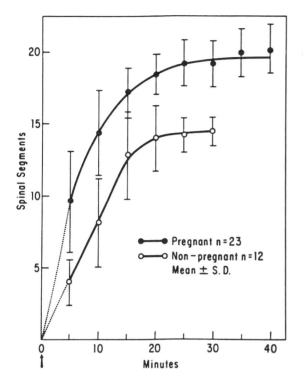

Figure 14.8. Rate of spread of epidural analgesia in nonpregnant and pregnant women in their first trimester. A line of best fit has been drawn. Injection time is denoted by the *arrow* at time zero. (Reprinted by permission from Fagraeus L, Urban BJ, Bromage PR: Spread of epidural analgesia in early pregnancy. Anesthesiology 53:184–187, 1983.)

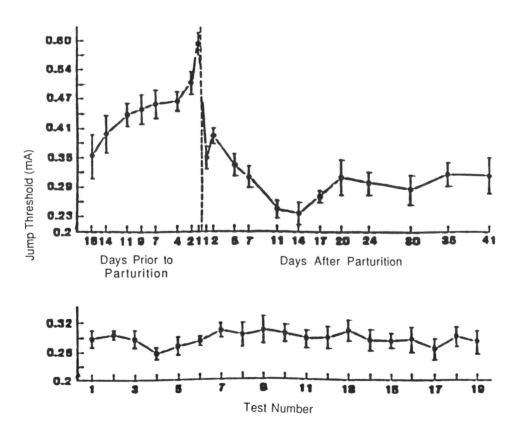

Figure 14.9. Mean jump threshold in pregnant rats as a function of days before and after parturition (*dashed line*). Each *point* represents the mean threshold of eight rats ± SE. (Reprinted by permission from Gintzler A: Endorphin-mediated increases in pain threshold during pregnancy. Science 210:193–195, 1980.)

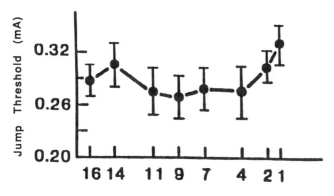

Figure 14.10. Mean jump thresholds of pregnant rats implanted with two naltrexone pellets, presented as a function of days before parturition. Testing was begin 1 day after implanation. Each *point* represents the mean threshold of seven rats ± SE. (Reprinted by permission from Gintzler A: Endorphin-mediated increases in pain threshold during pregnancy. Science 210:193–195, 1980.)

nant woman undergoing surgery during the third trimester or *any time during pregnancy if she has symptoms of esophagitis* should be intubated rapidly after induction of general anesthesia and pretreated with oral antacid.

TERATOGENICITY OF ANESTHETICS

Teratogenicity, either morphologic, biochemical, or behavioral, may be induced at any stage of gestation by exogenous agents and detected at birth or later. To produce a defect, a teratogenic drug must be given in an appropriate dosage, during a particular developmental stage of the embryo, in a species or individual with a particular genetic susceptibility (Fig. 14.11).

The critical stages of organ development in humans are illustrated in Fig. 14.12. Each organ and each system undergoes a critical stage of differentiation during which vulnerability to teratogens is greatest and specific malformations can be produced. For example, the period of sensitivity of the heart is 18 to 40 days and the limbs 24 to 34 days. Variations in genetic susceptibility may make interpretation of teratogenic studies difficult. Drugs may have a marked effect in one species and little teratogenic effect in another. Even in the same species different strains may respond differently. Thalidomide, which produces gross malformations in humans (Fig. 14.13) and rabbits, is safe in rats (22). Of the women who took thalidomide during the susceptible period, over 75% delivered normal babies (23).

Almost all commonly used anesthetics and premedicant drugs are teratogenic in some animal spe-

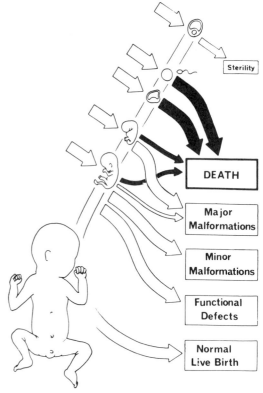

Figure 14.11. The influence of teratogenic factors on gametogenesis and various stages of embryonic and fetal development. During the preimplantation period strong teratogenic agents kill the embryo. During embryogenesis, from day 13 to day 60, teratogenic agents are embryotoxic or produce major congenital malformations. During the following fetal period minor morphologic and functional malformations can be produced. (Reprinted by permission from Tuchmann-Duplessis H: The effects of teratogenic drugs. In *Scientific Foundations of Obstetrics and Gynaecology.* E Phillipp, J Barnes, M Newton, eds. Davis, Philadelphia, 1970.)

cies. However, the applicability of these animal studies to humans has not been determined.

Systemic Medications

ANIMAL STUDIES

Numerous anomalies have been reported after pentobarbital or phenobarbital administration to mice, but not rats or rabbits (24–26). For example, a single dose of thiamylal caused teratogenic and growth-suppressing defects in the offspring of mice (25). Chlorpromazine, prochorperazine, imipramine, and amphetamines given to pregnant rats and rabbits have been shown to be teratogenic and produce permanent changes in brain levels of norepinephrine, dopamine, 5-hydroxytryptamine, and their metabolites in the offspring (27–29).

Methadone is teratogenic in mice (30) but not in rats or rabbits (31). In hamsters the number of ab-

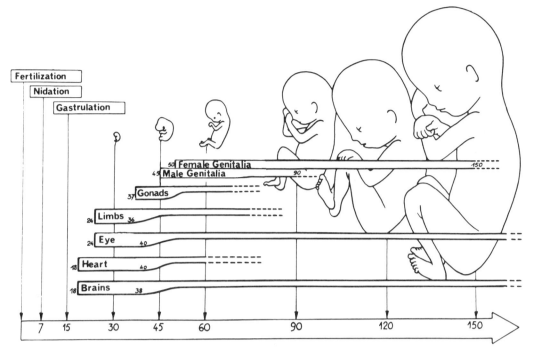

Figure 14.12. The timing of the morphogenesis of various organs, corresponding to the critical periods of teratogenic susceptibility. (Reprinted by permission from Tuchmann-Du-

plessis H: The effects of teratogenic drugs. In *Scientific Foundations of Obstetrics and Gynaecology*. E Phillipp, J Barnes, M Newton, eds. Davis, Philadelphia, 1970.)

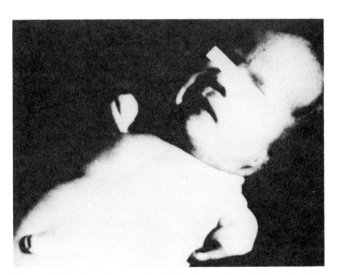

Figure 14.13. Phocomelia following maternal thalidomide ingestion between 24 and 34 days of gestation.

normal fetuses from females injected with a single dose of diacetylmorphine (heroin), phenazocine, pentazocine, propoxyphene, and methadone increased as the maternal dose increased (32). Morphine and meperidine produced an increase in the number of fetal anomalies only to a certain dose level. With multiple doses of diacetylmorphine and methadone the incidence of anomalies increased further.

Curiously, in this study, the narcotic antagonists, nalorphine, naloxone, and levallorphan blocked the teratogenic effects. The authors postulated that hypoxia and hypercarbia induced by the unantagonized narcotics may have actually been the teratogens rather than the narcotics per se.

This is supported by studies of the new narcotics: fentanyl, sufentanil, and alfentanil in rats in which respiratory depression did not develop (33, 34). Fentanyl in doses up to 500 µg/kg/day (from preconception to throughout pregnancy), sufentanil, 100 µg/kg/day, or alfentanil, 8000 µg/kg/day, (each from day 5 through day 20 of pregnancy) were not teratogenic.

HUMAN STUDIES

Three retrospective studies have suggested an association between ingestion of minor tranquilizers during pregnancy and an increased risk of congenital anomalies.

One study examined the prenatal records of over 19,000 live births to determine the incidence of severe anomalies in children whose mothers had taken either meprobamate (Equinal, Miltown), chlordiazepoxide (Librium), "other drugs," or no drugs (35). The incidence of anomalies when meprobamate or chlordiazepoxide was prescribed during the first 6 weeks of gestation was significantly higher (12.1% and 11.4%, respectively) than when one of the other drugs (4.6%) or no drug (2.6%) was given (Table 14.1). When the tranquilizers were administered later in pregnancy no differences were seen in the incidence of anomalies among the four groups. The study was not controlled for the presence of other risk factors for delivery of a child with congenital anomalies, and the findings for chlordiazepoxide were based on only four very different anomalies (duodenal atresia with Meckel's diverticulum, spastic diplegia with deafness, microcephaly, and mental deficiency) and did not reach the 5% level of statistical significance. However, the findings for meprobamate did reach a higher level of significance and, in addition, showed a preponderance of anomalies involving the heart (five of eight cases).

A second study from the Finnish Register of Congenital Malformations (1967–1971) reported an association of cleft palate with maternal ingestion of three groups of drugs: tranquilizers (diazepam and meprobamate), salicylates, and opiates (Table 14.2) (36). The study compared the usage of these drugs during the first trimester in mothers of 590 children with oral clefts and found that intake of these drugs was significantly greater in these mothers than in controls: antianxiety agents—6.2% in study mothers versus 2.9% in control mothers; opiates—6.7% versus 2.2%; and salicylates—14.9% versus 5.6%.

Table 14.1
Teratogenicity of Minor Tranquilizers in 19,044 Live Births[a]

Drug	Rate of Anomalies (per 100 Births)
No drug for anxiety	2.6
Meprobamate (Equanil, Miltown)	12.1
Chlordiazepoxide (Librium)	11.4
Other drugs	4.6

[a]Adapted from Milkovich L, van den Berg BJ: Effects of prenatal meprobamate and chlordiazepoxide hydrochloride on human embryonic and fetal development. N Engl J Med 291:1268–1271, 1974.

Table 14.2
Survey of 590 Children with Cleft Palate[a]

	Incidence of Cleft Palate	
	Drug Group	No Drug (Control) Group
Diazepam or meprobamate	6.2%	2.9%
Salicylates	14.9%	5.6%
Opiates	6.7%	2.2%

[a]Adapted from Saxen I, Saxen L: Association between maternal intake of diazepam and oral clefts. Lancet 2:498, 1975.

A third study was based on interviews of 278 mothers of children with selected birth defects who had been exposed to a variety of drugs during the first trimester of pregnancy (37). Mothers of infants with cleft lips with or without cleft palate reported use of diazepam four times more frequently than mothers of infants with other defects.

In contrast to these three studies a fourth investigation failed to find an increased risk of congenital malformation associated with the use of minor tranquilizers during early pregnancy (38). A total of 50,282 pregnancies were reviewed and the incidence of malformations in 1870 children exposed in utero to meprobamate or chlordiazepoxide was compared to the incidence in 48,412 unexposed children. No differences in the groups were found.

Nonetheless, the Food and Drug Administration (FDA Drug Bulletin September–November 1975) has stated that, "while these data do not provide conclusive evidence that minor tranquilizers cause fetal abnormalities they do suggest an association. Since the use of these drugs during the first trimester of pregnancy is rarely a matter of urgency, benefit-risk considerations are such that their use during this period should almost always be avoided."

Anesthetics

ANIMAL STUDIES

When **nitrous oxide** 80% was administered to chicken eggs for 6 hr on days 3, 4, or 5 of incubation, there was no increased rate of congenital anomalies (39). The combination of nitrous oxide and mild hypoxia (10% oxygen) for 6 hr produced more anomalies than mild hypoxia alone (39). When nitrous oxide 50% was administered to pregnant rats for 1 or 2 days a high incidence of intrauterine fetal death and a significant increase in skeletal malformations were found (40). When rats were exposed to 70 to 75% nitrous oxide, nitrogen, xenon (an anesthetic slightly more potent than nitrous oxide), or 0.6% halothane for 24 hr on day 9 of pregnancy, only nitrous oxide caused major anomalies (41, 42). On the other hand, continuous administration of 50 to 75% nitrous oxide for 24 hr on day 8 to 9 of gestation is teratogenic in rats (43). Mazze et al. (44) administered 50% nitrous oxide to mice for 4 hr each day on days 6 through 15 of pregnancy and did not show an increased incidence of anomalies. Similarly, Pope et al. (45) showed that, in rats, 50% nitrous oxide for 8 hr/day throughout gestation was not teratogenic. **These and other studies (46–49) indicate that, in chickens and rodents, exposure to nitrous oxide for up to 12 hr during each day of gestation is not teratogenic, but extreme conditions will produce teratogenic effects.**

One of the major concerns regarding the use of nitrous oxide for surgery during pregnancy relates to the adverse effects of nitrous oxide on DNA synthesis. In fact, some believe that nitrous oxide is contraindicated during the first two trimesters of pregnancy (43). Nitrous oxide inactivates vitamin B_{12}, the essential cofactor for the enzyme methionine synthetase. The temporary inactivation of methionine synthetase interferes with folate metabolism, the conversion of uridine to thymidine, and thereby impairs DNA synthesis (Fig. 14.14). While the temporary inactivation of methionine synthetase does not appear to be clinically significant in the nonpregnant surgical patient, there is concern that the use of nitrous oxide may be potentially deleterious to the developing fetus. Indeed, Baden et al. (55, 56) showed that in rats maternal exposure to nitrous oxide produced a marked decrease in fetal methionine synthetase activity. The decreased methionine synthetase activity persisted for up to 72 hr.

It has been suggested that nitrous oxide toxicity can be prevented by pretreatment with folinic acid (formyltetrahydrofolate) (50, 57–59). This suggestion has not been fully supported by animal studies. Indeed, the hypothesis that methionine synthetase inhibition is the mechanism of nitrous oxide teratogenicity has been questioned. One study showed that in rats, folinic acid administration reduced the incidence of skeletal abnormalities (but did not eliminate them) produced by exposure to 70 to 75% nitrous oxide on day 9 of pregnancy (59). Other studies

have failed to substantiate this (60–62). In these studies the volatile anesthetics, isoflurane and halothane, administered with N_2O prevented adverse reproductive effects in rats without preventing inhibition of methionine synthetase activity. Furthermore, treatment with folinic acid, which should have reversed the effects of N_2O on DNA production, did not prevent adverse reproductive effects (61, 62). It has been postulated that the adverse reproductive effects of nitrous oxide are due to decreased uterine blood flow but phenoxybenzamine, an α-1 adrenergic antagonist did not prevent nitrous oxide teratogenicity (63). Clearly, the etiology of nitrous oxide teratogenicity remains to be elucidated. **It should be emphasized that it is only teratogenic in animals under relatively extreme conditions not likely to be encountered clinically**.

Halothane in low concentrations for 12 to 48 hr produced numerous anomalies in rat fetuses (64). In mice, 3 hr of halothane 1.5% markedly increased the incidence of cleft palates and paw defects (65). In hamsters, 3 hr of halothane 0.6% in midgestation increased the number of abortions (66). The exposure of cell cultures to halothane produces marked inhibition in DNA synthesis, abnormal cell divisions, and bizarre multinucleated cells (67). Other investigators using rats, rabbits, and mice have not shown teratogenic effects of halothane (68–70).

Enflurane produces more cleft palates and other skeletal and visceral anomalies in fetuses of mice exposed to enflurane (1% vol) on days 6 and 15 of gestation (71).

Isoflurane (0.6%), in a similar study in mice, produced an incidence of cleft palate which was six times greater than that obtained with enflurane (12.2% versus 1.9%) (72). Because mice have a tendency to develop cleft palates following a large variety of treatments and manipulations, it is likely that the findings in the two previous studies were species specific and of questionable significance for humans. The same investigators, therefore, studied pregnant rats given 0.75 MAC of halothane, enflurane, isoflurane, and 0.55 MAC nitrous oxide for 6-hr periods at three different stages of gestation (70). There were no major or minor teratologic effects produced by any of the anesthetics. Nitrous oxide exposure did result in an increase in fetal resorptions.

Methoxyflurane 0.5% administered for 6 hr to incubating eggs resulted in a high incidence of embryonic deaths and multiple anomalies in the survivors. Methoxyflurane 0.3% given for 3 hr/day for 3 days produced up to a 40% incidence of anomalies (73).

Diethyl ether, cyclopropane, and **fluroxene** have been shown to be teratogenic in chick embryos (73, 74).

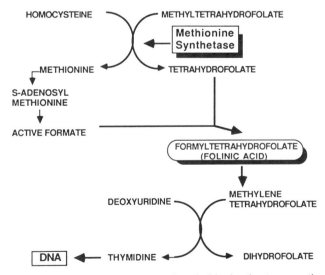

Figure 14.14. Nitrous oxide directly blocks the transmethylation reaction by which methionine is synthesized from homocystine and methyltetrahydrofolate. Nitrous oxide oxidizes vitamin B_{12}, the cofactor of the enzyme methionine synthetase. This action of nitrous oxide thus interferes with the production of DNA.

Muscle relaxants do not cross the placenta in significant amounts. Curare has been shown to cause musculoskeletal deformities when injected into the incubating chick embryo (75). Because of their respiratory effects, muscle relaxants are difficult to test in vivo. Using an in vitro rat whole embryo culture system d-tobcuranine, pancuronium, atracurium, and vecuronium were studied (76). Teratogenicity was only found at doses greater than 100 times the paralyzing dose in humans.

Local anesthetics act by stabilizing cell membranes and conceivably might affect cell mitosis and embryogenesis. The administration of lidocaine to pregnant rats did not result in an increased incidence of congenital anomalies or poor outcome (77). Cocaine, however, has been shown to be teratogenic in mice (78) and rats (79). The teratogenicity of cocaine in humans is discussed fully in Chapter 35.

HUMAN STUDIES

Human studies have consisted of large retrospective epidemiologic surveys of adverse reproductive outcomes either in groups chronically exposed to low levels of anesthetic gases or in women who have undergone surgery during their pregnancy. Both these approaches have significant limitations. Studies on the adverse effects of exposure to waste anesthetic gases are frequently deficient due to lack of comparable control groups, lack of confirmation and verification of reported adverse outcomes, low response rates to questionnaires, lack of details on duration and amounts of actual exposure to waste gases, and lack of information on other factors associated with people exposed to waste anesthetic gases, such as exposure to hepatitis B virus, radiation, and methylmethacrylate, all of which are potentially teratogenic. Shortcomings of surveys of women that have undergone surgery during pregnancy include many of the above limitations as well as relatively small sample sizes, a multiplicity of drugs administered, and the unknown implications of the surgical condition that necessitated the original need for anesthesia.

Table 14.3 summarizes the major studies of the effects of waste anesthetic gases on reproductive outcome. The most consistent finding is the increased risk of spontaneous abortion in female personnel exposed to waste anesthetic gases. The incidence of miscarriage among the exposed women is approximately 25 to 30% greater than in nonexposed women.

Buring et al. (86) noted that this increase is relatively small and well within the range that might be due to uncontrolled confounding variables. As noted by Mazze and Lecky (87), epidemiologists usually consider increases in incidence of less than 200 to 300% as possibly due to other factors. Furthermore a 30% increase is almost insignificant when one considers that the incidence of spontaneous abortions is increased at least 250% in women who consume more than three alcoholic drinks daily (88), and that cigarette smokers have an 80% increased risk of spontaneous abortions compared to nonsmokers (89).

The likelihood of exposure to waste anesthetic gases in operating rooms or dental offices producing major congenital anomalies is less certain. The studies with the most significant findings were the ASA Ad Hoc Committee on Occupational Diseases Among Operating Room Personnel (84) and the American Dental Association Survey (81). Both these studies showed borderline statistically significant increases in the incidence of congenital anomalies among some exposed personnel. These findings have been challenged, however (90). For example, the failure to find a dose-related effect of nitrous oxide in exposed dental assistants makes the alleged association between anesthetic gases and anomalies suspect. Furthermore, the incidence of anomalies in offspring of exposed assistants was no greater than that in the wives of unexposed (male) dentists. One might conclude, therefore, that other factors account for the results.

Several surveys of women who had received anesthesia for operations during pregnancy have failed to indict any anesthetic as a teratogen (1, 2, 4, 5, 91–94). Smith (2) retrospectively reviewed the neonatal outcomes of 67 women who had undergone surgery during pregnancy. Eleven of these women received an anesthetic during the first trimester. No congenital anomalies were found.

Shnider and Webster (1) reviewed the records of 147 women who received anesthesia for surgery during pregnancy: 47 during the first trimester, 58 during the second, and 42 during the third. These women were compared to 8926 women who delivered during this time period. The incidence of congenital anomalies was not significantly different in these groups. These investigators also reviewed the statistics from 61,000 patients who participated in the National Collaborative study. The incidence of birth defects in women who had not undergone surgery during pregnancy (60,000 women) was 5.02% compared to 6% in the 50 women undergoing appendectomy, a statistically insignificant difference.

Brodsky et al. (4) reported the incidence of anomalies in women having general anesthesia for surgery during pregnancy. Their survey was of 187 women having surgery and anesthesia during the first trimester and 100 women having surgery during the second trimester. These women were compared to a control group of 8654 women who had neither surgery during pregnancy nor occupational exposure to waste

Table 14.3
Results of Major Studies on Effects of Waste Anesthetic Gases on Reproductive Outcome

Study	Subjects	Number of Pregnancies	Miscarriage Rate (%)	Number of Live Births	Congenital Abnormality (%)
Cohen et al. (80)	Operating room nurses	36	27.7	26	NG[a]
	General duty nurses	34	5.2	31	NG
	Female anesthesiologists	37	37.8	23	NG
	Other female MDs	58	10.3	52	NG
Cohen et al. (81)	Dental chairside assistants				
	No N_2O exposure	3197	8.1	2882	3.6
	N_2O exposure	701	16.0[b]	579	5.5[b]
	N_2O + halogenate exposure	93	24.6[b]	68	7.7
	No N_2O exposure	3184	8.1	2882	3.6
	N_2O—light exposure	407	14.2[b]	341	5.7[b]
	N_2O—heavy exposure	400	19.1[b]	316	5.2
	Wives of dentists				
	No N_2O exposure	5709	6.7	5277	4.9
	N_2O—light exposure	2104	7.7[b]	1890	4.6
	N_2O—heavy exposure	1328	10.2[b]	1177	4.8
Knill-Jones et al. (82)	Female anesthetists	737	18.2	599	6.5
	Other female MDs	2150	14.7[b]	1817	4.9
Rosenberg and Kirves (83)	Operating room nurses	257	19.5	NG	NG
	Other nurses	150	11.4[b]	NG	NG
ASA Ad Hoc Committee (84)	Anesthesiologists	468	17.1	384	5.9
	Other MDs	308	8.9[b]	276	3.0
	Nurse anesthetists	1826	17.0	1480	9.6
	Other nurses	1948	15.1	1629	7.6[b]
Axelsson and Rylander (85)	Operating room & anesthesia nurses	139	15.1	114	4.4
	Other nurses	573	11.0	434	2.1

[a]Not given.
[b]$p < 0.05$.

anesthetic gases. Brodsky et al. found no association between surgery during early pregnancy and congenital anomalies in live-born offspring. They did find an increase in the incidence of spontaneous abortions. In the first trimester the incidence of miscarriage was 8.0% in anesthetized women and 5.1% in control women. In the second trimester the incidences were 6.5% for women having had anesthesia and surgery and 1.4% for women in the control group.

Duncan et al. (94) reviewed the incidence of congenital anomalies and spontaneous abortions in 2565 women who had undergone surgery during pregnancy. These women were matched to a similar number of control pregnancies by material age and area of residence.

There was no significant difference in the rate of congenital anomalies between study and control groups. There was a significant increase (two times) in spontaneous abortions in women undergoing surgery in the first or second trimesters with general anesthesia and having gynecologic procedures. The

risk was still increased (one and a half times) for procedures anatomically remote from the uterus. While it was concluded that general anesthesia was associated with a higher incidence of abortion, there were very few major procedures performed under regional anesthesia. It was not possible to determine from their data whether it was the magnitude or nature of the surgical procedure, rather than the anesthetic, which was responsible for the increased risk of abortion.

In the largest survey to date, Mazze and Källén (5) linked data from three Swedish health care registries, the Medical Birth Registry, the Registry of Congenital Malformations, and the Hospital Discharge Registry, for the years 1973 to 1981. Adverse outcomes examined were the incidences of (a) congenital anomalies, (b) stillborn infants, (c) infants dead at 168 hr, and (d) infants with very low and low birth weights. There were 5405 operations in the population of 720,000 pregnant women (operation rate, 0.75%). Of these, 2252 were performed in the first trimester, and

65% received general anesthetics, almost all of which included nitrous oxide. The results are summarized in Figure 14.15.

The incidences of congenital malformations and stillbirths were not increased in the offspring of women having an operation. However, the incidences of very low and low-birth-weight infants were increased; these were the result of both prematurity and intrauterine growth retardation. The incidence of infants born alive but dying within 168 hr was increased. No specific types of anesthesia or operation were associated with increased incidences of adverse reproductive outcomes. The cause of these outcomes was not determined. These adverse outcomes did not occur as a consequence of immediate delivery after operation because in most cases delivery was delayed by weeks to months. However, the incidence of premature birth was increased by 46% (7.4% versus 5.13%); intrauterine growth retardation was also a factor in reduced birth weight. Thus it is clear that there is significant risk to the fetus when an operation is performed during pregnancy, but it is unclear whether the hazard is due to the surgery, the pathology for which the surgery was necessary, or the anesthetic. Further indication of the safety of nitrous oxide comes from studies of in vitro fertilization procedures, in which ova were retrieved under general (nitrous oxide) or local anesthesia and showed no differences in pregnancy rates (95, 96). Two other reviews of exposure to nitrous oxide during cervical cerclage also showed no effects of the agent on fetal outcome (97, 98).

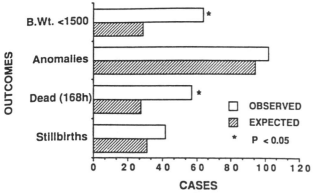

Figure 14.15. Total number of observed and expected adverse outcomes among women having nonobstetric operations during pregnancy. Incidence of infants with birth weights < 1500 gm and of infants born alive and dying within 168 hr of birth were significantly increased ($P < 0.05$) (Reprinted by permission from Mazze RI, Källén B: Reproductive outcome after anesthesia and operation during pregnancy: A registry study of 5405 cases. Am J Obstet Gynecol 161:1178–1185, 1989.)

Thus all studies to date indicate that surgery and anesthesia during pregnancy are not associated with an increased incidence of congenital anomalies but may produce a slightly increased risk of miscarriage. However, in all studies to date the number of women receiving an anesthetic during their pregnancy is in fact too small to state categorically that anesthetics are not teratogenic. Sullivan (99) has calculated the number of patients that must be exposed to a suspected teratogen to prove the drug's teratogenicity. For example, if an anesthetic doubled the incidence of an anomaly such as anencephaly, which has a spontaneous incidence of 1 per 1000, then 23,000 women would have to have been exposed to the anesthetic to have a statistically significant result. Of course, if an anesthetic had the teratogenicity of thalidomide, which increases the normal incidence of anomalies by 50,000 to 500,000 times, then a smaller number of anesthetic exposures would demonstrate teratogenicity. Clearly no anesthetic is such a potent teratogen.

Oxygen and Carbon Dioxide

Alterations in arterial blood gases frequently occur under anesthesia. In the experimental animal, hyperoxia, hypoxia, and hypercapnia may be teratogenic.

In mice (100), rabbits (101), rats (103) and chicks (102) congenital anomalies have been reported after exposure to hypoxia during organogenesis. The possible teratogenicity of hyperoxia is controversial. In hamsters, 100% oxygen at 2 atmospheres pressure for 3 hr, or 3 atmospheres pressure for 2 hr, resulted in a significant number of congenital anomalies (104). These defects included spina bifida, exencephaly, and limb defects. Hyperbaric oxygen administered to rabbits during late pregnancy resulted in retrolental fibroplasia, retinal detachment, microphthalmia, and stillbirth (105). Although it is clear from these studies that hyperbaric oxygen is teratogenic, high concentrations of oxygen at normal atmospheric pressure have not been found to be teratogenic in the experimental animal (106).

Prolonged periods of hypercarbia are associated with congenital anomalies in rats and rabbits. Carbon dioxide 6% and oxygen 20% administered to rats for 24 hr resulted in a high incidence of cardiac anomalies (107). In rabbits prolonged continuous inhalation of 10 to 13% carbon dioxide resulted in a high incidence of vertebral column malformations (106).

In humans, brief exposures of hypoxia, hyperoxia, hypercarbia, and hypocarbia have not been proven to be teratogenic, although isolated case reports alleging such an association have been published (108–110). Chronic hypoxemia, as occurs in people living at high altitude, is also not associated with an increased risk of anomalies.

Maternal Emotional Stress and Trauma

A number of factors that may be encountered in the pregnant patient having surgery have been suggested as being potentially teratogenic. Maternal anxiety and stress (111–117), maternal immobilization (118), and mechanical trauma such as falls, blows to the abdomen, automobile accidents, and bullet wounds (119–123) have all been implicated in case reports. The significance of these factors as teratogens is uncertain, because large epidemiologic studies have not been done.

Behavioral Teratology

The term "behavioral teratology" was first used by Werboff and Gottlieb (124) to describe the adverse action of a drug on "the behavior or functional adaptation of the offspring to its environment." Reserpine, chlorpromazine, and meprobamate administered to rats produced alterations of behavior in the offspring that persisted during adulthood (125–128). Other drugs such as bromides (192), barbiturates (130), and salicylates (131) all impaired maze-learning ability in rat offspring.

Halogenated agents have also been shown to produce behavioral effects in rodents. Smith et al. (132) reported the behavioral effects of halothane in rat offspring. Pregnant female rats were anesthetized with halothane 2.5% for 5 min followed by 1.2% for 115 min during either the first, second, or third trimester. Their offspring were then tested at approximately 75 days postdelivery, which developmentally corresponds to young adulthood in humans. Learning deficits and changes in foot-shock sensitivity were found in the litters of mothers exposed during the first and second trimesters but not during the third (Fig. 14.16).

Chalon et al. (133) have shown that mice twice exposed to halothane (1 or 2% for 30 min) or enflurane (2 or 4% for 30 min) in utero have significant learning defects. Second-generation offspring, born to dams exposed to 2% halothane in utero late in pregnancy and sired by normal unexposed males, also learned consistently slower than control mice (134).

The effect of lidocaine on postnatal development was studied in the rat (135). Injections of lidocaine, 6 mg/kg of body weight, were given intramuscularly daily, on days 10 and 11 of gestation. No clinical dysfunction or behavioral changes could be related to maternal lidocaine administration. No cognitive dysfunction was evident in the offspring of lidocaine-treated animals.

It seems that in subteratogenic doses, some psychoactive compounds produce behavioral deficits while not producing gross morphologic changes. The

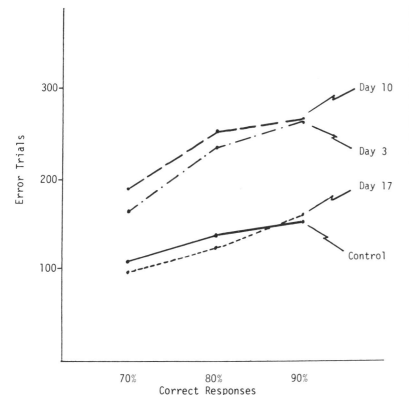

Figure 14.16. Total numbers of error trials on the maze task according to three increasingly difficult criteria. Control animals and animals who had received halothane during the third trimester of gestation behaved similarly. Behavioral abnormalities were seen in animals exposed to halothane during early pregnancy. (Reprinted by permission from Katz J, Smith RF, Bowman RE: Effects of single anesthetic exposure in utero on future nervous system performance. In *Abstracts of Scientific Papers*, American Society of Anesthesiologists, San Francisco, 1976, p 148.)

central nervous system, because of its prolonged period of development—which is not complete at the time of birth—may be susceptible to teratogens over an extended period. It has been alleged that even conventional doses of medications or anesthetics administered during childbirth may produce permanent central nervous system dysfunction in the offspring (136). These allegations are based on poorly controlled, improperly analyzed studies, but nevertheless, they are widely quoted. At present there is no evidence establishing the validity of the assertion that anesthesia administered to a pregnant woman adversely affects later mental and neurologic development of her infant (137).

Transplacental Carcinogenesis

Concern regarding the potential for anesthetic agents administered to a pregnant woman to induce cancer in her baby is based on a number of observations. Oral administration of large doses of chloroform (138, 139) or trichloroethylene (140) produced cancer of the liver or kidney in mice. Halothane has been shown to interfere with the synthesis of DNA (141, 142) and may also produce abnormal products of cell division.

Using an in vitro microbial assay system employing two histidine-dependent mutants of *Salmonella typhimurium* (143), Baden et al. (144, 145) showed that fluroxene was mutagenic but that halothane, enflurane, methoxyflurane, and isoflurane were not. In the experimental animal more than 30 different chemical compounds have been shown to be capable of inducing cancer in offspring when administered to the mother during gestation (147). It seems that the fetus is often more susceptible than the mother to carcinogenic compounds.

In a pilot study, Corbett (148) reported that isoflurane administered to mice during gestation produced hepatic neoplasms in the offspring. Because his studies had methodologic flaws (test and control animals were treated differently), the studies were repeated and expanded to include enflurane, halothane, nitrous oxide, and methoxyflurane (149). All treatment and control groups had a similar number of neoplastic lesions. *There was no indication that any anesthetic agent was carcinogenic.*

AVOIDANCE OF INTRAUTERINE FETAL ASPHYXIA

Intrauterine fetal asphyxia is avoided by maintaining normal maternal PaO_2, $PaCO_2$, and uterine blood flow. Fetal oxygenation is directly dependent on maternal arterial oxygen tension, oxygen-carrying capacity (hemoglobin content), oxygen affinity, and uteroplacental perfusion. Maternal hypoxia will result in fetal hypoxia and, if uncorrected, fetal demise.

Maternal Oxygenation

Common causes of maternal hypoxia during anesthesia for operations during pregnancy, as well as during childbirth include laryngospasm, airway obstruction, improperly positioned endotracheal tube, inadequate ventilation, and low inspired oxygen in the anesthetic gas mixture. Common causes of hypoxia during regional anesthesia include severe toxic reactions or excessively high spinal or epidural blocks with maternal hypoventilation. The usual careful anesthetic management should prevent the occurrence or continuation of significant maternal and fetal hypoxia.

Elevated maternal oxygen tensions commonly occur during anesthesia. In studies with isolated preparations of human placental and umbilical vessels, vasoconstriction occurs if high oxygen tensions are administered (149–151). Therefore it had been feared that elevated oxygen tensions would decrease uteroplacental blood flow and fetal oxygenation. Studies of fetal scalp capillary PO_2, measured by sampling fetal blood (152) or using a transcutaneous oxygen electrode (153) have shown that increasing maternal PaO_2 will increase fetal PO_2 (Fig. 14.17). If the normal placental-fetal circulation has been significantly compromised by conditions such as umbilical cord compression or maternal hypotension, then increasing maternal oxygenation will not be reflected in the fetus. In no studies has maternal hyperoxia resulted in fetal hypoxia (152–155).

A rise in maternal PaO_2 even to 600 torr seldom produces a fetal PaO_2 above 45 torr and never above 60 torr. The reasons for this large maternal-fetal oxygen tension gradient are high oxygen consumption of the placenta and uneven distribution of the maternal and fetal blood flow in the placenta. Thus maternal hyperoxia cannot produce in utero retrolental fibroplasia or premature closure of the ductus arteriosus.

Maternal Carbon Dioxide

Fetal $PaCO_2$ is also directly related to maternal $PaCO_2$ (Fig. 14.18). There is evidence that low maternal $PaCO_2$ or high maternal pH may be deleterious to the fetus for a number of reasons. Maternal hypocapnia produced by excessive positive pressure ventilation may increase mean intrathoracic pressure, decrease venous return to the heart, and lead to a fall in uterine blood flow (156) (see Fig. 3.22). Maternal respiratory or metabolic alkalosis also decreases umbilical blood flow because of direct vasoconstriction (Fig. 14.19) (157). In addition, maternal alkalosis shifts the maternal oxyhemoglobin dissociation curve to the left, thereby increasing the affinity of maternal hemoglobin for oxygen, resulting in the release of less oxygen

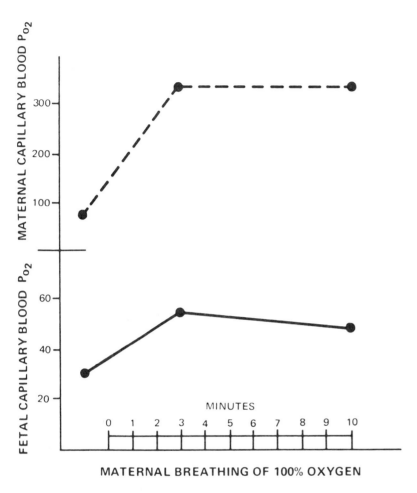

Figure 14.17. Effect of maternal inhalation of 100% oxygen in one case. At 3 and 10 min, fetal PO₂ was significantly above the basal level. (Reprinted by permission from Wood C: Use of fetal blood sampling and fetal heart rate monitoring. In *Diagnosis and Treatment of Fetal Disorders*. K Adamsons, ed. Springer-Verlag, New York, 1968, p 169.)

to the fetus at the placenta. Thus fetal hypoxia and metabolic acidosis can occur as a result of maternal hyperventilation during anesthesia.

Maternal hypercapnia, as may occur with spontaneous ventilation and deep levels of anesthesia, will be associated with fetal respiratory acidosis. Moderate elevations of fetal Pa_{CO_2} are probably not detrimental, but severe fetal acidosis may produce myocardial depression.

Maternal Hypotension

Maternal hypotension from deep general anesthesia, sympathectomy, hypovolemia, or vena caval compression will cause a fall in uterine blood flow and may lead to fetal asphyxia. Hypotension and regional anesthesia are discussed in Chapter 22. With a general anesthetic—for example, halothane—a small fall in blood pressure that may occur with light anesthesia is not associated with significant reductions in uterine blood flow because of the concomitant decrease in uterine vascular resistance (158). Deep levels of halothane anesthesia resulting in significant hypotension (30 to 40% below control) will produce a fall in uterine blood flow and fetal asphyxia. In monkeys, deep halothane anesthesia producing pro-

longed maternal hypotension to a mean arterial pressure of 40 torr or lower regularly produced fetal asphyxia, brain damage, or death (159). Fetal Pa_{O_2} fell from a normal control value of 30 torr to 15 torr, fetal pH fell from 7.30 to 7.10 or lower, fetal bradycardia occurred, and with severe asphyxia (pH 7) lasting several hours myocardial failure and fetal death occurred. With less severe asphyxia permanent brain damage occurred with lesions similar to those of human cerebral palsy.

Uterine Vasoconstriction and Hypertonus

Uterine vasoconstriction from endogenous or exogenous sympathomimetics increases uterine vascular resistance and decreases uterine blood flow (160–162). Sympathetic discharge and adrenal medullary activity may be encountered in the anxious unpremedicated patient or during light general anesthesia (163). Vasoactive drugs such as methoxamine, phenylephrine, or dopamine will reduce uterine blood flow (164–169). Uterine hypertonus is also associated with an increase in uterine vascular resistance and will decrease uterine blood flow. Drugs that increase uterine tone are ketamine in single intravenous doses above 1.1 mg/kg (Figs. 14.20 and 14.21)

Figure 14.18. Correlation of maternal capillary carbon dioxide tensions with fetal scalp blood carbon dioxide tensions in normal patients. *M* = maternal; *F* = fetal. (Reprinted by permission from Lumley J, Wood C: Effect of changes in maternal oxygen and carbon dioxide tensions on the fetus. In *Clinical Anesthesia Parturition and Perinatology*. G Marx, ed. Davis, Philadelphia, 1973, vol 10/2, p 128.)

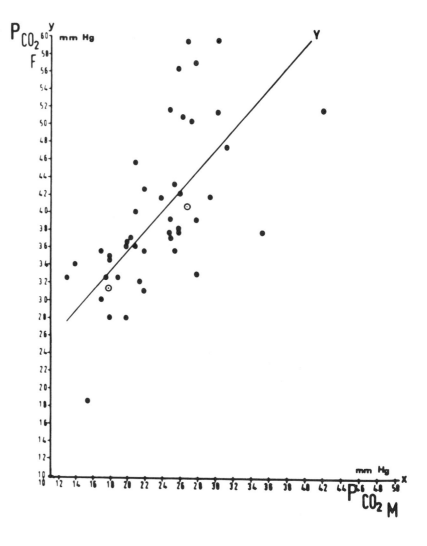

Figure 14.19. Effect of changes in maternal arterial pH on blood flow in one umbilical artery. All changes are expressed as percent change of initial flow. *Closed circles* and *triangles* represent values before and during changes in maternal pH, respectively. *Solid lines* indicate pH changes produced by respiratory alkalemia and acidemia; *broken lines* indicate pH changes produced by metabolic alkalemia. (Reprinted by permission from Motoyama EK, Rivard G, Acheson F, Cook CD: The effects of changes in maternal pH and P_{CO_2} on the P_{O_2} of fetal lambs. Anesthesiology 28:891–903, 1967.)

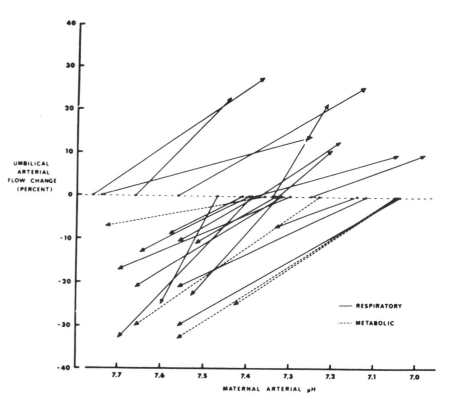

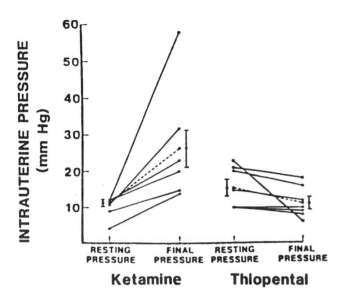

Figure 14.20. Changes in intrauterine pressure following administration of ketamine (2 mg/kg) or thiopental (4 mg/kg) to patients in the second trimester undergoing therapeutic abortions. *Solid lines* indicate individual patients; *dashed lines* are mean changes plus or minus standard error of the mean. (Reprinted by permission from Oats JN, Vasey DP, Waldron BA: Effects of ketamine on the pregnant uterus. Br J Anaesth 51:1163–1166, 1979.)

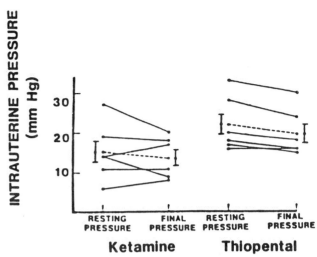

Figure 14.21. Changes in intrauterine pressure following administration of ketamine (2 mg/kg) or thiopental (4 mg/kg) to patients at term undergoing cesarean section. *Solid lines* indicate individual patients; *dashed lines* are mean changes plus or minus standard error of the mean. (Reprinted by permission from Oats JN, Vasey DP, Waldron BA: Effects of ketamine on the pregnant uterus. Br J Anaesth 51:1163–1166, 1979.)

(170, 171), toxic doses of local anesthetics (172) or α-adrenergic vasopressors.

PREVENTION OF PRETERM LABOR

Several anecdotal reports have suggested that anesthesia and operations during pregnancy may result in preterm labor during the postoperative period (173–175). In these reports intraabdominal procedures in which uterine manipulation or retraction was necessary most often resulted in preterm labor. Ovarian cystectomy, especially in the first trimester, has a high incidence of abortion. This is not inevitable; in many operations on the ovary, pregnancies have proceeded normally to term. Neurosurgical, orthopedic, thoracic, or plastic surgery procedures were not associated with preterm labor. In a review of 147 pregnant patients undergoing surgery, Shnider and Webster (1) reported that 8.8% (13 patients) went into labor shortly after surgery. This incidence was influenced by the number of preterm deliveries that occurred after Shirodkar procedures. (A Shirodkar operation is a repair of an incompetent cervix. The primary disease results in preterm labor.) In this series 28% of patients undergoing Shirodkar procedures had preterm deliveries; in a series reported by Smith (2) 40% of patients had preterm labor postoperatively. Therefore it is apparent that preoperative pathology plays a prominent role in cases of preterm labor.

Whether anesthetics can stimulate or inhibit the onset of preterm labor is unknown. There is little information on the effects of anesthesia on oxytocin, prostaglandins, follicle-stimulating hormone, estrogen, or progesterone levels in the uterus or blood. Some commonly used anesthetic agents, such as halothane and enflurane, decrease uterine tone and inhibit uterine contractions. On this basis, some have suggested that these agents be used during advanced pregnancy when uterine manipulation is anticipated. However, *in no study has any one anesthetic agent or technique been found to be associated with a higher or lower incidence of preterm delivery.*

As previously stated, some anesthetic agents—such as ketamine in doses greater than 1.1 mg/kg—and some vasopressors do increase uterine tone and should probably be avoided when possible. Rapid intravenous injection of anticholinesterase agents, such as neostigmine or edrophonium, may directly stimulate acetylcholine release and theoretically could increase uterine tone and stimulate preterm labor. Neostigmine, when used to reverse the effects of muscle relaxants, should be administered slowly and be preceded by adequate doses of atropine.

RECOMMENDATIONS FOR ANESTHETIC MANAGEMENT

1. *Elective surgery* should be deferred until after delivery when the physiologic changes of pregnancy

have returned toward normal. Women of childbearing age scheduled for elective surgery should be carefully queried regarding the possibility of pregnancy.

2. *Urgent surgery*—that is, operations that are essential but can be delayed without increasing the risk of permanent disability—should be deferred until the second or third trimester. *At present, no anesthetic drug—premedicant, intravenous induction agent, inhalation agent, or local anesthetic—has been PROVEN to be teratogenic in HUMANS.* However, despite the lack of proof, the authors consider it prudent to minimize or eliminate fetal exposure to drugs during the vulnerable first trimester.

3. *Emergency surgery*—that is, operations that cannot be delayed without increasing maternal morbidity or mortality—may be necessary during the first trimester. They are ideally performed under regional block if the contemplated surgery and maternal condition allow. Teratogenicity of local anesthetics in animals or humans has not been reported.

4. *With spinal anesthesia* fetal exposure to local anesthetic is much less than with other regional blocks.

5. *During the preoperative visit,* great effort should be made to allay maternal anxiety and apprehension. In describing risks and hazards to the parturients, the lack of documented teratogenicity can be presented. The likelihood of first trimester miscarriage increases from 5.1% without surgery to 8% with surgery (4), and the incidence of premature delivery increases from 5.13% without surgery to 7.47% with surgery (5). If pharmacologic premedication is necessary, barbiturates are preferable to minor tranquilizers such

as diazepam or meprobamate. Glycopyrrolate, unlike atropine and scopolamine, does not cross the placenta.

6. *If general anesthesia* is necessary during the first trimester there is no proof that any well-conducted technique is superior to any other. Adequate oxygenation and avoidance of hyperventilation are mandatory.

7. *During pregnancy* patients may be at increased risk of aspiration, and the usual safeguards to prevent aspiration pneumonitis should be performed.

8. *Aortocaval compression* during the second and third trimesters should be prevented by avoiding the supine position. The left lateral tilt position should be used whenever possible.

9. *Ideally, continuous fetal heart rate monitoring* during surgery should be employed after the 16th week of gestation. This may provide an indication of abnormalities in maternal ventilation or uterine perfusion (Fig. 14.22).

10. *Uterine activity* should be monitored continuously with an external tocodynamometer during the postoperative period to detect the onset of preterm labor. β-Mimetic therapy, instituted early, may prevent preterm delivery.

References

1. Shnider SM, Webster GM: Maternal and fetal hazards of surgery during pregnancy. Am J Obstet Gynecol 92:891–900, 1965.
2. Smith BE: Fetal prognosis after anesthesia during gestation. Anesth Analg 42:521–526, 1963.

TIME	9:58	10:05	10:32	10:55	13:45
	PRE-INDUCTION	POST-INDUCTION	POST-INCISION	POST-CORRECTION	RECOVERY ROOM
pH			7.25	7.30	7.37
PaCO$_2$ (TORR)			31	28	29
PaO$_2$ (TORR)			56	382	121
SaO$_2$			87%	100%	98%
% O$_2$			50	100	40

Figure 14.22.   Serial samples of fetal heart rate in a patient undergoing eye surgery. *A* and *B*, baseline fetal heart rate of 140 beats/min with normal beat-to-beat variability. *C*, fetal tachycardia and stabilization of the beat-to-beat interval during inadvertent maternal hypoxemia (maternal Pao$_2$ = 56 torr). *D*, after correction of maternal ventilation there is a return to baseline fetal heart rate and variability. *E*, normal baseline postoperatively. (Reprinted by permission from Katz JD, Hook R, Barash PG: Fetal heart rate monitoring in pregnant patients undergoing surgery. Am J Obstet Gynecol 125:267–269, 1976.)

3. Smith BE: Teratogenic capabilities of surgical anesthesia. Adv Teratol 3:127–179, 1968.

4. Brodsky JB, Cohen EN, Brown BW Jr, Wu ML, Whitcher C: Surgery during pregnancy and fetal outcome. Am J Obstet Gynecol 138:1165–1167, 1980.

5. Mazze RI, Källém B: Reproductive outcome after anesthesia and operation during pregnancy: A registry study of 5405 cases. Am J Obstet Gynecol 161:1178–1185, 1989.

6. Cugell DW, Frank NR, Gaensler EA, Badger TL: Pulmonary function in pregnancy. I. Serial observations in normal women. Am Rev Tuberc 67:568–597, 1953.

7. Prowse CM, Gaensler EA: Respiratory and acid-base changes during pregnancy. Anesthesiology 26:381–392, 1965.

8. Palahniuk RJ, Shnider SM, Eger EI II: Pregnancy decreases the requirement for inhaled anesthetic agents. Anesthesiology 41:82–83, 1974.

9. Strout CD, Nahrwold ML: Halothane requirement during pregnancy and lactation in rats. Anesthesiology 55:322–323, 1981.

10. Lees MM, Taylor SH, Scott DB, Kerr MG: A study of cardiac output at rest throughout pregnancy. J Obstet Gynaecol Br Commonw 74:319–328, 1967.

11. Lees MM, Scott DB, Kerr MG, Taylor SH: The circulatory effects of recumbent postural changes in late pregnancy. Clin Sci 32:453–465, 1967.

12. Ueland K, Novy MJ, Peterson EN, Metcalfe J: Maternal cardiovascular dynamics. IV. The influence of gestational age on the maternal cardiovascular response to posture and exercise. Am J Obstet Gynecol 104:856–864, 1969.

13. Pritchard JA: Changes in blood volume during pregnancy and delivery. Anesthesiology 26:393–399, 1965.

14. Ueland K: Maternal cardiovascular dynamics. VII. Intrapartum blood volume changes. Am J Obstet Gynecol 126:671–677, 1976.

15. Capeless EL, Clapp JF: Cardiovascular changes in the early phase of pregnancy. Am J Obstet Gynecol 161:1449–1453, 1989.

16. Fagraeus L, Urban B, Bromage P: Spread of epidural analgesia in early pregnancy. Anesthesiology 58:184–187, 1983.

17. Gintzler AR: Endorphin-mediated increases in pain threshold during pregnancy. Science 210:193–195, 1980.

18. Datta S, Lambert DH, Gregus J, Gissen AJ, Covino BG: Differential sensitivities of mammalian nerve fibers during pregnancy. Anesth Analg 62:1070–1072, 1983.

19. Attia RR, Eberd AM, Fischer JE: Gastrin: Placental, maternal and plasma cord levels: Its possible role in maternal residual gastric acidity. In Abstracts of Scientific Papers, American Society of Anesthesiologists, San Francisco, 1976, p 547.

20. Wyner MB, Cohen S: Gastric volume in early pregnancy. Anesthesiology 57:209–212, 1982.

21. Brock-Utne JG, Dow TGB, Dimopoulos GE, Welman S, Downing JW, Moshal MG: Gastric and lower oesophageal sphincter (LOS) pressures in early pregnancy. Br J Anaesth 53:381–384, 1981.

22. Tuchmann-Duplessis H: Influence of certain drugs on the prenatal development. Int J Gynaecol Obstet 8:777–797, 1970.

23. Eriksson M, Catz CS, Yaffe SJ: Drugs and pregnancy. Clin Obstet Gynecol 16:199–224, 1973.

24. Setala K, Nyyssonen O: Hypnotic sodium pentobarbital as a teratogen for mice. Naturwissenschaften 51:413, 1964.

25. Tanimura T: The effect of thiamylal sodium administration to pregnant mice upon the development of their offspring. Acta Anat Nippon 40:323, 1965.

26. Goldman AS, Yakovac WC: Prevention of salicylate teratogenicity in immobilized rats by central nervous system depressants. Proc Soc Exp Biol Med 115:693–696, 1964.

27. Roux C: Action teratogene de la prochlorperazine (Teratogenic action of prochlorperazine). Arch Franc Pediatr 16:968–971, 1959.

28. Robson JM, Sullivan FM: The production of foetal abnormalities in rabbits by imipramine. Lancet 1:638–639, 1963.

29. Tonge SR: Permanent alterations in catecholamine concentration in discrete areas of brain in the offspring of rats treated with methylamphetamine and chlorpromazine. Br J Pharmacol 47:425–427, 1973.

30. Jurand A: Teratogenic activity of methadone hydrochloride in mouse and chick embryos. J Embryol Exp Morphol 30:449–458, 1973.

31. Markham JK, Emmerson JL, Owen NV: Teratogenicity studies of methadone HCl in rats and rabbits. Nature 233:342–343, 1971.

32. Geber WF, Schramm LC: Congenital malformations of the central nervous system produced by narcotic analgesics in the hamster. Am J Obstet Gynecol 123:705–713, 1975.

33. Fujinaga M, Stevenson JB, Mazze RI: Reproductive and teratogenic effects of fentanyl in Sprague-Dawley rats. Teratology 34:51–57, 1986.

34. Fujinaga M, Mazze RI, Jackson EC, Baden JM: Reproductive and teratogenic effects of sufentanil and alfentanil in Sprague-Dawley rats. Anesth Analg 67:166–169, 1988.

35. Milkovich L, van den Berg BJ: Effects of prenatal meprobamate and chlordiazepoxide hydrochloride on human embryonic and fetal development. N Engl J Med 291:1268–1271, 1974.

36. Saxen I, Saxen L: Association between maternal intake of diazepam and oral clefts. Lancet 2:498, 1975.

37. Safra MJ, Oakley GP: Association between cleft lip with or without cleft palate and prenatal exposure to diazepam. Lancet 2:478–480, 1975.

38. Hartz SC, Heinomen OP, Shapiro S, Siskind V, Slone D: Antenatal exposure to meprobamate and chlordiazepoxide in relation to malformations, mental development, and childhood mortality. N Engl J Med 292:726–728, 1975.

39. Smith BE, Gaub MI, Moya F: Teratogenic effects of anesthetic agents: Nitrous oxide. Anesth Analg 44:726–732, 1965.

40. Fink BR, Shepard TH, Blandau RJ: Teratogenic activity of nitrous oxide. Nature 214:146–148, 1967.

41. Lane GA, Nahrwold ML, Tait AR, Taylor-Busch M, Cohen PJ: Anesthetics as teratogens: Nitrous oxide is fetotoxic, xenon is not. Science 210:899–901, 1980.

42. Lane GA, DuBoulay PM, Tait AR, Taylor-Busch M, Cohen PJ: Nitrous oxide is teratogenic: Halothane is not. Anesthesiology 55:A252, 1981.

43. Mazze RI, Wilson AI, Rice SA, Baden JM: Reproduction and fetal development in rats exposed to nitrous oxide. Teratology 30:259–265, 1984.

44. Mazze RI, Wilson AI, Rice SA, Baden JM: Reproduction and fetal development in mice chronically exposed to nitrous oxide. Teratology 26:11–16, 1982.

45. Pope WDB, Halsey MJ, Lansdown ABG, Simmonds A, Bateman PE: Fetotoxicity in rats following chronic exposure to halothane, nitrous oxide or methoxyflurane. Anesthesiology 48:11–16, 1978.

46. Coate WB, Kapp RW Jr, Lewis TR: Chronic exposure to low concentrations of halothane-nitrous oxide: Reproductive and cytogenetic effects in the rat. Anesthesiology 50:310–318, 1979.

47. Doenicke A, Wittmann R, Heinrich H, Pausch J: L'effet abortif de l'halothane (The abortive effect of halothane). Anesth Analg Rean 32:41–46, 1975.

48. Doenicke A, Wittman R: Effet teratogene de l'halothane sur le foetus de rat (Teratogenic effect of halothane on the fetus of the rat). Anesth Analg Rean 32:47–51, 1975.

49. Bussard DA, Stoelting RK, Peterson C, Ishaq M: Fetal changes in hamsters anesthetized with nitrous oxide and halothane. Anesthesiology 41:275–278, 1974.

50. Nunn JF, Chanarin I: Nitrous oxide inactivates methionine synthetase. In Nitrous Oxide/N₂O. EI Eger II, ed. Elsevier, New York, 1985, pp 211–233.

51. Eger EI II, Lampe GH, Wauk LZ, Whitendale P, Cahalan MK, Donegan JH: Clinical pharmacology of nitrous oxide: An argument for its continued used. Anesth Analg 71:575–585, 1990.

52. Lampe GH, Wauk LZ, Donegan JH, Pitts LH, Jackler RK, Litt LL, Rampil IJ, Eger EI II: Effect on outcome of prolonged

exposure of patients to nitrous oxide, Anesth Analg 71:586–590, 1990.

53. Koblin DD, Tomerson BW, Waldman FM, Lampe GH, Wauk LZ, Eger EI II: Effect of nitrous oxide on folate and vitamin B_{12} metabolism in patients. Anesth Analg 71:610–617, 1990.

54. Waldman FM, Koblin DD, Lampe GH, Wauk LZ, Eger EI II: Hematologic effects of nitrous oxide in surgical patients. Anesth Analg 71:618–624, 1990.

55. Baden JM, Rice SA, Serra M, Kelley M, Mazze RI: Thymidine and methionine syntheses in pregnant rats exposed to nitrous oxide. Anesth Analg 62:738–741, 1983.

56. Baden JM, Serra M, Mazze RI: Inhibition of fetal methionine synthetase by nitrous oxide. Br J Anaesth 56:523–526, 1984.

57. Deacon R, Chanarin I, Perry J, Lumb M: Impaired deoxyuridine utilization in the B_{12}-inactivated rat and its correction by folate analogues. Biochem Biophys Res Commun 93:516–520, 1980.

58. O'Sullivan H, Jannings F, Ward K, McCann S, Scott JM, Weir DG: Human bone marrow biochemical function and megaloblastic hematopoiesis after nitrous oxide anesthesia. Anesthesiology 55:645–649, 1981.

59. Keeling PA, Rocke DA, Nunn JF, Monk SJ, Lumb MJ, Halsey MJ: Folinic acid protection against N_2O teratogenicity in the rat. Br J Anaesth 58:524–534, 1986.

60. Fujinaga M, Baden JM, Yhap EO, Mazze RI: Reproductive and teratogenic effects of nitrous oxide, isoflurane and their combination in Sprague-Dawley rats. Anesthesiology 67:960–964, 1987.

61. Mazze RI, Fujinaga M, Baden JM: Halothane prevents nitrous oxide teratogenicity in rats, folinic acid does not. Teratology 38:121–127, 1988.

62. Fujinaga M, Baden JM, Mazze RI: Halothane and isoflurane prevent the teratogenic effects of nitrous oxide, folinic acid does not. Anesthesiology 67:A456, 1987.

63. Fujinaga M, Baden JM, Suto A, Myatt JK, Mazze RI: Preventive effects of phenoxybenzamine on N_2O-induced reproductive toxicity in Sprague-Dawley rats. Anesthesiology 73:A920, 1990.

64. Bashford AB, Fink BR: The teratogenicity of halothane in the rat. Anesthesiology 29:1167–1173, 1968.

65. Smith BE, Usubiaga LE, Lehrer SB: Cleft palate induced by halothane anesthesia in C-57 black mice. Teratology 4:242, 1971.

66. Bussard DA, Stoelting RK, Peterson C, Ishaq M: Fetal changes in hamsters anesthetized with nitrous oxide and halothane. Anesthesiology 41:275–278, 1974.

67. Sturrock JE, Nunn JF: Mitosis in mammalian cells during exposure to anesthetics. Anesthesiology 43:21–23, 1975.

68. Kennedy GL, Smith SH, Keplinger ML, Calandra JC: Reproductive and teratologic studies with halothane. Toxicol Appl Pharmacol 35:467–474, 1976.

69. Warton RS, Mazze RI, Baden JM, Hitt BA, Dooley JR: Fertility, reproduction and postnatal survival in mice chronically exposed to halothane. Anesthesiology 48:167–174, 1978.

70. Mazze RI, Fujinaga M, Rice SA, Harris SB, Baden JM: Reproductive and teratogenic effects of nitrous oxide, halothane, isoflurane and enflurane in Sprague-Dawley rats. Anesthesiology 64:339–344, 1986.

71. Wharton RS, Mazze RI, Wilson AI: Reproductive and fetal development in mice chronically exposed to enflurane. Anesthesiology 54:505–510, 1981.

72. Mazze RI, Wilson AI, Rice SA, Baden JM: Fetal development in mice exposed to isoflurane. Teratology 32:339–345, 1985.

73. Smith BE, Gaub MI, Moya F: Investigations into the teratogenic effects of anesthetic agents: The fluorinated agents. Anesthesiology 26:260–261, 1965.

74. Anderson NB: The teratogenicity of cyclopropane in the chicken. Anesthesiology 29:113–122, 1968.

75. Drachman DB, Coulombre AJ: Experimental clubfoot and arthrogryposis multiplex congenita. Lancet 2:523–526, 1962.

76. Fujinaga M, Baden JM, Mazze RI: Developmental toxicity of nondepolarizing muscle relaxants in cultured rat embryos. Anesthesiology 75:A850, 1991.

77. Fujinaga M, Mazze RI: Reproductive and teratogenic effects of lidocaine in Sprague-Dawley rats. Anesthesiology 65:626–632, 1986.

78. Mahalik MP, Gautieri RF, Mann DE: Teratogenic potential of cocaine hydrochloride in CF-1 mice. J Pharm Sci 69:703–706, 1980.

79. Fantel AG, MacPhail BJ: The teratogenicity of cocaine. Teratology 26:17–19, 1982.

80. Cohen EN, Bellville JW, Brown BW Jr: Anesthesia, pregnancy, and miscarriage. Anesthesiology 35:343–347, 1971.

81. Cohen EN, Brown BW Jr, Wu ML, Whitcher CE, Brodsky JB, Gift HC, Greenfield W, Jones TW, Driscoll EJ: Occupational disease in dentistry and chronic exposure to trace anesthetic gases. JADA 101:21–31, 1980.

82. Knill-Jones RP, Rodrigues LV, Moir DD, Spence AA: Anesthetic practice and pregnancy: Controlled survey of women anesthetists in the United Kingdom. Lancet 1:1326–1328, 1972.

83. Rosenberg P, Kirves A: Miscarriages among operating theatre staff. Acta Anaesthesiol Scand 53:S37–S42, 1973.

84. Ad Hoc Committee on the Effect of Trace Anesthetics on the Health of Operating Room Personnel (EN Cohen, Chairman), American Society of Anesthesiologists: Occupational disease among operating room personnel. Anesthesiology 41:321–340, 1974.

85. Axelsson G, Rylander R: Exposure to anesthetic gases and spontaneous abortion: Response bias in a postal questionnaire study. Int J Epidemiol 11:250–256, 1982.

86. Buring JE, Hennekens CH, Mayrent SL, Rosner B, Greenberg ER, Colton T: Health experiences of operating room personnel. Anesthesiology 62:325–330, 1985.

87. Mazze RI, Lecky JH: The health of operating room personnel (editorial). Anesthesiology 62:226–228, 1985.

88. Harlap S, Shiono PH: Alcohol, smoking and incidence of spontaneous abortions in the first and second trimester. Lancet 2:173–176, 1980.

89. Kline J, Stein ZA, Susser M, Warburton D: Smoking: A risk factor for spontaneous abortion. N Engl J Med 297:793–796, 1977.

90. Baden JM: Mutagenicity, carcinogenicity, and teratogenicity of nitrous oxide. In Nitrous Oxide/N_2O. EI Eger II, ed. Elsevier, New York, 1985, pp 235–247.

91. Lloyd TS: The safety of surgical operations during pregnancy. South Med J 58:179–184, 1965.

92. Jacobs WM, Cooley D, Goen GP: Cardiac surgery with extracorporeal circulation during pregnancy: Report of 3 cases. Obstet Gynecol 25:167–169, 1965.

93. Meffert WG, Stansel HC Jr: Open heart surgery during pregnancy. Am J Obstet Gynecol 102:1116–1120, 1968.

94. Duncan PG, Pope WDB, Cohen MM, Greer N: The safety of anesthesia and surgery during pregnancy. Anesthesiology 64:790–794, 1986.

95. Belaisch-Allart JC, Hazout A, Guillet-Rosso F, Glissant M, Testart J, Frydman R: Various techniques for oocyte recovery in an in vitro fertilization and embryo transfer program. J In Vitro Fert Embryo Transfer 2:99–104, 1985.

96. Rosen MA, Roizen MF, Eger EI II, Glass RH, Martin M, Dandekar PV, Dailey PA, Litt L: The effect of nitrous oxide on in vitro fertilization success rate. Anesthesiology 67:42–44, 1987.

97. Crawford JS, Lewis M: Nitrous oxide in early human pregnancy. Anaesthesia 41:900–905, 1986.

98. Aldridge LM, Tunstall ME: Nitrous oxide and the fetus: A review and the results of a retrospective study of 175 cases of anaesthesia for insertion of Sirodkhar suture. Br J Anaesth 58:1348–1356, 1986.

99. Sullivan FM: Animal tests to screen for human teratogens. Pediatrics 53(Suppl):822–823, 1974.

100. Ingalls TH, Curley FJ, Prindle RA: Anoxia as a cause of fetal death and congenital defect in the mouse. Am J Dis Child 80:34–45, 1950.

101. Degenhardt KH: Durch O_2-mangel induzierte fehlbildungen der axialgradienten bei kaninchen. Z Naturforsch 9:530, 1954.

102. Haring OM: The effects of prenatal hypoxia on the cardiovascular system in the rat. Arch Pathol 80:351–356, 1965.

103. Grabowski CT: Teratogenic significance of ionic and fluid imbalance. Science 142:1064–1065, 1963.

104. Ferm BH: Teratogenic effects of hyperbaric oxygen. Proc Soc Exp Biol Med 116:975–976, 1964.

105. Fujikura T: Retrolental fibroplasia and prematurity in newborn rabbits induced by maternal hyperoxia. Am J Obstet Gynecol 90:854–858, 1964.

106. Grote W: Storung der embryonalentwicklung bei erhohtem CO$_2$-und O$_2$-partialdruck und bei unterdruck. Z Morphol Anthropol 56:165, 1965.

107. Haring OM: Cardiac malformations in rats induced by exposure of the mother to carbon dioxide during pregnancy. Circ Res 8:1218–1227, 1960.

108. Ballabriga A, Samso Dies J, Bado JV: Estudios electro-encefalogradicos sobre la anoxia fetal y neonatal en los animales de experimentacion (Electroencephalographic studies on fetal and neonatal hypoxia in experimental animals). Med Clin 3:164, 1957.

109. Pitt DB: A study of congenital malformations. II. Aust N Z J Obstet Gynaecol 2:82–90, 1962.

110. Warkany J, Kalter H: Congenital malformations. N Engl J Med 265:1046–1052, 1961.

111. Abramson JH, Ansuyah RS, Mbambo V: Antenatal stress and the baby's development. Arch Dis Child 36:42–49, 1961.

112. Davis A, DeVault S, Talmadge M: Anxiety, pregnancy and childbirth abnormalities. J Consult Psychol 25:74–77, 1961.

113. Davis A, DeVault S: Maternal anxiety during pregnancy and childbirth abnormalities. Psychosom Med 24:464–470, 1962.

114. Crist T, Hulka JF: Influence of maternal epinephrine on behaviour of offspring. Am J Obstet Gynecol 106:687–691, 1970.

115. Ferreira AJ: Emotional factors in prenatal environment. J Nerv Ment Dis 141:108–118, 1965.

116. Geber WF: Developmental effects of chronic maternal audiovisual stress on the rat fetus. J Embryol Exp Morphol 16:1–16, 1966.

117. Geber WF, Anderson TA: Abnormal fetal growth in the albino rat and rabbit induced by maternal stress. Biol Neonate 11:209–215, 1967.

118. Goldman AS, Yakovac WC: The enhancement of salicylate teratogenicity by maternal immobilization in the rat. J Pharmacol Exp Ther 142:351–357, 1963.

119. Hinden E: External injury causing foetal deformity. Arch Dis Child 40:80–81, 1965.

120. Ozan HA, Gonzalez AA: Post-traumatic fetal epilepsy. Neurology 13:541–542, 1963.

121. Torpin R, Miller GT, Culpepper BW: Amniogenic fetal digital amputations associated with clubfoot. Obstet Gynecol 24:379–384, 1964.

122. Turner EK: Teratogenic effects of the human foetus through maternal emotional stress: Report of a case. Med J Aust 2:502–503, 1960.

123. Wiedemann HR: Schadigungen der frucht in der schwangerschaft. Med Monatsschr 9:141–148, 1955.

124. Werboff J, Gottlieb JS: Drugs in pregnancy: Behavioral teratology. Obstet Gynecol Surv 18:420–423, 1963.

125. Werboff J: Effects of prenatal administration of tranquilizers on maze learning ability. Am Psychol 17:397, 1962.

126. Hoffield DR, McNew J, Webster RL: Effect of tranquilizing drugs during pregnancy on activity of offspring. Nature 218:357–358, 1968.

127. Clarke CVH, Gorman D, Vernadakis A: Effects of prenatal administration of psychotropic drugs on behavior of developing rats. Dev Psychobiol 3:225–235, 1970.

128. Young RD: Effects of differential early experiences and neonatal tranquilization on later behavior. Psychol Rep 17:675–680, 1965.

129. Harned BK, Hamilton HC, Cole BB: The effect of administration of sodium bromide to pregnant rats on the learning ability of the offspring. II. Maze test. J Pharmacol Exp Ther 82:215, 1974.

130. Armitage SG: The effects of barbiturate on the behavior of rat offspring as measured on learning and reasoning situations. J Comp Physiol Psychol 45:146–152, 1952.

131. Butcher RE, Boorhees CV, Kimmel CA: Learning impairment from maternal salycylate treatment in rats. Nature New Biol 236:211–212, 1972.

132. Smith RF, Bowman RE, Katz J: Behavioral effects of exposure to halothane during early development in the rat: Sensitive period during pregnancy. Anesthesiology 49:319–323, 1978.

133. Chalon J, Tang C-K, Ramanathan S, Eisner M, Katz R, Turndorf H: Exposure to halothane and enflurane affects learning function of murine progeny. Anesth Analg 60:794–797, 1981.

134. Chalon J, Hillman D, Gross S, Eisner M, Tang C-K, Turndorf H: Intrauterine exposure to halothane increases murine postnatal autotolerance to halothane and reduces brain weight. Anesth Analg 62:565–567, 1963.

135. Teiling AKY, Mohammed AK, Minor BG, Torbjörn UC, Järbe, Hiltunen AJ, Archer T: Lack of effects of prenatal exposure to lidocaine on development of behavior in rats. Anesth Analg 66:533–541, 1987.

136. Kolata GB: Behavioral teratology: Birth defects of the mind. Science 202:732–734, 1978.

137. Committee on Drugs of the American Academy of Pediatrics and the Committee on Obstetrics and Maternal and Fetal Medicine of the American College of Obstetricians and Gynecologists: Effect of medication during labor and delivery on infant outcome. Pediatrics 62:402–403, 1978.

138. Eschenbrenner AB, Miller E: Induction of hepatomas in mice by repeated oral administration of chloroform with observations on sex differences. J Natl Cancer Inst 5:251, 1945.

139. Report of Carcinogenesis Bioassay of Chloroform. Carcinogenesis Program, Division of Cancer Cause and Prevention, National Cancer Institute, Bethesda, MD, 1976.

140. Carcinogenesis: Bioassay of Trichloroethylene. CAS No 90-01-6, NCI-CG-TR-Z. National Cancer Institute, Bethesda, MD, 1976.

141. Jackson SH: The metabolic effect of halothane on mammalian hepatoma cells in vitro. II. Inhibition of DNA synthesis. Anesthesiology 39:405–409, 1973.

142. Sturrock J, Nunn JF: Effects of halothane on DNA synthesis and the presynthetic phase (G1) in dividing fibroblasts. Anesthesiology 45:413–420, 1976.

143. Ames BN: The detection of chemical mutagens with enteric bacteria. In Chemical Mutagens: Principles and Methods for Their Detection. A Lollaender, ed. Plenum, New York, 1971, p 267.

144. Baden JM, Brinkenhoff BS, Wharton RS, Hitt BA, Simmon VF, Mazze RI: Mutagenicity of volatile anesthetics: Halothane. Anesthesiology 45:311–318, 1976.

145. Baden JM, Kelley M, Wharton RS, Hitt BA, Simmon VF, Mazze RI: Mutagenicity of halogenated ether anesthetics. Anesthesiology 46:346–350, 1977.

146. Tomatis L: Transplacental carcinogenesis. In Modern Trends in Oncology, RW Raven, ed. Butterworth, London, 1973, p 99.

147. Corbett TH: Cancer and congenital anomalies associated with anesthetics. Ann NY Acad Sci 271:58–66, 1976.

148. Eger EI II, White AE, Brown CL, Biana CG, Corbett LH, Stevens WC: A test of carcinogenicity of enflurane, isoflurane, halothane, methoxyflurane, and nitrous oxide in mice. Anesth Analg 57:678–694, 1978.

149. Nyberg R, Westin B: The influence of oxygen tension and some drugs on human placental vessels. Acta Physiol Scand 39:216–227, 1957.

150. Panigel M: Placental perfusion experiments. Am J Obstet Gynecol 84:1664–1683, 1962.

151. Tominaga T, Page EW: Accommodation of the human placenta to hypoxia. Am J Obstet Gynecol 94:679–691, 1966.

152. Khazin AF, Hon EH, Hahre FW: Effects of material hyperoxia on the fetus. I. Oxygen tension. Am J Obstet Gynecol 109:628–637, 1971.

153. Walker A, Madderin L, Day E, Renow P, Talbot J, Wood C: Fetal scalp tissue oxygen measurements in relation to maternal dermal oxygen tension and fetal heart rate. J Obstet Gynaecol Br Commonw 78:1–12, 1971.

154. Neuman W, McKinnon L, Phillips L, Paterson P, Wood C: Oxygen transfer from mother to fetus during labor. Am J Obstet Gynecol 99:61–70, 1967.

155. Gare DJ, Shime J, Paul WM, Hoskins M: Oxygen administration during labor. Am J Obstet Gynecol 105:954–961, 1969.

156. Levinson G, Shnider SM, deLorimier AA, Steffenson JL: Effects of maternal hyperventilation on uterine blood flow and fetal oxygenation and acid-base status. Anesthesiology 40:340–347, 1974.

157. Motoyama EK, Rivard G, Acheson F, Cook CD: The effect of changes in maternal pH and PCO_2 on the PO_2 of fetal lambs. Anesthesiology 28:891–903, 1967.

158. Palahniuk RJ, Shnider SM: Maternal and fetal cardiovascular and acid-base changes during halothane and isoflurane anesthesia in the pregnant ewe. Anesthesiology 41:462–472, 1974.

159. Brann AW, Myers RE: Central nervous system finding in the newborn monkey following severe in utero partial asphyxia. Neurology 25:327–338, 1975.

160. Adamsons K, Mueller-Heubach E, Myers RE: Production of fetal asphyxia in the rhesus monkey by administration of catecholamines to the mother. Am J Obstet Gynecol 109:248–262, 1971.

161. Rosenfeld CR, Baron MD, Meschia G: Effects of epinephrine on distribution of blood flow in the pregnant ewe. Am J Obstet Gynecol 124:156–163, 1976.

162. Shnider SM, Wright RG, Levinson G, Roizen MF, Wallis KL, Rolbin SH, Craft JB: Uterine blood flow and plasma norepinephrine changes during maternal stress in the pregnant ewe. Anesthesiology 50:524–527, 1979.

163. Shnider SM, Wright RG, Levinson G, Roizen MF, Rolbin SH, Biehl D, Johnson J, Jones M: Plasma norepinephrine and uterine blood flow changes during endotracheal intubation and general anesthesia in the pregnant ewe. In *Abstracts of Scientific Papers*, Annual Meeting, American Society of Anesthesiologists, Chicago, 1978, p 115.

164. James FM III, Greiss FC Jr, Kemp RA: An evaluation of vasopressor therapy for maternal hypotension during spinal anesthesia. Anesthesiology 33:25–34, 1970.

165. Shnider SM, de Lorimier AA, Asling JH, Morishima HO: Vasopressors in obstetrics. II. Fetal hazards of methoxamine administration during obstetric spinal anesthesia. Am J Obstet Gynecol 106:680–686, 1970.

166. Ralston DH, Shnider SM, de Lorimier AA: Effects of equipotent ephedrine, metaraminol, mephentermine and methoxamine on uterine blood flow in the pregnant ewe. Anesthesiology 40:354–370, 1974.

167. Callender K, Levinson G, Shnider SM, Feduska NJ, Beihl DR, Ring G: Dopamine administration in the normotensive pregnant ewe. Obstet Gynecol 51:586–589, 1978.

168. Eng M, Berges PU, Ueland K, Bonica JJ, Parer JT: The effects of methoxamine and ephedrine in normotensive pregnant primates. Anesthesiology 35:354–360, 1971.

169. Greiss FC Jr, Gobble FL Jr: Effect of sympathetic nerve stimulation on the uterine vascular bed. Am J Obstet Gynecol 97:962–967, 1967.

CHAPTER 15

Anesthesia for Fetal Procedures and Surgery

Mark A. Rosen, M.D.

Currently practiced fetal procedures originated with Liley's successful intraperitoneal blood transfusion to a fetus affected with erythroblastosis fetalis (1). Later poorly documented, unsuccessful attempts were made to effect complete exchange transfusions by directly accessing the fetal circulation with in utero fetal surgery (2). Treatment of fetal lung immaturity to avoid respiratory distress syndrome of prematurity was the next fetal disease treated; treatment consisted of administration of glucocorticoids to the fetus via the mother to increase fetal surfactant production. More recently, intrauterine blood transfusions for erythroblastosis fetalis have been commonly performed by an ultrasound-guided, direct, intravascular technique. Diagnosis of many other fetal disorders by sonography, chorionic villus sampling, amniocentesis, and fetal blood sampling (cordocentesis) had led to the potential use of other in utero therapeutic interventions, such as placement of a percutaneous vesicoamniotic shunt for bilateral hydronephrosis. Additionally, selective termination of an abnormal twin fetus is performed using a variety of techniques, including hysterotomy (sectio parva) for monochorionic twins.

Fetal therapy is still a very new field of medicine. Thus far it consists primarily of relatively noninvasive fetal treatments such as administration of medications, hormones, or blood. However, compelling rationale for prenatal correction of certain anatomic defects has led to the development of a Fetal Treatment Program at the University of California, San Francisco. In this program invasive fetal treatment has been undertaken via hysterotomy for surgical correction of bilateral hydronephrosis, diaphragmatic hernia, and congenital pulmonary cystic adenomatoid malformation. Success in these endeavors relies on a multidisciplinary team consisting of obstetricians, perinatologists, geneticists, sonologists, surgeons, anesthesiologists, neonatologists, specialized nurses, and many other support personnel. Special attention to the anesthetic management of both mother and fetus and to intraoperative fetal monitoring is mandatory for successful outcomes.

Although the future of fetal therapy remains uncertain, possibilities include attempts to correct other anatomic malformations, treat other prenatally diagnosed fetal diseases and correct genetic disorders prenatally. Liley wrote that "for a variety of disorders, the physician and the parents are no longer helplessly dependent on what time, luck, and intrauterine life present with at birth. . . . Some day, for a wider range of fetal illness, we may be able to offer a brighter prospect than the present dismal alternatives of neonatal death, abnormality or abortion" (3).

Advances in technology affecting fertilization, embryo transfer, and various types of fetal treatment continue to receive widespread publicity in both the scientific community and popular news media. At the core of this interest is a recognition of the fetus as a patient, an individual requiring medical treatment. Until relatively recently, the fetus was perceived as a medical isolate out of our sight and our reach in the womb. However, improvements in the diagnostic capabilities of high-resolution ultrasonography, fetoscopy, and cytogenetic and biochemical testing of amniotic fluid have increased our ability to recognize and delineate precisely fetal anatomy and anomalies. These and other advances in prenatal diagnostic techniques, such as early diagnosis by chorion biopsy and imaging by computed tomography and magnetic resonance imaging are changing our perception of the fetus as isolated from medical treatment.

Although, for some fetal malformations, known patterns of inheritance allow for specific diagnostic testing, many malformations are inadvertently discovered during maternal ultrasonography for obstetric indications. At one time prenatal diagnosis of fetal malformations raised only the question of aborting the fetus. Now a wide variety of therapeutic alternatives is being explored. The advent of one of these alternatives, invasive fetal intervention via hysterotomy (4), requires special attention to the management of anesthesia for both mother and fetus to prevent maternal and fetal morbidity.

THERAPEUTIC ALTERNATIVES FOR FETAL MANAGEMENT

Most correctable malformations that can be diagnosed in utero are best managed by appropriate medical and surgical therapy after delivery at term (Table 15.1). Although a diagnosis of correctable malformation may not suggest a therapeutic alternative, it does provide time to coordinate appropriate prenatal and postnatal care, including transportation of the fetus to a medical center while in utero rather than as a newly delivered, fragile neonate. Prenatal diagnosis of serious malformations that are neither correctable nor compatible with normal postnatal life provides the choice of terminating the pregnancy (Table 15.2).

Examples of fetal malformations that may benefit from intervention in utero include deficiencies in pulmonary surfactant, anemia caused by erythroblastosis, hypothyroidism, other nutritional and metabolic deficiencies, and potential single-gene defects (5, 6) (Table 15.3). However, correction of an anatomic malformation in utero is considerably more difficult than providing a missing substrate, hormone, or medication to the fetus.

Certain malformations may influence the timing of delivery, particularly when early correction of the malformation can help minimize progressive impairment (Table 15.4). In these cases, the abnormality becomes more severe with continued gestation. However, the risks of prematurity with preterm delivery must be evaluated against the risks of continued gestation. Elective cesarean delivery is appropriate for fetal malformations that cause dystocia but are correctable after delivery (Table 15.5). It is also appropriate when the fetal abnormality requires preterm delivery and adequate labor cannot be induced or cannot be tolerated by the fetus.

Tables 15.1
Fetal Malformations Detectable in Utero but Best Corrected after Delivery at Term[a]

Esophageal, duodenal, jejunoileal, and anorectal atresias
Meconium ileus (cystic fibrosis)
Enteric cysts and duplications
Small intact omphalocele
Small intact meningocele, myelomeningocele, and spina bifida
Unilateral hydronephrosis
Craniofacial, extremity, and chest wall deformities
Cystic hygroma
Small sacrococcygeal teratoma
Benign cysts: e.g., ovarian, mesenteric

[a] Modified from Harrison MR: Selection for treatment: Which defects are correctable? In Harrison MR, Golbus MS, Filly RA, eds. *The Unborn Patient: Prenatal Diagnosis and Treatment*, 2nd ed. WB Saunders, Philadelphia, 1991.

Table 15.2
Fetal Malformations Often Managed by Selective Abortion[a]

Anencephaly, porencephaly, encephalocele, and giant hydrocephalus
Severe anomalies associated with chromosomal abnormalities (e.g., trisomy 13, trisomy 18)
Renal agenesis or bilateral polycystic kidney disease
Inherited, nontreatable chromosomal, metabolic, and hematologic abnormalities (e.g., Tay-Sachs disease)
Lethal bone dysplasias (e.g., recessive osteogenesis imperfecta)

[a] Modified from Harrison MR: Selection for treatment: Which defects are correctable? In Harrison MR, Golbus MS, Filly RA, eds. *The Unborn Patient: Prenatal Diagnosis and Treatment*, 2nd ed. WB Saunders, Philadelphia, 1991.

Table 15.3
Fetal Deficiencies and Malfunctions That may Benefit from Medical Treatment in Utero[a]

Deficient pulmonary surfactant
Anemia
Endocrine deficiency (hypothyroidism, goiter, adrenal hyperplasia)
Metabolic block (B_{12}-dependent methylmalonic acidemia, biotin-dependent multiple carboxylase deficiency)
Nutritional deficiency (intrauterine growth retardation)
Cardiac arrhythmias
Hematopoietic defect
Single-gene defect

[a] Modified from Harrison MR: Selection for treatment: Which defects are correctable? In Harrison MR, Golbus MS, Filly RA, eds. *The Unborn Patient: Prenatal Diagnosis and Treatment*, 2nd ed. WB Saunders, Philadelphia, 1991.

Table 15.4
Fetal Malformations That may Benefit from Induced Preterm Delivery for Early Neonatal Correction[a]

Obstructive hydrocephalus
Obstructive hydronephrosis
Amniotic band malformations
Gastroschisis or ruptured omphalocele
Intestinal volvulus and meconium ileus causing intestinal ischemia and/or necrosis
Hydrops fetalis
Intrauterine growth retardation
Arrhythmias causing cardiac failure

[a] Modified from Harrison MR: Selection for treatment: Which defects are correctable? In Harrison MR, Golbus MS, Filly RA, eds. *The Unborn Patient: Prenatal Diagnosis and Treatment*, 2nd ed. WB Saunders, Philadelphia, 1991.

Table 15.5
Fetal Malformations That may Require Cesarean Delivery[a]

Conjoined twins
Giant omphalocele or gastroschisis
Large hydrocephalus, sacrococcygeal teratoma, cystic hygroma, meningomyelocele
Malformations requiring preterm delivery when labor is inadequate or in the presence of fetal distress

[a] Modified from Harrison MR: Selection for treatment; Which defects are correctable? In Harrison MR, Golbus MS, Filly RA, eds. *The Unborn Patient: Prenatal Diagnosis and Treatment*, 2nd ed. WB Saunders, Philadelphia, 1991.

Table 15.6
Anatomic Malformations That may Benefit from Prenatal Surgical Correction[a]

Bilateral obstructive hydronephrosis
Diaphragmatic hernia
Congenital cystic pulmonary adenomatoid malformation
Obstructive hydrocephalus
Cardiac abnormalities (ventricular outflow obstruction)
Sacrococcygeal teratoma
Complete heart block
Neural tube defects
Skeletal abnormalities
Craniosynostosis

[a] Modified from Harrison MR: Selection for treatment: Which defects are correctable? In Harrison MR, Golbus MS, Filly RA, eds. *The Unborn Patient: Prenatal Diagnosis and Treatment*, 2nd ed. WB Saunders, Philadelphia, 1991.

RATIONALE FOR INVASIVE INTRAUTERINE FETAL THERAPY

Intrauterine intervention is a reasonable therapeutic alternative for certain correctable fetal abnormalities, such as abnormalities that progress in utero and cause harm to the fetus before the development of fetal pulmonary maturity necessary for extrauterine survival (7). Fetal surgery is reasonable only when it will be more successful than therapy after birth. Before invasive therapy is considered, the fetus must be evaluated thoroughly to ensure an accurate diagnosis has been made, to assess the severity of the lesion, and to ensure the absence of associated congenital anomalies that may contraindicate invasive management.

Anatomic malformations to consider for invasive correction are those that significantly interfere with fetal organ development and that, if treated, would allow significant improvement in fetal development. Examples include congenital hydronephrosis, congenital diaphragmatic hernia, cystic pulmonary adenomatoid malformation, and obstructive hydrocephalus (Table 15.6). Correction of these anatomic malformations in utero may prevent irreversible organ damage. Malformations that cause high- or low-output cardiac failure such as complete heart block or large sacrococcygeal teratomas, structural cardiac defects, and craniofacial deformities also may benefit from prenatal correction. Similar hysterotomy techniques are useful for selective delivery (sectio parva) of an abnormal twin that jeopardizes the well-being of the normal twin, such as with an acardiac, anencephalic fetus that places the normal twin at risk of a high-output cardiac failure (8, 9).

The fetus may be an ideal surgical candidate because the in utero environment supports rapid postoperative healing without scarring (10); the umbilical circulation meets nutritional and respiratory needs without outside assistance; and during embryogenesis, limb buds retain the capacity for regeneration. Certain invasive procedures such as catheter placement may be facilitated by the poorly developed fetal immune-surveillance system.

Two classifications of anatomic fetal anomalies considered potentially correctable in utero include those resulting from failure of embryonic tissue closure and those resulting from obstructive phenomena (11). Correction in utero of congenital diaphragmatic hernia can prevent lung hypoplasia, allowing the fetal lung to develop normally before delivery (12–18). In the fetus with obstructive hydrocephalus, cephalocentesis may relieve intracranial pressure and protect development of the fetal brain by shunting spinal fluid (19). However, early attempts at percutaneous placement of ventricle-amniotic shunts have not resulted in improved outcome, and selection of appropriate cases remains an unsolved problem (20, 21). Other potentially correctable defects include certain cardiac abnormalities, gastroschisis, neural tube defects such as spina bifida, and skeletal anomalies correctable by allogenic bone grafting (22, 23). Treatment of these anomalies is being investigated in animal model studies of surgical correction in utero.

Congenital hydronephrosis caused by urethral obstruction is one example of an anatomically simple lesion with potentially devastating consequences for the developing fetus if uncorrected before birth (Fig. 15.1) (24–33). Hydronephrosis is now recognized with increasing frequency because fluid-filled masses are particularly easy to detect with sonography and because decreased fetal urine excretion results in oligohydramnios, a common obstetric indication for sonography. When prenatal findings suggest urinary tract obstruction, intervention may be necessary because persistent obstruction interferes with fetal renal development, with the severity of damage dependent on the degree and duration of obstruction. Oligohydramnios caused by fetal urinary tract obstruction is also associated with pulmonary hypoplasia and

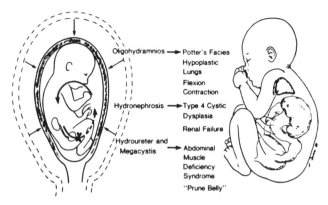

Figure 15.1. Developmental consequences of fetal urethral obstruction, with obstructed fetal urinary flow, hydrone-phrosis, hydroureter, megacystis, and oligohydramnios. (Reprinted by permission from Harrison MR, Filly RA, Parer JT, Faer MJ, Jacobson J, deLorimier AA: Management of the fetus with a urinary tract malformation.) JAMA 246:635–639, 1981.

skeletal, facial, and abdominal wall deformities. The pulmonary hypoplasia may be severe enough to prevent survival. Although one therapeutic approach might be preterm delivery of the fetus to allow for early urinary tract decompression ex utero, fetal pulmonary immaturity limits the efficacy of this approach. Physiologically, the ideal therapy is early decompression of the urinary tract with continued gestation in utero. This allows urine to drain from the bladder into the amniotic fluid, thereby decompressing the urinary tract and allowing for continued fetal renal and pulmonary development. It may also restore normal amniotic fluid dynamics and prevent the occurrence of the severe sequelae of oligohydramnios. Our clinical series in which fetal vesicostomy was performed via hysterotomy to decompress the fetal obstructive uropathy confirms that the development of fatal pulmonary hypoplasia can be prevented if amniotic fluid dynamics are restored and that relief of the obstruction may obviate further renal damage, allowing nephrogenesis to proceed normally (34).

ANESTHETIC CONSIDERATIONS

Many of the anesthetic considerations for fetal procedures and surgery are identical to those for nonobstetric surgery during pregnancy (Table 15.7). They include concern for maternal safety, avoidance of teratogenic drugs and of fetal asphyxia, and prevention of preterm delivery. The anesthesiologist must be familiar with the alterations in physiology induced by pregnancy and their clinical anesthetic implications. These basic considerations are extremely important, and are discussed in Chapter 14.

Fetal surgery is distinguished from other nonob-

Table 15.7
Anesthetic Considerations for Fetal Surgery

Basic objectives for pregnant women undergoing surgery
  Maternal safety
  Avoidance of teratogenic drugs
  Avoidance of intrauterine fetal asphyxia
  Prevention of preterm labor
Objectives unique to fetal surgery
  Fetal anesthesia and amnesia
  Increased requirement for fetal monitoring
  Increased likelihood of preterm labor
  Uterine relaxation for surgical exposure

stetric surgery during pregnancy by concerns for fetal anesthesia and fetal monitoring, an increased likelihood of preterm labor, and the need for surgical exposure through an open uterus (hysterotomy).

Unlike maternal surgery, during fetal procedures, the fetus is not an innocent bystander for whom we attempt the least anesthetic interference. Instead, the fetus is the primary patient and may benefit from anesthesia, with close monitoring of anesthetic effects to ensure well-being.

For many percutaneous procedures, such as fetal blood sampling or intrauterine blood transfusion, local anesthetic infiltration of the maternal abdominal wall is sufficient to reduce the mother's discomfort. When intravenous sedation and anxiolysis are required, opioids and benzodiazepines can be safely administered. We routinely administer supplemental oxygen during procedures involving intravenous sedation and have "stand-by" readiness for rapid intervention for fetal distress (i.e., induction of general anesthesia for emergency cesarean section) if the fetus is at a viable gestational age. Mothers fast overnight, receive an oral antacid before the procedure, and are monitored in a fashion suitable for general anesthetic administration. We use incremental doses of intravenous midazolam (0.5 mg) and/or fentanyl (25 μg) to achieve the desired level of sedation.

Fetal treatments that do not involve hysterotomy, such as placement of vesicoamniotic catheter shunts, involve procedures similar to those for intrauterine blood transfusion (Fig. 15.2) (21, 81). Despite sonographic guidance, however, larger sized needles or catheters and multiple placement attempts are often necessary. Adequate maternal anesthesia may be obtained with local anesthetic infiltration of the maternal abdomen, and the fetus may be sedated via placental transfer of drugs administered to the mother (including opioids and benzodiazepines). However, infiltration of the maternal abdomen with local anesthetic may be unsatisfactory for maternal comfort when needle placement requires multiple attempts.

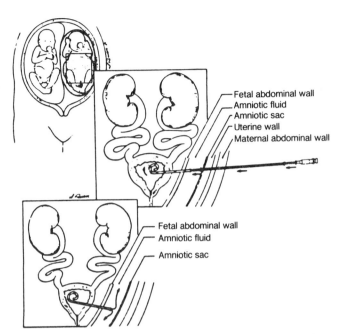

Figure 15.2. Shunt catheter placement for decompression of obstructed fetal urinary bladder. The catheter is pushed off the introducer needle so as to leave one end of the catheter in the fetal bladder and the other in the amniotic cavity. (Modified from Harrison MR, Golbus MS, Filly RA, Nakayama DK, deLorimier AA: Fetal surgical treatment. Pediatr Ann 11:896–903, 1982.)

Spinal, epidural, and general anesthetic techniques have been used as alternatives. In addition, fetal sedation by placental transfer of maternally administered medication does not ensure an immobile fetus, and excessive fetal activity may render the procedure technically difficult or infeasible.

Fetal movement can be dangerous to the fetus because displacement of a needle or catheter may lead to bleeding, trauma, or compromise to the umbilical circulation. When fetal movement is not controlled by placental transfer of maternally administered medication, general anesthesia may be used for both mother and fetus or control of fetal movement can be safely achieved by direct intramusclar or intravascular administration of a neuromuscular blocking agent to the fetus. Pancuronium (0.05 to 0.1 mg/kg IV or 0.3 mg/kg IM) has been used for fetal paralysis during intravascular transfusions (82–88). We have used vecuronium, in similar doses, to achieve paralysis of a shorter duration.

A variety of benefits and risks characterize the techniques for anesthesia during fetal procedures. For example, the necessity or benefit of fetal amnesia for surgical intervention is not documented. There has been widespread belief that the human neonate and fetus are not capable of perceiving pain (a subjective phenomenon) and that they possessed higher thresholds for nociceptive stimuli. This threshold would be adaptive for the pain associated with birth. Evidence of memories of pain in human neonates is only anecdotal. However, detailed hormonal studies in preterm neonates undergoing surgery under minimal anesthesia have revealed the marked release of catecholamines, growth hormone, glucagon, cortisol, aldosterone, and other corticosteroids and the suppression of insulin secretion (35–40). Furthermore, these endocrine and metabolic responses to stress are abolished by giving anesthetics to preterm neonates (41). In addition, surgical manipulation of an unanesthetized fetus results in varying degrees of autonomic nervous system stimulation, variations in heart rate, increased hormonal activity (42), and increased motor activity (43). Later in gestation, a fetus will respond to environmental stimuli such as noises, light, music, pressure, touch, and cold (44). Information about the development of perceptual mechanisms of pain (Fig. 15.3) and the response of human preterm neonates to pain provide a physiologic rationale to support the philosophic rationale of providing fetal anesthesia (45). Along with the requirement for fetal immobility during some procedures, amnesia may be an important goal of fetal anesthesia.

For procedures involving hysterotomy, such as repair of congenital cystic adenomatoid malformations, diaphragmatic hernia repair, or selective termination of an anencephalic, acardiac, monochorionic twin, we use general inhalational anesthetics (usually isoflurane) to produce maternal and fetal anesthesia and to provide the necessary uterine relaxation for surgery. Except for oral antacids, no premedication or adjuvant anesthetic agents are routinely used to supplement the inhalational agent, which allows for administration of maximal doses of isoflurane for uterine relaxation. The dose is limited by the stability of the maternal cardiovascular system. During uterine closure, magnesium sulfate therapy is started. After the initial bolus dose of magnesium sulfate is administered, the halogenated agent is discontinued and an anesthetic comprised of opioids and nitrous oxide in oxygen is administered. The regimen facilitates tracheal extubation when the patient is fully awake and capable of protecting her airway, without the coughing or straining with extubation that may jeopardize the integrity of the watertight uterine closure. Before the induction of anesthesia, we either place a lumbar epidural catheter to provide analgesia with opioids in the postoperative period or use patient-controlled analgesia (PCA) devised to administer opioids intravenously.

The danger of teratogenic effects from anesthetic drugs poses a potential risk. In genetically suscep-

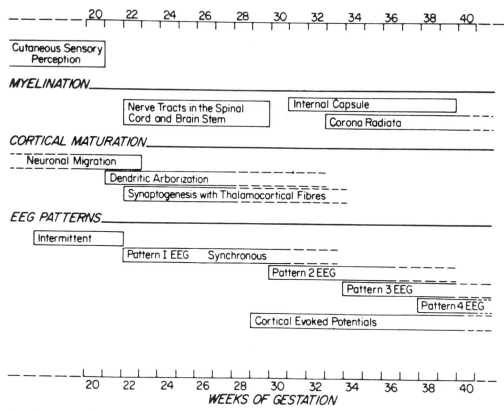

Figure 15.3. Development of cutaneous sensory perception, myelination of pain pathways, maturation of the fetal neocortex, and EEG patterns in the human fetus and neonate.

(Reprinted by permission from Anand KJS, Hickey PR: Pain and its effects in the human neonate and fetus. N Engl J Med 317:1321–1329, 1987.)

tible animal species, many of the commonly used anesthetic drugs induce teratogenic effects at specific stages of gestational development (see Chapter 14). In humans, however, no anesthetic agent appears to be safer or more teratogenic than another. However, the human studies are too few to confirm that anesthetic agents are nonteratogenic, and it is unlikely that such studies could ever be conducted to provide statistically significant results.

Various procedures and techniques may affect fetal physiologic functions. The relationship between these procedures and altered fetal physiology is not precisely understood. For example, uterine incision, fetal manipulation, and anesthetic management each may affect fetal and placental circulation by several mechanisms, sometimes producing fetal compromise. Increased uterine activity, maternal hypotension, maternal hypocarbia, or hyperventilation may interfere with uterine and umbilical blood flow. Fetal manipulation may affect umbilical blood flow by direct compression or by inducing responses that affect fetal circulation. The impact of some of these procedures on the fetal cardiovascular system, the distribution of fetal cardiac output, and the total fetal well-being is being investigated.

FETAL CARDIOVASCULAR CIRCULATION

The fetal cardiovascular circulation is adapted for use of the placenta as the organ for oxygen uptake and carbon dioxide elimination. Therefore it has a large placental blood flow and very small pulmonary blood flow. It is also adapted for existence in a low-oxygen environment and provides the cerebral circulation with blood that has a greater oxygen content than that perfusing the lower body. Fetal cardiovascular circulation allows for the mixing of blood between the right and left sides of the heart. Approximately one-third of the relatively well-oxygenated inferior vena caval blood (which includes the blood returning from the placenta) is deflected by the christa dividens in the right atrium and shunted through the foramen ovale into the left atrium. Two-thirds of the inferior vena caval blood passes from the right atrium to the right ventricle. Almost all poorly oxygenated superior vena caval blood also passes from the right atrium to the right ventricle. Approximately 90% of the right ventricular output, ejected into the pulmonary artery, is shunted by a conduit between the main pulmonary artery and the aorta, the ductus arteriosus. The left ventricular output, which includes

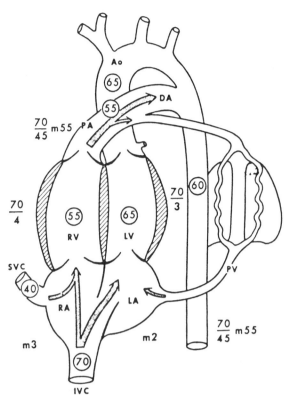

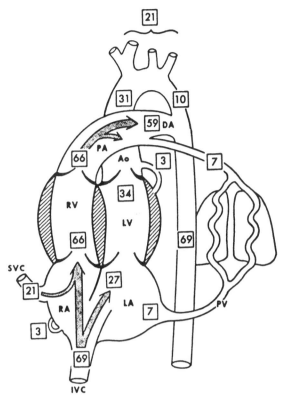

Figure 15.4. The fetal circulation. The *figures in circles* within the chambers and vessels represent percent oxygen saturation levels. The *figures alongside the chambers and vessels* are pressures in mm Hg relative to an amniotic pressure level of zero. *m* = mean pressure; *Ao* = aorta; *DA* = ductus arteriosus; *PA* = pulmonary artery; *RV, LV* = right and left ventricle; *RA, LA* = right and left atrium; *IVC* = inferior vena cava. Data are obtained from late-gestation lambs. (Reprinted by permission from Rudolph AM: *Congenital Diseases of the Heart*, Year Book Medical Publishers, Chicago, 1974, p 3.)

Figure 15.5. The fetal circulation. The *figure in squares* within the chambers and vessels represent percentages of the combined ventricular output that return to the fetal heart, percentages ejected by each ventricle, and percentages flowing through the main vascular channels. *SVC* = superior vena cava; *PV* = pulmonary vein; other abbreviations as in legend to Figure 15.4. Data are obtained from late gestation lambs. (Reprinted by permission from Rudolph AM: *Congenital Diseases of the Heart*, Year Book Medical Publishers, Chicago, 1974, p 8.)

the relatively well-oxygenated inferior vena caval blood (deflected through the foramen ovale) and the small amount of blood that perfuses the pulmonary circulation, is ejected into the aorta and perfuses the head and upper extremities. Figures 15.4 and 15.5 depict the circulation of the fetal lamb with normal blood pressures, oxygen saturations, and blood flows for the various vessels and cardiac chambers.

Cardiac output has two main determinants: heart rate and stroke volume. Fetal cardiac output, measured in terms of combined left and right ventricular output, is directly related to heart rate (46), which is probably the most important determinant of fetal cardiac output. Stroke volume is a function of preload, afterload, and myocardial contractility. Fetal myocardial contractility is probably maximally stimulated, with limited capacity to increase stroke volume. Fetal myocardial muscle strips are less compliant than those of adult hearts and have a greater

resting tension, but a diminished response for increasing myocardial tension when stimulated (47). In fetal lambs, augmentation of preload has little effect on increasing cardiac output. Volume loading increases cardiac output by only 15 to 20% (48).

To function properly, the fetal circulation depends on a high venous return (49). Because the heart rate is predominant in regulating fetal cardiac output, baroreceptor and chemoreceptor responsiveness have important regulatory roles. Baroreflex activity exists by midgestation and increases in sensitivity as gestation advances (50). Chemoreflex activity from the aortic and carotid chemoreceptors in fetal lambs has been elicited and studied in utero (51–54). However, most of the information about the chemoreceptor role in the regulation of circulation has been obtained from anesthetized or short-term studies in fetal animals. A method for selectively denervating the aortic and carotid chemoreceptor and baroreceptor in fetal lambs in utero has been developed. This will

Table 15.8
Fetal Anesthetic Requirement (MAC) for Halothane in Sheep (Mean ± SE)[a]

	Blood Concentration at MAC[b] (mg/liter)	Theoretical (Calculated) End-Tidal Concentration[b] (%)
Mothers	133 ± 5	0.69 ± 0.25
Fetuses	49 ± 28	0.33 ± 0.29

[a]Modified from Gregory GA, Wade JG, Biehl DR, Ong BY, Sitar D: Fetal anesthetic requirement (MAC) for halothane. Anesth Analg 62:9–14, 1983.
[b]Maternal and fetal values are significantly different (P < 0.001).

allow investigation of their roles in both normal fetal cardiovascular regulation and fetal response to stress (55, 56).

Because the fetus has a limited capacity to increase cardiac output in response to stress, oxygen delivery to vital organs must be maintained by redistribution of blood flow. Cerebral blood flow in the fetal lamb is twice that in the adult, although both cerebral metabolic rates are similar (57, 58). These characteristics of fetal blood flow may represent a protective advantage for the fetus.

Among the factors that may modulate cerebral blood flow are cerebral metabolic rate, arterial carbon dioxide tension ($PaCO_2$), arterial oxygen content, blood pressure, and autoregulation (59–61). In fetal lambs, increases in cerebral metabolic rate or $PaCO_2$ and decreases in arterial oxygen content are associated with increased cerebral blood flow. Cerebral blood flow autoregulation has been demonstrated to preserve cerebral blood flow in the normoxic fetal lamb when systemic blood pressures range 20% above or below normal values. However, autoregulation in response to hypotension may be incomplete, and the mechanism of autoregulation may depend on arterial oxygen concentration (62).

EFFECTS OF ANESTHESIA ON THE FETAL CARDIOVASCULAR CIRCULATION

The effects of inhalational anesthetic agents on the cardiovascular system of the fetus are being investigated and much is to be learned. In fetal lambs, the concentration of halothane required to prevent movement in response to painful stimuli is much lower than that for adult sheep or newborn lambs (Table 15.8) (63). Although placental transfer of inhaled agents occurs rapidly, fetal levels of the halogenated agents remain lower than do maternal levels for a significant period after administration of these agents to the mother (Figs. 15.6 and 15.7). Reports conflict on the effects in a fetus when the mother

has received halothane or isoflurane. In one study, maternal anesthesia with 0.7% halothane or 1% isoflurane (1 minimum alveolar concentration [MAC] for sheep) caused a mild decrease in fetal blood pressure with no change in fetal pulse rate, oxygen level, or acid-base status; however, anesthesia with 1.5% halothane or 2% isoflurane (i.e., deep anesthesia) caused decreases in fetal blood pressure, heart rate,

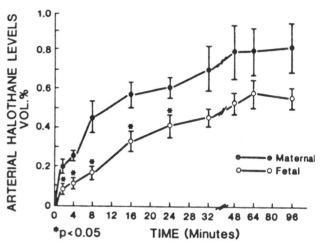

Figure 15.6. Maternal and fetal arterial halothane levels in sheep during maternal administration of 1.5% halothane (mean ± SE). (Reprinted by permission from Biehl DR, Cote J, Wade JG, Gregory GA, Sitar D: Uptake of halothane by the foetal lamb in utero. Can Anaesth Soc J 30:24–27, 1983.)

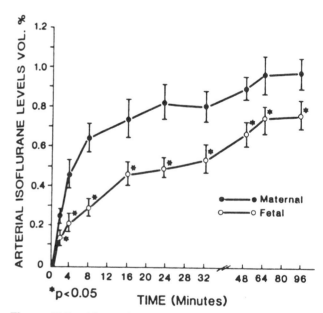

Figure 15.7. Maternal and fetal arterial isoflurane levels in sheep during maternal administration of 2.0% isoflurane (mean ± SE). (Reprinted by permission from Biehl DR, Yarnell R, Wade JG, Sitar D: The uptake of isoflurane by the foetal lamb in utero: Effect on regional blood flow. Can Anaesth Soc 30:581–586, 1983.)

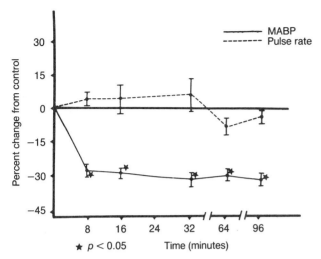

Figure 15.8. Changes in fetal sheep mean arterial blood pressure (*MABP*) and pulse rate during maternal administration of 1.5% halothane, expressed as percent change from control levels (mean ± SE). (Reprinted by permission from Biehl DR, Tweed WA, Cote J, Wade JG, Sitar D: Effect of halothane on cardiac output and regional flow in the fetal lamb in utero. Anesth Analg 62:489–492, 1983.)

oxygen saturation, and base access, with progressive fetal acidosis (64). Other studies demonstrated that maternal anesthesia with 1.5% halothane caused a decrease in fetal arterial pressure after a few minutes (primarily because of a decrease in peripheral vascular resistance), with no change in pulse rate, cardiac output, oxygen, acid-base status, or blood flow to the fetal brain or other major fetal organs (Figs. 15.8, 15.9, and 15.10) (65, 66). Yet, another study demonstrated that maternal anesthesia with 2.0% isoflurane produced no significant decline in fetal blood pressure, but did produce a decrease in fetal cardiac index and the development of progressive fetal acidosis (67). It appears that deep inhalation anesthesia (2 MAC) may result in progressive fetal acidosis, whereas light anesthesia (1 MAC) is safe for the fetus. However, the applicability of these studies is limited because the fetus was not studied while undergoing a surgical procedure capable of inducing stressful, noxious stimulation.

In unanesthetized experimental animals, fetal asphyxia induced by occlusion of the umbilical circulation results in fetal bradycardia and hypertension, with decreased cardiac output and increased cerebral blood flow mediated partially by the fetal α- and β-adrenergic systems (68–72). Reports on the effects of maternal halothane administration on the asphyxiated fetus are conflicting. In one study maternal halothane administration did not further compromise fetal well-being. The blood pressure of the anesthetized fetus declined to values that were nor-

mal compared with those of the awake asphyxiated fetus; however, because the pulse rate increased, the cardiac output remained unchanged. Oxygenation did not deteriorate and cerebral blood flow remained elevated (73). In another study, halothane administered to the mother of a severely acidotic fetus caused further aggravation of fetal acidosis and oxygen desaturation (74). Cerebral blood flow decreased as fetal blood pressure decreased.

MONITORING

Fetal asphyxia, hypoxia, or distress can be most effectively recognized, predicted, and avoided by fetal monitoring (75). Monitoring is also crucial to assess fetal response to corrective maneuvers. Methods for monitoring fetal well-being include fetal blood gas, pH, glucose, and electrolyte determinations and measurements of fetal heart rate, blood pressure, and umbilical blood flow. Invasive methods used in experimental fetal preparations require indwelling catheters that may have limited application for clinical fetal surgery. However, capillary blood samples can be obtained by the surgeon for blood gas determinations, and vascular access can be achieved for fluid, blood, or drug administration during prolonged procedures, such as correction of a diaphragmatic hernia. In the future, more information may be used from detailed waveform analysis of the fetal electrocardiogram (ECG). New devices will become available for monitoring the fetal electroencephalogram; for continuous monitoring of arterial oxygen saturation, P_{O_2} and P_{CO_2}; and for monitoring cerebral oxygenation, blood volume, and blood flow by near infrared spectroscopy and tissue pH (Figs. 15.11 and 15.12).

The author has used fetal heart rate monitoring, pulse oximetry, and intermittent blood gas determinations as relatively noninvasive methods of assessing fetal well-being during fetal surgery. The fetal heart rate can be monitored with a standard internal fetal electrode and a reference electrode on the maternal abdomen, both connected to a maternal ground plate and processed by a fetal heart rate cardiotachometer (76). However, the signal obtained is of low amplitude and is overwhelmed by movement artifact, rendering the conventional display of the beat-to-beat heart rate unreliable. The author has found that direct monitoring of the fetus by ECG is more reliable than the standard internal fetal electrode. Modified insulated atrial pacing wires are used as ECG leads. The bare wire at the distal end is sutured subcutaneously onto the fetal thorax for diaphragmatic hernia repair using the attached curved needles. The proximal end of the insulated wire is attached to a coaxial shielded cable, connecting the

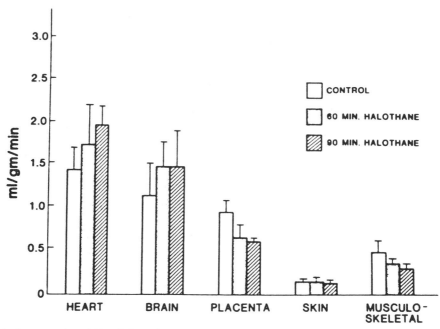

Figure 15.9. Fetal sheep regional blood flow during maternal administration of 1.5% halothane (mean ± SE). Values were obtained at control and after 60 and 90 min of halothane anesthesia using the labeled microsphere injection technique. (Reprinted by permission from Biehl DR, Tweed WA, Cote J, Wade JG, Sitar D: Effect of halothane on cardiac output and regional flow in the fetal lamb in utero. Anesth Analg 62:489–492, 1983.)

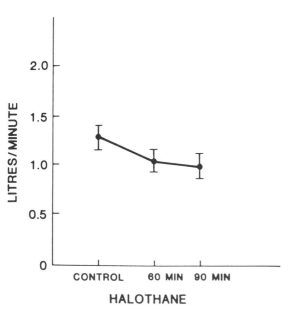

Figure 15.10. Fetal sheep cardiac output calculated using labeled microsphere injection technique during maternal administration of 1.5% halothane (mean ± SE). Values were obtained at control and after 60 and 90 min of halothane anesthesia. (Reprinted by permission from Biehl DR, Tweed WA, Cote J, Wade JG, Sitar D: Effect of halothane on cardiac output and regional flow in the fetal lamb in utero. Anesth Analg 62:489–492, 1983.)

three leads to a cardiotachometer. The cardiotachometer has been modified by an increased gain to allow for signal amplification and by the addition of a fixed low-pass frequency filter and variable high-pass frequency filter, which substantially reduces motion artifact. The ECG lead wires are stabilized to minimize capacitive coupling and changes in voltage offset between the fetal skin and the ECG lead wire. This allows for a more reliable display of the fetal ECG with visible P and QRS complexes. Alternatively, we have experimented with devices surgically implanted in the fetus (in a manner similar to cardiac pacemakers). These devices provide continuous radiosignal transmission to a portable receiver (antenna) adjacent to the mother. This latter technique enables fetal heart rate monitoring during the surgical procedure, in the recovery period, and during the remainder of gestation.

Plethysmography combined with spectrophotometric oximetry (pulse oximetry) has also proved very useful. A noninvasive sensor contains two low-voltage, low-intensity, light-emitting diodes as light sources and a photodiode as a light receiver. For diaphragmatic hernia repair and congenital cystic adenomatoid malformation excision, we use neonatal digital sensors—modified by waterproofing the light-emitting and photodetector diodes with clear, heat-shrunk plastic tubing—which are wrapped around the fetal arm, leg, or (preferably) palmar arch.

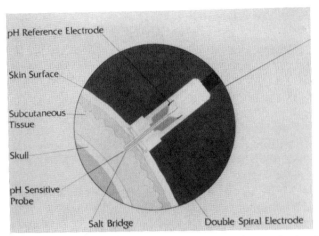

Figure 15.11. The Stamm tpH probe inserted into the fetal scalp subcutaneous tissue. The circuit consists of a Ag:AgCl pH reference electrode connected to the tissue fluids in the subcutaneous space by a Ag:AgCl-KCl solution. This forms an annular salt bridge near the pH sensitive probe, the special glass tip. A voltage is produced across the glass tip by the difference in hydrogen ion concentration between the subcutaneous tissue fluids and the electrolyte in the shaft supporting the tip. The circuit is completed by the wire inside the shaft, which goes through the cable into the electronics. The open liquid junction (salt bridge) provides slow flow of reference electrolyte, which in turn provides a large stable reference in the tissues. (Reprinted by permission from Hochberg HM: Tissue pH monitoring: Principles and practice. In *Clinical Perinatal Biochemical Monitoring*, NH Laursen, HM Hochberg, eds. Williams & Wilkins, Baltimore, 1981, pp 103–125.)

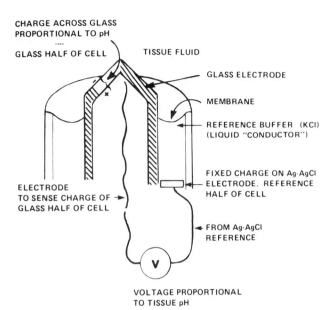

Figure 15.12. Principle of operation of the tissue pH electrode. The properties of the glass are such that it accumulates a charge in the presence of excessive or deficient hydrogen ion (i.e., if the pH is other than "neutral"). This charge is directly proportional to the pH. The pH is measured by using the charged glass to form one pole of a battery. The other pole, the Ag:AgCl electrode, does not change its charge with pH, and thus forms a reference electrode. A reference buffer allows connection to the tissue fluids without accumulating another charge and this completes the circuit. The "battery" voltage is a direct reflection of pH. (Reprinted by permission from Hochberg HM: Tissue pH monitoring: *Principles and practice in Clinical Perinatal Biochemical Monitoring*, NH Laursen, HM Hochberg, eds., Williams & Wilkins, Baltimore, 1981, pp 103–125.)

Alternatively, a flat sensor is placed over any exposed fetal parts so light can be measured predominantly by reflectance rather than transmission. Changes in the absorption of red light, relative to a change in the absorption of infrared light, indicate the arterial hemoglobin oxygen saturation (77). A Nellcor N-200 monitor, which has been modified by the addition of special circuits to reduce noise (low-noise amplifiers), is used. A computer data collection system is connected to the monitor to allow for visualization of both red and infrared pulse signals and their respective percentages of modulation. Thus qualitative and quantitative assessment of signal strength and reliability is possible.

Intraoperative sterile sonography is also important for monitoring the fetus. Fetal heart rate can be determined by visualization of the heart or by Doppler assessment of the flow of blood through the umbilical cord, and the quality of fetal cardiac contractility and volume can be determined. However, in most circumstances, the sterile transducer cannot be positioned continuously because it interferes with the surgical field.

PREVENTION OF PRETERM LABOR

The human uterine wall has a thick, muscular layer that is sensitive to stimulation or manipulation. Because uterine stimulation increases the likelihood of inducing uterine contraction, the risk of preterm labor accompanies invasive fetal intervention. After incision strong uterine contractions can occur; these have resulted in high incidences of postoperative abortion in experimental preparations using primate fetuses. Strong uterine contractions may impede uterine blood flow or induce partial placental separation, which interferes with umbilical-placental blood flow; both of these compromise fetal well-being. A uterine contraction can displace a percutaneous intrauterine needle placed for intrauterine transfusion or shunt catheter placement.

Prevention and treatment of preterm labor is critically important in the management of patients undergoing fetal intervention. Tocolytic therapy includes a variety of drugs. The agents most commonly used for tocolysis are β-adrenergic agonists and magnesium sulfate, which prevent or inhibit postoperative preterm labor. Although tocolysis is usually not necessary after simple percutaneous umbilical blood sampling or intrauterine transfusions, for more invasive percutaneous procedures (such as shunt catheter placement), low-dose β-adrenergic agonist tocolytic agents can be administered intravenously for prophylactic control of uterine irritability. For procedures involving hysterotomy, halogenated agents are used intraoperatively to inhibit uterine contractility and to provide the uterine relaxation necessary for surgical exposure through a small hysterotomy incision (4). We use a regimen of tocolysis that includes preoperative administration of indomethacin by suppository, intraoperative anesthetic by inhalation of halogenated agent, and (once closure of the uterus is begun) a bolus dose of magnesium sulfate administered over 20 min. A continuous intravenous magnesium sulfate infusion is initiated for postoperative tocolysis, supplemented by β-adrenergic agonists if necessary. The uterine relaxation provided by these agents can significantly increase the risk of maternal hemorrhage during incision. To reduce such risk, special surgical techniques employing a stapling device are used for vascular stasis during hysterotomy. Intraoperatively, intravenous fluids are restricted to minimize the risk of postoperative pulmonary edema associated with administration of magnesium sulfate and β-adrenergic agonists.

Prostaglandin synthetase inhibitors have been investigated as tocolytic agents (78) and used preoperatively for fetal surgical procedures. Although there have been case reports of prenatal closure of the ductus arteriosus and persistent fetal circulation associated with the use of prostaglandin synthetase inhibitors for tocolysis, more recent studies have not found these effects on the fetal cardiovascular system among neonates whose mothers were treated before 34 weeks' gestation (79). Indomethacin use has been associated with decreased fetal urine output caused by potentiation of the peripheral effects of antidiuretic hormone. In addition, neonatal bleeding and renal impairment could result from prolonged indomethacin therapy.

There is limited experience with the use of calcium-channel blockers for tocolysis. They are infrequently used for initial tocolytic management unless contraindications exist to the use of other agents. All tocolytic agents have maternal, fetal, and neonatal side effects. A more complete discussion of tocolytic agents and anesthetic interactions can be found in Chapter 18.

ETHICAL CONSIDERATIONS SURROUNDING FETAL SURGERY

The medical complexities associated with fetal surgery transcend the diagnosis and treatment of fetal disease. Fetal treatment presents technical options that have not yet been fully evaluated clinically. The options raise complex social, ethical, and legal issues that go beyond those customary for therapeutic intervention (89–96). Federal and state regulations governing this area of research are controversial. Although the rationale for and intent of improving fetal health by in utero procedures are within the scope of traditional medicine, we must distinguish innovative therapy from experimentation. To the usual issues of safety, efficacy, cost effectiveness (97), resource allocation, and expectations and availability of therapy are added the issues of sensitivity and specificity of diagnostic testing (including the ability to exclude other potentially associated anomalies), as well as the issue of the potential long-range applications, implications, and consequences of intervention.

Fetal treatment also raises unique and complicated ethical and legal questions about maternal rights and fetal needs. Some of these questions are medical. Treating a potentially viable fetus as a patient in its own right requires a consideration of the mother's medical interests, because it is her body that is the site of treatment. Who will act as medical advocate for each patient—mother and fetus—if preserving the health of one places the other at risk? Some of these questions must be resolved in the face of conflicting legal interpretations of the assumed responsibilities of parents, forced bodily intrusion, and legal termination of pregnancy. Could legal injunctions force fetal treatment in opposition to a mother's wishes, a situation analogous to overriding parental refusal of necessary treatment for a child? What are the liabilities (civil and criminal) once a therapy becomes established as safe and effective for intended purposes? Because these issues are complex, parents must be provided with complete information about the nature of the procedure, its potential benefits for the fetus, and the risks inherent for both patients before giving informed consent. Parents should also be offered alternative therapies, if any, and informed of their expected consequences.

THE FUTURE OF FETAL TREATMENT

Innovative treatment of the fetus must be tested in primate animal models, carefully evaluated in light of our uncertainties, and undertaken with caution. Before offering fetal procedures to patients, the University of California, San Francisco, (UCSF) Fetal Treatment Program established that intervention would not be considered until the natural history of the disease was defined (e.g., evaluating serial sonograms in untreated cases), the pathophysiology studied in an appropriate animal model, and the feasibility and safety of intervention established in primate models. Futhermore, researchers have an obligation to report all results to the medical profession so that the full merits and liabilities of fetal surgery can be established. For that purpose, members of the UCSF Fetal Treatment Program founded the International Fetal Medicine and Surgery Society, which sets general and specific guidelines for fetal treatment and maintains a voluntary registry of fetal surgical procedures.

Fetal surgical techniques and tocolytic management will undergo continued improvement. The risks and benefits of various anesthetic agents and techniques and the effectiveness and safety of fetal monitoring must continue to be evaluated. Possibilities for future therapy include in utero treatment for endocrine diseases, biochemical defects (98), thrombocytopenia (99), nonimmune hydrops (100), cardiac malformations (101), central nervous system malformations (102–107), genetic disorders (transplantation of hematopoietic stem cells or bone marrow) (108), allogenic bone transplantations for skeletal anomalies (22–23), transplantation of fetal cells (109), repair of craniofacial abnormalities (110), and nutritional supplementation for intrauterine growth retardation (111). We must learn, however, to distinguish fetuses that may benefit from invasive therapy from those that will not, intervening only when there is a reasonable probability of benefit.

References

1. Liley AW: Intrauterine transfusion of the foetus in haemolytic disease. Br Med J 2:1107–1109, 1963.
2. Adamsons K: Fetal surgery. N Engl J Med 275:204–206, 1966.
3. Liley AW: Foreword. In *The Unborn Patient: Prenatal Diagnosis and Treatment*, 2nd ed. MR Harrison, MS Golbus, RA Filly, eds. WB Saunders, Philadelphia, 1991, p XI.
4. Harrison MR, Golbus MS, Filly RA, Callen PW, Katz M, deLorimier AA, Rosen MA, Jonsen AR: Fetal surgery for congenital hydronephrosis. N Engl J Med 306:591–593, 1982.
5. Harrison MR, Golbus MS, Filly RA, Nakayama DK, deLorimier AA: Fetal surgical treatment. Pediatr Ann 11:896–903, 1982.
6. Harrison MR, Golbus MS, Filly RA: Management of the fetus: A correctable congenital defect. JAMA 246:774–777, 1981.
7. Pearson JF: Fetal surgery. Arch Dis Child 58:324–325, 1983.
8. Robie GF, Payne GG, Morgan MA: Selective delivery of an acardiac, acephalic twin. N Engl J Med 320:512–513, 1989.
9. Goldberg JD, Golbus MS: Personal communication.
10. Krummel TM, Longaker MT: Fetal Wound Healing. In *The Unborn Patient: Prenatal Diagnosis and Treatment*, 2nd ed. MR Harrison, MS Golbus, RA Filly, eds. WB Saunders, Philadelphia, 1991, pp 526–536.
11. Redwine F, Petres RE: Fetal surgery: Past, present and future. Clin Perinatol 10:399–410, 1983.
12. Harrison MR, Jester JA, Ross NA: Correction of congenital diaphragmatic hernia in utero. I. The model: Intrathoracic balloon produces fatal pulmonary hypoplasia. Surgery 88:174–182, 1980.
13. Harrison MR, Bressack MA, Churg AM, deLorimier AA: Correction of congenital diaphragmatic hernia in utero. II. Simulated correction permits fetal lung growth with survival at birth. Surgery 88:260–268, 1980.
14. Harrison MR, Ross NA, deLorimier AA: Correction of congenital diaphragmatic hernia in utero. III. Development of a successful surgical technique using abdominoplasty to avoid compromise of umbilical blood flow. J Pediatr Surg 16:934–942, 1981.
15. Harrison MR: The fetus with a diaphragmatic hernia: Pathophysiology, natural history and surgical management. In *The Unborn Patient: Prenatal Diagnosis and Treatment*, 2nd ed. MR Harrison, MS Golbus, RA Filly, eds. WB Saunders, Philadelphia, 1991, pp 295–313.
16. Harrison MR, Langer JC, Adzick NS, Golbus MS, Filly RA, Anderson RL, Rosen MA, Callen PW, Goldstein RB, deLorimier AA: Correction of congenital diaphragmatic hernia in utero. V. Initial clinical experience. J Pediatr Surg 25:47–57, 1990.
17. Harrison MR, Adzick NS, Longaker MT, Goldberg JD, Rosen MA, Filly RA, Evans MI, Golbus MS: Successful repair in utero of a fetal diaphragmatic hernia after removal of herniated viscera from the left thorax. N Engl J Med 322:1582–1584, 1990.
18. Harrison MR, Adzick NS, Jennings RW, Duncan BW, Rosen MA, Filly RA, Goldberg JD, deLorimier AA, Golbus MS: Antenatal intervention for congenital cystic adenomatoid malformation. Lancet 1:965–967, 1990.
19. Clewell WH, Johnson ML, Meier PR, Newkirk JR, Zide SL, Hendee RW, Bowes WA Jr, Hecht F, O'Keeffe D, Henry GP, Shikes RH: A surgical approach to the treatment of fetal hydrocephalus. N Engl J Med 306:1320–1325, 1982.
20. Hudgins RJ, Edwards MSB, Goldstein R, Callen PW, Harrison MR, Filly RA, Golbus MS: The natural history of fetal ventriculomegaly. Pediatrics 82:692–697, 1988.
21. Manning F, Harrison MR, Rodeck C, International Fetal Medicine and Surgery Society: Catheter shunts for fetal hydronephrosis and hydrocephalus: Report of the International Fetal Surgery Registry. N Engl Med J 315:336–340, 1986.
22. Michejda M, Hodgen GD: In utero diagnosis and treatment of non-human primate fetal skeletal anomalies. JAMA 246:1093–1097, 1981.
23. Hodgen GD: Antenatal diagnosis and treatment of fetal skeletal malformations: With emphasis on in utero surgery for neural tube defects and limb bud regeneration. JAMA 246:1079–1083, 1981.
24. Harrison MR, Filly RA, Parer JT, Faer MJ, Jacobson JB, deLorimier AA: Management of the fetus with a urinary tract malformation. JAMA 246:635–639, 1981.
25. Harrison MR, Ross NA, Noall RA, deLorimier AA: Correction of congenital hydronephrosis in utero. I. The model: Fetal urethral obstruction produces hydronephrosis and pulmonary hypoplasia in fetal lambs. J Pediatr Surg 18:247–256, 1983.
26. Harrison MR, Nakayama DK, Noall RA, Ross NA, deLorimier AA: Correction of congenital hydronephrosis in utero. II. Decompression reverses the effects of obstruction on the fetal lung and urinary tract. J Pediatr Surg 17:965–974, 1982.
27. Glick PL, Harrison MR, Noall RA, Villa RL: Correction of congenital hydronephrosis in utero. III. Early mid-trimester ureteral obstruction produces renal dysplasia. J Pediatr Surg 18:681–687, 1983.
28. Glick PL, Harrison MR, Adzick NS, Noall RA, Villa RL: Congenital hydronephrosis in utero. IV. In utero decompression prevents renal dysplasia. J Pediatr Surg 19:649–657, 1984.
29. Nakayama DK, Glick PL, Villa RL, Noall R, Harrison MR: Experimental pulmonary hypoplasia due to oligohydramnios and its reversal by relieving thoracic compression. J Pediatr Surg 18:347–353, 1983.

30. Sauer L, Harrison MR, Flake AW: Does an expanding fetal abdominal mass produce pulmonary hypoplasia? J Pediatr Surg 22:508–512, 1987.

31. Golbus MS, Harrison MR, Filly RA, Callen PW, Katz M: In utero treatment of urinary tract obstruction. Am J Obstet Gynecol 142:383–388, 1982.

32. Harrison MR, Golbus MS, Filly RA, deLorimier AA, Anderson RL, Flake AW, Huff RW, Rosen M: Fetal hydronephrosis: Selection and surgical repair. J Pediatr Surg 22:556–558, 1987.

33. Crombleholme TM, Harrison MR, Langer JC, Longaker MT, Anderson RL, Slotnik NS: Early experience with open fetal surgery for congenital hydronephrosis. J Pediatr Surg 3:1114–1121, 1988.

34. Harrison MR, Filly RA: The fetus with obstructive uropathy: Pathophysiology, natural history, selection and treatment. In *The Unborn Patient: Prenatal Diagnosis and Treatment*, 2nd ed. MR Harrison, MS Golbus, RA Filly, eds. WB Saunders, Philadelphis, 1991, pp 328–396.

35. Anand KJS: Hormonal and metabolic function of neonates and infants undergoing surgery. Curr Opin Cardiol 1:681–689, 1986.

36. Anand KJS: Brown MJ, Bloom SR, Aynsley–Green A: Studies on the hormonal regulation of fuel metabolism in the human newborn infant undergoing anaesthesia and surgery. Horm Res 22:115–128, 1985.

37. Milne EMG, Elliott MJ, Pearson DT, Holden MP, Orskov H, Alberti KGMM: The effect on intermediary metabolism of open-heart surgery with deep hypothermia and circulatory arrest in infants of less than 10 kilograms body weight. Perfusion 1:29–40, 1986.

38. Obara H, Sugiyama D, Maekawa N: Plasma cortisol levels in paediatric anaesthesia. Can Anaesth Soc J 31:24–27, 1984.

39. Srinivasan G, Jain R, Pildes RS, Kannan CR: Glucose homeostasis during anesthesia and surgery in infants. J Pediatr Surg 21:718–721, 1986.

40. Anand KJS, Brownk MJ, Causon RC, Cristofides ND, Bloom SR, Aynsley–Green A: Can the human neonate mount an endocrine and metabolic response to surgery? J Pediatr Surg 20:41–48, 1985.

41. Anand KJS, Sippell WG, Aynsley–Green A: Randomized trial of fentanyl anaesthesia in preterm neonates undergoing surgery: Effects on the stress response. Lancet 1:243–248, 1987.

42. Rose JC, Macdonald AA, Heymann MA, Rudolph AM: Developmental aspects of the pituitary-adrenal axis response to hemorrhagic stress in lamb fetuses in utero. J Clin Invest 61:424–432, 1978.

43. Liley AW: The foetus as a personality. Aust N Z J Psychol 6:99–105, 1972.

44. Smyth CN: Exploratory methods for testing the integrity of the foetus and neonate. J Obstet Gynaecol Br Commonw 72:920–935, 1965.

45. Anand KJS, Hickey PR: Pain and its effects in the human neonate and fetus. N Engl J Med 317:1321–1329, 1987.

46. Rudolph AM, Heymann MA: Cardiac output in the fetal lamb: The effects of spontaneous and induced changes of heart rate on right and left ventricular output. Am J Obstet Gynecol 124:183–192, 1976.

47. Friedman WF: The intrinsic physiologic properties of the developing heart. Prog Cardiovasc Dis 15:87–111, 1972.

48. Gilbert RD: Control of fetal cardiac output during changes in blood volume. Am J Physiol 238:H80–H86, 1980.

49. Gilbert RD: Determinants of venous return in the fetal lamb. Gynecol Invest 8:233–245, 1977.

50. Shinebourne EA, Vapaavuori EK, Williams RL, Heymann MA, Rudolph AM: Development of baroreflex activity in unanesthetized fetal and neonatal lambs. Circ Res 31:710–718, 1972.

51. Dawes GS, Duncan SLB, Lewis BV, Merlet CL, Owen-Thomas JB, Reeves JT: Hypoxaemia and aortic chemoreceptor function in foetal lambs. J Physiol 201:105–116, 1969.

52. Dawes GS, Duncan SLB, Lewis BV, Merlet CL, Owen-Thomas JB, Reeves JT: Cyanide stimulation of the systemic arterial chemoreceptors in foetal lambs. J Physiol 201:117–128, 1969.

53. Dawes GS, Lewis BV, Milligan JE, Roach MR, Talner NS: Vasomotor responses in the hind limbs of foetal and newborn lambs to asphyxia and aortic chemoreceptor stimulation. J Physiol 195:55–81, 1968.

54. Goodwin JW, Milligan JE, Thomas B. Taylor JR: The effect of aortic chemoreceptor stimulation on cardiac output and umbilical bloodflow in the fetal lamb. Am J Obstet Gynecol 116:48–56, 1973.

55. Itskovitz J, Rudolph AM: Denervation of arterial chemoreceptors and baroreceptors in fetal lambs in utero. Am J Physiol 242:H916–H920, 1982.

56. Itskovitz J, LaGamma EF, Rudolph AM: Baroreflex control of the circulation in chronically instrumented fetal lambs. Circ Res 52:589–596, 1983.

57. Jones MD, Rosenberg AA, Simmons MA, Molteni RA, Koehler RC, Traystman RJ: Oxygen delivery to the brain before and after birth. Science 216:324–325, 1982.

58. Makowski EL, Schneider JM, Tsoulos NG, Colwill JR, Battaglia FC, Meschia G: Cerebral blood flow, oxygen consumption and glucose utilization of fetal lambs in utero. Am J Obstet Gynecol 114:292–303, 1972.

59. Rosenberg AA, Jones MD, Traystman RJ, Simmons MA, Molteni RA: Response of cerebral blood flow to changes in PCO_2 in fetal, newborn and adult sheep. Am J Physiol 242:H862–H866, 1982.

60. Jones MD Jr, Sheldon RE, Peeters LL, Meschia G, Battaglia FC, Makowski EL: Fetal cerebral oxygen consumption at different levels of oxygenation. J Appl Physiol 43:1080–1084, 1977.

61. Tweed WA, Cote J, Wade JG, Gregory G, Mills A: Preservation of fetal brain blood flow relative to other organs during hypovolemic hypotension. Pediatr Res 16:137–140, 1982.

62. Tweed WA, Cote J, Pash M, Lou H: Arterial oxygenation determines autoregulation of cerebral blood flow in the fetal lamb. Pediatr Res 17:246–249, 1983.

63. Gregory GA, Wade JG, Biehl DR, Ong BY, Sitar DS: Fetal anesthetic requirement (MAC) for halothane. Anesth Analg 62:9–14, 1983.

64. Palahniuk RJ, Shnider SM: Maternal and fetal cardiovascular and acid-base changes during halothane and isoflurane anesthesia in the pregnant ewe. Anesthesiology 41:462–472, 1974.

65. Biehl DR, Tweed WA, Cote J, Wade JG, Sitar D: Effect of halothane on cardiac output and regional flow in the fetal lamb in utero. Anesth Analg 62:489–492, 1983.

66. Biehl DR, Cote J, Wade JG, Gregory GA, Sitar D: Uptake of halothane by the foetal lamb in utero. Can Anaesth Soc J 30:24–27, 1983.

67. Biehl DR, Yarnell R, Wade JG, Sitar D: The uptake of isoflurane by the foetal lamb in utero: Effect on regional blood flow. Can Anaesth Soc J 30:581–586, 1983.

68. Cohn HE, Sacks EJ, Heymann MA, Rudolph AM: Cardiovascular responses to hypoxemia and acidemia in fetal lambs. Am J Obstet Gynecol 120:817–824, 1974.

69. Peeters LLH, Sheldon RE, Jones MD, Makowski EL, Meschia G: Blood flow to fetal organs as a function of arterial oxygen content. Am J Obstet Gynecol 35:637–646, 1979.

70. Reuss ML, Parer JT, Harris JL, Krueger TR: Hemodynamic effects of alpha-adrenergic blockade during hypoxia in fetal sheep. Am J Obstet Gynecol 142:410–415, 1982.

71. Court DJ, Parer JT, Block BSB, Llanos AJ: Effects of beta-adrenergic blockade on blood flow distribution during hypoxaemia in fetal sheep. J Dev Physiol 6:349–358, 1984.

72. Johnson GN, Palahniuk RJ, Tweed WA, Jones MV, Wade JG: Regional cerebral blood flow changes during severe fetal asphyxia produced by slow partial umbilical cord compression. Am J Obstet Gynecol 135:48–52, 1979.

73. Yarnell R, Biehl DR, Tweed WA, Gregory GA, Sitar D: The effect of halothane anaesthesia on the asphyxiated foetal lamb in utero. Can Anaesth Soc J 30:474–479, 1983.

74. Palahniuk RJ, Doig GA, Johnson GN, Pash MP: Maternal hal-

othane anesthesia reduces cerebral blood flow in the acidotic sheep fetus. Anesth Analg 59:35–39, 1980.

75. Katz JD, Hook R, Barash PG: Fetal heart rate monitoring in pregnant patients undergoing surgery. Am J Obstet Gynecol 125:267–269, 1976.

76. Harrison MR, Anderson J, Rosen MA, Ross NA, Hendricks AG: Fetal surgery in the primate. I. Anesthetic, surgical, and tocolytic management to maximize fetal-neonatal survival. J Pediatr Surg 17:115–122, 1982.

77. Yelderman M, New W: Evaluation of pulse oximetry. Anesthesiology 59:349–352, 1983.

78. Novy MJ, Liggins GC: Role of prostaglandins, prostacyclin and thromboxanes in the physiologic control of the uterus and in parturition. Semin Perinatol 4:45–66, 1980.

79. Dudley DKL, Hardie MJ: Fetal and neonatal effects of indomethacin used as a tocolytic agent. Am J Obstet Gynecol 151:181–184, 1985.

80. Glick PL, Harrison MR, Golbus MS, Adzick NS, Filly RA, Callen PW, Mahoney BS, Anderson RL, deLorimier AA: Management of the fetus with congenital hydronephrosis. II. Prognostic criteria and selection for treatment. J Pediatr Surg 20:376–387, 1985.

81. Spielman FJ, Seeds JW, Corke BC: Anaesthesia for fetal surgery. Anaesthesia 39:756–759, 1984.

82. Seeds JW, Corke BC, Spielman FJ: Prevention of fetal movement during invasive procedures with pancuronium bromide. Am J Obstet Gynecol 155:818–819, 1986.

83. Moise KJ, Carpenter RJ, Deter RL, Kirshon B. The use of fetal neuromuscular blockade during intrauterine transfusions. Am J Obstet Gynecol 157:874–879, 1987.

84. Copel JA, Grannum PA, Harrison D, Hobbins JC: The use of intravenous pancuronium bromide to produce fetal paralysis during intravascular transfusion. Am J Obstet Gynecol 158:170–171, 1988.

85. Byers JW, Aubry RH, Feinstein SJ, Lodeiro JG, McLaren RA, Srinivasan JP, Sunderji S: Intravascular neuromuscular blockade for fetal transfusion. Am J Obstet Gynecol 158:677, 1988.

86. Pielet BW, Socol ML, MacGregor SN, Dooley SL, Minogue J: Fetal heart rate changes after fetal intravascular treatment with pancuronium bromide. Am J Obstet Gynecol 159:640–643, 1988.

87. Moise KJ, Deter RL, Kirshon B, Adam K, Patton DE, Carpenter RJ: Intravenous pancuronium bromide for fetal neuromuscular blockade during intrauterine transfusion for red-cell alloimmunization. Obstet Gynecol 74:905–908, 1989.

88. Chestnut DH, Weiner CP, Thompson CS, McLaughlin GL: Intravenous administration of d-tubocurarine and pancuronium in fetal lambs. Am J Obstet Gynecol 160:510–513, 1989.

89. Abram MB, Wolf SM: Public involvement in medical ethics: A model for government action. N Engl J Med 310:627–632, 1984.

90. Chervenak FA, Farley MA, Walters L, Hobbins JC, Mahoney MJ: When is termination of pregnancy during the third trimester morally justifiable? N Engl J Med 310:501–504, 1984.

91. AMA Council on Scientific Affairs: In utero fetal surgery, Resolution 73 (I-81). JAMA 250:1443–1444, 1983.

92. Barclay WR, McCormick RA, Sidbury JB, Michejda M, Hodgen GD: The ethics of in utero surgery. JAMA 246:1550–1555, 1981.

93. Fletcher JC: The fetus as patient: Ethical issues. JAMA 246:772–773, 1981.

94. Englehardt HT Jr: Current controversies in obstetrics: Wrongful life and forced fetal surgical procedures. Am J Obstet Gynecol 151:313–318, 1985.

95. Fletcher JC, Jonsen AR: Ethical considerations in fetal treat-
ment. In *The Unborn Patient: Prenatal Diagnosis and Treatment*, 2nd ed. MR Harrison, MS Golbus, RA Filly, eds. WB Saunders, Philadelphia, 1991, pp 14–18.

96. Robertson JA: Legal considerations in fetal treatment. In *The Unborn Patient: Prenatal Diagnosis and Treatment*, 2nd ed. MR Harrison, MS Golbus, RA Filly, eds. WB Saunders, Philadelphia, 1991, pp 19–24.

97. Korenbrot CC, Gardner L: Economic considerations in fetal treatment. In *The Unborn Patient: Prenatal Diagnosis and Treatment*, 2nd ed. MR Harrison, MS Golbus, RA Filly, eds. WB Saunders, Philadelphia, 1991, pp 25–38.

98. Shulman JD, Evan MI: The fetus with a biochemical defect. In *The Unborn Patient: Prenatal Diagnosis and Treatement*, 2nd ed. MR Harrison, MS Golbus, RA Filly, eds. WB Saunders, Philadelphia, 1991, pp 205–209.

99. Daffos F: The fetus at risk for thrombocytopenia. In *The Unborn Patient: Prenatal Diagnosis and Treatment*, 2nd ed. MR Harrison, MS Golbus, RA Filly, eds. WB Saunders, Philadelphia, 1991, pp 210–214.

100. Holgreve W: The fetus with nonimmune hydrops. In *The Unborn Patient: Prenatal Diagnosis and Treatment*, 2nd ed. MR Harrison, MS Golbus, RA Filly, eds. WB Saunders, Philadelphia, 1991, pp 228–248.

101. Verrier ED, Vlahakes GJ, Hanley FL, Bradley SM: Experimental fetal cardiac surgery. In *The Unborn Patient: Prenatal Diagnosis and Treatment*, 2nd ed. MR Harrison, MS Golbus, RA Filly, eds. WB Saunders, Philadelphia, 1991, pp 548–556.

102. Hudgins R, Edwards MSB: The fetus with a CNS malformation: Natural history and management. In *The Unborn Patient: Prenatal Diagnosis and Treatment*, 2nd ed. MR Harrison, MS Golbus, RA Filly, eds. WB Saunders, Philadelphia, 1991, pp 437–443.

103. Harrison MR, Duncan BW: Experimental fetal hydrocephalus. In *The Unborn Patient: Prenatal Diagnosis and Treatment*, 2nd ed. MR Harrison, MS Golbus, RA Filly, eds. WB Saunders, Philadelphia, 1991, pp 581–589.

104. Brodner RA, Markowitz RS, Lantner HJ: Feasibility of intracranial surgery in the primate fetus: Model and surgical principles. J Neurosurg 66:276–282, 1987.

105. Albright L: Techniques of spinal cord surgery in fetal rats. Neurosurg 20:240–242, 1987.

106. Glick PL, Harrison MR, Halks-Miller M, Adzick NS, Nakayama DK, Villa RL: Correction of congenital hydrocephalus in utero. II. Efficacy of in utero shunting. J Pediatr Surg 19:870–881, 1984.

107. Michejda M: Experimental repair of CNS lesions. In *The Unborn Patient: Prenatal Diagnosis and Treatment*, 2nd ed. MR Harrison, MS Golbus, RA Filly RA, eds. WB Saunders, Philadelphia, 1991, pp 565–580.

108. Karson EM, Anderson WF: Prospects for gene therapy. In *The Unborn Patient: Prenatal Diagnosis and Treatment*, 2nd ed. MR Harrison, MS Golbus, RA Filly, eds. WB Saunders, Philadelphia, 1991, pp 481–494.

109. Crumbleholme TM, Zanjani ED, Langer JC, Harrison MR: Transplantation of fetal cells. In *The Unborn Patient: Prenatal Diagnosis and Treatment*, 2nd ed. MR Harrison, MS Golbus, RA Filly, eds. WB Saunders, Philadelphia, 1991, pp 495–507.

110. Longaker MT, Kaban LB: Experimental craniofacial abnormalities. In *The Unborn Patient: Prenatal Diagnosis and Treatment*, 2nd ed. MR Harrison, MS Golbus, RA Filly, eds. WB Saunders, Philadelphia, 1991, pp 590–597.

111. Harding, JE, Charlton V: Experimental nutritional supplementation for intrauterine growth retardation. In *The Unborn Patient: Prenatal Diagnosis and Treatment*, 2nd ed. MR Harrison, MS Golbus, RA Filly, eds. WB Saunders, Philadelphia, 1991, pp 598–613.

CHAPTER 16

Anesthesia for Abnormal Positions and Presentations and Multiple Births

Gershon Levinson, M.D.
Sol M. Shnider, M.D.

The presenting part is that portion of the fetus that is felt through the cervix on vaginal examination. The presenting part determines the **presentation. Position** refers to the relation of an arbitrarily chosen portion of the fetus (occiput, chin, sacrum) to the left or right side of the mother. At delivery, approximately 90% of single gestation fetuses present as a cephalic presentation, either occiput transverse or anterior. All other positions (persistent occiput posterior, face, brow) and presentations (breech, shoulder) are considered abnormal. Compared to single gestation vertex deliveries, multiple gestations and single gestations with abnormal positions and presentations are associated with a higher risk of maternal, fetal, and neonatal morbidity and mortality (1–14). Management of these parturients involves several unique problems for the anesthesiologist and obstetrician.

PERSISTENT OCCIPUT POSTERIOR

Early in labor it is common for the occiput to be in the transverse or posterior position. During descent, or later during the active phase, the occiput usually undergoes normal internal rotation and comes to lie beneath the symphysis pubis. If this rotation does not occur, the persistent occiput posterior results in a more prolonged and painful labor than the occiput anterior position. The head does not fit well into the pelvis, resulting in prolonged or arrested descent and cervical dilation. The occiput exerts increasing pressure on the posterior sacral nerves, resulting in severe back pain. Spontaneous delivery requires more uterine and abdominal work. Cervical and perineal lacerations and postpartum bleeding are common (15). Although spontaneous delivery can occur, especially in the multipara with a large pelvis, usually manual or forceps rotation and extraction are performed. A prolonged second stage or a difficult midforceps rotation is associated with increased birth

trauma, intracranial hemorrhage, and birth asphyxia (16).

Anesthetic Considerations

If the vertex is known to be in the occiput posterior position during the first stage of labor and the parturient requests anesthesia, regional techniques that paralyze the perineal muscles are ideally avoided until spontaneous internal rotation occurs. Analgesia is best provided with a lumbar epidural block using low concentrations of local anesthetic usually combined with a lipid soluble opiate, i.e. bupivacaine 0.125% with fentanyl 1 μg/ml. If, despite an adequate T10-L1 block, severe back pain persists, the concentration of local anesthetic should be increased and either fentanyl (50 to 100 μg) or sufentanil (10 to 20 μg) administered epidurally. This block should not produce relaxation of the levator ani muscles, which play an important role in producing internal rotation. The epidural administration of fentanyl has not been associated with significant maternal or neonatal side effects (Chapters 9 and 10).

For delivery, if spontaneous rotation has not occurred and midforceps rotation is planned, it is ideal that complete analgesia and perineal relaxation be provided. Using a saddle block or caudal block or extending the existing lumbar epidural block to the perineum with 3% chloroprocaine or 1.5 to 2.0% lidocaine should provide the optimal conditions for an atraumatic delivery, thus minimizing maternal and neonatal morbidity. Midforceps delivery without adequate anesthesia is attended by increased fetal and maternal morbidity (lacerations and head trauma). In contrast, midvacuum application and delivery can be carried out safely with minimal or no anesthesia.

BREECH PRESENTATION

In approximately 3.5% of pregnancies the breech rather than the vertex presents first (17). There are three main types of breech presentations: frank, complete, and incomplete (Fig. 16.1). A frank breech is one in which the lower extremities are flexed at the hips and extended at the knees so that the feet are against the face. A complete breech is one in which the fetal lower extremities are flexed at both the hips and knees so that the buttocks with the feet along side them present at the cervix. Incomplete breech presentation is one in which one or both fetal lower extremities are extended and one or both feet present in the vagina or introitus. This type is also referred to as a single or double footling breech presentation. Frank breech is present in about 60% of breech deliveries, incomplete breech in about 30%, and complete breech in approximately 10%.

Etiology

All causes of breech presentation are unknown, but several associated abnormalities are thought to predispose to this presentation. During the first 35 weeks of pregnancy the fetus constantly changes its presentation, probably as a result of intrauterine fetal activity. It is believed that as the fetus approaches term it tends to accommodate to the shape of the uterine cavity, assuming a longitudinal lie with a vertex presentation. Breeches are more common in premature than full-term fetuses (6, 7, 17). When the fetus is premature, its smaller size requires less accommodation, and thus breech presentation is more frequent. Other factors that may interfere with the normal process of accommodation between the fetal head, uterine cavity, and maternal pelvis include placenta previa, uterine anomalies, pelvic tumors, fetal congenital anomalies—especially hydrocephalus and anencephaly—and uterine relaxation associated with great parity, multiple fetuses, and polyhydramnios (17).

Obstetric Management

The diagnosis of breech presentation is usually made by manual examination. There is a growing trend now to deliver all breeches by cesarean section. Consequently, the leading cause for primary elective cesarean section in many maternity units is breech presentation. However, many obstetricians believe it

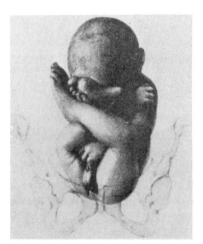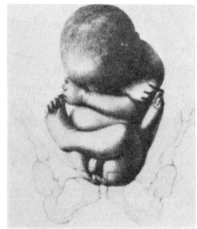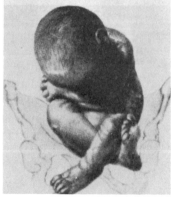

Figure 16.1 Types of breech presentation. *Upper left*, frank breech; *upper right*, complete breech; *lower*, incomplete breech. (Reprinted by permission from Cunningham FG, MacDonald PC, Gant NF: Attitude, the Presentation and Position of the Fetus. In *Williams Obstetrics*. 18th ed. Appleton & Lange, Norwalk, CT, 1989, pp 178–179.)

is safe to deliver selected breeches vaginally (10, 13, 17, 18). Their indications for cesarean section are listed in Table 16.1. Guidelines for consideration of vaginal delivery of a breech are listed in Table 16.2 (19).

In many centers external version prior to the expected date of confinement is attempted to convert a breech to a vertex presentation. Anesthesia is not recommended for this procedure lest it mask injury and possible rupture of the uterus. Version is usually performed with the aid of tocolytic agents (20–22).

METHODS OF BREECH DELIVERY

Breeches are delivered vaginally in one of four ways. During *spontaneous breech delivery* the entire infant is expelled by the mother without any traction or manipulation by the obstetrician other than support of the infant. *Partial breech extraction*—also called **assisted breech delivery**—refers to spontaneous delivery of the fetus as far as the umbilicus, with the obstetrician extracting the remainder of the body with or without forceps application to the aftercoming head. When the entire body of the infant is extracted with intrauterine manipulation by the obstetrician, the delivery is termed *total breech extraction. Breech decomposition and extraction* refers to the intrauterine conversion of a frank into an incomplete breech by flexion of the fetal knee(s) and extension of the hips prior to extraction.

MATERNAL, FETAL, AND NEONATAL HAZARDS

Breech deliveries are associated with increased maternal morbidity. Compared to vertex presentations there is greater likelihood of cervical lacerations, perineal injury, shock due to intrapartum and postpartum hemorrhage, retained placenta, and infection (17).

The neonatal prognosis is significantly worse in breech deliveries. Trauma to the term breech infant during vaginal delivery is 12 times higher than in vertex presentations (6–8). The perinatal mortality, corrected for prematurity and congenital anomalies is almost four times higher (7). With vaginal delivery, preterm breech infants have twice the rate of neurologic abnormalities at 1 year of age compared to vertex presentations (23). Preterm infants undergoing spontaneous breech delivery have a higher mortality than if delivered with Piper forceps. Large newborns (more than 3500 g) delivered vaginally have an increased neonatal mortality.

There are several reasons for the increased perinatal morbidity and mortality associated with breech presentations. These infants are more likely to suffer asphyxia from cord compression and intracranial hemorrhage from head trauma. Intrauterine manipulation may further increase fetal trauma and cord compression. During spontaneous breech delivery, the uncontrolled expulsion of the fragile fetal head can result in tentorial tears and brain damage.

Prolapse of the umbilical cord is a significant cause of increased fetal mortality. The gestational age of the baby has no effect on the incidence of cord prolapse, but the type of breech presentation does. The incidence of cord prolapse is 0.5% in vertex deliveries, 0.5% with frank breech presentations, and 10% with incomplete or complete breech presentations (17). The cause of increased frequency of prolapse of the umbilical cord is believed to be failure of the presenting part to fill the lower uterine segment.

Anesthetic Considerations in Breech Delivery

If the breech is to be delivered by elective primary cesarean section, either regional or general anesthesia may be used (see Chapter 12). With either spinal or epidural anesthesia difficulty extracting the infant through the uterine incision may be encountered. If uterine hypertonus is the primary cause, the anesthesiologist must be prepared to induce general anesthesia rapidly. Following endotracheal intubation halothane or isoflurane should be administered to relax the uterus. If emergency cesarean section is to

Table 16.1
Breech Presentation: Indications for Cesarean Section

Prematurity (infant less than 2500 g)
Large infant (greater than 3600 g)
Contracted or borderline pelvis
Abnormal first or second stage of labor
Elderly primipara
Hyperextension of the head
Prolapse of umbilical cord
Other obstetric complications not specific to breech
    presentation

Table 16.2
Guidelines for Consideration of Vaginal Delivery for Breech Presentation

Facilities: Capability of emergency cesarean delivery
Physician: Experience in vaginal breech delivery
Anesthesia: Personnel present for delivery
Type of breech: Frank; other types need further evaluation
Fetal size: Optimal estimated weight less than 4 kg
Head position and size: Exclusion of hyperextension and macrocephaly
Pelvimetry: Adequate pelvis
Labor: Adequate progression in dilation, effacement, and descent

From Management of the breech presentation. ACOG Tech Bull No. 95, 1986.

be performed for fetal distress or prolapsed umbilical cord, general anesthesia is usually indicated.

If the breech is to be delivered vaginally, an anesthesiologist must also be immediately available. Not only may he/she be required to provide adequate analgesia for labor and delivery, but he/she must also be prepared to provide perineal or uterine relaxation or sufficient anesthesia for emergency cesarean section rapidly. Preanesthetic preparations for breech presentations are listed in Table 16.3.

For vaginal breech delivery, partial breech extraction is the method of choice. At the end of the second stage of labor the parturient must be able to expel the fetus until the umbilicus is seen, whereupon the obstetrician can extract the arms and deliver the aftercoming head manually or with Piper forceps. Labor is often managed with narcotics and tranquilizers, and the delivery is managed with perineal infiltration of local anesthetic or pudendal block. Inhalation analgesia, if needed, may be administered by an anesthesiologist.

These techniques, on occasion, do not provide adequate analgesia or perineal muscle relaxation for delivery of the aftercoming head. Rapid induction of general anesthesia with thiopental, succinylcholine, endotracheal intubation, and nitrous oxide may be necessary and will provide optimal operating conditions. Halogenated agents are not necessary for the application of Piper forceps. Rarely, however, the lower uterine segment contracts and traps the aftercoming head and halothane or isoflurane must be added to relax the uterus and facilitate delivery.

Some obstetricians avoid major regional anesthesia because of concern over prolonging the first or second stages of labor, decreasing the ability of the mother to push effectively and thereby increasing the incidence of total breech extraction with its associated high fetal mortality. On the other hand, many find that spinal, epidural, or caudal anesthesia offers significant advantages.

Regional anesthesia allows for an alert, cooperative patient who, with proper coaching, can push effectively. It provides better pain relief compared to other methods of analgesia and provides maximal perineal relaxation for delivery of the aftercoming head. In addition, if there is a shortage of trained personnel, the anesthesiologist is more likely to be available for infant resuscitation. The incidence of complete breech extraction is not increased with regional anesthesia, although the second stage is lengthened slightly (24–26). Major regional anesthesia compared with no anesthesia, minor perineal local nerve blocks, or general anesthesia is not associated with an increased incidence of neonatal depression (Table 16.4) (24–31). In one study (26), 94 vaginal breech deliveries conducted with epidural anesthesia were compared to 277 vaginal breech deliveries managed without epidural anesthesia. Although the 1-min Apgar scores were lower in the full-term breech infants born under epidural anesthesia, the 5-min Apgar scores, perinatal morbidity, and maternal complications were similar in both groups.

If uterine relaxation is required for complete breech extraction, halothane or isoflurane anesthesia with rapid endotracheal intubation may be the preferred technique. However, if a major regional anesthetic has been used for labor, intrauterine manipulation can often be performed safely and easily between contractions. Intravenous nitroglycerine in 50-μg boluses has been suggested as a means of rapidly achieving uterine relaxation without general anesthesia (32, 33). If general anesthesia is to be used to provide uterine relaxation for intrauterine manipulation, then a rapid intravenous induction of anesthesia and endotracheal intubation with application

Table 16.3
Preanesthetic Preparations for Breech or Multiple Deliveries

Blood for emergency transfusion readily available (typed and screened, cross-matched or autologous).

Large-bore intravenous line in place. Fluid pumps, blood warmer, and equipment for second IV readily available.

Oxytocics readily available (pitocin, methergine, prostaglandin $F_{2\alpha}$).

Appropriate equipment and drugs for rapid-sequence induction of general anesthesia with possible uterine relaxation.

Equipment and personnel for newborn(s) resuscitation available.

Preanesthetic evaluation (including careful airway assessment) performed.

Table 16.4
Anesthesia for Breech Presentation (Infants over 2500 g and No Antepartum Obstetric or Medical Complications)[a]

	Number of Patients	Neonatal Depression at 1 Min of Age (% of Patients)	
		Moderate Depression	Severe Depression
Vaginal delivery and no epidural	79	42	20
Vaginal delivery with epidural	47	40	6

[a]Adapted by permission from Crawford JS: An appraisal of lumbar epidural blockade in patients with singleton fetus presenting by the breech. J Obstet Gynaecol Br Commonw 81:867–872, 1974.

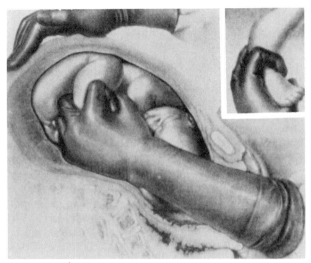

Figure 16.2. Internal podalic version. If at all possible, both feet are grasped because this technique makes the turning much easier. (Reprinted by permission from Pritchard JA, MacDonald PC, Gant NF: In *Williams Obstetrics*, 17th ed. Appleton-Century-Crofts, New York, 1985, p 865.)

of cricoid pressure is recommended. After intubation with thiopental and succinylcholine, halothane or isoflurane will provide uterine relaxation with rapid onset and reversibility. The parturient is especially susceptible to overdosage with inhalational anesthetics, and utmost caution must be exercised during controlled ventilation with potent agents.

FACE OR BROW POSITIONS OR SHOULDER PRESENTATION

Most infants with cephalic presentation and a face or brow position are delivered by cesarean section because of cephalopelvic disproportion. Either regional or general anesthesia may be used. Similarly, most infants in a transverse lie with a shoulder presentation are delivered by elective cesarean section. Rarely, internal podalic version and extraction (Fig. 16.2) are performed and the baby delivered vaginally as a breech presentation. Under these circumstances the intrauterine manipulation is best performed under general endotracheal halothane anesthesia (see Table 11.3).

MULTIPLE GESTATIONS

The incidence of twin gestation in the United States is approximately 1 in 90 births (30, 31). The incidence of twins is higher in blacks and lower in Orientals. Triplets occur in approximately 1 in 8000 (36) and quadruplets in 1 in 70,000 births.

Twin gestations may be single ovum (monozygous, identical twins) or double ovum (polyzygous). Heredity, maternal age, and increasing parity influence the incidence of double ovum twinning (34, 35).

Approximately 30% of twins are monozygotic (35, 37).

The Mother

Preeclampsia-eclampsia, anemia, premature labor, prolonged labor, and antepartum and postpartum hemorrhage are more common in multiple gestations (38, 39). Despite the fact that maternal blood volume increases earlier in pregnancy and reaches levels approximately 40% greater than in single gestation, anemia occurs more frequently and is more severe in multiple gestations (40). The larger uterus predisposes the parturient to more severe supine hypotension. The increase in uterine distension due to multiple gestation also leads to a more frequent occurrence of nausea and vomiting, dyspnea, leg edema, and varicosities (41). Blood loss during twin delivery is twice that of single gestation and manual extraction of the placenta is required twice as often (42). Maternal mortality is two to three times higher in multiple gestations.

The Fetus

There are two circumstances in monozygotic twinning that pose special hazards to the fetuses. An anastomosis may be present between the two vascular systems, resulting in transfusion of blood from one fetus to the other. In such cases one twin may receive most of the blood and become polycythemic with cardiomegaly and heart failure, while the other twin may not receive enough blood to survive. The other hazard of monozygotic twins involves being monoamniotic; this occurs in up to 4% of identical twins and is associated with an increased fetal mortality (50% chance of intrauterine death) due to intertwining and occlusion of the umbilical vessels (43).

The Neonate

Prematurity occurs six to ten times more frequently in multiple gestations compared to single births (5, 44, 45). Approximately 60% of twins are premature. The etiology of prematurity is not known but it has been attributed to overdistension of the uterus and an increased incidence of maternal complications such as preeclampsia-eclampsia. Fetal growth is independent of the number of fetuses in the uterus until 28 weeks' gestation, at which point a progressive weight lag develops when compared with single gestations. The neonatal death rate is higher in infants of multiple gestations, due mostly to prematurity. However, mature twins also have a higher mortality than mature single births; this is most likely due to a higher incidence of other factors, such as congenital anomalies, prolapse of umbilical cord, abnormal presentations and neonatal intracranial and visceral hemorrhage.

The second twin is likely to be more depressed and asphyxiated and require resuscitation more frequently than the first (38, 45–50). The most significant risk factor in the second twin is the period of hypoxemia caused either by contraction of the uterus or by premature separation of the placenta after the first infant is delivered.

Obstetric Management

Any combination of presentations of the fetuses can occur but the commonest are both vertex or one vertex and one breech (Table 16.5). Rarely, interlocking and interference with engagement or delivery of one infant by his/her twin may occur. Duration of labor is often shorter in multiple gestations because of the small fetal size and frequent effacement of the cervix before the onset of contractions. On the other hand, labor may be prolonged in some cases due to dysfunctional uterine contractions associated with an overdistended uterus.

Anesthetic Considerations

The major considerations in regard to choice of anesthesia for multiple gestations are the frequent occurrence of prematurity and breech presentation. The anesthesiologist may have to rapidly provide anesthesia for version, extraction, breech delivery, cesarean section, or midforceps delivery. Therefore an early preoperative evaluation and preparation of the parturient is essential. As described previously for a singleton breech delivery (Table 16.3), a large intravenous cannula should be placed, blood should be available, preparation for general anesthesia should be made, and personnel and equipment to resuscitate both infants should be available. Continuous fetal heart rate monitoring of both infants is recommended. If this is not feasible, after delivery of the first infant, the second infant should also have continuous monitoring for immediate recognition of acute fetal asphyxia.

Many obstetricians prefer pudendal block or local infiltration with or without inhalation analgesia. These techniques may provide adequate analgesia for de-

livery with minimum depression of the neonates. However, they do not provide analgesia during the first stage of labor and, for many women, do not provide satisfactory analgesia during the second stage. These techniques do not provide adequate perineal or uterine relaxation if these are necessary. The authors and others believe that, if analgesia is required, continuous epidural is ideal (51–53). Continuous regional blockade eliminates the need for administration of maternal narcotics and sedatives. Avoiding narcotics is of particular value in preterm infants. Reduced perinatal mortality for both mature and preterm twin infants whose mothers received conduction anesthesia (when compared with general anesthesia or local or no anesthesia) has been reported (5). With regional anesthesia, the first stage is not significantly prolonged, and the interval between the delivery of the first and second twin may be shortened (51). Forceps deliveries, which are more frequent with multiple gestations, are easier to accomplish with the good perineal relaxation found under epidural anesthesia. Even for version and extraction, some experts prefer conduction anesthesia, although most advise general anesthesia for uterine relaxation if intrauterine manipulations are necessary. When internal podalic version and complete extraction are performed under regional anesthesia, manipulations should be made between contractions. The anesthesiologist must be prepared for rapid induction of general anesthesia and uterine relaxation with halothane should difficulties arise.

Lumbar epidural anesthesia with dilute local anesthetic either alone or combined with fentanyl or sufentanil, provides complete pain relief but still ensures adequate strength in the abdominal muscles so the mother may push and thereby assist with delivery. Numerous reports have documented the safety of epidural anesthesia in twin deliveries (54–59).

With major conduction anesthesia, the parturient with a multiple gestation is at greater risk for developing hypotension. The larger gravid uterus produces more aortocaval compression and, together with the sympathetic block, increases the incidence and severity of maternal hypotension. Also, patients with sympathetic blockade will not vasoconstrict or maintain blood pressure in response to the increased blood loss at delivery. Left uterine displacement during labor and delivery and adequate fluid and blood replacement are essential.

On occasion, a cesarean section may be indicated. Either regional or general anesthesia may be used, the evidence available not favoring one method over the other. The choice of anesthesia for cesarean delivery of multiple gestation depends on the prefer-

Table 16.5
Presentation of Fetuses in Twin Delivery

	Approximate Percent of Deliveries
Both vertex	39
Vertex and breech	37
Both breech	10
Longitudinal and shoulder	8
Both shoulder	6

ence and experience of the anesthesiologist, the obstetrician, and the patient (60).

Reference

1. Cruikshank DP, White CP: Obstetric malpresentations: Twenty years' experience. Am J Obstet Gynecol 116:1097–1104, 1973.
2. Powers WF: Twin pregnancy: Complications and treatment. Obstet Gynecol 42:795–808, 1973.
3. Rementeria JL, Janakammal S, Hollander M: Multiple births in drug-addicted women. Am J Obstet Gynecol 122:958–960, 1975.
4. Scholtes G: Zum problem der zwillingsschwangerschaft (Problems in twin pregnancy). Arch Gynaekol 210:188–207, 1971.
5. Aaron JB, Halperin J: Fetal survival in 376 twin deliveries. Am J Obstet Gynecol 69:794–804, 1955.
6. Hall JE, Kohl S: Breech presentation: A study of 1,456 cases. Am J Obstet Gynecol 72:977–988, 1956.
7. Morgan HS, Kane SH: An analysis of 16,327 breech births. JAMA 187:262–264, 1964.
8. Potter MG Jr, Heaton CE, Douglas GW: Intrinsic fetal risk in breech delivery. Obstet Gynecol 15:158–162, 1960.
9. Abrams IF, Bresnan MJ, Zuckerman JE, Fisher EG, Strand R: Cervical cord injuries secondary to hyperextension of the head in breech presentations. Obstet Gynecol 41:369–378, 1973.
10. Bird CC, McElin TW: A six-year prospective study of term breech deliveries utilizing the Zatuchni-Andros prognostic scoring index. Am J Obstet Gynecol 121:551–557, 1975.
11. Brenner WE, Bruce RD, Hendricks CH: The characteristics and perils of breech presentation. Am J Obstet Gynecol 118:700–709, 1974.
12. Rovinsky JJ, Miller JA, Kaplan S: Management of breech presentation at term. Am J Obstet Gynecol 115:497–513, 1973.
13. Zatuchni GI, Andros GJ: Prognostic index for vaginal delivery in breech presentation at term. Am J Obstet Gynecol 93:237–242, 1965.
14. Sokol RJ, Roux JF, McCarthy S: Computer diagnosis of labor progression. VI. Fetal stress and labor in the occipitoposterior position. Am J Obstet Gynecol 122:253–260, 1975.
15. Cannell DE: The management of the occiput posterior. Am J Obstet Gynecol 60:496–503, 1950.
16. Cunningham FG, MacDonald PC, Gant NF: Dystocia due to abnormalities in presentation, position or development of the fetus. In *Williams Obstetrics*, 18th ed. Appleton & Lange, Norwalk, CT, 1989, pp 362–364.
17. Cunningham FG, MacDonald PC, Gant NF: Techniques for breech delivery. In *Williams Obstetrics*, 18th ed. Appleton & Lange, Norwalk, CT, 1989, pp 393–403.
18. Morley GW: Breech presentation: A 15 year review. Obstet Gynecol 30:745–751, 1967.
19. ACOG Technical Bulletin: Management of the breech presentation. 95:1, 1986.
20. Hofmeyr GJ: Effect of external cephalic version in late pregnancy on breech presentation and caesarean section rate: A controlled trial. Br J Obstet Gynaecol 90:392–399, 1983.
21. Dyson DC, Ferguson JE II, Hensleigh P: Antepartum external cephalic version under tocolysis. Obstet Gynecol 67:63–68, 1986.
22. Marchick R: Antepartum external cephalic version with tocolysis: A study of term singleton breech presentations. Am J Obstet Gynecol 158:1339–1346, 1988.
23. Bonica JJ, Nace FM: Breech delivery. In *Principles and Practice of Obstetric Analgesia and Anesthesia.* JJ Bonica ed. Davis, Philadelphia, 1969, pp 1223–1236.
24. Crawford JS: An appraisal of lumbar epidural blockade in patients with singleton fetus presenting by the breech. J Obstet Gynaecol Br Commonw 81:867–872, 1974.
25. Bowen-Simpkins P, Fergusson ILC: Lumbar epidural block and the breech presentation. Br J Anaesth 46:420–423, 1974.
26. Confino E, Ismajovich B, Rudick V, David MP: Extradural analgesia in the management of singleton breech delivery. Br J Anaesth 57:892–895, 1985.
27. Daily HI, Rogers SF: Saddle block anesthesia in breech delivery. Surg Gynecol Obstet 105:630–634, 1957.
28. Sears RT: Use of spinal analgesia in forceps and breech deliveries. Br Med J 1:755–758, 1959.
29. Boyson WA, Simpson JW: Breech management with caudal anesthesia. Am J Obstet Gynecol 79:1121–1130, 1960.
30. Gunther RE, Harer WB: Single-injection caudal anesthesia. Am J Obstet Gynecol 92:305–309, 1965.
31. Salvatore CA, Cicivizzo E, Turath S: Breech delivery with saddle block anesthesia. Obstet Gynecol 26:261–264, 1965.
32. Perg ATC, Gorman RS, Shulman SM, Demarchis E, Nyunt K, Blancato L: Intravenous nitroglycerin for uterine relaxation in patients with retained placenta. Anesthesiology 71:172–173, 1989.
33. DeSimone CA, Norris MC, Leighton BL: Intravenous nitroglycerin aids manual extraction of a retained placenta. Anesthesiology 73:787, 1990.
34. Guttmacher AF: The incidence of multiple births in man and some of the other unipara. Obstet Gynecol 2:22–35, 1953.
35. Gedda L: *Twins in History and Science.* Charles C Thomas, Springfield, IL, 1961.
36. Holcberg G, Biale Y, Lewenthal H, Inser V: Outcome of pregnancy in 31 triplet gestations. Obstet Gynecol 59:472–476, 1982.
37. Guttmacher AF, Kohl SG: The fetus of multiple gestations. Obstet Gynecol 12:528–541, 1958.
38. Bender S: Twin pregnancy: A review of 472 cases. J Obstet Gynaecol Br Emp 59:510–517, 1952.
39. Kotsalo K: Observations on the premature separation of the normally implanted placenta. Acta Obstet Gynecol Scand 37:155–194, 1958.
40. Rovinsky JJ, Jaffin H: Cardiovascular hemodynamics in pregnancy. I. Blood and plasma volumes in multiple pregnancy. Am J Obstet Gynecol 93:1–13, 1965.
41. Pritchard JA, MacDonald PC, Gant NF: *Williams Obstetrics,* ed 17. Appleton-Century-Crofts, New York, 1985, pp 503–524.
42. Pritchard JA, Baldwin RM, Dickey JC, Wiggins KM: Blood volume changes in pregnancy and the puerperium. Red blood cell loss and changes in apparent blood volume during and following vaginal delivery, cesarean section, plus total hysterectomy. Am J Obstet Gynecol 84:1271–1281, 1962.
43. Adams DM, Chervenak FA: Intrapartum management of twin gestation. Clin Obstet Gynecol 33:52–60, 1990.
44. Friedman EA, Sachtleben M: The effect of uterine overdistension on labor. I. Multiple pregnancy. Obstet Gynecol 23:164–172, 1964.
45. Little WA, Friedman EA: The twin delivery: Factors influencing second twin mortality—A review. Obstet Gynecol Surv 13:611–623, 1958.
46. Graves LR, Adams JQ, Schreier PC: The fate of the second twin. Obstet Gynecol 19:246–250, 1962.
47. Corston J McD: Twin survival: A comparison of mortality rates of the first and second twin. Obstet Gynecol 10:181–183, 1957.
48. Camilleri AP: In defense of the second twin. J Obstet Gynaecol Br Emp 70:258–262, 1963.
49. MacDonald RR: Management of the second twin. Br Med J 1:518–522, 1962.
50. Wyshak G, White C: Birth hazard of the second twin. JAMA 186:869–870, 1963.
51. Crawford JS: An appraisal of lumbar epidural blockade in labour in patients with multiple pregnancy. J Obstet Gynaecol Br Commonw 82:929–935, 1975.
52. James FM III, Crawford JS, Davies P, Naiem H: Lumbar epidural analgesia for labor and delivery of twins. Am J Obstet Gynecol 127:176–180, 1977.
53. Abouleish E: Caudal analgesia for quadruplet delivery. Anesth Analg 55:61–66, 1976.
54. Redick LF: Anesthesia for twin delivery. Clin Perinatol 15:107–122, 1988.

55. Crawford JS: A prospective study of 200 consecutive twin deliveries. Anaesthesia 42:33–43, 1987.

56. Rayburn WF, Lavin JP Jr, Miodovnik M, Varner MW: Multiple gestation: Time interval between delivery of the first and second twins. Obstet Gynecol 63:502–506, 1984.

57. Chervenak FA, Johnson RE, Youcha S, Hobbins JC, Berkowitz RL: Intrapartum management of twin gestation. Obstet Gynecol 65:119–124, 1985.

58. Young BK, Suidan J, Antonine C, Silverman F, Lustig I, Wasserman J: Differences in twins: The importance of birth order. Am J Obstet Gynecol 151:915–921, 1985.

59. Wessel J, Ralph G, Lichtenegger W, Schorer P: Specific obstetrical problems in the management of labor following cesarean section. Z Geburtshilfe Perinatol 193:134–138, 1989.

60. Craft JB Jr, Levinson G, Shnider SM: Anaesthetic considerations in caesarean section for quadruplets. Can Anaesth Soc J 25:236–239, 1978.

CHAPTER 17

Anesthetic Considerations in Preeclampsia-Eclampsia

Brett B. Gutsche, M.D.
Theodore G. Cheek, M.D.

Each year approximately 250,000 American women become hypertensive during pregnancy. Such hypertension is accompanied by a significantly higher incidence of maternal, fetal, and neonatal morbidity and mortality. Currently, the American College of Obstetricians and Gynecologists classifies hypertensive disorders of pregnancy as follows (1):

   I. Preeclampsia-eclampsia
   II. Chronic hypertension
   III. Chronic hypertension with superimposed preeclampsia (or eclampsia)
   IV. Gestational hypertension ("late or transient hypertension of the third trimester")

Preeclampsia is a disorder that does not manifest itself before the 20th week of gestation (and only rarely before the 24th week) except in the instance of hydatidiform mole. Preeclampsia is characterized by the triad of hypertension, generalized edema, and proteinuria. While not part of the triad, hyperreflexia is usually present. Recently some obstetricians have stated that edema is not a reliable sign of preeclampsia, pointing out that women with only hypertension and proteinuria develop eclamptic convulsions without having shown edema (2–4). These conditions usually abate within 48 hours of termination of pregnancy and delivery of the entire placenta. Preeclampsia becomes **eclampsia** when accompanied by a grand mal convulsion not related to other cerebral conditions. Although preeclampsia-eclampsia was referred to as "toxemia of pregnancy" this term is now in disfavor and should not be used.

Chronic hypertension is the presence of persistent hypertension, regardless of cause, before the 20th week of gestation or beyond 6 weeks after delivery. Gestational hypertension is hypertension not accompanied by proteinuria or generalized edema that develops during the last weeks of pregnancy or immediately after delivery. It dissipates within 2 weeks of delivery. Another term often used is "pregnancy-induced hypertension" (PIH). Although many health care workers use this term interchangeably with preeclampsia, it is more inclusive and covers not only preeclampsia-eclampsia but all hypertensive disorders (including gestational hypertension) that are associated with pregnancy. This chapter is concerned primarily with preeclampsia-eclampsia.

INCIDENCE AND ETIOLOGY OF PREECLAMPSIA-ECLAMPSIA

In the United States the incidence of preeclampsia complicating pregnancy is often stated to be 5 to 7%. However, recent reports have shown a lower incidence. Two large studies in the United States from the years 1959 to 1966 (6) and 1979–86 (7) reported the occurrence of preeclampsia as 32 per 1000 births and 26 per 1000 births, respectively. The incidence of eclampsia has been reported as 0.2 to 0.67 per 1000 births, with maternal mortality of 0.4 to 11.9% and perinatal mortality of 20 to 30% (7–12).

Preeclampsia-eclampsia most often occurs in young primigravidas, with those under age 20 years having five times the incidence of those over 20 years of age (7). There is no significant difference between its occurrence in blacks and whites, although there is a higher rate in unmarried vs. married women and in Medicaid vs. privately insured patients (7). There may also be variation in rates of both preeclampsia and eclampsia according to geographic location (7, 13). Although preeclampsia-eclampsia occurs most frequently in young primigravidas, it is by no means limited to this group. Several studies of eclamptic patients have indicated that maternal morbidity and mortality increase with both age and parity (9–11). From a series of 298 eclamptic patients, the onset of eclampsia occurred before delivery in 44%, during delivery in 37%, and after delivery in 19% (9). In hospitalized patients, eclampsia was manifested before delivery in 17%, during delivery in 52%, and after delivery in 34%. Of the last group, 43% had eclampsia within 4 hr of delivery, and 86% within 24 hr. The incidence of preeclampsia-eclampsia is markedly higher in conditions associated with rapid uterine enlargement, such as hydatidiform mole, multiple gestations, polyhydramnios, and diabetic mothers having macrosomic fetuses. A Canadian study found the incidence of preeclampsia to be 9.9% in 334 diabetic pregnancies compared to 4.3% in 16,534 nondiabetic controls (14). Perinatal mortality was 60 per 1000 births compared to 3.3 per 1000 births in nondiabetic preeclamptic mothers. The more severe the diabetes (as judged by the White classification) the higher the occurrence of preeclampsia.

Etiology of Preeclampsia-Eclampsia

The cause of preeclampsia-eclampsia, a disorder of only human gravidae, is yet to be elucidated. Whether the initiating factor of this disorder is immunologic, genetic, or simply a decrease in uterine blood flow is unknown. In normal pregnancy the spiral arteries of the myometrium lose their muscular wall and become distended. In preeclampsia some of these arteries do not lose their muscular wall and remain constricted (15). This results in increased uterine vascular resistance and causes as much as a 30 to 40% decrease in uterine blood flow, compared with that in normal pregnancies (16, 17). Several recent investigators have presented compelling evidence that damage to the vascular endothelial cells releases a peptide substance (fibronectin or endothelia) (18–23). The cause of endothelial cell damage resulting in the release of fibronectin has been postulated to be release of factors or mitogens from the poorly perfused placenta (19, 24). Endothelial cell injury, which may involve not only the maternal vascular endothelium but also the maternal myocardial endothelium (25) and the placental vascular endothelium (26), is associated with reduced synthesis of vasorelaxing substances, increased production of vasoconstrictors, and impaired synthesis of endogenous anticoagulants which favors platelet aggregation and activation of coagulation (20). Fibronectin or endothelia, the peptide released by damaged endothelial cells, causes vasoconstriction and loss of capillary endothelial integrity with leakage of fluid and protein and platelet aggregation (Fig. 17.1). Levels of fibronectin elevated in preeclampsia-eclampsia become markedly decreased by 48 hr after delivery, which could explain the rapid clinical improvement seen following delivery. Decreased colloid oncotic pressures and proteinuria are highly correlated to elevated fibronectin levels, which suggests that endothelial injury, not proteinuria, is the primary

DECREASED PLACENTAL PERFUSION

↓

Trophoblasts Release Substance Causing Vascular Endothelial Cell Injury

↓

RELEASE OF FIBRONECTIN
(Increased Blood Levels in Preeclamptics)

↓

FUTHER DAMAGE TO ALL VASCULAR ENDOTHELIAL CELLS CAUSING:

1. Loss of plasma protein (Decreased colloid oncotic pressure)
2. Renal damage
3. Vasoconstriction
4. Coagulation abnormalities
5. Myocardial and placental endothelial damage

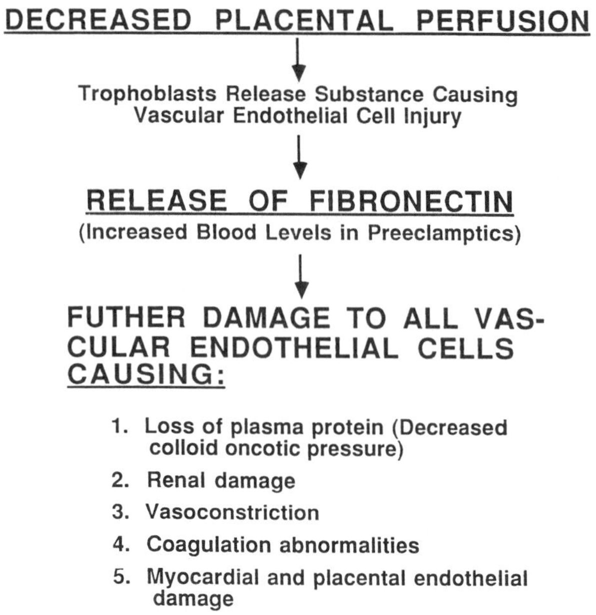

Figure 17.1. Hypothesis of capillary endothelial damage as the cause of preeclampsia-eclampsia. (Modified from Roberts JM, Musci TJ, Rogers GM, Hubel CA, McLaughlin MK: Preeclampsia: An endothelial cell disorder. Am J Obstet Gynecol 161:1200–1204, 1989.)

mechanism of hypoproteinuria and reduced colloid oncotic pressure in preeclampsia (27).

There is an imbalance in the production and circulating levels of two prostaglandins, prostacyclin and thromboxane, in preeclampsia-eclampsia (Fig. 17.2) (28). In addition, the production of thromboxane, associated with vasoconstriction, platelet aggregation, decreased uterine blood flow, and increased uterine activity, is increased, whereas the production of prostacyclin, which has the opposite effect, is decreased. This imbalance between thromboxane and prostacyclin may be related to endothelial cell injury (29) or placental trophoblastic production of thromboxane (20, 29, 39). Substances that decrease the production of thromboxane, such as aspirin (30–33) and thromboxane synthetase inhibitor (34), appear to decrease the incidence and severity of preeclampsia. Prostaglandin A_1, a vasodepressor prostaglandin with properties similar to prostacyclin, was very effective in reducing mean arterial pressure in severe preeclamptic women undergoing induction of labor (35). In preeclamptic mothers, an increase in placental production of progesterone was associated with decreased placental prostacyclin production (36).

As previously stated, hypertension, proteinuria, and generalized edema characterize preeclampsia. Hypertension is defined as an increase in systolic blood pressure of at least 30 torr (or to levels above

NORMAL PREGNANCY

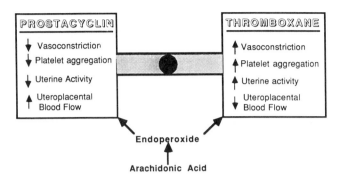

PREECLAMPSIA

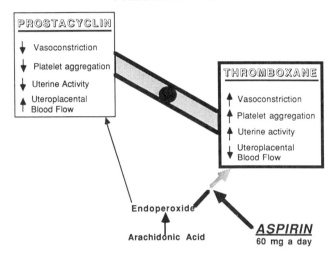

Modified from Walsh SW: Am J Obstet Gynecol 1985; 152: 335-40

Figure 17.2. Comparison of the balance in the biological actions of prostacyclin and thromboxane in normal pregnancy with the imbalance of increased thromboxane and decreased prostacyclin in the preeclamptic patient. If the patient at risk for the development of preeclampsia is given aspirin, 60 mg a day, from the end of the first trimester throughout the remaining gestation, it may block the production of thromboxane without significant effect on the formation of prostacyclin. This may attenuate the effects of preeclampsia. (Modified from Walsh SW: Preeclampsia: An imbalance in placental prostacyclin and thromboxane production. Am J Obstet Gynecol 152:335–340, 1985.)

140 torr); an increase in diastolic pressure of at least 15 torr (or to levels above 90 torr); or an increase in mean arterial pressure of at least 20 torr (105 torr). These blood pressure readings must be taken at least 6 hr apart while the subject is at rest in the lateral, not in the supine, position. Proteinuria is defined as the excretion of more than 0.3 g of protein per liter of urine in a 24-hr urine collection or the excretion of more than 1 g of protein per liter (+1 or +2 on "dipstick" test) in two catheterized or clean-catch

midstream samples taken more than 6 hr apart (1). Edema must be generalized and not limited to the ankles or legs, a normal condition frequently seen in late pregnancy. The presence of two of the three signs usually allows for the diagnosis of preeclampsia, provided the pregnancy has progressed beyond the 20th week or if the signs and symptoms develop earlier in a molar pregnancy.

Preeclampsia becomes "severe preeclampsia" if one of the following conditions exists: (a) systolic blood pressure of greater than 160 torr, diastolic blood pressure of greater than 110 torr, or mean blood pressure greater than 120 torr; (b) proteinuria in excess of 5 g/24 hr (+3 or +4 by "dipstick" test); (c) oliguria of less than 500 ml in 24 hr; (d) headache or cerebral disturbances; (e) visual disturbances; (f) epigastric pain; or (g) pulmonary edema or cyanosis (1). More recently, the development of the "HELLP" syndrome (hemolysis, elevated liver enzymes, low platelets) will also elevate the designation to severe preeclampsia. The development of preeclampsia in the early second trimester often indicates that it will rapidly progress to the severe category with significant perinatal mortality (37).

If one or more grand mal convulsions not related to other conditions occurs in preeclampsia, eclampsia is diagnosed and the prognosis for both mother and fetus worsens significantly.

PATHOPHYSIOLOGY OF PREECLAMPSIA

The pathophysiology of preeclampsia-eclampsia involves nearly every organ system of the body. In the past the primary pathophysiology was felt to be vasoconstriction and its consequences (38). Although vasoconstriction plays a major role, viewing the disorder as simply the result of vasoconstriction overly simplifies this complex disorder. Indeed, contrary to former beliefs, it appears that preeclampsia is associated with a hyperdynamic cardiovascular state (Table 17.1) (39). The cardiovascular findings can vary considerably between preeclamptic and hypertensive parturients. In severe preeclamptic patients near term (and often in labor) pulmonary artery catheterization has shown normal or high cardiac indexes (Fig. 17.3). Systemic vascular resistance itself was only slightly elevated, if at all, in two studies (40, 41), as compared with normal pregnant women at 36 to 38 weeks' gestation (Table 17.1). This indicates that the elevation in blood pressure observed in preeclampsia may be due more to an increased cardiac output than to an increased systemic vascular resistance, as previously thought. In both studies patients had normal or (more often) hyperdynamic left ventricular function (Fig. 17.4) (40, 41). Cardiac out-

Table 17.1
Comparison of Cardiovascular Parameter of Normal Nonpregnant, Normal Pregnant, and Severe Preeclamptic Women

	Normal Nonpregnant[a] (11–13 wks postpartum) ($n = 10$)	Normal Pregnancy[a] (36–38 wks gestation) ($n = 10$)	Severe PIH Before Delivery[b] ($n = 45$)	Severe Preeclampsia Before Delivery[c] ($n = 41$)	Severe Preeclampsia with Pulmonary Edema[d] ($n = 8$)
Mean arterial pressure (mm Hg)	86.4 ± 7.5	90.3 ± 5.8	138 ± 3	130 ± 2	136 ± 3
Central venous pressure (mm Hg)	3.7 ± 2.6	3.6 ± 2.5	4 ± 1	4.8 ± 0.4	11 ± 1
Pulmonary capillary wedge pressure (mm Hg)	6.3 ± 2.1	7.5 ± 1.8	10 ± 1	8.3 ± 0.3	18 ± 1
Cardiac output (liter/min)	4.3 ± 0.9	6.2 ± 1	7.5 ± 0.23	8.4 ± 0.2	10.5 ± 0.6
Systemic vascular resistance (dyne·cm·sec^{-3})	1530 ± 520	1210 ± 266	1496 ± 64	1226 ± 37	964 ± 50
Systemic vascular resistance index (dyne·cm·sec^{-3}·M^2)	—	—	2726 ± 120	2293 ± 65	—
Pulmonary vascular resistance (dyne·cm·sec^{-3})	119 ± 47	78 ± 22	70 ± 5	65 ± 3	71 ± 9
Left ventricular stroke work index (g·m·m^{-2})	41 ± 8	48 ± 6	81 ± 2	84 ± 2	87 ± 10

[a]Data are from 10 normal pregnancies at 36 to 38 weeks gestation and 11 to 13 weeks postpartum. (Adapted from Clark SL, et al.: Central hemodynamic assessment of normal term pregnancy. Am J Obstet Gynecol 161:1439–1442, 1989.)

[b]Data are taken from 45 patients with severe pregnancy-induced hypertension (PIH) near time of delivery. (Adapted from Cotton DB, Lee W, Huhta JC, Dorman KF: Hemodynamic profile of severe pregnancy-induced hypertension. Am J Obstet Gynecol 158:523–529, 1988.)

[c]Data are from 41 patients with severe preeclampsia but no pulmonary edema shortly before delivery. (Adapted from Mabie WC, Ratts TE, Sibai BM: The central hemodynamics of preeclampsia. Am J Obstet Gynecol 161:1443–1448, 1989.)

[d]Data are from eight patients with pulmonary edema superimposed on severe preeclampsia shortly before delivery. (Adapted from Mabie WC, Ratts TE, Sibai BM: The central hemodynamics of preeclampsia. Am J Obstet Gynecol 161:1443–1448, 1989.)

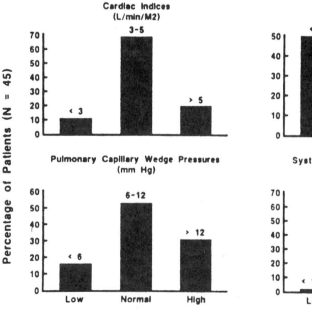
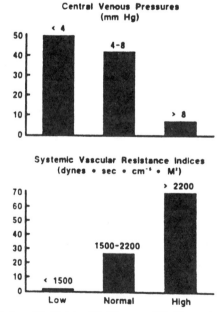
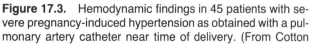

Figure 17.3. Hemodynamic findings in 45 patients with severe pregnancy-induced hypertension as obtained with a pulmonary artery catheter near time of delivery. (From Cotton DB, Lee W, Huhta JC, Dorman KF: Hemodynamic profile of severe pregnancy induced hypertension. Am J Obstet Gynecol 158:523–529, 1988.)

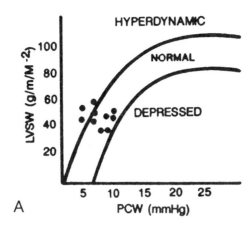

A

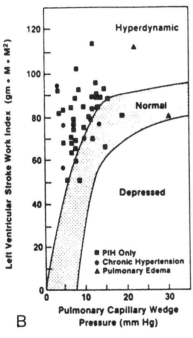

B

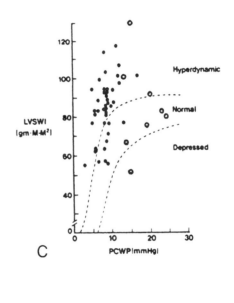

C

Figure 17.4. Left ventricular function expressed as pulmonary capillary wedge pressure (mm Hg) vs. left ventricular stroke work index (gm·M·M²). Note the vast majority of the patients afflicted with PIH or preeclampsia show a marked hyperdynamic left ventricular function. *A*, In normal gravid patients not in labor at 36 to 38 weeks' gestation. (From Clark SL, et al.: Central hemodynamic assessment of normal term pregnancy. Am J Obstet Gynecol 161:1439–1442, 1982.) *B*, In patients with severe pregnancy-induced hypertension shortly before delivery. (From Cotton DB, Lee W, Huhta JC, Dorman KF: Hemodynamic profile of severe pregnancy-induced hypertension (PIH). Am J Obstet Gynecol 158:523–529, 1988.) *C*, In patients with severe preeclampsia shortly before delivery. (From Mabie WC, Ratts TE, Sibai BM: The central hemodynamics of severe preeclampsia. Am J Obstet Gynecol 161:1443–1448, 1989.)

put is often considerably elevated in preeclampsia, and indeed this elevation may precede the hypertension and other findings associated with the disorder (39, 42). After delivery, left ventricular function may fall temporarily to within the normal range, then increase again (43). Although Joyce and coworkers (44) found that the central venous pressure

(CVP) was low and tended to fall as the severity of the disorder worsened (Fig. 17.5), in other more recent studies (40, 41) the CVP was essentially unchanged or very slightly elevated in patients with severe preeclampsia (Table 17.1). These findings may be different because Joyce et al. categorized their severe preeclamptics by diastolic pressures, whereas

MATERNAL DIASTOLIC PRESSURE (torr)

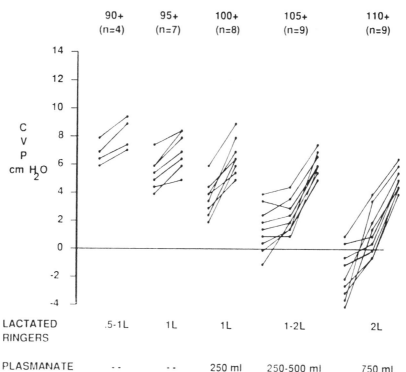

Figure 17.5. CVP measurements in five groups of preeclamptic women with different severity degrees of preeclampsia, classified by their initial diastolic pressure. The *first point* in each patient represents central venous pressure (CVP) before hydration; the *last point* represents the CVP following complete hydration and administration of epidural block. In the two most severe groups, the *second point* represents the CVP following crystalloid administration before hydration with colloid (plasmate, approximately equal to 5% albumin) and epidural block. NOTE: The more severe the disorder, the lower the CVP; the more hydration is required to bring it to the desired CVP of 6 to 8 cm water; and in the two most severe groups, colloid was required before this CVP level could be obtained. (Adapted by permission from Joyce TH III, Debnath K, Baker EA: Preeclampsia-relationship of CVP and epidural analgesia. Anesthesiology 51:S297, 1979.)

there was no such breakdown in the latter two studies. The CVP may not correlate well with the pulmonary capillary wedge pressure (PCWP), which tends to be normal (40). A low CVP may reflect better the decreased vascular volume than a low PCWP. Although the CVP and PCWP do show some correlation (Figs. 17.6 and 17.7) (40, 45), CVP is not reliable and has led some clinicians to discourage CVP monitoring in favor of PCWP monitoring (45–48). However, others think that CVP monitoring is a useful diagnostic and therapeutic tool, particularly when used to aid in vascular volume expansion (49–51). In most studies a CVP of 6 mm Hg or less has not been associated with serious elevations of PCWP.

Plasma volume is markedly reduced in preeclampsia compared with normal pregnancy. The plasma volumes of preeclamptic mothers having small-for-gestational-age fetuses may be decreased by 30%, as compared with normal pregnant women, whereas mildly preeclamptic patients with appropriate-for-gestation-age–sized fetuses had normal blood vol-

umes (52, 53). The failure of the plasma volume to expand in midpregnancy (20 to 24 weeks) may foretell the future development of preeclampsia with a small baby (52). In addition total plasma albumin is decreased, whereas total red blood cell mass is little affected (Table 17.2) (4, 54).

Colloid oncotic pressure may be decreased in preeclampsia and correlates with the decreased plasma protein levels (55, 56). An animal model, somewhat resembling the severe preeclamptic human, has been produced in the near-term gravid ewe by repeated plasmapheresis resulting in a lowering of the plasma oncotic pressure (57). The decreased plasma oncotic pressure, coupled with capillary endothelial damage and marked vasoconstriction, may well account for the development of pulmonary edema that occurs in 2.9% of preeclamptic patients (58). Usually associated with pulmonary edema are other complicating factors including disseminated intravascular coagulopathy, sepsis, abruptio placentae, preexisting chronic hypertension, and excessive intravenous infusion of

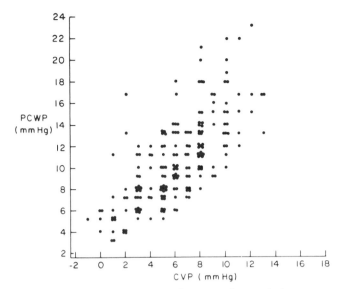

Figure 17.6. The relationship between the central venous pressure (CVP) and the pulmonary capillary wedge pressure (PCWP) in women with severe pregnancy-induced hypertension. Patients with the same data are represented by a single point. (Reprinted with permission from Cotton DB, Lee W, Huhta JC, Dorman KF: Hemodynamic profile of severe pregnancy-induced hypertension. Am J Obstet Gynecol 158:523–529, 1988.)

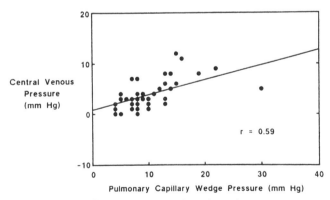

Figure 17.7. Cardiovascular alterations in severe pregnancy-induced hypertension. Relationship of central venous pressure to pulmonary capillary wedge pressure. (Reprinted with permission from Cotton DB, Gonik B, Dorman K, Harrist R: Am J Obstet Gynecol 151:762–764, 1985.)

crystalloid, colloid or both. Pulmonary edema usually occurs in the first few postpartum days and is seen more commonly in older multiparous patients with preexisting chronic hypertension. Increases in both the PCWP and CVP are associated with pulmonary edema (59, 60). The correlation between the two measurements is not constant and reliable in severe preeclampsia (61–63). However, those patients with pulmonary edema inevitably show a CVP of 6 mm Hg or greater. Not only are there increased circulating levels of renin, angiotensin, catechol-

amines, and atrial natriuretic factor in preeclampsia (38, 64, 65), but there is evidence that the response to vasoactive drugs may be heightened, as compared with the normal gravida (66). Although the intravascular volume may be decreased, salt and water are retained in tissues, causing edema. There is evidence of cerebral edema in eclamptic patients (67). Blood viscosity is elevated, thereby aggravating the problem of decreased uteroplacental perfusion (68). The cardiovascular pathophysiology associated with preeclampsia in the peripartum period have been well summarized by the studies of both Cotton et al. (40) and Mabie et al. (41).

Severe preeclampsia and eclampsia may have associated coagulation abnormalities that involve primarily decreases in platelet number and function (69, 70). Although some investigators have found a low incidence of thrombocytopenia (71), others found thrombocytopenia (defined as a platelet count of less than 150,000 per milliliter) in as many as 50% of preeclamptic patients in the third trimester (72). The cause of the thrombocytopenia appears to be an immune mechanism that causes increased destruction of platelets (72). Associated with a decreased platelet counts is an increased bleeding time (73). The thrombocytopenia usually is well resolved by the fourth postpartum day (74). Anecdotal reports of epidural or subarachnoid blocks inadvertently administered to patients with platelet counts of less than 100,000 per milliliter have not described epidural hematoma as a consequence (75). Nevertheless, most anesthesiologists are reluctant to administer a major regional block in patients with platelet counts of less than 100,000 per milliliter or who have clinical signs of a coagulopathy. Some anesthesiologists have suggested that measurements of bleeding time are a more reliable assessment of platelet function and should be routinely measured either in all severe preeclamptics or in those with platelet counts below 150,000. These clinicians believe that if the bleeding time is prolonged, regional anesthesia should be avoided. However, in a recent critical review (75a), it was concluded that bleeding time is not a useful predictor of the risk of hemorrhage. Indeed, a recent editorial in *Lancet* (75b) concluded that there was very little evidence to support the use of the bleeding time as a diagnostic test in individual patients before using regional anesthetic techniques.

A reduced platelet count may be associated with intrauterine growth retardation (76). Other less pronounced changes in coagulation include slightly prolonged partial thromboplastin time (statistically but not clinically significant) and an increased serum level of fibrin split products (Tables 17.3 and 17.4) (71, 77).

Table 17.2
Mean Plasma Volume, Albumin Levels, and Hematocrits in Nonpregnancy, Normal Pregnancy, and Preeclampsia

Study #1[a]	Nonpregnancy (n = 22)	Normal Pregnancy (n = 55)	Preeclampsia (n = 14)
Total blood volume (ml)	3675 ± 305	4723 ± 152	4250 ± 202
Plasma volume (ml)	2252 ± 271	3133 ± 97	2590 ± 108
RBC volume (ml)	1433 ± 99	1692 ± 67	1687 ± 92
Albumin (g/100 ml)	5.45 ± 0.01	3.92 ± 0.08	3.48 ± 0.08
Hematocrit (%)	39.0 ± 0.04	34.2 ± 0.54	39.3 ± 0.70

Study #2[b]	Nonpregnancy (n = 5)	Normal Pregnancy (n = 5)	Eclampsia (n = 5)
Total blood volume (ml)	3035	4425	3530
% Change from nonpregnant state	—	+47	+16
Hematocrit (%)	38.2	34.7	40.5

[a] Normal pregnant and preeclamptic women in third trimester of pregnancy. Note preeclamptic patients increased their RBC volume, but not their plasma volume compared to normal pregnant women. (Adapted from Bletka M, Hlavatj V, Trnkova M, Bendl J, Bendova L, Chytil M: Volume of whole blood and absolute amount of serum proteins in the early stages of late toxemia of pregnancy. Am J Obstet Gynecol 106:10–13, 1970.)

[b] Blood volumes measured with chromium 51 in five eclamptic women, after recovery in the nonpregnant state, then again in a subsequent normal pregnancy. Note the minimal elevation of the total blood volume, but the increased hematocrit concentration in the eclamptic patients. (Adapted from Prichard JA, Cunningham GA, Prichard SA: The Parkland Memorial Hospital protocol for the treatment of eclampsia: Evaluation of 245 cases. Am J Obstet Gynecol 148:951–963, 1984.)

Table 17.3
Coagulation Determinations in Eclampsia vs. Normal Pregnancy[a]

	Eclamptic Women (n = 62)	Normal Women (n = 24)	P Value
Platelets (10³/ml)	266 ± 89[b]	269 ± 54[b]	NS
−2 SD <161 × 10³	10/62	1/24	
<100 × 10⁵	1/62	1/24	
Fibrinogen (mg/dl)	405 ± 98[b]	437 ± 77[b]	NS
−2 SD <283 mg/dl	5/62	1/24	
Fibrin degradation products			
<10 μg/ml	44/62	22/24	<0.05
10–40 μg/ml	17/66	2/24	
>40 μg/ml	1/62	0/24	
Partial thromboplastin time (sec)	29.8 ± 6.6[b]	26.4 ± 1.8[b]	<0.001
Prothrombin time (sec)	11.2 ± 0.8[b]	11.2 ± 0.6[b]	NS

[a] Modified by permission from Sibai BM, Anderson GD, McCubbin JH: Eclampsia II: Clinical significance of laboratory findings. Obstet Gynecol 59:153–157, 1982.
[b] Mean ± SD; NS = not significant.

The "HELLP" syndrome which is associated with high maternal and fetal mortality and maternal morbidity, has been described in preeclampsia (78). It usually occurs before 36 weeks' gestation. Patients complain of malaise (90%), epigastric pain (90%), and nausea and vomiting (50%) with some having a nonspecific viral flu-like syndrome (79). Initially, hypertension and proteinuria may be very mild. The disorder is rapidly progressive, with development of disseminated intravascular coagulation and liver and renal failure. Its diagnosis calls for immediate delivery, regardless of gestation, if maternal and fetal death

are to be prevented (80). Patients developing thrombocytopenia below 50,000 per milliliter require as many as 11 postpartum days to achieve a platelet count in excess of 100,000 per milliliter. These severely affected patients require a longer period for diuresis to occur postpartum and may need plasma exchange. Those patients having platelet counts of more than 50,000 per milliliter experience a faster recovery and do not require plasma exchange (81). Commonly, platelet counts reach their lowest level by 24 to 48 hr after delivery (82). When delivery does not result in recovery, some authors advocate re-

Table 17.4
Coagulation Determinations in Normal Late Third–Trimester Pregnancies vs. Nulliparous Preeclampsia in Third Trimester with and without Thrombocytopenia (<150,000)[a,b]

	Normal Pregnant Controls ($n = 24$)	Nulliparous Preeclampsia with No Thrombocytopenia ($n = 22$)	Nulliparous Preeclampsia with Thrombocytopenia ($n = 22$)
Platelet count ($\times 10^3$ ml)	251.3 ± 60.6	199.6 ± 34	79.4 ± 40.6
Platelet associated IgG (fg IgG per platelet)	2.6 ± 1.1	3.9 ± 2.0	10.6 ± 12.2
Bleeding time (min)	4.4 ± 1.2	7.6 ± 4.6	13.0 ± 8.3
Thromboxane B_2 (ng/ml)	254.6 ± 135.0	120.4 ± 103.4	122.6 ± 94.3
Prothrombin time (sec)	12 ± 2	10.9 ± 0.6	10.5 ± 0.6
Activated partial thromboplastic time (sec)	33.5 ± 4.7	30.4 ± 4.4	33.5 ± 4.3
Fibrinogen (mg/dl)	449 ± 116	553.6 ± 199.0	452.8 ± 123

[a] Modified from Burrows RF, Hunter DJS, Andrew M, Kelton JG: A prospective study investigating the mechanism of thrombocytopenia in preeclampsia. Obstet Gynecol 70:334–338, 1987.
[b] Data expressed as mean ± SD.

placing the patient's plasma with fresh frozen plasma (83). Platelet counts frequently decrease to levels below 50,000 per milliliter following delivery; such levels have not been associated with epidural hematomas arising from previously administered epidural blocks for delivery (84).

The upper airway and laryngeal edema of normal pregnancy can be aggravated to the point of airway obstruction (85, 86). The lung volumes, capacities, and function are not significantly altered by preeclampsia (87). Respiratory depression from administration of magnesium, narcotics, or sedatives may lead to hypoxia and hypercarbia. Frank pulmonary edema with left ventricular failure is common following injudicious fluid hydration. The oxygen hemoglobin dissociation curve is shifted to the left, which may decrease oxygen availability to the fetus (88). This shift has been attributed to increased levels of carboxyhemoglobin resulting from an increased catabolism of circulating red blood cells occurring in the preeclamptic patient (89). Plasma pseudocholinesterase activity is decreased, as compared with both normal gravid and normal nongravid women (90). This decrease is not due to the effect of magnesium used to treat the disorder (91, 92). It may cause preeclamptic patients to be more sensitive to succinylcholine and to the toxicity of the "ester type" local anesthetics such as procaine, 2-chloroprocaine and tetracaine.

Renal function is adversely affected by preeclampsia-eclampsia (71). Glomerular filtration rate and creatinine clearance decrease. Blood uric acid levels increase and may correlate with the severity of the disease (93). Renal blood flow is compromised. Large amounts of all serum proteins may be lost through the urine. Renal lesions are common and are characterized by swelling of capillary endothelial cells

(a hallmark of the renal pathology in preeclampsia rarely seen in other conditions [94]), narrowing of glomerular capillaries, and deposition of fibrin within glomeruli. Acute renal failure with oliguria may occur in preeclampsia-eclampsia, especially in patients having other complicating factors such as abruptio placentae with disseminated intravascular coagulopathy and hemorrhage, the "HELLP" syndrome, and superimposed essential hypertension (95). Some clinicians believe that patients with preeclampsia will experience a complete reversal of these renal pathologic changes (94, 95), whereas others believe preeclampsia may be associated with the permanent lesions of focal glomerular sclerosis (96). Women with renal failure developing from preeclampsia superimposed on essential hypertension frequently suffer permanent renal damage, often requiring long-term dialysis (95). When renal failure occurs in the antepartum period, delivery is usually associated with its rapid resolution. Oliguria and renal failure may occur in the absence of hypovolemia and marked continued hydration can result in pulmonary edema (97). These patients may suffer either from selective renal artery vasospasm or from frank volume overload with cardiac dysfunction (98). Thus preeclamptic patients with oliguria who do not respond to a modest fluid load may require pulmonary artery catheterization for correct diagnosis and proper treatment (97, 98).

Hepatic involvement in preeclampsia is usually mild. However, in severe preeclampsia-eclampsia or when preeclampsia is complicated by the "HELLP" syndrome, periportal hemorrhages, ischemic lesions, generalized swelling, and even subcapsular hematoma sometimes occur in the liver. The hepatic swelling produces epigastric pain. An elevation in liver enzyme levels has been documented, and it is one of the hallmarks of the "HELLP" syndrome (71, 78). Hyperreflexia occurs, and central nervous system (CNS) irritability often increases. Coma may develop even without eclampsia. Many eclamptic patients have an increased intracranial pressure that can be exacerbated by hypercarbia, metabolic acidosis, and hypoxia (11, 67). Of patients becoming eclamptic 30% do so in the first 48 hr postpartum.

The uterus becomes hyperactive and markedly sensitive to oxytocin. Rapid labor with painful contractions are common. Preterm labor frequently occurs. Uterine and placental blood flow (intervillous blood flow) are markedly diminished by 50 to 70% (99) because of both increased vascular resistance and increased maternal blood viscosity secondary to the increased hematocrit (68). The placenta, which is often small, may show signs of premature aging and frequently exhibits infarcts, fibrin deposition, calcification, and abruption. The incidence of abruptio placentae is significantly increased in both preeclampsia-eclampsia and in mothers with pregnancies complicated by hypertension of other causes. The leading cause of maternal death in preeclampsia-eclampsia is intracranial hemorrhage (100). Other causes of morbidity and mortality include congestive heart failure with pulmonary edema, pulmonary aspiration of gastric contents, postpartum hemorrhage, disseminated intravascular coagulation, acute renal failure, ruptured liver, and septic shock (10).

In preeclampsia-eclampsia, the fetus is at great risk because of the marginal placental function, which may become inadequate, particularly in the presence of increased uterine activity. Aortocaval compression, induced hypotension from therapy or anesthesia, and the use of depressant drugs greatly increase the danger to the fetus. Both preterm and small-for-gestational-age neonates, born through thick meconium, are common. The leading causes of intrauterine mortality are placental infarction, followed by retardation of placental growth, abruptio placentae, and acute infection of amniotic fluid (101). In addition, severe maternal hypertension may be associated with an increased incidence of mental retardation and development of global and motor dysfunction (102). Perinatal morbidity and mortality are often related to preterm birth accompanied by respiratory distress, intracranial hemorrhage, small-for-gestational-age neonate, and aspiration of meconium.

THERAPY FOR PREECLAMPSIA-ECLAMPSIA

The definitive therapy for preeclampsia-eclampsia is delivery of the fetus and the placenta. Until this can be accomplished, the obstetric objective is control of the disease process. The pregnancy is allowed to continue as long as the intrauterine environment is adequate to support growth and maturation of the fetus without endangering the mother. In more severe preeclamptic patients, but in those who can be relatively well controlled, pregnancy may be continued until the fetus is of sufficient maturity and size to ensure survival following birth or until other factors indicate the need for delivery (103). In very severe preeclampsia, eclampsia, and the "HELLP" syndrome, the mother is quickly stabilized and the fetus delivered expeditiously, regardless of size and maturity. Prolonging gestation in these pregnancies is often disastrous, with a high fetal mortality and many maternal complications (104). As long as the fetus tolerates uterine contractions, induction and vaginal delivery is often possible and is not contraindicated in preeclampsia, despite a long, closed, "unripe" cervix. However, cesarean section is indicated if the fetus is markedly premature but viable; if there are signs of a significantly compromised or rapidly worsening intrauterine environment, a falling biophysical profile (105), or fetal distress; or if the mother's condition is rapidly deteriorating.

The general aims of therapy are to minimize vasospasm; to improve circulation, particularly to the uterus, placenta, and kidneys; to improve intravascular volume; to correct acid-base and electrolyte imbalances; and to decrease both CNS and reflex hyperactivity. Frequently, with early detection and proper therapy, the pathophysiologic changes of preeclampsia can be minimized and the pregnancy carried to near term. Therapy, as a rule, is symptomatic.

Hospitalization and bed rest in the lateral decubitus position (to prevent aortocaval compression and improve uterine blood flow) are often most effective. This therapy with adequate dietary intake frequently promotes diuresis and decreases blood pressure (106, 107). The upright and supine positions, which favor aortocaval compression, seem to aggravate the condition. Although preeclampsia is associated with water and salt retention and a few clinicians still favor fluid and salt restriction (on the basis it may be associated with pulmonary and cerebral edema (8, 108)), the predominant opinion is that adequate hydration and intravascular volume expansion with a balanced salt solution is beneficial from the standpoint of lowering maternal blood pressure and improving placental and fetal blood flow (109–112). In the past, severe sodium restriction was recommended, a practice that frequently led to sodium depletion and possibly increased production of renin, angiotensin, and aldosterone (113). Evidence now favors an adequate sodium intake with minimal, if any, sodium restriction (38, 114). Intravenous fluids should contain sodium, particularly if oxytocin is used, to prevent water intoxication and convulsions. The diet should be adequate and balanced with no attempt made at weight reduction.

Except for the teachings of a few authors (51, 115), the routine use of diuretics, particularly the thiazide derivatives, is generally discouraged (8, 116). These drugs produce diuresis at the expense of the already contracted blood volume. In addition they may cause electrolyte imbalance, increased blood viscosity, glucose intolerance in both mother and fetus, and (with thiazide diuretics) elevation of the already increased blood uric acid. They are seldom required for the therapy of hypertension in the gravid patient (53). Except for the acute treatment of pulmonary edema caused by congestive heart failure or other factors, diuretic drugs are rarely indicated in preeclampsia-eclampsia.

Magnesium Therapy

In North America and in many third world countries, parenterally administered magnesium is considered the first-line therapeutic drug in controlling preeclampsia-eclampsia. It is an effective anticonvulsant and tocolytic and a mild generalized vasodilator. The mechanism of its antiseizure activity is its depression of the central nervous system (117–119). Although many other anticonvulsants have been used, including barbiturates, diazepam, chlormethiazole, and phenytoin, none have proved superior to magnesium in either efficacy or lack of side effects (121). Magnesium's tocolytic action (see Chapter 18 on preterm labor) makes it useful in preeclampsia, in which the uterus is often hyperactive, frequently accompanied by a compromised intrauterine environment. Magnesium causes mild vasodilation by depressing smooth muscle contraction, and it depresses catecholamine release (122, 123). These properties explain its mild, but unreliable antihypertensive effects, its beneficial action on uterine blood flow, and its possible antagonism of cerebral vasospasm (124, 124a). The beneficial and detrimental effects of magnesium sulfate are summarized in Table 17.5. Therapeutic maternal plasma levels of magnesium are in the range of 4 to 6 mEq/liter, with toxicity occurring when plasma levels exceed 10 mEq/liter (Table 17.6).

Magnesium therapy is associated with both maternal and neonatal side effects. Serious toxicity may be the result of either absolute overdose or (more frequently) elevation of blood levels, following repeated doses or continuous infusions in the presence of decreased renal function. Overdose can lead to maternal weakness, respiratory insufficiency, and even cardiac failure. Fortunately, these complications do not usually arise until after the deep tendon reflexes are depressed. Therefore magnesium should be de-

Table 17.5
Various Actions of Magnesium Sulfate as Used in Preeclampsia-Eclampsia[a]

Beneficial effects for preeclampsia-eclampsia
1. Anticonvulsant
2. Vasodilation
   Increased uterine blood flow
   Increased renal blood flow
   Antihypertensive (not reliable)
3. Increased prostacyclin release by endothelial cells
4. Decreased plasma renin activity
5. Decreased angiotensin-converting enzymes
6. Attenuation of vascular responses to pressor substances
7. Reduced platelet aggregation
8. Bronchodilation
9. Tocolysis: improves uterine blood flow and antagonizes uterine hyperactivity

Detrimental effects
1. Tocolysis with prolonged labor and increased postpartum hemorrhage
2. Decreased fetal heart rate variability
3. Myoneural blocking effects
   Generalized muscle weakness
   Increased sensitivity to muscle relaxants, especially nondepolarizing muscle relaxants
4. Neonatal effects: lower Apgar scores and decreased muscle tone (only with maternal overdose)

[a] Modified from Sibai BM: Magnesium sulfate is the ideal anticonvulsant in preeclampsia-eclampsia. Am J Obstet Gynecol 162:1141–1145, 1990.

Table 17.6
Effects of Increasing Plasma Magnesium Levels

Plasma Mg (mEq/liter)	Effects
1.5–2.0	Normal plasma level
4.0–8.0	Therapeutic range
5.0–10	Electrocardiographic changes (P-Q interval prolonged, QRS complex widens)
10	Loss of deep tendon reflexes
15	Sinoatrial and atrioventricular block
15	Respiratory paralysis
25	Cardiac arrest

creased or discontinued when such deep tendon reflex depression occurs. Magnesium in therapeutic dosages is associated with abnormal neuromuscular transmissions, which correlates with increased serum magnesium levels and decreased serum calcium levels (125). Magnesium therapy increases the sensitivity of the mother to both the depolarizing and nondepolarizing relaxants (Fig. 17.8) (126–128) by decreasing (a) the amount of acetylcholine released by motor nerve terminals, (b) the depolarizing action of acetylcholine at the motor endplate, and (c) the

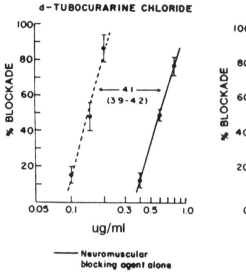

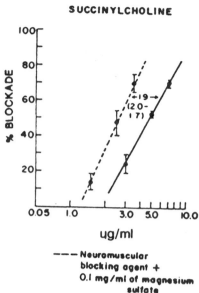

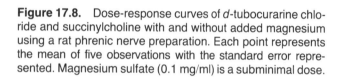

Figure 17.8. Dose-response curves of *d*-tubocurarine chloride and succinylcholine with and without added magnesium using a rat phrenic nerve preparation. Each point represents the mean of five observations with the standard error represented. Magnesium sulfate (0.1 mg/ml) is a subminimal dose.

The magnitude of the potentiation by magnesium is shown between the curves with their fiducial limits. (Reprinted with permission from Ghoneim MM, Long JP: Interaction between magnesium and other neuromuscular blocking agents. Anesthesiology 32:23–27, 1970.)

excitability of the muscle fiber membrane (126). Magnesium does not appear to affect plasma cholinesterase activity and its metabolism of succinylcholine (92). Similarly, studies in healthy women volunteers indicate that magnesium does not affect bleeding time (129).

Because magnesium rapidly crosses the placenta, it may affect the newborn. However, therapeutic levels in the mother are not associated with significant detrimental effects on the neonate (130–132). Hence, the cause of neonatal depression in mothers receiving magnesium is rarely due to the magnesium itself. When high maternal levels of magnesium are reached, the newborn may exhibit decreased muscle tone, respiratory depression, and apnea. Intravenously administered calcium may partially overcome the neuromuscular blocking properties of magnesium in both mother and newborn. Although the slow administration of calcium is safe in the newborn, its administration is a risk for the mother because calcium will antagonize the anticonvulsant effects of magnesium. Except in cases of gross magnesium overdose with cardiac depression, it is probably safer to support the mother's depressed respiration and avoid calcium. Because magnesium is excreted by the kidneys, it must be given with care and in reduced doses when urinary output is decreased or renal function impaired.

Magnesium therapy is usually initiated by intravenous administration of 4 to 6 g over 15 min. Two

to four grams given more rapidly during eclamptic convulsions frequently terminate the convulsion (8). In the past magnesium levels were maintained by following the intravenous loading dose with intramuscular injections every 3 to 4 hr. Because these injections are painful, it is now more common to maintain magnesium blood levels using a continuous intravenous infusion at the rate of 1 to 3 g/hour.

Antihypertensive Drugs

If, despite the administration of magnesium or other anticonvulsants and bed rest, the maternal blood pressure exceeds either 160 mm Hg systolic or 110 mm Hg diastolic, antihypertensives are indicated. Generally, lower blood pressures are not treated in preeclampsia-eclampsia. Antihypertensive therapy, although beneficial for the mother, does not appear to significantly improve fetal status or neonatal outcome (133–135). Veratrum alkaloids or reserpine, which were widely used in the past have been abandoned because of their prolonged latency and their tendency to cause neonatal nasal congestion, which interferes with respiration.

Until recently, the most widely used antihypertensive drug in preeclampsia was hydralazine. Its primary action is to decrease precapillary arteriolar resistance, but it is associated with an increased maternal cardiac output and tachycardia, which may interfere with its antihypertensive effect. Hydralazine is also associated with increased renal blood flow. Following intravenous administration, maximal effect is achieved in 20 to 30 min, with a duration of only 2 to 3 hr. Hydralazine was thought to increase placental blood flow (136). However, studies have shown that (a) in a significant number of women, it may decrease uterine blood flow (not necessarily related to placental blood flow) by as much as 25% (137, 138); (b) it has been associated with fetal distress (139); and (c) it may be associated with neonatal thrombocytopenia (140). Although still widely used in preeclampsia-eclampsia, hydralazine is being replaced by other antihypertensives. Methyldopa has been a popular antihypertensive in the treatment of preeclampsia-eclampsia, particularly in Europe. It may be useful in the chronically hypertensive patient after initial control of hypertension has been accomplished with hydralazine or for prolonged control of hypertension in the postpartum period. Its lack of ill effects on the fetus and newborn is well established (141). Clonidine and prazosin, two additional α_1 blockers have been used with good results in preeclampsia (142).

The use of β-blocking drugs in preeclampsia and hypertensive gravid patients is becoming more common. Initially it was feared that propanol, a nonselective β-blocker was associated with increased uterine activity, decreased uterine and placental blood flow, decreased fetal heart rate, decreased fetal tolerance to hypoxia, and adverse neonatal outcomes. Although well-controlled studies of β-blockers vs. placebo are frequently lacking, considerable clinical testing appears to demonstrate the safety of these drugs for the gravid mother and her fetus. Chronic use of cardioselective β_1-blockers during pregnancy, such as atenolol (143–145) and metropolol (146), appear to be effective maternal antihypertensives without causing ill effects on the fetus. Esmolol, a rapid ultrashort-acting cardioselective β_1-adrenergic blocker is effective in treating tachycardia and hypertension in nongravid patients (147) and has been used in isolated gravid patients with success. However, studies in the gravid ewe found it produced fetal β-adrenergic blockade and hypoxemia in the fetus (148). Hence, additional studies are required before its routine use can be recommended in the preeclamptic mother.

Labetalol is an effective antihypertensive that produces a nonselective β-blockade and a selective postsynaptic α_1-blockade with the β/α ratio of 3:1 to 7:1 following oral or intravenous administration, respectively (149). In addition, it may also produce vasodilation by β_2-receptor stimulation (150). Its onset is rapid after intravenous injection and, it has an elimination half-life of 1.7 hr following oral ingestion in gravid patients (151). Its administration in both gravid hypertensive animals (152, 153) and hypertensive mothers (134, 154–156) has not been associated with decreased uterine or placental perfusion, fetal bradycardia, fetal deterioration, or neonatal problems. It has a more rapid onset of action and lacks the side effects of tachycardia, nausea, headache, excessive hypotension, and decreased uterine blood flow associated with hydralazine (157, 158). Labetalol is becoming widely used for both the control of hypertension and for attenuation of acute hypertension associated with a rapid sequence induction of general anesthesia in the severely preeclamptic or eclamptic patient. Caution must be used in the administration of β-blockers to patients with bronchoconstrictive disorders and with compromised myocardial function because these drugs may cause bronchoconstriction and decreased ventricular function.

The calcium-channel blockers, particularly nifedipine, are gaining importance as safe and effective antihypertensives in pregnancy, particularly in preeclampsia-eclampsia. In addition to being relaxants of vascular smooth muscle (thus decreasing systemic vascular resistance), they also are potent uterine relaxants and increase renal blood flow. Because of its lack of associated tachycardia, nifedipine is usually preferred over verapamil. It is usually administered by the oral or sublingual routes. In norepinephrine rendered hypertensive ewes, nifedipine effectively lowers maternal blood pressure, while improving uterine blood flow and fetal oxygenation (159). In human studies its use in severe preeclampsia was shown to be more effective than that of hydralazine in lowering maternal blood pressure, prolonging pregnancy, and causing considerably less fetal distress (160, 161). Contrary to earlier reports, it is not associated with decreased uterine perfusion or fetal deterioration (162). Nifedipine has also been found to effectively increase urinary output in antepartum and postpartum severe preeclamptic patients (163). Nifedipine is a potent uterine muscle relaxant and is gaining popularity as a tocolytic; hence, postpartum hemorrhage may be more likely to occur if nifedipine is administered close to the time of delivery. When administered in the presence of magnesium, it is associated with a potentiated hypotensive response, which is possibly explained by the supposition that magnesium, like nifedipine, acts as a calcium-channel blocker (164, 165). Following oral ingestion in gravid patients with pregnancy-induced hypertension, peak blood levels were reached in 40 min, complete elimination occurred in 360 min, and a half-life of 54 minutes was found (166).

Other potent rapid-acting antihypertensives have been used primarily in acute hypertensive crises or to attenuate or treat the marked hypertensive response associated with laryngoscopy and intubation during induction of general anesthesia. Diazoxide, a thiazide derivative with no diuretic effect, has the disadvantage of often causing sudden uncontrolled hypotension associated with decreased uterine blood flow and fetal distress (167), particularly when given in the usual initial recommended dose of 300 mg IV. In addition, diazoxide interferes with glucose metabolism and uric acid excretion and is a potent uterine relaxant; thus it may be associated with significant postpartum hemorrhage. It is rarely used in obstetrics today. Ketanserin, a serotonergic antagonist with potent antihypertensive properties (not available in the United States) has shown promise in the acute treatment of the hypertension accompanying severe preeclampsia (168, 169). Given as an intravenous bolus, it rapidly lowered maternal blood pressure without affecting maternal heart rate. In addition, it had no apparent deleterious effects on the fetus; no adverse changes were noticed in beat-to-beat variability; and in 25% of the cases, it was associated with improvement in fetal heart rate patterns (169). The frequency, but not the amplitude, of contractions was decreased about a third with use of the drug.

Three other very potent and rapid-acting antihypertensives of short duration are trimethaphan, sodium nitroprusside (SNP), and trinitroglycerin (TNG). These are usually given as intravenous infusions for acute control of blood pressure during induction to and emergence from general anesthesia. Their use for this purpose is discussed later. When antihypertensives are given to the gravid patient with severe preeclampsia or eclampsia, the fetal heart rate should be closely monitored. Sudden decreases in maternal blood pressure can rapidly produce fetal distress as the uteroplacental circulation becomes further compromised. One usually aims to produce only a partial return of maternal blood pressure to normal levels and of diastolic pressure to below 110 torr until after delivery.

Control of Convulsions

In eclampsia, the first priority is to control grand mal convulsions. Until this is accomplished, no attempt is made to deliver the fetus. Maternal mortality increases according to the number of convulsions, the elevation of maternal blood pressure, and the age and parity of the patient (9–11). Initially, intravenous administration of a rapid-acting anticonvulsant—such as a thiobarbiturate (thiopental, 50 to 100 mg), a benzodiazepine (diazepam, 2.5 to 5 mg, or midazolam, 1 to 2 mg), or magnesium (2 to 4 g)—is used to terminate a convulsion. Further convulsions are prevented by continued intravenous administration of magnesium (2 to 4 g per hour) or another anticon-

vulsant, such as a benzodiazepine or chloromethiazole. Continued convulsions despite adequate magnesium therapy are often indicative of additional CNS pathology, such as venous thrombosis, intracerebral hemorrhage, or edema, and indicate the need for further evaluation (248). Oxygen should be administered during a seizure to protect the patient against hypoxia caused by diminished respiration and increased maternal metabolism. If convulsions do not terminate rapidly, administer succinylcholine and intubate the trachea to prevent pulmonary aspiration and to ensure adequate ventilation. Postictal depression may require the support of ventilation to ensure adequate oxygenation and to prevent hypercapnia and respiratory acidosis. Because convulsions are often associated with metabolic acidosis, bicarbonate may be indicated after determination of arterial blood gases and pH. In severe preeclampsia or eclampsia, frank congestive cardiac failure and pulmonary edema may occur, for which a rapidly acting, intravenously administered diuretic drug such as furosemide is given. Digitalization may be indicated. If cerebral edema is suspected, an osmotic diuretic drug such as mannitol may be administered, but only in the presence of adequate urinary output. Dexamethasone in a large dose (10 to 16 mg) may also be of use in this condition. Mechanical hyperventilation during the postpartum period may be initiated. Before birth, *excessive* maternal hyperventilation may result in fetal hypoxia and acidosis. Further therapy consists of controlling blood pressure. In severe preeclampsia or eclampsia, frank disseminated intravascular coagulation may develop but usually resolves promptly following delivery.

Pritchard and co-workers treated 245 eclamptic patients between 1955 and 1984 with only a single maternal death caused by an initial intravenous overdose of magnesium (77). All newborns in excess of 1501 g and alive when the mother was admitted survived. Essentially, only magnesium sulfate for convulsion control and the antihypertensive hydralazine were used. Fluids were restricted; diuretics were avoided; invasive maternal monitoring was rarely used; and once convulsions were controlled, rapid delivery was accomplished (usually by induction of labor and vaginal delivery). The authors disagree, however, with the philosophy of Pritchard et al. of the avoidance of major conduction analgesia and the required use of general anesthesia for cesarean section. This is discussed more fully later.

MONITORING THE SEVERE PREECLAMPTIC OR ECLAMPTIC PATIENT

Before anesthesia for delivery is initiated, convulsions must be controlled and severe hypertension in excess of 160/110 to 170/110 treated. Although patients with mild preeclampsia may not require any special monitoring, those severely afflicted with the disorder will require special considerations. Blood pressure should be monitored frequently. This usually is adequately accomplished noninvasively with the use of an automatic electronic device complete with recorder that employs the oscillometric method. Such equipment possesses good accuracy and, when necessary, can give readings every minute, although prolongation of such frequent readings is associated with patient discomfort and occasionally has been associated with radial nerve palsies. Invasive direct arterial blood pressure monitoring is rarely required. We reserve it for patients with pulmonary edema, those on ventilators, and others who may require frequent arterial specimens for pH and blood gas analysis. In addition, direct arterial monitoring may be indicated in very unstable patients receiving continuous infusions of potent vasoactive drugs such as sodium nitroprusside. *Central* venous monitoring is often indicated in severe preeclamptic or eclamptic patients, particularly in those with marked hypertension or oliguria and in those who are to have major conduction analgesia. As previously discussed, some obstetricians and anesthesiologists recommend the replacement of the CVP with the pulmonary artery catheter (43, 47, 48, 61–63). They argue that, in the presence of left ventricular failure or other cardiac disease, the CVP may not accurately reflect fluid replacement or left ventricular function. They also correctly state that, with only the CVP, one can not reliably diagnose the effects—the various components of the cardiovascular system contribute to the clinical picture found in a particular patient. For example, in a particular patient, is the severe hypertension observed caused by marked arterial vasoconstriction that is best treated with a vasodilator such as hydralazine or is it the result of a hyperdynamic left ventricle with an increased cardiac output that is treated best with a β_1-blocker? Although the advocates of pulmonary artery catheter monitoring claim few complications from its placement and use, the authors are personally aware of three deaths and several cases of severe morbidity with serious permanent sequelae that occurred in conjunction with placement of a pulmonary artery catheter by or under the direct supervision of an experienced physician. Because the vast majority of preeclamptic-eclamptic patients have adequate left ventricular function and normal pulmonary artery pressures, one must weigh the risk of pulmonary artery catheterization against the usefulness of any additional information gained beyond that obtained from central venous catheterization. For preeclamptic-eclamptic patients, the au-

Table 17.7
Indications for Pulmonary Artery Catheter Placement in the Severe Preeclamptic or Eclamptic Patient: Findings and Their Therapy

1. Unresponsive or refractory hypertension
   a. Increased systemic vascular resistance (Rx: vasodilators)
   b. Increased cardiac output (Rx: decrease preload with nitroglycerin or decrease cardiac output with a β-blocker)
2. Pulmonary edema
   a. Cardiogenic or left ventricular failure (Rx: afterload reduction or ionotrops)
   b. Increased systemic vascular resistance (Rx: afterload reduction)
   c. Noncardiogenic volume overload (Rx: diuretics, fluid restriction)
      Decreased colloid oncotic pressure (Rx: 25% albumin, fluid restriction)
3. Persistent arterial desaturation; unable to distinguish between cardiac or noncardiac origin
4. Oliguria unresponsive to modest fluid loading
   a. Low preload (Rx: crystalloid infusion)
   b. Severe increased systemic vascular resistance with low cardiac output (Rx: afterload reduction)
   c. Selective renal artery vasoconstriction

[a] Modified from Clark SB, Cotton DB: Clinical indications for pulmonary artery catheterization in the patient with severe preeclampsia. Am J Obstet Gynecol 158:453–458, 1988.

thors restrict the use of pulmonary artery catheterization to those patients with refractory oliguria, cardiac lesions, or signs of congestive heart failure. Then, if a central venous catheter gives insufficient information, a Swan-Ganz catheter can be inserted. Table 17.7 summarizes indications for pulmonary artery catheterization (47). Maternal urinary output and protein excretion are important indicators in the severe preeclamptic patient and need to be carefully monitored throughout the peripartum period. This requires an indwelling bladder catheter, especially during labor and for as long as several days following delivery. Continuous infusion of oxytocin has a marked antidiuretic effect, similar to antidiuretic hormone, and when infused at rates greater than 10 mu per minute, it may markedly decrease urinary output, cause retention of free water, and result in hyponatremia and water intoxication. When oxytocin is infused, all intravenous solutions should be isotonic in regard to electrolyte content.

The leading indication for cesarean section in preeclampsia-eclampsia is deterioration of the intrauterine environment or the development of fetal distress during labor. The severely preeclamptic patient frequently has diminished uterine and placental blood flows (16, 170), with a uterus that is hyperactive with prolonged and frequent contractions. Therefore, during labor, electronic fetal monitoring of fetal heart rate and uterine contractions is essential, especially with the use of labor induction, major conduction analgesia, or both. With the rupture of membranes, internal electronic fetal monitoring is often initiated. In addition, fetal blood analysis for pH may be indicated when significant fetal heart rate abnormalities occur.

Considerations for Delivery

Delivery of a preterm neonate may be necessitated by deterioration of either the intrauterine environment or the condition of the mother. When severe preeclampsia develops in the second trimester before 24 weeks' gestation despite aggressive obstetric management, the outcome of the fetus is dismal (less than 7% survival) and maternal complications are frequent (40%) (37). If the fetus is preterm, shows marked intrauterine growth retardation, or is in an unfavorable lie, delivery by cesarean section is usually chosen. If the fetus is dead or nonviable or if, conversely, it is of reasonable size (greater than 2500 g) and tolerates labor, vaginal delivery with induction (if necessary) is indicated. Because the uterus of the preeclamptic patient is markedly sensitive to oxytocin, induction and vaginal delivery are often possible even though the cervix is not "ripe."

Anesthesia and Analgesia for the Patient with Preeclampsia-Eclampsia

Because of his or her expertise in pain control, airway management, ventilatory care, and hemodynamic monitoring and because of the significant effects that preeclampsia-eclampsia and its management can have on anesthesia, the anesthesiologist should be consulted early in the care of these patients and should assume a major role in their medical management.

The preeclamptic-eclamptic patient requires a reliable means of intravenous drug administration, such as that provided by at least an 18-gauge indwelling catheter. Intravenously administered fluids should not consist of dextrose in water alone, especially if oxytocin is used, because of the danger of water intoxication. Rather, isotonic balanced salt solutions should be used. Rapid infusion of dextrose-containing solutions should be avoided or limited to a maximum of 125 ml/hour of 5% dextrose because neonatal hypoglycemia and hyperbilirubinemia are associated with maternal hyperglycemia (171). Urinary output should be monitored to help guide fluid replacement. In the severely preeclamptic or eclamptic patient, a CVP catheter may be of great value for determining fluid and blood replacement. To replenish intravascular volume before administration of an epidural block, balanced salt solutions or plasma expanders such as 5 or 25% albumin are given while the CVP is being monitored (44, 172). The choice of the hydrating solution is open to debate. Rapid infusion of 2 liters of balanced salt solution may significantly lower the colloid oncotic pressure for 24 hr (173). Although this is tolerated by the normal parturient (173), the preeclamptic patient with her often already lowered serum colloid oncotic pressure and damaged capillary endothelium may not tolerate such rapid crystalloid infusions, which can cause pulmonary edema (174–175). Infusion of 500 and 1000 ml of 5% albumin in severe preeclamptics has been found to increase cardiac output and decrease systemic vascular resistance with no effect or minimal lowering of mean arterial blood pressure (176). Hence, use of albumin infusions might be preferable in the severe preeclamptic patient. Certainly, rapid intravenous hydration, particularly with crystalloid solutions, should be done with care and with constant monitoring of the CVP and urinary output, while observing for early signs and symptoms of pulmonary edema. Blood should be readily available for transfusions. The patient should be encouraged to remain on her left side to avoid aortocaval compression. Supplemental oxygen during labor and delivery is indicated, especially because of the left-shifted maternal oxygen hemoglobin dissociation curve of the preeclamptic patient (88, 89). The choice of analgesia depends on the obstetric situation. For vaginal delivery, if narcotics are used, they should be given in minimal dosage and early in labor to minimize neonatal depression. Although narcotics provide analgesia, they have no anticonvulsant and little antihypertensive effect. Tranquilizers, often used with narcotics, particularly should be given in small doses, because no drugs are currently available to antagonize such adjuvants effectively. Patient-controlled analgesia (PCA) with fentanyl or meperidine may provide satisfactory analgesia during the active phase of labor. The initial intravenous loading dose of meperidine is 25 to 50 mg and of fentanyl is 50 to 100 μg. Additionally 10 to 15 mg of self-administered meperidine, 25 to 50 μg of fentanyl with hourly maximum of 50 mg of meperidine, or 50 μg of fentanyl for up to 6 hours may be given. For the late first stage of labor and delivery, continuous administration of 30 to 40% nitrous oxide in oxygen provides good analgesia, increases oxygenation, and incurs minimal cardiovascular depression or alterations and no measurable neonatal depression. At delivery, augmentation of nitrous oxide analgesia with a pudendal block or local infiltration of the perineum provides satisfactory analgesia for most forceps deliveries. Analgesia can be increased by the addition of 0.5 to

0.75% enflurane or 0.3 to 0.5% isoflurane to the nitrous oxide. The authors have found if maternal hypertension is well controlled, small (0.25 mg/kg) incremental intravenous doses of ketamine, not exceeding a total of 0.75 mg/kg before birth, may be used safely with 30 to 40% nitrous oxide in place of enflurane or isoflurane. Such small doses of ketamine provide short periods (2 to 5 min) of intense analgesia, which usually provides sufficient analgesia with a pudendal block or local infiltration of the perineum to allow for forceps or vacuum delivery. The above techniques of inhalation analgesia do not require endotracheal intubation, **providing maternal consciousness is not lost**. They are relatively simple to administer and provide rapid, intense analgesia, making them ideal for imminent delivery when time or the mother's condition do not permit major conduction analgesia. Unfortunately these techniques often may not provide ideal obstetric conditions. In addition they will not prevent the precipitous delivery of a small preterm infant that has a great risk of developing intracranial hemorrhage in an uncontrolled delivery.

In the unlikely event that general anesthesia is required for vaginal delivery, the technique described in Chapter 11 should be used. As described later in this chapter, care must be taken to avoid sudden severe maternal hypertension with intubation during a rapid-sequence intravenous induction. Such an event predisposes the mother to intracerebral hemorrhage and pulmonary hypertension with pulmonary edema. Paracervical block is associated with a high incidence of fetal bradycardia and acidosis: *Its use in the preeclamptic patient delivering a viable newborn is not recommended.* However, it provides excellent and safe first-stage maternal analgesia for a nonviable fetus, a postpartum dilation and evacuation (D&E), or repair of a cervical laceration.

Continuous Lumbar Epidural Analgesia

The use of major conduction analgesia, particularly continuous lumbar epidural analgesia, in preeclampsia-eclampsia has been much debated in the past. Today, the use of continuous lumbar epidural analgesia in the severe preeclamptic or eclamptic patient whose convulsions are under control is widely accepted and even recommended by both anesthesiologists and informed obstetricians (11, 12, 47, 177–183). When not contraindicated by gross coagulation abnormalities, maternal septicemia, or marked untreated hypovolemia, continuous lumbar epidural analgesia offers the preeclamptic-eclamptic parturient many advantages. It can provide complete pain relief for labor and delivery and affords maternal re-

Table 17.8
Blood Pressure and Intervillous Blood Flow (Means ± SD) before and after Epidural Block in Nine Patients with Severe Preeclampsia in Labor[a,b]

	Before Epidural	After Epidural	P Value
Systolic blood pressure (torr)	155 ± 15	155 ± 20	NS
Diastolic blood pressure (torr)	100 ± 16	100 ± 19	NS
Intervillous blood flow (ml/min/dl)	196 ± 120	320 ± 183	<0.01

[a] Reprinted by permission from Jouppila P, Jouppila R, Hollmén A, Koivula A: Lumbar epidural analgesia to improve intervillous blood flow during labor in severe preeclampsia. Obstet Gynecol 59:158–161, 1982.
[b] All Apgar scores at 1 and 5 min ≥8. Eight of nine patients had increases in intervillous blood flow following epidural block. One patient who gave birth to a 2200-g newborn at 39 weeks' gestation had a decrease in intervillous blood flow from 72 to 68 ml/min/dl after epidural block and no fetal distress. All patients were prehydrated with 500 ml Ringer's solution, were kept in 15-degree left lateral tilt, and had an epidural block initiated with 10 ml of 0.25% bupivacaine.

laxation without the need for various depressant drugs. Properly administered, epidural analgesia incurs no neonatal depression. It provides ideal obstetric conditions for vaginal delivery, especially of the preterm neonate. It is also suitable for operative vaginal delivery (vacuum extraction, forceps delivery) and can be extended rapidly for cesarean section. During labor and delivery, it decreases maternal oxygen requirements and prevents maternal hyperventilation associated with painful contractions (184, 185). This hyperventilation may further decrease uterine blood flow and cause maternal metabolic acidosis. Maternal circulating levels of catecholamines may be elevated in preeclampsia and may decrease uteroplacental perfusion: Epidural analgesia significantly decreases the circulating level of epinephrine (64). In fact, epidural analgesia has been shown to improve intervillous blood flow in severe preeclamptic patients (Table 17.8) (182), and it appears to protect against eclamptic convulsions (178, 180). Because epidural analgesia stabilizes blood pressure at modestly lower levels, sudden hypertensive events associated with rapid-sequence induction of general anesthesia and intubation are avoided (Fig. 17.9) (181, 186–189). Such sudden hypertensive events are associated with pulmonary edema, cerebral edema, and intracranial hemorrhage (10, 100, 190, 191). Finally, the risk of pulmonary aspiration of gastric contents is minimized because the patient remains awake.

Despite the above advantages of epidural analgesia, a few nonanesthesiologists still advocate its

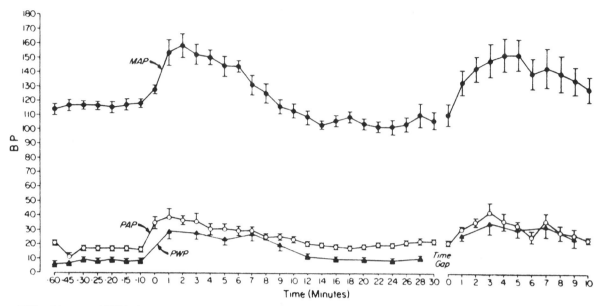

Figure 17.9. Mean and SEM of mean arterial pressure (MAP), mean pulmonary artery pressure (PAP), and pulmonary wedge pressure (PWP = PCWP) in eight patients with severe preeclampsia receiving general anesthesia for cesarean section. Anesthesia consisted of thiopental (3 mg/kg), succinylcholine (100 mg), nitrous oxide (40%), 0.5% halothane, and a 0.2% succinylcholine infusion. (Reprinted by permission from Hodgkinson R, Husain FJ, Hayashi RH: Systemic and pulmonary blood pressure during cesarean section in parturients with gestational hypertension. Can Anaesth Soc J 27:389–394, 1980.)

avoidance in the severe preeclamptic mother (5, 8, 140). They base their teachings on the following suppositions: (a) it may be associated with sudden maternal hypotension that rapidly leads to fetal deterioration (192) and may further decrease an already compromised intervillous blood flow; (b) the local anesthetics used may decrease the fetal heart rate beat-to-beat variability and thus impede the diagnosis of fetal hypoxia and distress (193, 194); and (c) it requires local anesthetics, which might predispose the mother to convulsions.

With proper technique, significant maternal hypotension and fetal distress can usually be avoided after lumbar epidural block (186). The percentage decrease in blood pressure is no greater in preeclamptic patients than it is in normal patients (Fig. 17.10) (177, 181, 186, 195, 196). When comparing parturients with mild to moderate preeclampsia who received epidural analgesia with those who did not receive epidural analgesia in the first stage of labor, no differences were noted in maximum blood pressures. However, those who received epidural blocks had slightly lower blood pressures than those who did not (197). Graham and Goldstein demonstrated that cardiac output was not decreased by epidural block in severe preeclamptic patients (198). Newsome and co-workers found that, in severe preeclamptic patients, although epidural block for either vaginal delivery or cesarean section lowered the mean arterial pressure from 121 mm Hg to 98 mm Hg, there

was no decrease in cardiac index, pulmonary vascular resistance, central venous pressure, or pulmonary capillary wedge pressure (63). Prevention of hypotension in patients with severe preeclampsia does not require large amounts of intravenous hydration (181, 182, 186, 199), but it does require the meticulous avoidance of aortocaval compression (200). Should hypotension occur, in addition to further uterine displacement and hydration, small intravenous doses of ephedrine (2.5–5 mg) are given as required to restore and maintain blood pressure. Hypotension associated with epidural block, if treated rapidly by the above means, was not associated with fetal and neonatal deterioration, even when the epidural block was used in cases of fetal distress for urgent cesarean section (201). Animal and human studies have shown no evidence of diminished uterine or intervillous blood flow during epidural analgesia unaccompanied by hypotension (202–206). Studies in preeclamptic parturients and parturients having essential hypertension showed that intervillous blood flow was maintained or improved with the use of epidural analgesia (Table 17.8) (182, 207). In contrast, induction of general anesthesia in normotensive animal and human mothers was associated with decreased uterine and intervillous blood flow (190, 208, 209). Although fetal heart rate beat-to-beat variability decreased slightly after an injection of lidocaine, fetal deterioration did not occur (193, 194). Bupivacaine used for epidural block is

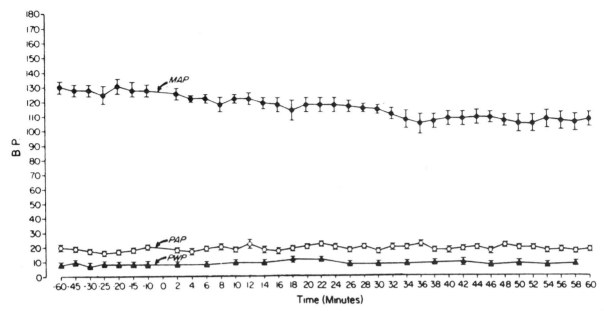

Figure 17.10. Mean and SEM of mean arterial pressure (MAP), mean pulmonary artery pressure (PAP), and pulmonary wedge pressure (PWP = PCWP) in 12 patients with severe preeclampsia receiving epidural analgesia for cesarean section. Bupivacaine, 0.75% (no longer recommended for use in obstetrics since 1983) was injected at time 0. (Reprinted with permission from Hodgkinson R, Husain FJ, Hagash RH: Systemic and pulmonary blood pressure during cesarean section. Can Anaesth Soc J 27:389–394, 1980.)

not associated with decreased fetal beat to beat variability (194a). It is well known that other drugs used to provide sedation and analgesia and to treat preeclampsia are associated with as great, if not greater, decreases in the fetal heart rate variability (210). These include narcotics, particularly those with the meperidine nucleus, phenothiazines, benzodiazepines, and magnesium sulfate. Finally, when local anesthetics are properly used, they are not associated with convulsions and are not contraindicated in seizure disorders (211). Indeed, local anesthetics have been used successfully to terminate clinical status epilepticus (212, 213). A comparison of epidurals for cesarean section using lidocaine showed similar neonatal outcomes in normal vs. preeclamptic pregnancies as judged by umbilical arterial and venous blood gases, Apgar scores, and early neurobehavioral scores at 4 and 24 hr, despite a modestly prolonged total body clearance of lidocaine in the neonates of preeclamptic mothers (18.5 ± 4.7 vs. 14.1 ± 1.3 μg-hr-ml^{-1}) (214).

In view of the vast favorable clinical experience and recent investgational work, the evidence supports the use of continuous lumbar epidural analgesia as the preferred method of analgesia for labor, vaginal delivery, and cesarean section in most mothers having severe preeclampsia or controlled eclampsia. Obviously, to obtain favorable results, lumbar epidural analgesia must be administered skillfully, the patient must receive constant care and monitor-

ing, and the technique must be avoided when contraindications exist. The authors strongly support the opinions of two recognized obstetric experts in the management of preeclampsia-eclampsia who state: "A cautiously administered epidural anesthetic is, in our opinion, not only justified but is *certainly the method of choice for anesthesia* in cesarean section or control of the pain of labor in the patient with severe preeclampsia" (47).

PATIENT PREPARATION

Before instituting a continuous lumbar epidural block in a severely preeclamptic patient, she should be under good medical management: Hypertension should be controlled, as demonstrated by a diastolic blood pressure of less than 110 torr. The absence of any severe coagulopathy must be confirmed. Blood pressure should be monitored frequently, using a noninvasive electronic oscillometric device with a recorder or, when indicated, an indwelling arterial catheter. The use of a pulse oximeter during labor is helpful and gives an early indication of developing pulmonary edema or inadequate circulation. Continuously recorded electronic monitoring of fetal heart rate and uterine contractions is mandatory because the mother's ability to judge the frequency, strength, and duration of contractions will be abolished. Although a decrease in systolic blood pressure of 25% is usually without consequence in normal pregnancy (provided the systolic blood pressure does not fall below 100 mm Hg), such a decrease may not be tolerated if placental function is already compromised, as it is in preeclampsia. The fetal heart tracing will provide rapid and reliable signs if hypotension is too great for the fetus to withstand. Before the block is initiated, prehydration should be provided to a positive CVP not exceeding 6 cm of water. This level may represent an acceptable improvement. Further rapid volume administration may cause excessive hydration and pulmonary edema. A pulmonary artery catheter is indicated in patients having (a) refractory hypertension, (b) oliguria not responding to a modest fluid load, (c) suspected left ventricular failure that is likely to progress to congestive heart failure, (d) signs of developing pulmonary edema, or (e) superimposed cardiac disease (Table 17.7).

Prehydration before an epidural or subarachnoid block in the severe preeclamptic patient must be performed with great caution. Her decreased colloid oncotic pressure and damaged capillary endothelial integrity predispose her to rapid development of pulmonary edema, especially when large amounts of crystalloid hydrating solution are used. Before an epidural block for labor, where only a T10 sensory level is sought, 500 ml of a full-strength balanced salt solution or 0.9% saline solution **without dextrose** is usually adequate to prevent hypotension, provided the mother is not dehydrated (182, 186, 199). When high epidural block for cesarean section is sought (which requires a minimum upper sensory level of T4) larger amounts of prehydration are indicated. In the mild preeclamptic patient, 1 to 2 liters of balanced salt solution is usually adequate. However, in more severe preeclamptic patients with diastolic blood pressures in excess of 100 mm Hg, such rapid prehydration with crystalloid alone may not be adequate to prevent hypotension and may subject the mother to pulmonary edema. A colloid such as albumin may be helpful. In these patients, the authors prefer to initiate rapid prehydration with 1000 ml of crystalloid. If the central venous pressure remains at 0 or less, we usually use either 5% or 25% albumin to elevate it to a positive pressure before initiating the block, then extend the block slowly in steps with further hydration, as required to prevent hypotension using a balanced salt solution, or albumin, or both. When such an epidural block is allowed to dissipate, the mother must be observed for signs indicating the development of pulmonary edema. A falling blood pressure following an epidural block is initially treated with a small intravenous injection of ephedrine (2.5 to 5 mg), then a bolus of 50 to 100 ml of 25% albumin usually stabilizes the blood pressure. A rapidly rising

central venous pressure, a falling oxygen saturation, or both are indicative of impending pulmonary edema.

Epidural Block for Vaginal Delivery

Because labor tends to be rapid and painful in the preeclamptic patient, early placement of the epidural catheter in established labor is indicated. This practice eliminates the need for narcotic analgesia, which has a depressant effect on the fetus. Following an appropriate test dose to detect unrecognized intravascular or subarachnoid injection, the block is initiated with a small volume of local anesthetic such as 5 to 8 ml of 2% 2-chloroprocaine, 1% lidocaine, or 0.25% bupivacaine through the epidural catheter. A bilateral segmental sensory block that includes the dermatomes T10–L1 will provide satisfactory pain relief from uterine contractions. If blood pressure remains stable, this block may be repeated and increased to provide complete pain relief throughout the first stage of labor. The authors prefer to increase the volume and concentration of the local anesthetic (i.e., 10 to 12 ml of 1.5% lidocaine or 0.375 to 0.5% bupivacaine) once the patient's blood pressure is stabilized to obtain a minimum of a solid T8–S5 sensory block, which is maintained without interruption throughout labor and delivery. The addition of fentanyl (50 μg) to this first repeat dose of lidocaine or bupivacaine (but not to 2-chloroprocaine) improves the quality and prolongs the duration of the block without apparent ill effects on the fetus or newborn. We also add 1:400,000 epinephrine to additional doses of local anesthetic, again to improve the quality and duration of the block. Despite the objections to its use in preeclampsia as summarized by Robinson (215), no ill effects of its use have been noted (216–218). Such a block ensures (a) that the mother will not suddenly bear down and precipitously deliver a small baby, (b) that adequate perineal analgesia will be available for a wide episiotomy and operative delivery if required, and (c) that sufficient analgesia will be present to allow for the start of an emergency cesarean section as the block is quickly elevated. Furthermore, if an emergency cesarean section is necessary, rapidly raising the block to a T4 sensory level in a parturient with the minimum T8 sensory block is less likely to be associated with maternal hypotension than when the patient has a block with a lower sensory level. The increase in the sympathetic block will be less pronounced than when a higher sensory level is maintained. Although an epidural block of such height and density will take away the maternal urge to bear down in the second stage of labor, because the mother is alert and pain free, she is usually cooperative and can be coached to bear down effectively and on command with her contractions.

With the onset of the second stage of labor, sufficient additional local anesthetic is injected through the epidural catheter, if needed, to ensure complete perineal analgesia. Total perineal analgesia is desirable because it allows for operative vaginal delivery: It prevents uncontrollable bearing down by the mother, an occurrence that is associated with sudden changes in the cardiovascular and the central nervous systems, and it minimizes the likelihood of a precipitous delivery of a preterm or small neonate, an event that is associated with neonatal intracerebral hemorrhage.

In the past, continuous caudal epidural analgesia was used and recommended for analgesia in the preeclamptic patient. Its disadvantages include the need for larger doses of local anesthetic, a greater difficulty in placing the catheters, and the frequent inability to extend the block to an adequate level to allow for cesarean section without using potentially toxic doses of local anesthetics.

Subarachnoid Block for Vaginal Delivery

If vaginal delivery is imminent, a modified saddle block to a T10 sensory level can safely provide rapid and complete analgesia for vaginal delivery (219). The problem of sudden maternal hypotension is usually not great if the sensory level does not exceed T10, if left uterine displacement is ensured, and if the block is preceded with hydration. The disadvantages of modified saddle block are that it cannot be increased if the need for cesarean section arises and that postlumbar puncture headache occasionally occurs. This latter side effect can be minimized by using a 25- or 26-gauge spinal needle and entering the dura with the bevel facing the side or, alternatively, using a pencil-point needle such as the Whitacre or the newly designed Sprotte needle. To produce the required T10 sensory level, hyperbaric lidocaine (35 to 50 mg), bupivacaine (5 to 7.5 mg) or tetracaine (4 to 6 mg) are all satisfactory. The addition of 15 to 25 μg of fentanyl to the above solutions will improve the quality and prolong the duration of the block.

Cesarean Section

Cesarean section is often indicated in preeclampsia-eclampsia because of the deterioration of the intrauterine environment or the worsening of the mother's condition. If time allows and no contraindications (such as coagulation disorders) exist, the authors use continuous lumbar epidural anesthesia. The authors do not consider eclampsia to be a contraindication to the use of epidural anesthesia for either vaginal delivery or cesarean section, if convulsions are controlled and the mother is responsive. Medical therapy is continued, the mother is monitored and prehydrated, and left uterine displacement is ensured. Following placement of the epidural catheter and injection of a suitable test dose(s), a T10 sensory level is obtained by injection of 8 to 10 ml of 1.5 to 2% lidocaine or 0.5% bupivacaine. After the initial block is obtained and the maternal arterial and central venous pressures are stabilized, the sensory level is raised to a minimum T4 level in one or two stages by administering additional doses of local anesthetics. In the severely preeclamptic or eclamptic patient, an epidural block produced as described will require 30 min or longer to achieve, but it is rarely associated with severe maternal hypotension or fetal deterioration. The addition of 50 to 75 μg of fentanyl to the local anesthetic will (a) speed the onset of the block; (b) improve the quality of the block; (c) decrease visceral discomfort associated with uterine exteriorization, uterine interiorization, and peritoneal retraction; and (d) prolong the duration of the block without demonstrable ill effects on the fetus. At the conclusion of surgery, epidural injection of preservative-free morphine (3.5 to 5 mg) will provide up to 24 hr of excellent postoperative analgesia. After delivery and during closure, small amounts of intravenous narcotics and midazolam or diazepam are given if required for maternal sedation and comfort. In addition to the advantages discussed earlier, epidural anesthesia for cesarean section in preeclampsia-eclampsia eliminates the sudden maternal hypertension associated with induction to and emergence from general anesthesia, provides maternal cardiovascular and CNS stability (Fig. 17.10), and provides effective postoperative analgesia without producing significant maternal depression by infusions of low concentrations of local anesthetics or epidural narcotics.

Because subarachnoid block for cesarean section requires a minimum of a T4 sensory level, its use often is associated with a sudden and profound sympathetic block. Even when left uterine displacement and prehydration precede the block, sudden and marked maternal hypotension is common unless ephedrine is given prophylactically, a practice that may be risky in preeclampsia. Because of the risk of hypotension, which can be minimized by raising the sensory level of a continuous epidural block in stages, the authors prefer continuous lumbar epidural anesthesia for cesarean section in patients with severe preeclampsia or eclampsia. However, in the true emergency situation in which time does not permit initiation of a lumbar epidural for cesarean section and when it is not contraindicated by other factors, we strongly prefer the initiation of a subarachnoid block to the rapid sequence induction of general anesthesia for the severe preeclamptic patient. With great attention to detail, continuous monitoring of maternal blood pressure, and the use of small, repeated doses of intravenous ephedrine following adequate prehydration, one can safely use spinal anesthesia. Hyperbaric 5% lidocaine (70 to 80 mg), 0.75% bupivacaine (12 to 15 mg), or 0.5% tetracaine (9 to 11 mg) with epinephrine 100 to 200 μg are all satisfactory and will reliably produce a minimum T4 sensory level. The addition of 15 to 25 μg of fentanyl and 0.15 to 0.25 mg of preservative-free morphine to the local anesthetic solution will improve the quality of the block, diminish visceral discomfort, and provide prolonged continuous pain relief in the postoperative period (see Chapter 10). The problems of general anesthesia in severe preeclampsia-eclampsia and the means by which these problems can be overcome are discussed later.

A truly emergent cesarean section in preeclampsia is often required for severe, acute fetal distress. If the mother's blood pressure is stable, she is not severely hypovolemic, she has a functioning lumbar epidural catheter in place, and she has a sensory block, this block can be quickly increased by injecting a rapid-acting local anesthetic (i.e., 3% 2-chloroprocaine or 1.5 to 2% lidocaine) as the patient is being prepared, without delaying surgery. The administration of pH-adjusted, 2-chloroprocaine or lidocaine with 0.25 to 0.5 ml of 7.5 or 8.4% sodium bicarbonate per 10 ml and the addition of 50 to 75 μg fentanyl to the lidocaine may decrease the latency and prolong the duration of the block. As previously stated, in the true emergency, including nonominous fetal distress with no epidural catheter in place, the authors do not hesitate to use subarachnoid block in the severe preeclamptic patient if not contraindicated by other factors.

On rare occasions, general anesthesia is required for cesarean section in the severe preeclamptic mother. Its use usually indicates poor planning by the obstetrician, anesthesiologist or patient, unless used because other factors contraindicate lumbar epidural or subarachnoid block. Because of the markedly increased risks associated with the use of general anesthesia, it is essential for the mother to be adequately evaluated and monitored and for the anesthesiologist to have capable assistance before induction. The cry of "fetal distress, take her down" to save the baby is completely unjustified if it results in serious harm to or the death of the mother. The technique of general anesthesia described in Chapter 11 must be mod-

ified in the severe preeclamptic patient to allow for (a) increased upper airway edema; (b) interactions of anesthetic drugs with drugs used by the obstetrician, particularly magnesium; and (c) marked hypertensive responses to intubation, surgical stimulation, and later, extubation under light general anesthesia.

The increased upper airway edema associated with normal pregnancy is usually exacerbated in preeclampsia, at times to an extent that may seriously compromise the patient's airway (85, 86, 200–223, 249). Cases have been reported in which awake intubation or tracheostomy were required to maintain an open airway (86, 249). Severe uvular edema obstructing vision of the posterior pharynx has also been observed (86, 223). Before induction of general anesthesia, the airway must be thoroughly evaluated. If dysphonia, dysphoria, dyspnea, or respiratory distress are present, inspection of the larynx and vocal cords is mandatory with possible awake intubation or tracheostomy required. Unless the mucosa is decongested with phenylephrine or another vasoconstrictor (not recommended in preeclampsia-eclampsia), nasal suction, nasal intubation, or placement of a nasal airway or a nasogastric tube should be avoided to prevent brisk and often difficult to control epistaxis.

Because of the interaction of magnesium and muscle relaxants, the latter must be used with caution in preeclampsia. Defasciculation with a nondepolarizing relaxant is unnecessary, because magnesium usually accomplishes this (224). For endotracheal intubation, succinylcholine (1.5 mg/kg, not exceeding 120 mg) ensures rapid and complete relaxation. Additional relaxants should not be given unless the surgical field and response to a nerve stimulator indicate the need. When necessary, the authors prefer to use small (5 to 10 mg) bolus injections of succinylcholine rather than a succinylcholine infusion, which may result in overdose because of the significantly decreased levels of pseudocholinesterase found in the preeclamptic patient and the myoneural blocking properties of magnesium itself (90, 91, 125). The sensitivity to nondepolarizing muscle relaxants, including the intermediate-acting vecuronium, is markedly increased in patients receiving magnesium (126, 128, 225–227), and reversal at the conclusion of surgery may be prolonged. Hence, we avoid these relaxants. If nondepolarizing relaxants are used, only very small doses are given (e.g., vecuronium 1 to 2 mg) while monitoring the mother with a nerve stimulator. If, following delivery, one continues to administer two-thirds of the minimum alveolar concentration (MAC) of a potent inhalational agent combined with 60 to 70% nitrous oxide, supplemented as required with small doses of narcotic, additional doses of muscle relaxants are usually not required.

Endotracheal intubation, surgical stimulation, and emergence from light-balanced general anesthesia in normal patients are accompanied by significant increases in blood pressure, maternal heart rate, and circulating catecholamines (228). These increases can be extreme in the mother who has severe pregnancy-induced hypertension (Fig. 17.9) (181). In one study, elevation of the systolic pressure in hypertensive parturients averaged more than 56 mm Hg (187). Multiparous parturients older than 25 years of age appear to be at greatest risk for this severe blood pressure elevation (Fig. 17.11) (187). Means used to attenuate this response have included pretreatment with narcotics, magnesium, lidocaine, or (more frequently) antihypertensives. A recent study found that pretreatment with 1.5 mg/kg intravenous lidocaine before intubation was not effective in decreasing the hypertensive response in the preeclamptic patient when the injection of magnesium sulfate 40 mg/kg was for intubation but not for skin incision or extubation (229). Lawes and co-workers (188) found intravenous fentanyl (200 μg) and droperidol (5 mg) effective in the attenuation of the hypertensive response to intubation in 19 of 25 hypertensive parturients, without ill effects on the neonate. Allen and co-workers observed that the administration of alfentanil (10 μg/kg) 60 sec before intubation prevented significant hypertension in 24 preeclamptic patients; however, 17 of the neonates required naloxone and four neonates had low 1-min Apgar scores (152). Various antihypertensive drugs (i.e., hydralazine, β-blockers [labetalol, esmolol], trimethaphan, nitroglycerin, and nitroprusside) have been used to prevent acute hypertension during general anesthesia in the parturient, particularly during induction and endotracheal intubation. Table 17.9 outlines the advantages and disadvantages associated with each drug. The anesthetist must be prepared to prevent and immediately treat any severe hypertension or (on occasion) hypotension that occurs during general anesthesia.

Cesarean section with the patient receiving nitrous oxide and a muscle relaxant alone is often associated with maternal hypertension and recall of surgery. This practice also does not allow for administration of high concentrations of inspired oxygen ($FIO_2 > 0.5$), which is shown to be beneficial for both normal and asphyxiated fetuses during general anesthesia (243, 244). Adding up to two-thirds MAC of a potent inhalational drug (e.g., 0.5% halothane, 0.75% isoflurane, or 1.0% enflurane) overcomes these problems and ensures maternal analgesia and amnesia. Indeed, in cases of severe fetal distress using the potent inhalation anesthetics, initially at one and ½ MAC for the first minute, then at two-thirds MAC in oxygen alone until delivery, ensures adequate maternal amnesia and analgesia and maintains maternal oxygen saturation near 100%, desirable because of the left shift of the maternal oxygen hemoglobin dissociation curve in the preeclamptic patient (88, 89). The use of such low concentrations of potent inhalational drugs is not associated with decreased uterine activity, increased uterine bleeding, or neonatal depression (245–247). Ketamine, which is recommended for induction of general anesthesia in bleeding or asthmatic patients, is best avoided in preeclampsia because of its tendency to produce hypertension when full anesthetic doses (0.75 to 1 mg/kg) are used for induction. Throughout general or regional anesthesia those patients receiving magnesium should continue to receive it. Antihypertensive drugs should be given as required. During general anesthesia, monitoring the mother with a pulse oximeter and capnograph is becoming routine, with efforts made to keep the maternal oxygen saturation at 100% and not to allow the maternal end-tidal carbon dioxide level to fall below 25 mm Hg before delivery, which may be associated with a further leftward shift of the maternal oxygen-hemoglobin curve, predisposing to additional fetal hypoxia and fetal acidosis.

Postpartum Care of Mother and Neonate

As indicated previously, the neonate born of a preeclamptic-eclamptic mother is at higher risk for prematurity, for small-for-gestational-age size, for asphyxiation, drug-depression and for meconium aspiration (Table 17.10). If such a neonate is to survive intact, prompt and proper resuscitation is required. Respiratory distress, instability of body temperature, poor feeding, hypoglycemia, and hypocalcemia are all problems confronting these neonates. In the first days of life, intensive therapy is often required to ensure adequate monitoring and support. If available, it is prudent to admit the newborn of a severely preeclamptic or eclamptic mother directly to a neonatal intensive care unit rather than to the well-baby nursery.

The severely preeclamptic-eclamptic patient is prone to convulse or develop pulmonary edema within 24 hr of delivery. These events may occur as an epidural block dissipates (177, 180). If magnesium has been given, it should be continued, usually for 48 hr postpartum, or other longer acting oral anticonvulsants may be substituted. Similarly antihypertensive therapy is continued (as necessary) with longer act-

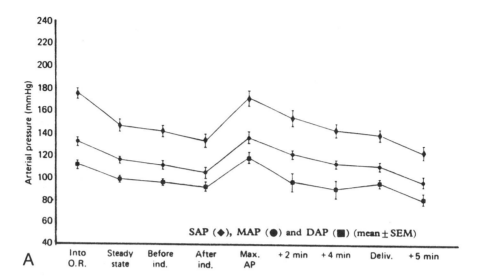

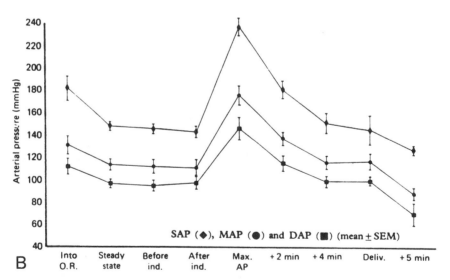

Figure 17.11. Responses of systolic arterial pressure (SAP), mean arterial pressure (MAP), and diastolic arterial pressure (DAP) in women undergoing cesarean section with general anesthesia, as follows: induction with lidocaine (1 mg/kg), etomidate (0.2 mg/kg), and suxamethonium (100 mg); intubation and maintenance with 50% nitrous oxide and 0.5% halothane. A, In 13 young (mean age, 20 years), low-parity women. B, In seven older (mean age, 30 years) multiparous women. Note the greater degree of hypertension in the group of older multiparous mothers. (Reprinted with permission from Connell H, Dalgleish JG, Downing JW: General anaesthesia in mothers with severe preeclampsia-eclampsia. Br J Anaesth 59:1375–1380, 1987.)

Table 17.9
Antihypertensive Drugs Used to Prevent or Treat Episodes of Hypertension during General Anesthesia

	Administration and Dose	Onset and Duration of Action	Effect on Uterine and Placental Blood Flow	Special Properties	
				Advantages	Disadvantages
Hydralazine Arteriolar vasodilator MW: 160 (References 136, 138, 139, 140, 158)	IV bolus: 5–10 mg IV infusion: 20 mg/500 ml (0.04 mg/ml)	Maximum effect requires 20–30 min after IV administration; duration about 2 hr	Originally thought to improve, this is now questioned	1. Easy to administer; no special equipment or monitoring required 2. Maintains maternal cardiac output 3. Long history of safe use in obstetrics	1. Slow unreliable onset 2. Maternal tachycardia 3. Decreased placental blood flow; fetal distress 4. Neonatal thrombocytopenia 5. Maternal nausea, vomiting, headache
Labetalol β_1 and α blocker; ?—β_2 agonist MW: 365 (References 134, 153, 154, 155, 158)	IV boluses: 10–20 mg up to total of 1–3 mg/kg	IV onset, 1–2 min; duration 2–3 hr	Improves uterine and placental blood flow	1. Easy to administer; no special equipment or monitoring required 2. Little risk of overshoot 3. No associated fetal bradycardia or distress 4. Improved placental blood flow 5. Few maternal side effects 6. Rapid onset 7. Becoming widely used by obstetricians and anesthesiologists	1. Large variation in effective dose 2. Alone, may not effectively decrease BP 3. Use with caution in patients with asthma, COPD, or compromised ventricular function
Trimethaphan Ganglionic blocker MW: 597 (References 230, 231, 232)	IV infusion: 1 mg/ml IV boluses: 1–4 mg	IV onset less than 1 min; duration less than 5 min	Minimal, if no severe maternal hypotension	1. Reliable—rapid acting 2. Large molecular weight limits fetal transfer 3. Rapid dissipation	1. May require arterial line for BP monitoring 2. Interferes with action of pseudocholinesterase, resulting in prolonged duration of succinylcholine 3. Histamine release (?) 4. May cause mydriasis
Nitroglycerin Venodilator MW: 227 (References 46, 175, 230, 233, 234, 235, 236)	Constant IV infusion: 5–50 μg/min Infusion: 25–50 mg/500 ml (50–100 μg/ml)	Onset less than 2 min; duration only a few minutes	Questionable, depends on state of maternal hydration; has been associated with fetal deterioration	1. Rapid onset and dissipation	1. Need IV pump to administer 2. Should make up in glass 3. May need arterial line 4. Great variation in response; if well-hydrated, not very effective (>60% failure rate)

Table 17.9
Antihypertensive Drugs Used to Prevent or Treat Episodes of Hypertension during General Anesthesia— Continued

	Administration and Dose	Onset and Duration of Action	Effect on Uterine and Placental Blood Flow	Special Properties	
				Advantages	Disadvantages
					5. Increased intra-cranial pressure
					6. Frequent nausea and vomiting
					7. Decreases cardiac index and oxygen delivery
Nitroprusside Direct-acting arterial vasodilator MW: 298 (References 186, 235, 237, 238, 239, 240, 241, 242)	Constant IV infusion: 0.05–10 μg/kg/hr Infusion: 50 mg/500 ml 5% dextrose in water (50 μg/ml)	Onset less than 1 min; duration only a few minutes	Dilates uterine artery in vitro; no ill effects unless severe hypotension present	1. Rapid onset and dissipation 2. Potent reliable antihypertensive 3. No ill effects on fetus	1. Unstable solution must protect from light 2. Easy to over-shoot; need A-line 3. Difficult to regulate 4. Increased intra-cranial pressure 5. Cyanide = toxicity; not a problem with short-term use and infusion <3 μg/k/hr 6. Tachyphylaxis

Table 17.10
Effect of Preeclampsia on Fetal and Neonatal Parameters[a]

Severity of Preeclampsia	Number of Cases	Prematurity (%)	Small for Gestational Age	Apgar Score <6 (%)	Meconium-Stained Amniotic Fluid (%)	Perinatal Death (%)
Mild	63	13	23	24	29	9
Moderate	67	16	39	39	38	16
Severe	38	45	48	48	29	37

[a] Reprinted by permission from Muller G, Philippe E, Lefakis P, M deMot-Leclair, Dreyfus J, Nusynowicz G, Renand R, Gandor R: Les lésions placentaires de la gestose: étude anatomoclinique. Gynecólogie Et Obstétrique 70:309, 1971.

ing preparations replacing intravenous infusions. The first 48 hr are as critical for such a patient as any other period of her prenatal course. Thus, in the severely preeclamptic or eclamptic patient, intensive care with continued monitoring, therapy, and pain relief are required if convulsions and other problems are to be avoided. Because of their expertise in pain relief and monitoring, anesthesiologists should have an important role in the postpartum management of severe preeclamptic or eclamptic mothers.

References

1. American College of Obstetricians and Gynecologists, Committee on Terminology. In Obstetric-Gynecologic Terminology. EC Hughes, ed. FA Davis, Philadelphia, 1972, pp 442–443.
2. Chesley LC: Diagnosis of preeclampsia (editorial). Obstet Gynecol 65:423–425, 1985.
3. Davey DA, MacGillivray I: The classification and definition of the hypertensive disorders of pregnancy. Am J Obstet Gynecol 158:892–898, 1988.
4. Sibai BM: Pitfalls in the diagnosis and management of preeclampsia (editorial). Am J Obstet Gynecol 159:1–5, 1988.

. Cunningham FG, MacDonald PC, Gant NF: Hypertensive disorders in pregnancy. In *Williams' Obstetrics*, 18th ed. Appleton & Lange, Norwalk, CT, 1989, pp 653–694.

6. U.S. Department of Health, Education, and Welfare: *The Collaborative Study on Cerebral Palsy, Mental Retardation and other Neurological and Sensory Disorders of Infancy and Childhood (Manual)*. U.S. Department of Health, Education and Welfare, Public Health Service, Bethesda, MD, 1966.

7. Saftlas AF, Olson DR, Franks AL, Atrash HK, Pokras R: Epidemiology of preeclampsia and eclampsia in the United States, 1979–1986. Am J Obstet Gynecol 163:460–465, 1990.

8. Pritchard JA, Cunningham FG, Prichard SA: The Parkland Memorial Hospital protocol for the treatment of eclampsia: Evaluation of 245 cases. Am J Obstet Gynecol 148:951–963, 1984.

9. Porapakkham S: An epidemiologic study of eclampsia. Obstet Gynecol 54:26–30, 1979.

10. Lopez-Liera M: Complicated eclampsia: Fifteen years' experience in a referral medical center. Am J Obstet Gynecol 142:28–35, 1982.

11. Moodley J, Naicker RS, Mankowitz E: Eclampsia—A method of management. S Africa Med J 63:530–535, 1983.

12. Hibbard BM, Rosen M: The management of severe preeclampsia and eclampsia. Br J Anaesth 49:3–9, 1977.

13. World Health Organization: WHO international collaborative study of hypertensive disorders of pregnancy: Geographic variation in the incidence of hypertension in pregnancy. Am J Obstet Gynecol 158:80–83, 1988.

14. Garner PR, D'Alton ME, Dudley DK, Huard P, Hardie M: Preeclampsia in diabetic pregnancies. Am J Obstet Gynecol 163:505–508, 1990.

15. Khong TY, DeWolfe F, Robertson WB, Brosens I: Inadequate maternal vascular response to placentation in pregnancies complicated by preeclampsia and by small-for-gestational-age infants. Br J Obstet Gynecol 93:1049–1059, 1986.

16. Ducey J, Schulman H, Farmakides G: A classification of pregnancy based on Doppler velocimetry. Am J Obstet Gynecol 157:860–864, 1987.

17. Kaar K, Jouppila P, Kuikka J, Luotola H, Toivanen J, Rekonen A: Intervillous blood flow in normal and complicated late pregnancy measured by means of an intravenous ^{133}Xe method. Acta Obstet Gynecol Scand 59:7–10, 1980.

18. Saleh AA, Bottoms SF, Welch RA, Abdelkarim MA, Mariona FG: Preeclampsia, delivery and the hemostatic system. Am J Obstet Gynecol 157:331–336, 1987.

19. Rogers GM, Taylor RN, Roberts JM: Preeclampsia is associated with a serum factor cytotoxic to human endothelial cells. Am J Obstet Gynecol 159:908–914, 1988.

20. Roberts JM, Taylor RN, Musci TJ, Rodgers GM, Hubel CA, McLaughlin MK: Preeclampsia: An endothelial cell disorder. Am J Obstet Gynecol 161:1200–1204, 1989.

21. Taylor RN, Varma M, Teng NH, Roberts JM: Women with preeclampsia have higher plasma endothelin levels than women with normal pregnancies. J Clin Endocrin Metab 71:1675–1677, 1990.

22. Liston WA, Kilpatrick DC: Preeclampsia—An endothelial cell disorder plus "something else" (letter). Am J Obstet Gynecol 163:1365–1366, 1990.

23. Schrier RW, Briner VA: Peripheral arterial vasodilation and water retention in pregnancy: Implications for pathogenesis of preeclampsia-eclampsia. Obstet Gynecol 77:632–639, 1991.

24. Musci TJ, Roberts JM, Rodgers GM, Taylor RN: Mitogenic activity is increased in the sera of preeclamptic women before delivery. Am J Obstet Gynecol 159:1446–1451, 1988.

25. Barton JR, Hiett AK, O'Connor WN, Nissen SE, Greene JW Jr: Endomyocardial ultrastructural findings in preeclampsia. Am J Obstet Gynecol 165:389–391, 1991.

26. Shanklin DR, Sibai BM: Ultrastructural aspects of preeclampsia. I. Placental bed and uterine boundary vessels. Am J Obstet Gynecol 161:735–741, 1989.

27. Bhatia RK, Bottoms SF, Saleh AA, Norman GS, Mammen EF, Sokol RJ: Mechanisms for reduced colloid osmotic pressure in preeclampsia. Am J Obstet Gynecol 157:106–108, 1987.

28. Walsh SW: Preeclampsia: An imbalance in placental prostacyclin and thromboxane production. Am J Obstet Gynecol 152:335–340, 1985.

29. Goodman RP, Killam AP, Brash AR, Branch RA: Prostacyclin production during pregnancy: Comparison of production during normal pregnancy and pregnancy complicated by hypertension. Am J Obstet Gynecol 142:817–822, 1982.

30. Nelson DM, Walsh SW: Aspirin differentially affects thromboxane and prostacyclin production by trophoblast and villous core compartments of human placental villi. Am J Obstet Gynecol 161:1593–1598, 1989.

31. Wallenburg HCS, Dekker CA, Makovitz JW, Rotmans D: Low-dose aspirin prevents pregnancy-induced hypertension and preeclampsia in angiotensin-sensitive primagravidae. Lancet 1:1–3, 1986.

32. Benigni A, Gregorini G, Frusca T, Chiabrando C, Ballerini S, Valeamonico A, Orisio S, Piccinell A, Pineiroli V, Fanelli R: Effect of low dose aspirin on fetal and maternal generation of thromboxane by platelets in women at high risk of pregnancy-induced hypertension. N Engl J Med 321:357–362, 1989.

33. Lubbe WF: Prevention of preeclampsia by low-dose aspirin. N Z Med J 103:237–238, 1990.

34. Keith JC Jr, Thatcher CD, Schaub RG: Beneficial effects of U-63, 557A, a thromboxane synthetase inhibitor, in an ovine model of pregnancy-induced hypertension. Am J Obstet Gynecol 157:199–203, 1987.

35. Toppodaza MK, Ismail AAA, Hegab HM, Kamel MA: Treatment of preeclampsia with prostaglandin A₁. Am J Obstet Gynecol 159:160–165, 1988.

36. Walsh SW, Coulter S: Increased placental progesterone may cause decreased placental prostacyclin production in preeclampsia. Am J Obstet Gynecol 161:1586–1592, 1989.

37. Sibai BM, Akl S, Fairlie F, Moretti M: A protocol for managing severe preeclampsia in the second trimester. Am J Obstet Gynecol 163:733–738, 1990.

38. Speroff L: Toxemia of pregnancy: Mechanism and therapeutic management. Am J Cardiol 32:582–591, 1973.

39. Easterling TR, Benedetti TJ: Preeclampsia: A hyperdynamic disease model. Am J Obstet Gynecol 160:1447–1453, 1989.

40. Cotton DB, Lee W, Huhta JC, Dorman KF: Hemodynamic profile of severe pregnancy-induced hypertension. Am J Obstet Gynecol 158:523–529, 1988.

41. Mabie WC, Ratts TE, Sibai BM: The central hemodynamics of severe preeclampsia. Am J Obstet Gynecol 161:1443–1448, 1989.

42. Easterling TR, Benedetti TD, Schmucker BC: Maternal cardiac output in preeclamptic pregnancies: A longitudinal study. In *Abstracts of Scientific Papers*, Society for Obstetric Anesthesia and Perinatology, 1989, Seattle, p 4.

43. Phelan JP, Yurth DA: Severe preeclampsia. I. Peripartum hemodynamic observations. Am J Obstet Gynecol 144:17–22, 1982.

44. Joyce TH III, Debnath KS, Baker EA: Preeclampsia-relationship of CVP and epidural analgesia. Anesthesiology 51:S297, 1979.

45. Tellez R, Curiel R: Relationship between central venous pressure and pulmonary capillary wedge pressure in severely toxemic patients (letter). Am J Obstet Gynecology 165:487, 1991.

46. Cotton DB, Longmire S, Jones MM, Dorman KF, Tessem J, Joyce TH III: Cardiovascular alterations in severe pregnancy-induced hypertension: Effects of intravenous nitroglycerin coupled with blood volume expansion. Am J Obstet Gynecol 154:1053–1059, 1986.

47. Clark SL, Cotton DB: Clinical indications for pulmonary artery catheterization in the patient with severe preeclampsia. Am J Obstet Gynecol 158:453–458, 1988.

48. Clark SL: Reliance on central venous pressure with regard

to fluid management in preeclampsia deemed dangerous (letter). Am J Obstet Gynecol 162:598, 1990.

49. Fliegner JR: Correction of hypovolemia and central venous pressure monitoring in the management of severe preeclampsia and eclampsia. Am J Obstet Gynecol 156:1041–1042, 1987.

50. Woodward DG, Romanoff ME: Is central venous pressure monitoring "contraindicated" in patients with severe preeclampsia (letter)? Am J Obstet Gynecol 161:837–839, 1989.

51. Goodlin RC: Pulmonary artery catheterization in severe preeclampsia (letter). Am J Obstet Gynecol 162:601–603, 1990.

52. Hays PM, Cruikshank DP, Dunn LJ: Plasma volume determination in normal and preeclamptic pregnancies. Am J Obstet Gynecol 151:958–966, 1985.

53. Sibai BM, Abdella TN, Anderson GD, Dilts PV Jr: Plasma findings in pregnant women with mild hypertension: Therapeutic considerations. Am J Obstet Gynecol 145:539–544, 1983.

54. Bletka M, Hlavatj V, Trnková M, Bendl J, Bendova L, Chytil M: Volume of whole blood and absolute amount of serum proteins in the early stages of toxemia of pregnancy. Am J Obstet Gynecol 106:10–13, 1970.

55. Nguyen NH, Clark SL, Greenspoon J, Diesfield P, Wu PYK: Peripartum colloid osmotic pressure: Correlation with serum proteins. Obstet Gynecol 68:807–810, 1986.

56. Benedetti TJ, Carlson RW: Studies of colloid osmotic pressure in pregnancy-induced hypertension. Am J Obstet Gynecol 135:308–311, 1979.

57. Joyce TH III, Longmire S, Tessem JH, Baker BW, Jones MM: Creation of pregnancy induced hypertension model in the pregnant ewe. Anesthesiology 67:A455, 1987.

58. Sibai BM, Mabie BC, Harvey CJ, Gonzalez AR: Pulmonary edema in severe preeclampsia-eclampsia: Analysis of 37 consecutive cases. Am J Obstet Gynecol 156:1174–1179, 1987.

59. Strauss RG, Keefer JR, Burke T, Civetta JH: Hemodynamic monitoring of cardiogenic pulmonary edema complicating toxemia of pregnancy. Obstet Gynecol 55:170–174, 1980.

60. Keefer JR, Strauss RJ, Civetta JM, Burke T: Non-cardiogenic pulmonary edema and invasive cardiac monitoring. Obstet Gynecol 58:46–51, 1981.

61. Benedetti TJ, Cotton DB, Read JC, Miller FC: Hemodynamic observations in severe pre-eclampsia with a flow-directed pulmonary artery catheter. Am J Obstet Gynecol 136:465–470, 1980.

62. Cotton DB, Gonik B, Dorman K, Harrist R: Cardiovascular alterations in severe pregnancy-induced hypertension: Relationship of central venous pressure to pulmonary capillary wedge pressure. Am J Obstet Gynecol 151:762–764, 1985.

63. Newsome LR, Bramwell RS, Curling PE: Severe preeclampsia: Hemodynamic effects of lumbar epidural analgesia. Anesth Analg 65:31–36, 1986.

64. Abboud T, Artal R, Sarkis F, Henriksen EH, Kammula RK: Sympathoadrenal activity, maternal, fetal and neonatal responses after epidural anesthesia in the preeclamptic patient. Am J Obstet Gynecol 144:915–918, 1982.

65. August P, Lenz T, Ales KL, Druzin ML, Edersheim TG, Hutson JM, Müller FB, Laragh JH, Sealey JE: Longitudinal study of the renin-angiotensin aldosterone system in hypertensive pregnant women: Deviations related to the development of superimposed preeclampsia. Am J Obstet Gynecol 163:1612–1621, 1990.

66. Leighton BL, Norris MC, DeSimone CA, Darby MJ, Menduke H: Pre-eclamptic and healthy term pregnant patients have different chronotropic responses to isoproterenol (letter). Anesthesiology 72:392–393, 1990.

67. Richards N, Noodley J, Graham DJ, Bullock MRR: Active management of the unconscious eclamptic patient. Br J Obstet Gynaecol 93:554–562, 1986.

68. Buchan PC: Preeclampsia: A hyperviscosity syndrome. Am J Obstet Gynecol 142:111–112, 1982.

69. Kelton JG, Hunter DJS, Neame P: A platelet function defect in preeclampsia. Obstet Gynecol 65:107–109, 1985.

70. deBoer K, Leconder I, ten Cate JW, Borm JJJ, Treffers PE: Placenta-type plasminogen activator inhibitor in preeclampsia. Am J Obstet Gynecol 158:518–522, 1988.

71. Sibai BM, Anderson CD, McCubbin JH: Eclampsia. II. Clinical significance of laboratory findings. Obstet Gynecol 59:153–157, 1982.

72. Burrows RF, Hunter DJF, Andrew M, Keltow JG: A prospective study investigating the mechanism of thrombocytopenia in preeclampsia. Obstet Gynecol 70:334–338, 1987.

73. Ramanathan J, Sibai BM, Vu T, Chauhan D: Correlation between bleeding times and platelet counts in women with preeclampsia undergoing cesarean section. Anesthesiology 71:188–191, 1991.

74. Katz VL, Thorp JM, Rozas LS, Bowes WA Jr: The natural history of thrombocytopenia associated with preeclampsia. Am J Obstet Gynecol 163:1142–1143, 1990.

75. Rasmus KT, Rottman RL, Kotelko DM, Wright WC, Stone JJ, Rosenblatt RM: Unrecognized thrombocytopenia and regional anesthesia in parturients: A retrospective review. Obstet Gynecol 73:943–946, 1989.

75a. Channing-Rogers RP, Levin J: A critical review of the bleeding time. Semin Thromb Hemost 16:1–20, 1990.

75b. The bleeding time (editorial). Lancet 337:1447–1448, 1991.

76. Trudinger BJ: Platelets and intrauterine growth retardation in preeclampsia. Br J Obstet Gynaecol 83:284–286, 1976.

77. Prichard JA, Cunningham FG, Mason RG: Coagulation changes in eclampsia, their frequency and pathogenesis. Am J Obstet Gynecol 124:855–864, 1976.

78. Weinstein L: Syndrome of hemolysis, elevated liver enzymes and low platelet count: A severe consequence of hypertension in pregnancy. Am J Obstet Gynecol 142:159–167, 1982.

79. Sibai BM: The HELLP syndrome (hemolysis, elevated liver enzymes and low platelets): Much ado about nothing. Am J Obstet Gynecol 162:311–316, 1990.

80. VanDam PA, Renier M, Baekelandt TM, Buytaert P, Ugttenbroeck F: Disseminated intravascular coagulation and the syndrome of hemolysis, elevated liver enzymes and low platelets in severe preeclampsia. Obstet Gynecol 73:97–102, 1989.

81. Martin JN Jr, Blake PE, Lowry SI, Perry KG, Files JC, Morrison JC: Pregnancy complicated by preeclampsia-eclampsia with the syndrome of hemolysis, elevated liver enzymes, and low platelet count: How rapid is postpartum recovery? Obstet Gynecol 76:737–741, 1990.

82. Martin JN, Blake PG, Perry KG Jr, McCaul JF, Hess LW, Martin RW: The natural history of HELLP syndrome: Patterns of disease progression and regression. Am J Obstet Gynecol 164:1500–1513, 1991.

83. Martin JN Jr, Files JC, Blake PG, Norman PH, Martin RW, Hess LW, Morrison JC, Wiser WL: Plasma exchange for preeclampsia. I. Postpartum use for presently severe preeclampsia-eclampsia with HELLP syndrome. Am J Obstet Gynecol 162:126–137, 1990.

84. Ramanathan J, Khalil M, Sibai BM, Chauhan D: Anesthetic management of the syndrome of hemolysis, elevated liver enzymes, and low platelet count (HELLP) in preeclampsia, a retrospective study. Reg Anesth 13:20–24, 1988.

85. Seager SJ, MacDonald R: Laryngeal edema and preeclampsia, a case report. Anaesthesia 35:360–362, 1980.

86. Heller PJ, Scheider EP, Marx GF: Pharyngolaryngeal edema as a presenting symptom in preeclampsia. Obstet Gynecol 62:523–524, 1983.

87. Rees GB, Pipkin FB, Symonds EM, Patrick JM: A longitudinal study of respiratory changes in normal human pregnancy with cross-sectional data on subjects with pregnancy-induced hypertension. Am J Obstet Gynecol 162:826–830, 1990.

88. Kambam JR, Handte RE, Brown WV, Smith BE: Effect of normal and preeclamptic pregnancies on oxyhemoglobin dissociation. Anesthesiology 65:426–427, 1986.

89. Kambam JR, Entman S, Mouton S, Smith BE: Effect of preeclampsia on carboxyhemoglobin levels: A mechanism for a decrease in P_{50}. Anesthesiology 68:433–434, 1988.

90. Kambam JR, Mouton S, Entman S, Sastry BVR, Smith BE:

Effect of preeclampsia on plasma cholinesterase activity. Can J Anaesth 34:509–511, 1987.

91. Kambam JR, Perry SM, Entman S, Smith BE: Effect of magnesium on plasma cholinesterase activity. Am J Obstet Gynecol 69:A697, 1988.

92. Kambam JR, Perry SM, Entman S, Smith BE: Effect of magnesium on plasma cholinesterase activity. Am J Obstet Gynecol 159:309–311, 1988.

93. Fay RA, Bromham DR, Brooks JA, Chir B, Gebski VJ: Platelets and uric acid in the prediction of preeclampsia. Am J Obstet Gynecol 152:1038–1039, 1985.

94. Gaber LW, Spargo BH, Lindheimer MD: Renal pathology in preeclampsia. Clin Obstet Gynaecol 1:971–995, 1987.

95. Sibai BM, Villar MA, Mabie BC: Acute renal failure in hypertensive disorders of pregnancy: Pregnancy outcome and remote prognosis in thirty-one consecutive cases. Am J Obstet Gynecol 162:777–783, 1990.

96. Nochy D, Hinglais N, Jacquot C, Gaudry C, Remy P, Bariety J: De novo focal glomerular sclerosis in preeclampsia. Clin Nephrol 24:221–227, 1986.

97. Lee W, Gonik B, Cotton DB: Urinary diagnostic indices in preeclampsia-associated oliguria: Correlation with invasive hemodynamic monitoring. Am J Obstet Gynecol 156:100–103, 1987.

98. Clark SL, Greenspoon JS, Aldahl D, Phelan JP: Severe preeclampsia with persistent oliguria: Management of hemodynamic subsets. Am J Obstet Gynecol 154:490–494, 1986.

99. Sibai BN, Spinnato JA, Anderson GD: Eclampsia. V. The incidence of nonpreventable eclampsia. Am J Obstet Gynecol 154:581–590, 1986.

99a. Lunell NO, Nylund NE, Lewander R, Sarby B: Uteroplacental blood flow in preeclampsia: Measurements with indium 133m and a computer linked gamma camera. Clin Exp Hypertens 1:105–117, 1982.

100. Hibbard LT: Maternal mortality due to acute toxemia. Obstet Gynecol 42:263–270, 1973.

101. Naeye RL, Friedman EA: Causes of perinatal death associated with gestational hypertension and proteinuria. Am J Obstet Gynecol 133:8–10, 1979.

102. Taylor DJ, Howie PW, Davidson J, Davidson D, Drillien CM: Do pregnancy complications contribute to neurodevelopmental disability? Lancet 1:713–716, 1985.

103. Odendaal HJ, Pattinson RC, Bam R, Grove D, Kotze TJW: Aggressive or expectant management for patients with severe preeclampsia between 28–34 weeks' gestation: A randomized controlled trial. Obstet Gynecol 76:1070–1075, 1990.

104. Sibai BM, Taslimi M, Abdella TN, Brooks TF, Spinnato JA, Anderson G: Maternal and perinatal outcome of conservative management of severe preeclampsia in midtrimester. Am J Obstet Gynecol 152:32–37, 1985.

105. Platt LD, Walla CA, Paul RH, Trujillo ME, Loesser CV, Jacobs ND, Broussard PM: A prospective trial of the fetal biophysical profile versus the nonstress test in the management of high risk pregnancies. Am J Obstet Gynecol 153:624–633, 1985.

106. Atkinson SM Jr: Salt water and rest as a preventative for toxemia of pregnancy. J Reprod Med 9:223–228, 1972.

107. Sullivan JM: Blood pressure elevation in pregnancy. Prog Cardiovasc Dis 16:375–393, 1974.

108. Lindheimer MD, Katz AI: Preeclampsia: Pathophysiology, diagnosis and management. Ann Rev Med 40:233–250, 1989.

109. Sehgal NN, Hitt JR: Plasma volume expansion in the treatment of preeclampsia. Am J Obstet Gynecol 138:165–168, 1980.

110. Gallery ED, Mitchell MD, Redman CW: Fall in blood pressure in response to volume expansion in pregnancy associated hypertension (pre-eclampsia): Why does it occur? J Hypertens 2:177–182, 1984.

111. Siekmann U, Heilmann L, Klosa W, Quaas L, Schilliniger H: Simultaneous investigations of maternal cardiac output and fetal blood flow during hypervolemic hemodilution in preeclampsia: Preliminary observations. J Perinat Med 14:59–69, 1986.

112. Kirskon B, Moise KJ, Cotton DB, Longmire S, Jones M, Tessem J, Joyce TA III: Role of volume expansion in severe preeclampsia. Surg Gynecol Obstet 167:367–371, 1988.

113. Page EW: On the pathogenesis of preeclampsia and eclampsia. J Obstet Gynaecol Br Commonw 79:833–894, 1972.

114. Sims EAH: Pre-eclampsia and related complications of pregnancy. Am J Obstet Gynecol 107:154–181, 1970.

115. Ferris TF: Toxemia and hypertension. In *Medical Complications of Pregnancy*. GN Burrows, TF Ferris, eds. Saunders, Philadelphia, 1988, pp 1–33.

116. Davidson JM, Lindheimer MD: Hypertension in pregnancy. In *Diseases of the Kidney*, 4th ed. RW Schrier, CW Gottschalk, eds. Little Brown, Boston, 1988, pp 1653–1688.

117. Borges LF, Gucer G: Effects of magnesium on epileptic foci. Epilepsia 19:81, 1978.

118. Shelly WC, Gutsche BB: Magnesium and seizure control (letter). Am J Obstet Gynecol 136:146–147, 1980.

119. Thurnau GR, Kemp DB, Jarvis A: Cerebrospinal fluid levels of magnesium in patients with preeclampsia after treatment with magnesium sulfate: A preliminary report. Am J Obstet Gynecol 157:1435–1438, 1987.

120. Mokriski BLK, Malinow AM, Martz DG, Matjasko MJ: MgSO$_4$ and EEG effects in preeclampsia. Anesthesiology 69:A696, 1988.

121. Sibai BM: Magnesium sulfate is the ideal anticonvulsant in preeclampsia-eclampsia. Am J Obstet Gynecol 162:1141–1145, 1990.

122. Lipman J, James MFM, Erskine J, Plit ML, Eidelman J, Esser JD: Autonomic dysfunction in severe tetanus: Magnesium sulfate as an adjunct to deep sedation. Crit Care Med 15:987–988, 1987.

123. James MEM, Beer RE, Esser JD: Intravenous magnesium sulfate inhibits catecholamine release associated with tracheal intubations. Anesth Analg 68:772–776, 1989.

124. Cotton DB, Gonik B, Dorman KF: Cardiovascular alterations in severe pregnancy-induced hypertension: Acute effects of intravenous magnesium sulfate. Am J Obstet Gynecol 148:162–165, 1984.

124a. Sadeh M: Action of magnesium sulfate in the treatment of preeclampsia-eclampsia. Stroke 20:1273–1275, 1989.

125. Ramanathan J, Sibai BM, Pillai R, Angel JJ: Neuromuscular transmission studies in preeclamptic women receiving magnesium sulfate. Am J Obstet Gynecol 158:40–46, 1988.

126. Ghoneim MM, Long JP: Interaction between magnesium and other neuromuscular blocking agents. Anesthesiology 32:23–27, 1970.

127. Giesecke AG, Morris RE, Dalton MD, Stephen CR: On magnesium muscle relaxants, toxemic parturients and cats. Anesth Analg 47:689–695, 1980.

128. Sinatra RS, Philip BK, Naulty JS, Ostheimer JS: Prolonged neuromuscular blockade with vecuronium in a patient treated with magnesium sulfate. Anesth Analg 64:1220–1222, 1985.

129. Kelleher JF, Millar WL, Reisner LS: The effect of intravenous magnesium sulfate on the bleeding time in healthy volunteers. Anesthesiology 71:A887, 1989.

130. Stone SR, Prichard JA: Effect of maternally administered magnesium sulfate on the neonate. Obstet Gynecol 35:574–577, 1970.

131. Green KW, Key TC, Coen R, Resnik R: The effects of maternally administered magnesium sulfate on the neonate. Am J Obstet Gynecol 146:29–33, 1983.

132. Pruett KM, Kirshon B, Cotton DB, Adam K, Doody KJ: The effects of magnesium sulfate therapy on Apgar scores. Am J Obstet Gynecol 159:1047–1048, 1988.

133. Naden RP, Redman CWG: Antihypertensive drugs in pregnancy. Clin Perinatol 12:521–538, 1985.

134. Sibai BM, Gonzalez AR, Mabie WC, Moretti M: A comparison of labetalol plus hospitalization versus hospitalization alone in the management of preeclampsia remote from term. Obstet Gynecol 70:323–327, 1987.

135. Sibai BM, Mabie WC, Shamson F, Villar MA, Anderson GD: A comparison of no medication versus methyldopa or la-

betalol in chronic hypertension during pregnancy. Am J Obstet Gynecol 162:960–967, 1990.

136. Jouppila P, Kirkinen P, Koivula A, Ylikorkala O: Effects of dihydralazine infusion on the fetoplacental blood flow and maternal prostanoids. Obstet Gynecol 65:115–118, 1985.

137. Lunell NO, Lewander R, Nylund L, Sarby B, Thornstrom S: Acute effect of dihydralazine on uteroplacental blood flow in hypertension during pregnancy. Gynecol Obstet Invest 16:274–282, 1983.

138. Lipshitz J, Ahokas RA, Reynolds SL: The effect of hydralazine on placental perfusion in the spontaneously hypertensive rat. Am J Obstet Gynecol 156:356–359, 1987.

139. Vink GJ, Moodley J: The effect of low-dose dihydralazine on the fetus in the emergency treatment of hypertension in pregnancy. S Afr Med J 62:475–477, 1982.

140. Lindheimer MD, Katz AI: Current concepts: Hypertension in pregnancy (medical intelligence). N Engl Med J 313:675–680, 1985.

141. Cockburn J, Moar VA, Olmstead M, Redman CW: Final report of study on hypertension during pregnancy: The effects of specific treatment on the growth and development of the children. Lancet 1:647–649, 1982.

142. Horvath JS, Phippard A, Korda A, Henderson-Smart DJ, Child A, Tiller DJ: Clonidine hydrochloride: A safe and effective antihypertensive in pregnancy. Obstet Gynecol 66:634–638, 1985.

143. Rubin PC, Butters L, Clark DM, Reynolds B, Summer DJ, Steedman D, Low RA, Reid JL: Placebo-controlled trial of atenolol in treatment of pregnancy induced hypertension. Lancet 1:431–434, 1983.

144. Rubin PC: Beta blockers in pregnancy (editorial). Br J Obstet Gynaecol 94:292–293, 1987.

145. Mouton S, Liedholm H, Lingman G, Marsal K, Sjoborg NO, Solum T: Fetal and uteroplacental haemodynamics during short term atenolol treatment of hypertension in pregnancy. Br J Obstet Gynaecol 94:312–317, 1987.

146. Liedholm H, Melander A: Drug selection in treatment of pregnancy hypertension. Acta Obstet Gynecol Scand 118(Suppl):49–55, 1984.

147. Gold MI, Sacks DJ, Grosnoff DB, Herrington C, Skillman CA: Use of esmolol during anesthesia to treat tachycardia and hypertension. Anesth Analg 68:101–104, 1989.

148. Eisenach JB, Castro MI: Maternally administered esmolol produces fetal β-adrenergic blockade and hypoxemia in sheep. Anesthesiology 71:718–722, 1989.

149. MacCarthy PE, Bloomfield SS: Labetalol: A review of its pharmacology, pharmacokinetics, clinical uses and adverse effects. Pharmacotherapy 3:193–219, 1983.

150. Baum T, Sybertz EJ: Pharmacology of labetalol in experimental animals. Am J Med 75(Suppl):15–23, 1983.

151. Rogers RC, Sherif AKL, Sibai BM: Nifedipine pharmacokinetics in pregnancy-induced hypertension. In Abstracts of Scientific Papers, Society of Perinatal Obstetricians, Houston, 1990, p 63.

152. Ahokas RA, Mabie WC, Sibai BM, Anderson GD: Labetalol does not decrease placental perfusion in the hypertensive term-pregnant rat. Am J Obstet Gynecol 160:480–484, 1989.

153. Eisenach JC, Mandell G, Dewan DM: Maternal and fetal effects of labetalol in pregnant ewes. Anesthesiology 74:292–297, 1991.

154. Jouppila P, Kirkinew PS, Koivula A, Ylikorkala O: Labetalol does not alter the placental and fetal blood flow or maternal prostanoids in preeclampsia. Br J Obstet Gynaecol 93:543–547, 1986.

155. Ramanathan J, Sibai BM, Mabie WC, Chauhan D, Ruiz AG: The use of labetalol for attenuation of the hypertensive responsive to endotracheal intubation in preeclampsia. Am J Obstet Gynecol 159:650–654, 1988.

156. Pickles CJ, Symonds EM, Pipkin FB: The fetal outcome in a randomized double-blind controlled trial of labetalol versus placebo in pregnancy induced hypertension. Br J Obstet Gynaecol 96:38–43, 1989.

157. Davey DA, Dommisse J, Garden A: Intravenous labetalol and intravenous dihydralazine in severe hypertension in pregnancy. In The Investigation of Labetalol in the Management of Hypertension in Pregnancy. A Riley, EM Symonds, eds. Exerpta Medica, Oxford-Princeton, Amsterdam, 1982, pp 51–61.

158. Mabie WC, Gonzalez AR, Sibai BM, Amon E: A comparative trial of labetalol and hydralazine in the acute management of severe hypertension complicating pregnancy. Obstet Gynecol 70:328–333, 1987.

159. Norris MC, Rose JC, Dewan DM: Nifedipine or verapamil counteracts hypertension in gravid ewes. Anesthesiology 65:254–258, 1986.

160. Walters BNJ, Redman CWG: Treatment of severe pregnancy associated hypertension with the calcium antagonist nifedipine. Br J Obstet Gynaecol 91:330–336, 1984.

161. Fenakel K, Fenakel G, Appelman Z, Lurie S, Katz Z, Shoham Z: Nifedipine in the treatment of severe preeclampsia. Obstet Gynecol 77:331–337, 1991.

162. Moretti MM, Fairlie FM, Akl S, Khoury AD, Sibai BM: The effect of nifedipine therapy on fetal and placental Doppler waveforms in preeclampsia remote from term. Am J Obstet Gynecol 163:1844–1848, 1990.

163. Barton JR, Hiett AK, Conover WB: The use of nifedipine during the postpartum period in patients with severe preeclampsia. Am J Obstet Gynecol 162:788–792, 1990.

164. Waisman GD, Magorga LM, Camera MI, Vignolo CA, Martinotti A: Magnesium plus nifedipine: Potentiation of hypotensive effect in preeclampsia. Am J Obstet Gynecol 159:308–309, 1988.

165. Lindeman KS, Hirshman CA, Freed AN: Magnesium sulfate resembles a calcium channel blocker in airway smooth muscle. Anesthesiology 69:A699, 1988.

166. Rogers RC, Sibai BM, Whybrew WD: Labetalol pharmacokinetics in pregnancy induced hypertension. Am J Obstet Gynecol 162:362–366, 1990.

167. Neuman J, Weiss B, Rabello Y, Cabalt L, Freeman RK: Diaxide for the acute control of severe hypertension complicating pregnancy: A pilot study. Obstet Gynecol 53:50S–55S, 1979.

168. Weiner CP, Socol ML, Vaisrub N: Control of preeclamptic hypertension by ketanserin, a new serotonin receptor antagonist. Am J Obstet Gynecol 149:496–500, 1984.

169. Hulme VA, Odendaal HJ: Intrapartum treatment of preeclamptic hypertension by Katanserin. Am J Obstet Gynecol 155:260–263, 1986.

170. Jacobson SL, Imhof R, Manning N, Manniou V, Little D, Rey E, Redman C: The value of Doppler assessment of the uteroplacental circulation in predicting preeclampsia or intrauterine growth retardation. Am J Obstet Gynecol 162:110–114, 1990.

171. Kenepp NE, Kumar S, Shelley WC, Stanley CA, Gabbe SA, Gutsche BB: Fetal and neonatal hazards of maternal hydration with 5% dextrose before cesarean section. Lancet 1:1150–1152, 1982.

172. Joyce TH III, Loon M: Preeclampsia: Effect of albumin 25% infusion. Anesthesiology 55:A313, 1981.

173. Jones MM, Longmire S, Cotton DB, Dorman KF, Skjonsby BS, Joyce TH III: Influence of crystalloid versus colloid infusion on peripartum colloid osmotic pressure changes. Obstet Gynecol 66:659–661, 1986.

174. Benedetti TJ, Kates R, Williams V: Hemodynamic observations in severe preeclampsia complicated by pulmonary edema. Am J Obstet Gynecol 152:330–334, 1985.

175. Cotton DB, Jones MM, Longmire SS, Dorman KF, Tessem J, Joyce TH III: Role of intravenous nitroglycerin in the treatment of severe pregnancy-induced hypertension complicated by pulmonary edema. Am J Obstet Gynecol 154:91–93, 1986.

176. Wasserstrum N, Kirshon B, Willis RS, Morse KJ Jr, Cotton DB: Quantitative hemodynamic effects of acute volume expansion in severe preeclampsia. Obstet Gynecol 73:545–550, 1989.

177. Moir DD, Victor-Rodriquez L, Willocks J: Extradural anal-

gesia during labour in patients with preeclampsia. J Obstet Gynaecol Br Commonw 79:465–469, 1972.

178. Bigler von R, Stamm O: Die periduralanasthesis zur Verhinderung des eklamptischen Anfalls und als Therapie des eklamptischen Comas. Gynaecologia 158:228–233, 1964.

179. Benedetti TJ, Benedetti JK, Steuchever MA: Severe preeclampsia: Maternal and fetal outcome. Part B. Hypertension in Pregnancy. Clin Exper Hypertens 2/3:401–416, 1982.

180. Merrell DA, Koch MAT: Epidural anaesthesia as an anticonvulsant in the management of hypertensive and eclamptic patients in labour. S Afr Med J 58:875–877, 1980.

181. Hodgkinson R, Husain FJ, Hayashi RH: Systemic and pulmonary blood pressure during caesarean section in parturients with gestational hypertension. Can Anaesth Soc J 27:389–394, 1980.

182. Jouppila P, Jouppila R, Hollmén A, Koivula A: Lumbar epidural analgesia to improve intervillous blood flow during labor in severe preeclampsia. Obstet Gynecol 59:158–161, 1982.

183. Gutsche BB: The Experts Opine: The role of epidural anesthesia in preeclampsia. Surv Anesthesiol 30:304–311, 1986.

184. Sangoul F, Fox GS, Houle GL: Effect of regional anesthesia on maternal oxygen consumption during the first stage of labor. Am J Obstet Gynecol 121:1080–1083, 1975.

185. Hagerdal M, Morgan CW, Sumner AE, Gutsche BB: Minute ventilation and oxygen consumption during labor with epidural analgesia. Anesthesiology 59:425–427, 1983.

186. Moore TR, Key TC, Reisner LS, Resnik R: Evaluation of the use of continuous lumbar epidural anesthesia for hypertensive pregnant women in labor. Am J Obst Gynecol 152:404–412, 1985.

187. Connell H, Dalgleish JG, Downing JG: General anaesthesia in mothers with severe pre-eclampsia/eclampsia. Br J Anaesth 59:1375–1380, 1987.

188. Lawes EG, Downing JW, Duncan PW, Bland B, Lavies N, Gane GAC: Fentanyl droperidol supplementation of rapid sequence induction in the presence of severe pregnancy-induced and pregnancy-aggravated hypertension. Br J Anaesth 59:1381–1391, 1987.

189. Lavies NG, Meiklejohn BH, May AE, Achola KJ, Fell D: Hypertensive and catecholamine response to tracheal intubation in patients with pregnancy-induced hypertension. Br J Anaesth 63:429–434, 1989.

190. Fox EJ, Sklar GS, Hill CH, Villaneuva R, King BD: Complications related to the pressor response to endotracheal intubation. Anesthesiology 47:524–525, 1977.

191. Lopez-Llera M, Rubio Linares G, Hernandez Horla JL: Maternal mortality rates in eclampsia. Am J Obstet Gynecol 124:149–155, 1976.

192. Hon EH, Reid BL, Hehre FW: The electronic evaluation of fetal heart rate. II. Changes with maternal hypotension. Am J Obstet Gynecol 79:209–215, 1960.

193. Hehre FW, Hook R, Hon E: Continuous lumbar peridural anesthesia in obstetrics. Anesth Analg 48:909–913, 1969.

194. Boehm F, Woodruff L, Growdon J: The effect of lumbar epidural analgesia on the fetal heart rate baseline variability. Anesth Analg 54:779–782, 1975.

194a. Lavin JP: The effects of epidural anesthesia on electronic fetal heart rate monitoring. Clin Perinatol 9:55–62, 1982.

195. James FM III, Davis P: Maternal and fetal effects of lumbar epidural analgesia for labor and delivery in patients with gestational hypertension. Am J Obstet Gynecol 126:195–201, 1976.

196. Crawford JS: Epidural analgesia in pregnancy hypertension. Clin Obstet Gynaecol 4:735–744, 1977.

197. Greenwood PA, Lilford RJ: Effect of epidural analgesia on maximum and minimum blood pressures during first stage of labour in primigravidae with mild/moderate gestational hypertension. Br J Obstet Gynaecol 93:260–263, 1986.

198. Graham C, Goldstein A: Epidural analgesia and cardiac output in severe preeclampsia. Anaesthesia 35:709–712, 1980.

199. Wright JP: Anesthetic considerations in preeclampsia-eclampsis (review article). Anesth Analg 62:590–601, 1982.

200. Marx GF, Hodgkinson R: Anesthesia in the presence of complications of pregnancy. Clin Obstet Gynecol 2:609–633, 1975.

201. Brizgys RV, Dailey PA, Shnider SM, Kotelko DM, Levinson G: The incidence and neonatal effects of maternal hypotension during epidural anesthesia for cesarean section. Anesthesiology 67:782–786, 1987.

202. Wallis KH, Shnider SM, Hicks JS, Spivey HT: Epidural anesthesia in the normotensive pregnant ewe: Effects on uterine blood flow and fetal acid base status. Anesthesiology 44:481–487, 1976.

203. Jouppila R, Jouppila P, Kuikka J, Hollmén A: Placenta blood flow during cesarean section under lumbar extradural analgesia. Br J Anaesth 50:275–278, 1978.

204. Jouppila R, Jouppila P, Hollmén A: Effect of segmental extradural analgesia on placental blood flow during normal labour. Br J Anaesth 50:563–567, 1978.

205. Husemeyer RP, Crawley JCW: Placental intervillous blood flow measured by inhaled ^{133}Xe clearance in relation to induction of epidural analgesia. Br J Obstet Gynaecol 86:426–431, 1979.

206. Houvinen K, Lehtovirta P, Forss M, Kivalo I, Teramo K: Changes in placental intervillous blood flow measured by the 133 Xenon method during lumbar epidural block for elective cesarean section. Acta Anaesthesiol Scand 23:529–533, 1979.

207. Jouppila R, Jouppila P, Hollmén A, Koivula A: Epidural analgesia and placental blood flow during labour in pregnancies complicated by hypertension. Br J Obstet Gynaecol 86:969–972, 1979.

208. Jouppila P, Kuikka J, Jouppila R: Effects of induction of general anesthesia for cesarean section on intervillous blood flow. Acta Obstet Gynecol Scand 58:249–253, 1979.

209. Palahniuk RJ, Cumming M: Foetal deterioration following thiopentone-nitrous oxide anaesthesia in the pregnant ewe. Can Anaesth Soc J 24:361–370, 1977.

210. Petrie R, Yeh S, Murata Y, Paul RH, Hon EH, Barron BA, Johnson RJ: The effects of drugs on fetal heart rate variability. Am J Obstet Gynecol 130:294–299, 1978.

211. deJong RH: *Physiology and Pharmacology of Local Anesthesia.* Charles C Thomas, Springfield, IL, 1970, p 211.

212. Bernhard CG, Bohm E: *Local Anaesthetics as Anticonvulsants.* Almqvist & Wiksel, Stockholm, 1966.

213. Ritchie JM, Greene NM: Local Anesthetics. In *The Pharmacological Basis of Therapeutics,* 6th ed. AG Gilman, LS Goodman, A Gilman, eds. Macmillan, New York, 1980, p 307.

214. Ramanathan J, Bottorff M, Jeter JN, Khalil M, Sibai BM: The pharmacokinetics and maternal and neonatal effects of epidural lidocaine in preeclampsia. Anesth Analg 65:120–126, 1986.

215. Robinson DA: Epinephrine should not be used with local anesthetics for epidural anesthesia in pre-eclampsia (letter). Anesthesiology 66:577–578, 1987.

216. Heller PJ, Goodman C: Use of local anesthetics with epinephrine for epidural anesthesia in preeclampsia. Anesthesiology 65:224–226, 1986.

217. Heller PJ: Epinephrine should not be used with local anesthetics for epidural anesthesia in pre-eclampsia (letter). Anesthesiology 66:578–579, 1987.

218. Dror A, Abboud TK, Moore N, Swart F, Mosaad P, Davis H, Gangolly J, Mantilla M, Makar A, Zaki N: Maternal hemodynamic responses to epinephrine containing solutions in mild preeclampsia. Reg Anesth 13:107–111, 1988.

219. Smith BE, Cavanagh D, Moya F: Anesthesia for vaginal delivery of the patient with toxemia of pregnancy. Anesth Analg 45:853–861, 1966.

220. Brock-Utne JC, Downing JW, Seedat F: Laryngeal oedema associated with preeclamptic toxemia. Anaesthesia 32:556–580, 1977.

221. MacKenzie AL: Laryngeal oedema complicating obstetric anaesthesia (letter). Anaesthesia 33:271, 1978.

222. Jouppila R, Jouppila P, Hollmén A: Laryngeal oedema as an

obstetric anaesthesia complication. Acta Anaesthesiol Scand 24:97–98, 1980.

223. Perlow JH, Kirz DS: Severe preeclampsia presenting as dysphonia secondary to uvular edema: A case report. J Reproduct Med 35:1059–1062, 1990.

224. DeVore JS, Asrani R: Magnesium sulfate prevents succinylcholine-induced fasciculations in toxemia parturients. Anesthesiology 52:76–77, 1980.

225. Lee C, Nguyen NB, Tran BK, Katz R: Quantification of magnesium-pancuronium interaction in the diaphragm and tibialis anterior. Anesthesiology 57:A392, 1982.

226. Tran B, Nguyen B, Chung H, Murad S, Lee C: Interaction between magnesium and vecuronium in rabbits. Anesthesiology 61:A403, 1984.

227. Baraka A, Yazigi A: Neuromuscular interaction of magnesium with succinylcholine-vecuronium sequence in the eclamptic parturient. Anesthesiology 67:806–808, 1987.

228. Loughran PG, Moore J, Dundee JW: Maternal stress response associated with caesarean delivery under general and epidural anesthesia. Br J Obstet Gynaecol 93:943–949, 1986.

229. Allen RW, James MFM, Uys PF: Attenuation of the pressor response to tracheal intubation in the hypertensive proteinuric pregnant patient by lignocaine, alfentanyl and magnesium sulfate. Br J Anaesth 66:216–223, 1991.

230. Hood DD, Dewan DM, James FM III, Floyd HM, Bogard TD: The use of nitroglycerine in preventing the hypertensive response to tracheal intubation in severe preeclampsia. Anesthesiology 63:329–332, 1985.

231. Paulton TJ, James FM III, Lockridge O: Prolonged apnea following trimethaphan and succinylcholine. Anesthesiology 50:54–56, 1979.

232. Sosis M, Leighton B: In defense of trimethaphan for use in preeclampsia (letter). Anesthesiology 64:657–658, 1986.

233. Craft JB Jr, Co EG, Yonekura ML, Gilman RM: Nitroglycerin therapy for phenylephrine-induced hypertension in pregnant ewes. Anesth Analg 59:494–499, 1980.

234. Snyder SW, Wheeler AS, James FM III: The use of nitroglycerin to control severe hypertension of pregnancy during cesarean section. Anesthesiology 51:563–564, 1979.

235. Wheeler AS, James FM III, Meis PJ, Rose JC, Fishburne JL, Dewan DM, Urban RB, Greiss FC Jr: Effects of nitroglycerin and nitroprusside on the uterine vasculature of gravid ewes. Anesthesiology 52:390–394, 1980.

236. Longmire S, Leduc L, Jones MM, Hawkins JL, Joyce TH III, Cotton DB: The hemodynamic effects of intubation during nitroglycerin infusion in severe preeclampsia. Am J Obstet Gynecol 164:551–556, 1991.

237. Leib SM, Zugaib M, Nuwayhid B, Tabsh K, Erkkola R, Ushioda E, Brinkman CR III, Assali NS: Nitroprusside induced hemodynamic alterations in normotensive and hypertensive pregnant sheep. Am J Obstet Gynecol 139:925–931, 1981.

238. Naulty J, Cefalo RC, Lewis PE: Fetal toxicity of nitroprusside in the pregnant ewe. Am J Obstet Gynecol 139:708–711, 1981.

239. Stempel JE, O'Grady JP, Morton MJ, Johnson KA: Use of sodium nitroprusside in complications of gestational hypertension. Obstet Gynecol 60:533–538, 1982.

240. Ellis SC, Wheeler AS, James FM III, Rose JC, Meis PJ, Shihabi Z, Greiss FC Jr, Urban RB: Fetal and maternal effects of sodium nitroprusside used to counteract hypertension in gravid ewes. Am J Obstet Gynecol 143:766–770, 1982.

241. Nelson SH, Suresh MS: Comparison of nitroprusside and hydralazine in isolated uterine arteries from pregnant and nonpregnant patients. Anesthesiology 68:541–547, 1988.

242. Rigg D, McDonogh A: Use of sodium nitroprusside for deliberate hypotension during pregnancy. Br J Anaesth 53:985–987, 1981.

243. Marx GF, Mateo CV: Effects of different oxygen concentrations during general anaesthesia or elective caesarean section. Can Anaesth Soc J 18:587–593, 1971.

244. Morishima HO, Daniels SS, Richards RT, James LS: The effect of increased maternal PaO$_2$ upon the fetus during labor. Am J Obstet Gynecol 123:257–264, 1975.

245. Moir DD: Anaesthesia for caesarean section. An evaluation of a method using low concentrations of halothane and 50 per cent of oxygen. Br J Anaesth 42:136–142, 1970.

246. Marx GF, Kim YI, Lin CC, Halevy S, Schulman H: Postpartum uterine pressures under halothane or enflurane anesthesia. Obstet Gynecol 51:695–698, 1978.

247. Warren TM, Datta S, Ostheimer GW, Naulty JS, Weiss JB, Morrison JA: Comparison of maternal and neonatal effects of halothane, enflurane and isoflurane for cesarean section delivery. Anesth Analg 62:516–520, 1983.

248. Dunn R, Lee W, Cotton DB: Evaluation by computerized axial tomography of eclamptic women with seizures refractory to magnesium sulfate therapy. Am J Obstet Gynecol 155:267–268, 1986.

249. Keeri-Szanto M: Laryngeal oedema complicating obstetric anaesthesia (letter). Anaesthesia 33:272, 1978.

250. Clark SL, Cotton DB, Lee W, Bishop C, Hill T, Southwick T, Pivarnik J, Spillman T, DeVore GR, Phelan J, Hankins GVD, Benedetti TJ, Trolley D: Central hemodynamic assessment of normal term pregnancy. Am J Obstet Gynecol 161:1439–1442, 1989.

CHAPTER 18

Anesthesia for Preterm Labor and Delivery

David H. Chestnut, M.D.
Patricia A. Dailey, M.D.

PHARMACOLOGIC THERAPY FOR PRETERM LABOR

Preterm labor occurs in as many as 14% of all deliveries (1) and is the leading cause of perinatal mortality in the United States (2–4). Currently 7 to 8% of deliveries in the United States occur preterm, but such deliveries are responsible for over 60% of perinatal morbidity and mortality (2–4). Thus the high incidence of preterm delivery is largely responsible for the relatively high perinatal mortality in the United States, as compared with other Western countries.

As gestational age or birth weight increases, the survival rate increases (2, 5). Thus the prevention of preterm labor or the recognition and *successful* treatment of preterm labor has a significant impact on perinatal survival. Based on data from 1979 to 1981, an infant born alive at 26 weeks' gestational age and weighing 500 to 750 g had a predicted survival rate of 36%, whereas an infant born at 32 weeks' gestational age and weighing 1000 to 1250 g had a predicted survival rate of near 100% (Fig. 18.1) (5). During the last decade, survival has improved for infants weighing 750 to 1000 g at birth. Such infants now have a 70% chance of survival if they have access to neonatal intensive care (6).

The cost effectiveness of prenatal drug treatment to arrest preterm labor is controversial. One study showed such therapy to be cost effective when provided between 26 and 33 weeks of gestation (7). In 1981 dollars, for patients receiving tocolytic treatment initiated at 28 to 29 weeks of gestation, the combined maternal and neonatal charges per survivor were $25,640 vs. $47,030 if mothers were not treated and their infants were born without gestational delay (Fig. 18.2). Leveno et al. (8) recently estimated that more than 100,000 United States women are given ritodrine for treatment of preterm labor. Unfortunately, they concluded that tocolytic therapy has had "minimal if any impact on the incidence of low birth weight in this country."(8)

Investigators currently are attempting to better define the causes of preterm labor. Concurrently, clinicians are giving emphasis to providing intensive antenatal care and education for patients at high risk for preterm labor. Preterm labor-prevention programs typically include weekly visits to the obstetrician and nurse-educator for a review of early symptoms and for examination of the cervix. The primary goal is the prevention of preterm labor, and a secondary goal is the early recognition and treatment of preterm labor (9). Several studies have noted conflicting results regarding the efficacy of specialized preterm birth-prevention programs (10–14). Some obstetricians have advocated the use of home uterine-activity monitoring, but the role of such monitoring is unclear. In 1989 the American College of Obstetricians and Gynecologists noted that such monitoring "has not been shown to add independently to the value of frequent provider-initiated phone contact"(15). They concluded that the use of home uterine-activity monitoring remains investigational.

The currently accepted definition of **preterm labor** is as follows: (a) pregnancy between 20 and 37 completed weeks from the last menstrual period; (b) regular uterine contractions of at least 30-sec duration occurring at least once every 10 min; and (c) cervical effacement and/or dilation. The term **premature infant** has been replaced by **preterm infant**. A preterm infant has been defined as an infant delivered between 20 and 37 weeks after the first day of the last menstrual period (i.e., at least 3 weeks before the expected date of term delivery). In the past any infant weighing less than 2500 g at delivery was considered to be preterm. But it is now recognized that some of these neonates are **small for gestational age (SGA)** and are not preterm. An infant who weighs less than 2500 g at birth is now labeled as a **low–birth-weight infant**, regardless of gestational age. A **very low–birth-weight infant** is an infant that weighs less than 1500 g at delivery.

A history of a previous preterm delivery, mul-

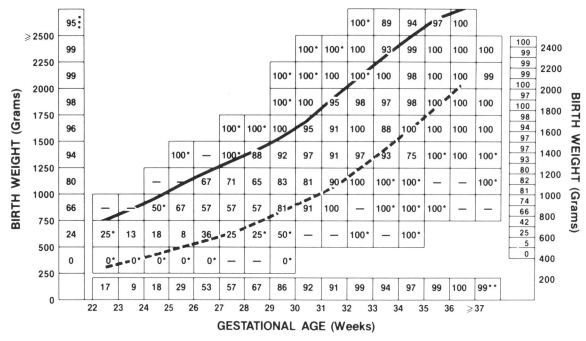

Figure 18.1. The survival rate by birth weight and gestational age at the University of Alabama in Birmingham from 1979 to 1981. The *dotted line* represents the 10th percentile of birth weight for gestational age and the *solid line* represents the 90th percentile. * = <5 values; ** = >37 weeks but <2500 g; *** = >2500 g but <37 weeks. (Reprinted by permission from Goldenberg RL, Nelson KG, Hale CD, Wayne J, Bartolucci AA, Koski J: Survival of infants with low birth weight and early gestational age, 1979 to 1981. Am J Obstet Gynecol 149:508–511, 1984.)

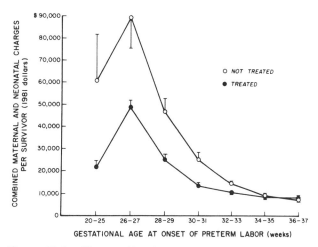

Figure 18.2. The combined maternal and neonatal charges per surviving infant (±SEM) relative to gestational age at onset of preterm labor. Charges were based on hospital charges and physicians' fees. Patients in the *treated* group received intravenous terbutaline or isoxsuprine. Patients in the *not treated* group received no β-adrenergic therapy and were allowed to deliver without gestational delay. (Reprinted by permission from Korenbrot CC, Aalto LH, Laros RK: The cost effectiveness of stopping preterm labor with beta-adrenergic treatment. N Engl J Med 310:691–696, 1984.)

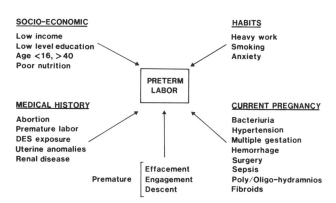

Figure 18.3. Obstetric and social factors associated with preterm labor. (Reprinted with modification from Creasy RK: Preterm Labor and Delivery. *Maternal-Fetal Medicine, Principles and Practice.* RK Creasy, R Resnik, eds. WB Saunders, Philadelphia, 1984, p 419.)

tiple gestation, or both represent two of the most significant risk factors for preterm labor and delivery (4). Many other obstetric and social factors are associated with preterm labor (Fig. 18.3). These associations do not necessarily represent cause-and-effect relationships. But in some cases infection probably represents the cause of preterm labor. For example, pyelonephritis significantly increases the risk of preterm labor. Similarly, subclinical chorioamnionitis may represent the cause of preterm

Table 18.1
Criteria for Inhibition of Preterm Labor

Long-term treatment
  1. Intact membranes
  2. Fetus <2500 g; 20–30 weeks
  3. Documented contractions
  4. Cervical change and >80% effacement, or cervical
     dilation >2 cm but less than 4 cm
Short-term treatment
  1. Postoperative
  2. Patient transfer
  3. Corticosteroid treatment
  4. Fetal distress: preparation for immediate delivery
Relative contraindications to treatment
  1. Ruptured amniotic membranes (long term)
  2. Fever of unknown origin/amnionitis
  3. Severe hemorrhage
  4. Fetal anomalies incompatible with life
  5. Maternal cardiac disease

labor in some patients (4). Unfortunately, in most cases the cause of preterm labor is unclear, and approximately 50% of preterm deliveries occur in women with no risk factors (4). Furthermore, not all preterm births result from preterm labor. As many as 20 to 25% of all preterm deliveries are performed electively, for maternal or fetal indications. For example, the obstetrician may electively deliver the preterm patient with severe preeclampsia. Likewise, he or she may deliver the patient whose fetus has hemolytic anemia secondary to Rh sensitization. Unfortunately, some infants are delivered electively before term because of an error in the estimation of gestational age.

By identifying patients with factors that place them at increased risk for preterm labor, it is possible to suspect and diagnose preterm labor early. Once preterm labor has been diagnosed, a decision of whether to attempt inhibition of preterm labor must be made (Table 18.1). There are some situations in which the inhibition of preterm labor is relatively contraindicated. For example, most obstetricians have avoided *tocolytic therapy* in women with ruptured membranes because of uncertainty regarding efficacy, as well as concern that such therapy might increase the risk of maternal and/or fetal infection. Two studies evaluated the use of tocolytic therapy in such patients (16, 17). Tocolytic therapy did not increase maternal or neonatal infectious complications in either study. Tocolytic therapy also did not result in improved neonatal outcome when compared with expectant management. However, one study (17) suggested that a subgroup of patients with ruptured membranes at less than 28 weeks' gestation might benefit from tocolytic therapy.

The benefits of attempting to delay delivery of the preterm infant must be weighed against the maternal and fetal risks of therapy. Although the prognosis for preterm infants has improved during recent years, these infants are still at high risk for intrapartum death, neonatal respiratory failure, and intraventricular hemorrhage. If inhibition of preterm labor is attempted, it may be for the *short term* to allow glucocorticoids administered to the mother to accelerate fetal lung maturity or to allow for arrangement of the proper delivery setting (e.g., patient transport and assembly of neonatal specialists). *Long-term* inhibition of preterm labor will allow further maturation of the fetus for weeks to months.

Tocolytic agents are occasionally used to manage intrapartum fetal distress while preparations are made for immediate delivery. Uterine contractions, by reducing placental blood flow, may exceed the reserve of an already compromised fetoplacental unit. Tocolytic agents may improve uteroplacental blood flow and fetal oxygenation by decreasing myometrial activity. Terbutaline (18), ritodrine (19), and magnesium sulfate (20) havé been used to manage intrapartum fetal distress; they appear most useful when there is evidence of increased uterine activity.

Maternal, fetal, and neonatal side effects of drugs currently used for treating preterm labor are listed in Table 18.2. It is obvious that these drugs have important implications for the anesthesiologist because of their varying effects on fluid and electrolyte balance, as well as on the cardiovascular and respiratory systems. Despite aggressive tocolysis, preterm labor may still occur. Indeed it is not unusual for an attempted inhibition of labor to be unsuccessful and for labor to progress rapidly. The anesthesiologist may be asked to provide analgesia for labor or for an operative delivery by forceps or cesarean section. Thus an understanding of the effects of tocolytic drugs on anesthetic management is important.

Physiology of Uterine Contractions

The physiology of uterine contractions is reviewed in detail elsewhere (21, 22). Briefly, contraction of smooth muscle depends on the interaction of filaments of actin and myosin. The energy for this interaction comes from the hydrolysis of adenosine triphosphate (ATP), and the interaction depends on the phosphorylation of myosin by the enzyme myosin light-chain kinase. This enzyme requires activation by calmodulin, which in turn depends on a relatively high level of intracellular calcium ions for activation. There are a number of steps in this cascade at

Table 18.2
Side Effects of Drugs Used to Stop Labor

Drug	Maternal Effects	Fetal and Neonatal Effects

β-Adrenergic agents	Hypotension
	Tachycardia
	Chest pain/tightness
	Pulmonary edema
	Congestive heart failure
	Arrhythmias (atrial and
	  ventricular)
	Anxiety, nervousness
	Nausea and vomiting
	Headache
	Hyperglycemia
	Metabolic (lactic) acidosis
		Tachycardia
		Hyperglycemia
		Increased free fatty acids
		Fetal asphyxia with large doses due to
		  maternal hypotension or increased
		  uterine vascular resistance resulting in
		  decreased uterine blood flow
		Decreased incidence of respiratory
		  distress syndrome (?)

Magnesium sulfate	Pulmonary edema Chest pain/tightness Nausea and vomiting Flushing Drowsiness Blurred vision Increased sensitivity to muscle relaxants	Hypotonia Drowsiness Decreased gastric motility Hypocalcemia
Prostaglandin synthetase inhibitors	Gastrointestinal irritation Inhibition of platelet function Reduced factor XII Depressed immune system	Premature closure of the ductus arteriosus Pulmonary hypertension
Calcium entry-blocking agents	Hypotension Reduced cardiac contractility Reduced cardiac conduction Inhibition of platelet aggregation	

which smooth muscle contraction can be inhibited (Fig. 18.4). β-Adrenergic agonists, prostaglandin synthetase inhibitors, and ethanol produce increased levels of cyclic AMP. Magnesium sulfate and calcium entry-blocking drugs probably prevent the increase in intracellular Ca^{++} levels needed for the activation of calmodulin, which is necessary for activation of myosin light-chain kinase.

Inhibition of smooth muscle contraction is discussed in more detail in the sections on the mechanisms of action of specific tocolytic agents.

Prevention and Treatment of Preterm Labor

EFFICACY OF PHARMACOLOGIC THERAPY

The use of pharmacologic therapy to inhibit or prevent preterm labor has become a standard obstetric practice. However, there are few prospective, randomized studies in which tocolytic agents are compared to placebo. Thus it is difficult to evaluate the efficacy and overall safety of tocolytic therapy. A review (23) of studies published between 1971 and 1979 noted that the mean effectiveness of drug ther-

apy was 70% (with a range of 29 to 87%), whereas the mean effectiveness of placebo was 49% (27 to 71% range). In addition, the various clinical series have varying criteria for inclusion in the study and varying definitions of success of therapy. The high rate of success with placebo underscores the fact that not all preterm women with uterine contractions need pharmacologic tocolytic therapy. Some patients will experience cessation of contractions with bed rest and hydration alone. The use of real-time ultrasonography may help the obstetrician determine which patients need tocolytic therapy. Castle and Turnbull (24) reported their experience with real-time ultrasonography to establish the presence or absence of fetal breathing movements in patients with a diagnosis of preterm labor. Delivery occurred within 48 hr in 19 of 20 patients with no detectable fetal breathing, whereas pregnancy continued for at least 1 week in 25 of 34 patients with fetal breathing movements. Subsequently, others have confirmed the predictive value of fetal breathing movements in the diagnosis and assessment of preterm labor (25, 26).

Tocolytic agents used in modern obstetric practice

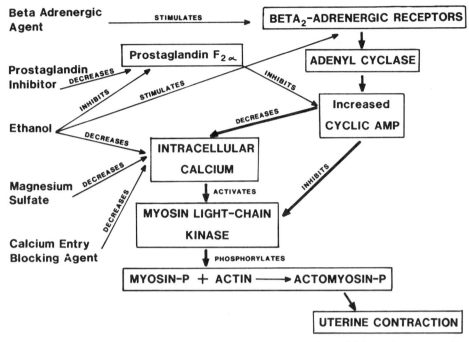

Figure 18.4. Principle site of pharmacologic action of drugs used to inhibit uterine contractility and stop preterm labor.

include: (a) β-adrenergic agents; (b) magnesium sulfate; (c) prostaglandin synthetase inhibitors; and (d) calcium-entry blocking agents. The use of ethanol to treat preterm labor has been abandoned by most obstetricians in the United States and is not discussed in this chapter. Interested readers may refer to Chapter 18 on this subject published in the second edition of this text (27).

β-Adrenergic Agents

β-Adrenergic agents are the most commonly used drugs for the treatment of preterm labor. These agents may be administered intravenously, subcutaneously, or orally. All β-agonists have combined β_1 and β_2 effects (Table 18.3). The desired uterine tocolytic activity is a result of stimulation of β_2-receptors in uterine smooth muscle. Unfortunately, stimulation of β_1-receptors may result in marked increases in maternal heart rate and cardiac output. Hyperglycemia and hypotension are the major undesirable β_2-receptor effects (Fig. 18.5).

Until 1980 when **ritodrine** was approved by the Food and Drug Administration for the treatment of preterm labor, isoxsuprine and **terbutaline** were the drugs most commonly used for this purpose. Other β-adrenergic agents that have been evaluated in the treatment of preterm labor include hexoprenaline, fenoterol, salbutamol, orciprenaline, and isoproterenol. Ritodrine and terbutaline are more β_2-receptor

Table 18.3
Selective β-Adrenergic Receptor Stimulation[a]

	β_1	β_2
Uterine muscle	No effect	Relaxation
Cardiovascular		
Blood vessels	No effect	Vasodilation
Heart rate	Increase	No effect
Heart muscle (strength of contraction)	Stimulation	No effect
Cardiac output	Increase	No effect
Respiratory		
Bronchial muscle	No effect	Relaxation
Secretions	No effect	Slight increase
Central nervous system	?	Stimulation
Gastrointestinal	?	Relaxation
Metabolic		
Pancreas β cells	No effect	Insulin secretion
Liver	No effect	Glycogenolysis
Fat cells	Lipolysis	Gluconeogenesis

[a] All β-agonists when given systemically have combined β_1 and β_2 effects.

specific than all of these agents, with the possible exception of hexoprenaline (28). At the present time, only ritodrine is specifically approved for treatment of preterm labor.

Mechanism of Action. Through the action of cyclic AMP and the calcium pump, the β-adrenergic agents inhibit the cellular regulatory mechanisms of myosin light-chain phosphorylation, resulting in relaxation

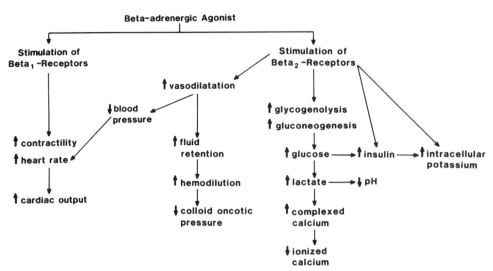

Figure 18.5. The cardiovascular and metabolic effects of β-adrenergic receptor stimulation. (Reprinted with modification from Cotton DB, Strassner HT, Lipson LG, Goldstein DA: The effects of terbutaline on acid base, serum electrolytes, and glucose homeostasis during the management of preterm labor. Am J Obstet Gynecol 141:617–624, 1981.)

of the smooth muscle of the uterus (Fig.18.4) (21, 22). β-Agonists interact with β-adrenergic receptors located on the outer surface of the target cell. This complex then activates adrenyl cyclase, an enzyme located on the internal surface of the plasma membrane of the target cell. This stimulates the conversion of ATP to cyclic AMP (cAMP). Increased cAMP concentration diminishes myosin light-chain kinase activity through reduced intracellular calcium levels. When myosin phosphorylation is reduced, the actin-myosin interaction diminishes and the myometrium relaxes. cAMP also affects ion transport across cellular and mitochondrial membranes by acting on the $Na^+ - K^+$ pump, resulting in hypokalemia caused by increased pumping of Na^+ out of the cell and K^+ into the cell.

Treatment Regimen. β-Adrenergic therapy should be initiated only after (a) obtaining baseline maternal weight, blood pressure, heart rate, and respiratory rate measurements; (b) performing a physical examination with emphasis on the heart and lungs; and (c) collecting urine for microscopic examination and culture. It is prudent to obtain a blood sample for complete blood count and serum electrolyte determination. Some clinicians routinely obtain a baseline electrocardiogram. This allows for detection of an undiagnosed arrhythmia, which may be worsened by β-adrenergic therapy. It also provides a baseline electrocardiogram for comparison should the patient experience a cardiovascular complication of β-adrenergic therapy. However, in practice, the baseline electrocardiogram rarely affects the management of patients with no history of cardiovascular disease and no cardiovascular abnormality on physical examination.

Usual initial intravenous infusion rates are 0.05 to 0.1 mg/min for ritodrine, and 0.01 mg/min for terbutaline. Usual maximal infusion rates are 0.35 mg/min for ritodrine and 0.08 mg/min for terbutaline. Maternal blood pressure and heart rate are monitored closely.

Side Effects of β-Adrenergic Agents

Widespread use of β-adrenergic agents has resulted in cases of pulmonary edema, hypotension, myocardial ischemia, cardiac arrhythmia, cerebral vasospasm, and rarely maternal death (29). Isoxsuprine is more likely to cause maternal hypotension than is ritodrine or terbutaline. Fortunately, isoxsuprine has been abandoned by most obstetricians in the United States.

Pulmonary Edema. Pulmonary edema is the most frequent serious complication of β-adrenergic tocolytic therapy. This complication occurs in approximately 1% of those patients who receive parenteral β-adrenergic therapy. Prolonged exposure to β-adrenergic therapy appears to be a risk factor for the development of pulmonary edema. The majority of published case reports have noted the development of pulmonary edema only after 24 hr, and in many cases after 48 hr, of therapy (30–34). Earlier case reports suggested that concurrent corticosteroid (e.g., dexamethasone, betamethasone) administration predisposed patients to pulmonary edema (30, 35). However, these glucocorticoids have little mineralocorticoid activity,[a] and at least one prospective study

---

[a]As an aside, two doses of glucocorticoid, administered 12 to 24 hr apart, do not render a patient steroid dependent.

has not confirmed that glucocorticoid therapy is a risk factor for development of pulmonary edema (36).

Pulmonary edema may develop on a cardiogenic basis as the result of fluid overload and myocardial failure or on a noncardiogenic basis as the result of "capillary leak" with increased protein in the pulmonary edema fluid (29, 30, 37, 38). The circulatory effects of β-adrenergic receptor stimulation have been studied in unanesthetized chronically instrumented pregnant sheep (39, 40). Ritodrine produces a significant increase in maternal heart rate and cardiac output and a decrease in systemic vascular resistance. Pulmonary arterial and pulmonary capillary wedge pressures tend to increase, despite a slight fall in the pulmonary vascular resistance (Fig. 18.6) (40). The shortened systolic ejection and diastolic filling times associated with the β-adrenergic-induced tachycardia may result in myocardial ischemia, an increase in pulmonary capillary wedge pressure, or both.

Patients receiving β-adrenergic therapy are at significant risk for fluid overload. Fluid overload can occur as a result of injudicious hydration before and during tocolytic therapy, of sodium and water retention secondary to β-adrenergic receptor stimulation, or of both. β-Adrenergic activation stimulates antidiuretic hormone release (40, 41) and exerts a direct action on renal tubular handling of sodium, resulting in enhanced tubular reabsorption of sodium (42). Because of the antinatriuretic effects of β-adrenergic

stimulation, the amount of fluid retained during β-adrenergic therapy is greater when isotonic saline is administered than when dextrose is administered (36, 40). In a study comparing glucose and saline solutions as vehicles for ritodrine (36), patients who received isotonic saline retained at least 1 liter of fluid more than did the glucose-treated patients. Seven of twelve patients in the saline group, but none in the glucose group, developed pulmonary congestion requiring treatment. Pregnant baboons (43, 44), who were given ritodrine and lactated Ringer's solution retained 61% of administered fluid, as compared with 23% retained by animals who received lactated Ringer's solution alone. Ritodrine-treated animals also retained more sodium than did animals not treated with ritodrine. Ritodrine-treated animals had a significant increase in cardiac index, pulmonary capillary wedge pressure, and heart rate and a significant decrease in systemic vascular resistance. Colloid oncotic pressure decreased in both groups during a period of increased volume infusion. In ritodrine-treated animals, the lowest colloid oncotic pressures were seen concurrently with maximal wedge pressures, resulting in a colloid oncotic pressure-to-pulmonary capillary wedge pressure gradient favoring a net flux of water from pulmonary vasculature to pulmonary interstitium.

However, Benedetti (45) noted that there are few data that confirm that β-adrenergic tocolytic therapy

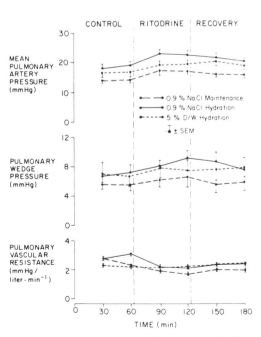

Figure 18.6. The effects of β-adrenergic receptor stimulation on systemic and pulmonary hemodynamics in unanesthetized, chronically instrumented pregnant sheep. Values represent mean ± 1 SEM and are for the three different types of hydration. (Reprinted by permission from Kleinmen G, Nuwayhid B, Rudelstorfer R, Khoury A, Tabsh K, Murad S, Brinkman CR, Assali NS: Circulatory and renal effects of beta-adrenergic-receptor stimulation in pregnant sheep. Am J Obstet Gynecol 149:865–874, 1984.)

actually results in myocardial failure. He also noted that pulmonary edema during tocolytic therapy is not unique to β-adrenergic therapy. He reviewed 12 patients who had pulmonary edema during tocolytic therapy between 1978 and 1985. Nine patients received either β-adrenergic therapy alone or in combination with magnesium sulfate. But three patients received magnesium sulfate alone. He hypothesized that "in patients who are at high risk for the development of pulmonary edema, there is an underlying infection associated with if not causing the preterm labor" (45). Such infections might include unrecognized amniotic fluid or urinary tract infection and may be associated with the release of endotoxin. Endotoxin has been shown to increase lung capillary permeability and to affect lung balance (46). Noncardiogenic pulmonary edema may occur secondary to increased lung capillary permeability. After *Escherichia coli* endotoxin administration, lung extravascular fluid volume increases at lower pulmonary capillary pressure minus plasma oncotic pressure, as compared with control sheep or sheep receiving ritodrine infusion only. β-Adrenergic agents do not increase permeability. An increase in pulmonary capillary wedge pressure caused by β-adrenergic therapy, combined with the increased pulmonary capillary permeability caused by endotoxin, would predispose patients receiving β-adrenergic agents to pulmonary edema (30). A recent retrospective study (47) confirmed that tocolytic therapy for preterm labor was associated with an increased incidence of pulmonary edema in the presence of maternal infection. It is recommended that clinicians rule out underlying infection in patients receiving tocolytic therapy, even in those without clinical symptoms.

Hypoxia during pulmonary edema may be exacerbated by the inhibition of hypoxic pulmonary vasoconstriction by β-adrenergic agents. A study in dogs has demonstrated that ritodrine significantly inhibits hypoxic pulmonary vasoconstriction, the normal mechanism for diverting blood flow away from areas of hypoventilation (48). Thus the patient who develops pulmonary edema with gas exchange defects during ritodrine therapy may develop hypoxia out of proportion to the degree of radiologically apparent pulmonary edema as a result of the failure of the lung to autoregulate and effectively redistribute pulmonary perfusion.

To avoid pulmonary edema during β-adrenergic therapy, total fluid intake (intravenous and oral) should be limited to 1.5 to 2.5 liters/24 hr. One approach is to administer the β-adrenergic agonist in a solution of 0.45 sodium chloride. Dextrose is not included in the intravenous fluids because of the hyperglycemia induced by the β-adrenergic agents. Daily weights, strict intake and output measurements, and hematocrits are closely observed. The frequency of cardiovascular complications may be decreased by carefully limiting the dose of the β-adrenergic agent. Specifically, there is little tocolytic efficacy to be gained by giving more β-agonist than that necessary to increase the maternal heart rate by 20 to 30%. The authors also recommend the use of the pulse oximeter in patients receiving parenteral β-adrenergic tocolytic therapy. The pulse oximeter may facilitate early diagnosis of pulmonary edema by allowing the physician to detect early decreases in hemoglobin oxygen saturation.

If pulmonary edema develops, the drug infusion should be discontinued and supplemental oxygen administered. An arterial blood gas should be obtained to determine the degree of hypoxemia. Frequently, these measures are sufficient and no further intervention is necessary (30, 38). In a recent review of 58 cases of pulmonary edema associated with tocolytic therapy, the clinical response to conservative therapy was prompt (38). Only 4 of the 58 patients required intubation and mechanical ventilation.

With the discontinuation of β-adrenergic therapy, heart rate and blood pressure usually return toward pretherapy values over a 30- to 90-min time period (Fig. 18.6) (39, 40, 49). If hypoxemia persists, further intervention including diuretics, chest radiographic examination, positive pressure ventilation, and central venous and pulmonary artery pressure monitoring may be necessary. The possibility of an unrecognized site of infection should be investigated, particularly if pulmonary arterial and pulmonary capillary wedge pressures are normal. Serum potassium values should be closely monitored if diuretics are administered.

Myocardial Effects. β-Adrenergic agents, including the $β_2$-selective agents, have potent inotropic and chronotropic effects on the maternal heart. Ritodrine therapy increases heart rate, stroke volume, left ventricular ejection fraction, and cardiac output, resulting in a greatly increased myocardial oxygen demand (39, 50). Premature ventricular contractions, premature nodal contractions, and atrial fibrillation have occurred in patients receiving β-adrenergic therapy (29). There have been some reports of myocardial ischemia, which appears to be subendocardial in location, usually manifesting as chest pain or tightness and ST-segment and T-wave changes on electrocardiogram, and resolving shortly after discontinuation of β-adrenergic therapy (34, 50–54). However, not all ST-segment and T-wave changes represent myocardial ischemia. Two recent studies noted frequent electrocardiographic changes during ritodrine therapy in asymptomatic patients (55, 56). Both studies concluded that these changes may represent "a physiologic expression of ritodrine-induced tachycardia or hypokalemia" (55).

Metabolic Effects. β-Adrenergic therapy produces a number of metabolic changes related to glucose, insulin, and potassium (Fig. 18.7) (29, 57–62). By stimulating adenyl cyclase on the membranes of liver cells, ritodrine activates hepatic phosphorylase, which mediates the production of glucose from stored glycogen. *Hyperglycemia* occurs rapidly, even in nondiabetic patients. Patients who are receiving dextrose-containing solutions or concurrent corticosteroid therapy or who are known to be diabetic are at increased risk for significant hyperglycemia and may require insulin. Insulin-dependent diabetic patients usually require a concomitant insulin infusion to prevent the development of diabetic ketoacidosis (29).

Both direct stimulation of pancreatic β cells by the β-adrenergic agent and increased levels of glucose result in increased serum insulin levels. *Hypokalemia* occurs as the result of the insulin-mediated movement of potassium, together with glucose, from the extracellular to the intracellular space and to direct stimulation of β_2-receptors in skeletal muscle leading to activation of $Na^+ - K^+$ ATPase (59). Urinary excretion of potassium during β-adrenergic therapy is not increased. **Total body potassium levels appear to be maintained.** The influence of intravenous solution content on ritodrine-mediated metabolic changes in 25 patients who received ritodrine for treatment of preterm labor was evaluated (63). The use of the following was compared: (*a*) 5% dextrose in water; (*b*) 5% dextrose in 0.9 sodium chloride; (*c*) 5% dextrose in Ringer's lactate; (*d*) 0.9 sodium chloride; and (*e*) Ringer's lactate. Dextrose enhanced the ritodrine-mediated decrease in the serum concentration of potassium. The researchers concluded that, of the five solutions evaluated in their study, Ringer's lactate appeared to be the best solution, whereas 5% dextrose in water was the least desirable.

The administration of supplemental potassium is controversial. Although it is postulated that hypokalemia results in hyperpolarization of nerve and conducting systems as the result of the alteration of the intracellular to extracellular potassium concentration ratio, no adverse effects caused by the hypokalemia have been reported. Restoration of serum potassium to normal levels is not recommended (29, 61, 62, 64). Rapid intravenous infusion of potassium

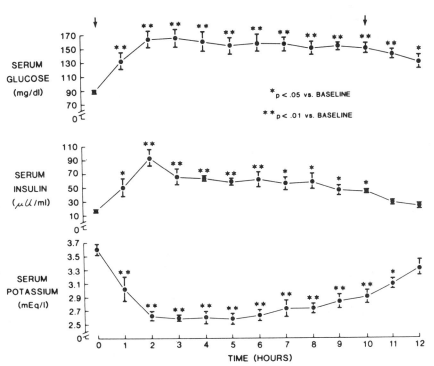

Figure 18.7. The levels of mean serum glucose, insulin, and potassium at baseline (*left arrow*), during 10 hr of infusion of terbutaline, and 2 hr after the infusion (*right arrow*) in 6 patients in preterm labor. (Reprinted by permission from Cotton DB, Strassner HT, Lipson LG, Goldstein DA: The effects of terbutaline on acid base, serum electrolytes, and glucose homeostasis during the management of preterm labor. Am J Obstet Gynecol 141:617–624, 1981.)

can cause significant complications. Serum potassium concentrations usually return to normal within 3 hr of discontinuing β-adrenergic therapy (54, 62).

Anesthetic Considerations. Patients who have recently received β-adrenergic agents to treat preterm labor or to acutely treat fetal distress before delivery may require anesthesia. Unfortunately, the half-lives of ritodrine and terbutaline in pregnant women are prolonged. For example, Kuhnert et al. (65) noted that the distribution phase and equilibrium phase half-lives for ritodrine in pregnant women are 32 ± 20 min and 17 ± 10 hr, respectively. As noted earlier, the cardiovascular effects of ritodrine and terbutaline persist for 30 to 90 min after their discontinuation (39, 40, 49). When anesthesia is required after administration of a β-adrenergic tocolytic agent, a delay to allow the tachycardia to subside is ideal. However, women with failed tocolysis frequently require urgent induction of anesthesia. A long delay may compromise the fetus.

There are no prospective clinical studies of anesthetic management after administration of a β-adrenergic tocolytic agent. The literature is limited to case reports (66–70), retrospective studies published in letter (71) and abstract form (72), and review articles and textbook chapters. Ravindran et al. (69) presented one case each of intraoperative pulmonary edema, sinus tachycardia, and ventricular arrhythmia after perioperative administration of terbutaline. They recommended that induction of general anesthesia be delayed at least 10 min after discontinuation of β-adrenergic infusion.

Shin and Kim (72) retrospectively noted that maternal hypotension occurred in two of three women who received ***epidural anesthesia*** within 30 min of discontinuation of ritodrine vs. one of eight women in whom there was a delay of greater than 30 min (*P* = 0.15). They recommended that epidural anesthesia should "be deferred at least 30 minutes following discontinuation of ritodrine . . . provided that such a delay does not jeopardize the fetus" (72). However, Chestnut et al. (73) recently observed that prior administration of ritodrine did not worsen maternal hypotension during epidural lidocaine anesthesia in gravid ewes (epinephrine was not included in the lidocaine solution) (Fig. 18.8). The inotropic and chronotropic activity of ritodrine seemed to protect cardiac output and uterine blood flow during epidural lidocaine anesthesia in that study. In practice, a delay of 15 min often will result in sufficient slowing of the maternal heart rate to allow the physician to proceed with slow induction of epidural anesthesia. Epidural anesthesia, with its slower onset and greater flexibility, is usually preferred over spinal anesthesia, except when vaginal delivery is immi-

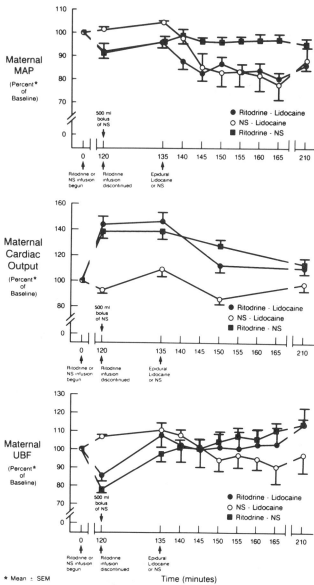

Figure 18.8. Response over time of maternal mean arterial pressure (MAP), cardiac output, and uterine blood flow after intravenous infusion of ritodrine or normal saline (NS)-control for 2 hr, followed by epidural administration of lidocaine or NS-control in gravid ewes. (Reprinted with permission from Chestnut DH, Pollack KL, Thompson CS, DeBruyn CS, Weiner CP: Does ritodrine worsen maternal hypotension during epidural anesthesia in gravid ewes? Anesthesiology 72:315–321, 1990.)

nent. One should avoid aggressive hydration before induction of epidural anesthesia in patients who have received long-term β-adrenergic tocolytic therapy. Frequently, these patients have a positive fluid balance and are at risk for the development of pulmonary edema if presented with a large fluid bolus. Instead, a modest fluid bolus (e.g., 250 to 500 ml of Ringer's lactate) should be given, followed by the slow establishment of epidural anesthesia. The volume of crystalloid should be titrated to maintain normal blood pressure.

If hypotension occurs, what vasopressor should be given? Ephedrine, a mixed α- and β-agonist, is the preferred vasopressor in most cases of hypotension in obstetric anesthesia practice. The conventional wisdom is that ephedrine's β-agonist activity helps to maintain maternal cardiac output and uterine perfusion. Chestnut et al. (74, 75) hypothesized that, in a patient already receiving a β-agonist, any vasopressor effect from ephedrine should result from α-receptor stimulation. The accompanying uterine vasoconstriction would then result in decreased uterine blood flow. However, they noted that ephedrine aided restoration of uterine blood flow velocity in gravid guinea pigs rendered hypotensive by acute hemorrhage during terbutaline infusion (Fig. 18.9)

(74). Ephedrine seemed to restore cardiac output despite the presence of preexisting β-receptor stimulation. Subsequently, they evaluated the prophylactic administration of various vasopressors to normotensive gravid guinea pigs after ritodrine infusion (75). Epinephrine and phenylephrine each significantly worsened uterine blood flow velocity (Fig. 18.10). Ephedrine clearly preserved uterine blood flow velocity, and mephentermine resulted in an intermediate response. Collectively these studies suggest that ephedrine produces greater venoconstriction than arterial constriction (76). One should use caution before extrapolating laboratory data to clinical practice. Nonetheless, these results suggest that ephedrine remains a satisfactory choice of vasopressor in patients who have recently received a β-adrenergic tocolytic agent. Alternatively, if one is concerned that ephed-

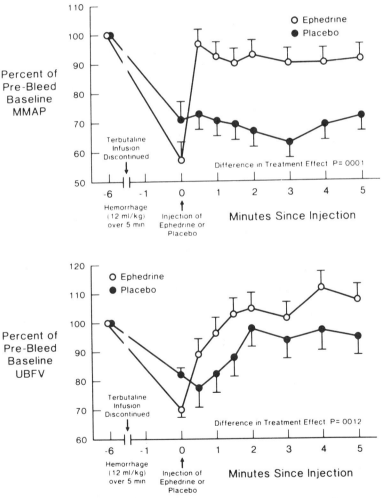

Figure 18.9. Response over time of maternal mean arterial pressure (MMAP) and uterine artery blood flow velocity (UBFV) after hemorrhage and intravenous administration of ephedrine, 1 mg/kg, or placebo (saline, 0.2 ml) in gravid guinea pigs. All values are expressed as mean (± SEM) percentage of the prebleed baseline. (Reprinted with permission from

Chestnut DH, Weiner CP, Wang JP, Herrig JE, Martin JG: The effect of ephedrine upon uterine artery blood flow velocity in the gravid guinea pig subjected to terbutaline infusion and acute hemorrhage. Anesthesiology 66:508–512, 1987.)

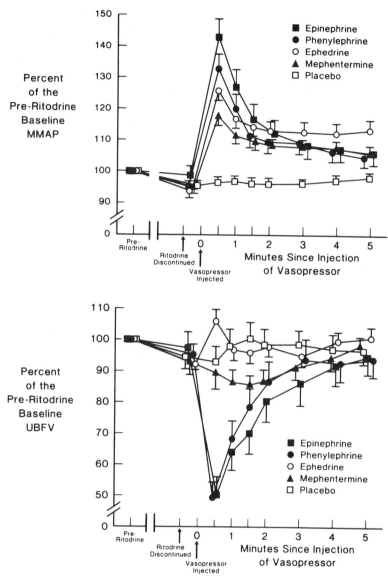

Figure 18.10. Response over time of maternal mean arterial pressure (MMAP) and uterine artery blood flow velocity (UBFV) after intravenous infusion of ritodrine and subsequent injection of epinephrine (0.001 mg/kg), phenylephrine (0.01 mg/kg), mephentermine (1 mg/kg), ephedrine (1.0 mg/kg), or placebo (saline, 0.2 ml) in gravid guinea pigs. Each value is expressed as the mean (± SEM) percentage of the preri-todrine baseline for that vasopressor. (Reprinted with permission from Chestnut DH, Ostman LG, Weiner CP, Hdez MJ, Wang JP: The effect of vasopressor agents upon uterine artery blood flow velocity in the gravid guinea pig subjected to ritodrine infusion. Anesthesiology 68:363–366, 1988.)

rine may worsen tachycardia or precipitate arrhythmia, administration of small doses of phenylephrine may represent a safe alternative (77, 78). Of course, prophylaxis of hypotension is preferable to treatment of hypotension. Shin and Kim (70) recently reported one case in which ventricular tachycardia and fibrillation developed after administration of ephedrine for treatment of hypotension (during epidural anesthesia for cesarean section) 30 min after discontinuation of ritodrine infusion.

If general anesthesia is required after discontin-uation of the β-adrenergic agent, one should remember that tachycardia as a result of β-adrenergic therapy makes it difficult to estimate the depth of anesthesia and fluid status. The tachycardia may be interpreted as a sign of inadequate analgesia, which may result in an overdosage of anesthetics. It may be interpreted as a sign of hypovolemia, which may result in excess fluid replacement. One should avoid using agents that exacerbate the tachycardia (e.g., atropine, glycopyrrolate, pancuronium) (79). Severe tachycardia and systolic hypertension have been reported in patients given ritodrine followed shortly thereafter with atropine premedication (79). Patients receiving β-adrenergic agonists have an increased incidence of arrhythmias. Thus it seems prudent to avoid halothane, which sensitizes the myocardium to catecholamine-induced ventricular arrhythmias, more than do enflurane and isoflurane. An intravenous bolus of lidocaine (1 mg/kg) administered at the time of rapid intravenous induction of anesthesia with thiopental and succinylcholine may reduce the incidence of ventricular ectopy. Hyperventilation should be avoided because this will increase the movement of potassium intracellularly and potentiate the hyperpolarization of the cell membrane (62).

In a prospective, randomized study terbutaline pretreatment shortened the onset time and recovery of succinylcholine-induced neuromuscular blockade in nonpregnant patients (80). The researchers concluded that "those patients receiving terbutaline require close monitoring of neuromuscular function and may need early intubation to mitigate possible risk of aspiration."

Magnesium Sulfate

For a long time obstetricians have administered magnesium sulfate for seizure prophylaxis in preeclamptic women. Recently magnesium sulfate has emerged as the tocolytic agent of choice in some centers. The tocolytic effects of magnesium sulfate were reported by Hall et al. (81) in 1959. They demonstrated that strips of myometrium excised from gravid human uteri exhibited reduced contractility in the presence of magnesium ion. They also reported that patients with pregnancy-induced hypertension who were treated with magnesium sulfate had a greater incidence of labor prolonged beyond 24 hr than did controls. Since the initial report of prolonged labor associated with magnesium sulfate, there have been a number of other reports of intravenous magnesium sulfate slowing uterine contractions, both when it is used for seizure prophylaxis in preeclampsia (82) and when it is used in the treatment of preterm labor (83–92). Although chest pain and pulmonary edema may occur, these complications occur less often with magnesium sulfate therapy than with β-adrenergic therapy.

Mechanism of Action. **Magnesium** probably works at a cellular level and a nerve transmission level to decrease uterine activity. The mechanism for the inhibitory effect of magnesium sulfate on smooth muscle activity remains uncertain. Like calcium, magnesium is intimately involved in the regulation of muscle contraction (interaction of actin and myosin) and neuromuscular transmission (release of acetylcholine at the neuromuscular junction). Extracellular

Table 18.4
Serum Magnesium Levels Obtained after Intravenous Bolus Followed by Constant Infusion[a]

MgSO$_4$ Therapy	No. of Samples	Magnesium in Serum (mg/dl)	
		Mean ± SD	Range
Baseline	17	1.8 ± 0.4	1.3–2.9
After 4-g bolus	35	3.5 ± 0.7	1.6–4.8
1 g/h	74	4.0 ± 0.8	2.3–5.7
2 g/h	536	5.1 ± 0.8	2.9–7.5
3 g/h	28	6.4 ± 1.4	4.1–12.0

[a] MgSO$_4$ intravenous bolus of 4 g followed by infusion started at 2 g/h with the rate changed on the basis of the patient's clinical response. (Reprinted by permission from Elliott JP: Magnesium sulfate as a tocolytic agent. Am J Obstet Gynecol 147:277–284, 1983.)

magnesium affects uptake, binding, and distribution of cellular calcium in vascular smooth muscle (93). Iseri and French (94) described magnesium as "nature's physiologic calcium blocker." By competing with calcium for surface-binding sites on smooth muscle membranes, magnesium probably prevents the increase in the free intracellular calcium concentration that is necessary for myosin light-chain kinase activity. In addition, there is evidence that an increased magnesium ion concentration activates adenyl cyclase and synthesis of cAMP (93).

Magnesium also acts at the neuromuscular junction by decreasing the release of acetylcholine (by competing with calcium for binding sites on the acetylcholine vesicle) and by decreasing the sensitivity of the endplate to acetylcholine. In unanesthetized preeclamptic women receiving magnesium sulfate neuromuscular transmission is abnormal (95). The intensity of the abnormality correlates with increased serum concentrations of magnesium.

Treatment Regimen. Several clinical protocols have been described for the tocolytic use of magnesium sulfate (83–86). Serum magnesium concentrations between 5 and 7 mg/100 ml are usually sufficient to inhibit the contractions of patients in preterm labor (86). Table 18.4 lists serum magnesium concentrations obtained after intravenous administration of magnesium sulfate at various dosages.

Side Effects. Magnesium sulfate tocolysis has also been associated with some of the same side effects associated with β-adrenergic tocolysis, including pulmonary edema, chest pain, chest tightness, and nausea (86, 97). Simultaneous administration of magnesium sulfate with a β-adrenergic agent may increase the likelihood of these side effects. Ferguson et al. (87) compared ritodrine alone with ritodrine and magnesium sulfate for tocolysis. Serious side effects (chest pain with or without electrocardiogram changes, chest pressure, adult respiratory distress syndrome) occurred more often in the magnesium sulfate-ritodrine group (46% of patients) than in the ritodrine-alone group (6% of patients). Of note was the fact that, in most of these patients, ritodrine was discontinued and magnesium sulfate alone was continued for tocolysis without sequelae.

Serum magnesium concentrations greater than 7 mg/dl may result in sedation, profound muscle weakness, respiratory paralysis, impaired myocardial conduction and function, and even death. In the presence of impaired renal function, serum magnesium concentrations may rapidly reach toxic levels.

The conventional wisdom is that administration of magnesium sulfate incurs little risk of cardiovascular side effects. Indeed, bolus administration of magnesium sulfate typically results in only transient decreases in systemic vascular resistance and mean arterial pressure in preeclamptic women (96). These changes typically are not maintained by continuous magnesium sulfate infusion. Thus many clinicians consider magnesium sulfate to be the tocolytic agent of choice in patients at risk for hemorrhage (e.g., placenta previa). Benedetti (29) reported one case of prolonged hypotension after terbutaline therapy in a bleeding parturient. He concluded that use of β-adrenergic agents should be avoided in bleeding patients. Subsequently, he stated that "In most instances of suspected clinical abruption and documented placenta previa, magnesium sulfate is an effective and safe alternative to betamimetic therapy. This agent has no significant vasodilatory properties and will not work against the body's own compensatory mechanisms in handling volume loss" (45).

Chestnut et al. (98) evaluated whether the intravenous infusion of ritodrine or magnesium sulfate altered the hemodynamic response to maternal hemorrhage in gravid ewes. They noted that magnesium sulfate, but not ritodrine, worsened the maternal hypotensive response to hemorrhage (Fig. 18.11). They speculated that Mg^{2+} attenuated the compensatory cardiovascular response to hemorrhage. They also speculated that ritodrine's inotropic and chronotropic activity helped maintain maternal cardiac output and mean arterial pressure during hemorrhage.

Anesthetic Considerations. Should there be a delay between the discontinuation of magnesium sulfate and the administration of regional anesthesia? Suresh and Lawson (99) opined that magnesium sulfate "should be discontinued prior to initiation of lumbar epidural analgesia because magnesium can increase the likelihood of hypotension through its generalized vasodilating properties." However, many anesthesiologists safely give epidural anesthesia to preeclamptic women who *continue* to receive mag-

nesium sulfate during anesthesia and surgery. Magnesium sulfate decreased maternal blood pressure but not uterine blood flow or fetal oxygenation during epidural lidocaine anesthesia in gravid ewes (Fig. 18.12) (100). If applicable to humans, this study suggests that hypermagnesemia may interfere with maintenance of maternal blood pressure and increase the risk of modest hypotension during regional anesthesia in normotensive parturients. In the author's judgement, it is not necessary for the anesthesiologist to withhold epidural anesthesia from women who have recently received magnesium sulfate for tocolysis. But the slower onset of epidural anesthesia seems preferable to the faster onset of spinal anesthesia.

Patients who are receiving magnesium sulfate therapy are more sensitive to both the depolarizing and nondepolarizing muscle relaxants (101). These patients should not be "pretreated" with a nondepolarizing agent before receiving succinylcholine. However, because of individual patient variation, the dose of succinylcholine used for endotracheal intubation should not be decreased below 1 mg/kg. If additional muscle relaxation is required, muscle relaxants should be administered in small increments and neuromuscular blockade monitored (102).

Thompson et al. (103) observed that parturients receiving magnesium sulfate often appear sedated. They evaluated the anesthetic effects of magnesium sulfate and ritodrine on the minimum alveolar anesthetic concentration (MAC) of halothane in pregnant and nonpregnant rats. Increased plasma magnesium concentrations were associated with nonlinear reductions of halothane MAC that were unrelated to sex or pregnancy. They observed a 20% decrease in MAC with plasma magnesium concentrations of 7 to 11 mg/dl.

Prostaglandin Synthetase Inhibitors

Prostaglandin synthetase inhibitors (PGSIs) have been suggested as an alternative to β-adrenergic agents for inhibition of preterm labor, particularly in patients with cardiac disease or hyperthyroidism (104). PGSIs alone have been shown to be effective in postponing preterm delivery (104–107), and PGSIs have been used to potentiate the tocolytic effects of β-adrenergic drugs (105, 106). However, some obstetricians avoid these agents because of concern regarding potential adverse effects on the fetus (Table 18.2).

Mechanism of Action. Prostaglandins $F_2\alpha$ and $E_2\alpha$ have a potent stimulatory action on the uterus. They not only activate myometrial contraction but also cause softening of the cervix (108). Prostaglandins are present in blood and amniotic fluid in low concentrations during pregnancy. However, during

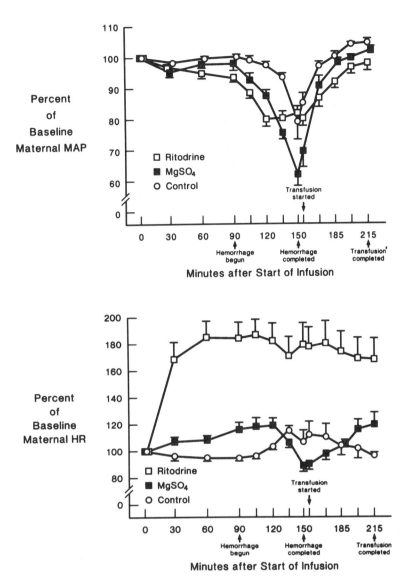

Figure 18.11. Response over time of maternal heart rate (HR) and mean arterial pressure (MAP) during intravenous administration of ritodrine (0.004 mg/kg/min), magnesium sulfate (4 gm/hour), or saline-control, and maternal hemorrhage in gravid ewes. All values are expressed as mean (± SEM) percentage of baseline. (Reprinted with permission from Chestnut DH, Thompson CS, McLaughlin GL, Weiner CP: Does the intravenous infusion of ritodrine or magnesium sulfate alter the hemodynamic response to hemorrhage in gravid ewes? Am J Obstet Gynecol 159:1467–1473, 1988.)

labor and spontaneous abortion, blood and amniotic fluid prostaglandin concentrations increase (109).

Nonsteroidal anti-inflammatory analgesics such as aspirin, *indomethacin*, naproxen, and others inhibit the synthesis of prostaglandins by preventing the metabolic conversion of arachidonic acid (110). Of these drugs, indomethacin has received the most extensive evaluation as a tocolytic agent. Indomethacin may be administered either orally or rectally.

Side Effects. Prostaglandins are involved in maintaining prenatal patency of the ductus arteriosus. There is concern that the administration of PGSIs to the mother in preterm labor will produce premature closure of the ductus arteriosus in utero and result in neonatal pulmonary hypertension. This appears to be related to the gestational age of the fetus. Most adverse effects have been associated with use of PGSIs after 34 weeks' gestation. Studies (111, 112) have shown that the administration of PGSIs to pregnant rats in late gestation produces contraction of the fetal ductus arteriosus in utero; however, there was less decrease in ductal diameter as gestational age decreased. Administration of acetylsalicylic acid to fetal lambs in late gestation caused increased fetal pulmonary artery pressure as well as increased resistance to flow across the ductus arteriosus. These changes did not occur in early gestation (113, 114). Indomethacin is now frequently used to cause clo-

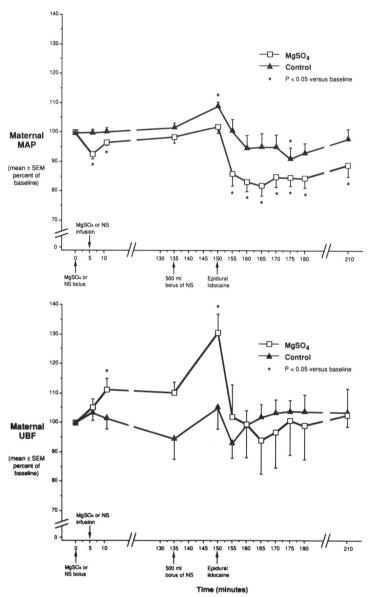

Figure 18.12. Response over time of maternal mean arterial pressure (MAP) and uterine blood flow after intravenous administration of magnesium sulfate (MgSO₄), followed by epidural administration of lidocaine in gravid ewes. (Reprinted with permission from Vincent RD, Chestnut DH, Sipes SL, Weiner CP, DeBruyn CS, Bleuer SA: Magnesium sulfate decreases maternal blood pressure but not uterine blood flow during epidural anesthesia in gravid ewes. Anesthesiology 74:77–82, 1991.)

sure of patent ductus arteriosus in preterm infants; however, it appears to be less effective in infants under 1000 g. These observations collectively suggest that PGSIs might be safer to use earlier (24 to 28 weeks) than later in gestation. Niebyl and Witter (115) concluded that adverse neonatal effects are unlikely if indomethacin is used in short courses, is restricted to patients at less than 34 weeks' gestation, and is stopped at an appropriate interval before delivery. Other studies (116, 117) have also suggested that short-term administration of indomethacin before 34 weeks' gestation is safe for the fetus. Moise et al. (118) per-

formed serial fetal echocardiography in 13 pregnant women who received indomethacin for treatment of preterm labor between 26 and 31 weeks' gestation. Evidence of ductal constriction in seven of fourteen fetuses led the authors to discontinue indomethacin. The authors concluded that indomethacin causes transient constriction of the ductus arteriosus in some fetuses, even after short-term maternal use.

PGSIs also affect renal function. Indomethacin has been shown to decrease the glomerular filtration rate and to lower plasma renin activity. Long-term indomethacin administration to pregnant monkeys resulted in decreased fetal kidney size and increased fetal liver size (119). Oligohydramnios was common, probably resulting from renal vasoconstriction and antidiuretic effect associated with decreased renal prostaglandin $E_2\alpha$ synthesis. Kirshon et al. (120) observed that maternal administration of indomethacin results in decreased fetal urine output. Indeed, some obstetricians give indomethacin specifically to treat polyhydramnios. However, Wurtzel (121) observed that maternal administration of indomethacin does not significantly alter neonatal renal function.

PGSIs inhibit cyclooxygenase, the first enzyme in prostaglandin synthesis. In platelets the major product of prostaglandin synthesis is thromboxane A_2, a potent stimulator of platelet aggregation and a vasoconstrictor. Aspirin permanently inactivates the enzyme; the effect of aspirin remains for the lifetime of exposed platelets, and aggregation is abnormal up to 7–10 days following ingestion of aspirin. In contrast, indomethacin and most other PGSIs reversibly inhibit cyclooxygenase and only transiently interfere with platelet function (122).

Anesthetic Considerations. Aspirin may result in prolongation of the bleeding time (123, 124). Some anesthesiologists perform a bleeding time test before initiating regional anesthesia in patients who have recently received a PGSI to treat preterm labor. Williams et al. (125) reported one case of cervical epidural hematoma after steroid injection into the cervical epidural space of a patient who had been receiving indomethacin. This complication occurred after the seventh epidural steroid injection over a 2-year period. However, epidural hematoma is a very rare complication in obstetric patients, and the authors are unaware of any case of epidural hematoma after administration of epidural anesthesia to a parturient who was taking a PGSI. Further, it may be difficult to obtain a bleeding time measurement with sufficient speed to help the anesthesiologist select the anesthetic technique. The anesthesiologist should assess all risks and benefits of regional anesthesia vs. alternatives. In the absence of other risk factors for abnormal bleeding and coagulation, the authors perform regional anesthesia without first obtaining a bleeding time measurement in selected patients who have received a PGSI. Finally, PGSIs should be considered a potential factor in postoperative or postpartum bleeding resulting from inhibition of myometrial contraction (126).

Calcium Entry-Blocking Drugs

Calcium entry-blocking drugs are primarily used in the treatment of ischemic heart disease, hypertension, and paroxysmal supraventricular tachycardia, but they are potentially useful as tocolytic agents.

Among the calcium-entry blocking drugs, nifedipine has received the most extensive evaluation for use as a tocolytic agent. *Nifedipine* has fewer effects on cardiac conduction and has more specific effects on myometrial contractility than some of the other calcium-entry blocking drugs. Ulmsten et al. (127) administered nifedipine to 10 patients in preterm labor with a gestational age of 33 weeks or less. The primary aim of treatment was to postpone delivery for 3 days to allow glucocorticoid treatment to accelerate fetal lung maturation. Delivery was postponed in all patients for at least 3 days. Nifedipine regularly caused transient facial flush and a moderate increase in heart rate; headache and dizziness sometimes occurred. However, no other serious side effects were observed in the mother, fetus, or neonate. Others (128–130) have reported that nifedipine seems both efficacious and safe when given for tocolysis in pregnant women. These studies have consistently noted that nifedipine is associated with less frequent and less severe cardiovascular side effects than occur with ritodrine. Using Doppler ultrasound, Mari et al. (131) observed that short-term oral administration of nifedipine did not affect either the fetal or uteroplacental circulation in pregnant women. Pirhonen et al. (132) noted that a single oral dose of nifedipine decreased uterine vascular resistance and did not affect fetal vascular resistance in pregnant women. These studies conflict with other studies (133, 134), which noted that administration of nifedipine or nicardipine decreased uterine blood flow and resulted in fetal hypoxemia and acidosis in laboratory animals. Further studies are needed before there is widespread clinical use of these agents for tocolysis in pregnant women. Given that the calcium entry blockers are a diverse group of drugs with different mechanisms of action, it is possible that some but not all of these agents are safe and appropriate for tocolysis.

Mechanism of Action. The contractility of smooth muscle (including myometrium) is directly related to the concentration of free calcium within the cytoplasm; a decrease in cytoplasmic free calcium decreases contractility. Calcium entry blockers act by altering net calcium uptake through cellular membranes by blockade of the aqueous voltage-dependent membrane channels selective for calcium or by affecting intracellular uptake and release mechanisms. The calcium entry blockers form a chemically diverse group, with unrelated chemical structure and differing pharmacologic and electrophysiologic profiles; thus it is unlikely that there is a single site of action (135, 136).

Anesthetic Considerations. Experience with the calcium entry-blocking drugs suggests that the drugs may be continued until surgery (137). However, the effects of these drugs in combination with inhalation anesthetic agents (e.g., halothane, enflurane, isoflurane) may exacerbate myocardial depression, conduction defects, and vasodilation (138). In addition, postpartum uterine atony may occur and may be unresponsive to oxytocin and prostaglandin $F_2\alpha$, leading to postpartum hemorrhage. The administration of the calcium entry-blocking drug nicardipine to rats has been shown to arrest labor; however, oxytocin and prostaglandin $F_2\alpha$ were ineffective in restoring uterine activity (139).

THE PRETERM INFANT

The preterm fetus, especially the fetus of less than 30 weeks' gestation and weighing less than 1500 g, is physiologically less well adapted than the fully mature full-term fetus to tolerate the stress of labor and delivery (140). The preterm fetus is more vulnerable to asphyxia during labor and delivery than is the term fetus, because of a lower hemoglobin concentration and thus a lower oxygen-carrying capacity. The preterm fetus is more susceptible to intracranial hemorrhage resulting from a soft, poorly calcified cranium and fragile dura mater, germinal matrix, and subependymal veins; the cerebral distortion resulting from molding of the fetal head may result in stretching and tearing of intracranial structures and hemorrhage. Preterm fetuses also have a relative deficiency of clotting factors that may accentuate their susceptibility to intraventricular hemorrhage; coagulation abnormalities are further exacerbated by hypoxia.

Cesarean Section or Vaginal Delivery

The safest method of delivery of the preterm infant, particularly one of less than 30 weeks' gestation and less than 1500 g, is controversial. In the past only a minority of obstetricians performed a cesarean section before 30 weeks' gestation because of the poor prognosis for survival in the face of increased risk of maternal morbidity and mortality. Current obstetric management of the preterm infant includes intrapartum electronic fetal heart rate monitoring and aggressive attempts at minimizing delivery-related trauma. Obstetricians now perform cesarean delivery of very low–birth-weight infants for a variety of indications (e.g., fetal distress, breech presentation, intrauterine growth retardation, failure of labor to progress, and maternal conditions such as severe preeclampsia and antepartum hemorrhage). In some cases obstetricians face the dilemma of deciding whether or not to perform cesarean section for fetal distress in patients with uncertain gestational age or in patients whose fetuses are on the borderline of extrauterine viability. For example, the obstetrician must decide whether or not to recommend cesarean sec-

tion to a patient with fetal distress at 25 weeks' gestation. In that case is it appropriate to subject the mother to the increased risk of cesarean section, recognizing the borderline viability of the fetus? In some cases of uncertain gestational age, the obstetrician may use ultrasound to obtain an estimated fetal weight. For example, the obstetrician may decide to perform cesarean section for fetal distress if the estimated fetal weight is greater than 750 g, but may avoid cesarean section if the estimated fetal weight is less than 750 g.

Some but not all studies suggest that liberal or even routine performance of cesarean section may increase the survival of preterm infants (141–149), presumably because cerebral trauma and the intermittent hypoxia of labor are avoided. But most studies on the method of delivery of very low–birth-weight infants are retrospective and not well controlled. In a retrospective study of 109 singleton neonates with birth weights of 1000 g or less, there was no difference in the frequency of neonatal morbidity or mortality between infants delivered vaginally and those delivered by cesarean section among those with birth weights from 751 to 1000 g (141). Among the newborns with birth weights between 501 and 750 g, the vaginally delivered infants had an increased frequency of intraventricular hemorrhage, as compared with those born by cesarean section, but this was not statistically significant. Anderson et al. (148) performed a prospective study, evaluating the effects of the active phase of labor and the method of delivery on the frequency of germinal layer/intraventricular hemorrhage in 89 neonates with ultrasound-estimated fetal weights less than or equal to 1750 g. They noted an increased incidence of germinal layer/intraventricular hemorrhage within 1 hour after delivery in the infants of women who experienced the active phase of labor, regardless of the method of delivery. The incidence of germinal layer/intraventricular hemorrhage beyond 1 hour after delivery and the overall incidence of these complications were both similar in the vaginal delivery and the cesarean delivery groups. Thus they concluded that "The infant of the woman delivered by cesarean section before the active phase of labor is not protected from developing germinal layer/intraventricular hemorrhage; only the time at which the infant will develop hemorrhage is shifted to later in neonatal life." They also noted that there was an increased incidence of progression to more severe grades of hemorrhage (i.e., grades III and IV), regardless of the method of delivery, in those infants whose mothers experienced the active phase of labor. Thus they speculated that "abdominal delivery before the active phase of labor may prevent the most serious form of germinal layer/intraventricular hemorrhage rather than the overall frequency of hemorrhage" (148).

It is clear that obstetricians now deliver a large percentage of preterm infants by cesarean section. Malloy et al. (149) examined birth and death certificate data from Missouri for the years 1980 to 1984. The cesarean section rate for infants weighing 2500 to 7000 g increased from 14 to 18% between 1980 and 1984. Meanwhile, the cesarean section rate for 1500 to 2499 g infants increased from 21 to 26%, and the cesarean section rate for very low–birth-weight infants (i.e., 500 to 1499 g) increased from 24 to 44%. The first-day death rate was higher in those infants delivered vaginally; however, this difference was nullified by an excess of deaths in the next 6 days of life in the cesarean section group. Overall, there was no significant difference between the vaginal and cesarean section groups in survival beyond the 1 week. The authors concluded that "There is little evidence that the use of cesarean section for the delivery of very low birth-weight infants, independent of maternal or fetal compromise, improves overall survival" (149). That is, this study suggests that there is no benefit to performing cesarean section *just because the patient is preterm.*

However, there is an increased risk of fetal distress during preterm labor. Also, patients with a preterm **breech presentation** are at risk for prolapse of the umbilical cord, entrapment of the fetal head behind an incompletely dilated cervix, or both. Entrapment of the head appears to be more common in infants weighing less than 1500 g because the head is relatively larger than the buttocks or trunk. Many authors have recommended the routine use of cesarean section for delivery of breech infants weighing less than 1500 g (142, 145–147, 150–152), resulting in an increase in the use of cesarean section for preterm breech delivery. In a retrospective study (147) of infants born between 1974 and 1978, the risk of neonatal death was significantly higher for breech infants delivered vaginally than for those delivered by cesarean section. For the 1000- to 1500-g birth-weight group the neonatal mortality for vaginal and cesarean breech deliveries was 433 and 170 neonatal deaths per 1000 live births, respectively. However, there is no prospective controlled study demonstrating that abdominal delivery of a fetus in breech presentation is safer than vaginal delivery. The apparent improvement in survival with cesarean section may be related to the change in the mode of delivery or may be due to other factors and perinatal maneuvers (153–159).

The controversy persists regarding the importance of continuous **electronic fetal heart rate (FHR) monitoring** of the preterm fetus. Luthy et al. (160) compared continuous electronic FHR monitoring and fe-

tal blood gas sampling with periodic auscultation of the FHR in a multicenter randomized study of preterm singleton pregnancies with fetal weights between 700 and 1750 g. They noted no significant difference between the two groups in the incidence of perinatal or infant death, in the prevalence of low 5-min Apgar scores, intrapartum acidosis, or intracranial hemorrhage, or in the frequency of cesarean section. In a follow-up study of the surviving children, Shy et al. (161) observed that the incidence of cerebral palsy was higher in the electronic FHR monitored group than in the group that was monitored by auscultation (20% vs. 8%, $P < 0.03$). The authors concluded that "as compared with a structured program of periodic auscultation, electronic fetal monitoring does not result in improved neurologic development in children born prematurely" (161).

Maternal Anesthesia

There are no well-controlled, prospective clinical studies on the use of analgesia and anesthesia during labor and delivery of the preterm fetus. In a Canadian study of 10 university teaching hospitals, the perinatal death rate for premature infants was 440 per 1000 when no anesthesia was administered, as compared with 140 per 1000 when conduction anesthesia was administered (162). These differences may reflect a large number of precipitous or poorly controlled deliveries with subsequent injury of the fetal head.

Wright et al. (163) retrospectively reviewed the neonatal outcome for 339 consecutive parturients who underwent preterm vaginal delivery over a 10-year period at their hospital. The study was limited to women who delivered singleton fetuses in a vertex presentation, with no congenital anomalies, between 25 and 36 weeks' gestation. The authors divided these 339 patients into those who received epidural or spinal anesthesia and those who received pudendal block, local perineal infiltration, or no anesthesia (i.e., the control group). They also divided the infants into three groups according to gestational age: 25 to 28 weeks, 29 to 32 weeks, and 33 to 36 weeks. Within these groups the authors noted no statistically significant differences between the regional and the control group in umbilical cord venous and arterial blood gas and pH values, Apgar scores, or time to sustained respiration. There was a tendency toward more vigorous neonates in the 25 to 28 weeks' gestation group when regional anesthesia was used, but this difference was not statistically significant.

In selecting an analgesic technique it must be remembered that the preterm fetus and newborn are particularly susceptible to the depressant effects of transplacentally acquired systemic medications and local and general anesthetic agents as a result of: (a) less protein available for drug binding (164) and decreased drug affinity by the protein that is present (165, 166); (b) increased levels of bilirubin (167–169), which may compete with the drug for protein binding; (c) increased likelihood that the drug may attain high concentrations in the central nervous system because of a poorly developed blood-brain barrier (170); (d) a higher incidence of asphyxia during labor and delivery (164, 171, 172); and (e) a decreased ability to metabolize and excrete drugs.

However, the capability of the fetus to metabolize drugs is greater than originally thought. In contrast to fetuses of other species, liver microsomes of human fetuses have significant amounts of cytochrome P-450, detectable as early as the 14th week of gestation (173–175), to catalyze the oxidation of various drugs (176, 177). For example, even the preterm human fetus has the capability of metabolizing both ester- and amide-type local anesthetics (178–182). In fact, two studies noted that preterm fetal lambs are more resistant to toxic reactions than are term fetuses. Teramo et al. (183, 184) administered lidocaine to preterm fetal lambs either by continuous intravenous infusion or by bolus injection and found that, as long as the fetal arterial concentration of lidocaine remained below 7 μg/ml, there were no fetal cardiovascular changes. On the other hand, concentrations of lidocaine of 11.6 μg/ml produced transient episodes of epileptiform high-voltage activity recorded in the electroencephalogram, followed immediately by hypertension associated initially with tachycardia (Fig. 18.13). Only with the bolus injection of 30 to 50 mg of lidocaine did they observe an initial fetal bradycardia and hypotension (Fig. 18.14) (183). The amounts of lidocaine necessary to produce convulsive episodes depended on fetal gestational age: younger fetuses required far more lidocaine than did older fetuses (Fig. 18.15) (184). Gestational age also influenced the fetal cardiovascular response: increases in blood pressure and heart rate in response to lidocaine were greater with advancing gestational age. Teramo et al. suggested that the greater toxicity of local anesthetics in the older fetuses could be related to an increased propensity of the drug to enter the neural tissues or to the increased number and sensitivity of individual neurons.

Pedersen et al. (185) performed a study to evaluate whether gestational age affects the pharmacokinetics and pharmacodynamics of lidocaine in gravid ewes and fetal lambs. They gave lidocaine intravenously to gravid ewes for 180 min, to reach a steady-state maternal plasma lidocaine concentration of approximately 2 μg/ml. There were no significant differences in steady-state plasma lidocaine concentrations between preterm (119 ± 1 days gestation or 0.8 of term pregnancy) and term (138 ± 1.2 days) fetuses. Tissue uptake of lidocaine tended to be higher in the preterm mothers than in the term mothers, but these differences were significant only in the brain and the adrenal glands. Tissue uptake of lidocaine was similar in both groups of fetal lambs, except that it was higher in the lungs and liver in the term fetuses. Transplacental passage of lidocaine did not adversely affect fetal cardiac output, organ blood flow, or blood gas and acid-base values. The authors concluded that the pharmacokinetics and pharmacodynamics of lidocaine in the maternal and fetal sheep did not differ between the two gestational ages studied.

However, as mentioned previously, preterm fetuses may still be at great risk for developing toxic reactions to local anesthetics and for experiencing increased depression after maternally administered opioid, sedative, and general anesthetic drugs because of low protein-binding capacities (165, 166, 186–188), a poorly developed blood-brain barrier (170), and a higher incidence of asphyxia during labor and delivery (164, 171, 172). In fact, asphyxia: (a) reduces the protein-binding capacity (188–190); (b) increases the normal maternal-fetal hydrogen ion difference, thereby causing "trapping" (i.e., weak bases, such as amide local anesthetics, and opioids administered to the mother, concentrate on the fetal side of the placental circulation when the fetal pH drops) (166, 190–194); (c) increases the blood-brain barrier permeability (195–197); and (d) enhances the myocardial depressant effects of local anesthetics (198–202). Recently Morishima et al. (203) subjected preterm fetal lambs (i.e., 119 ± 2 days gestation, or 0.8 of term pregnancy) to modest asphyxia by producing partial umbilical cord occlusion. They then gave either lidocaine or saline-control intravenously to the mothers for 180 min. At steady state, maternal and fetal plasma lidocaine concentrations were 2.32 ± 0.12 and 1.23 ± 0.17 μg/ml, respectively, similar to those obtained during epidural anesthesia in humans. Asphyxia resulted in the typical fetal compensatory response (i.e., decreased fetal heart rate and increased blood flow to the fetal brain, heart, and adrenal glands). Asphyxia and saline did not result in additional deterioration of the fetal lamb, but asphyxia and lidocaine resulted in a significant increase in $PaCO_2$ and significant decreases in fetal pH, mean arterial pressure, and blood flows to the brain, heart, and adrenal glands. These responses differed from the responses to lidocaine in the asphyxiated mature fetal lamb, as observed in an earlier study by the same group of investigators (204). The authors concluded that the

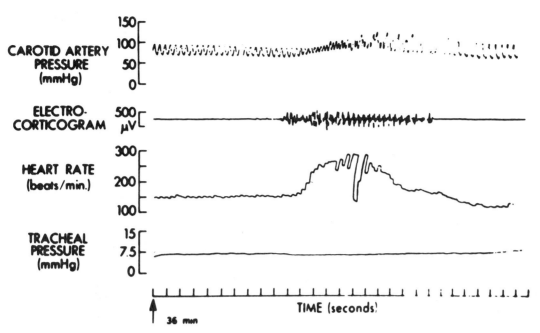

Figure 18.13. Fetal arterial pressure, electrocorticogram, heart rate, and tracheal pressure during one epileptiform burst following fetal infusion of 1.98 mg/min/kg of lidocaine. The epileptiform activity precedes increases in blood pressure and heart rate by approximately 2 sec. The fetus had been paralyzed with succinylcholine. Thirty-six minutes indicates the time from the beginning of the infusion. (Reprinted by permission from Teramo K, Benowitz N, Heymann MA, Rudolph AM: Effects of lidocaine on heart rate, blood pressure, and electrocorticogram in fetal sheep. Am J Obstet Gynecol 118:935–949, 1974.)

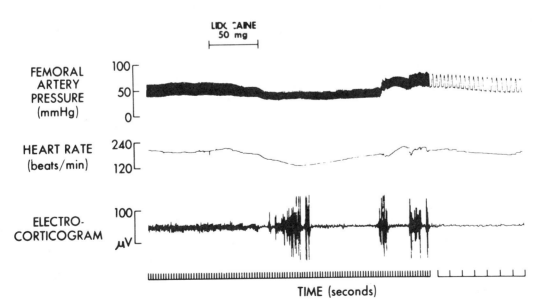

Figure 18.14. Effect of 50 mg (22.2 mg/kg) of lidocaine injected as a bolus into the femoral vein of the fetal lamb in utero. (Reprinted by permission from Teramo K, Benowitz N, Heymann MA, Rudolph AM: Effects of lidocaine on heart rate, blood pressure, and electrocorticogram in fetal sheep. Am J Obstet Gynecol 118:935–949, 1974.)

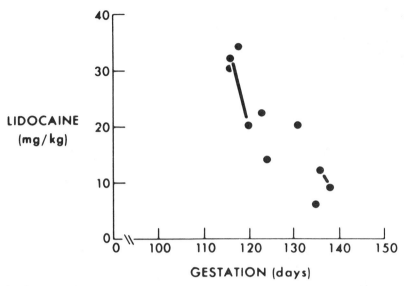

Figure 18.15. Correlation between the convulsive dose of lidocaine (mg/fetal weight) and gestational age in the lamb fetus. *Points connected with a line* represent data from the same fetus. (Reprinted by permission from Teramo K. Be-nowitz N, Heymann MA, Rudolph AM: Gestational differences in lidocaine toxicity in the fetal lamb. Anesthesiology 44:133–138, 1976.)

preterm, immature fetal lamb "loses its cardiovascular adaptation to asphyxia when exposed to clinically acceptable plasma concentrations of lidocaine obtained transplacentally from the mother." Of course, one should keep in mind that the authors did not compare the fetal response to lidocaine with the fetal response to other anesthetic, analgesic, or sedative drugs. Also the authors evaluated the effects of lidocaine-alone on the fetal response to asphyxia. That is, they did not consider the other potential benefits of epidural anesthesia, such as the decreased maternal stress response and the ability of epidural anesthesia to facilitate a smooth, controlled, atraumatic delivery of the preterm fetal head.

During labor, systemic analgesics should be avoided or given with caution. Bilirubin is competitively displaced by water-soluble organic anions that also bind to albumin, such as salicylates, sulfonamides, and benzoates (205). Preterm infants are already predisposed to the development of hyperbilirubinemia as a result of a decreased albumin-binding capacity for bilirubin (206).

During the latent phase of labor, emotional support and reassurance are often sufficient. If analgesia is necessary during the active phase, continuous lumbar epidural anesthesia is the anesthetic of choice. Minimal doses of local anesthetic can be used to provide segmental analgesia during the first stage, then extended to provide perineal relaxation and anesthesia during the second stage. 2-Chloroprocaine is rapidly metabolized and bupivacaine is highly protein bound, so fetal toxicity is minimal with either

agent. Kuhnert et al. (207) observed no difference in the elimination of 2-chloroaminobenzoic acid (a major metabolite of 2-chloroprocaine) between preterm and term neonates.

The anesthesiologist should remember that patients in preterm labor may have a rapid active phase of the first stage of labor; these patients often deliver precipitously. Specific anesthetic requirements or vaginal delivery of the preterm infant include: (a) inhibition of inappropriate maternal expulsive efforts before complete cervical dilation, especially with a breech presentation; (b) avoidance of precipitous delivery, which results in rapid decompression of the fetal head and increased risk of intracranial bleeding; and (c) provision of a relaxed pelvic floor and perineum, which will facilitate a smooth, controlled delivery of the infant's head. This last factor is especially important in cases of breech presentation. Unfortunately, appropriate timing of regional anesthesia is more difficult with preterm labor than with term labor. The preterm parturient may have a latent phase of labor that is prolonged for hours or days by administration of a tocolytic agent. When tocolytic therapy fails, the patient typically is in advanced labor. For example, after a few strong contractions, she may have a cervical dilation of 5 or 6 cm, and delivery may be imminent. The anesthesiologist should remember that full cervical dilution represents the dilation sufficient to allow for retraction of the cervix over the fetal head. In the preterm parturient, 7 cm may constitute full cervical dilation, rather than 10 cm as at term. Thus the anesthesiologist may be asked to provide epidural anesthesia immediately.

When patients are admitted in preterm labor, if analgesia is not yet required but rapid progress of labor is anticipated, an epidural catheter can be placed early in labor and local anesthetic can be injected when needed. On occasion, when it appears that tocolysis has failed or delivery is imminent, one may begin epidural anesthesia in a preterm patient and labor may cease (208). If the original goal was to stop the labor, this is not a source of concern. One should not view epidural anesthesia as primary tocolytic therapy. Indeed, it is not clear that there is a cause and effect relationship between epidural anesthesia and cessation of labor, even in preterm parturients. But the authors consider it preferable to start epidural anesthesia early in preterm patients, recognizing that one may discontinue the epidural anesthesia (and in some cases even remove the catheter) when labor stops in some of those patients. Chestnut tells his residents: "If you do not occasionally discontinue epidural anesthesia in a preterm patient whose labor has stopped, you probably are not starting epidural anesthesia sufficiently early in your preterm patients." In other words, if you wait until it is clear that preterm delivery is imminent, you will wait too long in some patients.

In cases where vaginal delivery is imminent, low spinal anesthesia most rapidly provides maximal perineal relaxation and analgesia. While pudendal block or even simple local infiltration of the perineum provides some analgesia for delivery, neither produces profound relaxation of the pelvic floor. Relaxation of the levator ani and bulbocavernous muscles helps reduce soft tissue resistance of the lower birth canal.

Most obstetricians agree that episiotomy is indicated in the vaginal delivery of a preterm infant and that the episiotomy should be performed before the fetal vertex begins to distend the perineum (209). Delivery of the head should be controlled to avoid rapid decompression of the head and intracranial bleeding. There is controversy regarding the role of forceps in the delivery of the preterm infant. Excessive compression with forceps or malplacement of forceps may fracture the fetal skull or tear the falx or tentorium. Many obstetricians use forceps only if there is a need to shorten the second stage of labor.

For cesarean section either lumbar epidural or spinal anesthesia is preferred to avoid the potential neonatal central system depression associated with general anesthesia.

After delivery the preterm neonate often requires extensive resuscitation as outlined in Chapter 39. These infants have a high incidence of birth as-phyxia, respiratory distress, hypovolemia, hypoglycemia, anemia, and temperature instability.

References

1. Bakketeig LS, Hoffman HJ: Epidemiology of preterm birth: Results from a longitudinal study of births in Norway. In *Obstetrics and Gynecology I: Preterm Labor*. MG Edler, CH Hendricks, eds. Butterworth, London, 1981, pp 17–46.
2. Brans YW, Escobedo MB, Hayashi RH, Huff RW, Kagan-Hallet KS, Ramamurthy RS: Perinatal mortality in a large perinatal center: Five-year review of 31,000 births. Am J Obstet Gynecol 148:284–289, 1984.
3. Gonik B, Creasy RK: Preterm labor: Its diagnosis and management. Am J Obstet Gynecol 154:3–8, 1986.
4. American College of Obstetricians and Gynecologists Technical Bulletin. Preterm labor. No. 133, 1989.
5. Goldenberg RL, Nelson KG, Hale CD, Wayne J, Bartolucci AA, Koski J: Survival of infants with low birth weight and early gestational age, 1979 to 1981. Am J Obstet Gynecol 149:508–511, 1984.
6. Ehrenhaft PM, Wagner JL, Herdman RC: Changing prognosis for very low birth weight infants. Obstet Gynecol 74:528–535, 1989.
7. Korenbrot CC, Aalto LH, Laros RK: The cost effectiveness of stopping preterm labor with beta-adrenergic treatment. N Engl J Med 310:691–696, 1984.
8. Leveno KJ, Little BB, Cunningham FG: The national impact of ritodrine hydrochloride for inhibition of preterm labor. Obstet Gynecol 76:12–15, 1990.
9. Iams JD: Current status of prematurity prevention. JAMA 262:265–266, 1989.
10. Herron MA, Katz M, Creasy RK: Evaluation of a preterm birth prevention program: Preliminary report. Obstet Gynecol 59:452–456, 1982.
11. Creasy RK: Prevention of preterm birth: Birth Defects 19:97–102, 1983.
12. Konte JM, Creasy RK, Laros RK: California North Coast preterm birth prevention project. Obstet Gynecol 71:727–730, 1988.
13. Main DM, Richardson DK, Hadley CB, Gabbe SG: Controlled trial of a preterm labor detection program: Efficacy and costs. Obstet Gynecol 74:873–877, 1989.
14. Goldenberg RL, Davis RO, Copper RL, Corliss DK, Andrews JB, Carpenter AH: The Alabama preterm birth prevention project. Obstet Gynecol 75:933–939, 1990.
15. American College of Obstetricians and Gynecologists Committee on Obstetrics: Maternal and Fetal Medicine Committee Opinion. *Strategies to Prevent Prematurity: Home Uterine Activity Monitoring*, No. 74. Washington, D.C., 1989.
16. Garite TJ, Keegan KA, Freeman RK, Nageotte MP: A randomized trial of ritodrine tocolysis versus expectant management in patients with premature rupture of membranes at 25 to 30 weeks of gestation. Am J Obstet Gynecol 157:388–393, 1987.
17. Weiner CP, Renk K, Klugman M: The therapeutic efficacy and cost-effectiveness of aggressive tocolysis for premature labor associated with premature rupture of the membranes. Am J Obstet Gynecol 159:216–222, 1988.
18. Arias F: Intrauterine resuscitation with terbutaline: A method for the management of acute intrapartum fetal distress. Am J Obstet Gynecol 131:39–43, 1978.
19. Sheybany S, Murphy JF, Evans D, Newcombe RG, Pearson JF: Ritodrine in the management of fetal distress. Br J Obstet Gynaecol 89:723–726, 1982.
20. Reece EA, Chervenak FA, Romero R, Hobbins JC: Magnesium sulfate in the management of acute intrapartum fetal distress. Am J Obstet Gynecol 148:104–106, 1984.
21. Huszar G: Biology and biochemistry of myometrial contractility and cervical maturation. Semin Perinatol 5:216–235, 1981.

22. Huddleston JF: Preterm labor. Clin Obstet Gynecol 25:123–136, 1982.
23. Hendricks CH: The case for nonintervention in preterm labor. In Obstetrics and Gynecology I: Preterm labor. MG Elder, CH Hendricks, eds. Butterworth, London, 1981, p 98.
24. Castle BM, Turnbull AC: The presence or absence of fetal breathing movements predicts the outcome of preterm labour. Lancet 2:472–473, 1983.
25. Agustsson P, Patel NB: The predictive value of fetal breathing movements in the diagnosis of preterm labour. Br J Obstet Gynaecol 94:860–863, 1987.
26. Schreyer P, Caspi E, Natan NB, Tal E, Weinraub Z: The predictive value of fetal breathing movement and Bishop score in the diagnosis of "true" preterm labor. Am J Obstet Gynecol 161:886–889, 1989.
27. Dailey PA: Anesthesia for preterm labor. In Anesthesia for Obstetrics, 2nd ed. SM Shnider, G Levinson, eds. Williams & Wilkins, Baltimore, 1987, pp 243–262.
28. Lipshitz J, Baillie P, Davey DA: A comparison of the uterine beta$_2$-adrenoreceptor selectivity of fenoterol, hexoprenaline, ritodrine, and salbutamol. S Afr Med J 50:1969–1972, 1976.
29. Benedetti TJ: Maternal complications of parenteral β-sympathomimetic therapy for premature labor. Am J Obstet Gynecol 145:1–6, 1983.
30. Benedetti TJ, Hargrove JC, Rosene KA: Maternal pulmonary edema during premature labor inhibition. Obstet Gynecol 59:33S–37S, 1982.
31. Elliott HR, Abdulla U, Hayes PJ: Pulmonary oedema associated with ritodrine infusion and betamethasone administration in premature labour. Br Med J 2:799–800, 1978.
32. Stubblefield PG: Pulmonary edema occurring after therapy with dexamethasone and terbutaline for premature labor: A case report. Am J Obstet Gynecol 132:341–342, 1978.
33. Jacobs MM, Knight AB, Arias F: Maternal pulmonary edema resulting from betamimetic and glucocorticoid therapy. Obstet Gynecol 56:56–59, 1980.
34. Katz M, Robertson PA, Creasy RK: Cardiovascular complications associated with terbutaline treatment for preterm labor. Am J Obstet Gynecol 139:605–608, 1981.
35. Tinga DJ, Aarnoudse JG: Post-partum pulmonary oedema associated with preventive therapy for premature labor. Lancet 1:1026, 1979.
36. Philipsen T, Eriksen PS, Lynggard F: Pulmonary edema following ritodrine-saline infusion in premature labor. Obstet Gynecol 58:304–308, 1981.
37. Wheeler AS, Patel KF, Spain J: Pulmonary edema during beta$_2$-tocolytic therapy. Anesth Analg 60:695–696, 1981.
38. Pisani RJ, Rosenow EC: Pulmonary edema associated with tocolytic therapy. Ann Intern Med 110:714–718, 1989.
39. Nuwayhid BS, Cabalum MT, Lieb SM, Zugaib M, Brinkman CR, Tabsh KM, Assali NS: Hemodynamic effects of isoxsuprine and terbutaline in pregnant and nonpregnant sheep. Am J Obstet Gynecol 137:25–29, 1980.
40. Kleinman G, Nuwayhid B, Rudelstorfer R, Khoury A, Tabsh K, Murad S, Brinkman CR, Assali NS: Circulatory and renal effects of β-adrenergic-receptor stimulation in pregnant sheep. Am J Obstet Gynecol 149:865–874, 1984.
41. Schrier RW, Lieberman R, Ufferman RC: Mechanism of antidiuretic effect of beta-adrenergic stimulation. J Clin Invest 51:97–111, 1972.
42. Bello-Reuss E: Effect of catecholamines on fluid reabsorption by the isolated proximal convoluted tubule. Am J Physiol 238:F347–F352, 1980.
43. Hauth JC, Hankins GD, Kuehl TJ, Pierson WP: Ritodrine hydrochloride infusion in pregnant baboons. I. Biophysical effects. Am J Obstet Gynecol 146:916–924, 1983.
44. Hankins GD, Hauth JC, Kuehl TJ, Brans YW, Cunningham FG, Pierson W: Ritodrine hydrochloride infusion in pregnant baboons. II. Sodium and water compartment alterations. Am J Obstet Gynecol 147:254–259, 1983.
45. Benedetti TJ: Life-threatening complications of betamimetic therapy for preterm labor inhibition. Clin Perinatol 13:843–852, 1986.
46. Gabel JC, Drake RE: Effect of endotoxin on lung fluid balance in unanesthetized sheep. J Appl Physiol 56:489–494, 1984.
47. Hatjis CG, Swain M: Systemic tocolysis for premature labor is associated with an increased incidence of pulmonary edema in the presence of maternal infection. Am J Obstet Gynecol 159:723–728, 1988.
48. Conover WB, Benumof JL, Key TC: Ritodrine inhibition of hypoxic pulmonary vasoconstriction. Am J Obstet Gynecol 146:652–656, 1983.
49. Barden TP: Effect of ritodrine on human uterine motility and cardiovascular responses in term labor and the early postpartum state. Am J Obstet Gynecol 112:645–652, 1972.
50. Hosenpud JD, Morton MJ, O'Grady JP: Cardiac stimulation during ritodrine hydrochloride tocolytic therapy. Obstet Gynecol 62:52–58, 1983.
51. Michalak D, Klein V, Marquette GP: Myocardial ischemia: A complication of ritodrine tocolysis. Am J Obstet Gynecol 146:861–862, 1983.
52. Ron-El R, Caspi E, Herman A, Schreyer P, Algom M, Schlezinger Z: Unexpected cardiac pathology in pregnant women treated with beta-adrenergic agents (ritodrine). Obstet Gynecol 61:10S–12S, 1983.
53. Tye K-H, Desser KB, Benchimol A: Angina pectoris associated with use of terbutaline for premature labor. JAMA 244:692–693, 1980.
54. Ying Y-K, Tejani NA: Angina pectoris as a complication of ritodrine hydrochloride therapy in premature labor. Obstet Gynecol 60:385–388, 1982.
55. Hendricks SK, Keroes J, Katz M: Electrocardiographic changes associated with ritodrine-induced maternal tachycardia and hypokalemia. Am J Obstet Gynecol 154:921–923, 1986.
56. Faidley CK, Dix PM, Morgan MA, Schechter E: Electrocardiographic abnormalities during ritodrine administration. South Med J 83:503–506, 1990.
57. Cotton DB, Strassner HT, Lipson LG, Goldstein DA: The effects of terbutaline on acid base, serum electrolytes, and glucose homeostasis during the management of preterm labor. Am J Obstet Gynecol 141:617–624, 1981.
58. Spellacy WN, Cruz AC, Buhi WC, Birk SA: The acute effects of ritodrine infusion on maternal metabolism: Measurements of levels of glucose, insulin, glucagon, triglycerides, cholesterol, placental lactogen, and chorionic gonadotropin. Am J Obstet Gynecol 131:637–642, 1978.
59. Brown MJ, Brown DC, Murphy MB: Hypokalemia from beta$_2$-receptor stimulation by circulating epinephrine. N Engl J Med 309:1414–1419, 1983.
60. Kauppila A, Tuimala R, Ylikorkala O, Haapalahti J, Karppanen H, Viinikka L: Effects of ritodrine and isoxsuprine with and without dexamethasone during late pregnancy. Obstet Gynecol 51:288–292, 1978.
61. Moravec MA, Hurlbert BJ: Hypokalemia associated with terbutaline administration in obstetrical patients. Anesth Analg 59:917–920, 1980.
62. Hurlbert BJ, Edelman JD, David K: Serum potassium levels during and after terbutaline. Anesth Analg 60:723–725, 1981.
63. Perkins RP, Varela-Gittings F, Dunn TS, Argubright KF, Skipper BJ: The influence of intravenous solution content on ritodrine-induced metabolic changes. Obstet Gynecol 70:892–895, 1987.
64. Chestnut DH: Anesthesia for preterm delivery. In Problems in Anesthesia. DD Hood, ed. JB Lippincott, Philadelphia, 3:32–44, 1989.
65. Kuhnert BR, Gross TL, Kuhnert PM, Erhard P, Brashar WT: Ritodrine pharmacokinetics. Clin Pharmacol Ther 40:656–664, 1986.
66. Knight RJ: Labour retarded with β-agonist drugs: A therapeutic problem in emergency anesthesia. Anaesthesia 32:639–641, 1977.
67. Schoenfeld A, Joel-Cohen SJ, Duparc H, Levy E: Emergency obstetric anaesthesia and the use of β$_2$-sympathomimetic drugs. Br J Anaesth 50:969–971, 1978.
68. Crowhurst JA: Salbutamol, obstetrics and anaesthesia: A re-

view and case discussion. Anaesth Intensive Care 8:39–43, 1980.

69. Ravindran R, Viegas OJ, Padilla LM, LaBlonde P: Anesthetic considerations in pregnant patients receiving terbutaline therapy. Anesth Analg 59:391–392, 1980.

70. Shin YK, Kim YD: Ventricular tachyarrhythmias during cesarean section after ritodrine therapy: Interaction with anesthetics. South Med J 81:528–530, 1988.

71. Suppan P: Tocolysis and anaesthesia for caesarean section (letter). Br J Anaesth 54:1007, 1982.

72. Shin YK, Kim YD: Anesthetic considerations in patients receiving ritodrine therapy for preterm labor. Anesth Analg 65:S140, 1986.

73. Chestnut DH, Pollack KL, Thompson CS, DeBruyn CS, Weiner CP. Does ritodrine worsen maternal hypotension during epidural anesthesia in gravid ewes? Anesthesiology 72:315–321, 1990.

74. Chestnut DH, Weiner CP, Wang JP, Herrig JE, Martin JG: The effect of ephedrine upon uterine artery blood flow velocity in the gravid guinea pig subjected to terbutaline infusion and acute hemorrhage. Anesthesiology 66:508–512, 1987.

75. Chestnut DH, Ostman LG, Weiner CP, Hdez MJ, Wang JP: The effect of vasopressor agents upon uterine artery blood flow velocity in the gravid guinea pig subjected to ritodrine infusion. Anesthesiology 68:363–366, 1988.

76. Lawson NW, Wallfisch HK: Cardiovascular pharmacology: A new look at the "pressors." In *Advances in Anesthesia*. RK Stoelting, PG Barash, TJ Gallagher, eds. Year Book Medical Publishers, Chicago, 1986, pp 195–270.

77. Ramanathan S, Grant GJ: Vasopressor therapy for hypotension due to epidural anesthesia for cesarean section. Acta Anaesthesiol Scand 32:559–565, 1988.

78. Moran DH, Perillo M, Bader AM, Datta S: Phenylephrine in treating maternal hypotension secondary to spinal anesthesia. Anesthesiology 71:A857, 1989.

79. Sheybany S: Ritodrine in the management of fetal distress. Br J Obstet Gynaecol 89:723–726, 1982.

80. From RP, Slater RM, Sum-Ping ST, Choi WW, Pank JR: Onset and recovery of succinylcholine induced neuromuscular blockade in patients receiving terbutaline. Anesthesiology 71:A885, 1989.

81. Hall DG, McGaughey HS Jr, Corey EL, Thornton WN Jr: The effects of magnesium therapy on the duration of labor. Am J Obstet Gynecol 78:27–32, 1959.

82. Hutchinson HT, Nichols MM, Kuhn CR, Vasicka A: Effects of magnesium sulfate on uterine contractility, intrauterine fetus, and infant. Am J Obstet Gynecol 88:747–758, 1964.

83. Steer CM, Petrie RH: A comparison of magnesium sulfate and alcohol for the prevention of premature labor. Am J Obstet Gynecol 129:1–4, 1977.

84. Spisso KR, Harbert GM Jr, Thiagarajah S: The use of magnesium sulfate as the primary tocolytic agent to prevent premature delivery. Am J Obstet Gynecol 142:840–845, 1982.

85. Valenzuela G, Cline S: Use of magnesium sulfate in premature labor that fails to respond to β-mimetic drugs. Am J Obstet Gynecol 143:718–719, 1982.

86. Elliott JP: Magnesium sulfate as a tocolytic agent. Am J Obstet Gynecol 147:277–284, 1983.

87. Ferguson JE, Hensleigh PA, Kredenster D: Adjunctive use of magnesium sulfate with ritodrine for preterm labor tocolysis. Am J Obstet Gynecol 148:166–171, 1984.

88. Petrie RH: Tocolysis using magnesium sulfate. Semin Perinatol 5:266–274, 1981.

89. Harbert GM, Spisso KR: The management of preterm labor: Use of magnesium sulfate. In *Reid's Controversy in Obstetrics and Gynecology*, 3rd ed. FP Zuspan, CD Christian, eds. WB Saunders, Philadelphia, 1983, pp 73–79.

90. Beall MH, Edgar BW, Paul RH, Smith-Wallace T: A comparison of ritodrine, terbutaline, and magnesium sulfate for the suppression of preterm labor. Am J Obstet Gynecol 153:854–859, 1985.

91. Hollander DI, Nagey DA, Pupkin MJ: Magnesium sulfate and ritodrine hydrochloride: A randomized comparison. Am J Obstet Gynecol 156:631–637, 1987.

92. Wilkins IA, Lynch L, Mehalek KE, Berkowitz GS, Berkowitz RL: Efficacy and side effects of magnesium sulfate and ritodrine as tocolytic agents. Am J Obstet Gynecol 159:685–689, 1988.

93. Altura BM, Altura BT: Magnesium ions and contraction of vascular smooth muscles: Relationship to some vascular diseases. Fed Proc 40:2672–2679, 1981.

94. Iseri LT, French JH: Magnesium: Nature's physiologic calcium blocker. Am Heart J 108:188–193, 1984.

95. Ramanathan J, Sibai BM, Pillai R, Angel JJ: Neuromuscular transmission studies in preeclamptic women receiving magnesium sulfate. Am J Obstet Gynecol 158:40–46, 1988.

96. Cotton DB, Gonik B, Dorman KF: Cardiovascular alterations in severe pregnancy-induced hypertension: Acute effects of intravenous magnesium sulfate. Am J Obstet Gynecol 148:162–165, 1984.

97. Elliot JP, O'Keefe DF, Greenberg P, Freeman RK: Pulmonary edema associated with magnesium sulfate and betamethasone administration. Am J Obstet Gynecol 134:717–719, 1979.

98. Chestnut DH, Thompson CS, McLaughlin GL, Weiner CP: Does the intravenous infusion of ritodrine or magnesium sulfate alter the hemodynamic response to hemorrhage in gravid ewes? Am J Obstet Gynecol 159:1467–1473, 1988.

99. Suresh MS, Lawson NW: Anesthesia for parturients with toxemia of pregnancy. In *Common Problems in Obstetric Anesthesia*. SJ Datta, GW Ostheimer, eds. Year Book Medical Publishers, Chicago, 1987, pp 332–347.

100. Vincent RD, Chestnut DH, Sipes SL, Weiner CP, DeBruyn CS, Bleuer SA: Magnesium sulfate decreases maternal blood pressure but not uterine blood flow during epidural anesthesia in gravid ewes. Anesthesiology 74:77–82, 1991.

101. DeVore JS, Asrani R: Magnesium sulfate prevents succinylcholine induced fasciculations in toxemic parturients. Anesthesiology 52:76–77, 1980.

102. Skaredoff MN, Roak ER, Datta SJ: Hypermagnesaemia and anaesthetic management. Can Anaesth Soc J 29:35–41, 1982.

103. Thompson SW, Moscicki JC, DiFazio CA: The anesthetic contribution of magnesium sulfate and ritodrine hydrochloride in rats. Anesth Analg 67:31–34, 1988.

104. Neibyl JR: Prostaglandin synthetase inhibitors. Semin Perinatol 5:274–287, 1981.

105. Gamissans O, Cararach V, Serra J: The role of prostaglandin-inhibitors, beta-adrenergic drugs and glucocorticoids in the management of threatened pre-term labor. In *Beta-mimetic Drugs in Obstetrics and Perinatology: Third Symposium on Beta-mimetic Drugs*. Aachen, November 1980, H Jung, G Lamberti, eds. Thieme-Stratton, New York, 1982, pp 71–84.

106. Gamissans O, Canas E, Escofet J, Figueras J, Lecumberri J, Jimenez R: Prostaglandin synthetase inhibitors in the managment of premature labor. In *Proceedings of the Ninth World Congress of Gynecology and Obstetrics, Tokyo, 1979*. Excerpta Medica, Amsterdam, 1979, pp 914–918.

107. Zuckerman H, Reiss U, Rubinstein I: Inhibition of human premature labor by indomethacin. Obstet Gynceol 44:787–792, 1974.

108. Grieves S, Liggins GC: Phospholipase A activity in human and ovine uterine tissue. Prostaglandins 12:229–241, 1976.

109. Karim SMM: Appearance of prostaglandin F$_2\alpha$ in human blood during labor. Br Med J 4:618–621, 1968.

110. Vane JR: Inhibition of prostaglandin synthesis as a mechanism of action for aspirin-like drugs. Nature New Biol 231:232–235, 1971.

111. Sharpe GL: Indomethacin and closure of the ductus arteriosus. Lancet 1:693, 1975.

112. Sharpe GL, Larsson KS, Thalme B: Studies on closure of the ductus arteriosus. XII. In utero effect of indomethacin in rats and rabbits. Prostaglandins 9:585–596, 1975.

113. Rudolph AM, Heymann MA: Hemodynamic changes induced by blockers of prostaglandin synthesis in the fetal lamb in utero. Adv Prostaglandin Thromboxane Leukotriene Res 4:231–237, 1978.

114. Heymann MA, Rudolph AM: Effects of acetylsalicylic acid on the ductus arteriosus and circulation in fetal lambs in utero. Circ Res 38:418–422, 1976.

115. Niebyl JR, Witter FR: Neonatal outcome after indomethacin treatment for preterm labor. Am J Obstet Gynecol 155:747–749, 1986.

116. Dudley DKL, Hardie MJ: Fetal and neonatal effects of indomethacin used as a tocolytic agent. Am J Obstet Gynecol 151:181–184, 1985.

117. Morales WJ, Smith SG, Angel JL, O'Brien WF, Knuppel RA: Efficacy and safety of indomethacin versus ritodrine in the management of preterm labor: A randomized study. Obstet Gynecol 74:567–572, 1989.

118. Moise KJ, Huhta JC, Sharif DS, Ou C-N, Kirshon B, Wasserstrum N, Cano L: Indomethacin in the treatment of premature labor. Effects on the fetal ductus arteriosus. N Engl J Med 319:327–331, 1988.

119. Novy MJ: Effects of indomethacin on labor, fetal oxygenation, and fetal development in Rhesus monkeys. Adv Prostaglandin Thromboxane Leukotriene Res 4:285–300, 1978.

120. Kirshon B, Moise KJ Jr, Wasserstrum N, Ou C-N, Huhta JC: Influence of short-term indomethacin therapy on fetal urine output. Obstet Gynecol 72:51–53, 1988.

121. Wurtzel D: Prenatal administration of indomethacin as a tocolytic agent: Effect on neonatal renal function. Obstet Gynecol 76:689–692, 1990.

122. Kocsis JJ, Hernandovich J, Silver MJ, Smith JB, Ingerman C: Duration of inhibition of platelet prostaglandin formation and aggregation by ingested aspirin or indomethacin. Prostaglandins 3:141–144, 1973.

123. Bick RL, Adams T, Schmalhorst WR: Bleeding times, platelet adhesion, and aspirin. Am J Clin Pathol 65:69–72, 1976.

124. Benigni A, Gregorini G, Frusca T, Chiabrando C, Ballerini S, Valcamonico A, Orisio S, Piccinelli A, Pinciroli V, Fanelli R, Gastaldi A, Remuzzi G: Effect of low-dose aspirin on fetal and maternal generation of thromboxane by platelets in women at risk for pregnancy-induced hypertension. N Engl J Med 321:357–362, 1989.

125. Williams KN, Jackowski A, Evans PJD: Epidural haematoma requiring surgical decompression following repeated cervical epidural steroid injections for chronic pain. Pain 42:197–199, 1990.

126. Lewis RB, Schulman JD: Influence of acetylsalicylic acid, an inhibitor of prostaglandin synthesis, on the duration of human gestation and labour. Lancet 2:1159–1161, 1973.

127. Ulmsten U, Andersson K-E, Wingerup L: Treatment of premature labor with the calcium antagonist nifedipine. Arch Gynecol 229:1–5, 1980.

128. Read MD, Wellby DE: The use of a calcium antagonist (nifedipine) to suppress preterm labour. Br J Obstet Gynaecol 93:933–937, 1986.

129. Ferguson JE, Dyson DC, Holbrook RH, Schutz T, Stevenson DK: Cardiovascular and metabolic effects associated with nifedipine and ritodrine tocolysis. Am J Obstet Gynecol 161:788–795, 1989.

130. Ferguson JE, Dyson DC, Schutz T, Stevenson DK: A comparison of tocolysis with nifedipine or ritodrine: Analysis of efficacy and maternal, fetal, and neonatal outcome. Am J Obstet Gynecol 163:105–111, 1990.

131. Mari G, Kirshon B, Moise KJ, Lee W, Cotton DB: Doppler assessment of the fetal and uteroplacental circulation during nifedipine therapy for preterm labor. Am J Obstet Gynecol 161:1514–1518, 1989.

132. Pirhonen JP, Erkkola RU, Ekblad UU, Nyman L: Single dose of nifedipine in normotensive pregnancy: Nifedipine concentrations, hemodynamic responses, and uterine and fetal flow velocity waveforms. Obstet Gynecol 76:807–811, 1990.

133. Ducsay CA, Thompson JS, Wu AT, Novy MJ: Effects of calcium entry blocker (nicardipine) tocolysis in rhesus macaques: Fetal plasma concentrations and cardiorespiratory changes. Am J Obstet Gynecol 157:1482–1486, 1987.

134. Harake B, Gilbert RD, Ashwal S, Power GG: Nifedipine: Ef-

fects on fetal and maternal hemodynamics in pregnant sheep. Am J Obstet Gynecol 157:1003–1008, 1987.

135. Forman A, Andersson KE, Ulmsten U: Inhibition of myometrial activity by calcium antagonists. Semin Perinatol 5:288–294, 1981.

136. Struyker-Boudier HAJ, Smits JFM, DeMey JGR: The pharmacology of calcium antagonists: A review: J Cardiovasc Pharmacol 15:S1–S10, 1990.

137. Reves JG, Kissin I, Lell WA, Tosone S: Calcium entry blockers: Uses and implications for anesthesiologists. Anesthesiology 57:504–518, 1982.

138. Tosone SR, Reves JG, Kissin I: Hemodynamic response to nifedipine in dogs anesthetized with halothane. Anesth Analg 62:903–908, 1983.

139. Csapo AI, Puri CP, Tarro S, Henzl MR: Deactivation of the uterus during normal and premature labor by the calcium antagonist nicardipine. Am J Obstet Gynecol 142:483–491, 1982.

140. Bowes WA Jr: Delivery of the very low birth-weight infant. Clin Perinatol 8:183–195, 1981.

141. Barrett JM, Boehm FH, Vaughn WK: The effect of type of delivery on neonatal outcome in singleton infants of birth weight of 1,000 g or less. JAMA 250:625–629, 1983.

142. Smith ML, Spencer SA, Hull D: Mode of delivery and survival in babies weighing less than 2000 g at birth. Br Med J 281:1118–1119, 1980.

143. Stewart AL, Reynolds EOR: Improved prognosis for infants of very low birthweight. Pediatrics 54:724–735, 1974.

144. Stewart AL, Turcan DM, Rawlings G, Reynolds EOR: Prognosis for infants weighing 1000 grams or less at birth. Arch Dis Child 52:97–104, 1977.

145. Goldenberg RL, Nelson KG: The premature breech. Am J Obstet Gynecol 127:240–244, 1977.

146. Ingemarsson I, Westgren M, Svenningsen NW: Long-term follow-up of preterm infants in breech presentation delivered by caesarean section. Lancet 2:172–175, 1978.

147. Sachs BP, McCarthy BJ, Rubin G, Burton A, Terry J, Tyler CW Jr: Cesarean section: Risk and benefits for mother and fetus. JAMA 250:2157–2159, 1983.

148. Anderson GD, Bada HS, Sibai BM, Harvey C, Korones SB, Magill HL, Wong SP, Tullis K: The relationship between labor and route of delivery in the preterm infant. Am J Obstet Gynecol 158:1382–1390, 1988.

149. Malloy MH, Rhoads GG, Schramm W, Land G: Increasing cesarean section rates in very low-birth-weight infants: Effect on outcome. JAMA 262:1475–1478, 1989.

150. Lewis BV, Seneviratne HR: Vaginal breech delivery or cesarean section. Am J Obstet Gynecol 134:615–618, 1979.

151. Duenhoelter JH, Wells CE, Reisch JS, Santos-Ramos R, Jimenez JM: A paired controlled study of vaginal and abdominal delivery of the low birth weight breech fetus. Obstet Gynecol 54:310–313, 1979.

152. Main DM, Main EK, Maurer MM: Cesarean section versus veginal delivery for the breech fetus weighing less than 1500 grams. Am J Obstet Gynecol 146:580–584, 1983.

153. Karp LE, Doney JR, McCarthy T, Meis PJ, Hall M: The premature breech: Trial of labor or cesarean section? Obstet Gynecol 53:88–92, 1979.

154. Fairweather DUI, Stewart AL: How to deliver the under 1500-gram infant. In Reid's Controversy in Obstetrics and Gynecology, 3rd ed. FP Zuspan, CD Christian, eds. WB Saunders, Philadelphia, 1983, pp 154-164.

155. Woods JR Jr: Effects of low-birth-weight breech delivery on neonatal mortality. Obstet Gynecol 53:735–740, 1979.

156. Mann LI, Gallant JM: Modern management of the breech delivery. Am J Obstet Gynecol 134:611–614, 1979.

157. Bowes WA Jr, Taylor ES, O'Brien M, Bowes C: Breech delivery: Evaluation of the method of delivery on perinatal results and maternal morbidity. Am J Obstet Gynecol 135:965–973, 1979.

158. Effer SB, Saigal S, Hunter DJS, Stoskopf B, Harper AC, Nimrod C, Milner R: Effect of delivery method on outcomes in the very low-birth weight breech infant: Is the improved

survival related to cesarean section or other perinatal maneuvers? Am J Obstet Gynecol 145:123–128, 1983.

159. Rosen MG, Chik L: The effect of delivery route on outcome in breech presentation. Am J Obstet Gynecol 148:909–914, 1984.

160. Luthy DA, Shy KK, van Belle G, Larson EB, Hughes JP, Benedetti TJ, Brown ZA, Effer S, King JF, Stenchever MA: A randomized trial of electronic fetal monitoring in preterm labor. Obstet Gynecol 69:687–695, 1987.

161. Shy KK, Luthy DA, Bennett FC, Whitfield M, Larson EB, van Belle G, Hughes JP, Wilson JA, Stenchever MA: Effects of electronic fetal-heart-rate monitoring, as compared with periodic auscultation, on the neurologic development of premature infants. N Engl J Med 322:588–593, 1990.

162. Ontario Perinatal Mortality Study Committee: Second Report of the Perinatal Mortality Study in Ten University Teaching Hospitals, Three Reports, Sec. 1, 1961, Suppl. to 2nd report, Department of Health, Toronto, 1967. Tables 108–124.

163. Wright RG, Shnider SM, Thirion A-V, Messer CP, Rosen MA: Regional anesthesia for preterm labor and vaginal delivery: Effects on the fetus and neonate. Anesthesiology 69:A654, 1988.

164. Cook LN: Intrauterine and extrauterine recognition and management of deviant fetal growth. Pediatr Clin North Am 24:431–454, 1977.

165. Mather LE, Long GJ, Thomas J: The binding of bupivacaine to maternal and foetal plasma proteins. J Pharm Pharmacol 23:359–365, 1971.

166. Thomas J, Long G, Moore G, Morgan D: Plasma protein binding and placental transfer of bupivacaine. Clin Pharmacol Ther 19:426–434, 1976.

167. Boggs TR, Hardy JB, Frazier FM: Correlation of neonatal serum total bilirubin concentration and developmental status at age eight months. J Pediatr 71:553–560, 1967.

168. Chez RA, Fleischman AR: Fetal therapeutics: Challenges and responsibilities. Clin Pharmacol Ther 14:754–761, 1973.

169. Cashore WJ, Stern L: Neonatal hyperbilirubinemia. Pediatr Clin North Am 24:509–527, 1977.

170. Himwich WA: Physiology of the neonatal central nervous system. In Physiology of Perinatal Period. U Stave, ed. Appleton-Century-Crofts, New York, 1970, pp 725–728.

171. Jones MD Jr, Battaglia FC: Intrauterine growth retardation. Am J Obstet Gynecol 127:540–549, 1977.

172. Low JA, Wood SL, Killen HL, Pater EA, Karchmar EJ: Intrapartum asphyxia in the preterm fetus < 2000 gm. Am J Obstet Gynecol 162:378–382, 1990.

173. Rane A, Sjoqvist F, Orrenius S: Cytochrome P-450 in human fetal liver microsomes. Chem Biol Interact 3:305, 1971.

174. Yaffe SJ, Juchau MR: Perinatal pharmacology. Ann Rev Pharmacol 14:219–238, 1974.

175. Alvares AP, Schilling G, Levin W, Kuntzman R, Brand L, Mark LC: Cytochromes P-450 and b5 in human liver microsomes. Clin Pharmacol Ther 10:655–659, 1969.

176. Pelkonen O, Vorne M, Arvela P, Jouppila P, Karki NT: Drug metabolizing enzymes in human fetal liver and placenta in early pregnancy. Scand J Clin Lab Invest 27(Suppl):S116–S117, 1971.

177. Rane A, Sjoqvist F, Orrenius S: Drugs and fetal metabolism. Clin Pharmacol Ther 14:666–672, 1973.

178. Vallner JJ: Binding of drugs by albumin and plasma protein. J Pharm Sci 66:447–465, 1977.

179. Magno R, Berlin A, Karlsson K, Kjellmer I: Anesthesia for cesarean section. IV. Placental transfer and neonatal elimination of bupivacaine following epidural analgesia for elective cesarean section. Acta Anaesth Scand 20:141–155, 1976.

180. Shnider SM, Way EL: The kinetics of transfer of lidocaine (Xylocaine) across the human placenta. Anesthesiology 29:944–950, 1968.

181. Meffin P, Long GL, Thomas J: Clearance and metabolism of mepivacaine in the human neonate. Clin Pharmacol Ther 14:218–225, 1973.

182. Brown WU Jr, Bell GB, Lurie AO, Weiss JB, Scanlon JW, Alper MH: Newborn blood levels of lidocaine and mepiva-

caine in the first postnatal day following maternal epidural anesthesia. Anesthesiology 42:698–707, 1975.

183. Teramo K, Benowitz N, Heymann MA, Rudolph AM: Effects of lidocaine on heart rate, blood pressure, and electrocorticogram in fetal sheep. Am J Obstet Gynecol 118:935–949, 1974.

184. Teramo K, Benowitz N, Heymann MA, Rudolph AM: Gestational differences in lidocaine toxicity in the fetal lamb. Anesthesiology 44:133–138, 1976.

185. Pedersen H, Santos AC, Morishima HO, Finster M, Plosker H, Arthur GR, Covino BG: Does gestational age affect the pharmacokinetics and pharmacodynamics of lidocaine in mother and fetus? Anesthesiology 68:367–372, 1988.

186. Burt RAP: The foetal and maternal pharmacology of some of the drugs used for the relief of pain in labour. Br J Anaesth 43:824–836, 1971.

187. Scott DB: Analgesia in labour. Br J Anaesth 49:11–17, 1977.

188. Tucker GT, Mather LE: Pharmacokinetics of local anaesthetic agents. Br J Anaesth 47:213–224, 1975.

189. Tucker GT: Plasma binding and disposition of local anesthetics. Int Anesthesiol Clin 13:33–59, 1975.

190. Shnider SM, Way EL: Plasma levels of lidocaine (Xylocaine) in mother and newborn following obstetrical conduction anesthesia: Clinical applications. Anesthesiology 29:951–958, 1968.

191. Ralston DH, Shnider SM: The fetal and neonatal effects of regional anesthesia in obstetrics. Anesthesiology 48:34–64, 1978.

192. Brown WU Jr, Bell GC, Alper MH: Acidosis, local anesthetics, and the newborn. Obstet Gynecol 48:27–30, 1976.

193. Dodson WE: Neonatal drug intoxication: Local anesthetics. Pediatr Clin North Am 23:399–411, 1976.

194. Biehl D, Shnider SM, Levinson G, Callender K: Placental transfer of lidocaine: Effects of fetal acidosis. Anesthesiology 48:409–412, 1978.

195. Lending M, Slobody LB, Mestern J: Effect of hyperoxia, hypercapnia and hypoxia on blood-cerebrospinal fluid barrier. Am J Physiol 200:959–962, 1961.

196. Evans CAN, Reynolds JM, Reynolds ML, Saunders NR: The effect of hypercapnia and hypoxia on a blood-brain barrier mechanism in fetal and newborn sheep. J Physiol 255:701–714, 1976.

197. Ritter DA, Kenny JD, Norton HJ, Rudolph AJ: A prospective study of free bilirubin and other risk factors in the development of kernicterus in premature infants. Pediatrics 69:260–266, 1982.

198. Asling JH, Shnider SM, Margolis AJ, Wilkinson GL, Way EL: Paracervical block anesthesia in obstetrics. II. Etiology of fetal bradycardia following paracervical block anesthesia. Am J Obstet Gynecol 107:626–634, 1970.

199. Rosefsky JB, Petersiel ME: Perinatal deaths associated with mepivacaine paracervical block anesthesia in labor. N Engl J Med 278:530–533, 1968.

200. Anderson KE, Gennser G, Nilsson E: Influence of mepivacaine on isolated human foetal hearts at normal or low pH. Acta Physiol Scand 353(Suppl):34–47, 1970.

201. Morishima HO, Heymann MA, Rudolph AM, Barrett CT, James LS: Transfer of lidocaine across the sheep placenta to the fetus: Hemodynamic and acid-base responses of the fetal lamb. Am J Obstet Gynecol 122:581–588, 1975.

202. Rosen MA, Thigpen JW, Shnider SM, Foutz SE, Levinson G, Koide M: Bupivacaine cardiotoxicity in hypoxic-acidotic sheep. Anesth Analg 64:1089–1096, 1985.

203. Morishima HO, Pedersen H, Santos AC, Schapiro HM, Finster M, Arthur GR, Covino BG: Adverse effects of maternally administered lidocaine on the asphyxiated preterm fetal lamb. Anesthesiology 71:110–115, 1989.

204. Morishima HO, Santos AC, Pedersen H, Finster M, Tsuji A, Hiraoka H, Arthur GR, Covino BG: Effect of lidocaine on the asphyxial responses in the mature fetal lamb. Anesthesiology 66:502–507, 1987.

205. Seligman JW: Recent and changing concepts of hyperbi-

lirubinemia and its management in the newborn. Pediatr Clin North Am 24:509–527, 1977.
206. Kapitulnik J, Valaes T, Kaufman NA, Blondheim SH: Clinical evaluation of Sephadex gel filtration in estimation of bilirubin binding in serum in neonatal jaundice. Arch Dis Child 49:886–894, 1974.
207. Kuhnert BR, Kuhnert PM, Reese ALP, Philipson EH, Rosen MG: Maternal and neonatal elimination of CABA after ep-

idural anesthesia with 2-chloroprocaine during parturition. Anesth Analg 62:1089–1094, 1983.
208. Melsen NC, Noreng MF: Epidural blockade in the treatment of preterm labour. Anaesthesia 43:126–127, 1988.
209. Bishop EH, Israel SL, Briscoe CL: Obstetric influences on the infant's first year of life. Obstet Gynecol 26:628–634, 1965.

CHAPTER 19

Coagulation Disorders and Hemoglobinopathies in the Obstetric and Surgical Patient

Russell K. Laros, Jr., M.D.

On occasion the obstetrician-gynecologist and anesthesiologist are confronted by the need to anesthetize and deliver or operate on a patient with a coagulation disorder or hemoglobinopathy. The diagnosis for patients with a hemoglobinopathy will have been made during the antepartum period. However, when the history suggests an undiagnosed abnormality of coagulation, a preoperative laboratory screen (bleeding times, platelet count, prothrombin time, partial thromboplastin time and thrombin time) will usually indicate either normalcy or the need for further studies to specifically identify the abnormality. Although most bleeding disorders can be anticipated and diagnosed preoperatively by history and laboratory evaluation, on occasion they may present themselves dramatically for the first time during surgery. In either instance, a clear understanding of the coagulation mechanism, the laboratory evaluation of coagulation, and therapy of the common disorders of hemostasis is essential.

THE COAGULATION MECHANISM

The initial coagulation mechanism for thrombus formation in vivo is adhesion of platelets to the injured vessel walls (1). Exposed subendothelium in the injured tissue initiates adhesion, which is promptly followed by a change in shape of the platelet:

$$\text{Injury + platelets} \xrightarrow[\text{aggregation}]{\text{adhesion}} \text{platelet factors + ADP}$$

Both the platelet membrane and release of the contents of δ-, α- and λ-granules are involved in platelet adhesion and aggregation as well as in the initiation of the plasma phase of coagulation.

The ADP released from platelets attracts more platelets to the area, resulting in *platelet aggregation*. The aggregation phenomenon tends to perpetuate itself, because newly attracted platelets in turn release ADP and attract additional platelets.

Increasingly large amounts of platelet factor III become available for initiation of the plasma phase of coagulation.

Table 19.1 details some of the properties of the coagulation factors (2). With the exception of fibrinogen, prothrombin, and calcium, the coagulation factors are trace proteins. Factor III is not listed in the table and is, in fact, the tissue factor thromboplastin. The preferred descriptive name and several common synonyms for the coagulation factors are as follows: V, proaccelerin, or labile factor; VII, proconvertin, or serum prothrombin conversion accelerator; VIII, antihemophilic factor or antihemophilic globulin; IX, plasma thromboplastin component, or Christmas factor; X, Stuart factor, or Prower factor; XI, plasma thromboplastin antecedent; XII, Hageman factor, or glass or contact factor; and XIII, fibrin stabilizing factor.

The third column in the table indicates the site of biosynthesis for each factor. It is noteworthy that prothrombin, factor VII, factor IX, and factor X depend on vitamin K for their synthesis and thus are the factors that are depleted when a patient is receiving a vitamin K antagonist such as sodium warfarin. The biologic half-life is also listed for each factor and can be used to estimate roughly the frequency of replacement therapy needed during an acute bleeding problem.

The remainder of the coagulation process can be broadly divided into three phases: the extrinsic, intrinsic, and common pathways. The pathway of function for each of the plasma factors is also noted in Table 19.1.

The total coagulation scheme can be summarized by the following schematized seven formulas:

1. $\text{Injury + platelets} \xrightarrow[\text{aggregation}]{\text{adhesion}} \text{platelet factors + ADP}$

2. $\text{Tissue thromboplastin + VII} \xrightarrow{\text{Ca}^{++}} \text{extrinsic activator}$

3. $\text{XII + XI + IX + PF3 + VIII} \xrightarrow{\text{Ca}^{++}} \text{intrinsic activator}$

Table 19.1
Some Properties of Coagulant Factors

Factor	Biochemistry	Biosynthesis	Biologic Half-life (hr)	Function
Fibrinogen (I)	Glycoprotein; MW[a] 340,000; three globular subunits	Liver	72–120	Common pathway; fibrin precursor
Prothrombin (II)	Monomeric glycoprotein, MW 71,600	Liver; vitamin K[b]	67–106	Common pathway; proenzyme precursor of thrombin
Calcium (IV)	Ionic calcium	—	—	Extrinsic, intrinsic, and common pathways
Factor V	Multimeric; MW 200,000–400,000	Liver	12–36	Common pathway
Factor VII	Monomeric glycoprotein; MW 50,000	Liver; vitamin K	4–6	Extrinsic pathway; proenzyme
Factor VIII	Multimeric glycoprotein; MW 330,000; circulates bound to multimeric von Willebrand factor	Probably by liver	10–14	Intrinsic pathway
Factor IX	Monomeric glycoprotein; MW 56,800	Liver; vitamin K	24	Intrinsic pathway; proenzyme
Factor X	Two-chain glycoprotein; MW 58,000	Liver; vitamin K	24–60	Common pathway; proenzyme
Factor XI	Two-chain glycoprotein; MW 143,000	Liver	48–84	Intrinsic pathway; proenzyme
Factor XII	Monomeric glycoprotein; MW 78,000	Unknown	52–60	Intrinsic pathway; proenzyme
Factor XIII	Tetrameric glycoprotein; MW 320,000; 4 subunits	Liver; megakaryocytes	72–168	Common pathway; proenzyme; transglutaminase
von Willebrand	Series of macromolecules; MW $1\text{-}15 \times 10^6$	Endothelial cells and megakaryocytes	12–36	Intrinsic pathway; forms a stable complex with factor VIII

[a] MW = molecular weight.
[b] Vitamin K required for synthesis.

4. $X + V + PF3 + Ca^{++} \xrightarrow[\text{intrinsic activator}]{\text{extrinsic activator}}$ common activator

5. Prothrombin $\xrightarrow[Ca^{++}]{\text{common activator}}$ thrombin

6. Fibrinogen $\xrightarrow{\text{thrombin}}$ fibrin polymer

7. Fibrin polymer + VIII $\xrightarrow{Ca^{++}}$ stabilized fibrin

The basic feature of coagulation is the conversion of circulating fibrinogen into a stabilized fibrin clot; it occurs in two steps. First, fibrinogen is enzymatically converted to fibrin monomer by the action of thrombin, and the fibrin monomeric units polymerize (formula 6). Next, the resulting fibrin clot is strengthened and further rendered insoluble by the action of factor XIII (formula 7).

For fibrinogen to be converted to fibrin, thrombin must be generated from its precursor prothrombin. This reaction is catalyzed by a complex, common activator, which consists of the activated form of factor X, factor V, calcium, and platelet factors (formula 5). The production of the common activator can occur as a result of two different pathways, the intrinsic and extrinsic. The intrinsic is so named because all its components are present in the circulating plasma (formula 3). This pathway is probably triggered by both endothelial damage and platelet factors. The extrinsic pathway is so named because it is triggered by tissue thromboplastin (formula 2).

Finally, the fibrinolytic system must be briefly considered. Fibrinolysis is the major physiologic means by which fibrin is disposed of after its hemostatic function has been fulfilled. The mechanism of fibrinolysis is schematically summarized by formulas 8 and 9:

8. Plasminogen $\xrightarrow{\text{activators}}$ plasmin

9. $\left.\begin{array}{l} \text{Fibrin} \\ \text{Fibrinogen} \\ \text{Complement} \\ \text{Factor VIII} \end{array}\right\} \xrightarrow{\text{plasmin}}$ degradation products

Plasminogen is a β-globulin with a molecular mass of 81,000 daltons. It circulates in the plasma in concentrations of 10 to 20 mg/dl. It is activated by a heterogeneous group of substances termed *plasminogen activators* (formula 8). Activators reside within the lysozyme of most cells, and urokinase and streptokinase are samples of specifically identified activators. The activated form of plasminogen, plasmin, is a proteolytic enzyme with a wide spectrum of activity. It cleaves arginyl-lysine bonds in a large variety of substrates, including fibrinogen, fibrin, factor VIII, and various components of complement (formula 9). It has a very short life in plasma, owing to its inactivation by humoral antiplasmins.

There are also a number of plasma proteases that function as inhibitors of coagulation and fibrinolysis. They serve to control both the speed and extent of coagulation and fibrinolysis. The major inhibitor of the extrinsic phase is C1 inhibitor, which inactivates factor VII_a and kallikrein. The major inhibitor of the intrinsic phase is antithrombin III which inhibits factor IX_a, factor X_a, and thrombin. Other inhibitors are α_1-antitripsin, α_2-macroglobulin and α_2-antiplasmin. Protein C is also a potent inhibitor of coagulation. Activated protein C (with its cofactor, protein S) reacts with factors V and VIII to destroy their coagulation property.

LABORATORY METHODS FOR STUDY OF BLOOD COAGULATION

There is no single test that is suitable as an overall laboratory screening study of hemostasis and blood coagulation. Commonly, the combination of bleeding time, platelet count, activated partial thromboplastin time (aPTT), prothrombin time (PT), and thrombin time are used as a screening battery. Table 19.2 indicates which factors are measured by each study and gives the normal value for the study in question. There are a large number of additional studies that define specific abnormalities of platelet function or allow measurements of a specific plasma clotting factor. The Rumpel-Leede test, platelet adhesiveness, platelet aggregation, whole blood prothrombin activation rate, and clot retraction are all examples of studies that further define abnormalities of platelet function.

Precise levels of each circulating plasma factor can be defined by either the thromboplastin generation test or cross-correction studies with normal plasma and plasma known to be deficient in the factor being assayed. A specific assay for factor XIII is also available. Several accurate methods are now available for the quantitative assay of plasma fibrinogen. Normal values range from 160 to 415 mg/dl and are abnormal in acquired hypofibrinogenemia secondary to disseminated intravascular coagulation and in the hereditary afibrinogenemias and dysfibrinogenemias.

Studies used in the evaluation of fibrinolysis include the euglobulin clot lysis time and the demonstration of fibrin-fibrinogen degradation products by a variety of techniques.

It is important to remember that the screening coagulation studies do not provide a specific etiologic diagnosis. Such a diagnosis is important because only then is it possible to optimally treat excessive bleeding should it occur during surgery. Furthermore, the presence of an adequate coagulation screen in a patient suspected of having a coagulation abnormality does not diminish the necessity of pursuing a specific diagnosis and making available specific therapy should it be needed.

In the past the bleeding time has been proported to be useful in predicting severe bleeding during surgical procedures and delivery. Several extensive reviews indicate that the use of the bleeding time has not been enhanced by standardization of the method, that there is no clinically useful correlation between the bleeding time and platelet count in thrombocytopenic individuals, and that there is no evidence the bleeding time is a predictor of the risk of either spontaneous or surgically induced hemorrhage (3, 4).

TREATMENT OF COAGULATION ABNORMALITIES

The author will not attempt to discuss all possible congenital and acquired coagulation disorders but only considers those most commonly seen by the obstetrician-gynecologist and anesthesiologist dealing with obstetric patients. Acquired disorders are far more common than congenital, and those seen most frequently include idiopathic thrombocyto-

Table 19.2
Screening Coagulation Tests

Study	Measures	Normal Values
Bleeding time	Platelets and vascular integrity	1 − 5 min (Ivy)
Platelet count	Number of platelets	$140 - 440 \times 10^9$/liter
Partial thromboplastin time	II, V, VIII, IX, X, XI	24 − 36 sec
Prothrombin time	II, V, VII, X	11 − 12 sec
Thrombin time	I, II, circulating split products, heparin	16 − 20 sec

penic purpura, disseminated intravascular coagulation, liver disease, and anticoagulant therapy. The congenital disorders seen most frequently are von Willebrand's disease and factor XI deficiency.

Platelet Disorders

Thrombocytopenia is the most common platelet disorder and is due to either diminished production or increased destruction of platelets. The severity of bleeding in thrombocytopenia is roughly proportional to the degree to which the platelet count has been lowered.

A specific diagnosis is obviously essential for the proper total management of a patient with thrombocytopenia. However, when hemorrhage is due to thrombocytopenia, platelet transfusions are frequently of value (5). The success of platelet transfusion therapy is dependent on the functional integrity of the transfused platelets, the underlying cause of the platelet defect in the recipient, and the presence and level of antiplatelet antibodies. Platelet transfusions are available both as platelet-rich plasma and platelet concentrates. When platelet concentrates are used, a relatively large number of platelets remain in the bag and can be harvested by adding a small amount of normal saline solution after evacuation of each bag to resuspend platelets remaining in the bag. One can expect an increase in platelet count of $5 - 10 \times 10^9$/liter/unit of platelets transfused. The exact incremental rise and the length of platelet survival depend both on the underlying disease process and the freshness of the platelets.

The complications of platelet transfusion are less common and less serious than those accompanying transfusion of whole blood. They include bacterial contamination, infectious hepatitis, febrile transfusion reaction and posttransfusion purpura.

Management of *idiopathic thrombocytopenic purpura* (ITP) during pregnancy requires concern for both mother and fetus (6, 7). ITP is an autoimmune disorder in which antiplatelet immunoglobulin (Ig)G is produced. The reticuloendothelial system is responsible for platelet destruction with the spleen being the primary site for both antibody production and platelet destruction. The diagnosis of ITP is made according to established criteria that include a normal blood count except for thrombocytopenia, a normal bone marrow analysis result with adequate or increased megalokaryocytes, a blood smear result showing an increased percentage of large platelets, normal coagulation study results, increased levels of platelet-associated IgG, and no other obvious cause of thrombocytopenia.

The goal of treatment for patients with ITP is remission, not cure. Thus therapy is stepwise corti-

costeroids, then splenectomy, and following that, consideration of immunosuppressive therapy or plasmapheresis. Each step is determined by the severity of the clinical situation. The management of ITP in pregnancy requires special consideration because the human placenta is known to have receptors for the F_c portion of the IgG molecule. Active transfers of IgG and antibodies from the mother to the fetus occur and cause neonatal thrombocytopenia in from 50 to 70% of neonates.

Most obstetricians and hematologists would agree that the overall management of pregnant women with this disorder should be similar to that of a nonpregnant individual. Initially one should employ corticosteroids such as prednisone in a dose of 0.5 to 1 mg/kg. Corticosteroids have been used for the last 30 years and owe their efficacy to both an immunosuppressive effect and a slowing of the rate of platelet destruction by the reticuloendothelial systems. By themselves, corticosteroids produce a transient remission in 75% of cases in adults, but a sustained remission in only 14 to 33% of cases. More recently immunosuppression with high-dose serum immune globulin has been found to be useful and now is often used during pregnancy before resorting to splenectomy. Other agents include danazol, cyclophosphamide, azathioprine, vincristine and vinblastin. Danazol is relatively contraindicated if the patient is carrying a male fetus, and the various chemotherapeutic agents are only used as a last resort.

The major controversial issue in the management of ITP has been the mode of delivery. Because of the theoretic risks of intracranial hemorrhage to thrombocytopenic fetuses, many investigators have advocated cesarean section for all women with ITP. A review summarizes data on 165 cases (6). Of the 134 infants delivered vaginally, 50 (37%) either had or developed platelet counts below 100×10^9/liter and 28 (21%) had counts below 30×10^9/liter. Only one infant was described as having intracerebral bleeding and this was nonfatal. By contrast, of the 31 infants delivered by cesarean section, 17 (55%) had platelet counts below 10×10^9/liter and 9 (29%) below 30×10^9/liter. There were three serious hemorrhages, one of which was intracranial hemorrhage at 3 days of age. These data do not support the premise that delivery by cesarean section is beneficial for thrombocytopenic infants of women with ITP. A more recent report describing 31 pregnancies from 25 women with immune thrombocytopenic purpura managed at a single institution also concluded that the route of delivery may not affect the incidence of intracranial hemorrhage in infants with thrombocytopenia (8). In an attempt to define those fetuses really at risk, Scott and associates (9) have suggested the use of fetal platelet counts obtained by fetal scalp blood sampling in early labor. They documented the reliability of the technique and suggest cesarean section only for those infants with platelet counts proven to be below 30×10^9/liter. An alternative technique is percutaneous umbilical cord blood sampling performed at 38 weeks' gestation (10, 11). Similarly, Samuels and associates (12) and Kelton and associates (13) have studied the value of platelet-associated IgG in predicting the significantly thrombocytopenic infant.

Because there is no evidence substantiating that cesarean section offers benefits to a thrombocytopenic infant, the author believes that the decision on route of delivery should be based on obstetric indications alone.

Three recent reports concern the use of epidural catheters in 14 patients with platelet counts $< 100 \times 10^9$/liter without any neurologic sequelae (14–16). Hew-Wing and associates conclude that "the current belief, that epidural anesthesia is contraindicated in patients whose platelet counts are below 100×10^9/liter has no supporting data" (17).

Acquired and Congenital Plasma Factor Disorders

Von Willebrand's disease (vWD) is inherited as an autosomal dominant trait and is characterized by abnormal bleeding of varying severity. The pathophysiologic basis for the disease is a marked decrease or absence of both clottable and antigenic factor VIII. Criteria for laboratory diagnosis are as yet not completely satisfactory but include slight to moderate reduction in the aPTT, a clottable factor VIII level 15 to 30% of normal, a prolonged bleeding time, abnormal platelet adhesiveness, a lack of ristocetin-induced platelet aggregation, and a factor VIII coagulant activity-to-factor VIII antigen ratio of 1 (18, 19).

The factor VIII level should be checked periodically during the antenatal course and pretreatment reserved for patients with levels < 25% of normal. DDAVP (l-deamino-8-D-argenine vasopressin) should be used instead of cryoprecipitate for cases known to be responsive (type I and some IIa). Treatment is begun when the patient presents in labor. A dose of 0.3 µg/kg of DDAVP is given over 30 min with the total dose not greater than 25 µg. Treatment is repeated every 12 hr with infusions being progressively less effective.

The specific treatment for serious hemorrhagic manifestations in patients with vWD who are not responsive to DDAVP is cryoprecipitate or fresh frozen plasma. Serious bleeding (and thus treatment) is rare if the factor VIII level is > 25% of normal, if the

bleeding time is <15 min or both. If cesarean section is required for obstetric reasons, treatment is indicated if the level is 40%. Cryoprecipitate, given in a dose 24 to 36 U/kg (0.24 to 0.39 bags/kg) is followed by one-half the dose every 12 hr for 3 to 8 days. If possible, treatment should be begun 24 hr preoperatively to allow new factor VIII synthesis in addition to the elevation obtained from the therapeutic material. When unanticipated acute bleeding is encountered or immediate cesarean section is planned, the initial therapeutic dose should be increased by approximately 50% and a second dose should be given approximately 12 hr later (20). Levels should be checked daily after vaginal delivery or cesarean section and therapy given if the level falls below 25% or bleeding occurs (21–24). The various glycine-precipitated antihemophiliac factors available for treatment of classical hemophilia should not be used in vWD. Although they are effective at raising factor VIII levels, they do not correct the bleeding time, ristocetin-platelet aggregation defect, or, in fact, clinical bleeding.

In *liver disease* virtually every hemostatic function may be impaired. Deficiencies of prothrombin and of factors VII, IX, and X generally result from decreased synthesis by the damaged liver. Factor V and fibrinogen are also synthesized by the liver; however, their levels are usually not so severely depressed. The diversity of the coagulation abnormality will be reflected in the laboratory studies by abnormalities in the aPTT, PT, and fibrogen levels and by abnormal fibrinolysis.

Treatment consists of both vitamin K administration and procoagulant replacement therapy. Vitamin K can be administered as vitamin K_1 in a dose of 50 mg intramuscularly; it will produce improvement in approximately 30% of patients with liver disease. Replacement therapy is accomplished with fresh frozen plasma in a dose of 10 to 20 ml/kg (25).

Factor XI deficiency (plasma thromboplastin antecedent deficiency) is a hereditary disorder transmitted as an incompletely recessive autosomal trait manifested either as a major defect in homozygous individuals with factor XI levels below 20% or as a minor defect in heterozygous individuals with levels ranging from 30 to 65% of normal (26). However, severity of bleeding does not always correlate with the level of factor XI (27–28). The aPTT is usually prolonged in individuals with factor XI deficiency, and the specific diagnosis is confirmed by demonstrating a factor XI level that is below 65% of normal.

Despite the fact that factor XI normally decreases during pregnancy (29); most gravidas do not encounter bleeding problems. In one series nine women went through 17 pregnancies without a major hemorrhage (30). Therapy is based on maintaining the Factor XI level above 40% for minor procedures (including delivery) and above 50% for major procedures. Treatment consists of a loading dose of fresh frozen plasma of 10 ml/kg followed by a maintenance dose of 5 mg/kg/day.

Disseminated intravascular coagulation is really a syndrome produced as part of an underlying disease that in some way leads to initiation of the clotting mechanisms (31). In obstetrics and gynecology, disseminated intravascular coagulation is seen in association with placental abruption (3), the dead fetus syndrome (32), amniotic fluid embolism (33), gram-negative sepsis (34), saline abortions (35), and severe preeclampsia-eclampsia (36–37).

Laboratory diagnosis is based on demonstrating consumption of procoagulants: (*a*) a decrease in fibrinogen, a decrease in platelet count, and variable prolongation of the PT and aPTT; (*b*) demonstration of circulating fibrin-fibrinogen degradation products [prolongation of the total clotting time (TCT) and a positive study of fibrin degradation products]; and (*c*) indirect evidence of obstruction of the microcirculation, such as abnormal red blood cell morphology (increased red cell fragmentation).

Treatment consists of: (*a*) treatment of the underlying disease, that is, removal of the source of thromboplastin whenever possible; (*b*) administration of procoagulants to replace factors that have been consumed; and (*c*) anticoagulant therapy with heparin to stop consumption and generation of split products. Heparin is administered in a dose of 500 to 1000 units/hr intravenously after a loading dose of 5000 units. Laboratory control of heparin therapy may be difficult. However, unless the fibrinogen level is very low, an adequate end-point can usually be obtained consisting of an increased TCT or activated clotting time to approximately 1.5 times the control value. Procoagulants can be administered in the form of fresh, platelet-rich plasma following the guidelines above for platelet transfusions. Platelet transfusions are particularly indicated if heparin is to be administered in the face of significant thrombocytopenia ($< 30 \times 10^9$/liter).

Finally, surgery or delivery in the *anticoagulated patient* must be considered. Patients receiving coumarin anticoagulants will generally withstand minor surgery if the PT is less than 35 sec and major surgery if the PT is less than 13 sec. Correction of a bleeding disorder secondary to coumarin therapy is accomplished by withholding the drug and administering vitamin K_1 in a dose of 5 to 50 mg intravenously. Although the larger doses of vitamin K_1 will speed the rate of return to normal, this is accomplished at

the cost of making reanticoagulation with coumarin difficult for a week or more. When prompt correction is required, it can also be accomplished by administering fresh frozen plasma as outlined above.

In a number of situations it is desirable to have a patient fully anticoagulated with heparin during delivery or a surgical procedure. If adequate hemostasis becomes a problem, heparin can be discontinued and instantly counteracted by the administration of protamine sulfate in a dose of 50 mg intravenously. If bleeding continues following this dose and the thrombin time or activated clotting time is still prolonged, a second dose of 50 mg should be given and this regimen repeated as needed until correction is obtained.

HEMOGLOBINOPATHIES

Our understanding of the molecular genetics of the hemoglobinopathies and the ability to make specific diagnosis has unfolded rapidly over the past three decades (39–41). The hemoglobinopathies can be broadly divided into two general types. In the thalassemia syndromes normal hemoglobin is synthesized at an abnormally slow rate. In contrast, the structural hemoglobinopathies occur because of a specific change in the amino acid content of hemoglobin. These structural changes may have either no effect or profound effects on the function of hemoglobin, including instability of the molecule, reduced solubility, methemoglobinemia, and increased or decreased oxygen affinity.

Thalassemia Syndromes

The thalassemia syndromes are named and classified by the type of chain that is inadequately produced. The two most common are α- and β-thalassemia, both of which affect the synthesis of hemoglobin A. Reduced synthesis of γ- or δ-chains and combinations in which two or more globin chains are affected are relatively rare. In each instance, the thalassemia is a quantitative disorder of globin synthesis.

α-THALASSEMIA

In α-thalassemia one or more structural genes are physically absent from the genome. In the homozygous stage all four genes are deleted and no α-chains are produced. Thus the fetus is unable to synthesize normal hemoglobin F or any adult hemoglobins. This deficiency results in high output cardiac failure, hydrops fetalis, and stillbirth (42).

The most severe form of α-thalassemia compatible with extrauterine life is hemoglobin H disease, which results from deletion of three α-genes. In these patients abnormally high quantities of both hemoglobin

H (β_4) and hemoglobin Barts (γ_4) accumulate. Because hemoglobin H precipitates within the red blood cell, the cell is removed by the reticuloendothelial system, leading to a moderately severe hemolytic anemia.

In α-thalassemia minor (α-thalassemia 1) two genes are deleted, leading to a mild, hypochromic, microcytic anemia that must be differentiated from iron deficiency. A single gene deletion (α-thalassemia 2) is clinically undetectable and is called the "silent carrier" state.

Thus the α-thalassemias present in the adult as mild, hypochromic, microcytic anemias. Diagnosis is presumptive by exclusion of iron deficiency and β-thalassemia. A specific diagnosis of α-thalassemia trait can be made with restriction endonuclease techniques. However, these studies would only be applicable under special circumstances. Although α-thalassemia does not present a hazard to the adult, it does have serious genetic implications when a mating of two individuals with α-thalassemia trait occurs. Under these circumstances a specific diagnosis must be made using restriction endonuclease techniques or a DNA probe before undertaking antenatal diagnosis (43–44).

β-THALASSEMIA

In β-thalassemia no gene deletions have been demonstrated. The best evidence to date suggests that underproduction of β-globulin chains is caused by a quantitative reduction in messenger RNA leading to a decreased rate of transcription. In the homozygous β-thalassemia condition, α-chain production is unimpeded and these highly unstable chains accumulate and eventually participate. Markedly ineffective erythropoiesis and severe homolysis result in a condition known as thalassemia major or Cooley's anemia. The fetus is protected from severe disease by γ-chain production. However, this protection disappears rapidly after birth, with the affected infant becoming anemic by 3 to 6 months of age. The infant has splenomegaly and requires blood transfusions every 3 to 4 weeks. Death generally occurs by the third decade of life and is usually secondary to myocardial hemochromatosis. Those female infants surviving until puberty are usually amenorrheic with severely impaired fertility (45–46).

β-Thalassemia minor results in a variable degree of illness depending on the rate of β-chain production. The characteristic findings include a relatively high red blood cell count (RBC), moderate to marked microcytosis, and a peripheral smear resembling iron deficiency. Hemoglobin electrophoresis characteristically shows an elevation of hemoglobin A_2.

β-Thalassemia trait does not impair fertility, and the incidences of prematurity, low–birth-weight infants, and infants of abnormal size for gestational age are identical to those in normal women (47, 48).

Again, the mating of two individuals both heterozygous for β-thalassemia is an indication for antenatal diagnosis. A detailed program of prenatal identification and antenatal diagnosis has been described by Alger and associates (47). The clinical characteristics and hematologic findings of the various thalassemias are summarized in Table 19.3.

Structural Hemoglobinopathies

To date several hundred variants of α-, β-, γ-, and δ-chains have been identified. Most differ from normal chains by only one amino acid. The nomenclature and frequency of the commonest hemoglobinopathies in American blacks are depicted in Table 19.4 (49). Diagnosis of a specific hemoglobinopathy requires identification of the abnormal hemoglobin using hemoglobin electrophoresis.

SICKLE CELL TRAIT

Women with sickle cell trait do well during pregnancy and labor but caution must be observed when using anesthesia to ensure good oxygenation. Because there is a twofold increase in the rate of urinary tract infection, prenatal patients should be screened for asymptomatic bacteriuria (50–52). These patients may become iron deficient, and supplementation during pregnancy is indicated.

SICKLE-CELL ANEMIA

Patients with sickle cell anemia (SCA) suffer from lifelong complications in part caused by the markedly shortened life span of their red blood cells. Most observers feel that the prepregnancy course of an individual is a good index of how she will do during pregnancy. Although series reported before 1979 indicated a high perinatal mortality and incidence of infants weighing less than 2500 g (53, 54), recent series showed generally good fetal outcomes (55, 56).

Virtually all of the signs and symptoms of SCA are secondary to either hemolysis, vasoocclusive disease, or an increased susceptibility to infection. Clinical manifestations may affect growth and development, with growth retardation and skeletal changes secondary to expansion of the marrow cavity. Painful crises may occur in the long bones, abdomen, chest, or back. The cardiovascular manifestations are those of a hyperdynamic circulation, and pulmonary signs may be secondary either to infection or vasoocclusion. In addition to painful vasoocclusive episodes, patients may exhibit hepatomegaly, signs and symptoms of hepatitis, cholecystitis, and painful splenic

Table 19.3
Hematologic and Clinical Aspects of the Thalassemia Syndromes

Condition	Hemoglobin (Hb) Pattern[a]				Clinical Severity
	Hb Level	HbA$_2$	HbF	Other Hb	
Homozygotes					
α-Thalassemia	↓↓↓↓	0	0	80% Hb Barts, remainder Hb H and Hb Portland	Hydrops fetalis
β$^+$-Thalassemia	↓↓↓	Variable	↑↑↑	Some Hb A	Moderately severe features of Cooley's anemia
β°-Thalassemia	↓↓↓↓	Variable	↑↑↑	No Hb A	Severe Cooley's anemia
δβ°-Thalassemia	↓↓	0	100%	No Hb A	Thalassemia intermedia
Heterozygotes					
α-Thalassemia silent carrier	N	N	N	1–2% Hb Barts in cord blood at birth	N
α-Thalassemia trait	↓	N	N	5% Hb Barts in cord blood at birth	Very mild
Hb H disease	↓↓	N	N	4–30% Hb H in adults; 25% Hb Barts in cord blood	Thalassemia intermedia
β$^+$-Thalassemia	↓ to ↓↓	↑	↑	None	Mild
β°-Thalassemia	↓ to ↓↓	↓	↑↑↑	None	Mild

[a] ↑ = increase; ↓ = decrease; N = normal. Number of arrows indicates relative intensity.

Table 19.4
Nomenclature and Frequency of the Most Common Hemoglobinopathies in Adult U.S. Blacks

Hemoglobinopathy	Abbreviated Name	Frequency
Sickle cell trait	Hb SA	1:122
Sickle cell anemia	Hb SS	1:708
Sickle cell–hemoglobin C disease	Hb SC	1:757
Hemoglobin C disease	Hb CC	1:4790
Hemoglobin C trait	Hb CA	1:41
Hemoglobin S–β-thalassemia	Hb Sβ-thal	1:1672
Hemoglobin S–high F	Hb S–HPFH	1:3412

Table 19.5
Protocol for Partial Exchange Transfusion[a]

I. Begin: at 24–28 weeks' gestation
II. Baseline laboratory studies
  A. Hb, Hct, WBC, reticulocyte count
  B. Hb electrophoresis
III. Type and cross-match blood: 4 units of fresh, buffy coat—poor, Hb S—free, washed, packed RBCs
IV. Exchange
  A. In morning
    1. Infuse 500 ml crystalloid over 1–2 hr
    2. Remove 500 ml by phlebotomy over same time period
    3. Infuse 2 units of packed RBCs over 1–2 hr
  B. In afternoon: Repeat morning procedure
V. Repeat laboratory evaluation following morning
  A. Hb, Hct
  B. Hb electrophoresis
VI. Additional exchange (2–4 units) if
  A. Hct < 35%
    or
  B. Hb A level < 40%

[a] Hb = hemoglobin; Hct = hematocrit; WBC = white blood cell count; RBC = red blood cell.

infarcts. Genitourinary signs include hyposthenuria, hematuria, and pyelonephritis (57).

Treatment for patients with SCA has been largely symptomatic, with the major objective being to end a painful crisis and combat infection. Urinary tract and pulmonary infections should be promptly diagnosed and vigorously treated with appropriate antibiotics. During the third trimester, fetal surveillance with either nonstress or stress tests should be carried out regularly.

Transfusion therapy has been used widely for years in the treatment of symptomatic patients with SCA. More recently, partial exchange transfusions and/or prophylactic transfusions have been advocated (51, 58). The transfusion protocol used at the author's institution is outlined in Table 19.5. The objective of the partial exchange transfusion is to achieve a hematocrit of >35% and a hemoglobin A level of >40%. Exchange transfusion is repeated when the hematocrit falls to less than 25%, the hemoglobin A level to less than 20%, or crisis or labor occur. A prospective, randomized study of 72 patients with SCA showed no significant difference in perinatal outcome between women treated with prophylactic transfusion and those transfused only if their hemoglobin fell below 6 g/dl or hematocrit below 18% (59). Sixty-six patients with sickle cell-hemoglobin C disease and 23 with sickle cell–β-thalassemia were only transfused for hematologic reasons and experienced similar perinatal outcomes. Prophylactic transfusion significantly reduced the incidence of painful crises and other sickle cell disease-related complications. However, the benefits attained must be balanced against a 25% incidence of alloimmunization and 20% delayed transfusion reaction.

During labor and delivery care must be taken to ensure that the patient is well oxygenated and well hydrated. Anesthesia-related hypovolemia, hypoxia, or both, are contraindicated. In an untransfused patient, regional anesthesia should be administered with great caution (60, 61). Careful fetal monitoring should be performed throughout labor. However, if an exchange transfusion protocol has been used and the hemoglobin A level is >40%, painful crises are distinctly unusual (62).

SICKLE CELL HEMOGLOBIN SICKLE CELL DISEASE

Women who are doubly heterozygous for both the hemoglobin S and the hemoglobin C genes are referred to as having hemoglobin sickle cell (SC) disease (Hb SCD). Hemoglobin electrophoresis reveals approximately 60% hemoglobin C and 40% hemoglobin S. Patients with Hb SCD generally have a normal habitus, a healthy childhood, and a normal life span. If a systematic screening program has not been utilized, many women are first diagnosed during the latter part of pregnancy when a complication occurs. At the beginning of pregnancy, most women are mildly anemic and splenomegaly is present. Examination of a peripheral blood smear will show numerous target cells. Hemoglobin electrophoresis will ensure the correct diagnosis (63, 64).

During pregnancy, 40 to 60% of patients with Hb SCD behave as if they had sickle cell anemia. In contrast to patients with SCA, they frequently experience rapid and severe anemic crises caused by splenic sequestration. Also, they have a greater tendency to experience bone marrow necrosis with the release of fat-forming marrow emboli. The clinical manifestations of Hb SCD are otherwise similar to SCA but are milder. The general management of symptomatic patients with Hb SCD is identical to that for patients with SCA. While several authors have reported good results with vigorous transfusion protocols for all patients with Hb SCD, the author has reserved exchange transfusion for those patients who are either symptomatic or whose hematocrit is <25%. Considerations for the management of labor are the same as with SCA.

HEMOGLOBIN S-β-THALASSEMIA

In this condition the patient is heterozygous for the sickle cell and the β-thalassemia gene. In addition to decreased β-chain production, there is a variably increased production of hemoglobin F and hemoglobin A_2. Because of this variable production rate, hemoglobin electrophoresis reveals a spectrum of hemoglobin concentrations. Hemoglobin S may account for 70 to 95% of the hemoglobin present, with hemoglobin F rarely exceeding 20% (65). Because of the thalassemia influence, hemoglobin S concentration exceeds hemoglobin A concentration. This is in sharp contrast to patients with sickle cell trait, in whom hemoglobin A levels exceed the concentration of hemoglobin S.

The diagnosis is made in an anemic patient by demonstrating increased hemoglobin A_2 and hemoglobin F levels in association with level of hemoglobin S exceeding that of hemoglobin A. The peripheral smear reveals hypochromia and microcytosis with anisocytosis, poikilocytosis, basophilic stippling, and target cells. The clinical manifestation of this disorder parallel SCA but are generally milder. Painful crises may occur; however, these patients have a normal body habitus and frequently enjoy an uncompromised life span. The author believes that the role of exchange transfusion should be similar to that in patients with Hb SCD. That is, exchange transfusion is reserved for the woman who experiences painful crises or whose anemia leads to a hematocrit of <25%.

HEMOGLOBIN C TRAIT AND DISEASE

Hemoglobin C trait is an asymptomatic trait without reproductive consequences. Target cells are found in the peripheral smear but anemia is not present. Hemoglobin C disease is the homozygous state and is a mild disorder usually discovered during a medical evaluation. Mild hemolytic anemia with a hematocrit in the range of 15 to 35% is characteristic. The red blood cells show microspherocytes and characteristic targeting. There is no increased morbidity or mortality associated with pregnancy and no specific therapy is indicated.

HEMOGLOBIN E DISEASE

The recent resettlement of individuals of Southeast Asian extraction has resulted in an increase in the number of persons with hemoglobin E trait and disease. The clinical and laboratory manifestations of the various hemoglobin E syndromes are outlined in Table 19.6 (66–67). Most individuals have a mild microcytic anemia that is of no clinical significance and requires no treatment. Those individuals homozygous for hemoglobin E have a greater degree of microcytosis and are frequently anemic. Target cells are prominent. Like hemoglobin C trait and disease, no specific therapy is required and reproductive outcome is normal.

Table 19.6
Various Genotypes of Hemoglobin E and Their Phenotypic Expression

Hemoglobin Genotype	Degree of Anemia[a]	MCV[b]	Electrophoresis (%)				Phenotypic Expression
			A + A$_2$	E	F	S	
A/E	0	↓	68	30	<2	0	None
E/E	0 to +	↓ ↓	<4	94	<2	0	None
E/α-thal	+ to + +	↓	50	15	35	0	None
S/E	+ +	↓	0	40	0	60	None
E/β + -thal	+ +	↓ ↓	10	60	30	0	Splenomegaly
E/$\beta°$-thal	+ + +	↓ ↓	0	60	40	0	Splenomegaly

[a] Number of + symbols indicates relative severity.
[b] MCV = mean corpuscular volume; number of arrows indicates relative amount of decrease.

References

1. Shattil SJ, Bennett JS: Platelets and their membranes in hemostasis: Physiology and pathophysiology. Ann Intern Med 94:108–118, 1981.
2. Colman RW, Hirsh J, Marder VJ, Salzman EW: *Hemostasis and Thrombosis.* JB Lippincott, Philadelphia, 1987.
3. Rodgers RPC, Levin J: A critical reappraisal of the bleeding time. Semin Thromb Hemost 16:1–20, 1990.
4. Lind SE: The bleeding time does not predict surgical bleeding. Blood 77:2547–2552, 1991.
5. Cash JD: Platelet transfusion therapy. Clin Hematol 1:395–411, 1972.
6. Kagan R, Laros RK Jr: Immune thrombocytopenia. Clin Obstet Gynecol 26:537–546, 1983.
7. Laros RK Jr, Kagan R: Route of delivery for patients with immune thrombocytopenia purpura. Am J Obstet Gynecol 148:901–908, 1984.
8. Cook RL, Miller RC, Katz VL, Cefalo RC: Immune thrombocytopenic purpura in pregnancy. A reappraisal of management. Obstet Gynecol 78:578–583, 1991.
9. Scott JR, Gruikshank DP, Kochenour NK, Pitkin R, Warenski JC: Fetal platelet counts in the obstetric management of immunologic thrombocytopenic purpura. Am J Obstet Gynecol 136:495–499, 1980.
10. Moise KL Jr, Carpenter RJ Jr, Cotton DB, Wasserstrum N, Kirshon B, Cano L: Percutaneous umbilical cord blood sampling in the evaluation of fetal platelet counts in pregnant patients with autoimmune thrombocytopenia purpura. Obstet Gynecol 72:346–350, 1988.
11. Scioscia AL, Grannum PAT, Copel JA, Hobbins JC: The use of percutaneous umbilical blood sampling in immune thrombocytopenic purpura. Am J Obstet Gynecol 159:1066–1068, 1988.
12. Samuels P, Bussel JB, Braitman LE, Tomaski A, Druzin ML, Mennuti MT, Cines DB: Estimation of the risk of thrombocytopenia in the offspring of pregnant women with presumed immune thrombocytopenic purpura. N Engl J Med 323:229–235, 1990.
13. Kelton JG, Inwood MJ, Barr RM, Effer SB, Hunter D, Wilson WE, Ginsburg DA, Powers PJ: The prenatal prediction of thrombocytopenia in infants of mothers with clinically diagnosed immune thrombocytopenia. Am J Obstet Gynecol 144:449–454, 1982.
14. Waldman SD, Feldstein GS, Waldman HJ, Waldman KA, Allen ML: Caudal administration of morphine suflate in anticoagulated and thrombocytopenic patients. Anesth Analg 66:267–271, 1987.
15. Rolbin SH, Abbott D, Musclow E, Papsin F, Lie LM, Freedman J: Epidural anesthesia in pregnant patients with low platelet counts. Obstet Gynecol 71:918–920, 1988.
16. Rasmus KT, Rottman RL, Kotelko DM, Wright WC, Stone JJ, Rosenblatt RM: Unrecognized thrombocytopenia in parturients: A retrospective review. Obstet Gynecol 71:943–946, 1989.

17. Hew-Wing R, Rolbin SH, Hew E, Amato D: Epidural anesthesia and thrombocytopenia. Anesthesia 44: 775–782, 1989.
18. Veltkamp JJ, van Tilberg NH: Autosomal haemophilia. Br J Haematol 26:141–152, 1974.
19. Weiss HJ, Hoyer LW, Rickles FR, Varma A, Rogers J: Quantitative assay of a plasma factor deficient in von Willebrand's disease that is necessary for platelet aggregation. J Clin Invest 52:2708–2716, 1973.
20. Shulman NR: The physiologic basis for therapy of classic hemophilia and related disorders. Ann Intern Med 67:856–882, 1967.
21. Noller KL, Bowie EJW, Kempers RD, Owen CA Jr: Von Willebrand's disease in pregnancy. Obstet Gynecol 41:865–872, 1973.
22. Krishanamurth M, Miotti AB: Von Willebrand's disease and pregnancy. Obstet Gynecol 49:244–247, 1977.
23. Lipton RA, Ayromlooi J, Coller BS: Severe von Willebrand's disease during labor and delivery. JAMA 248:1355–1357, 1982.
24. Cohen S, Goldiner PL: Epidural analgesia for labor and delivery in a patient with von Willebrand's disease. Reg Anesth 14:95–97, 1989.
25. Spector I, Corn M: Laboratory tests of hemostasis: The relation to hemorrhage in liver disease. Arch Intern Med 119:577–582, 1967.
26. Leiba H, Ramot B, Many A: Heredity and coagulation studies in ten families with Factor XI deficiency. Br J Haematol 11:654–665, 1965.
27. Rimon A, Schiffman S, Feinstein D, Rapaport SI: Factor XI activity and Factor XI antigen in homozygous and heterozygous factor XI deficiency. Blood 48:165–174, 1976.
28. Purcell G, Nossel HL: Factor XI (PTA) deficiency. Obstet Gynecol 35:69–74, 1970.
29. Phillips LL, Rosano L, Skrodelis V: Changes in Factor XI levels during pregnancy. Am J Obstet Gynecol 116:1114–1116, 1973.
30. Rapaport SI, Proctor RR, Patch MJ, Yettra M: The mode of inheritance of PTA disease. Blood 18:149–174, 1961.
31. Laros RK Jr (ed): *Blood Disorders in Pregnancy*, Lea & Febiger, Philadelphia, 1986.
32. Sutton DMC, Hauser R, Kulaping S, Bachmann F: Intravascular coagulation in abruptio placentae. Am J Obstet Gynecol 109:604–614, 1971.
33. Phillips LL, Skrodelis V, Kers TA: Hypofibrinogenemia and intrauterine fetal death. Am J Obstet Gynecol 89:903–914, 1964.
34. Phillips LL, Davidson EC: Procoagulant properties of amniotic fluid. Am J Obstet Gynecol 113:911–919, 1972.
35. Phillips LL, Skrodelis V, Quigley JH: Intravascular coagulation in septic abortion. Obstet Gynecol 30:350, 1967.
36. Laros RK Jr, Penner JA: Pathophysiology of disseminated intravascular coagulation in saline-induced abortion. Obstet Gynecol 48:353–356, 1976.
37. Davidson EC, Phillips LL: Coagulation studies in the hypertensive toxemias of pregnancy. Am J Obstet Gynecol 113:905–910, 1972.

38. Pritchard JA, Cunningham FG, Mason RA: Coagulation changes in eclampsia. Am J Obstet Gynecol 124:855–864, 1976.

39. Bunn HF, Forget BJ: *Human Hemoglobins*, WB Saunders, Philadelphia, 1986.

40. Weatherall DJ, Clegg JB: *The Thalassemia Syndromes*, 2nd ed. Blackwell Scientific, Oxford, 1981.

41. Steinberg MH, Adams JG: Thalassemia: Recent insights into molecular mechanisms. Am J Hematol 12:81–92, 1982.

42. Higgs DR, Vickers MA, Wilkie AOM, Pretorius AP, Weatherall DJ: A review of the molecular genetics of the human α-globin gene cluster. Blood 73:1081–1104, 1989.

43. Miller JM: Alpha thalassemia minor in pregnancy. J Reprod Med 27:207–209, 1982.

44. Kan YW, Golbus MS, Dozy AM: Prenatal diagnosis of alpha-thalassemia. N Engl J Med 295:1165–1167, 1976.

45. Kazazian HH, Boehm CD: Molecular basis and prenatal diagnosis of β-thalassemia. Blood 72:1107–1116, 1988.

46. Fosburg MT, Nathan DG: Treatment of Cooley's anemia. Blood 76:435–444, 1991.

47. Alger LS, Golbus MS, Laros RK Jr: Thalassemia and pregnancy. Am J Obstet Gynecol 134:662–673, 1979.

48. Fleming AF, Lynch W: Beta-thalassemia minor during pregnancy with particular reference to iron status. J Obstet Gynaecol Br Common 76:451–457, 1967.

49. Motulsky AG: Frequency of sickling disorders in U.S. Blacks. N Engl J Med 288:31–33, 1973.

50. Whalley PJ, Pritchard JA, Richards JR: Sickle cell trait and pregnancy. JAMA 186:1132–1135, 1963.

51. Blattner P, Dar H, Nitowski HM: Pregnancy outcome in women with sickle cell trait. JAMA 238:1392–1394, 1977.

52. Whalley PJ, Martin FG, Pritchard JA: Sickle cell trait and urinary trait infections during pregnancy. JAMA 189:903–906, 1964.

53. Horger E: Sickle cell and sickle cell-hb C disease during pregnancy. Obstet Gynecol 39:873–876, 1972.

54. Pritchard JA, Scott DE, Whalley PJ, Cunningham FG, Mason RA: The effects of maternal sickle cell hemoglobinopathies and sickle cell trait on reproductive performance. Am J Obstet Gynecol 117:662–670, 1973.

55. Morrison JC, Wiser WL: The use of prophylactic partial transfusion in pregnancies associated with sickle cell hemoglobinopathies. Obstet Gynecol 48:516–520, 1976.

56. Cunningham FG, Pritchard JA, Mason RA: Pregnancy and sickle cell hemoglobinopathies. Obstet Gynecol 62:419–424, 1983.

57. Francis RB, Johnson CS: Vascular occlusion in sickle cell disease: Current concepts and unanswered questions. Blood 77:1405–1414, 1991.

58. Cunningham FG, Pritchard JA, Mason RA, Chase G: Prophylactic transfusion of normal red blood cells during pregnancy complicated by sickle cell hemoglobinopathies. Am J Obstet Gynecol 135:994–1003, 1979.

59. Koshy M, Burd L, Wallace D, Moawad A, Baron J: Prophylactic red-cell transfusion in pregnant patients with sickle cell disease. N Engl J Med 319:1447–1452, 1988.

60. Maduska AL, Guinee WS, Heaton AJ, North WC, Barreras LM: Sickling dynamics of red blood cells and other physiologic studies during anesthesia. Anesth Analg 54:361–364, 1975.

61. Finer P, Blair J, Rowe P: Epidural analgesia in the management of labor pain and sickle cell crisis: A case report. Anesthesiology 68:799–800, 1988.

62. Morrison JC, Whybrew WD, Bucovary ET: Use of partial exchange transfusion preoperatively in patients with sickle cell hemoglobinopathies. Am J Obstet Gynecol 132:59–63, 1978.

63. Maberry MC, Mason RA, Cunningham FG, Pritchard JA: Pregnancy complicated by hemoglobin CC and C-β-thalassemia disease. Obstet Gynecol 76:324–327, 1990.

64. Laros RK Jr: Sickle cell hemoglobin C disease in pregnancy. PA Med 70:73–77, 1967.

65. Laros RK Jr, Kalstone C: Sickle cell beta-thalassemia and pregnancy. Obstet Gynecol 37:67–71, 1971.

66. Wong SC, Ali MAM: Hemoglobin E disease. Am J Hematol 13:15–21, 1982.

67. Ferguson JE, O'Reilly RA: Hemoglobin E and pregnancy. Obstet Gynecol 6:136, 1985.

CHAPTER 20

Amniotic Fluid Embolism

Dennis M. Kotelko, M.D., F.R.C.P.(C.)

Amniotic fluid embolism is a rare but often fatal obstetric complication caused by sudden infusion of "abnormal" amniotic fluid into the maternal circulation. The classic presentation is that of dyspnea, cyanosis, cardiovascular collapse, and coma, followed frequently by profuse uncontrollable hemorrhage secondary to uterine atony and severe coagulation disorders. Previously, amniotic fluid embolism was thought to occur only during labor and delivery and was considered universally fatal. Today, with invasive cardiac monitoring and immediate treatment of left ventricular failure, frequent survival is reported. Because the anesthesiologist is usually present when amniotic fluid embolism occurs, his or her understanding of the pathophysiologic derangements of this complication, and the subsequent aggressive guiding of the initial resuscitation, can increase the likelihood of successful patient outcomes.

HISTORY AND INCIDENCE

Entry of amniotic fluid into the maternal circulation was first reported by Meyer in 1926 (1). During a postmortem examination, he noticed the presence of fetal debris in the pulmonary blood vessels of a young woman. Although the syndrome was experimentally induced in animals the following year (2), the clinical entity went unrecognized until 1941, at which time amniotic fluid embolism was described by Steiner and Lushbaugh (3) as a distinct clinical entity. By careful postmortem examination, and confirmation by animal experimentation, they showed that sudden infusion of amniotic fluid produced "anaphylactoid shock," pulmonary edema, and death.

Although the incidence of amniotic fluid embolism averages 1 in 20,000, various extremes (1 in 1250 to 1 in 80,000) have been reported (3–9). Undoubtedly, many cases of minor embolism pass unnoticed and fatal nonautopsied cases are misdiagnosed.

Although overall maternal mortality has decreased in recent decades, amniotic fluid embolism has increased as a cause of death. The mortality for this condition is very high: Of 272 cases reviewed by Morgan (10), survival occurred in only 39 (i.e., mortality was 86%). In some obstetric centers (12) amniotic fluid embolism and thromboembolism are the leading causes of death; these complications generally account for 7 to 20% of all maternal mortality (12–15) (see also Chapter 25).

PATHOGENESIS

Mode of Infusion of Amniotic Fluid

For amniotic fluid to enter the maternal circulation, the membranes must be ruptured at some point and abnormal open sinusoids at the uteroplacental site or lacerations of endocervical veins must exist. In normal labor (16) and especially with rapid cervical dilation, tears of the endocervical veins may result (17); these are the most common routes of entry. Once the membranes are ruptured and the fetal head tamponades the cervix, ensuing uterine contractions push amniotic fluid upward between the membranes and the uterine wall, thereby creating a route of entry to the traumatized endocervical veins (18). Other authors (19–21) believe that the main route of entry of amniotic fluid is at the uteroplacental site or placental margin, as might occur with placental abruption, placenta previa, or placenta accreta, retained placenta, or ruptured uterus (22) or during cesarean section. Shotton and Taylor (23) postulated that uterine contractions increase intrauterine pressure, thereby forcing amniotic fluid into the circulation at these placental sites. However, during uterine contractions, intramyometrial pressure may exceed 120 mm Hg. This pressure would minimize the entry of the amniotic fluid into the vessels of the muscular uterine upper segment. Observations that some fetal squamous cells may routinely enter the venous circulation of pregnant women further support the contention that it is not amniotic fluid per se but an abnormal amniotic fluid that causes the clinical syndrome of amniotic fluid embolism (24–26).

When abnormal amniotic fluid enters the maternal circulation, the resulting syndrome is often a clini-

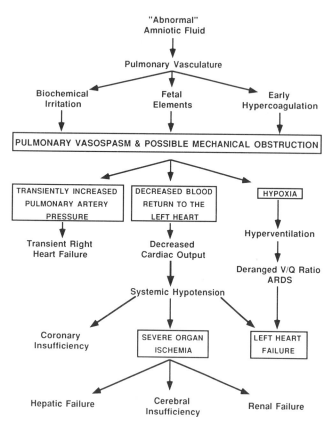

Figure 20.1. Cardiopulmonary effects and sequelae of amniotic fluid embolism.

cally biphasic process (26). Initially, the pulmonary embolism causes profound changes in hemodynamics and oxygenation. Uterine atony is common, and usually within an hour severe left ventricular failure ensues. In 40% of cases this is accompanied by disseminated intravascular coagulation (DIC).

Pulmonary Embolism

The entry of abnormal amniotic fluid into the pulmonary circulation causes cardiorespiratory collapse (Fig. 20.1). Biochemical vasospasm of the pulmonary vessels produces three acute and transient cardiopulmonary effects:

1. *A sudden decrease in blood return* to the left atrium that decreases left ventricular output, thereby producing peripheral vascular collapse and hypotension.

2. *A sudden development of pulmonary hypertension* acute cor pulmonale, and right ventricular failure.

3. *A severe derangement of the ventilation-perfusion ratio*, resulting in low arterial oxygen tension, marked tissue hypoxia, and organ ischemia.

Various animal studies have concluded that particulate matter in amniotic fluid (3, 27, 28), the number of fetal squamous cells (29), the presence of placental extracts (30), and even filtered amniotic fluid

(17, 31) (implying a humoral vasoactive substance) are responsible for these obstructive changes in the pulmonary vessels. However, major interspecies differences exist in the physiologic response to amniotic fluid embolism (26). Prostaglandins, especially $F_{2\alpha}$, have been suspected of chemically irritating the epithelium and thus producing precapillary pulmonary vasospasm (32). "Metabolites of arachidonic acid, including the prostaglandins and leukotrienes, have many of the hemodynamic and hematologic effects present in patients with clinical amniotic fluid embolism" (26). Azegami and Mori (33) showed that pretreatment of rats with an inhibitor of leukotriene synthesis prevented the otherwise fatal hemodynamic collapse observed in experimental amniotic fluid embolism in this species. Although Steiner and Lushbaugh (3) and early authors (6, 8, 34, 35) likened the effects of amniotic fluid embolism to those of anaphylactic shock, the evidence for the latter is slight. A true anaphylactic reaction requires prior sensitization, and during pregnancy, amniotic fluid normally does not enter the maternal circulation. In addition, bronchospasm, which is associated with true histamine-mediated reactions, occurs only rarely during amniotic fluid embolism.

Disseminated Intravascular Coagulation

A brief period of hypercoagulability (36) is followed by hypofibrinogenemia (37, 38), resulting in a state of profound hypocoagulability and severe hemorrhage from all traumatized sites, especially the uterus. When DIC develops, fibrin degradation products increase and circulating platelets decrease (5, 15, 34, 37–42).

Mechanics by which hypocoagulability of blood may develop include:

1. *Liberation of thromboplastin substances* into the circulation, causing depletion of plasma fibrinogen (43). Both placental tissues and amniotic fluid (44, 45) have high concentrations of thromboplastin-like materials.

2. *Destruction of fibrin and fibrinogen* by plasma fibrinolysins (46, 47).

3. *Release of a heparin-like substance* present in amniotic fluid into the circulation. This substance blocks the conversion of prothrombin to thrombin and inactivates thrombin (34, 48).

Uterine Atony

Uterine atony, a consistent feature of amniotic fluid embolism, is caused by hypotension and decreased uterine perfusion. Amniotic fluid can also have a direct depressant effect on uterine muscles (19); subsequently, both factors cause further hemorrhage.

ASSOCIATED CONDITIONS

Clinical features and patient characteristics associated with amniotic fluid embolism are presented in Table 20.1. Some of these conditions contrast with the classic view of amniotic fluid embolism, in which elderly multiparous patients have large babies following a short, tumultuous labor facilitated by administration of oxytocin. In fact, this complication often occurs in relatively young primiparous patients, and uterine stimulants are used in only a small percentage of patients. Also, babies had a mean weight of 3.3 kg, certainly a value within normal limits.

Although amniotic fluid embolism usually occurs during labor and delivery, it has also occurred after intraamniotic injection of hypertonic saline for abortion (49) and during suction and curettage in the first or second trimester (50–53). In an unusual case reported by Quance of a patient undergoing cesarean section, the oxygen saturation level fell to 71% (detected by pulse oximetry) within 1 min of delivery of the infant (54). Although the patient felt clinically well, she continued to have abnormal arterial blood gas test results and underwent pulmonary artery catheterization in an intensive care unit. Thirty minutes after insertion of the pulmonary artery catheter and 3 hr after delivery, she complained of feeling "unwell" during external uterine massage by the nurse and immediately had a generalized seizure and asystole episode. Despite aggressive treatment, she died of amniotic fluid embolism.

CLINICAL FEATURES AND DIAGNOSIS

Recent case reports suggest that amniotic fluid embolism presents as a clinically biphasic process (26) recognized initially by its sudden onset and its four cardinal features: dyspnea, cyanosis, cardiovascular collapse, and coma, followed later by left ventricular failure. A sudden severe drop in maternal oxygen saturation detected by pulse oximetry may be the first and most sensitive clinical sign of impending amniotic fluid embolism. In addition, prodromal chills, sweating, coughing, hyperreflexia, and convulsions occasionally occur (5, 6). Although the classic opinion holds that a hemorrhagic tendency is likely only

if the patient survives beyond the first hour, abnormal bleeding was the presenting feature in 12% of cases reviewed by Morgan (10). A documented case of amniotic fluid embolism that first presented as acute fetal distress manifested by severe fetal bradycardia also has been reported (55).

It was once thought that a definitive diagnosis of amniotic fluid embolism could only be made by finding fetal elements in the maternal circulation, but detection of squamous cells in the maternal pulmonary artery circulation is a common finding in patients without evidence of amniotic fluid embolism (24, 25). There is no single laboratory or clinical finding by which amniotic fluid embolism can be diagnosed.

Although not diagnostic, blood samples should be aspirated from the right side of the heart through a central venous pressure catheter (8, 15, 18, 56) or a pulmonary artery catheter (39–41, 57–59). When the blood is centrifuged, the sediment may contain fetal squamous cells, amorphous debris, bile-containing meconium, fat from vernix caseosa, fetal gut mucin, or lanugo hairs. The pathologist must be notified that amniotic fluid embolism is suspected so that special stains (Attwood's [18, 60], Giemsa [15], Wright's [57], Papanicolaou's [40], or oil red [41]) can be used when examining the smear (Fig. 20.2).

Conventional chest radiographs are not specific for amniotic fluid embolism and do not always show diffuse alveolar infiltrates. Radiographs may even be normal despite severe clinical features. Ventilation-perfusion lung scanning may aid in documenting the diagnosis (61). The electrocardiograph (ECG) may show evidence of acute right ventricular strain in the first few minutes after cardiovascular collapse (15, 57). Echocardiography has helped to confirm severe left ventricular failure and to guide the treatment and slow resolution in a patient who survived (62).

In fulminant DIC, laboratory tests confirm the clinical diagnosis and aid in treatment. Findings consistent with DIC (63) are presented in Table 20.2.

Table 20.1
Clinical Features and Patient Characteristics in Two Reviews of Amniotic Fluid Embolism

	Peterson and Taylor (13) (n = 40)	Morgan (10) (n = 272)
Patient's mean age	32 years	32 years (15–48 years)
Parity: multiparity	90%	88%
Gestational age	35–42 wk	—
In labor	90%	90%
Tumultuous contractions	28%	28%
Uterine stimulation	7%	22%
Fetal death	40%	—
Meconium staining of amniotic fluid	35%	—
Premature placental separation	45%	—

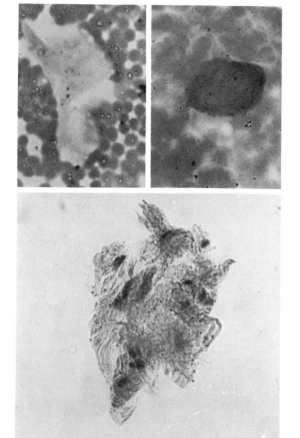

Figure 20.2. Composite of three groups of cells in blood films prepared from central venous blood removed during critical episode in a survivor. *Top left* is mucus and cellular debris, *top right* is squamous debris, both in Giemsa-stained films. *Bottom* photograph represents a cluster of squamous cells staining red in Attwood's stain. (×640) (Reprinted by permission from Resnik R, Swartz WH, Plumer MH, Benirschke K, Stratthaus ME: Amniotic fluid embolism with survival. Obstet Gynecol 47:295–298, 1976.)

At postmortem examination, marked dilatation of the right ventricle is typical (6), and amniotic fluid embolic material can usually be found in the coronary arteries, kidneys, and brain (13). On gross examination the lungs are edematous (13), and microscopic examination of lung tissue always reveals fetal elements (13, 18). Although not pathognomonic, the absence of blood clots may also be a finding at autopsy (5, 8, 23).

DIFFERENTIAL DIAGNOSIS

Amniotic fluid embolism must be differentiated from other conditions causing acute cardiorespiratory failure or excessive hemorrhage in the obstetric patient, including (a) other types of pulmonary embolism; (b) aspiration pneumonitis; (c) toxicity caused by local anesthetics; (d) eclampsia; (e) intracranial hemorrhage; (f) hemorrhagic shock; and (g) acute heart failure. These conditions are described in more detail in other chapters in this text. The following remarks suggest ways of distinguishing such conditions from amniotic fluid embolism.

Thrombotic pulmonary embolism usually occurs later in the postpartum period and is accompanied by chest pain (5). Air embolism is rare but may occur with placenta previa, following blood transfusion under pressure, or during cesarean section when large venous sinuses are open and air is entrained. When a Doppler system is placed over the precordium, the detection of a characteristic erratic roaring noise (as opposed to regular swishing sounds) should help identify intravascular air embolism (64).

Aspiration pneumonitis usually is preceded by regurgitation, vomiting or both and is usually accompanied by bronchospasm.

With the increasing use of epidural anesthesia in obstetrics, ***toxic reactions*** caused by accidental intravascular or subarachnoid injection or rapid absorption of local anesthetics are now more frequent. Bupivacaine has recently been implicated in maternal deaths, and some reports indicate that this local anesthetic may possess inherent cardiotoxic effects when injected intravascularly (65, 66). Noticing the relationship between drug administration and maternal symptoms should differentiate these causes of cardiovascular collapse.

Eclampsia differs from amniotic fluid embolism in several ways; the associated hypertension, proteinuria, and peripheral edema usually indicate the reason for the convulsions and coma.

Intracranial hemorrhage causes lateralizing signs and unconsciousness, but rarely central cyanosis or hypotension, and can be confirmed by cerebrospinal fluid examination, computed tomography, or magnetic resonance imaging.

In obstetrics, ***hemorrhagic shock*** is most commonly associated with uterine atony, retained placenta, placenta previa, placental abruption, uterine rupture, or laceration of the cervix (67). A careful history and physical examination and a low value for central venous pressure usually confirm the diagnosis.

Acute heart failure in pregnancy may result from acute myocardial infarction, rheumatic heart disease (68), cardiomyopathy (68, 69), or tocolytic therapy with β-mimetic drugs (70–72). Findings on ECG, history, and physical examination (e.g., murmurs) aid in distinguishing the acute heart failure causing respiratory distress, cyanosis, and hypotension from amniotic fluid embolism.

Table 20.2
Blood Coagulation and Laboratory Tests in Disseminated Intravascular Coagulation

	Normal Values during Pregnancy	DIC
Plasma fibrinogen	400–650 mg/dl	<150 mg/dl
Platelet count	150,000–300,000/mm^3	<50,000/mm^3
Thrombin time	15–20 sec	>100 sec
Prothrombin time	10–12 sec	>100 sec
Partial thromboplastin time	35–50 sec	>100 sec
Fibrin degradation products	<16 μg/ml	>200 μg/ml
Fibrin degradation product dilution	1:4	>1:128
Red blood cell fragmentation	No	Yes

MONITORING, MANAGEMENT, AND TREATMENT

Once amniotic fluid embolism has occurred, rapid and aggressive cardiopulmonary resuscitation is mandatory for patient survival (Table 20.3). The sequence of therapeutic interventions and the priority assigned to each will of course depend on the clinical presentation of the amniotic fluid embolus and the judgment of the physicians caring for the patient. The uterus and its contents should be evacuated as quickly as possible. Delivery of a live infant is possible in up to 40% of cases (13), even when postmortem cesarean section is necessary. When the uterus is empty, aortocaval compression is no longer present; thus closed chest cardiac massage is more effective (73). Based on case reports of patient survival since the mid-1980s, (39–41, 56–58, 62, 74) and a review (26), it is now well established that left ventricular failure is the principal finding in patients with amniotic fluid embolism who survive initial oxygenation and resuscitation (Table 20.4). Guided by invasive hemodynamic monitoring, therapy directed toward treatment of the failing left ventricle using inotropic drugs and afterload reduction is likely to be successful.

Cardiopulmonary Resuscitation

To assess the effectiveness of cardiopulmonary resuscitation, one must monitor the ECG, blood pressure (arterial line), and urinary output (bladder catheter) continuously. Monitoring hemodynamic status with a pulmonary artery catheter provides critical information. Specific therapy includes the following:

1. *To alleviate the severe hypoxia*, intubate the patient and ventilate the lungs with 100% oxygen through an endotracheal tube. Correction of hypoxia relieves pulmonary vasoconstriction, and the addition of positive end-expiratory pressure (PEEP) to control ventilation helps to reduce or prevent pulmonary edema.

2. *Two large intravenous cannulas* should be inserted for drug injection and in anticipation of blood replacement if DIC develops.

3. *Adequate tissue perfusion must be ensured.* If

Table 20.3
Monitoring and Treatment of Amniotic Fluid Embolism: A Suggested Approach

1. Intubate and ventilate with 100% O$_2$ and maintain positive end-expiratory pressure (PEEP).
2. If there is no pulse, start external cardiac massage.
3. Insert two large-bore intravenous cannulas, a pulmonary artery catheter, a bladder catheter, and if possible an arterial line.
4. Monitor oxygen saturation, ECG and heart rate, pulmonary and systemic blood pressures, cardiac indices, and neurologic function.
5. Aspirate blood from the right side of the heart for pathologic examination.
6. Draw blood for baseline coagulation studies, cross-matching, and arterial blood analysis. Notify the blood bank of the diagnosis and the probable need for red blood cells, fresh frozen plasma, and platelets.
7. Administer NaHCO$_3$ to correct acidosis.
8. Fetus and placenta should be delivered as soon as is feasible.
9. Administer sympathomimetic drugs to treat left ventricular failure and augment cardiac output and peripheral perfusion.
   Dopamine, 2–5 μg/kg/min
   Dobutamine, 15–30 μg/kg/min
   Isoproterenol, 0.05–0.10 μg/kg/min
   Norepinephrine/epinephrine, 0.1–0.4 μg/kg/min/0.15–0.30 μg/kg/min
10. If CVP is rising, digoxin (0.5 mg) or deslanoside (0.8 mg) and furosemide (10–40 mg) may be administered intravenously.
11. Administer hydrocortisone in 1-g intravenous boluses every 6 hr for 48 hr.
12. Transfer the patient to the ICU as soon as possible for invasive monitoring and therapy.
13. Maintain vascular volume by infusing crystalloid. Treat disseminated intravascular coagulation (DIC) and bleeding with red blood cells, fresh frozen plasma, and platelets, depending on the patient's clinical condition and serial coagulation results.

Table 20.4
Hemodynamic Indices in Patients with Amniotic Fluid Embolism[a]

Case	MPAP[b] (mmHg)	PCWP[b] (mmHg)	PVR[b] (dynes/s/cm^{-5})	LVWSI[b] (g/m/M^2)
1	20	14	83	Clinical LVF
2	31	26	206	Clinical LVF
3	27	21	86	33
4	23	14	277	Nuclear scan: LVF
5	27*	18		Clinical LVF
6	29	19	138	19
7	18	16	133	3
8	42	31	215	12
9	21	16	137	31

[a]Reprinted with permission from Clark SL: Amniotic fluid embolism. In *Critical Care Obstetrics*, SL Clark, JP Phelan, DB Cotton, ed. Medical Economics Books, Oradell, NJ, 1987, p 320.
[b]*MPAP* = mean pulmonary artery pressure; *PCWP* = pulmonary capillary wedge pressure; *PVR* = pulmonary vascular resistance; *LVSWI* = left ventricular stroke work index. *LVF* = left ventricular failure.

peripheral pulses cannot be felt, closed chest cardiac massage should be initiated, even though electrical activity is present on the cardiac monitor. Serial analyses of arterial blood gases are useful in confirming the adequacy of resuscitation. Occasionally, sodium bicarbonate must be administered to correct any acidosis.

4. *Monitoring of central venous pressure* is important for regulating fluid infusion. After aspirating a blood sample from the right side of the heart for microscopic examination for amniotic fluid debris, intravenous fluids should be administered with care because of possible right ventricular overload.

5. *Administering cardiac stimulants and vasopressors* especially dopamine and dobutamine has been effective (26, 62 75, 76). Dopamine increases cardiac output and peripheral and renal perfusion (75). An infusion rate of 2 to 5 μg/kg/min is recommended. In the first 24 hr while in the intensive care unit, patients often exhibit episodes of deterioration and cardiovascular collapse. Dobutamine in doses of up to 30 μg/kg/min has been used to maintain left ventricular output (62).

6. *Digitalization may lessen ventricular failure,* especially if central venous pressure is rising. Deslanoside (0.8 to 1.6 mg) or digoxin (0.5 mg) may be given intravenously.

7. *Some reports have advocated the use of furosemide* in treating the pulmonary edema that frequently occurs with ongoing therapy (39–41, 56). Determining pulmonary capillary wedge pressure and cardiac output with a pulmonary artery catheter will aid in diagnosing acute left ventricular failure from fluid overload and will direct appropriate therapy with digitalization and diuresis. Positive pressure ventilation, PEEP, or both could be finely tuned by calculating venous admixture from hemodynamic studies (39) using a pulmonary artery catheter and peripheral arterial line.

8. *In nearly all survivors of amniotic fluid embolism, 1- to 2-g boluses of hydrocortisone* were administered intravenously. Hydrocortisone may help to reduce pulmonary edema and to decrease endothelial swelling and chemical irritation.

Treatment of Bleeding and DIC

Following amniotic fluid embolism, treatment of DIC should be directed at blood volume replacement and circulatory support after the fetus and placenta have been delivered expeditiously. Once the initiating stimulus (amniotic fluid, placental thromboplastin, or both) is removed, DIC should be self-limiting. Within 24 hr after the uterus has been emptied, levels of coagulation factors are usually adequate for hemostasis, even if agents specifically directed at correction of abnormal coagulation are not administered (77, 78).

Although both crystalloids or colloids can restore blood volume, in ongoing hemorrhage, transfusion of packed red blood cells is necessary to restore oxygen-carrying capacity. Stored blood is deficient in factor V, factor VIII, and platelets. These deficiencies can be overcome by giving fresh frozen plasma and platelets. When possible, single-donor platelets and fresh frozen plasma collected by apheresis techniques should be given. Both are better blood components, and because the patient is exposed to single rather than multiple donors, the risks of transmitting infectious agents are reduced.

The outcome of DIC is determined by dynamic interactions between pathologic depletion and compensatory repletion of coagulation factors and platelets. Serial laboratory tests used to guide ongoing therapy must be interpreted while keeping the clinical findings in mind.

Although mentioned in previous reports, transfusion of fibrinogen (5, 6, 10, 16, 63) is usually unnecessary, and administration of heparin (10, 41, 79) or inhibitors of fibrinolysis (ϵ-aminocaproic acid) (6, 10) may be dangerous. Although heparin has antithrombin effects, no controlled studies have shown heparin to be valuable in treating DIC from amniotic fluid embolism. If bleeding in DIC is due more to anticoagulant breakdown products of fibrinogen than to depletion of clotting factors, the use of fibrinogen may precipitate generalized clotting. Likewise, antifibrinolytic agents, which block the thrombin-limiting action of plasmin, may also produce generalized thrombosis.

Massage of the uterus, administration of oxytocics and prostaglandin $F_{2\alpha}$ (56), and uterine packing (17) can be attempted to increase uterine tone. However, uterine atony is resistant to most therapy and is terminated only with restoration of circulatory status.

Possible late sequelae after amniotic fluid embolism and DIC include (a) renal failure caused by cortical necrosis; (b) neurologic deficits and convulsions usually of central origin; (c) myocardial ischemic injury and infarction; and (d) liver damage.

Although the mortality is still very high, maternal death from amniotic fluid embolism and DIC need not be inevitable if the syndrome is recognized promptly and treated appropriately.

References

1. Meyer JR: Embolis pulmonar amnio-caseosa. Brazil-Medico 2:301, 1926.
2. Warden MR: Amniotic fluid as possible factor in etiology of eclampsia. Am J Obstet Gynecol 14:292–300, 1927.
3. Steiner PE, Lushbaugh CC: Maternal pulmonary embolism by amniotic fluid as a cause of obstetric shock and unexpected death in obstetrics. JAMA 117:1245–1254, 1340–1345, 1941.
4. Abouleish E: Amniotic fluid embolism: Report of a fatal case. Anesth Analg 53:549–553, 1974.
5. Shnider SM, Moya F: Amniotic fluid embolism. Anesthesiology 22:108–119, 1961.
6. Courtney LD: Amniotic fluid embolism. Obstet Gynecol Surv 29:169–177, 1974.
7. Barno A, Freeman DW: Amniotic fluid embolism. Am J Obstet Gynecol 77:1199–1210, 1959.
8. Gross P, Benz EJ: Pulmonary embolism by amniotic fluid: Report of 3 cases with a new diagnostic procedure. Surg Gynecol Obstet 85:315–320, 1947.
9. Lewis TLT: *Progress in Clinical Obstetrics and Gynecology*, 2nd ed. Churchill, London, 1964, p 48.
10. Morgan M: Amniotic fluid embolism. Anaesthesia 34:20–32, 1979.
11. Guha-Ray DK: Maternal mortality in an urban hospital: A fifteen-year survey. Obstet Gynecol 47:430–433, 1976.
12. Kaunitz AM, Hughes JM, Grimes DA, Smith JC, Rochat RW, Kafrissen ME: Causes of maternal mortality in the United States. Obstet Gynecol 65:605–612, 1985.
13. Peterson EP, Taylor MB: Amniotic fluid embolism: An analysis of 40 cases. Obstet Gynecol 35:787–793, 1970.
14. Department of Health and Social Security. *Report on Confidential Enquiries into Maternal Deaths in England and Wales 1970–1972*. Report on Health and Social Subjects, No. 11. Her Majesty's Stationery Office, London, 1975.
15. Resnik R, Swartz WH, Plumer MH, Bernischke K, Stratthaus ME: Amniotic fluid embolism with survival. Obstet Gynecol 47:295–298, 1976.
16. Reid DE, Weiner AE, Roby CC: Intravascular clotting and afibrinogenemia, presumptive lethal factors in syndrome of amniotic fluid embolism. Am J Obstet Gynecol 66:465–474, 1953.
17. Reis RL, Pierce WS, Behrendt DM: Hemodynamic effects of amniotic fluid embolism. Surg Gynecol Obstet 129:45–48, 1969.
18. Attwood HD: Fatal pulmonary embolism by amniotic fluid. J Clin Pathol 9:38–46, 1956.
19. Courtney LD: Amniotic fluid embolism. Br Med J 1:545, 1970.
20. Kistner RW, Graf WR, Johnstone RE: Pulmonary embolism by particulate matter of the amniotic fluid: A report of two cases with a review of the literature. Obstet Gynecol Surv 5:629–647, 1950.
21. Cawley LP, Douglass RC, Schneider CL: Nonfatal pulmonary amniotic fluid embolism: An unusual transplacental path of entry. Obstet Gynecol 14:615–620, 1959.
22. Josey WE: Hypofibrinogenemia complicating uterine rupture: Relationship to amniotic fluid embolism. Am J Obstet Gynecol 94:29–34, 1966.
23. Shotton DM, Taylor CW: Pulmonary embolism by amniotic fluid: A report of a fatal case, together with a review of the literature. J Obstet Gynaecol Br Emp 56:45–53, 1949.
24. Clark SL, Pavlova A, Greenspoon J, Horenstein J, Phelan JP: Squamous cells in the maternal pulmonary circulation. Am J Obstet Gynecol 154:104–106, 1986.
25. Lee W, Ginsburg KA, Cotton DB, Kaufman R: Squamous and trophoblastic cells in the maternal pulmonary circulation identified by invasive hemodynamic monitoring during the peripartum period. Am J Obstet Gynecol 155:999–1001, 1986.
26. Clark SL: New concepts in amniotic fluid embolism: A review. Obstet Gynecol Surv 45:360–368, 1990.
27. Halmagyi DF, Starzecki B, Shearman RP: Experimental amniotic fluid embolism: Mechanism and treatment. Am J Obstet Gynecol 84:251–256, 1962.
28. Attwood HD, Downing SE: Experimental amniotic fluid and meconium embolism. Surg Gynecol Obstet 120:255–262, 1965.
29. Macmillan D: Experimental amniotic fluid infusion. J Obstet Gynaecol Br Commonw 75:849–852, 1968.
30. Spence MR, Mason KG: Experimental amniotic fluid embolism in rabbits. Am J Obstet Gynecol 119:1073–1078, 1974.
31. Rodgers BM, Staroscik RN, Reis RL: Effects of amniotic fluid on cardiac contractility and vascular resistance. Am J Physiol 220:1979–1982, 1971.
32. Kitzmiller JL, Lucas WE: Studies on a model of amniotic fluid embolism. Obstet Gynecol 39:626–627, 1972.
33. Azegami M, Mori N: Amniotic fluid embolism and leukotrienes. Am J Obstet Gynecol 155:1119–1124, 1986.
34. Stefanini M, Turpini RA: Fibrinogenopenic accident of pregnancy and delivery: A syndrome with multiple etiological mechanisms. Ann NY Acad Sci 75:601–625, 1959.
35. Eastman NJ: Editorial comment. Obstet Gynecol Surv 3:35–37, 1948.
36. Bowman JA Jr: Amniotic fluid embolism: Case report. Am J Obstet Gynecol 69:905–907, 1955.
37. Ratnoff OD, Vosburgh GJ: Observations on the clotting defect in amniotic-fluid embolism. N Engl J Med 247:970–973, 1952.
38. Tuller MA: Amniotic fluid embolism, afibrinogenemia, and disseminated fibrin thrombosis: Case report and review of the literature. Am J Obstet Gynecol 73:273–287, 1957.
39. Moore PG, James OF, Saltos N: Severe amniotic fluid embolism: Case report with haemodynamic findings. Anaesth Intensive Care 10:40–44, 1982.
40. Masson RG, Ruggieri J, Siddiqui MM: Amniotic fluid embolism: Definitive diagnosis in a survivor. Am Rev Respir Dis 120:187–192, 1979.
41. Duff P, Engelsgjerd B, Zingery LW, Huff RW, Montiel MM: Hemodynamic observations in a patient with intrapartum amniotic fluid embolism. Am J Obstet Gynecol 146:112–115, 1983.
42. Lumley J, Owen R, Morgan M: Amniotic fluid embolism: A report of three cases. Anaesthesia 34:33–36, 1979.
43. Fulton LD, Page EW: Nature of refractory state following sub-

lethal dose of human placental thromboplastin. Proc Soc Exp Biol Med 68:594, 1948.

44. Weiner AE, Reid DE, Roby CC: The hemostatic activity of amniotic fluid. Science 110:190–191, 1949.

45. Weiner AE, Reid DE: Pathogenesis of amniotic-fluid embolism. III. Coagulant activity of amniotic fluid. N Engl J Med 243:597–598, 1950.

46. Albrechtsen OK, Storm O, Trolle D: Fibrinolytic activity in the circulating blood following amniotic fluid infusion. Acta Haematol 14:309–313, 1955.

47. Beller FK: Disseminated intravascular coagulation and consumption coagulopathy in obstetrics. Obstet Gynecol Ann 3:267, 1974.

48. Schneider CL: Coagulation defects in obstetric shock: Meconium embolism and heparin—Fibrin embolism and defibrination. Am J Obstet Gynecol 69:758–775, 1955.

49. Ballas MD, Lessing JB, Michowitz M: Amniotic fluid embolism and disseminated intravascular coagulation complicating hypertonic saline-induced abortion. Postgrad Med J 59:127–129, 1983.

50. Stromme WB, Fromke VL: Amniotic fluid embolism and disseminated intravascular coagulation after evacuation of missed abortion. Obstet Gynecol 52:76S–80S, 1978.

51. Lees DE, Shin Y, Macnamara TE: Probable amniotic fluid embolism during curettage for a missed abortion: A case report. Anesth Analg 56:739–742, 1977.

52. Cromey MG, Taylor PJ, Cumming DC: Probable amniotic fluid embolism after first-trimester pregnancy termination. J Reprod Med 28:209–211, 1983.

53. Mainprise TC, Maltby JR: Amniotic fluid embolism: A report of four probable cases. Can Anaesth Soc J 33:382–387, 1986.

54. Quance D: Amniotic fluid embolism: Detection by pulse oximetry. Anesthesiology 68:951–952, 1988.

55. Barrows JJ: A documented case of amniotic fluid embolism presenting as acute fetal distress. Am J Obstet Gynecol 143:599–600, 1982.

56. Schaerf RHM, de Campo T, Civetta JM: Hemodynamic alterations and rapid diagnosis in a case of amniotic-fluid embolus. Anesthesiology 46:155–157, 1977.

57. Dolyniuk M, Orfei E, Vania H, Karlman R, Tomich P: Rapid diagnosis of amniotic fluid embolism. Obstet Gynecol 61:28S–30S, 1983.

58. Clark SL, Montz FJ, Phelan JP: Hemodynamic alterations associated with amniotic fluid embolism: A reappraisal. Am J Obstet Gynecol 151:617–621, 1985.

59. Shah K, Karlman R, Heller J: Ventricular tachycardia and hypotension with amniotic fluid embolism during cesarean section. Anesth Analg 65:533–535, 1986.

60. Attwood HD: Amniotic fluid embolism. Pathol Annu 7:145–172, 1972.

61. Gregory MG, Clayton EM Jr: Amniotic fluid embolism. Obstet Gynecol 42:236–244, 1973.

62. Girard P, Mal H, Laine JF, Petitpretz P, Rain B, Duroux P: Left heart failure in amniotic fluid embolism. Anesthesiology 64:262–265, 1986.

63. Abouleish E: amniotic fluid embolism and disseminated intravascular coagulopathy. In Pain Control in Obstetrics. E Abouleish, ed., JB Lippincott, Philadelphia, 1977, p 160.

64. Shapiro HM, Drummond JC: Neurosurgical anesthesia and intracranial hypertension. In Anesthesia, Vol 2. RD Miller, ed. Churchill Livingstone, New York, 1990, pp 1743–1746.

65. Marx GF: Cardiotoxicity of local anesthetics: The plot thickens. Anesthesiology 60:3–5, 1984.

66. Kotelko DM, Shnider SM, Dailey PA, Brizgys RV, Levinson G, Shapiro WA, Koike M, Rosen MA: Bupivacaine-induced cardiac arrhythmias in sheep. Anesthesiology 60:10–18, 1984.

67. Cunningham FG, MacDonald PC, Gant NF: Obstetrical hemorrhage. In Williams Obstetrics, 18th ed. FG Cunningham, PC MacDonald, NF Gant, eds. Appleton & Large, Norwalk, CT, 1989, p 697.

68. Metcalf J, Mc Anulty JH, Ueland K, eds: Heart Disease and Pregnancy. Little Brown, Boston, 1986, pp 185–222, 295–305.

69. Demakis JG, Rahimtoola SH: Peripartum cardiomyopathy. Circulation 44:964–968, 1971.

70. Nagey DA, Crenshaw MC: Pulmonary complications of isoxuprine therapy in the gravida. Obstet Gynecol 59:38S–42S, 1982.

71. Katz M, Robertson PA, Creasy RK: Cardiovascular complications associated with terbutaline treatment for preterm labor. Am J Obstet Gynecol 139:605–608, 1981.

72. Barden TP, Peter JB, Merkatz IR: Ritodrine hydrochloride: A betamimetic agent for use in preterm labor. I. Pharmacology, clinical history, administration, side effects, and safety. Obstet Gynecol 56:1–6, 1980.

73. Marx GF: Cardiopulmonary resuscitation of late-pregnant women (letter). Anesthesiology 56:156, 1982.

74. Clark SL, Cotton DB, Gonik B, Greenspoon J, Phelan JP: Central hemodynamic alterations in amniotic fluid embolism. Am J Obstet Gynecol 158:1124–1126, 1988.

75. Goldberg LI: Dopamine: Clinical uses of an endogenous catecholamine. N Engl J Med 291:707–710, 1974.

76. Ricou B, Reper P, Suter PM: Rapid diagnosis of amniotic fluid embolism causing severe pulmonary failure. Intensive Care Med 15:129–131, 1989.

77. Kelton JG, Cruickshank M: Hematologic disorders of pregnancy. In Medical Complications during Pregnancy, 2nd ed. GN Burrow, TR Ferris, eds. WB Saunders, Philadelphia, 1988, p 85–86.

78. Plumer MH: Bleeding problems. In Obstetric Anesthesia: The Complicated Patient. FM James III, AS Wheeler, DM Dewan, eds. Davis, Philadelphia, 1988, p 336–338.

79. Chung AF, Merkatz IR: Survival following amniotic fluid embolism with early heparinization. Obstet Gynecol 42:809–814, 1973.

CHAPTER 21

Antepartum and Postpartum Hemorrhage

Diane R. Biehl, M.D.

Hemorrhage in the obstetric patient is no longer a major cause of maternal mortality on the North American continent (1, 2). Better prenatal care, more accurate diagnostic methods, and the availability of intensive care during parturition accounts for this. The precipitating factors for obstetric hemorrhage have not been eliminated, however. Thus a complete understanding of the causes and management of obstetric hemorrhage is important for all anesthesiologists.

ANTEPARTUM HEMORRHAGE

A patient may bleed at any time during her pregnancy, but the most severe bleeding usually occurs in the third trimester. The major causes are placenta previa and abruptio placentae.

Placenta Previa

The incidence of placenta previa varies between 1:345 and 1:53 deliveries (3, 4) and is higher in multiparous patients and in patients undergoing repeat cesarean sections (5). The recurrence risk is approximately 5%.

Placenta previa varies in degree and may be complete (37%), partial (27%), or low lying (46%) (Fig. 21.1). The main symptom is painless vaginal bleeding. The patient may bleed, then bleeding may stop spontaneously (the usual situation); however, sudden severe hemorrhage may recur at any time.

Although placenta previa is the cause of vaginal bleeding in only about one-third of antepartum hemorrhages (6), all patients who present with vaginal bleeding in the third trimester should be considered to have placenta previa until disproved. If the diagnosis of placenta previa is suspected, the placenta may be located by means of B-scan ultrasonography (Figs. 21.2 and 21.3). The recent development of gray imaging has provided for even more accurate localization of placental position in low-lying or marginal implantation. The accuracy of this technique in the third trimester is 95%. If the ultrasound examination is inconclusive, definitive diagnosis is made by direct examination of the cervical os. This procedure is usually done in the delivery room only after all preparations have been made to perform a cesarean section (i.e., "the double set-up") (Table 21.1). A vaginal examination is carried out to determine whether the placenta is covering or encroaching on the lower segment of the uterus.

Before term the patient is usually managed with bed rest in the hope that the bleeding will cease spontaneously. Once the patient is near term, fetal maturity is assessed by amniocentesis (Chapter 35), and the mother is delivered by cesarean section. In most instances a vaginal examination is still performed immediately before cesarean section to confirm the diagnosis. If, during pregnancy, the patient begins to bleed and does not stop spontaneously, emergency cesarean section must be carried out despite the gestational age of the fetus. The fetus becomes compromised quickly if maternal hypotension occurs (Fig. 21.4) (7). It is also possible for the placental bleeding to cause fetal exsanguination. The fetus becomes asphyxiated and, if delivered prematurely, usually succumbs to a combination of asphyxia and hyaline membrane disease.

ANESTHETIC MANAGEMENT

"Double Set-Up"

Before the double set-up, if the patient has bled profusely as manifested by postural or obvious hypotension, blood volume should be restored. A central venous pressure line is especially useful in evaluating and treating hypovolemia.

During the vaginal examination for the diagnosis of placenta previa, sudden and severe maternal hemorrhage may occur, necessitating immediate emergency cesarean section. Therefore, with the patient in the lithotomy position, the abdomen is prepared and draped and all preparations for cesarean section are completed. It is mandatory that at least one and preferably two intravenous lines be established with 16- or 18-gauge intravenous catheters. The patient's blood type must be crossmatched and at least 2 units of packed red blood cells must be immediately available before examination of the patient.

Preparation for general anesthesia should include administration of a nonparticulate oral antacid within 15 to 30 min of the examination. A trained assistant should be present to provide cricoid pressure. The examination of the cervical os is then performed, and the diagnosis is made.

Placenta Previa—Actively Bleeding

If the diagnosis of placenta previa is confirmed and the patient is actively bleeding, an emergency

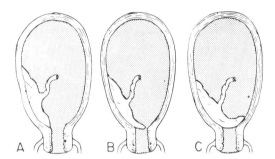

Figure 21.1. Types of placenta previa. *A*, Low implantation of placenta. *B*, Partial placenta previa. *C*, Total placenta previa. (Reprinted by permission from Bonica JJ, Johnson WL: Placenta praevia, abruptio placentae or rupture of the uterus. In *Principles and Practice of Obstetric Analgesia and Anesthesia, Vol 2*. Davis, Philadelphia, 1969, p 1164.)

cesarean section under general anesthesia is performed immediately.

When the mother is bleeding copiously and may be in hemorrhagic shock, resuscitation of the mother may be extremely difficult. Unlike some anesthetic emergencies, it may not be possible to correct completely the blood loss before surgery, because the hemorrhaging will continue until the placenta is removed. Packed red blood cells and crystalloid or colloid should, nevertheless, be infused as rapidly as possible.

Induction of anesthesia is accomplished with either an appropriate dose of thiopental (usually less than 100 mg) or ketamine (0.5–1 mg/kg) plus succinylcholine (1.5 mg/kg) and endotracheal intubation. Ketamine stimulates the sympathetic nervous system centrally to increase heart rate and blood pressure. In the severely hypovolemic patient in whom peripheral vasoconstriction is already maximal, ketamine will not cause any increase in blood pressure. In fact, in these patients the direct cardiac depressant effect of ketamine may actually produce a decrease in blood pressure. In these severe situations, endotracheal intubation should be facilitated with succinylcholine alone. The possibility of maternal recall should be disregarded to provide maximal maternal safety.

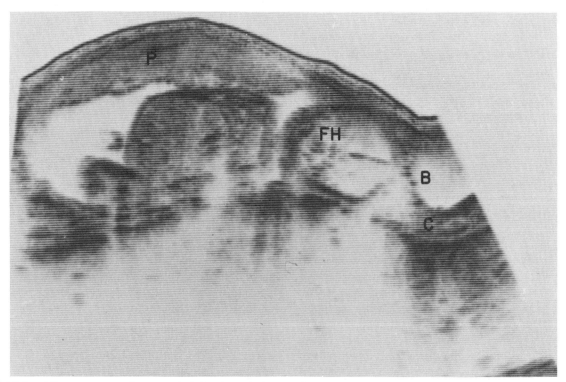

Figure 21.2. Ultrasonogram of an anteriorly implanted placenta. *P* = placenta, *FH* = fetal head; *B* = maternal bladder; *C* = cervix. (Courtesy of Dr. R. Filly, University of California, San Francisco.)

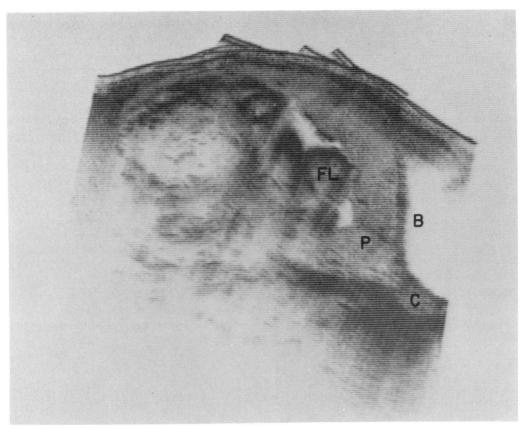

Figure 21.3. Ultrasonogram of a complete placenta previa. P = placenta; FL = fetal limb; B = maternal bladder; C = cervix. (Courtesy of Dr. R. Filly, University of California, San Francisco.)

Table 21.1
Antepartum Hemorrhage: "The Double Set-Up"

Preparation
  Two 16- or 18-gauge plastic catheters
  Blood pump IV set
  Blood for transfusion
  Oral antacid (nonparticulate)
  Oxygen
  Skilled assistant
Bleeding and cesarean section
  Treat hypovolemia
  Induce ketamine (1 mg/kg) plus succinylcholine
    (1.5 mg/kg)
  Intubate: provide cricoid pressure
  O_2 or 50% N_2O and O_2 until baby delivered
  Awake extubation

Maintenance of anesthesia before delivery depends on the clinical condition of the mother. Vecuronium, atracurium, or pancuronium will provide optimum operating conditions. Initially, 100% oxygen is administered. Nitrous oxide up to 50% may be added as tolerated by the patient. A halogenated agent in a low dose may be used to supplement nitrous oxide to decrease the incidence of maternal recall if the cardiovascular system is stable.

If the placenta is easily removed intact, the threat to the mother is much less. Blood volume—as assessed by blood pressure, central venous pressure, and urine output—is restored to normal, and anesthesia is maintained with either the inhalational agent or narcotics and muscle relaxants.

The neonate may require intensive resuscitation at birth. These infants may be asphyxiated, acidotic, and hypovolemic. Immediate intubation and ventilation with 100% oxygen should be instituted, and an umbilical venous catheter should be placed for administration of fluids. An umbilical arterial catheter is also useful for monitoring blood pressure and blood gases (Chapter 38). Ideally, another anesthesiologist or a neonatologist should be present to attend to the neonate. Transfer to an intensive care nursery for further close observation and treatment should be accomplished as soon as possible.

Placenta Previa—Not Bleeding

If the diagnosis of placenta previa is confirmed by double set-up and the patient is not bleeding, cesarean section is still performed at this time. Despite

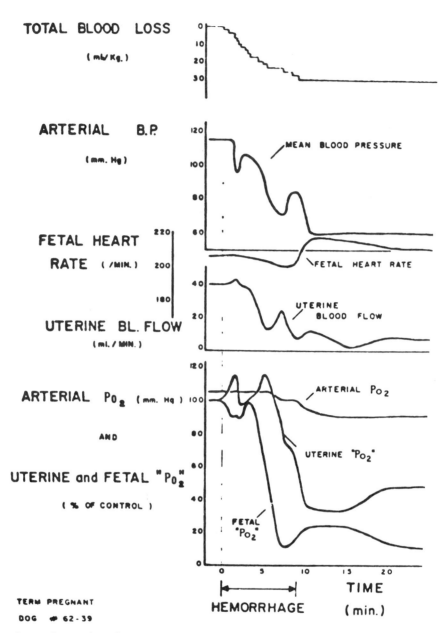

Figure 21.4. Effects of acute hemorrhage in pregnant dogs. Rapid bleeding produced a prompt fall in mean material arterial blood pressure, a comparable fall in uterine blood flow, decreased fetal tissue Po_2, and fetal bradycardia. (Modified by permission from Romney SL, Gabel PV, Takeda Y: Experimental hemorrhage in late pregnancy. Am J Obstet Gynecol 87:636, 1963.)

the preparation of the patient for a general anesthetic as part of the double set-up, some believe that spinal or epidural anesthesia may be used if the patient requests it and if no evidence of hypovolemia is present. Others believe that general anesthesia is still preferable because of the possible increased blood losses in these patients. If the placenta is anterior in the lower uterine segment the uterine incision will cut through the placenta. Tears in the lower uterine segment may also occur, which increases maternal blood loss.

Placenta Previa and Placenta Accreta

Placental implantation directly onto or into the myometrium gives rise to one of three conditions: *placenta accreta* is *onto* the myometrium; *placenta increta* is *into* the myometrium; and *placenta percreta* is *penetration through* the full thickness of the myometrium (Fig. 21.5) (8). Any of these may produce a markedly adherent placenta, which cannot be removed without tearing the myometrium.

These abnormal placental implantations occur more freqeuently in patients with placenta previa. In the general obstetric population the incidence of placenta accreta is approximately 1:2500 (8). In patients with *placenta previa* and no prior cesarean sections, the incidence is 5 to 7% (5, 9, 10). However, the risk of placenta accreta in patients with placenta previa who have had a prior cesarean delivery is much greater (Table 21.2). With one prior uterine incision, the incidence of placenta accreta has been reported to be between 24 and 31%, and with two or more prior uterine incisions, the incidence rises to about 50%.

In patients with placenta previa and accreta, massive intraoperative blood loss is common. Reported average blood loss has ranged from 2000 to 5000 ml with some patients requiring more than 30 units of blood. Approximately 20% of these patients develop coagulopathies (11). Between 30 and 72% have required cesarean hysterectomy (5, 9–11).

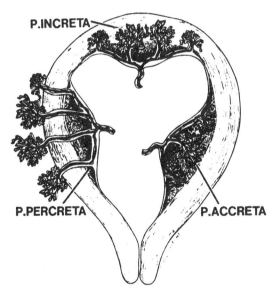

Figure 21.5. Classification of placenta accreta based on degree of penetration of myometrium. (Reprinted by permission from Kamani AAS, Gambling DR, Christilaw J, Flanagan ML: Anaesthetic management of patients with placenta accreta. Can J Anaesth 34:613–617, 1987.)

Placenta accreta is not reliably diagnosed until the uterus is open. The anesthesiologist must keep in mind this possibility and be prepared to treat sudden massive blood loss. Despite the serious risks, the type of anesthesia chosen for patients with placenta previa and repeat cesarean is still open to debate. Reviews suggest that epidural anesthesia does not contribute to increased maternal morbidity (9, 12), and one review (9) suggested that regional anesthesia actually decreases blood loss.

Abruptio Placentae

The term *abruptio placentae* refers to the separation of a normally implanted placenta after 20 weeks' gestation and before the birth of the fetus. The term *marginal separation* of the placenta refers to a mild form of abruptio placentae. The incidence of abruptio placentae varies from 0.2 to 2.4% (6). Maternal mortality is significant, probably 1.8 to 2.8% (6, 13). Perinatal mortality may be as high as 50% (13).

The etiology of abruptio placentae is not well defined but is associated with hypertensive disorders of pregnancy, high parity, uterine abnormalities (e.g., tumors), and previous placental abruption (6, 15). The clinical manifestations of this disease depend primarily on the site and degree of placental separation (Fig. 21.6) and the amount of blood loss. Bleeding from the abruption may appear through the vagina (external or revealed hemorrhage) or remain concealed in the uteroplacental unit (internal or concealed hemorrhage). The degree of revealed vaginal bleeding is often misleading, and concealed hemorrhage (retroplacental clot) provides one of the main problems for the anesthesiologist in coping with these patients on an emergency basis. The amount of blood loss is commonly underestimated, and as much as 4000 ml of blood may be sequestered in the uterus. Abruptio placentae is classified as mild, moderate, or severe. In mild or moderate abruption there is usually no maternal hypotension or coagulopathies and no fetal distress. Severe abruption is characterized by maternal hypotension, uterine irritability,

Table 21.2
Placenta Previa with Prior Uterine Incision(s)—Effect on Incidence of Placenta Accreta[a]

Prior Cesarean Sections (No.)	Patients with Placenta Previa (n = 286)	Placenta Previa/Accreta (n = 29)	%
0	238	12	5
1	25	6	24
2	15	7	47
3	5	2	40
4	3	2	67

[a] Reprinted by permission from Clark SL, Koonings PP, Phelan JP: Placenta previa/accreta and prior cesarean section. *Obstet Gynecol* 66:89–92, 1985.

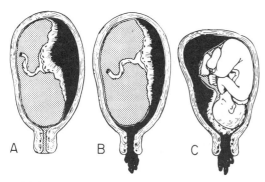

Figure 21.6. Abruptio placentae. *A*, Internal or concealed hemorrhage. *B*, External hemorrhage. *C*, Prolapse of the placenta. (Reprinted by permission from Bonica JJ, Johnson WL: Placenta praevia, abruptio placentae or rupture of the uterus. In *Principles and Practice of Obstetric Analgesia and Anesthesia, Vol 2*. Davis, Philadelphia, 1969, p 1166.)

hypertonicity and pain, fetal distress or death, and clotting abnormalities. Of all abruptions, the mild to moderate types account for 85 to 90% and severe types account for 10 to 15%.

CLOTTING ABNORMALITIES ASSOCIATED WITH ABRUPTIO PLACENTAE

Besides the problem of hemorrhage in the mother, severe abruptio placentae may result in blood coagulation defects (16, 17). Two theories have evolved to explain the observed clotting defects:

1. ***Placental abruption causes circulating plasminogen to be activated***, which enzymatically destroys circulating fibrinogen (fibrinolysis).

2. ***Thromboplastin from placenta and decidua triggers the activation of the extrinsic clotting pathway***, causing thrombin to convert fibrinogen to fibrin (disseminated intravascular coagulation).

It is unlikely that either mechanism operates exclusively. In the clinical situation, the end result is hypofibrinogenemia, platelet deficiency, and decreased factors V and VIII. Once the clotting mechanism has been activated, degeneration products of the fibrin-fibrinogen system also appear in the circulation. The patient then manifests widespread bleeding from the intravenous sites, gastrointestinal tract, and subcutaneous tissues, as well as the uterus.

In all patients suspected of having abruptio placentae, clotting parameters should be determined. With sophisticated laboratory equipment, actual amounts of the clotting factors present in the blood and degradation products can be measured. However, the clinical situation is often acute, and treatment must be instituted before test results are known. For this reason, a simple clot observation test that can be performed in the delivery suite is often preferred. In this test, 5 ml of maternal venous blood are drawn into a clean glass test tube, shaken gently, and allowed to stand. If a clot does not form within

6 min or the clot is lysed within 1 hr, a clotting defect is present. If the clot fails to form within 30 min, the fibrinogen level is probably less than 100 mg/dl.

When the blood sample is drawn for the clot observation test, a sample should also be sent to the laboratory for complete analysis, including hemoglobin, hematocrit, platelet count, prothrombin time, partial thromboplastin time, fibrinogen level, and fibrin degradation product analyses. The complete results will be useful for the management of these patients both intrapartum and postpartum. Analyses should be repeated frequently to monitor treatment, because the clotting parameters may take several days to return to normal.

MANAGEMENT OF ABRUPTIO PLACENTAE

The definitive management of abruptio placentae is to empty the uterus. The method by which this is done depends on: (*a*) the degree of abruption; (*b*) the time in gestation at which abruption occurs; (*c*) the stability of the maternal cardiovascular and hematologic systems; and (*d*) the status of the fetus.

The diagnosis of mild or moderate abruption is usually made by excluding placenta previa at a double set-up. After the diagnosis, if the fetus is mature, an amniotomy is performed; labor is induced or augmented with oxytocin if necessary; and the fetus is monitored continuously by electronic means. Baseline clotting studies are obtained. If there are no signs of maternal hypovolemia or uteroplacental insufficiency and if clotting studies are normal, continuous lumbar epidural, caudal, or subarachnoid block may be used for labor and vaginal delivery.

In severe abruption, if emergency cesarean section is performed to save the life of the fetus or the mother, general anesthesia should be used. Regional anesthesia is contraindicated in patients with hypovolemic shock, severe coagulation abnormalities, or both. The induction and maintenance of general anesthesia are similar to the procedures used for actively bleeding placenta previa, as outlined earlier.

If the infant is alive at delivery, intensive resuscitation is usually required. These infants are usually severely asphyxiated and severely hypovolemic. In addition, they may also be premature.

After delivery of the infant and removal of the placenta, subsequent management of the mother may continue to be difficult. If blood has extravasated into the myometrium, the uterus may not contract and bleeding may continue. Oxytocin by infusion (20 to 40 units in 500 ml of normal saline) should be started as soon as the infant is delivered. If this is not effective, intravenous ergot preparations may be tried or prostaglandin $F_{2\alpha}$ may be injected into the uterus. As a last resort, internal iliac artery ligation or hysterectomy may be required as a life-saving procedure for the mother (18).

Massive and rapid blood transfusion restores the depleted blood volume, maintains tissue perfusion, and prevents renal damage. If blood is not immediately available, crystalloid, albumin, or plasmanate should be used to maintain the circulating blood volume. When necessary, fresh frozen plasma will restore the factor V and VIII components, and in severe situations, platelet concentrate may also be required (6 to 12 units). Cryoprecipitate contains 23% of the fibrinogen in a unit of plasma and thus provides a concentrated fibrinogen and factor VIII in a small volume. Infusion of fibrinogen is no longer recommended because: (a) it may only aggravate the disseminated intravascular coagulation and (b) it carries a high risk of transmitting serious viral illnesses.

During an apparently normal vaginal delivery, abruptio placentae may occur just before the birth of the infant. In this situation, the problems are maternal hemorrhage and fetal asphyxia. Clotting deficits do not usually become manifest. The anesthesiologist should resuscitate the mother by establishing intravenous lines, monitoring vital signs, and supporting the circulation with crystalloid solution and blood when available. Intravenous infusion of oxytocin should be begun as soon as the infant and placenta are delivered. General anesthesia may be required if extraction of the infant is necessary. The technique of rapid induction, previously described, should be used.

These patients, regardless of the mode of delivery, are extremely susceptible to postpartum hemorrhage resulting from uterine atony. Frequent monitoring of maternal vital signs, urine output, and fundal firmness is necessary.

Other Causes of Antepartum Hemorrhage

Placenta previa and abruptio placentae account for one-half to two-thirds of all cases of antepartum hemorrhage. The remainder are due to cervical polyps, carcinoma, vaginal and vulvar varicosities, circumvallate placenta, and vasoprevia. The latter two causes do not present as much of a threat to the mother as to the fetus, because the bleeding is primarily from fetal vessels. Other obstetric problems may give rise to hemorrhage as a result of derangement of the clotting mechanisms (Chapter 19). Severe preeclampsia, maternal infection, amniotic fluid embolism, and intrauterine death may all result in disseminated intravascular coagulation and hemorrhage if the diagnosis is not established quickly and treatment instituted.

UTERINE RUPTURE

Uterine rupture is an uncommon but potentially catastrophic obstetric complication that may occur antepartum, intrapartum or postpartum. The incidence of uterine rupture has declined significantly in the past decade, and in the United States maternal mortality is calculated to be 0.1% (19) when rupture occurs. This is most likely the result of improved diagnostic and treatment facilities and the decline in grand multiparity. Causes include: (a) separation of the uterine scar; (b) rupture of the myomectomy scar; (c) previous difficult deliveries; (d) rapid, spontaneous, tumultuous labor; (e) prolonged labor in association with excessive oxytocin stimulation or cephalopelvic disproportion; (f) weak or stretched uterine muscles, such as might be found in the grand multipara, in multiple gestation, or in polyhydramnios; and (g) traumatic rupture (iatrogenic) occurring from intrauterine manipulations, difficult forceps applications, and excessive suprafundal pressure.

Although the uterine rupture is usually found at the site of a previous operation or injury, reviews (19, 20) have indicated that maternal mortality is low in these circumstances because rupture is recognized and promptly treated. With traumatic rupture or spontaneous rupture and no uterine scar, maternal mortality from obstetric hemorrhage was 26 and 66%, respectively (21). Maternal death from rupture apparently occurs because the possibility is not considered, and blood transfusions are inadequate and laparotomy is delayed or not done.

Signs and symptoms depend on the extent of the rupture and include vaginal bleeding, severe uterine or lower abdominal pain, shoulder pain from subdiaphragmatic irritation by blood, disappearance of fetal heart tones, and severe maternal hypotension and shock. Anesthetic management for the laparotomy, uterine repair, hysterectomy, or hypogastric ligation is similar to that outlined above for the actively bleeding, acutely hypovolemic patient.

TRIAL OF LABOR FOLLOWING CESAREAN SECTION

In 1978 in the United States, 98% of all women who had cesarean sections were delivered by cesarean in subsequent pregnancies. Since then a marked change has occurred. In 1982 the American College of Obstetricians and Gynecologists (ACOG) published specific guidelines on a trial of labor following cesarean section (11). This abrupt change in attitude has, in part, been due to the tremendous increase in cesarean sections in the last decade. The guidelines specifically exclude patients who have had classic cesarean sections, but recommend that many patients who have lower segment transverse scars be considered candidates for a trial of labor in subsequent pregnancies.

Dehiscence of the lower segment transverse scar has been shown to be much less catastrophic than rupture of the classical scar or spontaneous rupture of the uterus. Maternal hemorrhage, hypotension, and fetal demise are associated with rupture through the uterine muscle. In contrast the lower uterine segment consists predominantly of connective tissue after 36 weeks' gestation. In addition, this part of the uterus does not contain placental tissue under normal circumstances. Dehiscence of a lower segment scar, at least initially, does not produce maternal instability. We are unaware of any maternal deaths recorded in the past 30 years with dehiscence of a lower segment scar.

Fetal compromise with scar dehiscence is also much less frequent than with classic rupture. In a survey, Lavin suggested that perinatal mortality is 0.93:1000 (23).

The safety of both mother and fetus during a trial of labor can only be ensured, however, if the patient is carefully monitored in a hospital that is equipped to perform cesarean sections. Appropriate selection of patients for a trial of labor is necessary for a reasonable chance of successful vaginal delivery. Patients with a singleton fetus and vertex presentation are candidates, if no other maternal risk factors such as a placenta previa, marginal separation of the placenta, hypertension, or diabetes are present. A previous diagnosis of cephalopelvic disproportion or failure to progress is not considered an absolute contraindication: 33% of patients with these diagnoses in previous pregnancies deliver vaginally after a trial of labor. With such nonrecurrent indications for cesarean as placenta previa, breech presentation, or preeclampsia, the success rate for vaginal delivery is 74% (23).

The advantages of delivery over cesarean section include decreased maternal blood loss, decreased febrile morbidity, and more rapid ambulation after delivery, as well as less well-defined psychologic benefits in terms of maternal-infant bonding and maternal sense of success and well-being. Therefore we will most likely see a great increase in trial of labor for parturients in many labor and delivery suites. This has implications for the anesthesiologist as to what type of analgesia or anesthesia is best for these patients.

Initially, when the recommendations for the management of a trial of labor were being developed, regional anesthetic techniques were considered to be contraindicated because it was believed that regional anesthesia might mask the hallmark sign of uterine rupture—pain. Subsequent experience showed that dehiscence of the lower segment scar frequently did not cause pain. The most reliable method of detecting dehiscence was by the change in uterine tone and contraction pattern. Several reports (23–25) have demonstrated that epidural anesthesia can be used safely in patients undergoing a trial of labor. It is

prudent in this patient group to use the lowest effective concentrations and volumes of local anesthetic with continuous electronic monitoring of uterine contractions and fetal heart rate.

The anesthesiologist and obstetrician must be readily available should complications occur. An added advantage of epidural anesthesia is that, following delivery, the obstetrician may do an internal pelvic examination to assess the uterine scar.

If a trial of labor is judged to be a failure and cesarean section is required, the epidural block may be used for the cesarean section if both mother and fetus are stable. In the emergency situation with suspected uterine scar rupture, fetal distress, or other maternal complications, a general anesthetic to effect a rapid delivery is indicated. The anesthesiologist must also anticipate that cesarean hysterectomy may be required if a complicated rupture has occurred. The incidence of hysterectomy for uncontrollable hemorrhage in this group of patients is 0.001% (23).

POSTPARTUM HEMORRHAGE

The postpartum period is typically defined as the 6-week period after delivery of the infant. The main causes of hemorrhage in this group of women (3 to 5% of all deliveries) occur within minutes of birth: retained products of conception; uterine atony; cervical, vaginal, or uterine lacerations; or bleeding from the episiotomy site. Twenty percent of all patients who have antepartum hemorrhage will also bleed postpartum. Severe postpartum hemorrhage often occurs with little or no warning. For this reason, immediately after delivery the anesthesiologist must observe the patient closely and be prepared to institute resuscitation of the mother and to give an anesthetic at a few seconds' notice.

Retained Placenta

The incidence of retained placenta is approximately 1% of all vaginal deliveries, and retained products of conception usually require a manual exploration of the uterus. In the multiparous patient, this can sometimes be done without an anesthetic, but usually the mother is severely distressed and the obstetrician may encounter difficulty in exploring a uterus that is partially contracted. For these reasons, analgesia is usually necessary. If the mother has an epidural or spinal block encompassing T10 to S4, manual removal of the placenta can be accomplished. The anesthesiologist must remember, however, that, should severe bleeding occur, the sympathectomy imposed by the block may make resuscitation more difficult and may result in severe maternal hypotension.

If the parturient has not received a regional block before delivery, other maneuvers may be tried before administering general anesthesia. Administration of 50 to 100 µg (26) or 500 µg of nitroglycerin intravenously has been reported to result in uterine relaxation sufficient to remove the placenta (27). Because of the side effects of hypotension and headache, careful monitoring of maternal vital signs is required both during and after administration of nitroglycerin. Nitroglycerin is preferable to inhalation of amyl nitrite, however, as the administration is more controlled.

Intravenous sedation with ketamine (0.1 mg/kg), inhalation analgesia, or judicious use of narcotics such as alfentanil or fentanyl may also be tried, but careful observation of the mother is essential to prevent oversedation both during and after removal of the placenta.

If the uterus remains firmly contracted around the placenta and cervical relaxation is required, this is best accomplished under general endotracheal anesthesia. Following the usual technique for rapid induction and intubation, the patient is given sufficient halothane or isoflurane in oxygen, with or without nitrous oxide, to provide adequate uterine relaxation (see Table 11.3). The halogenated agent should be discontinued as soon as the uterus has relaxed enough to allow manual removal. An oxytocin infusion should be initiated immediately after removal of the placenta. If removal of the placenta is extremely difficult, the possibility of placenta accreta should be considered. This problem was discussed in association with placenta previa.

Another difficulty rarely encountered is uterine inversion when the removal is attempted by traction on the umbilical cord without careful pressure applied to the uterus through the abdomen (25, 26). The uterus and placenta appear at the introitus, and severe hypotension and bradycardia may occur in the mother. This initial response is thought to be a vasovagal reflex, but hemorrhage from the placental site and endometrium also occur. The treatment is to replace the uterus as quickly as possible with steady pressure before the cervix constricts and prevents replacement. This will require a general anesthetic and uterine relaxation with a halogenated agent. Once the uterus is replaced, an infusion of oxytocin is started to keep the uterus contracted and to prevent a recurrence of the inversion.

Uterine Atony

Uterine atony, in varying degrees, occurs in approximately 2 to 5% of all vaginal deliveries (30). A completely atonic uterus may result in a loss of 2 liters of blood in less than 5 min. In one report of 502 maternal deaths, postpartum uterine atony was the leading cause of death in the parturient (31).

Uterine atony is increased with high parity, multiple births, polyhydramnios, large infants, retained placenta, or operative intervention, such as internal version and extraction. It may occur immediately or several hours after delivery of the infant.

Resuscitation of the mother necessitates: (a) replacement of blood loss initially with crystalloid and colloid solution, then with packed red blood cells as soon as possible; (b) intravenous infusion of oxytocin to cause contraction of the uterus; (c) general supportive measures (i.e., oxygen by face mask) with the patient in the Trendelenburg position; and (d) close monitoring of vital signs, including central venous pressure, when practical, and urine output.

The obstetric maneuvers involved for uterine atony include uterine massage through the abdominal wall and packs placed through the cervix into the uterus to control bleeding. Administration of ergot intravenously or directly into the myometrium may also improve uterine contractility. Prostaglandin $F_{2\alpha}$ is now available commercially and is administered directly into the uterus by injection into the paracervical areas or through the abdominal wall (32). The anesthesiologist should be aware that both ergot compounds and prostaglandins are associated with a high incidence of maternal nausea and vomiting. In addition, prostaglandin $F_{2\alpha}$ may be associated with bronchospasm, hypotension, or hypertension. Cardiovascular collapse has been documented with this agent (33).

If the above measures are not successful, emergency hysterectomy or internal iliac artery ligation may be required. The considerations here are very similar to those for placenta previa or abruptio placenta, except that there is no infant to influence management. The patient in an unstable condition before surgery can be expected to lose anywhere from 2 to 18 liters of blood before completion of the hysterectomy (12).

Cervical and Vaginal Lacerations

Both of these conditions may result in hemorrhagic shock. One of the main problems with lacerations is that they may be undiagnosed because of other complications. Blood loss may also go undetected if it occurs after the patient has been removed from the delivery room. In these situations, resuscitation should be started and the patient should be transferred back to the delivery room. A careful search for the source of the bleeding may require a general anesthetic to allow the obstetrician to explore the uterus and examine the cervix and vaginal vault. If the bleeding source is not found, in rare cases laparotomy may be required.

Blood Loss and Cesarean Section

In most high-risk obstetric units, the incidence of cesarean sections is now 15 to 25%. Regardless of the indication for cesarean section, the obstetric anesthesiologist must remember that sudden hemorrhage may occur with any manipulation of the highly vascular full-term uterus. Blood loss at "elective" cesarean sections is estimated to be between 800 and 1200 ml, which is 10 to 15% of the circulating blood volume of the normal pregnant woman at term. Any further bleeding may result in a compromised patient. With repeat cesarean sections, adhesions, varicosities in the uterus, or rupture of the previous scar, sudden and severe hemorrhage may occur. The anesthesiologist in any obstetric unit must be prepared to institute suddenly any of the measures previously discussed to resuscitate a parturient in hemorrhagic shock.

In the future, patients who are undergoing repeat cesareans or who are at risk for bleeding complications during delivery may elect autologous blood donation during pregnancy (34). Because of the risk of transmission of serious viral illnesses in homologous blood transfusions, many patients are donating their own blood before surgery. One study of 48 pregnant patients who made autologous donations suggests that this is a low-risk procedure for the pregnant patient (35). The procedure merits consideration for use in obstetrics.

CONCLUSION

Hemorrhage in the obstetric patient is still a potential cause of maternal death in modern obstetrics and contributes heavily to perinatal mortality. The pregnant patient often bleeds unexpectedly and may exsanguinate in a matter of minutes. Because of this, no obstetric patient should be treated "routinely," and every anesthesiologist should be prepared to diagnose and treat hemorrhagic shock immediately.

References

1. Rochat RW, Koonin LM, Atrash RS, Jewett JF: Maternal mortality in the United States: Report from the Maternal Mortality Collaborative. Obstet Gynecol 72:91–97, 1988.
2. Sachs BP, Brown DA, Driscoll SG, Schulman E, Acker D, Ransil BJ, Jewett JF: Maternal mortality in Massachusetts: Trends and prevention. N Engl J Med 316:667–672, 1987.
3. Hibbard LT: Placenta previa. Am J Obstet Gynecol 104:172–184, 1969.
4. Green-Thompson RW: Antepartum haemorrhage. Clin Obstet Gynecol 9:479–515, 1982.
5. Clark SL, Koonings PP, Phelan JP: Placenta previa/accreta and prior cesarean section. Obstet Gynecol 66:89–92, 1985.
6. Willson RJ: Bleeding during late pregnancy. In *Obstetrics and Gynecology*, 7th ed. RJ Wilson, ER Carrington, WJ Ledger, eds. CV Mosby, St. Louis, 1983, pp 356–371.
7. Romney SL, Gabel PV, Takeda Y: Experimental hemorrhage in late pregnancy: Effects on maternal and fetal hemodynamics. Am J Obstet Gynecol 87:636–649, 1963.
8. Breen JL, Neubecker RT, Gregori CA, Franklin JE Jr: Placenta accreta, increta and percreta: A survey of 40 cases. Obstet Gynecol 49:43–47, 1977.
9. Arcario T, Greene M, Ostheimer GW, Datta S, Naulty JS: Risks of placenta previa/accreta in patients with previous cesarean deliveries. Anesthesiology 69:A659, 1988.
10. Singh PN, Rodrigues C, Gupta AN: Placenta previa and previous cesarean section. Acta Obstet Gynecol Scand 60:367–368, 1981.
11. Read JA, Cotton DB, Miller FC: Placenta accreta: Changing clinical aspects and outcomes. Obstet Gynecol 56:31–34, 1980.
12. Chestnut DH, Dewan DM, Redick LF, Caton D, Spielman FJ: Anesthetic management for obstetric hysterectomy: A multi-institution study. Anesthesiology 70:607–610, 1989.
13. Hibbard BM, Jeffcoate TNA: Abruptio placenta. Obstet Gynecol 27:155–167, 1966.
14. Abdul-Karin RW, Chevli RN: Antepartum hemorrhage and shock. Clin Obstet Gynecol 19:533–539, 1976.
15. Abdella TN, Sibal BM, Hays JM Jr, Anderson GD: Relationship of hypertensive disease to abruptio placentae. Obstet Gynecol 64:365–370, 1984.
16. Gilabert J, Estelles A, Aznar J, Galbis M: Abruptio placentae and disseminated intravascular coagulation. Acta Obstet Gynecol Scand 64:35–39, 1985.
17. Pritchard JA: Hematological problems associated with delivery, placental abruption, retained dead fetus and amniotic fluid embolism. Clin Haematol 2:563–586, 1973.
18. Evans S, McShane P: The efficacy of internal iliac artery ligation in obstetrical hemorrhage. Surg Obstet Gynecol 160:250, 1985.
19. Megafu U: Factors influencing maternal survival in ruptured uterus. Int J Obstet Gynecol 23:475–480, 1985.
20. Schrinsky DC, Benson RC: Rupture of the pregnant uterus: A review. Obstet Gynecol Surv 33:217–232, 1978.
21. Ware HH Jr: Rupture of the uterus. Clin Obstet Gynecol 3:637–645, 1960.
22. ACOG Committee on Obstetrics, Maternal Fetal Medicine: American College of Obstetricians and Gynecologists' guidelines for vaginal delivery after cesarean childbirth. ACOG Newsl 26:1, 1982.
23. Lavin JP Jr: Vaginal delivery after cesarean birth: Frequently asked questions. Clin Perinatol 10:439–453, 1983.
24. Uppington J: Epidural analgesia and previous cesarean section. Anaesthesia 38:336–341, 1983.
25. Rudnick V, Niv D, Hetman-Peri M, Geller E, Avni A, Golan A: Epidural analgesia for planned vaginal delivery following previous cesarean section. Obstet Gynecol 64:621–623, 1984.
26. DeSimone CA, Norris MC, Leighton BL: Intravenous nitroglycerin aids manual extraction of a retained placenta. Anesthesiology 73:787, 1990.
27. Peng ATC, Gorman RS, Shulman SM, DeMarchis E, Nyunt K, Blancato LS: Intravenous nitroglycerin for uterine relaxation in the postpartum patient with retained placenta. Anesthesiology 71:172–173, 1989.
28. Platt LD, Druzing ML: Acute puerperal inversion of the uterus. Am J Obstet Gynecol 141:187–190, 1981.
29. Watson P, Besch N, Bowes WA Jr: Management of acute and subacute puerperal inversion of the uterus. Obstet Gynecol 55:12–16, 1980.
30. Herbert WNP, Afalo RC: Management of postpartum hemorrhage. Clin Obstet Gynecol 27:139–148, 1984.
31. Gibbs CE, Locke WE: Maternal deaths in Texas, 1969–1973: A report of 501 consecutive deaths from the Texas Medical Association's Committee on Maternal Health. Am J Obstet Gynecol 126:687–692, 1976.
32. Buttino L Jr, Garite TJ: The use of 15 methyl F_2 alphaprostaglandin (Prostin 15 M) for the control of postpartum hemorrhage. Am J Perinatol 3:241–243, 1986.
33. Douglas MJ, Farquharson DR, Ross PL, Renwich SE: Cardiovascular collapse following an overdose of prostaglandin F_2 alpha: A case report. Can J Anaesth 36:466–469, 1989.
34. Palmer RH, Kane JG, Churchill WH, Goldman L, Komaroff AL: Cost and quality in the use of blood bank service for normal deliveries, cesarean sections and hysterectomies. JAMA 256:219–223, 1986.
35. Kruskall MS, Leonard S, Klapholz H: Autologous blood donation during pregnancy: Analysis of safety and blood use. Obstet Gynecol 70:938–941, 1987.

ANESTHETIC COMPLICATIONS

CHAPTER 22

Hypotension and Regional Anesthesia in Obstetrics

Richard G. Wright, M.D.
Sol M. Shnider, M.D.

Arterial hypotension is the most common complication of spinal or epidural anesthesia in the parturient. Mild to moderate reductions in maternal blood pressure that do not adversely affect the mother may have profound effects on uterine blood flow and fetal well-being.

ETIOLOGY

Despite an increase in blood volume of 40% above prepregnant levels, the parturient at term is particularly susceptible to hypotension during major conduction anesthesia (1, 2). Partial or complete inferior vena cava and aortic occlusion from compression by the gravid uterus is present in the majority of parturients lying in the supine position (Figs. 22.1 and 22.2) (3–7). Vena caval obstruction not only impedes venous return to the heart, thereby causing hypotension (Fig. 22.3), but also increases uterine venous pressure, further decreasing uterine blood flow. In most parturients, an increase in resting sympathetic tone compensates for the effects of caval compression, and blood pressure is maintained (Fig. 22.4). However, when sympathetic tone is abolished acutely, as with spinal or epidural anesthesia, marked falls in blood pressure may result. It is generally believed that hypotension occurs less frequently and may be less severe with epidural than with spinal anesthesia. This is likely due, in large part, to the gradual onset of epidural anesthesia, allowing time for compensatory mechanisms to modify the anesthetic's cardiovascular effects. The addition of sodium bicarbonate to local anesthetics to increase the speed of onset of epidural blockade has become increasingly popular (8). Associated with this faster onset may be a greater incidence of hypotension (9). In general, the higher the level of sympathetic blockade, the greater the incidence and severity of hypotension. A diminished intravascular volume—as is frequently found with preeclampsia, antepartum bleeding, or dehydration—may further promote maternal hypotension.

SIGNIFICANCE

Many healthy individuals, including most parturients, tolerate systolic blood pressures of 80 to 90 mm Hg without ill effects to their brain, heart, and kidneys. The fetus, however, is highly sensitive to decreases in maternal arterial blood pressure. In contrast to other vital organs, with acute falls in maternal blood pressure there is no autoregulation of blood flow to the uterus. With spinal or epidural hypotension, uterine blood flow falls linearly with blood pressure (10–12).

The fetal consequences of the reduced uterine blood flow depend on the degree and duration of the fall and the preexisting status of the uteroplacental circulation. When uterine blood flow is inadequate, fetal asphyxia will develop (13–17). The precise degree and duration of hypotension necessary to cause fetal distress seems to be variable. Ebner et al. (18) reported that with conduction anesthesia a maternal systolic blood pressure of less than 70 mm Hg consistently produced sustained fetal bradycardia. When maternal systolic blood pressure was between 70 and 80 mm Hg for 4 min or longer, some fetuses developed sustained bradycardia. Hon et al. (19) and Bonica and Hon (20) found that, with maternal systolic blood pressure less than 100 mm Hg for about 5 min, abnormal fetal heart rate patterns developed. Zilianti (21) reported that a systolic pressure of less than 100 mm Hg for 10 to 15 min usually leads to fetal acidosis and bradycardia. In all these studies fetal heart rate returned to normal with correction of hypotension. Moya and Smith (22) reported an increased incidence of low Apgar scores when maternal systolic blood pressure fell to between 90 and 100 mm Hg for longer than 15 min (Fig. 22.5). Women who had

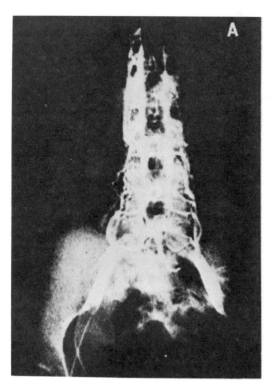

Figure 22.1. *A,* Venogram in the supine position just before cesarean section. Dye has been injected into both femoral veins but does not reach the inferior vena cava, traversing instead the paravertebral veins. *B,* Same patient just after cesarean section. The dye now easily reaches the inferior vena cava. (Reprinted by permission from Kerr MG, Scott DB, Samuel E: Studies of the inferior vena cava in late pregnancy. Br Med J 1:532–533, 1964.)

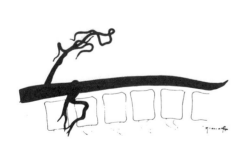

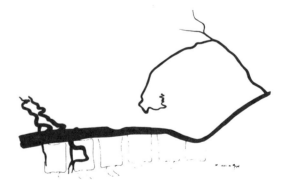

Figure 22.2. Schematic of lateral angiograms obtained from two women lying in the supine position. In the nonpregnant woman (*left*) there is a clear gap between the vertebral column and the aorta. Note the uniform width of the aorta. In the pregnant patient near term (*right*) the aorta is clearly displaced in the dorsal direction, encroaching on the shadow of the spine. The aorta is narrowed at the level of the lumbar lordosis. (Reprinted by permission from Bieniarz J, Crottogini JJ, Curuchet E, Romero-Salinas G, Yoshida T, Posiero JJ, Caldeyro-Barcia R: Aortocaval compression by the uterus in late human pregnancy. Am J Obstet Gynecol 100:203–217, 1978.)

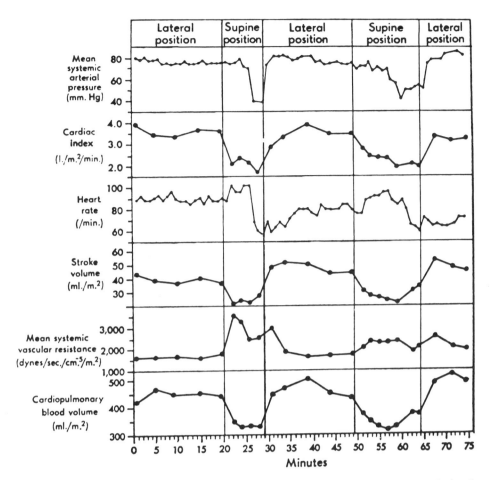

Figure 22.3. Serial hemodynamic studies in a patient who exhibited supine hypotension. After the patient was lying supine for 6 min, a profound fall in arterial pressure and pulse rate was seen. (Reprinted by permission from Kerr MG: Cardiovascular dynamics in pregnancy and labour. Br Med Bull 24:19–24, 1968.)

even greater falls in blood pressure but were promptly treated delivered vigorous neonates.

Several investigators (23–25) have shown that when the hypotension (defined as a systolic blood pressure lower than 100 mm Hg or a greater than 30% decrease from baseline) associated with regional anesthesia is promptly corrected, it has no effect on the clinical condition of the newborn as assessed by Apgar score at 1 and 5 min of age or the Neurologic Adaptive Capacity Score (NACS) at 15 min, 2 hr, and 24 hr of age (Fig. 22.6) (25). However, hypotension does appear to be associated with an increase in base deficit and a decrease in pH in umbilical cord blood. These changes are small (pH value change of 0.02 to 0.04 with epidural and slightly greater with spinal hypotension) and thought to be of little clinical significance. In summary, hypotension is best prevented. It seems that systolic blood pressures of less than 100 mm Hg in a previously normotensive parturient should be treated. In the hypertensive patient, a fall of 20 to 30% of her control pressure should probably be treated.

PREVENTION

Several preventive measures can be taken to minimize the incidence and severity of hypotension following conduction anesthesia in obstetrics. For routine spinal or epidural blocks the following measures have been recommended.

1. ***Intravenous infusion of 1500 to 2000 ml of balanced, nondextrose-containing solution should be administered within 30 min of high spinal or epidural anesthesia*** (dermatome level of T4 for cesarean section) ***or 500 ml before a low epidural or saddle block*** (dermatome level of T10 for labor and delivery).

Initial recommendations for prehydration of healthy women about to undergo cesarean section under regional anesthesia recommended 1000 ml of balanced electrolyte solution (26). Although prehydration with 1000 ml of crystalloid decreases the incidence of hypotension with high regional blockade, hypotension remains a frequent event. Investigators attempted to further decrease the frequency through more aggres-

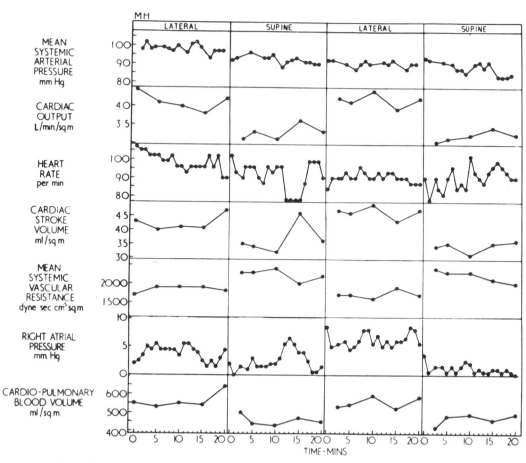

Figure 22.4. Hemodynamic parameters in a patient during late pregnancy who developed a reduced cardiac output in the supine position. The patient was asymptomatic. Note that the changes could be reproduced by turning the patient a second time. (Reprinted by permission from Scott DB: Inferior vena caval occlusion in late pregnancy. In *Parturition and Perinatology*. GF Marx, ed. Davis, Philadelphia, 1973, p 42.)

Figure 22.5. In a series of babies delivered by cesarean section under spinal anesthesia, maternal systolic blood pressures below 90 mm Hg were treated immediately. Mothers with blood pressures between 90 and 99 mm Hg were not considered to be hypotensive and were not treated. Note that even this mild degree of hypotension, when uncorrected, resulted in neonatal depression. (Reprinted by permission from Lichtiger M, Moya F: *Introduction to the Practice of Anesthesia*. Harper & Row, Hagerstown, MD, 1974, p 313.)

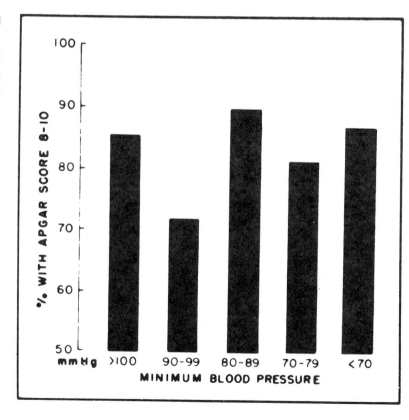

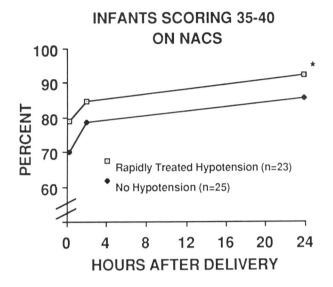

INFANTS SCORING 35-40 ON NACS

* No Significant Differences

Figure 22.6. Percentage of infants scoring 35 to 40 on the NACS at 15 min, 2 hr, and 24 hr of age after spinal anesthesia (no hypotension versus rapidly treated hypotension). (From Abboud TK, Blikian A, Noueihid R, Nagappala S, Afrasiabi A, Henriksen EH: Neonatal effects of maternal hypotension during spinal anesthesia as evaluated by a new test. Anesthesiology 59:A421, 1983.)

sive fluid administration. Some investigators increased the volume of crystalloid to 2000 ml, whereas others continued with about 1000 ml of fluid but included some colloid in that volume. Since colloids remain in the vascular compartment for a much longer time period than do crystalloids, it is said to require only one-third to one-fourth as much colloid as crystalloid for an equivalent amount of venous expansion. Although studies with colloid prehydration have produced conflicting results, their use does appear to decrease the incidence of hypotension (27–29). However, colloid solutions are considerably more expensive than crystalloids and, depending on the product, have other significant disadvantages, including anaphylaxis. Lewis et al. (30) found that the incidence of hypotension with epidural anesthesia for cesarean section could be substantially reduced by increasing crystalloid prehydration to 2000 ml.

Although dextrose-containing solutions may be useful in reducing maternal ketosis (31), they are undesirable in the large volumes required for acute intravenous loading prior to regional anesthesia. Adverse effects include maternal hyperglycemia (often associated with an osmotic diuresis) fetal hyperglycemia and subsequent neonatal hyperinsulinemia and hypoglycemia (32–34). Evidence that hyperglycemia increases the brain's susceptibility to anoxic injury

is further cause for avoiding it during labor and delivery (35).

2. *Prophylactic vasopressor administration is recommended with spinal anesthesia for cesarean section.* A predominantly centrally acting vasopressor such as 25 to 50 mg of ephedrine administered intramuscularly within 30 min of instituting a high subarachnoid block is effective in decreasing the incidence of hypotension (36). An increasingly popular alternative to intramuscular prophylaxis is intravenous ephedrine just prior to the block (boluses of 10 to 15 mg (24) or titration of an infusion with 50 mg in 500 ml of crystalloid [37]) administered when *any* fall in systolic blood pressure occurs. With this approach, spinal hypotension can be prevented. While prophylactic intramuscular ephedrine is effective in lowering the incidence of hypotension with high spinal anesthesia, it is not similarly effective with epidurals (23), and in the high dose range, it may result in maternal hypertension and mild fetal acidosis (38). Intravenous prophylaxis with epidural anesthesia has not been studied. Vasopressor prophylaxis is not recommended for low epidural or saddle block. The frequency of hypotension is not great if other preventative measures are taken; when it does occur, it is usually mild and easily treated. Furthermore, ephedrine may increase fetal heart rate and variability making interpretation of the fetal heart rate tracing during labor more difficult (Figs. 22.7 and 22.8) (39).

3. *Continuous left uterine displacement should be applied to minimize aortocaval compression.* Aortocaval compression results in changes in uteroplacental blood flow, which can be deleterious to the fetus. During labor, fetal oxygenation can fall rapidly when a mother assumes the supine position, even in the absence of maternal hypotension or hypoxemia (Fig. 22.9) (40). During the second stage of labor, a time-related decrease in fetal pH has been reported when the mother is delivered in the supine lithotomy position. This fetal acidosis is not seen if the mother is tilted to the left (41). With cesarean section, better fetal oxygenation, less fetal acidosis, and higher Apgar scores have been reported when left uterine displacement is established as soon as the mother is placed on the operating table (42). Laboring patients should remain in the lateral or semilateral position with a wedge under the right hip. Aortocaval compression can be reduced in the patient undergoing cesarean section by tilting the operating table 15 to 30 degrees to the left, placing a wedge under the right hip, manually displacing the uterus, or using a mechanical uterine displacing device (43, 44).

4. *Frequent monitoring of arterial blood pressure after institution of the block is mandatory.*

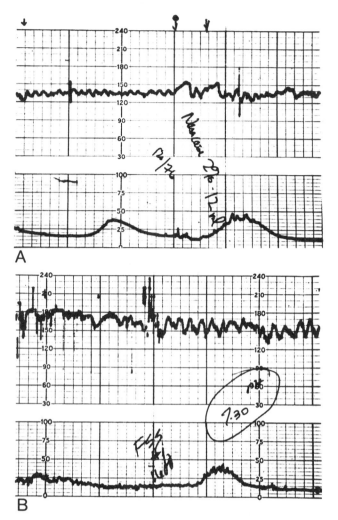

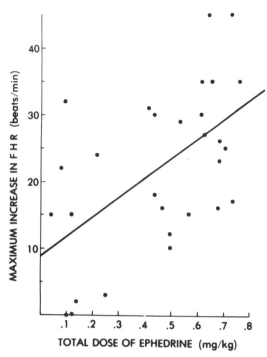

Figure 22.8. Least-squares regression of maximum increase in fetal heat rate (FHR) on total dose of ephedrine therapy for hypotension. Regression line slope = 28.7. Regression line y intercept = 8.697; x intercept = 0.303; r = 0.57; P < 0.05. (Reprinted by permission from Wright RG, Shnider SM, Levinson G, Rolbin SH, Parer JT: The effect of maternal administration of ephedrine on fetal heart rate and variability. Obstet Gynecol 57:734–738, 1981.)

Figure 22.7. *A,* Epidural administration of 240 mg of chloroprocaine (Nesacaine). Baseline fetal heart rate is approximately 135 beats/min. *B,* Fetal tachycardia and marked increase in heart rate variability (saltatory pattern) in the same patient as in *A.* The tracing was obtained approximately 1 hr after ephedrine therapy (10 mg intravenously, 25 mg intramuscularly) for mild epidural hypotension. The fetal scalp blood pH at this time was 7.3. (Reprinted by permission from Wright RG, Shnider SM, Levinson G, Rolbin SH, Parer JT: The effect of maternal administration of ephedrine on fetal heart rate and variability. Obstet Gynecol 57:734–738, 1981.)

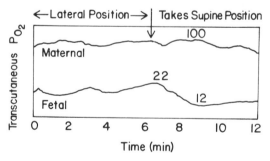

Figure 22.9. Continuous monitoring of maternal and fetal transcutaneous Po_2 during labor. Fetal Po_2 was monitored using a fetal scalp transcutaneous oxygen electrode. When mother turned from the lateral to the supine position, fetal Po_2 promptly fell. (Modified from Huch A, Huch R: Transcutaneous noninvasive monitoring of Po_2. Hosp Pract 11:43–52, 1976.)

Measurements should be made at 1 min intervals for the first 20 min after the local anesthetic is injected and then every 5 to 10 min until anesthesia is terminated. This will allow early recognition and prompt therapy of hypotension.

SAFETY OF PROPHYLAXIS

The safety of the above measures as prophylaxis for hypotension is well established (26, 30, 45). Acute hydration of the normal parturient with 1000 ml of balanced salt solution has no significant effect on central venous pressure, even in the absence of sym-

pathetic blockade (Fig. 22.10) (26). The effect of acute volume loading with 2000 ml of crystalloid solution on the central venous pressure has also been studied, but not in the absence of sympathectomy. Lewis et al. (30) administered 2000 ml of balanced salt solution at the same time as epidural local anesthetic to healthy women receiving epidural anesthesia for cesarean section. A small mean rise in venous pressure occurred with simultaneous epidural blockade and fluid administration. In patients with significant cardiac disease, acute hydration should only be performed with monitoring of central venous or pulmonary arterial pressures.

In a study on the prophylactic administration of vasopressors in pregnant ewes, Ralston and co-workers (46) found that ephedrine or mephentermine in doses sufficient to raise the mean arterial blood pressure 40 to 50% above control values had no significant effects on uterine blood flow (see Fig. 3.16). Although ephedrine may cross the placenta and has been reported to increase fetal heart rate and beat-to-beat variability, no adverse fetal or neonatal effects have been noted (39, 47). In general, it appears that vasopressors with a mixture of both α- and β-adrenergic activity exert as much, if not more, effect on the venous capacitance as on the arteriolar resistance system and, as a result, restore blood pressure to a large extent by increasing central venous return and cardiac output. Pure α-agents, on the other hand, work mostly on the arterioles and, when used to treat spinal hypotension, will not return cardiac output or vital organ blood flow to preanesthetic values (49). Studies in pregnant sheep made hypotensive with spinal anesthesia show that ephedrine, mephentermine, and metaraminol, vasopressors with mixed α- and β-adrenergic activity, returned uterine blood flow

toward control while restoring maternal arterial blood pressure (48, 50). Fetal deterioration was, in fact, arrested and often reversed (48). Vasopressors with primarily peripheral α-adrenergic action, such as methoxamine or phenylephrine, may be harmful to the fetus because they produce further uterine vasoconstriction (51, 52).

Extreme care must be exercised in administering oxytocics, and most especially ergot alkaloids, to any patient who has received a vasopressor, especially an α-adrenergic agent, during labor or delivery. The combination of the two drugs can produce severe hypertension and stroke. If an ergot alkaloid is deemed necessary in a patient who has received a vasopressor, the dose must be reduced and the blood pressure monitored frequently.

THERAPY

Therapy for epidural or spinal hypotension includes more left uterine displacement, rapid fluid infusion, the Trendelenburg position to increase venous return, intravenous ephedrine, and oxygen administration (Table 22.1). Administration of oxygen to the mother may not necessarily raise the fetal PaO_2 until the hypotension is corrected. After spinal hypotension in pregnant ewes, fetal PaO_2 returned to normal only after maternal arterial blood pressure was restored (Fig. 22.11) (48).

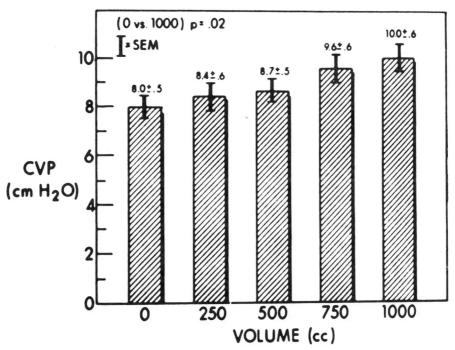

Figure 22.10. Response of central venous pressure (*CVP*) to rapid (14- to 20-min) infusion of 1000 ml of 5% dextrose in lactated Ringer's solution. (Reprinted by permission from Wollman SB, Marx GF: Acute hydration for prevention of hypotension of spinal anesthesia in parturients. Anesthesiology 29:374–380, 1968.)

Two investigators (53, 54) have recently compared the safety and efficacy of ephedrine and phenylephrine in the treatment of maternal hypotension associated with regional anesthesia for cesarean section. Healthy women undergoing elective cesarean section under either epidural (53) or spinal (54) anesthesia were prehydrated with intravenous crystalloid. Decreases in blood pressure were promptly treated with small intravenous doses of either ephedrine or phenylephrine. There were no differences in outcome as assessed by umbilical cord blood gases or Apgar scores. Uterine blood flow was not measured in these studies. However, maternal stroke volume and end-diastolic volume did not differ following ephedrine or phenylephrine therapy, indicating that both drugs worked by augmenting venous re-

turn. In spite of these recent papers, we believe that ephedrine is the vasopressor of choice for the treatment of anesthesia-induced hypotension in obstetrics. It is clearly superior in most animal studies and has a long record of safety in clinical obstetrics. Nevertheless, in clinical situations in which the parturient may not tolerate ephedrine's potential β-mimetic effects or when ephedrine is ineffective, phenylephrine may be an acceptable alternative.

In a classic study published in 1969, Marx and co-workers (55) found both better fetal biochemical and neonatal clinical conditions when spinal hypotension was prevented rather than treated. However, direct application of these results to today's practice should be made with caution because preventive measures for and treatment of hypotension have changed significantly since that time. Also, other investigators (23–25, 56) have more recently demonstrated no significant difference in Apgar scores or blood gases between neonates of mothers who become hypotensive and those who do not (see Fig. 12.3 and Table 12.22), provided hypotension is detected early and treated quickly. Thus, with appropriate monitoring and prompt therapy, the deleterious effects of hypotension on the fetus can be prevented.

Table 22.1
Treatment of Hypotension

Increase left uterine displacement
Increase intravenous fluid infusion
Place patient in 10- to 20-degree Trendelenburg position
   If no response in 1 min:
Administer ephedrine 5 to 10 mg IV
Administer oxygen by face mask

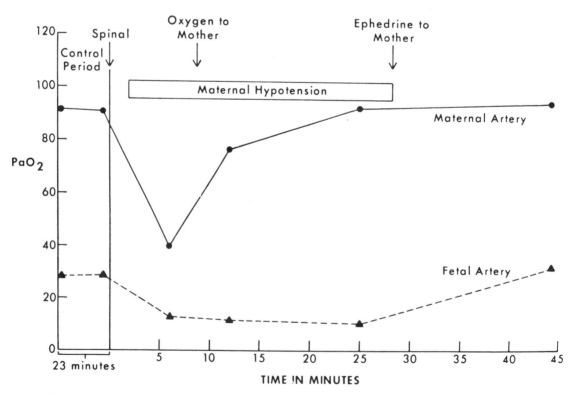

Figure 22.11. Changes in fetal arterial oxygen tension after maternal spinal hypotension, maternal hypoxia, oxygen administration, then ephedrine administration to the mother. (Reprinted by permission from Shnider SM, deLorimier AA, Holl JW, Chapler FK, Morishima HO: Vasopressors in obstetrics. I. Correction of fetal acidosis with ephedrine during spinal hypotension. Am J Obstet Gynecol 102:911–919, 1968.)

References

1. Bromage PR: Physiology and pharmacology of epidural analgesia: A review. Anesthesiology 28:592–622, 1967.
2. Marx GF: Shock in the obstetric patient. Anesthesiology 26:423–434, 1965.
3. Eckstein KL, Marx GF: Aortocaval compression and uterine displacement. Anesthesiology 40:92–96, 1974.
4. Goodlin RC: Aortocaval compression during cesarean section: A cause of newborn depression. Obstet Gynecol 37:702–705, 1971.
5. Holmes F: The supine hypotensive syndrome: Its importance to the anaesthetist. Anaesthesia 15:298–306, 1960.
6. Bieniarz J, Crottogini JJ, Curuchet E, Romero-Salinas G, Yoshida T, Posiero JJ, Caldeyro-Barcia R: Aortocaval compression by the uterus in late human pregnancy. An arteriographic study. Am J Obstet Gynecol 100:203–217, 1968.
7. Kerr MG, Samuel E: Studies on the inferior vena cava in late pregnancy. Br Med J 1:532–533, 1964.
8. DiFazio CA, Carron H, Grosslight KR, Moscicki JC, Bolding WR, Johns RA: Comparison of pH-adjusted lidocaine solutions for epidural anesthesia. Anesth Analg 65:760–764, 1986.
9. Parnass SM, Curran MJA, Becker GL: Incidence of hypotension associated with epidural anesthesia using alkalinized and nonalkalinized lidocaine for cesarean section. Anesth Analg 66:1148–1150, 1987.
10. Greiss FC Jr, Crandell DL: Therapy for hypotension induced by spinal anesthesia during pregnancy. JAMA 191:793–796, 1965.
11. Greiss FC Jr: Pressure flow relationship in the gravid uterine vascular bed. Am J Obstet Gynecol 96:41–47, 1966.
12. Martin CB Jr, Gingerick B: Uteroplacental physiology. JOGNN 5(suppl):16–25, 1976.
13. Adams FH, Assali N, Cushman M, Westersten A: Interrelationships of maternal and fetal circulations. Pediatrics 27:627–635, 1961.
14. Adamsons K, Myers RE: Circulation in the intervillous space: Obstetrical considerations in fetal deprivation. In The Placenta, P Grunewald, ed. University Park Press, Baltimore, 1975, p 158.
15. Lucas WE, Kirschbaum T, Assali NS: Spinal shock and fetal oxygenation. Am J Obstet Gynecol 93:583–587, 1965.
16. Moya F, Thorndike V: Maternal hypotension and the newborn. In Proceedings of the Third World Congress of Anesthesiology, Sao Paulo, Brazil, 1964.
17. Myers RE: Two patterns of perinatal brain damage and their condition of occurrence. Am J Obstet Gynecol 112:246–276, 1972.
18. Ebner H, Barcohana J, Bartoshuk AK: Influence of postspinal hypotension on the fetal electrocardiogram. Am J Obstet Gynecol 80:569–576, 1960.
19. Hon EH, Reid BL, Hehre FW: The electronic evaluation of the fetal heart rate. II. Changes with maternal hypotension. Am J Obstet Gynecol 79:209–215, 1960.
20. Bonica JJ, Hon EH: Fetal distress. In Principles and Practice of Obstetric Analgesia and Anesthesia. JJ Bonica, ed. Davis, Philadelphia, 1964, p 1252.
21. Zilianti M, Salazar JR, Aller J, Aguero O: Fetal heart rate and pH of fetal capillary blood during epidural analgesia in labor. Obstet Gynecol 36:881–886, 1970.
22. Moya F, Smith B: Spinal anesthesia for cesarean section: Clinical and biochemical studies of effects on maternal physiology. JAMA 179:609–614, 1962.
23. Brizgys RV, Dailey PA, Shnider SM, Kotelko DM, Levinson G: The incidence and neonatal effects of maternal hypotension during epidural anesthesia for cesarean section. Anesthesiology 67:782–786, 1987.
24. Datta S, Alper MH, Ostheimer GW, Weiss JB: Method of ephedrine administration and nausea and hypotension during spinal anesthesia for cesarean section. Anesthesiology 56:68–70, 1982.
25. Abboud TK, Blikian A, Noueihid R, Nagappala S, Afrasiabi A, Henriksen EH: Neonatal effects of maternal hypotension during spinal anesthesia as evaluated by a new test. Anesthesiology 59:A421, 1983.
26. Wollman SB, Marx GF: Acute hydration for prevention of hypotension of spinal anesthesia in parturients. Anesthesiology 29:374–380, 1968.
27. Mathru M, Rao TLK, Kartha RK, Shanmugham M, Jacobs KH: Intravenous albumin administration for prevention of spinal hypotension during cesarean section. Anesth Analg 59:655–658, 1980.
28. Ramanathan S, Masih A, Rock I, Chalon J, Turndorf H: Maternal and fetal effects of prophylactic hydration with crystalloids or colloids before epidural anesthesia. Anesth Analg 62:673–678, 1983.
29. Hallworth D, Jellicoe JA, Wilkes RG: Hypotension during epidural anesthesia for caesarean section: A comparison of intravenous loading with crystalloid and colloid solutions. Anaesthesia 37:53–56, 1982.
30. Lewis M, Thomas P, Wilkes RG: Hypotension during epidural analgesia for caesarean section. Anaesthesia 38:250–253, 1983.
31. Evans SE, Crawford JS, Stevens ID, Durbin GM, Daya H: Fluid therapy for induced labour under epidural analgesia: Biochemical consequences for mother and infant. Br J Obstet Gynaecol 93:329–333, 1986.
32. Kenepp NB, Shelley WC, Gabbe SG, Kumar S, Stanley CA, Gutsche BB: Fetal and neonatal hazards of maternal hydration with 5% dextrose before caesarean section. Lancet 1:1150–1152, 1982.
33. Mendiola J, Grylack LJ, Scanlon JW: Effects of intrapartum maternal glucose infusion on the normal fetus and newborn. Anesth Analg 61:32–35, 1982.
34. Morton KE, Jackson MC, Gillmer MDG: A comparison of the effects of four intravenous solutions for the treatment of ketonuria during labour. Br J Obstet Gynaecol 92:473–479, 1985.
35. Lanier WL, Stangland KJ, Scheithauer BW, Milde JH, Michenfelder JD: The effects of dextrose infusion and head position on neurologic outcome after complete cerebral ischemia in primates: Examination of a model. Anesthesiology 66:39–47, 1987.
36. Gutsche BB: Prophylactic ephedrine preceding spinal analgesia for cesarean section. Anesthesiology 45:462–465, 1976.
37. Kang YG, Abouleish E, Caritas S: Prophylactic intravenous ephedrine infusion during spinal anesthesia for cesarean section. Anesth Analg 61:839–842, 1982.
38. Rolbin SH, Cole AFD, Hew EM, Pollard A, Virgint S: Prophylactic intramuscular ephedrine before epidural anaesthesia for caesarean section: Efficacy and actions on the foetus and newborn. Can Anaesth Soc J 29:148–153, 1982.
39. Wright RG, Shnider SM, Levinson G, Rolbin SH, Parer JT: The effect of maternal administration of ephedrine on fetal heart rate and variability. Obstet Gynecol 57:734–738, 1981.
40. Huch A, Huch R: Transcutaneous noninvasive monitoring of PO₂. Hosp Pract 11:43–52, 1976.
41. Humphrey MD, Chang A, Wood EC, Morgan S, Hounslow D: A decrease in fetal pH during the second stage of labor when conducted in the dorsal position. J Obstet Gynaecol Br Commonw 81:600–602, 1974.
42. Crawford JS, Burton M, Davies P: Time and lateral tilt at caesarean section. Br J Anaesth 44:447–484, 1972.
43. Kennedy RL: An instrument to relieve inferior vena cava occlusion. Am J Obstet Gynecol 107:331–333, 1970.
44. Colon-Morales MA: A self-supporting device for continuous left uterine displacement during cesarean section. Anesth Analg 49:223–224, 1970.
45. Caritas SN, Abouleish E, Edelstone DI, Mueller-Heubach E: Fetal acid-base state following spinal or epidural anesthesia for cesarean section. Obstet Gynecol 56:610–615, 1980.
46. Ralston DH, Shnider SM, deLorimier AA: Effects of equipotent ephedrine, metaraminol, mephentermine, and methoxamine on uterine blood flow in the pregnant ewe. Anesthesiology 40:354–370, 1974.
47. Hughes SC, Ward MG, Levinson G, Shnider SM, Wright RG,

Gruenke LD, Craig JC: Placental transfer of ephedrine does not affect neonatal outcome. Anesthesiology 63:217–219, 1985.

48. Shnider SM, deLorimier AA, Holl JW, Chapler FK, Morishima HO: Vasopressors in obstetrics. I. Correction of fetal acidosis with ephedrine during spinal hypotension. Am J Obstet Gynecol 102:911–919, 1968.

49. Butterworth JF IV, Piccione W Jr, Berrizbeitia LD, Dance G, Shemin RJ, Cohn LW: Augmentation of venous return by adrenergic agonists during spinal anesthesia. Anesth Analg 65:612–616, 1986.

50. James FM III, Greiss FC Jr, Kemp RA: An evaluation of vasopressor therapy for maternal hypotension during spinal anesthesia. Anesthesiology 33:25–34, 1970.

51. Shnider SM, deLorimier AA, Asling JH, Morishima HO: Vasopressors in obstetrics. II. Fetal hazards of methoxamine administration during obstetric spinal anesthesia. Am J Obstet Gynecol 106:680–686, 1970.

52. Greiss FC Jr, Van Wilkes D: Effects of sympathomimetic drugs and angiotensin on the uterine vascular bed. Obstet Gynecol 23:925–930, 1964.

53. Ramanathan S, Grant GJ: Vasopressor therapy for hypotension due to epidural anesthesia or cesarean section. Acta Anaesthesiol Scand 32:559–565, 1988.

54. Moran DH, Perillo M, Bader AM, Datta S: Phenylephrine in treating maternal hypotension secondary to spinal anesthesia. Anesthesiology 71:A857, 1989.

55. Marx GF, Cosmi RV, Wollmen SB: Biochemical status and clinical condition of mother and infant at cesarean section. Anesth Analg 48:986–994, 1969.

56. Norris MC: Hypotension during spinal anesthesia for cesarean section: Does it affect neonatal outcome? Reg Anesth 12:191–193, 1987.

CHAPTER 23

Pulmonary Aspiration of Gastric Contents

Theodore G. Cheek, M.D.

Brett B. Gutsche, M.D.

The avoidance of gastric content aspiration in the pregnant patient remains a major concern of the anesthesiologist. The most reliable data from England and Wales suggest that, over the last 20 years, the two leading causes of maternal anesthetic death remain anoxial loss of airway control and aspiration of gastric contents (1). The most recent triennial mortality report shows five anesthetic deaths from anoxia and one from aspiration (ranitidine given) (Table 23.1). The apparent decrease in death from aspiration may represent either statistical periodicity or, alternatively, may provide evidence that increased awareness of maternal risk and improved attention to safety precautions and prophylaxis at induction of anesthesia have resulted in fewer deaths from this disaster. One large series estimated the overall incidence of aspiration during cesarean anesthesia to be 4 in 2643 (Table 23.2) (2). Estimates of the incidence of aspiration as a cause of maternal death vary widely and range from an earlier 100 times a year in the United States (3) to less than 1 in 1 million deliveries in a more recent survey (1). Although some would suggest that the risk of maternal aspiration is not as great as once believed (4–6), most authors agree (7) that it remains one of the most devastating threats to maternal well-being. A recent survey of the Society for Obstetric Anesthesia and Perinatology membership (8) portrays the circumstances surrounding aspiration during obstetric anesthesia and suggests some old but still valid conclusions: "1) General anesthesia for emergency cesarean section is particularly hazardous, 2) A difficult or failed intubation increases the risk of aspiration, 3) Even when accomplished with ease, endotracheal intubation per se does not prevent aspiration." Maternal death after aspiration has been estimated to occur in 10 to 25% of reported cases of aspiration (9, 10) and in 33% of those who develop a severe pulmonary acid aspiration syndrome (10). Faced with these alarming facts, it is imperative that all anesthesiologists be thoroughly familiar with the risk factors, prevention, and appropriate management of maternal aspiration.

FACTORS THAT INCREASE THE RISK OF ASPIRATION

The parturient is predisposed to the catastrophe of aspiration for many reasons. Food is frequently ingested shortly before the onset of labor. Stomach emptying is decreased in pregnancy. In women at 12 to 14 weeks' gestation, 71 min were required to reach peak paracetamol absorption compared with 45 min in nonpregnant controls (11). This is thought to be caused by the combined effects of increased plasma levels of progesterone (12), decreased plasma levels of the hormone motilin (13), and mechanical displacement of the pylorus by the gravid uterus later in pregnancy. These findings are disputed by investigators using epigastric external impedance monitors (14). Yet most authors acknowledge gastric activity in pregnancy is attenuated. Labor clearly further retards stomach emptying (14, 15). Pregnant women suffering from heartburn, which may indicate gastroesophageal junction dysfunction, have the longest delay in gastric emptying (13). The stress response activated by fear, apprehension, pain, starvation, and ketosis such as experienced by the parturient in labor has been shown to delay stomach emptying (14, 16).

Drugs and Stomach Emptying

The use of drugs, particularly narcotics and sedatives, retards stomach emptying. Meperidine prolongs gastric emptying time by 5 hr or more in 70% of patients in labor (17, 18), which is antagonized by naloxone (21). Parenteral meperidine prolongs the antacid effect of sodium citrate because of decreased gastric emptying (19) but decreases the effectiveness of metoclopramide (20–22). Epidural analgesia during labor has little effect on gastric emptying (21). Ritodrine and other mixed β-agonists employed as tocolytics for premature la-

Table 23.1
Anesthesia Factors as a Cause of Maternal Death[a]

	1973–1975	1976–1978	1979–1981	1982–1984	1985–1987	1973–1987
Pulmonary aspiration	13	11 (3)	8	7	1	40 (3)
Anoxia (failed intubation)	7	16	8	8	5	44
Drug misuse	4	4	3	1	0	12
Apparatus	2	2	0	1	0	5
Epidural	2	4	1	1	1	9
Miscellaneous	7	9	9	1	1	27
TOTAL	35	46	29	19	8	137

[a] Adapted from *Confidential Inquiries into Maternal Deaths in England and Wales, 1985–1987*. Her Majesty's Stationery Office, London, 1991.

Table 23.2
Incidence of Pulmonary Aspiration during Anesthesia[a]

Authors	Type Surgery	Anesthesia	Aspiration	Aspiration per 10,000
Mendelson (1946)	Obstetric	44,016	66	15.0
Olsson, et al. (1986) (2)	Cesarean	2,643	4	15.0
Olsson, et al. (1986) (2)	Nonobstetric and obstetric	185,358	87	4.7

[a] Adapted with permission from James CF: Maternal mortality. Semin Anesth 11:76–82, 1992.

bor may inhibit gastrointestinal motility (23). Intravaginal prostaglandin E_2 does not appear to affect gastric emptying (24).

Gastric Acidity

Increased gastric acid secretion occurs during pregnancy (25, 26), caused by the markedly elevated plasma levels of the hormone gastrin (27). The elevated plasma levels of gastrin, together with the very high placental tissue concentration, suggest placental production and/or storage of the hormone. Dehydration and starvation ketosis during labor may also increase gastric acid secretions. Intravenous alcohol, now rarely used as a tocolytic, and oral alcohol, sometimes abused, markedly increases gastric secretions and acidity.

Combined Risk of Volume and pH

The exact gastric volume for each pH at which parturients are at risk for acid aspiration has not been determined. Mendelson (28) was one of the first to suggest that both volume and pH play a role in the severity of aspiration sequelae. Teabeaut suggested a gastric pH below 2.5 was associated with a high incidence of acute symptoms of aspiration pneumonitis (29). Roberts and Shirley described a human "threshold volume" of 0.4 ml/kg gastric fluid (~25 ml) and a pH lower than 2.5 that caused aspiration pneumonitis. Using these criteria, Roberts and Shirley (30, 31) found that, regardless of the time of last meal or the time between the last meal and the onset of labor, 25% of parturients were at risk. They also found that 70% of women who were fasted before

elective cesarean section were still at high risk for the complication of aspiration.

James et al. (32) found all mothers undergoing tubal ligation within 9 hr of delivery had gastric aspirates with a pH less than 2.5, and 60% had gastric volumes greater than 26 ml (Table 23.3). In rats it has been shown that the percentage mortality can be estimated if the specific pH and volume of the aspirate is known, with the highest death rates seen below a pH of 1.5 to 2 (Fig. 23.1) (33). More recently Raidoo has suggested that the volume of liquid pH 2.5 required to cause pneumonia in primates is two times higher than once thought (34). These efforts suggest that pH is the dominant factor in producing pulmonary lesions. Unfortunately, the one maternal death from aspiration in England between 1984 and 1987 occurred in a woman who had received ranitidine 2 hr before the event, which suggests that an alkaline aspirate does not always protect these patients from death (1). High pH gastric fluid with particulate matter can also predispose patients to severe pneumonia (33).

In recent years the concept of a critical or "threshold" volume has been questioned (4–6). It is clear that the incidence and intensity of aspiration pneumonitis increases as pH decreases and volume increases (28, 29, 33). Unfortunately, the understandable lack of precise volume/pH outcome studies in humans has led to extreme reactions among practicing anesthesiologists, ranging from rigid adherence to strict NPO and gastric emptying protocols in patients admitted in labor to the rejection of any pro-

Table 23.3
Gastric pH and Volume Found in Patients Undergoing Postpartum Tubal Ligation[a]

	Group I (1–8 hr)	Group II (9–23 hr)	Group III (24–45 hr)	Group IV (control)[b]
Mean DSI (hr)[c]	4.8 ± 2.1	17.3 ± 4.7	32.6 ± 6.9	—
Mean pH (range)	1.53 (1.2–2.2)	1.48 (1.1–2.1)	1.40 (0.1–2.8)	1.56 (1.1–6.5)
pH <2.5 (%)	100	100	80	80
pH <1.4 (%)	33	40	46	26
Mean volume (ml) (range)	39.1 (7–73)	24.0 (6–56)	40.9 (8–73)	38.1 (10–82)
Volume >25 ml (%)	73	40	73	67
High risk for pH <2.5 + vol >25 ml (%)	73	40	67	60

[a]Adapted with permission from James CF, Gibbs CP, Banner T: Postpartum perioperative risk of aspiration pneumonia. Anesthesiology 61:756–759, 1984.
[b]Nonpregnant patients undergoing general surgical procedures.
[c]DSI = Delivery-to-surgery interval, time elapsed in hours from delivery to anesthesia for postpartum tubal ligation.

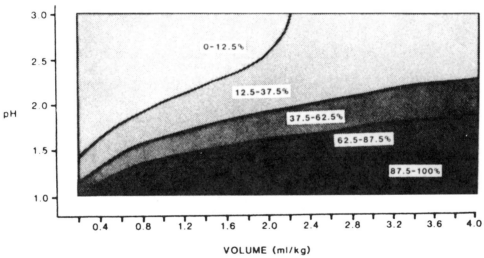

Figure 23.1. Predicted mortality (%) after aspiration. Each *shaded area* represents the mortality interval predicted for a specific pH and volume of solution aspirated. (Reprinted by permission from James CF, Modell JH, Gibbs CP, Kuck EJ, Ruiz BC: Pulmonary aspiration effects of volume and pH in the rat. Anesth Analg 63:655–668, 1984.)

phylaxis guidelines. Without doubt early definitions were based on studies with designs and methods fraught with small numbers, inappropriate statistics, and unverified assumptions that make the use of a volume/pH cutoff criteria scientifically questionable, as pointed out by Gorback (5). Although we agree it is appropriate in clinical practice to approach patient risk as a continuum, it is often necessary when conducting an investigation to assign a cutoff value—however, arbitrary—to obtain clinically useful information. For example, humans can tolerate a sustained cerebral blood flow of 25 ml/100 gm brain tissue without experiencing ischemia (35). Although this correlates with a mean blood pressure of about 40 mm Hg, most anesthesiologists arbitrarily choose 50 mm Hg as the lowest

allowable sustained MAP to assure a margin of safety (36). Likewise, the volume and pH cutoff values of 25 ml and 2.5 although not a precise LD 50, continue to serve as clinically useful investigational tools. To paraphrase Greenburg: Just because the methods or design of older studies were wrong or flawed, it does not follow that the conclusions drawn were wrong (37). This opinion is reinforced by ongoing confidential mortality reports and outcome studies that indicate the continued devastating risk of aspiration in parturition.

Fasting and Gastric Volume

For many years, most patients in labor have received orders to take nothing by mouth once labor starts until after delivery. These recommendations were based both on intuitive reasoning and observation that parturients having recently ingested food had larger gastric volumes than those who were fasted. It is interesting to note that in some hospitals pregnant women are still offered full meals during labor (38), whereas in others, prolonged labor, fasting, and glucose restriction are associated with maternal ketosis and possible hypotension (39, 40). The interesting work of O'Sullivan suggests gastric emptying may not be as slow as once believed in pregnancy (14). An array of investigators suggest small volumes of oral liquid are not associated with increased gastric volume or lower pH prior to surgery in pregnant and nonpregnant patients (41–46). Lewis and Crawford (47) compared patients who were given a light breakfast less than 4 hr before elective cesarean section to those who fasted. They found the gastric volume was 73.4 ml and 33 ml, respectively, with a lower pH in the fed versus the fasted parturients. We believe that it is well advised for anesthesiologists to continue the practice of presurgical fasting of 6 to 8 hr in pregnancy, especially if there is a probability of general anesthesia and no functioning epidural is present (48). In our practice, women in labor with a functioning epidural block are allowed ice chips and limited sips of clear liquids. After 15 years and more than 8000 cesarean sections we have not had an aspiration.

Gastroesophageal Tone, Reflux, and Gastric Pressure

Heartburn during pregnancy occurs in 45 to 70% of women (49), with 27% of these having hiatal hernias (50). The heartburn is caused by gastric reflux as a result of a decreased competence of the lower esophageal sphincter (LES) (51, 52). Gastroesophageal reflux decreases markedly by the second postpartum day (52). The presence of heartburn indicates an increased risk of regurgitation, particularly when the supine position is assumed.

During pregnancy the upward force of the uterus increases gastric pressure from 7.3 cm H_2O (normal) to 17.2 cm H_2O (53, 54). Lithotomy and Trendelenburg positions can cause a further rise in gastric pressure of 5.6 to 8.8 cm H_2O (53). The presence of twins, hydramnios, or gross obesity may be associated with intragastric pressures greater than 40 cm H_2O (53). Both fundal pressure (Fig. 23.2) and succinylcholine fasciculations can raise intragastric pressure significantly. During pregnancy the LES tone usually rises from 35 to 44 cm H_2O, providing some protection from rising intragastric pressures. However, Lind et al. (54) found that parturients with heartburn experienced an average fall in LES tone to 24 cm H_2O and

required only a small rise in gastric pressure of 7.3 cm H_2O to cause LES opening and regurgitation. All pregnant women studied by Brock-Utne and co-workers (55) had decreased LES tone.

Medications that reduce LES tone include narcotics, diazepam, and anticholinergics such as atropine and glycopyrrolate (56–61). Whereas metoclopramide, 10 mg IV, and domperidone, 10 mg IV, increase LES tone in the narcotized or atropinized nonpregnant patient (61, 62), they effectively increase LES tone in the parturient (55, 63); only domperidone counteracts the effect of atropine (64, 65).

Other Risk Factors

Nausea and vomiting are common during labor and are frequently exacerbated by various factors. Hypotension resulting from aortocaval compression, hemorrhage, or sympathetic block can result in nausea, vomiting, and loss of consciousness, predisposing the patient to pulmonary aspiration. Narcotics predispose parturients to nausea and vomiting and, along with sedatives and tranquilizers, depress consciousness and upper airway reflexes, predisposing parturients to aspiration. Various medications given to treat a variety of obstetric conditions—such as magnesium, prostaglandins, tocolytics, ergot derivatives, and others—are often associated with nausea and vomiting. In pregnancy the upper airway is swollen, airway obstruction occurs easily, and airway management is considerably more challenging, further increasing the risk of aspiration during inhalational analgesia or the induction of general anesthesia.

Gastric material can reach the lungs following either active vomiting or passive regurgitation. If the protective airway reflexes are lost during the process of vomiting or regurgitation from (a) development of hypotension with cerebral hypoxia, (b) general anesthesia or excessive premedication, or (c) the onset of muscle paralysis, aspiration may occur. These many factors place every parturient at risk for the catastrophe of pulmonary aspiration and require that she be managed as a patient with a full stomach.

PATHOPHYSIOLOGY AND TREATMENT OF PULMONARY ASPIRATION OF GASTRIC CONTENTS

The morbidity and mortality following aspiration depend on both the amount and the nature of aspirated matter. Three types of gastric material can be aspirated, each of which will cause a different clinical picture: (a) material of a pH of less than 2.5, causing a chemical pneumonitis or acid aspiration syndrome; (b) solid or particulate matter; or

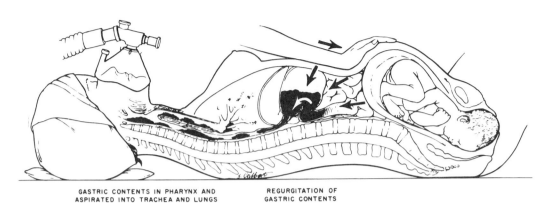

GASTRIC CONTENTS IN PHARYNX AND
ASPIRATED INTO TRACHEA AND LUNGS

REGURGITATION OF
GASTRIC CONTENTS

Figure 23.2. Regurgitation of gastric contents caused by marked increase in intraabdominal and intragastric pressure from an attempt to place pressure on the uterus during de-

livery. (Reprinted by permission from Bonica JJ: *Principles and Practice of Obstetric Analgesia and Anesthesia, Vol 1.* Davis, Philadelphia, 1967, p 676.)

(c) fecal or other bacterially contaminated material, usually as a result of intestinal obstruction, perforation, or bowel infarct. In the parturient the most common forms of pulmonary aspiration are those of acid and particulate aspiration; fecal aspiration is rare.

Diagnostic and Therapeutic Considerations

Aspiration of gastric material should be suspected if the patient shows any of the following signs and symptoms: (a) the presence of foreign material in the mouth or posterior pharynx; (b) sudden coughing or laryngospasm; (c) dyspnea, tachypnea, hyperpnea, or apnea; (d) bronchospasm, wheezing, or rales; (e) chest retraction or obvious airway obstruction; (f) cyanosis, particularly if not relieved by oxygen; (g) tachycardia and signs of shock; and (h) the development of a pink frothy exudate. Signs and symptoms usually occur within the first hour of aspiration in most patients (Table 23.4) (66), although latency periods of 6 to 8 hr have been reported, especially during general anesthesia (67).

If aspiration is witnessed or suspected, particularly in an obtunded patient, she should be turned on her side and placed in the head-down position; the mouth and posterior pharynx should be suctioned; and the trachea should be intubated with a cuffed endotracheal tube. The trachea should be suctioned several times immediately after intubation. Ventilation with 100% oxygen between suctioning is recommended to prevent hypoxia. Except in the aspiration of particulate matter, saline or bicarbonate tracheal lavage should not be performed because it may spread the material and extend the lung damage (67). When particulate matter has been aspirated, bronchoscopy for removal of solid material and reexpansion of atelectatic segments of lung should be done as soon as initial resuscitation is accomplished.

Table 23.4
Clinical Signs after Aspiration of Gastric Contents in 50 Patients[a]

	Number	Percentage
Latent period		
0–1 hr	48	96
2 hr	2	4
Fever, total	47	94
99–102°F	24	48
>102°F	23	46
Tachypnea	39	78
Rales	36	72
Cough	18	36
Cyanosis	16	32
Wheezing	16	32
Apnea	15	30
Shock	12	24

[a] Reprinted with permission from Bynum LJ, Pierce AK: Pulmonary aspiration of gastric contents. Am Rev Respir Dis 114:1129–1136, 1976.

A specimen of gastric contents should be obtained and examined for the presence of particulate matter, analyzed for pH, and cultured for the presence of bacteria and their antibiotic sensitivities. Serial arterial blood gas determinations will indicate the need for increased inspired oxygen concentrations, ventilation, and the use of positive end-expiratory pressure (PEEP). Chest x-rays taken as soon as possible after the incident and at regular intervals as the clinical picture indicates will aid in determining the extent and progress of the pathologic process. A record of urinary output and continuous central venous pressure (CVP) measurement will aid in fluid management. Any patient suspected of aspirating gastric material, particularly if symptoms of aspiration are present, should be placed in an intensive care environment for close monitoring and ventilatory care until resolution of the process. Rapid early therapy is essential to minimize morbidity and mortality. A recent report of aggressive ventilation and rapid crystalloid volume restoration in 38 severe aspiration victims resulted in the survival of 30 (79%), with 5 deaths from cerebral hemorrhage and only 3 from respiratory complications (68).

Acid Gastric Material

The most common form of pulmonary aspiration in the parturient is that of acid material resulting in a chemical pneumonitis characterized by bronchospasm, the development of a high alveolar-arterial oxygen gradient, and a pulmonary exudate resembling pulmonary edema fluid. This syndrome was described by Mendelson in 1946 (27) and now bears his name. Teabeaut (28) showed in rabbits that, once the pH of aspirated material fell below 2.5, the typical clinical syndrome developed. Both Mendelson (27) and Bosomworth and Hamelberg (69) demonstrated that the pH of the aspirate, not gastric or enteric enzymes, was responsible for the development of the syndrome. Roberts and Shirley (29, 30) have suggested that the aspiration of 25 ml (0.4 ml/kg) or more of gastric juice with a pH of 2.5 or less will produce symptoms. A recent study in small monkeys disputes these criteria based on results that, at a pH of 1, 1 ml/kg of pooled gastric aspirate (or approximately 50 ml in humans) resulted in a 50% mortality (33). Aspiration of large volumes of material with a pH greater than 2.5 has also been reported to result in Mendelson's syndrome (44). Although no patients died in Mendelson's original study, later reports suggest a mortality as high as 70% (71–75). Lewis et al. (72) found a 100% mortality in humans who aspirated gastric contents with a pH of less than 1.75.

Symptoms of acid aspiration may have a rapid onset heralded by sudden bronchospasm or may be delayed for several hours after the insult, as described earlier. Despite the frequent clinical picture of pulmonary edema, left ventricular failure is rarely present, as indicated by a low or normal pulmonary wedge pressure and a decreased plasma volume averaging 500 ml or more, accompanied by hemoconcentration (Fig. 23.3) (72, 76, 77). The CVP may be slightly elevated due to an increased pulmonary vascular resistance (78).

Blood gases frequently show a marked hypoxemia with a PaO_2 of less than 50 torr on room air. With the administration of high inspired oxygen concentrations, a marked alveolar-arterial gradient (PA-aO_2) is found (Fig. 23.4). This is thought to represent impaired diffusion, pulmonary shunting, and pulmonary arteriolar vasoconstriction (72, 77). Initially the $PaCO_2$ may be normal or slightly below normal, but with the progession of the process, this may become slightly elevated. A metabolic acidosis is often seen as the condition worsens.

The chest x-ray shows soft mottled densities widely distributed over the peripheral areas but especially pronounced in the dependent lung areas, particularly of the right side. The initial picture resembles that of a "snow storm" over the lung fields (Fig. 23.5), usually assuming an alveolar pattern and occasionally a reticular pattern (66). Mediastinal shift is rare. As the process continues, an x-ray picture typical of pulmonary edema may develop. Atelectasis and pleural effusion may also be present.

The pathologic picture is best described as a severe chemical burn of the lung. Initially, there is decreased pulmonary compliance. Acid aspiration is followed by interstitial edema, transudation of a plasma-like substance, and disruption of the alveolar-capillary membrane. There is acute bronchitis and bronchiolitis, sloughing of mucosa, intraalveolar edema, and intraalveolar hemorrhage. Type I and II alveolar cells undergo necrosis, and free laminated inclusion bodies are seen in the pulmonary transudate. Lung weight may be two or three times normal. Initially no signs of infection are present, but with progression there may be an increase in polymorphonuclear leukocytes. Kennedy and co-workers (79) recently observed a biphasic pattern to acid pulmonary injury at 1 and 4 hr in a rat model. This suggested an initial direct physiochemical interaction or capsaicin-sensitive afferent nerve–mediated response. A second phase of acute inflammatory response 2 to 3 hr later is mediated by neutrophils. In 24 to 36 hr after the initial insult, alveolar consolidation and airway damage are observed and may result in mucosal sloughing (80). Organization of a hyaline membrane may be seen (81).

Resolution of the lesion begins by about 72 hr, and by 2 to 3 weeks lung weight has returned to near normal. Permanent damage is usually minimal and may include scarring, bronchiolitis obliterans, and atypical bronchial degeneration (82). When infection occurs it may be Gram-positive, Gram-negative, or a mixture of bacteria. The pathophysiologic picture of pulmonary acid aspiration has been well reviewed by a number of authors (66, 77, 83).

Therapy for severe acid aspiration pneumonitis has often been reported to be ineffective. Although morbidity and mortality are reported to be high, early and aggressive initiation of therapy will do much to lessen them. The primary object of therapy is to ensure adequate oxygenation and ventilatory function

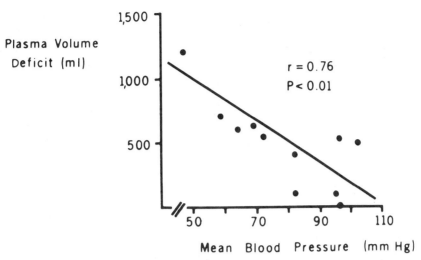

Figure 23.3. Plasma volume deficits 12 to 18 hr after aspiration in 11 patients. There is significant correlation between moderate deficits and mean systemic blood pressure. (Reprinted by permission from Lewis RT, Burgess JH, Hampson LG: Cardiorespiratory studies in critical illness: Changes in aspiration pneumonitis. Arch Surg 103:335–340, 1971.)

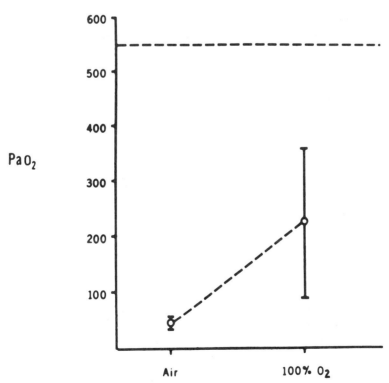

Figure 23.4. Response of mean PaO_2 to breathing 100% oxygen for 15 min in 12 patients. In all cases the rise fell short of the generally accepted normal value of 500 mm Hg, indicating a right-to-left shunt-like effect. (Reprinted by permission from Lewis RT, Burgess JH, Hampson LG: Cardiorespiratory studies in critical illness: Changes in aspiration pneumonitis. Arch Surg 103:335–340, 1971.)

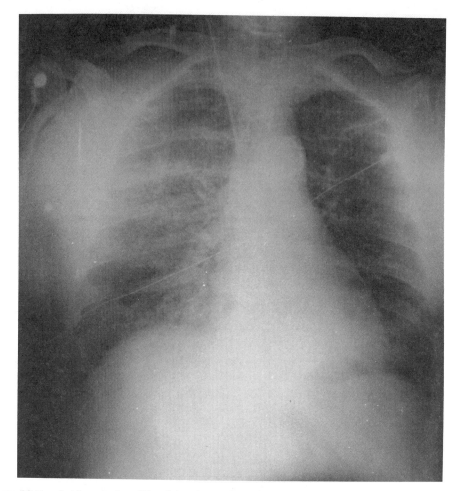

Figure 23.5.   Acid aspiration (Mendelson's syndrome) with marked involvement of the right lung.
Note the generalized soft, mottled densities and the absence of mediastinal shift.

and to restore and maintain blood volume until the damaged lungs can recover.

In the event that one actually witnesses pulmonary aspiration, such as during the induction of anesthesia, the patient should be intubated at once with a cuffed endotracheal tube. This should be followed by immediate tracheal suction. Unless particulate matter is retrieved from the trachea, the instillation of saline into the trachea is contraindicated. Hamelberg and Bosomworth (67) observed that 60 ml of material containing methylene blue dye instilled in the tracheae of dogs, both in vivo and in vitro, reached the lung periphery in 12 to 18 sec. Saline lavage with even small quantities of fluid only spread the process and caused further damage. Attempts to dilute or neutralize acid instilled into the lungs of rabbits with saline or sodium bicarbonate solution created more lung damage than the acid instillation alone (84). Tracheal instillation of steroids in animals subjected to acid aspiration did not decrease the severity of the lung lesions, and such instillations of steroids alone produced lung lesions (85).

Particulate and Antacid Aspiration

Gastric contents are often a combination of fluid and particulate food stuffs. The pulmonary response to aspiration of gastric particulate matter differs from aspiration of acid alone. The response to small food particles is a combination of hemorrhage and edema occurring soon after aspiration, followed more slowly by a granulomatous reaction with bronchiolar and alveolar damage (86, 87).

Aspiration of large particles or a large amount of particulate material can lead to immediate and complete obstruction of the airway with suffocation, unless the material can be removed by rapid intubation, suction, and possibly bronchoscopy. Instillation of small amounts (3 to 5 ml) of physiologic saline solution before suction may help dislodge particles. Aspiration of a smaller amount of material with small particulates can produce obstruction of bronchi or bronchioles, which results in atelectasis of the affected lobe or segment. Clinically, this may be accompanied by coughing, tachypnea, cyanosis, and tachycardia. Breath sounds may be decreased over the involved areas. Chest x-ray initially shows atelectasis with homogeneous densities in affected areas. If involvement is sufficiently great, there will be mediastinal shift. If the condition is untreated, pulmonary abscess may develop. Initial treatment includes immediate and repeated tracheobronchial suction, oxygenation, ventilation, and tracheal instillation of small amounts of saline to help dislodge material. Encouragement of coughing may help dislodge the material. Except in cases in which only minimal amounts of material are aspirated, bronchoscopy should be performed as soon as possible after the incident for diagnosis and removal of foreign material. Initially the fiberoptic bronchoscope may be used through the endotracheal tube to diagnose the presence of foreign material and to remove very small particulate matter under direct vision. The presence of large particulate matter or the development of atelectasis requires immediate bronchoscopy to remove this material and allow reinflation of the atelectatic segments. Tracheal aspirates should be obtained at regular intervals, especially with the development of fever, for Gram stain, culture, and sensitivity to allow rational antibiotic therapy.

The concept that severe lung lesions occur below a threshold of pH 2.5 has led many to conclude the nonacidic aspirates are relatively benign (29). Although the effects are transient and less severe, aspiration of clear liquids such as saline and water can produce signs of pulmonary edema, epithelial damage, and a widening alveolar-arterial oxygen gradient. Of particular concern is the aspiration of insoluble particulate antacids such as magnesium and aluminum hydroxides, carbonates, and trisilicates. Because of their widespread use in obstetrics (in some instances 30 ml every 2 hr [88]), many women may be unwittingly placed at risk for dangerous, even lethal aspiration of antacids, a situation where the prevention is potentially worse than the disease. Aspiration of gastric fluids containing particulate antacids has been shown in humans to result in a clinical picture similar to that of acid aspiration (70) with pulmonary edema, impaired oxygenation, and pulmonary shunting, even when the pH of the aspirate was 6.5 (89, 90). Gibbs et al. (90) and others (91) have shown that aspiration of insoluble particulate antacids (e.g., Kolantyl gel, Riopan, Mylanta) in animals results in pulmonary lesions that are more severe and of longer duration than those produced by aspiration of similar volumes of hydrochloric acid (pH 1.6). Numerous reports of maternal death (92–94) following aspiration of insoluble antacid preparations indicate that such prophylaxis is an ineffective, as well as potentially dangerous, medical practice.

Fecal or Bacterial Material

Aspiration of even small amounts of any fecal or bacterially contaminated material is associated with close to 100% mortality. Severe generalized pneumonia involving primarily the dependent portion of the lungs develops, along with symptoms of septic or endotoxic shock. Therapy includes massive doses of antibiotics, particularly those effective against Gram-negative bacteria. Tracheal cultures for sensitivity may help in choosing appropriate antibiotics. Massive doses of intravenous steroids are not of value, especially in the presence of sepsis (105). Support of the cardiovascular system with fluids, both colloid and crystalloid, and with appropriate inotropic cardiac drugs is indicated. Adequate oxygenation and ventilatory support are required. Fortunately this type of aspiration is rarely seen in the parturient.

Positive Pressure Ventilation

Following suction, the patient should be ventilated with high concentrations of oxygen. Questions arise as to (a) which patients should be ventilated, (b) when it should be started, and (c) how long it should be continued. There is abundant evidence from animal studies that positive pressure ventilation markedly decreases mortality from acid aspiration (69, 73, 95, 96). Cameron and co-workers (97) demonstrated in dogs that the immediate initiation of positive pressure ventilation after an insult of 2 ml/kg of 0.1 N HCl placed in the right mainstem bronchus resulted in a 100% survival rate. When ventilation was delayed 24 hr, only 40% survived, suggesting the efficacy of early ventilation, even in the absence of severe symptoms. If aspiration is suspected but not witnessed, ventilation should be begun as soon as any signs or symptoms become apparent—for example, dyspnea, bronchoconstriction, moist rales, or an x-ray that shows acid aspiration pneumonitis. During spontaneous respirations a PaO_2 of less than 50 torr on room air or less than 200 torr on 100% oxygen is indication for intubation and ventilatory therapy (78). Inspired oxygen tension should be adequate to maintain the PaO_2 above 70 torr. One should not wait for the development of pulmonary edema before starting ventilation. Roberts (98) recommended immediate intubation and ventilation with blood gas monitoring of all patients who have aspirated gastric material with a pH of less than 3. Ventilation is continued at least 8 hr after the aspiration.

The type of ventilation (i.e., assisted, controlled, or intermittent mandatory) is not of great importance, provided that adequate oxygenation and carbon dioxide elimination are maintained. The use of PEEP may allow lower inspired oxygen concentrations, decreasing the risk of pulmonary oxygen toxicity, but it increases the chance of pneumothorax and decreases cardiac output, particularly at higher pressures. High humidity of inspired gases and frequent tracheobronchial toilet are necessary. Initially, control of bronchospasm with bronchodilators such as aminophylline, isoproterenol, or terbutaline may be beneficial, although these drugs have tocolytic properties that can be associated with postpartum uterine bleeding. The time of extubation should be governed by pulmonary function studies, arterial blood gas determinations, and the patient's clinical picture. Chapman (78) recommended a 15-min trial of spontaneous respiration before extubation when (a) a PaO$_2$ of greater than 60 torr is maintained on 30% inspired oxygen, (b) there is no evidence of a respiratory acidosis, (c) the vital capacity is greater than 15 ml/kg, (d) the inspiratory force is more than 20 cm H$_2$O, and (e) the PA-aO$_2$ is less than 300 torr on 100% oxygen.

Pulmonary Edema

The development of pulmonary edema is an ominous sign. Therapy includes sedation, tracheal suction, high oxygen administration, and positive pressure ventilation with the possible addition of PEEP. Because the plasma volume is low and cardiac failure is rare (72, 73, 76, 77), rotating tourniquets and administering digitalis and diuretics are not usually indicated. By the same token overhydration with crystalloid may add to the fluid outpouring across the damaged alveolar-capillary membrane. In the past, recommendations have been made for the use of colloid and/or furosemide (72, 76). Geer and co-workers (99) studied the effect of furosemide and 25% albumin, both alone and in combination, in rabbits subjected to a controlled nonfatal acid aspiration. Lung water, extravascular lung albumin, and PA-aO$_2$ were significantly decreased (improved) with the combination but were not changed or were increased (made worse) with the use of either furosemide or albumin alone. The use of fluids, albumin, and diuretics should be monitored with at least a CVP, but a pulmonary artery wedge pressure is more reliable because the CVP may not reflect the normally increased pulmonary artery pressure (78).

Studies by Broe et al. (100) found that the magnitude of lung injury response is in part a function of rising pulmonary artery pressures. Infusion of pulmonary vasodilators (e.g., isoproterenol, nitroprusside) resulted in a significant decrease in lung injury response as reflected in less lung weight gain and pulmonary shunting (101). Kobayashi (102) and Lamm (103) have reported improved survival in rabbits that were lavage-treated with artificial surfactant after hy-

drochloric acid aspiration. Its use in humans has not been reported to our knowledge.

Steroid Therapy

The routine use of steroids following gastric aspiration remains controversial. Many authorities now discourage steroid administration following gastric aspiration, reporting that it has no benefit for treatment (66, 72, 80). Steroids have been shown in animals (86, 87, 104–107) and humans (66) to (a) have no beneficial short-term effect on mortality, (b) interfere with the healing process, (c) increase morbidity due to Gram-negative and anaerobic pneumonias, and (d) provide no improvement in oxygenation, prevention of pulmonary edema, radiologic resolution, and length of hospital stay. Nevertheless, some authorities advocate steroid therapy in the management of Mendelson's syndrome based on favorable reports of its efficacy after aspiration (76, 108–111). Dudley and Marshall (112) showed that very small doses of dexamethasone (0.08 mg/kg) produced the greatest decrease in lung water in animals aspirating hydrochloric acid (pH 1.5), although this has been recently challenged by Wynn and co-workers (87). If used, steroids should be started early and administered in physiologic doses—for example, hydrocortisone, 200 mg intravenously immediately and 100 mg intramuscularly or intravenously every 6 hr until clearing on the chest x-ray is seen. The steroid chosen does not appear to be critical, as long as equivalent doses are used. Inhaled steroids are not considered effective therapy (113).

Antibiotic Therapy

Immediate treatment with broad-spectrum antibiotics following pulmonary acid aspiration has been suggested as a prophylaxis against infection, particularly when steroids are used (67, 109). Prophylactic antibiotics were widely used in the past. Most clinicians today oppose initiation of prophylactic antibiotic therapy at the time of acid aspiration (66, 77, 78, 80, 114). Lewis et al. (72) showed that sputum cultures were negative in 12 of 15 patients at the time of initial aspiration. With prophylactic antibiotics, 13 of 15 patients developed positive cultures with resistant organisms. If the material aspirated is grossly contaminated, initial antibiotics may be indicated. Otherwise, regular cultures should be taken of the tracheal aspirate for Gram stain, culture, and sensitivity. Appropriate antibiotics can then be rationally started on the basis of this information.

PREVENTION OF PULMONARY ASPIRATION IN THE OBSTETRIC PATIENT

"That which cannot be easily treated had better be prevented." These words by the British anaesthetist J. Alfred Lee summarize well the circumstances that surround pulmonary aspiration in the parturient. The first and most important step in the prevention of pulmonary aspiration is the recognition that every parturient is at risk for this catastrophe. Since pulmonary aspiration is usually associated with the use of general anesthesia, many claim general anesthesia is best avoided in the obstetric patient. Such a rigid policy not only denies the use of general anesthesia when it is indicated, but in addition gives no guarantee that aspiration will not occur. Nevertheless, the routine use of general anesthesia in obstetrics is best replaced by other forms of analgesia that preserve maternal consciousness. Clearly these forms of analgesia are not without risk of aspiration. Heavy maternal sedation with systemic narcotics, tranquilizers, and sedatives may obtund the airway reflexes. Narcotics are associated with nausea and vomiting. Regional anesthesia can lead to (a) local anesthetic toxicity with convulsions, followed by central nervous system depression; (b) hypotension from sympathetic block compounded by aortocaval compression, also causing central nervous system depression; and (c) abdominal and intercostal muscle weakness, depressing the ability of the patient to cough and clear the airway. Inhalation analgesia, although it avoids neonatal depression and maintains upper airway reflexes, may accidentally advance to the stage of airway obstruction and airway reflex obtundation. The anesthetist must be aware that the patient may vomit, and if the mask is not removed and the mouth suctioned, the vomitus can be inhaled. In reality all parturients in labor, especially those who receive any form of pharmacologic analgesia, require continuous monitoring and observation by qualified medical personnel if the disaster of aspiration is to be avoided.

General Anesthesia

When general anesthesia is required for the obstetric patient, her airway must be protected with a cuffed endotracheal tube expertly placed either immediately after consciousness is lost or, less commonly, before induction. Although a intravenous rapid-sequence induction is usually employed, inhalation induction is not absolutely contraindicated.

The authors take strong exception to the belief that general anesthesia in the parturient without intubation may be safer than with intubation, particularly in the hands of an inexperienced or untrained anesthetist. Such inexperienced people should never give general anesthesia to any patient, much less to the parturient, who is at high risk for this life-threatening catastrophe. It is rare that general anesthesia is required for vaginal delivery. Even difficult forceps deliveries can usually be accomplished with a pudendal block supplemented by inhalation analgesia. If general anesthesia is required, it is in the mother's best interest to delay delivery until a competent anesthetist or anesthesiologist is available, just as this would be demanded for the surgical patient. General anesthesia for the parturient without intubation, except under the most unusual circumstances, is not acceptable practice. A rapid intravenous induction of anesthesia with thiopental and succinylcholine, followed by immediate intubation of the trachea (as described in Chapters 11 and 12), is recommended.

To successfully accomplish a safe induction, the anesthetist requires at least one trained assistant to administer intravenous drugs, to apply cricoid pressure, and to stand by with suction should regurgitation of gastric contents occur. A rapid-sequence induction technique must not be used if the anesthetist has any doubt concerning his or her ability to rapidly intubate the patient's trachea. Although awake intubation before the induction of anesthesia may in theory seem ideal, it is impractical in most parturients because it is time consuming, is associated with trauma and bleeding in the parturient due to upper airway edema, and is unpleasant to both the mother and anesthetist. On the other hand, awake intubation by direct visualization after topical anesthesia, fiberoptic bronchoscopy, or the blind nasal route following adequate shrinking of the nasal mucosa is recommended in any patient in whom difficult laryngoscopy and intubation is anticipated—that is, in those with morbid obesity, hypoplastic mandible, limited range of neck motion, limited temporomandibular joint mobility, and the like.

Position During Induction

The authors do not recommend the use of any form of a "head-up tilt" position as suggested by some authors (115–117) because it renders laryngoscopy and intubation more difficult. The head-up position increases the danger of hypotension, and pulmonary aspiration is more likely should vomiting occur just before muscle relaxation takes place. The patient is placed in the supine position on the delivery table and the right hip is elevated 10 to 12 cm with folded sheets, a foam wedge, or inflatable bag or the table is tipped 15 degrees to the left to minimize aortocaval compression. The head should be supported on a small pillow in the "sniffing" position and not be in full extension, such as used for bronchoscopy. The sniffing position will give better visualization during laryngoscopy and will facilitate intubation.

Prevention of Fasciculations

The depolarizing muscle relaxant succinylcholine causes generalized muscle fasciculations and an im-

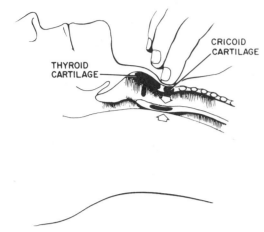

Figure 23.6. The technique of posterior pressure on the cricoid cartilage to occlude the esophagus can be effective in blocking regurgitation but not active vomiting. (Modified from Hamelberg W, Bosomworth PB: *Aspiration Pneumonitis*. Charles C Thomas, Springfield, IL, 1968.)

mediate rise in intragastric pressure (118–120). Pretreatment with a small dose of a nondepolarizing muscle relaxant, such as curare (3 mg), will prevent the fasciculations and associated rise in intragastric pressure, thereby reducing the risk of passive regurgitation. Precurarization also avoids fasciculation-induced increases in maternal oxygen consumption prior to intubation, a potential benefit in the parturient with a decreased oxygen reserve (121). However, the use of a nondepolarizing relaxant to prevent fasciculations results in a longer latency period and requires a larger dose of succinylcholine to ensure adequate relaxation for laryngoscopy and intubation. The effects of fasciculations on lower esophageal sphincter tone and the possibility that fasciculations may actually prevent passive regurgitation are discussed in Chapter 12.

Cricoid Pressure (Sellick's Maneuver)

Pressing the cricoid cartilage dorsally and cephalad against the body of the sixth cervical vertebra will occlude the esophagus and prevent passive regurgitation of stomach contents during intubation (Fig. 23.6) (122). Cricoid pressure has been shown to be effective in preventing reflux of gastric contents into the posterior pharynx with gastric pressures as high as 50 to 94 (mean 74) cm H_2O (123). Potential hazards of the maneuver are excessive pressures with possible trauma to the larynx and lateral displacement of the larynx making intubation more difficult. When cricoid pressure is applied, support of the neck (usually with the operator's other hand) is essential to prevent flexion of the head and neck, which may render laryngoscopy and laryngeal visualization impossible (Figs. 23.7 and 23.8). Training is essential to properly execute cricoid

pressure. An assistant can be easily trained by applying cricoid pressure to himself or herself while he or she attempts to swallow a mouthful of water. Adequate cricoid pressure is applied when the trainee finds swallowing impossible (M. Rosen, M.B., Ch.B., F.R.C.A., personal communication).

The Relationship Between the Difficult Airway and Aspiration

A growing body of evidence points to general anesthesia as the greatest risk factor contributing to maternal anesthetic death (124–129) and to failed intubation and inability to control the airway as highly associated with the catastrophe of gastric content aspiration (124, 130). In Sweden between 1971 and 1980, 12 of 13 maternal deaths were associated with emergency cesarean section (131). The anesthesiologist must be prepared to avoid or manage the failed intubation. There are a number of suggested approaches. These include avoidance of general anesthesia whenever possible in the obstetric patient. This is highly desirable, especially in the high-risk parturient in whom a continuous lumbar epidural block is initiated early and continued throughout labor. Most obstetric emergencies requiring rapid initiation of anesthesia can be managed with an expeditiously placed subarachnoid block if a functioning continuous epidural is not in place. At the University of Pennsylvania Medical Center in a large percentage of high-risk parturients, less than 5% of those having cesarean sections receive general anesthesia and less than 0.1% of those having vaginal deliveries are administered general anesthesia.

However, when an obstetric emergency is of such urgency as to prohibit any delay required for regional block or if conduction analgesia itself is strongly contraindicated, a rapid-sequence induction to general oral tracheal anesthesia is indicated, unless there are conditions that would make intubation difficult. Awake intubation must be increasingly considered as an important alternative to "crash" induction or a failed regional block. Pregnancy appears to increase the risk for failed intubation. A recent series reported 1 failed intubation in 283 women (132), whereas there were only 6 failures in 13,380 nonpregnant patients receiving general anesthesia (133). A combination of several recent studies suggests that the incidence of failed intubation in obstetrics is as high as 1 in 500 anesthetics (Table 23.5).

PREVENTION OF DIFFICULT AIRWAY COMPLICATIONS

Regardless of the urgency of the situation, a thorough airway evaluation is done! It rarely requires more than a minute. Signs of potentially difficult

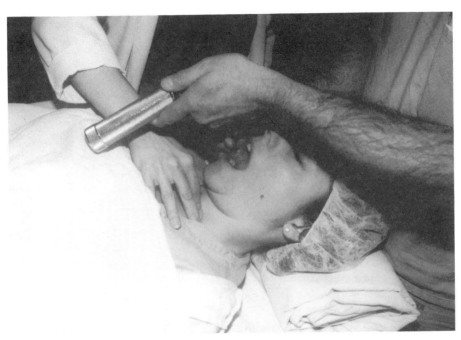

Figure 23.7. Cricoid pressure applied without neck support causes flexion of chin and hinders insertion of laryngoscope and visualization of retropharynx.

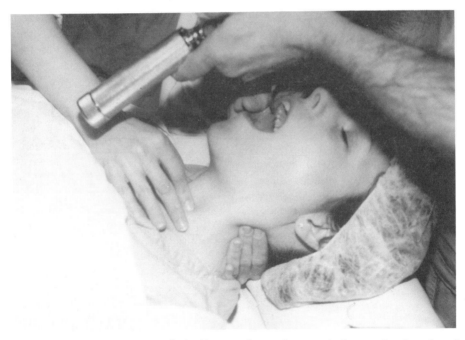

Figure 23.8. Cricoid pressure applied with posterior neck support allows extension of neck and promotes easier insertion of laryngoscope and visualization of retropharynx.

intubation include: short bull neck, small mouth that cannot open at least two fingerbreadths between teeth, protruding or partially missing upper incisors, limited neck extension, receding or protruding chin, high anterior larynx (<3 fingerbreaths between mentum and Adam's apple), large floppy tongue, inability of examiner to see tip of uvula or posterior pharynx (134), inability of patient to touch chin with tongue (gives a good view of posterior pharynx) (135), a history of diabetes (136), or a previous history of difficult glottic visualization (132). It is also important on physical examination to remember those conditions associated with laryngeal and upper airway edema, including pregnancy, pregnancy-induced hy-

Table 23.5
Difficult Airway in Obstetrics (Estimates)[a]

Author	Incidence of Failed Intubation
Lyons (1985) (212)	1/291
Lyons and MacDonald (1985) (213)	1/2,130
Cormack and Lehane (1984) (214)	1/283
Overall obstetric average	1/500
Surgical: Samsoon and Young (1987) (132)	1/2,230 (6/13,380)

[a] Adapted with permission from James CF: Maternal mortality. Semin Anesth 11:76–82, 1992.

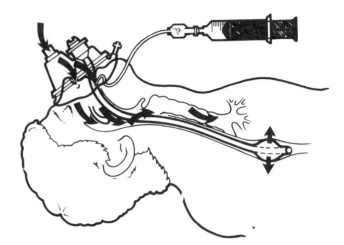

Figure 23.9. Esophageal Gastric Tube Airway in place. (Used with permission from: Tunstall ME, Geddes C: Failed intubation in obstetric anaesthesia. An indication for the use of the 'esophageal gastric tube airway'. Br J Anaesth 56:659–661, 1984.)

pertension, tocolytic drugs and tocolysis, overhydration, and trauma, such as repeated attempts at intubation. If it appears that intubation will be difficult, a rapid-sequence induction should be avoided. Our first choice is major conduction analgesia, subarachnoid block, or lumbar epidural. Surgery is not allowed until adequacy of the block is assured. If regional block is contraindicated or extremely difficult, awake intubation is planned. This is accomplished with a combination of mild sedation and topicalization of the airway. Shrinkage of the edematous upper airway may also be required by adding a vasoconstrictor such as phenylephrine or oxymetazoline to the topical local anesthetic solution. Unfortunately, the use of such topical vasoconstrictors may increase the mother's blood pressure. We believe this approach will facilitate control of the airway with less chance of vomiting and aspiration than in the unsedated uncooperative patient. The methods for acceptable airway control by awake intubation include: direct visualization with a laryngoscope; fiberoptic oral bronchoscopy (137); blind awake nasal intubation only after adequate membrane shrinkage with lidocaine and phenylephrine; or a retrograde catheter though the larynx as a guide to the tracheal tube. Regardless of the urgency of the situation from the fetal standpoint, the welfare of the mother must take priority. Preparation for the induction of general anesthesia should include: placing the patient's head in "sniffing" position; presence of a skilled and reliable assistant; adequate and functioning anesthetic equipment and supplies; patient preoxygenation (at least four deep breaths of 100% oxygen at high flow); adequate relaxation with succinylcholine 1.5 mg/kg (100 mg minimum); proper cricoid pressure; antacid prophylaxis; and a plan if failure to intubate becomes a reality.

UNABLE TO INTUBATE

When unable to intubate a patient, the first rule is not to panic: One can almost always oxygenate the patient until recovery. Do not repeatedly try to intubate. Continued attempts will cause trauma and further decrease the chance of successful intubation or airway maintenance. Maintain cricoid pressure; perform a triple airway maneuver (138); use an oral airway; and attempt gentle ventilation, which in most cases will allow adequate exchange. Although the obstetric patient is at great risk for aspiration, one must not get "hung up" on the need to intubate when this is difficult or impossible. If cricoid pressure is maintained and a clear airway can be maintained, aspiration is unlikely, particularly if the patient is breathing on her own in stage III of general anesthesia. We suggest that surgery not begin until successful tracheal intubation has been verified. In the vast majority of nonemergent cases, the mother is allowed to recover and an alternate induction plan undertaken. In cases in which fetal distress is present and the airway is clear and easily maintained, the safest course may be to continue with mask anesthesia in a well anesthetized patient. In the very rare case where ventilation is not possible, there is no choice but to recover the patient. If this does not occur before hypoxia develops, either the use of an esophageal gastric tube airway (EGTA) (Fig. 23.9) (139, 140) or a method of trans-tracheal ventilation must be available and used until the patient regains consciousness (141). It has been suggested that the use of a laryngeal mask airway in the presence of difficult intubation may reduce the incidence of aspiration, not because it directly protects against regurgitated contents but because it facilitates maintenance of the airway: the lack of which is an important precursor to aspiration (Fig. 23.10) (142). In addition, a fiber-

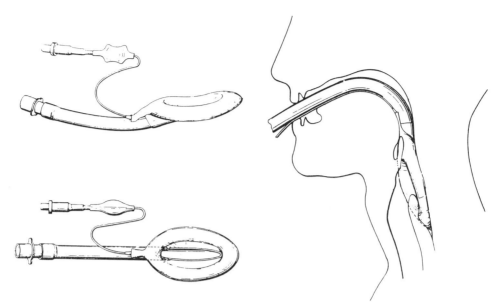

Figure 23.10. View of Laryngeal Airway and Airway in Place. (Used with permission from: Brain AIJ: The laryngeal mask— A new concept in airway management. Br J Anaesth 55:801–805, 1983.)

optic-guided, small (5.0 O.D.) endotracheal tube can be advanced through a #4 laryngeal mask airway. It is well advised to have and rehearse a failed intubation plan such as the one described by Tunstall (Table 23.6) (143, 144).

Awake Extubation

After emergence from anesthesia the endotracheal tube must be left in place until the patient is awake, is completely responsive to commands, and has no signs of muscle weakness. The patient should be placed in the lateral head-down (Trendelenburg) position. The mouth and posterior pharynx are suctioned. Extubation should take place with the patient breathing 100% oxygen. The lungs are inflated, and during inflation, the cuff is deflated and the tube immediately removed. Deflation of the cuff and removal of the tube during positive pressure inflation of the lungs will tend to blow material that may have collected above the cuff up and out of the trachea. In the supine position some patients, even when fully reactive, will be unable to protect their airway from vomited or regurgitated gastric contents. Therefore we recommend placing the patient on her side during and following extubation.

ISSUES IN ASPIRATION PNEUMONITIS PROPHYLAXIS

Several forms of prophylaxis against pulmonary pneumonitis aspiration have been advocated, but these are at best of limited value and may not be relied upon to prevent aspiration pneumonitis.

Oral Antacid Therapy

After Taylor and Pryse-Davies (25) first showed the efficacy of oral magnesium trisilicate BPC to increase the gastric pH above 2.5, it became a widespread practice to administer suspensions of insoluble oral antacids every 3 to 4 hr in 15- to 30-ml doses to laboring women (88). Fortunately this practice, widely recommended in the 1970s, has been abandoned (145). Aspiration of insoluble antacids may result in severe and persistent lung pathologic conditions, as described earlier in this chapter. An alternative oral antacid, 0.3 M sodium citrate, was first recommended by Lahiri and co-workers (146), who found that 15 ml resulted in a very rapid neutralization of stomach contents. Gibbs and co-workers (147) showed that aspiration of sodium citrate in dogs produced a pulmonary histologic lesion that was much less severe and resolved within a month, as compared with those lesions produced by aspiration of equal volumes of emulsion antacids or acid. Arterial blood gas impairment and shunting, although present after aspiration of sodium citrate, are not as severe as compared with that with acid aspiration (148). Thirty milliliters of 0.3 M sodium citrate is capable of neutralizing up to 255 ml of hydrochloric acid with a pH of 1 (149). Neutralization of gastric acid by sodium citrate has been reported to last 40 min to 1 hr (149–153). The time required for this elevation is usually less than 5 min as compared with 30 min for the insoluble antacids.

Sodium citrate is available commercially in buffered solutions such as Polycitra, flavored Bicitra (a buffer of sodium citrate and citric acid) (Willens)

Table 23.6
Failed Intubation Protocol of Tunstall

1. Maintain cricoid pressure, avoid aortocaval compression.
2. Place patient in complete lateral position with help from obstetrician. If changing position is not possible use esophageal gastric tube airway (EGTA) and go to step #9.
3. Tilt table head down.
4. Suction larynx as required.
5. Apply IPPB—100% O_2 with face mask. Close respiratory valve and use "face mask leak."
6. Maintain airway with "triple airway maneuver," have assistant squeeze bag or use ventilator.
7. If obstruction remains, try various airways, try releasing cricoid pressure, but only if patient is in head down lateral position.
8. If airway obstruction still exists but there are signs of returning ventilation, persist with IPPB until recovery. If no recovery, use EGTA with 100% O_2.
9. If clear airway exists, in a serious emergency consider allowing surgery to start and go to spontaneous respiration.
10. If oxygenation is not possible, puncture cricoid thyroid membrane and ventilate.

Shortened Protocol
1. Call for help.
2. Maintain cricoid pressure.
3. Left lateral position.
4. Head down tilt.
5. Bag and mask 100% oxygen.
6. If necessary improve airway with
   a) triple airway maneuver
   b) release cricoid pressure
   c) EGTA
7. Airway?
   If clear—classical mask and airway anesthesia if true emergency.
   If partially obstructed—allow to recover.
   If total obstruction—transtracheal ventilation.

(154), and Alka Seltzer Effervescent "Gold" (155). These compounds have been found to be as effective as pure sodium citrate (156). The limitations of sodium citrate include systemic absorption and metabolic alkalosis after multiple doses, a laxative effect, and disagreeable taste requiring the addition of flavoring, which may decrease its effectiveness. Gillett and co-workers (157) found that 17% of both elective and emergency cesarean section patients still had a gastric pH <3 after receiving 30 ml of oral 0.3 M sodium citrate. These findings may be explained by the excessive gastric volume or inadequate gastric mixing that is more prone to occur in the pregnant patient (158).

The properties of rapid mixing, effective neutralization of gastric acid, and lack of pulmonary damage if aspirated make sodium citrate 0.3 M (30 ml) the preferred antacid to give before induction of general

anesthesia in the obstetric patient. Its absorption from the gastrointestinal tract and its unpleasant taste contradicts its routine use in every obstetric patient throughout labor. We have abandoned routine oral antacid prophylaxis in all obstetric patients and give only sodium citrate (15 min prior to induction) to those obstetric patients who are to undergo **general** anesthesia in elective cases and immediately upon learning general anesthesia will be required in emergency cases. Others, including the editors, administer antacid to **all** patients having a cesarean section.

Although some authors recommend oral sodium bicarbonate as an effective antacid (159), others have found that 20 ml of 8.4% sodium bicarbonate is not completely effective as a sole preanesthetic antacid (160). Sodium bicarbonate (20 ml) will also release about 0.4 liters intragastric gas (7), which may distend the stomach and increase the risk of regurgitation. Although helpful, antacid prophylaxis is not a panacea and will not protect all obstetric patients. It will not prevent the aspiration of solid or bacterially contaminated material. It produces a false sense of security. In addition it may not effectively neutralize gastric material when large volumes are present (70).

H_2-Receptor Antagonists

Pharmacologic suppression of gastric acid production by histamine receptor inhibition as a form of aspiration prophylaxis in obstetrics was first studied by Pickering and co-workers (161). Thorough reviews of H_2-receptor antagonists in anesthesia are available (162, 163). Both cimetidine and ranitidine, when given orally the night before surgery and again 1 to 2 hr before anesthesia induction, are effective in reliably elevating gastric pH above 2.5 in most but not all parturients (164, 165). When these drugs are combined with metoclopramide, gastric volume is consistently less than 25 ml (166, 167).

When given just before emergency general anesthesia, the H_2 blockers are not effective in rapidly elevating gastric pH. However, giving the H_2 blocker intramuscularly or intravenously along with 30 ml of oral 0.3 M sodium citrate has been shown to reliably maintain the gastric pH above 2.5 for much longer than citrate alone. From studies evaluating neonatal neurobehavior, the acute use of the H_2 blockers does not appear to have any ill effects on the newborn (164). Likewise, the occasional CNS side effects seen in patients receiving chronic cimetidine are not seen in mothers after short-term administration. Rarely, the rapid intravenous use of both cimetidine and ranitidine may be associated with cardiovascular depression or arrhythmia (168–170), which is not seen when these drugs are given orally or by intramuscular injection. The administration of both cimetidine and ranitidine have been reported to alter hepatic metabolic activity and to prolong the metabolism and elevate the blood levels of a number of drugs by inhibiting P450 oxidation and redistribution. These drugs include amide local anesthetics, anticoagulants, propranolol, benzodiazepines, and theophylline (171–173). Recently, investigators have questioned these earlier reports as they have found preoperative H_2 blockers have little or no effect on drug disposition in pregnancy (174–177). In the presence of H_2 blockers, the above drugs are given with the awareness that the recommended therapeutic doses may be excessive and may produce more side effects. Suspension of oral antacids has been shown to inhibit the bioavailability of both cimetidine and ranitidine (178). Earlier reports that H_2 blockers inhibited anticholinesterase activity (179) are not clinically relevant. H_2 inhibitors have been shown not to affect the duration of neuromuscular block after depolarizing or nondepolarizing drugs (180–184).

Famotidine, an amidine derivative H_2 receptor antagonist, is reported to have negligible effects on hepatic blood flow, drug enzyme induction, and cholinesterase activity (185–187). It is also said to have no adverse hemodynamic effects (188–189). Famotidine, 20 mg (2 hr orally; 1 hr intramuscularly), prior to general anesthesia will maintain pH between 5.7 and 7.2 and gastric volume below 10 ml in nonpregnant patients (190). Comparison of new generation H_2 inhibitors have been made in parturients without revealing important individual drug advantages (191, 192). In practice, it has been suggested by some authors that all mothers in labor receive intramuscular ranitidine every 6 hr (157). This therapy appears to be effective after several hours in elevating gastric pH and lowering gastric volume. We do not subscribe to this view because (a) the vast majority of parturients will not require general anesthesia and, hence, are not at great risk for aspiration of gastric contents; (b) those requiring emergency general anesthesia can be adequately treated with 30 ml 0.3 M sodium citrate and an intravenous H_2 blocker plus metoclopramide shortly before induction; (c) the cost of routine H_2 blocker administration would be significant; and (d) there is growing evidence that the elevated pH associated with presurgical prophylactic H_2 antagonists causes increased intragastric bacterial growth (193, 194). If such material is aspirated, we may be "exchanging the aspiration of acid for the aspiration of colonized gastric contents" (195). In our opinion the risks of such prophylaxis outweigh the benefits.

In our practice, H_2 inhibitor therapy is limited to elective cesarean section under general anesthesia or to the parturient who has known gastric reflux or peptic ulcer disease. Because of their latency, H_2 blockers administered shortly before induction of anesthesia will do little to protect against acid aspiration during induction. In an obstetric emergency requiring general anesthesia, a combination of an H_2 inhibitor, metoclopramide, and sodium citrate prior to induction may be a sensible choice. Short-term protection is provided by sodium citrate, and longer term protection is afforded by cimetidine against aspiration during emergence if gastric contents are removed intraoperatively with an oral-gastric tube (108).

Emptying the Stomach

The dopamine antagonists, characterized by metoclopramide, have come into clinical use. These increase gastroesophageal sphincter pressure and are effective antiemetics (37, 56, 60–62, 197). Although these drugs do not block gastric acid secretion, they inhibit dopaminergic receptors, thus promoting gastric emptying and decreasing gastric volume in normal patients and in patients undergoing cesarean section (198). It appears these drugs act on postganglionic nerves intrinsic to the wall of the intestinal tract, thereby releasing acetylcholine, which promotes peristalsis and increases lower esophageal sphincter tone. Centrally, metoclopramide blocks dopamine receptors and induces secretion of prolactin. Metoclopramide (10 mg), a derivative of procaine, increases stomach emptying over a 40- to 60-min period. Wyner and Cohen (199) studied gastric volumes in early pregnancy and found that gravidas receiving 10 mg of metoclopramide 15 to .30 min before anesthesia had significantly lower gastric volumes (15 versus 28 ml) and fewer volumes exceeding 25 ml (13 versus 51%) than did controls. Unfortunately, the effectiveness of metoclopramide in increasing gastroesophageal sphincter tone is decreased by anticholinergics such as glycopyrrolate. Despite narcotic antagonism to the gastric emptying effects of metoclopramide, recent studies have shown the drug still to have considerable efficacy in decreasing the gastric volume in laboring patients who have received narcotics (198–200). Metoclopramide crosses the blood-brain barrier and the placenta (201). As a dopamine antagonist, metoclopramide is unlikely to produce sedation. However, in high doses it can produce extrapyramidal effects (which respond readily to diphenhydramine) and perhaps stress-induced tachycardia (202). Some authors have found that metoclopramide (10 mg) may exert a small but clinically insignificant inhibitory effect on pseudocholinesterase (203). Combined with an H_2 blocker, the dopamine antagonists reliably elevate gastric pH above 2.5 and lower gastric volume below 25 ml in normal nonpregnant patients undergoing elective surgery (166, 167). The usual dose of metoclopram-

Table 23.7
Ranitidine, Na Citrate, and Gastric Status in Obstetrics[a]

Group	Gastric Vol		Gastric pH			
	Mean	Range	>25	Mean	Range	<2.5
1—Elective, ranitidine 150 po and 50 IM (20)	9 ± 7.2	0–23	0	6.5 ± 0.8	4.5–7.7	0
2—In labor, ranitidine 150 po and 50 IM q 6 hr (30)	31 ± 27	0–127	14	5.3 ± 2.1	1.8–7.7	5
3—In labor, ranitidine (50 IM and 50 IM q 6 hr and Na citrate (15 or 30 ml) po (30)	43 ± 38	4–150	9	6.0 ± 1.0	3.9–7.4	0
4—In labor Na citrate (15–30 ml) po; no ranitidine (30)	123 ± 98	10–450	29	5.3 ± 1.1	1.8–7.6	1

[a] Reprinted with permission from Colman RD, Frank M, Loughnan BA, Cohen DG, Cattermole R: Use of i.m. ranitidine for the prophylaxis of aspiration pneumonitis in obstetrics. Br J Anaesth 61:720–729, 1988.

Table 23.8
Effective Means of Preventing Pulmonary Aspiration

I. Avoid oversedation.
II. Avoid excessive depth during inhalation analgesia.
III. Avoid significant hypotension.
IV. Avoid local anesthetic toxicity.
V. Maintain proper general anesthesia technique:
   A. Trained assistant on induction of anesthesia
   B. Defasciculation with curare (3 mg IV)
   C. Cricoid pressure from loss of consciousness until successful intubation
   D. Rapid production of relaxation with succinylcholine 1.5 mg/kg IV
   E. Extubation only when patient completely reversed, responsive, and in lateral position
   F. Intubation of all obstetric patients beyond the first trimester of pregnancy who receive general anesthesia
VI. Continuously observe all obstetric patients receiving analgesia or anesthesia, including postpartum.
VII. Assume that all women beyond the first trimester and for several days postpartum are at risk for gastric content aspiration.

ide is 10 mg (po or IM) about 1 hr prior to the induction of anesthesia. In an emergency, 10 mg IV injected slowly will have an effect within 1 to 3 min.

Domperidone, also a dopamine antagonist, is an effective antiemetic but does not pass the blood-brain barrier; thus it does not subject the patient to extrapyramidal effects. However, it can reach the chemoreceptor trigger zone. Theoretically, domperidone (0.2 mg/kg) should function as an effective gastric emptier (55). Domperidone, unlike metoclopramide, is effective in antagonizing the relaxant effect of atropine on the lower esophageal sphincter and maintains its gastric emptying properties following narcotic administration (64). The performance of dom-

peridone in pregnancy and labor has not yet been thoroughly studied. Acute usage of dopamine antagonists prior to cesarean section has not produced adverse effects in either mother or newborn.

The use of emetics (i.e., apomorphine) or nasogastric tubes will not guarantee an empty stomach. The duration of apomorphine's emetic effect is unpredictable; it may continue into the induction period. If the stomach is distended, which is rare in the parturient, it may be decompressed by a orogastric tube before extubation.

Combination Antacid Prophylaxis

In recent years, most anesthestists have adopted a variation of H_2 receptor antagonist, dopamine receptor inhibitor and clear oral liquid antacid, such as that earlier recommended by Moir (204). Although there is disagreement regarding the most effective combination (205–209) and the arbitrary use of cutoff values for pH and volume (5, 6), a majority of surveyed anesthetists use some combination of the above (Table 23.7) (145).

Anticholinergic Therapy

It has been suggested that the use of anticholinergics (atropine, scopolamine, glycopyrrolate) protect against acid aspiration by decreasing the volume of gastric secretions and decreasing the amount of gastric acid secreted. Human studies have failed to demonstrate the effectiveness of anticholinergics in decreasing either the acidity or volume of gastric contents (29, 106, 210). An undesirable anticholinergic side effect is the decrease in lower esophageal sphincter resting tone, which could increase the incidence of gastric reflux in an already high-risk population (56, 58). Anticholinergic therapy is not recommended for routine preoperative use during pregnancy and should be reserved for specific medical or anesthetic indications.

CONCLUSION

Pulmonary aspiration of stomach contents remains a leading cause of maternal morbidity and mortality. Most cases of aspiration in the parturient are preventable by careful observation and expert anesthesia care during labor and delivery (Table 23.8 and Appendix). All parturients must be assumed to have a full stomach. Avoidance of general anesthesia, oversedation, and hypotension will do much to eliminate pulmonary aspiration. When general anesthesia is required, a skilled anesthetist and a trained assistant are required. Should pulmonary aspiration occur, prompt and proper therapy with continuous monitoring is required and is best accomplished in an intensive care situation if high mortality is to be avoided. The parturient requires and deserves the same degree of competence in anesthesia as the patient undergoing emergency surgery. It is well known that, until the last confidential maternal mortality reports, anesthesia was the third most common cause of maternal death (48). On a positive note, it is observed that the number of anesthetic deaths in relation to the number of anesthetics given is a far more important number (129). If one considers the threefold increase of cesarean section and the millions of legal abortions performed in the last 20 years, then in Morgan's words, "there has been an *enormous* reduction in anesthetic related maternal mortality, of which obstetric anesthetists, and pioneers in the field in particular can be justly proud" (211). We believe that the struggle to reduce the incidence of maternal mortality from aspiration to zero must continue.

References

1. Tindall VR, Beard RW, Sykes MK, Tighe JR, Hibbard BM, Rosen M, Knight BH, Gordon G, McClure JH, Cameron HM, Pinkerton JHM, Moore J, Toner PG: *Confidential Enquiries into Maternal Deaths in the United Kingdom, 1985–1987.* Her Majesty's Stationery Office, London 1991.
2. Olsson GL, Hallen B, Hambraeus-Jonzon K: Aspiration during anaesthesia: A computer-aided study of 185,358 anaesthetics. Acta Anaesth Scand 30:84–92, 1986.
3. Merrill RB, Hingson RA: Studies of the incidence of maternal mortality from the aspiration of vomitus during anesthesia occurring in major obstetric hospitals in the United States. Anesth Analg 30:121–135, 1951.
4. Conklin K: Maternal physiological adaptations during gestation, labor and the puerperium. Semin Anesth 10:221–234, 1991.
5. Gorback MS: Cut-off values and aspiration risk [letter]. Anesth Analg 69:417, 1989.
6. Gorback MS: What we still don't know about the risk of aspiration. Curr Rev Clin Anesth 11:215–219, 1991.
7. Gutsche BB, Domurat MF, Marx G, Crawford JS, Moir DD, Cheek TG, Gibbs CP, Hodgkinson R: Should parturients in labor receive prophylaxis to elevate gastric pH and decrease

gastric volume? The Expert's Opine. Surv Anesth 29:196–198, 1986.
8. Gibbs CP, Rolbin SH, Norman P: Cause and prevention of maternal aspiration. Anesthesiology 61:111–112, 1984.
9. Crawford JS, Oppit LJ: A survey of anesthetic services to obstetrics in the Birmingham Hospital. Reg Anesth 31:56–59, 1976.
10. Hutchinson BR, Newson AJ: Preoperative neutralization of gastric acidity. Anaesth Intensive Care 3:198–203, 1975.
11. Simpson KH, Stakes AF, Miller M: Pregnancy delays paracetamol absorption and gastric emptying in patients undergoing surgery. Br J Anaesth 60:24–27, 1988.
12. Csapo A: Progesterone block. Am J Anat 98:273–291, 1956.
13. Christofides ND, Ghatei MA, Bloom SR, Barbog C, Gillmer MDG: Decreased plasma motilin concentrations in pregnancy. Br Med J 285:1453–1454, 1982.
14. O'Sullivan GM, Sutton AJ, Thompson SA, Carrie LE, Bullingham RE: Noninvasive measurement of gastric emptying in obstetric patients. Anesth Analg 66:505–511, 1987.
15. Davison JS, Davison MC, Hay DM: Gastric emptying time in late pregnancy and labour. J Obstet Gynaecol Br Commonw 77:37–41, 1970.
16. Simpson KH, Stakes AF: Effect of anxiety on gastric emptying in preoperative patients. Br J Anaesth 59:540–544, 1987.
17. LaSalvia LA, Steffen EA: Delayed gastric emptying time in labor. Am J Obstet Gynecol 59:1075–1081, 1950.
18. Nimmo WS, Wilson J, Prescott LF: Narcotic analgesics and delayed gastric emptying during labour. Lancet 1:890–893, 1975.
19. O'Sullivan GM, Bullingham RE: Noninvasive assessment by radiotelemetry of antacid effect during labor. Anesth Analg 64:95–100, 1985.
20. Nimmo WS, Wilson J, Prescott LF: Narcotic analgesics and delayed gastric emptying during labour. Lancet 1:890–893, 1975.
21. Wilson J: Gastric emptying in labour: Some recent findings and their clinical significance. J Int Med Res 6(suppl):54–62, 1978.
22. Holdsworth JD: Relationship between stomach contents and analgesia in labour. Br J Anaesth 50:1145–1148, 1978.
23. Creasy RK: Preterm parturition. Semin Perinatol 3:191–302, 1981.
24. O'Sullivan GM, Bullingham RE: Noninvasive assessment by radiotelemetry of antacid effect during labor. Anesth Analg 64:95–100, 1985.
25. Murray FA, Erskine JP, Fielding J: Gastric secretion in pregnancy. J Obstet Gynaecol Br Commonw 64:373, 1957.
26. Taylor G, Pryse-Davies J: The prophylactic use of antacids in the prevention of the acid-pulmonary aspiration syndrome (Mendelson's syndrome). Lancet 1:288–291, 1966.
27. Attia RR, Ebeid AM, Fischer JE, Goudsouzian NG: Maternal, fetal and placental gastrin concentrations. Anaesthesia 37:18–21, 1982.
28. Mendelson CL: Aspiration of stomach contents into lungs during obstetric anesthesia. Am J Obstet Gynecol 52:191–205, 1946.
29. Teabeaut JR: Aspiration of gastric contents: An experimental study. Am J Pathol 28:51–67, 1952.
30. Roberts RB, Shirley MA: Reducing the risk of acid aspiration during cesarean section. Anesth Analg 53:859–868, 1974.
31. Roberts RB, Shirley MA: The obstetrician's role in reducing the risk of aspiration pneumonitis with particular reference to the use of oral antacids. Am J Obstet Gynecol 124:611–617, 1976.
32. James C, Gibbs CP, Banner T: Postpartum perioperative risk of aspiration pneumonia. Anesthesiology 61:756–759, 1984.
33. James CF, Modell JH, Gibbs CP, Kuck EJ, Ruiz BC: Pulmonary aspiration: Effects of volume and pH in the rat. Anesth Analg 63:665–668, 1984.
34. Raidoo DM, Rocke DA, Brock-Utne JG, Marszalek A, Engelbrecht HE: Critical volume for pulmonary acid aspiration: reappraisal in a primate model. Br J Anaesth 65:248–250, 1990.

35. Sundt TM, Sharbrough FW, Anderson RE, Michenfelder JD: Cerebral blood flow measurements and electroencephalograms during carotid endarterectomy. J Neurosurg 41:310–320, 1974.

36. Tinker J: Deliberate hypotension: How and when? In *ASA Refresher Course Lectures*, Lippincott, Philadelphia, 1980, pp 1–7.

37. Greenburg AG: Is the emperor really without clothes [editorial]? Crit Care Med 17:967, 1989.

38. Cheek DBC: Personal communication, 1987.

39. Marx GF, Domurat MF, Costin M: Potential hazards of hypoglycaemia in the parturient. Can J Anaesth 34:400–402, 1987.

40. Marx GF, Desai PK, Habib NS: Detection and differentiation of metabolic acidosis in parturients. Anesth Analg 59:929–931, 1980.

41. Miller M, Wishart HY, Nimmo WS: Gastric contents at induction of anaesthesia: Is a 4-hour fast necessary? Br J Anaesth 55:1185–1187, 1983.

42. Hutchinson A, Maltby JR, Reid CRG: Gastric fluid volume and pH in elective inpatients: Coffee or orange juice versus overnight fast. Can J Anaesth 35:12–15, 1988.

43. McGrady EM, MacDonald AG: Effect of the preoperative administration of water on gastric volume and pH. Br J Anaesth 60:803–805, 1988.

44. Sutherland AD, Maltby JR, Sale JP, Reid CRG: The effect of preoperative oral fluid and ranitidine on gastric fluid volume and pH. Can J Anaesth 34:117–121, 1987.

45. Lewis P, Maltby JR, Sutherland LR: Unrestricted oral fluid until three hours preoperatively: Effect on gastric fluid volume and pH. Can J Anaesth 37:S132, 1990.

46. Shevde K, Trivedi N: Effects of clear liquids on gastric volume and pH in healthy volunteers. Anesth Analg 72:528–531, 1991.

47. Lewis M, Crawford JS: Can one risk fasting the obstetric patient for less than 4 hours? Br J Anaesth 59:312–314, 1987.

48. James CF: Maternal mortality. Semin Anesth 11:76–82, 1992.

49. Hart DM: Heartburn in pregnancy. J Int Med Res 6(suppl):1–5, 1978.

50. Mixson WJ, Woloshin HJ: Hiatus hernia in pregnancy. Obstet Gynecol 8:249–260, 1956.

51. Castro L de P: Reflux esophagitis as the cause of heartburn in pregnancy. Am J Obstet Gynecol 98:1–10, 1967.

52. Vanner RG, Goodman NW: Gastro-oesophageal reflux in pregnancy at term and after delivery. Anaesthesia 44:808–811, 1989.

53. Spence AA, Moir DD, Finlay WEI: Observations on intragastric pressure. Anaesthesia 22:249–256, 1967.

54. Lind JF, Smith A, McIver DR, Coopland AT, Crispin JS: Heartburn in pregnancy: A manometric study. Can Med Assoc J 98:571–574, 1968.

55. Brock-Utne JG, Downing JW, Dimopoulos GE, Rubin J, Moshal MG: Effect of domperidone on lower esophageal sphincter tone in late pregnancy. Anesthesiology 52:321–323, 1980.

56. Brock-Utne JG, Rubin J, Downing JW, Dimopoulos CE, Moshal MG, Naicker M: The administration of metoclopramide with atropine. Anaesthesia 31:1186–1190, 1976.

57. Brock-Utne JG, Rubin J, Welman S, Dimopoulos GE, Moshal MG, Downing JW: The action of commonly used antiemetics on the lower oesophageal sphincter. Br J Anaesth 50:295–298, 1978.

58. Brock-Utne JG, Rubin J, Welman S, Dimopoulos GE, Moshal MG, Downing JW: The effect of glycopyrrolate (Robinul) on the lower oesophageal sphincter. Can Anaesth Soc J 25:144–146, 1978.

59. Hall AW, Moossa AR, Clark J, Cooley GR, Skinner DB: The effects of premedication drugs on the lower oesophageal high pressure zone and reflux status of rhesus monkeys and man. Gut 16:347–352, 1975.

60. Hey UMF, Ostick DG, Mazumder JK, Lord WD: Pethidine, metoclopramide and the gastro-esophageal sphincter: A study in healthy volunteers. Anaesthesia 36:173–176, 1981.

61. Cotton BR, Smith G: Comparison of the effects of atropine and glycopyrrolate on the lower oesophageal sphincter pressure. Br J Anaesth 53:875–879, 1981.

62. McNeill MJ, Ho ET, Kenny GNC: Effect of I.V. metoclopramide on gastric emptying after opioid premedication. Br J Anaesth 64:450–452, 1990.

63. Brock-Utne JG, Dow TGB, Welman S, Dimopoulos GE, Moshal MG: The effect of metoclopramide on lower oesophageal sphincter tone. Anaesth Intensive Care 6:26–29, 1978.

64. Brock-Utne JG: Domperidone antagonizes the relaxant effect of atropine on the lower esophageal sphincter. Anesth Analg 59:921–924, 1980.

65. Brock-Utne JG, Rusin J, Downing JW, Dimopoulos GE, Moshal MG, Naicker M: The administration of metoclopramide with atropine. Anaesthesia 31:1186–1190, 1976.

66. Bynum LJ, Pierce AK: Pulmonary aspiration of gastric contents. Am Rev Resp Dis 114:1129–1136, 1976.

67. Hamelberg W, Bosomworth PP: Aspiration pneumonitis: Experimental studies and clinical observations. Anesth Analg 43:669–677, 1964.

68. Hickling KG, Howard R: A retrospective survey of treatment and mortality in aspiration pneumonia. Intensive Care Med 14:617–622, 1988.

69. Bosomworth PP, Hamelberg W: Etiologic and therapeutic aspects of aspiration pneumonitis: Experimental study. Surg Forum 13:158–159, 1962.

70. Taylor G: Acid pulmonary aspiration syndrome after antacids: A case report. Br J Anaesth 47:615–617, 1975.

71. Morton HJV, Wylie WD: Anaesthetic deaths due to regurgitation or vomiting. Anaesthesia 6:190–205, 1951.

72. Lewis RT, Burgess JH, Hampson LG: Cardiorespiratory studies in critical illness: Changes in aspiration pneumonitis. Arch Surg 103:335–340, 1971.

73. Awe WC, Fletcher WS, Jacob SW: The pathophysiology of aspiration pneumonitis. Surgery 60:232–239, 1966.

74. Cameron JL, Mitchell WH, Zuidema GD: Aspiration pneumonia: Clinical outcome following documented aspiration. Arch Surg 106:49–52, 1973.

75. Bartlett JG, Gorbach SL: The triple threat of aspiration pneumonia. Chest 68:560–566, 1975.

76. Baggish MS, Hooper S: Aspiration as a cause of maternal death. Obstet Gynecol 43:327–336, 1974.

77. Morgan JG: Pathophysiology of gastric aspiration. Int Anesthesiol Clin 15:1–11, 1977.

78. Chapman RL: Treatment of aspiration pneumonitis. Int Anesthesiol Clin 15:85–96, 1977.

79. Kennedy TP, Johnson KJ, Kunkel RG, Ward PA, Knight PR, Finch JS: Acute acid aspiration lung injury in the rat: Biphasic pathogenesis. Anesth Analg 69:87–92, 1989.

80. Modell JH: Aspiration pneumonitis. In *ASA Refresher Course Lectures*. Lippincott, Philadelphia, 1983, pp 163–170.

81. Greenfield LJ, Singleton RP, McCaffree DR, Coalson JJ: Pulmonary effects of experimental graded aspiration of hydrochloric acid. Ann Surg 170:74–86, 1969.

82. Moran TJ: Experimental aspiration pneumonia. IV. Inflammatory and reparative changes produced by intratracheal injection of autologous gastric juice and hydrochloric acid. Arch Pathol 60:122–129, 1955.

83. Dal Santo G: Acid aspiration: Pathophysiological aspects, prevention, and therapy. Int Anesth Clin 24:31–52, 1986.

84. Bannister WK, Sattilaro AJ, Otis RD: Therapeutic aspects of aspiration pneumonitis in experimental animals. Anesthesiology 22:440–443, 1961.

85. Taylor G, Pryse-Davies J: Evaluation of endotracheal steroid therapy in acid pulmonary aspiration syndrome (Mendelson's syndrome). Anesthesiology 29:17–21, 1968.

86. Churg A: Aspiration of gastric contents. Anesthesiology 51:2–3, 1979.

87. Wynn JW, Reynolds JC, Hood DI, Auerbach D, Ondrasick J: Steroid therapy for pneumonitis induced in rabbits by aspiration of food stuff. Anesthesiology 51:11–19, 1979.

88. Crawford JS: *Principles and Practice of Obstetric Anaesthesia*. London, Blackwell, 1971, p 96.

89. Bond VR, Stoelting RK, Gupta CD: Pulmonary aspiration syndrome after inhalation of gastric contents containing antacids. Anesthesiology 51:452–453, 1979.
90. Gibbs CP, Schwartz DJ, Wynne JW, Hood CI, Ruck EJ: Antacid pulmonary aspiration in the dog. Anesthesiology 51:380–385, 1979.
91. Eyler SW, Cullen BF, Welch WD, Murphy M: Antacid aspiration in rabbits. Anesth Analg 61:183–184, 1982.
92. Tompkinson J, Turnbull A, Robson G, Cloake E, Adelstein AM, Weatherall JAC: Report on Confidential Enquiries into Maternal Deaths in England and Wales, 1973–1975. Her Majesty's Stationery Office, London, 1979, pp 79–80.
93. Heaney GAH, Jones HD: Aspiration syndromes in pregnancy. Br J Anaesth 51:266–267, 1979.
94. Whittington RM, Robinson JS, Thompson JM: Fatal aspiration (Mendelson's) syndrome despite antacids and cricoid pressure. Lancet 2:228–230, 1979.
95. Booth DJ, Zuidema GD, Cameron JL: Aspiration pneumonia: Pulmonary arteriography after experimental aspiration. J Surg Res 12:48–52, 1972.
96. Chapman RL, Modell JH, Ruiz BC, Calderwood HW, Hood CI, Graves SA: Effects of continuous positive-pressure ventilation and steroids on aspiration of hydrochloric acid (pH 1.8) in dogs. Anesth Analg 53:556–562, 1974.
97. Cameron JL, Sebor J, Anderson RP, Zuidema GD: Aspiration pneumonia: Results of treatment by positive-pressure ventilation in dogs. J Surg Res 8:447–457, 1968.
98. Roberts RB: Aspiration and its prevention in obstetric patients. Int Anesthesiol Clin 15:49–70, 1977.
99. Geer RT, Soma LR, Barnes C, Leatherman JL, Marshall BE: Effects of albumin and/or furosemide therapy on pulmonary edema induced by hydrochloric acid aspiration in rabbits. J Trauma 16:788–791, 1976.
100. Broe PJ, Toung TJK, Permutt S, Cameron JL: Aspiration pneumonia: Treatment with pulmonary vasodilators. Surgery 94:95–99, 1982.
101. Huval WV, Lelcuk S, Feingold H, Valeri CR, Shepro D, Hechtman HB: Effects of nitroprusside and ketanserin upon pulmonary edema after acid injury. Surg Gynecol Obstet 166:527–534, 1988.
102. Kobayashi T, Ganzuka M, Taniguchi J, Nitta K, Murakami S: Lung lavage and surfactant replacement for hydrochloric acid aspiration in rabbits. Acta Anaesthesiol Scand 34:216–221, 1990.
103. Lamm WJ, Albert RK: Surfactant replacement improves lung recoil in rabbit lungs after acid aspiration. Am Rev Respir Dis 142:1279–1283, 1990.
104. Giesecke AH Jr: Anesthesia for trauma surgery. In Anesthesia. RD Miller, ed. Churchill Livingston, New York, 1981, p 1253.
105. Bone RC, Fisher CJ Jr, Clemmer TP, Slotman GJ, Metz CA, Balk RA: A controlled clinical trial of high-dose methylprednisolone in the treatment of severe and septic shock. N Engl J Med 317:653–658, 1987.
106. Downs JB, Chapman RL, Modell JH, Hood CI: An evaluation of steroid therapy in aspiration pneumonitis. Anesthesiology 40:129–135, 1974.
107. Lowrey LD, Anderson M, Calhoun J, Edmonds H, Flint LM: Failure of corticosteroid therapy for experimental acid aspiration. J Surg Res 32:168–172, 1982.
108. Kennedy RL: General analgesia and anesthesia in obstetrics. Clin Obstet Gynecol 17:227–239, 1974.
109. Lawson DW, DeFalco AJ, Phelps JA: Corticosteroids as treatment for aspiration of gastric contents: An experimental study. Surgery 59:845–852, 1966.
110. Ashe JR Jr: Pulmonary aspiration: A life-threatening complication in obstetrics. NC Med J 37:655–657, 1976.
111. Sukumaran M, Granada MJ, Berger HW, Lee L, Reilly TA: Evaluation of corticosteroid treatment in aspiration of gastric contents: A controlled clinical trial. Mount Sinai J Med 47:335–340, 1980.
112. Dudley WR, Marshall BE: Steroid treatment for acid-aspiration pneumonitis. Anesthesiology 40:136–141, 1974.
113. Warriner CB, Brooks L, Pare PD: The effect of inhalation of nebulized steroid on the acid aspiration syndrome. Can Anaesth Soc J 28:436–441, 1981.
114. Murray HW: Antimicrobial therapy in pulmonary aspiration. Am J Med 66:188–190, 1979.
115. Snow RG, Nunn JF: Induction of anaesthesia in the foot down position for patients with a full stomach. Br J Anaesth 31:493–497, 1959.
116. Hodges RJH, Tunstall ME, Bennett JR: Vomiting and the head-up position. Br J Anaesth 32:619–620, 1960.
117. Stark DCC: Aspiration in the surgical patient. Int Anesthesiol Clin 15:13–48, 1977.
118. Andersen N: Changes in intragastric pressure following administration of suxamethonium: Preliminary report. Br J Anaesth 34:363–367, 1962.
119. Miller RD, Way WL: Inhibition of succinylcholine-induced increased intragastric pressure by nondepolarizing muscle relaxants and lidocaine. Anesthesiology 34:185–188, 1971.
120. Muravchick S, Burkett L, Gold MI: Succinylcholine-induced fasciculations and intragastric pressure during induction of anesthesia. Anesthesiology 55:180–183, 1981.
121. Marx GF, Bassell GM: In defense of the use of d-tubocurarine prior to succinylcholine in obstetrics. Anesthesiology 59:157, 1983.
122. Sellick BA: Cricoid pressure to control regurgitation of stomach contents during induction of anaesthesia. Lancet 2:404–406, 1961.
123. Fanning GL: The efficacy of cricoid pressure in regurgitation of gastric contents. Anesthesiology 32:553–555, 1970.
124. Scott DB: Mendelson's syndrome. Br J Anaesth 50:977–978, 1978.
125. Conklin KA: Can anesthetic-related mortality be reduced? Am J Obstet Gynecol 163:253–254, 1990.
126. Morgan M: Anesthetic contribution to maternal mortality. Br J Anaesth 59:842–855, 1987.
127. Endler GC, Mariona FG, Sokol RJ, Stevenson LB: Anesthesia-related maternal mortality in Michigan, 1972 to 1984. Am J Obstet Gynecol 159:187–193, 1988.
128. May WJ, Greiss FW: Maternal mortality in North Carolina: A forty year experience. Am J Obstet Gynecol 161:555–561, 1989.
129. Sachs BP, Oriol NE, Ostheimer GW, Weiss JB, Driscoll S, Acker D, Brown AJ, Jewett JF: Anesthetic-related maternal mortality, 1954 to 1985. J Clin Anesth 1:333–338, 1989.
130. Rubin GL, Peterson HB, Rochat RW, McCarthy BJ, Terry JS: Maternal death after cesarean section in Georgia. Am J Obstet Gynecol 139:681–685, 1981.
131. Hogberg U: Maternal deaths in Sweden, 1971–1980. Acta Obstet Gynecol Scand 65:161–167, 1986.
132. Samsoon GLT, Young JRB: Difficult tracheal intubation: A retrospective study. Anaesthesia 42:487–490, 1987.
133. Wilson ME, Spiegelhalter D, Robertson JA, Lesser P: Predicting difficult intubation. Br J Anaesth 61:211–216, 1988.
134. Mallampati SR, Gatt SP, Gugino LD, Desai SP, Waraksa B, Freiberger D, Liu PL: A clinical sign to predict difficult tracheal intubation: A prospective study. Can Anaesth Soc J 32:429–434, 1985.
135. Joyce T: Personal communication, 1988.
136. Salzarulo HH, Taylor LA: Diabetic "stiff joint syndrome" as a cause of difficult endotracheal intubation. Anesthesiology 64:366–368, 1986.
137. Ovassapian A, Krejcie TC, Yelich SJ, Dykes MHM: Awake fibreoptic intubation in the patient at high risk of aspiration. Br J Anaesth 62:13–16, 1989.
138. Safar P: Cardiopulmonary Cerebral Resuscitation. Saunders, Philadelphia, 1981, p 240.
139. Tunstall ME, Geddes C: "Failed intubation" in obstetric anaesthesia: An indication for the use of the "esophageal gastric tube airway". Br J Anaesth 56:659–661, 1984.
140. Williamson R: Emergency caesarean section: Tracheal intubation or oesophageal gastric tube airway? Br J Anaesth 60:476, 1988.

141. Benumoff JL, Scheller JS: The importance of transtracheal jet ventilation in the management of the difficult airway. Anesthesiology 71:769–778, 1989.

142. Brain AIJ: The laryngeal mask: A new concept in airway management. Br J Anaesth 55:801–805, 1983.

143. Tunstall ME, Sheick A: Failed intubation protocol: Oxygenation without aspiration. Clin Anaesthesiol 4:171–188, 1986.

144. Tunstall ME: Failed intubation drill. Anaesthesia 31:850, 1976.

145. Tordoff SG, Sweeney BP: Acid aspiration prophylaxis in 288 obstetric anaesthetic departments in the United Kingdom. Anaesthesia 45:776–780, 1990.

146. Lahiri SK, Thomas TA, Hodgson RMH: Single-dose antacid therapy for the prevention of Mendelson's syndrome. Br J Anaesth 45:1143–1146, 1973.

147. Gibbs CP, Hempling RE, Wynne JW, Hood CI: Antacid pulmonary aspiration. Anesthesiology 51:S290, 1979.

148. Eyler SW, Cullen BF, Murphy ME, Welch WD: Antacid aspiration in rabbits: A comparison of Mylanta and Bicitra. Anesth Analg 61:288–292, 1982.

149. Gibbs CP, Spohr L, Schmidt D: The effectiveness of sodium citrate as an antacid. Anesthesiology 57:44–46, 1982.

150. Abboud TR, Curtis JP, Shnider SM, Earl S, Henriksen EH: Comparison of the effects of sodium citrate and Gelusil on gastric acidity and volume. Anesth Analg 61:167, 1982.

151. Viegas OJ, Ravindran RS, Stoops CA: Duration of action of sodium citrate as an antacid. Anesth Analg 61:624, 1982.

152. Dewan DM, Floyd HM, Thistlewood JM, Bogard TD: Sodium citrate premedication for elective cesarean section. Anesth Analg 63:S205, 1984.

153. O'Sullivan GM, Bullingham RE: Does twice the volume of antacid have twice the effect in pregnant women at term? Anesth Analg 63:752–756, 1984.

154. Gibbs CP, Banner TC: Effectiveness of Bicitra as a preoperative antacid. Anesthesiology 61:97–99, 1984.

155. Chen CT, Toung TJR, Haupt HM, Hutchins GM, Cameron JL: Evaluation of Alka Seltzer Effervescent in gastric acid neutralization. Anesth Analg 63:325–329, 1984.

156. Conklin KA, Ziadlou-Rad F: Buffering capacity of citrate antacids. Anesthesiology 58:391–392, 1983.

157. Gillett GB, Watson JD, Langford RM: Prophylaxis against acid aspiration syndrome in obstetric practice. Anesthesiology 60:525, 1984.

158. Holdsworth JD, Johnson K, Mascall G, Gwynne Roulston R, Tomlinson PA: Mixing of antacids with stomach contents. Anaesthesia 35:641–650, 1980.

159. Faure EAM, Lim HS, Block BS, Tan PL, Roizen MF: Sodium bicarbonate buffers gastric acid during surgery in obstetric and gynecologic patients. Anesthesiology 67:274–277, 1987.

160. Mathews HM, Moore J: Sodium bicarbonate as a single dose antacid in obstetric anaesthesia. Anaesthesia 44:590–591, 1989.

161. Pickering BG, Palahniuk RJ, Cumming M: Cimetidine premedication in elective cesarean section. Can Anaesth Soc J 27:33–35, 1980.

162. Williams JG: H$_2$ receptor antagonists and anaesthesia. Can Anaesth Soc J 30:264–269, 1983.

163. Manchikanti L, Kraus JW, Edds SP: Cimetidine and related drugs in anesthesia. Anesth Analg 61:595–608, 1982.

164. Hodgkinson R, Glassenberg R, Joyce TH III, Coombs DW, Ostheimer GW, Gibbs CP: Comparison of cimetidine (Tagamet) with acidity before elective cesarean section. Anesthesiology 59:86–90, 1983.

165. McAuley DM, Moore J, Dundee JW, McCaughey W: Oral ranitidine in labor. Anaesthesia 39:433–438, 1984.

166. Manchikanti L, Marrero TC, Roush JR: Preanesthetic cimetidine and metoclopramide for acid aspiration prophylaxis in elective surgery. Anesthesiology 61:48–54, 1984.

167. Manchikanti L, Colliver JA, Marrero TC, Roush JR: Ranitidine and metoclopramide for prophylaxis of aspiration pneumonitis in elective surgery. Anesth Analg 63:903–910, 1984.

168. Camarri E, Chirone E, Fanteria G, Zocchi M: Ranitidine induced bradycardia. Lancet 2:160, 1982.

169. Mangiameli A, Condorelli G, Dato A: Cardiovascular response to the acute intravenous administration of the H$_2$ receptor antagonists ranitidine and cimetidine. Curr Therap Res 36:13–17, 1984.

170. Shaw RC, Marshford ML, Desmond PV: Cardiac arrest after intravenous injection of cimetidine. Med J Aust 2:629–630, 1980.

171. Freely J, Wilkinson GR, Wood AJJ: Reduction of liver blood flow and propranolol metabolism by cimetidine. N Engl J Med 304:692–695, 1981.

172. Feely J, Guy E: Ranitidine also reduces liver blood flow. Lancet 1:169, 1982.

173. Feely J, Wilkinson GR, McAllister CB, Wood AJ: Increased toxocity and reduced clearance of lidocaine by cimetidine. Ann Intern Med 96:592–594, 1982.

174. Flynn RJ, Moore J, Collier PS, Howard PJ: Effect of intravenous cimetidine on lignocaine disposition during extradural caesarean section. Anaesthesia 44:739–741, 1989.

175. Flynn RJ, Moore J, Collier PS, Howard PJ: Single dose oral H$_2$-antagonists do not affect plasma lidocaine levels in the parturient. Acta Anaesthesiol Scand 33:593–596, 1989.

176. O'Sullivan GM, Smith M, Morgan B, Brighouse D, Reynolds F: H$_2$ antagonists and bupivacaine clearance. Anaesthesia 43:93–95, 1988.

177. Dailey PA, Hughes SC, Rosen MA, Healy K, Cheek DBC, Shnider SM: Effect of cimetidine and ranitidine on lidocaine concentrations during epidural anesthesia for cesarean section. Anesthesiology 69:1013–1017, 1988.

178. Mihaly GW, Marino AT, Webster LK, Jones DB, Louis WJ, Smallwood RA: High dose antacid (Mylanta II) reduces the bioavailability of ranitidine. Br Med J 285:998–999, 1982.

179. Cheah LS, Lee HS, Gwee MC: Anticholinesterase activity of and possible ion-channel block by cimetidine, ranitidine and oxmetidine in the toad isolated rectus abdominis muscle. Clin Exp Pharmacol Physiol 12:353–357, 1985.

180. Turner DR, Kao YJ, Bivona C: Neuromuscular block by suxamethonium following treatment with histamine type 2 antagonists or metoclopramide. Br J Anaesth 63:348–350, 1989.

181. Kambam JR, Franks JJ: Cimetidine does not affect plasma cholinesterase activity. Anesth Analg 67:69–70, 1988.

182. Hawkins JL, Adenwala J, Camp C, Joyce TH III: The effect of H$_2$-receptor antagonist premedication on the duration of vecuronium-induced neuromuscular blockade in postpartum patients. Anesthesiology 71:175–177, 1989.

183. McCarthy G, Mirakhur RK, Elliott P, Wright J: Effect of H$_2$-receptor antagonist pretreatment on vecuronium and atracurium induced neuromuscular block. Br J Anaesth 66:713–715, 1991.

184. Woodworth GE, Sears DH, Grove TM, Ruff RH, Kosek PS, Katz RL: The effect of cimetidine and ranitidine on the duration of action of succinylcholine. Anesth Analg 68:295–297, 1989.

185. Ohnishi K, Saitoh N, Nomura F, Okuda K, Suzuki N, Ohtsuki T, Goto N, Takashi M: Effect of famotidine on hepatic hemodynamics and peptic ulcer. Am J Gastroenterol 82:415–418, 1987.

186. Chermos AN: Pharmacodynamics of famotidine in humans. Am J Med 81(suppl):3–7, 1986.

187. Takeda M, Tagaki T, Fujiwara A, Kamato T, Tachikawa S: Pharmacology of famotidine: Comparison with cimetidine and ranitidine. Clin Reports 18:6125–6133, 1984.

188. Omote K, Namiki A, Sumita S, Takashi T, Ujike Y, Hagiwara T: Comparative studies on hemodynamic effects of intravenous cimetidine, ranitidine and famotidine in intensive care unit patients. Jpn J Anesthesiol 36:940–947, 1987.

189. Miyata K, Fujiwara A: Effect of famotidine on cardiovascular system and bronchoresistance in anesthetized dogs. Clin Reports 21:221–230, 1987.

190. Abe K, Shibata M, Demizu A, Hazano S, Sumikawa K, Enomoto H, Mashimo T, Tashiro C, Yoshiya I: Effect of oral famotidine on pH and volume of gastric contents. Anesth Analg 68:541–544, 1989.

191. McAllister JD, Moote CA, Sharpe MD, Manninen PH: Ran-

dom double-blind comparison of nizatidine, famotidine, ranitidine and placebo. Can J Anaesth 37:S22, 1990.

192. Moore J, Flynn RJ, Sampaio M, Wilson CM, Gillon KR: Effect of single-dose omeprazole on intragastric acidity and volume during obstetric anaesthesia. Anaesthesia 44:559–562, 1989.

193. Lehot JJ, Deleat-Besson R, Bastien O, Brun Y, Adeleine P, Robin J: Should we inhibit gastric acid secretion before cardiac surgery? Anesth Analg 70:185–190, 1990.

194. Laws HL, Palmer MD, Donald JM Jr, Bryant JW, Boudreaux A, Wheeler AS: Effects of preoperative medications on gastric pH, volume and flora. Ann Surg 203:614–619, 1986.

195. Gorback MS: Preoperative H₂-receptor antagonists. Anesth Analg 71:205–206, 1990.

196. Gonzalez ER, Kallar SK, Dunnavant BW: Single-dose intravenous H₂ blocker prophylaxis against aspiration pneumonitis: Assessment of drug concentration in gastric aspirate. AANA J 57:238–243, 1989.

197. Chestnut DH, Vandewalker GE, Owen CL, Bates JN, Choi WW: Administration of metoclopramide for prevention of nausea and vomiting during epidural anesthesia for elective cesarean section. Anesthesiology 66:563–566, 1987.

198. Murphy DF, Nally B, Gardiner J, Unwin A: Effect of metoclopramide on gastric emptying before elective and emergency caesarean section. Br J Anaesth 56:1113–1116, 1984.

199. Wyner MB, Cohen S: Gastric volume in early pregnancy. Anesthesiology 57:209–212, 1982.

200. McNeill MJ, Ho ET, Kenny GNC: Effect of IV metoclopramide on gastric emptying after opioid premedication. Br J Anaesth 64:450–452, 1990.

201. Bylsma-Howell M, McMorland GH, Rurak DW, Ongley R, McEvlane B, Axelson JE: Placental transport of metoclopramide: Assessment of maternal and neonatal side effects. Can Anaesth Soc J 30:487–492, 1983.

202. Eisenach JC, Rose JC, Castro MI, Dewan DM: Metoclopramide exaggerates stress-induced tachycardia. Anesthesiology 69:A678, 1988.

203. Turner DR, Kao YJ, Bivona C: Neuromuscular block by suxamethonium following treatment with histamine type 2 antagonists or metoclopramide. Br J Anaesth 63:348–350, 1989.

204. Moir D: Cimetidine, antacids and pulmonary aspiration. Anesthesiology 59:81–83, 1983.

205. Maltby JR, Elliott RH, Warnell I, Fairbrass M, Sutherland LR, Shaffer EA: Gastric fluid volume and pH in elective surgical patients: Triple prophylaxis is not superior to ranitidine alone. Can J Anaesth 37:650–655, 1990.

206. Colman RD, Frank M, Loughnan BA, Cohen DG, Cattermole R: Use of i.m. ranitidine for the prophylaxis of aspiration pneumonitis in obstetrics. Br J Anaesth 61:720–729, 1988.

207. Mathews HML, Wilson CM, Thompson EM, Moore J: Combination treatment with ranitidine and sodium bicarbonate prior to obstetric anesthesia. Anaesthesia 41:1202–1206, 1986.

208. Pond W, Lindsey R, Cowan J: Preoperative ranitidine and metoclopramide. Anesth Analg 66:1202, 1987.

209. Ormezzano X, Francois TP, Viaud JY, Bukowski JG, Bourgeonneau MC, Cottron D, Ganansia MF, Gregoire FM, Grinand MR, Wessel PE: Aspiration pneumonitis prophylaxis in obstetric anaesthesia: Comparison of effervescent cimetidine-sodium citrate mixture and sodium citrate. Br J Anaesth 64:503–506, 1990.

210. Christensen V, Skovsted P: Effects of general anaesthetics on pH of gastric contents of man during surgery: A survey of halothane, fluroxene and cyclopropane anesthesia. Acta Anaesthesiol Scand 19:49–74, 1975.

211. Morgan M: The confidential enquiry in maternal deaths (editorial). Anaesthesia 41:689–691, 1986.

212. Lyons G: Failed intubation. Anaesthesia 40:759–762, 1985.

213. Lyons G, MacDonald R: Difficult intubation in obstetrics. Anaesthesia 40:1016, 1985.

214. Cormack RS, Lehane J: Difficult tracheal intubation in obstetrics. Anaesthesia 39:1105–1111, 1984.

Labor Unit Guidelines: Prevention of Aspiration at the University of Pennsylvania

1. Most women in active labor and all who undergo anesthesia receive an intravenous infusion. Rigid NPO is not enforced; rather, limited oral clear liquids (up to 200 ml/hr)—such as ice chips, flavored ice (popsicles, water ice), ginger ale, lemon/lime soda, jello, and hard candy—are allowed.

2. Patients with uncomplicated normal or augmented labor, with or without labor analgesia, do not receive routine prophylactic medication (antacids, H_2 blockers, gastric emptiers). If an uncomplicated parturient has heartburn or a history of reflux and requests treatment, 30 ml of sodium citrate is given po. If this is ineffective, cimetidine 150 mg is injected IM.

3. High-risk parturients in labor
   Maternal disorders
   Pregnancy induced hypertension; diabetes; maternal infection; cardiac or pulmonary disease; ITP; previous cesarean section for trial of labor
   Fetal disorders
   Prematurity; signs of fetal stress (thick meconium, low scalp pH, persistent tachycardia, severe variable decelerations, late decelerations); congenital anomalies; Rh isoimmunization
   Utero Placental
   Postmaturity; placental infarct; abruption; previa; hyperactivity
   Labor Complications
   Prolonged labor; prolonged ruptured membranes; multiple gestation; difficult forceps delivery anticipated; abnormal presentation, e.g., breech or transverse lie
   A. If effective epidural analgesia is used for labor (most parturients at Hospital of University of Pennsylvania) antacids, Zantac (rantidine), Tagamet (cimetidine), Reglan (metoclopramide) are not used.
   B. If epidural analgesia is refused or not used
      i. 150 mg Zantac (ranitidine) or 300 mg Tagamet (cimetidine) po is given at first visit. Then 150 mg ranitidine or 300 mg cimetidine po is given with sip water in 6 hr. We do not routinely give H_2 blockers for >6 hr.
      ii. If general anesthesia is to be given, administer 30 ml of sodium citrate 0.3 M (Bicitra or Citra pH) po up to 20 min before induction.
      iii. If general anesthesia is planned and time exists, 10 mg Reglan (metoclopramide) IV 1 hr before induction may accelerate gastric emptying even in the presence of systemic narcotics.

4. Elective cesarean section
   A. *Regional block planned (>99%)*
   Antacids or gastric emptiers are not routinely used
   B. *General anesthesia planned*
   Pharmacologic aspiration prophylaxis is used. The protocol is similar to that described under 3.B.ii. above except that the parturient receives one dose of H_2 blocker the night before HS and one dose of H_2 blocker po with sip water in the morning, two hours before surgery.

5. Emergency cesarean section
   A. If effective lumbar epidural catheter is functioning, the level of anesthesia is rapidly raised and pharmacologic prophylaxis is not routinely used.
   B. If effective spinal anesthesia is given, pharmacologic prophylaxis is not routinely used.
   C. If general anesthesia is chosen and anesthesia is notified with sufficient time (1 hour), Zantac (ranitidine) 50 mg IV or Tagamet (cimetidine) 150 mg IV is administered; Reglan (metoclopramide) 10 mg IV is given and sodium citrate 30 ml po given 5 to 10 min prior to induction.
   D. If cesarean section is very urgent and anesthesia induction is urgent (i.e., in cases of cord prolapse, sustained fetal bradycardia, severe maternal hemorrhage), a rapid po dose of 30 ml Bicitra is given just prior to induction of anesthesia. H_2 blockers and gastric emptiers will not be as effective in this situation, but are given after induction to decrease the risk of aspiration on emergence with extubation.

Note

A patient who, on physical examination, appears to be very difficult to intubate does not receive a rapid induction of general anesthesia. This may lead to airway loss and make it difficult, if not impossible, to sustain maternal life. The obstetrician and anesthetist must ***not*** focus on the welfare of the fetus at the expense of maternal well-being.

In the presence of a very difficult airway, either awake intubation or regional block is performed, despite the slightly longer time required, in order to avoid the devastating consequences of loss of the maternal airway.

CHAPTER 24

Neurologic Complications of Regional Anesthesia for Obstetrics

Philip R. Bromage, M.B., B.S., F.F.A.R.C., F.R.C.P.(C)

The severity of neurologic sequelae to regional anesthesia ranges from mild and transient to catastrophic and permanent. Fatal complications appear to be extremely rare. Their precise incidence is unknown because of incomplete recording requirements in different countries, but it is probably of the same magnitude as or less than the incidence of deaths attributable to general anesthesia. At the time of writing the most recent and complete estimate comes from the 1989 *Report on Confidential Enquiries into Maternal Deaths in England and Wales* for the triennium 1982–1984 (1). This report lists 19 anesthetic deaths out of 1,903,096 births. Of these 19 maternal deaths, 18 were attributable to general anesthesia and 1 to unnoticed spinal anesthesia following an epidural top-up dose given by a midwife. However, a more recent retrospective survey by the English Colleges of Obstetrics and Gynecology and Anaesthesia for the 5-year period of 1982–1986 reports three cardiac arrests (one with permanent brain damage) out of a total of 506,000 epidural-assisted deliveries—that is, an incidence of 1:168,700 near-fatal complications (2).

The process of childbirth itself also carries its own intrinsic burden of neurologic sequelae, ranging from mild to catastrophic, again with the precise incidence unknown beyond approximate estimates gathered from independent, limited series collected under widely differing conditions of obstetric practice. Clearly, there are cogent medical and medicolegal reasons to distinguish between intrinsic and iatrogenic causes of postpartum palsies; thus this chapter attempts not only to review the causes and avoidance of neurologic sequelae to regional anesthesia, but also to set the risks of regional anesthesia in perspective against the background of intrinsic maternal obstetric palsy. Without this perspective, regional anesthesia is often mistakenly blamed for adverse neurologic events that have little or nothing to do with the anesthetic itself. Moreover, in rare instances the wrong etiologic diagnosis may deprive the mother of appropriate treatment that might contribute to partial or complete recovery from a potentially permanent intrinsic postpartum paralysis.

To sketch this perspective, three important causes of maternal obstetric paralysis are summarized before discussing adverse neurologic outcomes caused by regional anesthesia. One of these is common and well recognized; the other two are less common and less well known, but important causes. For a more comprehensive survey and greater detail, the reader is referred to Donaldson's *Neurology of Pregnancy* (3).

INTRINSIC MATERNAL OBSTETRIC PALSY

Pressure by Fetal Head on Nerve Structures in the Pelvis

Major neurologic sequelae may follow general anesthesia (4). However, in childbirth, neurologic complications may occur without any anesthetic at all.

The first well-documented report of maternal obstetric palsy in the English language comes from what is now the Rotunda Hospital in Dublin and dates from 1838, before general and regional anesthesia were developed (5). That report describes in vivid terms how a young primagravida suffered foot-drop and loss of sensation in the right leg after a normal delivery. Partial recovery took place and her foot-drop was improving by the tenth postpartum week, when she contracted a fever and died of what appears to have been septic pericarditis (5).

As time went by many more cases of lower motor neuron injury were reported, some after natural childbirth and some following instrumental delivery (6). Later, intraspinal compression from prolapsed intervertebral discs, spinal tumors, spontaneous epidural hematoma, and abscess were added to the reports (3, 7, 8). Scattered in the literature were also rare, unexplained instances of permanent paraplegia involving sacral, lumbar and sometimes lower thoracic segments (3).

Pressure of Fetal Head on Spinal Nutrient Arteries in the Pelvis

In the early 1960s the etiologic spectrum of maternal birth palsy was suddenly widened by the studies of Lazorthes and his colleagues on the arterial supply to the spinal cord and, particularly, to the lumbosacral enlargement (9, 10). They demonstrated a dual blood supply to the conus medullaris, with the primary source coming from the long descending branch of the artery of Adamkiewicz (radicularis magna or arteria magna) and a secondary supply from the internal iliac arteries ascending via the iliolumbar and laterosacral arteries (Fig. 24.1). Lazorthes also showed that a reciprocal contribution is made by

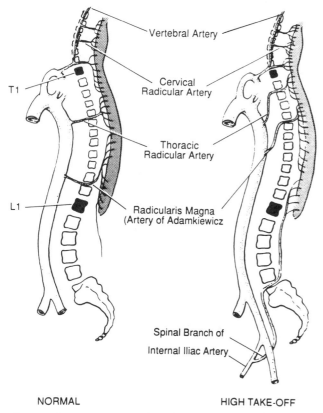

Figure 24.1. Diagram showing blood supply of the spinal cord. In about 85% of cases the radicularis magna originates between T9 and L2 and provides the major blood supply to the thoracolumbar region. In about 15% of cases the radicularis magna originates at about T5 (high take-off), and the lower thoracolumbar region is supplied by a branch of the internal iliac artery entering by way of the intervertebral foramen between L5 and the sacrum. (Modified from Bromage PR: Anatomy. In *Epidural Analgesia*. WB Saunders, Philadelphia, 1978, p 52; Lazorthes G, Poulhes J, Bastide G, Chancolle AR, Zadel O: La vascularisation de la moelle épinière (etude anatomique et physiologique). Rev Neurol 106:535, 1962; and Lazorthes G, Gouaze A, Bastide G, Soutoul J-H, Zadeh O, Santini J-J: La vascularisation artérielle du renflement lombaire. Etude des variations et des suppléances. Rev Neurol (Paris) 114:109, 1966.

these two sources, depending on the vertebral level at which the artery of Adamkiewicz originates from the aorta. In approximately 85% of the population this artery arises between T9 and L3 and supplies the bulk of the conus medullaris, whereas the ascending contribution from the internal iliac arteries is relatively tenuous and probably expendable without causing permanent ischemic damage to the conus. However, in the remaining 15% of the population the artery of Adamkiewicz originates in the middle to upper thoracic region (average level: T5), and then the respective contributory roles of the two arterial supplies are reversed. A relatively slender supply descends from above, and a larger and relatively more important component ascends from branches of the internal iliac artery that lie along the posterior wall of the pelvis and cross in front of the ala of the sacrum. It is in this 15% minority that the conus may be in danger of ischemic necrosis from prolonged compression by the fetal head, especially if any degree of disproportion exists and if labor is protracted and complicated by difficult instrumental delivery.

More than a decade later in 1980 an interesting survey of maternal obstetric palsy from Nigeria corroborated the clinical implications of Lazorthes' work to a remarkably precise degree (11). Bademosi and his colleagues reviewed 34 cases of maternal palsy arising out of their obstetric population at the University of Ibadan in the 10-year period of 1966–1976 (11). Of these 34 mothers, 29 recovered within 1 to 2 years. The remaining five mothers (i.e., 15%) did not recover and remained permanently paraplegic.

Bademosi's initial report did not mentioned whether these sequelae could have arisen as complications of regional anesthesia rather than from intrinsic obstetric causes, either in the 29 women who recovered or in the unfortunate 5 who remained permanently paralysed. Subsequent personal correspondence with the senior author revealed that none of the 34 patients had received subarachnoid or epidural anesthesia, thus eliminating the possibility that regional anesthesia might have contributed to the catastrophic outcome of the 5 permanently paralysed patients (12).

Vascular Anomalies Causing Ischemia of the Conus Medullaris

In the meantime, advances in the manufacture of nonionic injectable radiopaque contrast media and in neuroradiologic techniques expanded opportunities to visualize engorged subarachnoid blood vessels, as well as the inflow and outflow vasculature of the spinal cord itself, first by epidural phlebography and later by selective arteriography of the cord. These advances, which were shortly followed by the introduction of magnetic resonance imaging (MRI), have opened a whole new field of hitherto unknown vascular pathologic conditions contributing to postpartum paralysis and that may be curable by surgery or invasive radiologic techniques (13–17).

In the 15 years between 1975 and 1990, more than 500 cases of paralysis due to arteriovenous malformations have been published. Some of these were clinically manifest for the first time as a neurologic consequence of childbirth and, in one instance, as quadraplegia following epidural analgesia for vaginal delivery (17).

Incidence of Maternal Obstetric Paralysis

The task of estimating the incidence of these intrinsic cases of maternal obstetric palsy is enormously difficult, especially against the background of evolving obstetric practice.

In the current increasingly active management of childbirth, it is almost impossible to obtain a large but pure control series of "natural childbirth" that is free of obstetric interference. Much of the data that we do have stems from series gathered in the four decades between 1930 and 1970, with estimates of intrinsic obstetric maternal paralysis and adverse neurologic outcomes ranging between 1:2100 and 1:3000 (Fig. 24.2) (18–20).

A contemporary and carefully conducted survey at the University of Manitoba reviewed 23,827 de-liveries during the 9-year period between 1975–1983. The overall incidence of transient sensory and motor dysfunction was 1:529, but all of these cases resolved within 72 hr. It is noteworthy that the incidence of these transient occurrences was almost exactly the same in patients who received epidural anesthesia (1:276) as in those who received general anesthesia (1:289). Only two patients suffered prolonged neurologic deficits; one of these developed foot-drop after a difficult Kjelland's forceps rotation under epidural anesthesia, and the other had bladder dysfunction after a pudendal nerve infiltration. Thus, out of the 9403 patients who received epidural anesthesia, only one experienced a prolonged neuropraxia, and that was associated with a difficult forceps extraction that was undoubtedly the real cause of the unilateral foot-drop (21).

A more recent retrospective survey from Britain reviewed the serious nonfatal complications associated with epidural analgesia in obstetric practice from a population of 2,580,000 deliveries (2). Of these, 506,000 were conducted under epidural analgesia and 108 adverse events were reported. Approximately 73 of those adverse events were prolonged neurologic complications that included 38 cases of neuropathy of a single spinal nerve, which in the light of the preceding discussion *could* have been of obstetric rather than anesthetic origin. Thus, on the basis of these figures, the present incidence of ad-

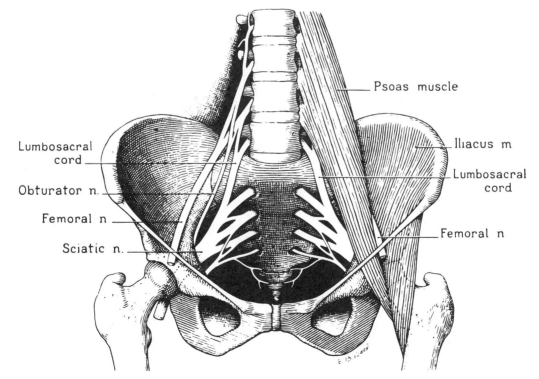

Figure 24.2. The relationship of the lumbosacral cord to the pelvis and the psoas major muscle. (Reprinted by permission from Cole JT: Maternal obstetric paralysis. Am J Obstet Gynecol 52:374, 1946.)

verse neurologic sequelae to obstetric analgesia may lie somewhere between 1:7000 and 1:14,000. Unfortunately, this survey did not examine the incidence of neurologic sequelae in the one and one-half million deliveries without regional anesthesia; thus, the background incidence of maternal obstetric paralysis in a control population of the Western world is still unknown.

However, based on the existing evidence available, rough estimates of the etiologic incidence of *intrinsic* maternal paralyses and their prognoses are outlined in Table 24.1. It is against these background estimates that we must formulate our judgments of the true cause of any case of neurologic deficit that arises after regional anesthesia for childbirth. For this reason it is most important for the profession and the insurance industry to address the long delayed task of acquiring accurate contemporary data on the incidence and etiology of adverse neurologic outcomes after *natural* childbirth.

DIRECT COMPLICATIONS OF REGIONAL ANESTHESIA

Backache

A well-known gynecologist used to begin his lectures by saying, "A woman is a constipated biped with backache." This unflattering and inaccurate generalization nevertheless focused attention on the fact that postpartum backache is so common it tends to be dismissed as a complication of the lordosis of pregnancy and to be ignored as a dependent variable of anesthetic interventions.

A recent survey of postpartum backache in a population of 11,701 deliveries from one hospital in Britain found that backache lasting for more than 6 weeks arose in 10.5% of women delivered by natural childbirth. A similar incidence of backache occurred after delivery by elective cesarean section, regardless of whether general or epidural anesthesia was used (22). However, in those women who received epidural analgesia for labor and delivery or for cesarean section following a failed trial of labor, the incidence of prolonged backache rose to 18.9%. This highly signifi-

cant difference was attributed to the combination of active labor and epidural anesthesia and to the possibility of ligamentous damage arising from tolerance of potentially damaging postures and straining movements in the presence of segmental analgesia.

To explain the surprisingly powerful influence of epidural analgesia on the incidence of prolonged backache, it is important to understand the historic and pharmacologic implications of these figures, which were gathered during an 8-year period commencing in 1978. At that time many British anesthetists were still employing more concentrated solutions of local anesthetics for labor than were colleagues elsewhere. It was common for 0.375% or even 0.5% bupivacaine to be used throughout labor, although the 0.25% solution was more favored in North America and the 0.125% dilution was encouraged in Belgium (23).

Surgical concentrations of local anesthetics for epidural analgesia in labor cause an inappropriate degree of motor blockade in the affected parts, resulting in loss of tone in muscles of the pelvic floor once analgesia has spread downwards to involve the sacral segments. A relaxed and deafferentated pelvic gutter impairs normal flexion and rotation of the fetal head so that a high incidence of malrotation results and the second stage of labor becomes unduly prolonged (24). Throughout the protracted second stage, intense analgesia permits the mother to adopt and maintain postures that may place excessive strain on vertebral and sacroiliac joints and that are likely to result in prolonged postpartum backache and disability. Recent trends towards more selective deafferentation with very low concentrations of local anesthetic mixed with potent lipid-soluble opiates preserve motor tone and result in more normal mechanics of labor that may lessen the incidence of backache after epidural-assisted deliveries.

Chloroprocaine (Nesacaine) Backache

In 1989 reports of severe backache after epidural analgesia with 2% or 3% 2-chloroprocaine began to appear in the literature (25). In all cases the solution used was the newly formulated methylparaben-free

Table 24.1
Estimated Incidence and Prognosis of Intrinsic Maternal Obstetric Paralysis

Cause	Estimated Incidence	Prognosis
Neuropraxia from pelvic neural compression	1:3000	Recoverable within weeks to 2 years
Herniated intervertebral disc	1:10,000	Recoverable with early surgical treatment
Compressive arterial ischemia of conus medullaris	1:15,000	Permanent paraplegia
Arteriovenous malformation with venous congestion of lumbosacral enlargement	1:20,000	Variable, ranging from complete recovery to permanent paralysis; prognosis improved by occlusion of arterial feeder to arteriovenous fistula

(MPF) preparation by Astra, from which the former antioxidant sodium bisulphite had been eliminated, but in which 0.01% disodium ethylenediaminetetraacetic acid (EDTA) had replaced calcium EDTA as a chelating agent to exclude metal impurities. In most reported cases the total epidural volume of 2% or 3% 2-chloroprocaine was relatively large. Although one subject reported back pain after as little as 15 ml, the average dose that evoked pain was 29.9 ± 5.1 ml in one series (25) and 24.0 ± 3.9 ml in another (26). In a third study doses in excess of 30 ml were used, and four out of five of these subjects reported very severe pain (27).

The backache had the following characteristics (26):

1. An unrelenting and incapacitating deep ache of a severity ranging from 2.5 to 9 on a visual analogue pain scale of 0 to 10 and lasting 24 to 36 hr.

2. Incidence and severity of pain related to the volume of Nesacaine-MPF formulation injected, but no incidences were reported with volumes of less than 15 ml.

3. Pain temporarily relieved by a second epidural injection of 3-chloroprocaine, but only for the duration of the subsequent analgesic block.

4. Pain promptly and completely relieved by epidural fentanyl (100 to 200 μg).

It is speculated that the pain may be caused by the chelating action of disodium EDTA in the new MPF formulation and to lowering of free calcium in spinal or paraspinal structures. It also has been suggested that replacement of sodium EDTA with calcium EDTA may correct this problem. Meanwhile, it is prudent to limit the total dose of epidural 2-chloroprocaine to less than 25 ml.

Postdural Puncture Headache

Typically, postdural puncture headache is relieved by recumbency and is exacerbated by standing, sitting, or walking. It is due to leakage of cerebrospinal fluid (CSF) through the puncture hole, resulting in diminished hydraulic support for intracranial structures. Tension on these structures results in headache as a symptom and rarely as oculomotor or trigeminal nerve paresis as a sign (28). In very rare instances the tension may be sufficient to rupture an intracranial vein leading to life-threatening subdural hematoma with a mortality of approximately 30% (29–31). Thus severe, prolonged postpuncture headache must be treated as a potentially serious complication.

Severity of the headache is related to the rate of loss of CSF. This in turn is determined by the degree of pressure exerted by distended veins inside and outside the dural tube and by the size of the puncture hole through which CSF escapes (32, 33). Parturients are twice as likely to suffer spinal headaches as are normal patients of the same age. The expulsive efforts of the second stage of labor contribute to this difference by engorging the azygos venous system and the extradural veins, which squeeze the dural tube and express CSF through the needle hole. This difference in incidence may not be significant after puncture with needles smaller than 22 gauge or when bearing down efforts are restricted to 10 to 12 "pushes" (34). However, after 18-gauge punctures, the incidence doubles from 54% with elective cesarean section in which no straining has occurred to 95% with active labor and forceful expulsive efforts (35). Because the size of the dural hole is related to the caliber of the needle used, the incidence of postpuncture headache drops from about 70% after puncture with a 16-gauge needle to about 2% when a 25-gauge needle is used and no straining occurs. In addition, the size of the hole is larger and the incidence of headache higher when the cutting edges of a Quincke or Tuohy-type needle are orientated at right angles to the longitudinal fibers of the dura than when the needle is turned to align the cutting edges with the axis of the dural tube so that the longitudinal fibers are pushed apart rather than cut (36–38).

In one teaching institution reporting a high accidental dural puncture rate of 2.6% with 17-gauge or 18-gauge Tuohy needles the incidence of postpuncture headache was reduced from 70% to 26% by the following maneuver. Needles were advanced into the epidural space with the orifice directed laterally and the cutting edges parallel to the dural fibers, in case the dura should be punctured. Once the epidural space was safely entered and no CSF appeared, the needle was rotated 90 degrees to point the orifice cephalady and in line with the axis of the spinal canal for passage of the epidural catheter (39). However, for more experienced anesthesiologists, this technique is controversial on two counts. First, the method does not reduce the incidence of dural puncture but only the incidence of headache that may follow. Second, rotation of the bevel within the epidural space introduces the danger of incising the dura with the arcing needle tip, thus increasing the more subtle risk of accidental subdural cannulation (considered later) (40, 41).

Finally, a wide-angled lateral approach has been recommended for subarachnoid puncture, so that the needle will penetrate the dura obliquely and create a track with a flap-valve effect that tends to close under the pressure of CSF (42). A zero incidence of headache has been reported from a series of more than 600 subarachnoid punctures performed with this approach using 20-gauge needles. However, in most hands the technical difficulties of an exaggerated paramedian approach are likely to outweigh its theoretical advantages.

OTHER CRANIAL CAUSES OF POSTDURAL PUNCTURE HEADACHE

Treatment of postdural puncture headache should always be preceded by a routine history and physical examination to exclude causes other than low CSF pressure. The cardinal sign of headache due to CSF hypotension is unremitting cephalgia in the sitting or standing posture that is promptly relieved by recumbency. Failure to obtain relief on lying down is the signal to intensify a search for other possibly more urgent causes.

Paranasal Sinusitis

This usually follows an upper respiratory infection, with tenderness to pressure over the frontal, ethmoidal, or maxillary sinuses and possibly a low fever.

Cortical Vein Thrombosis

The estimated incidence ranges between 1:3000 and 1:6000 deliveries. Headache is throbbing and unrelieved by bed rest, with sweating, nausea, and occasionally focal seizures (43–45).

Subdural Hematoma

This is a rare but potentially fatal result of prolonged and excessively low CSF pressure. It has been reported after lumbar puncture for myelography (46), after spinal anesthesia (47, 48), and after accidental "wet tap" with 16-gauge and 18-gauge epidural needles (29–31).

Occasionally the bleed may be intracerebral (49). Both of these conditions call for urgent diagnosis with computed tomography (CT) scan or magnetic resonance imaging (MRI).

TREATMENT OF LOW-PRESSURE POSTDURAL PUNCTURE HEADACHE

Because postdural puncture headache is brought on by standing or sitting and is relieved by recumbency, 24-hr bed rest used to be enforced as a logical prophylactic measure after spinal anesthesia or accidental dural puncture. Enforced recumbency as an effective prophylactic measure was challenged as long ago as 1947. Cullen and Griffith studied the incidence of headache in 200 women after spinal anesthesia with a 22-gauge needle for delivery. The incidence (20%) and intensity of headache were precisely the same whether the mothers were allowed to adopt their position of choice or whether recumbency was strictly enforced (50). This observation went unnoticed until rediscovered in 1974 when the subject was again addressed in the same journal 27 years later (51). Since 1974 increasing evidence has accumulated that posture is not a factor influencing the incidence of headache, regardless of other variables such as needle size, age, and pregnancy (Fig.

24.3) (51–53). One recent study using 25- and 26-gauge needles for subarachnoid anesthesia for vaginal delivery showed a 36% incidence of headache in patients kept at rest for 24 hr and a 22% incidence in those allowed out of bed after 6 hr (54). Contemporary obstetric practice favors adoption of the patient's position of choice during the first 6 hr, followed by early ambulation and a return to bed rest if headache arises—possibly with a trial of caffeine therapy, then active treatment with epidural blood patch, if the headache persists.

Caffeine Therapy

The theoretical support for using systemic caffeine is based on primate studies showing that acutely lowered CSF pressure causes venodilation (55). Caffeine redresses the balance by inducing cerebral vasoconstriction and reduction of cerebral blood flow in postdural puncture patients (56). However, the palliative effects are transient (57). Because many postspinal headaches resolve spontaneously in 2 to 3 days, the results of palliative treatment depend on timing. False-positive results are likely to arise if caffeine treatment is started too early or too late (when the headache is beginning to wane spontaneously). One preliminary study reported 14 successful results in 18 patients receiving caffeine (58). However, in a more recent series of 106 patients undergoing myelography with 22-gauge needles, the incidence of headache was not significantly different between those receiving and those not receiving caffeine (59).

Epidural Saline Infusions

Epidural saline infusions to bolster a sagging low-pressure dural tube have had a long but relatively

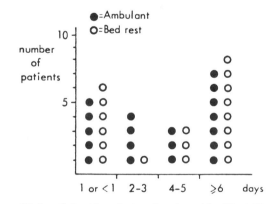

Figure 24.3. Spinal headache developed in 19 of 50 neurology patients following diagnostic lumbar puncture (18-gauge needle) who were allowed to ambulate at will immediately following the block. In a similar group of patients kept at bed rest for 24 hr spinal headache developed in 18 of 50. Duration of the headache was also similar in both groups. (Reprinted by permission from Carbaat PAT, van Crevel H: Lumbar puncture headache: Controlled study on the preventive effect of 24 hours' bed rest. Lancet 2:1133–1135, 1981.)

unsuccessful history over the past 40 years. Following accidental dural puncture, an epidural catheter is left in place and 1 to 1.5 liters of isotonic Ringer's or Hartmann's solution are infused over 24 hr (60). Relief is usually satisfactory for the first day, but continued infusion may give rise to severe interscapular pain and headache often returns by the third or fourth day (61).

In contemporary practice, epidural blood patch is the treatment of choice, and epidural saline infusions are seldom employed, except when epidural blood patch is contraindicated.

Epidural Dextran

One preliminary report of epidural dextran-40 in volumes of 20 to 30 ml claimed it relieved postdural puncture headache in 56 patients after other methods had failed. Relief occurred rather slowly—within 5 to 30 min in most patients, but up to 2 hours for others (62). If substantiated by similar studies, dextran may have promise as an alternative to epidural blood patch in situations in which an intraspinal injection of autologous blood should be avoided, such as in septic patients.

Epidural Blood Patch

Since its introduction by Gormley in 1960, autologous epidural blood patch has become recognized as the definitive treatment for postdural puncture headache (63). Three requirements are necessary for success. First, a normal clotting profile. Second, the blood should be introduced close to or at the site of puncture. Introduction of the blood one space *below* the dural rent ensures that the normal negative intrapleural pressure transmitted to the epidural space will draw the blood cephalad and spread it effectively over the hole. Third, a sufficient volume of blood must be injected to accomplish two aims: (*a*) to seal the hole and (*b*) to exert enough pressure around the dural tube to restore CSF pressure and relieve headache immediately. The instant relief characteristic of a successful blood patch seems to depend on the administration of rather generous volumes of autologous blood—in the range of 15 to 20 ml (64, 65).

Controversy still exists over the choice between delayed and prophylactic blood patch when a functioning epidural catheter is in place, although a large dural hole is known to exist from an earlier accidental dural puncture. In obstetrics the wait-and-see school of thought may anticipate a 35 to 85% chance of headache, which will require active blood patch treatment sooner or later. The preventive school prefers to lessen the odds by injecting autologous blood through the catheter an hour or so after the epidural block has worn off and fluid has had an opportunity to resorb from the epidural space (66).

Evidence is accumulating that the prophylactic school may be correct, with an incidence of post–blood patch headache in the range of 10 to 21% (67–69). The minority of patients who suffer a headache after a prophylactic blood patch usually respond satisfactorily to a second blood patch.

However, like so many other interventions, prophylactic blood patch at the end of satisfactory epidural anesthesia is not without its own inherent complications. One case of immediate total spinal anesthesia has been reported following a 15-ml prophylactic epidural blood patch given at the conclusion of operation in which the upper segmental level of analgesia did not rise above T4. Presumably, the compressive effects of the epidural blood on the outside of the dural tube forced local anesthetic-laden CSF up to medullary and midbrain levels (70).

To summarize, current practice favors early ambulation after dural puncture with a trial of palliative treatment, which may include oral or intravenous caffeine sodium benzoate, if headache arises. Specific treatment with an autologous blood patch is usually held in reserve for severe persistent headache, after causes other than CSF pressure have been excluded. Preemptive epidural blood patch should be given sooner if large dural holes are known to exist from inadvertent dural puncture with an 18- to 16-gauge needle. Epidural dextran may be held in reserve as a rational alternative to autologous blood in septic patients.

Shivering

Shivering is a trivial but annoying accompaniment of about 10% of normal labors. The incidence rises to 20 to 75% in patients receiving epidural blocks for labor or cesarean section. The resulting rise of oxygen consumption and cardiac output is rarely a concern unless serious cardiac disease exists. The neurologic etiology of shivering remains unclear. Warming the epidural anesthetic solutions to body temperature in an effort to prevent local cooling of the spinal contents does not reduce the incidence (71). However, two other steps can be taken with some success. First, warming the intravenous fluids in an attempt to maintain total body temperature is reported to be highly successful (72, 73). Second, epidural opiates also effectively reduce the incidence, and high doses of epidural sufentanil (50 to 100 μg) are reported to eliminate shivering completely (74). Epidural meperidine (Demerol) in small doses of 25 mg appears to be equally successful, as well as safer from the point of view of respiratory depression (75).

However, prevention of shivering by epidural opiates is accomplished at the cost of lowering the body temperature. Moderate hypothermia to below 34°C may be expected when sufentanil is used in doses larger than 50 μg (74).

ENHANCED LOCAL ANESTHETIC ACTION IN PREGNANCY

Horner's Syndrome

Several reports have drawn attention to the unexpected appearance of Horner's syndrome during epidural analgesia at term, even when the upper segmental level of anesthesia is below the fifth thoracic dermatome and the dorsal outflow of the cranial sympathetic motor pathways (76, 77). The cause of this neurologic oddity is probably due to two factors: (a) to the very superficial anatomic location of the descending spinal sympathetic fibers lying just below the spinal pia of the dorsolateral funiculus and within easy diffusion range of subanesthetic dilutions of local anesthetics in the CSF (78) and (b) to the general enhancement of local anesthetic nerve-blocking action that becomes evident from the first trimester onwards (79) and that is related to rising tissue concentrations of progesterone, which reach their peak just before term (80, 81).

The space-occupying effect of dilated epidural veins was formerly considered a major factor in this phenomenon of enhanced cephalad spread of local anesthetics. However, it is probably of minor importance compared with the hormonal effects of pregnancy on local anesthetic susceptibility.

Overdose

Because of hormonal enhancement of local anesthetic action in pregnancy, obstetric patients require 25 to 30% less local anesthetic than does the normal population. Failure to allow for this enhanced susceptibility will lead to relative overdose and excessively high-segmental blockade, with undue vasomotor and muscular paralysis. Nevertheless, the need for caution must be balanced against the pragmatic clinical observation that effective regional anesthesia for cesarean section requires a segmental block to T4 if the mother is to be pain-free throughout the operation. This is particularly important if the surgical technique entails the added trauma of exteriorizing the uterus, instead of the lesser stimulation that accompanies repair of the uterus in situ.

Prolonged Neural Blockade

The remote possibility of prolonged residual anesthesia (lasting up to 48 hr) is a third corollary of the enhanced neural susceptibility of pregnancy. Formerly, prolonged local anesthetic blockade was associated with repeated epidural injections of concentrated local anesthetics for relief of pain in labor. Table 24.2 summarizes nine cases reported from the literature before 1978 (82–84). It should be noted that in all nine cases the epidural solutions were unnecessarily concentrated for the task of providing pain relief during labor. Although current practice would not permit the prolonged use of such concentrated epidural solutions for control of labor pain, these cases still have significance. The same sort of phenomenon may arise with the increasingly popular use of continuous subarachnoid anesthesia for labor if local anesthetics are not in suitable dilution and administered under careful observation to avoid excessive motor block.

Techniques that carry a risk of prolonged anesthetic blockade should be avoided because the persistent block may be difficult to distinguish from paralysis due to pathologic causes (such as epidural hematoma), which must be excluded by expensive imaging procedures and which may demand urgent surgical intervention if a compressive lesion is found to exist.

Massive Misplaced Injection

The most serious immediate neurologic complication is massive injection of local anesthetic into the wrong site—either subdural, subarachnoid, or intravenous. Accidental misplaced injections may be immediate, yielding dramatic and potentially life-threatening effects, or delayed for many hours or days as an epidural catheter migrates into one or more of the wrong anatomic areas. Because catheter migration is a constant but remote possibility, the segmental level of analgesia should be checked and documented at regular intervals during continuous epidural infusions.

Table 24.2
Prolonged Blockade after Epidural Analgesia in Labor followed by Complete Recovery

Author	Drug	Cases (n)	Duration of Residual Analgesia (hr)
Bromage (3)	Tetracaine 0.5% + epinephrine	3	9–48
	Bupivacaine 0.5% + epinephrine	1	10
Pathy and Rosen (4)	Bupivacaine 0.5% + epinephrine	1	48
Cuerden et al. (5)	Bupivacaine 0.5% + epinephrine	4	23–48

Massive Subdural Injection

A potential space exists between the dura mater and the pia-arachnoid membrane. Rough handling of the needle, or unnecessary rotation of the bevel during induction of epidural blockade are factors that may cause a breach in the dura, with the possibility of injecting solutions or passing a catheter directly into the subdural space (85–87). However, subdural cannulation has been documented in the absence of needle rotation (88).

Attempted subarachnoid injections frequently enter the subdural space with a proven incidence of 4 to 13% in radiologic practice when 18- and 19-gauge needles are used (89, 90) and a suspected rate of 1 to 3% with the smaller bore spinal needles employed in anesthetic practice (91). An accidental single-shot subdural injection, instead of an intended subarachnoid dose, causes no ill effects beyond a poorly functioning spinal anesthetic. However, large-volume injections intended for the epidural space produce bizarre spread of analgesia, characterized by slow onset of extensive but asymmetric sensory and motor blockade following a negative aspiration test for CSF (92). Fortunately, the onset of high-subdural anesthesia may be relatively slow over a period of 10 to 20 min; thus there is usually time to correct the hemodynamic effects before severe hypotension occurs (93).

Massive Subarachnoid Injection

In vitro studies of human dura mater show that epidural catheters are very unlikely to penetrate uninjured dura (94). However, damage by the needle point may leave a weak spot through which a catheter may enter the subdural space as described above (95) and then pass into the subarachnoid space, either at the time of insertion or hours later after body movements have carried the catheter a few millimeters further (93, 96). Therefore recognition of dural puncture and the possibility of delayed intrathecal cannulation with massive subarachnoid spread is not always revealed by routine aspiration tests at the time of catheter insertion (61).

Table 24.3 shows the distribution of diagnostic signs of dural puncture in one series, with a 0.6% incidence of unintentional dural taps in 3500 attempted epidurals (61). One-third of the accidental punctures were not revealed by commonly accepted routine tests at the time of catheter insertion. These data reemphasize the need for regular measurements and documentation of the upper and lower segmental levels of analgesia during continuous epidural infusions for labor to ensure that accidental subarachnoid spread of analgesia does not go unrecognized and untreated.

Table 24.3
Diagnostic Signs in 21 Cases of Unintentional Dural Puncture Among 3500 Epidural Blocks for Labor (0.6%)[a]

CSF drip from needle	9/21
CSF aspirated from needle	3/21
Hypotension after test dose	2/21
No discernible sign of dural puncture at time of catheter insertion (retrospective diagnosis: postpuncture headache)	7/21

[a]Reprinted by permission from Okell RW, Sprigge JS: Unintentional dural puncture: A survey of recognition and management. Anaesthesia 42:1110–1113, 1987.

Toxic Intravenous Injection

Accidental intravascular injection is a potential hazard in any form of regional anesthesia. Epidural venous cannulation occurs in 4 to 5% of epidural catheter insertions during labor (97). Rapid intravenous injection may result in convulsions and cardiovascular depression. It is standard to teach that needles should be kept moving during infiltration anesthesia to avoid the danger of inadvertent intravenous injection. This precaution is obviously impossible in epidural analgesia because of the narrowness of the space; thus it is especially important to perform tests to ensure that large-bolus doses of local anesthetic are not accidentally injected into the vascular system.

Two sites of accidental intravenous injection are relatively common. First, needles passed into the caudal canal may pierce the cortical layer of a sacral vertebra and enter cancellous bone. Subsequent injections into the marrow cavity enter the circulation as rapidly as by direct intravenous injection, and toxic reactions may result (98). Second, cannulation of a lumbar epidural vein is more likely to occur if epidural puncture is made in the lateral part of the space, where the veins are more plentiful, than in the midline. Due to partial occlusion of the inferior vena cava, pressure and flow in the extradural and azygos system is higher at term than in the normal population. Azygos flow is likely to rise in proportion to the degree of caval obstruction, and this is greatest when the mother is lying on her back. Hence, extradural intravenous injections in the dorsal position travel fast and reach the heart as a bolus, so that quite small quantities of local anesthetic produce disproportionately large effects. Convulsions have arisen from as little as 15 mg of etidocaine, with a toxic equivalence of about 60 mg of lidocaine.

Prevention lies in:

1. Insertion of the catheter in the midline of the epidural space rather than in the lateral extremities of the space, where epidural veins are most plentiful.

2. Careful aspiration through the epidural catheter before it is taped in place.

3. Use of appropriate test doses through the catheter, both at the initial induction and with each succeeding "top-up" injection (97).

4. Injection of "top-up" doses in the lateral position or in marked pelvic tilt, but not with the mother lying on her back.

Ideally, test doses should contain ingredients that will give early warning if the epidural needle or catheter is either in the vascular or the subarachnoid compartment. A small dose of rapidly acting local anesthetic (e.g., lidocaine) is appropriate for warning of accidental subarachnoid injection. Test doses to exclude accidental intravascular injection are more controversial. In the past the α and β effect of epinephrine in doses of 15 to 20 μg were considered to cause sufficiently large changes in pulse and blood pressure and subjective pounding of the pulse to warn of intravenous injection without causing fetal distress (99). It has been argued that false positives may arise from intercurrent uterine contractions and that transient fetal distress may be caused by the small dose of epinephrine (99, 100).

However, continuous tracings of maternal heart rate do indicate that transient but significant tachycardia is reliably evident after an intravenous test dose injection (even when the patient is unaware of any symptoms) if 10 ml of 0.125% bupivacaine with 1:800,000 epinephrine (i.e., 12.5 mg bupivacaine and 12.5 μg epinephrine) are injected slowly over 30 to 60 sec. This test dose procedure has been shown to avoid fetal distress and to fulfill the requirements of an effective warning against accidental intravenous or subarachnoid injection (101).

Whether test doses are used with epinephrine, or not, careful fractionation of the main induction dose will allow for premonitory warning signs of toxicity to develop if accidental intravascular injection has occurred; so that the procedure can be halted and revised before an overwhelmingly toxic bolus has been administered.

Treatment of convulsions from extradural venous injection is along standard lines with (a) turning of mother into lateral posture; (b) hyperventilation with oxygen; (c) intravenous diazepam; (d) succinylcholine and endotracheal intubation if convulsions do not immediately subside; (e) vasopressor therapy if arterial hypotension occurs; and (f) electrical defibrillation if ventricular fibrillation occurs. Relatively modest intravenous doses of the lipid-soluble agents etidocaine and bupivacaine may cause resistant cardiac arrest, and resuscitative measures may have to be continued for as long as 45 min. One such prolonged, but eventually successful, resuscitation in a male is reported after a caudal injection of 250 mg of 1% plain etidocaine (103).

Resuscitation must be carried out with full left-lateral pelvic tilt to ensure adequate venous return through the inferior vena cava, otherwise efforts may not overcome the fatal combination of a toxic myocardium and poorly filled cardiac chambers.

CHRONIC NEUROLOGIC COMPLICATIONS

Trauma

Trauma to nerve pathways may occur during labor from causes unrelated to regional anesthesia, as reviewed earlier in this chapter. The incidence of direct neurologic trauma from spinal or epidural needles and catheters is extremely rare. Pressure on the cord or spinal roots by a needle point is accompanied by severe lancinating pain, and this is a signal to withdraw the needle immediately. Trauma to the spinal cord can be avoided by making spinal or epidural puncture below the termination of the conus medullaris. The cord usually ends at the level of the first lumbar intervertebral disc, but occasionally it may extend lower to the level of the disc between the second and third lumbar vertebrae (Fig. 24.4). Therefore selection of the third or fourth interspace is a prudent initial step in performing subarachnoid or epidural puncture.

Epidural catheters have been suspected of causing trauma to spinal nerve roots. Transient paresthesia occurs relatively frequently during insertion of an epidural catheter, but is harmless and attributable to the catheter tip gliding past a dural root sleeve. Persistent paresthesia is very rare and usually indicates that the catheter tip may have lodged against a root sleeve in an intervertebral foramen, where much of the injected anesthetic may escape into the paravertebral space and be wasted. The catheter should be withdrawn and resited. In cases in which it was suspected that an epidural catheter may have caused root trauma, there were always alternative and more likely causes, and there is no objective evidence of neurologic trauma caused by a modern epidural catheter inserted in awake patients when the puncture has been in the lumbar region and below the termination of the spinal cord.

Stiff intrathecal catheters for continuous subarachnoid analgesia may be capable of damaging the soft spinal cord. During experiments in dogs in which percutaneous intracisternal catheters were passed downwards in the subarachnoid space, some catheters could penetrate the cord with surprising ease and could travel some distance in it without any appreciable sense of resistance being transmitted to the operator's fingers.

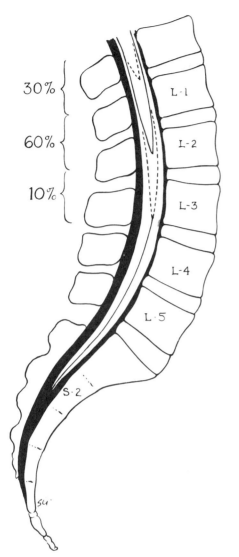

Figure 24.4. Variations of the level of termination of the spinal cord. The figures (*left*) indicate the approximate percentage of each level that was found among 129 specimens. Extradural space is shown in *black* and subarachnoid space in *white*. (Reprinted by permission from Bonica JJ: *Principles and Practice of Obstetric Anesthesia, Vol 1*. FA Davis, Philadelphia, 1969, p 552; adapted from data by Reimann AE, Anson BJ: Vertebral level of termination of the spinal cord with a report of a case of sacral cord. Anat Rec 88:127, 1944.)

There is a current resurgence of interest in continuous subarachnoid anesthesia for surgery and obstetrics, especially now that the risk of postspinal headache has been reduced by the manufacture of fine microcatheters of 32-gauge diameters, designed to pass through 26-gauge spinal needles (104). However, significant technical difficulties have been reported with these catheters (105), and it is premature to assess their association with neurologic sequelae.

Complications of Vascular Origin

HEMATOMA

Subarachnoid or epidural puncture is sometimes associated with a little blood-stained reflux in the needle or catheter. Thus it must be assumed that minor injuries to the large, thin-walled epidural veins are common. Under normal circumstances, bleeding stops and no untoward effects occur. However, coagulopathies may be associated with spontaneous pathologic bleeding in any of the three spaces surrounding the spinal cord: (*a*) the epidural space; (*b*) the subdural space, between the dura mater and pia-arachnoid; or (*c*) the subarachnoid space. Subsequent pressure on the cord may cause permanent paralysis. Clearly, passage of a spinal needle or catheter in the presence of a coagulopathy increases the danger of intraspinal bleeding. The epidural space is the most commonly reported site for hemorrhage within the spinal cord (106, 107). The subarachnoid space is the next most common site (108–110), whereas hemorrhage in the subdural space is exceedingly rare (111–114).

Subarachnoid or epidural blockade should be avoided in the presence of clotting abnormalities or a low platelet count or when anticoagulants are being administered to the mother. However, difficult decisions in anesthetic management may have to be made when the mother and child would benefit from continuous epidural blockade and yet, reasonable grounds exist for suspecting the development of a coagulopathy, such as in preeclamptic toxemia. Under these circumstances, relative risks and benefits should be carefully discussed with all concerned and should be well documented in the patient's chart.

The obstetric anesthesiologist, called at short notice with a request to administer epidural or subarachnoid anesthesia, is often faced with a difficult decision when there are grounds to suspect that the clotting mechanisms may not be functioning adequately to seal off any venous trauma caused by his epidural needle or catheter. Coagulopathies are dealt with in Chapter 19, and this section will merely review the salient features of platelet function and clotting tests that are immediately relevant to appropriate anesthetic decisions.

The preanesthetic interview may give a hint of long-standing clotting deficiencies if there is a history or evidence of easy bruising of the ankles or other exposed parts. Mild bleeding of the gums after dental toilet is a frequent and normal accompaniment of late pregnancy and is not a reliable indicator of a coagulation defect. The diagnosis of toxemia should raise a strong suspicion of possible deficiencies in the coagulation profile, especially in the presence of a recently depressed platelet count and a prolonged bleeding time. The relevance of the bleeding time to intraspinal bleed is controversial and some authorities consider it unhelpful as a single definitive test (115a). However, I believe an accurately performed bleeding time provides one of the most relevant answers to the question of whether a patient is likely to bleed intraspinally, provided the test is regarded as only one of several signs to guide appropriate decisions (115b, 115c).

In preeclampsia, platelet deficiencies are characterized by increased platelet consumption and shortened platelet life span, leading to a decreased platelet count, with the surviving platelets suffering from some degree of impaired function (116). Platelet counts of over 100×10^9/liter probably indicate normal platelet function and may not require an immediate bleeding time as a confirmatory test for the suitability of regional anesthesia (117). However, counts between 50 to 100×10^9/liter or a count that is falling towards 100×10^9/liter may indicate some dysfunction, and I believe a bleeding time test should be performed. Counts of less than 50×10^9/liter have predictably prolonged bleeding times (115–117); thus the test becomes unnecessary, since subarachnoid and epidural injections are probably contraindicated at this low level of platelet competence. Isolated reports of successful and uncomplicated epidural anesthesia in the presence of profound thrombocytopenia should not be regarded as a license to undertake the risk of spinal puncture if there is clinical or laboratory evidence of significant platelet suppression (118).

Bleeding times are most conveniently and reliably performed by the modified and standardized Ivy technique using a spring-operated, disposable device, such as the Simplate-II (Organon Teknika Corporation, Durham, NC), which delivers two small cuts 5-mm long and 0.5-mm deep. This device is painless, leaves no scar, and is easy to operate. Normal bleeding times with an arm cuff pressure of 40 mm Hg average about 5 min, with an upper acceptable limit of 9½ min. In this author's opinion the device should be available in every obstetric unit, and anesthesiologists should be willing and able to perform the test with reasonable accuracy at the bedside, if laboratory response times are likely to be longer than 30 min. The decision of whether to perform epidural (or subarachnoid) anesthesia without undue risk of hematoma formation can then be made with improved confidence, based on the objective evidence of a recent and acceptable platelet count *and* the immediate bedside bleeding time. If bleeding times cannot be obtained at short notice, it is prudent to set the lowest acceptable platelet count at 100×10^9/liter and to defer epidural or subarachnoid punc-

tures, rather than expose the patient to the possible risk of intraspinal hematoma.

Paralysis from intraspinal hematoma is a dire emergency, and urgent surgical decompression of the cord is indicated. Recovery is likely if this is done within 6 hours, but permanent paralysis usually follows if surgery is delayed (119). However, very rarely a patient may make a spontaneous partial recovery in spite of severe neurologic deficits lasting for several hours (120a, 120b).

OTHER VASCULAR LESIONS

Other vascular lesions, such as the anterior spinal artery syndrome, are rare possibilities in an elderly population, but they may also be seen in women of childbearing age if severe arterial hypotension occurs in the peripartum period (120c). Vascular lesions unrelated to regional anesthesia, such as arteriovenous malformations, have been discussed earlier in this chapter.

INFECTION

Infection of the epidural or subarachnoid space is an extremely rare event, but it is devastating when it does occur. Infection in the spinal canal is usually secondary to infection elsewhere in the body, and only very rarely is it introduced from an exogenous source (121). Nevertheless, there is a temptation to lower aseptic standards in the hurly-burly conditions of a busy delivery suite, and this temptation must be resisted by all concerned. The anesthesiologist and all those in close attendance should wear face masks during the performance of subarachnoid or epidural blocks and during the performance of epidural blood patch for relief of postdural puncture headache.

It is extremely unlikely that single subarachnoid or epidural injections will introduce exogenous infection, but continuous epidural and caudal techniques establish multiple opportunities for contamination. Micropore filters have been recommended as a protection against both particulate and microbial invasion of the epidural space, but the pore size must be 0.2 μm or less to exclude common bacterial contaminants. Some disposable epidural trays include a filter of 1-μm pore size. However, these large pores are not of any benefit in excluding bacteria, although they can keep out microscopic particles of broken glass that often contaminate solutions from glass ampoules (122, 123).

EPIDURAL ABSCESS

Baker and her associates (124) reviewed 39 cases of pyogenic spinal epidural abscess over a period of 27 years at the Massachusetts General Hospital. In 38 of these, the abscess was secondary to endogenous infection elsewhere in the body. Only one case was associated with an epidural catheter, and this patient did not suffer any permanent sequelae. A more recent 12-year survey of 35 cases of epidural abscess from the New York Hospital did not include a single case following epidural analgesia.

One case of puerperal spinal epidural abscess and paraplegia has been reported (125). This followed an attack of infectious hepatitis. However, membranes had not ruptured prematurely; there was no prodromal fever or chorioamnionitis; and no intraspinal regional anesthesia had been administered. Several furuncular spots were found that had apparently been present before delivery. The authors pointed out the potentially adverse medicolegal implications that would have arisen if an epidural anesthetic had been given, a situation in common with any coincidental adverse neurologic outcome following administration of epidural or spinal anesthesia under any circumstances (126).

Symptoms and signs of acute epidural abscess develop rapidly and inexorably, and anesthesiologists should be familiar with the cardinal signs. Four signs are almost always present: (a) severe back pain, (b) local overlying tenderness, (c) fever, and (d) leukocytosis. Treatment is by urgent spinal decompression. Paraplegia is almost inevitable unless laminectomy is done at an early stage.

Because there is a risk of metastatic epidural infection from established infectious processes elsewhere in the body, the question arises of whether it is safe to induce epidural analgesia in the presence of preexisting infection and bacteremia. For example, what policy should be adopted in the face of prematurely ruptured membranes and signs of developing amnionitis?

Anesthetic practice has been divided on this point. Some authors are sanguine about inducing epidural blockade in the presence of chorioamnionitis (127, 128), whereas others have been more cautious and have advised against it (129, 130). The issue may be clarified and a middle ground met by briefly summarizing some of the relevant evidence to date.

1. Despite the widespread use of epidural anesthesia in the presence of prematurely ruptured membranes and mild fever, no case of epidural abscess has been reported following this practice. In one retrospective study, 115 major conduction blocks (113 epidurals and 2 spinals) were performed in patients who had developed signs of bacteremia from chorioamnionitis. None of these patients developed signs or symptoms of epidural abscess or meningitis, but it must be noted that all of them received antibiotics before or after performance of the blocks (131).

2. Epidural abscess can arise spontaneously in the presence of bacteremia, as indicated earlier, and is probably more likely to occur if free blood is present to act as a nidus of culture medium in the epidural space.

3. One study in rats made bacteremic with *Escherichia coli* found no CNS complications if the dura was intact, whereas 30% of the animals developed meningitis if the dura was punctured (132).

4. Epidural puncture carries a risk of accidental dural puncture that varies between less than 0.5% to greater than 5%, depending on the expertise of the operator.

5. Fortunately, the bacteremia of chorioamnionitis is usually controllable by appropriate antibiotic therapy (133, 134).

On the basis of this summary, the prudent middle course, which avoids maternal danger while providing the benefits of conduction blockade, would seem to be the following:

1. In the presence of signs of systemic infection from chorioamnionitis (Table 24.4) ensure that antibiotic coverage is started *before* proceeding to epidural blockade.

2. Perform the block as meticulously and gently as possible.

3. If in doubt about the feasibility of an atraumatic puncture, abandon regional anesthesia and proceed to systemic analgesia for labor and to general anesthesia for cesarean section.

4. If a block is performed, it is wise to instruct the patient and her partner in the premonitory symptoms and signs of epidural abscess, so that valuable time can be saved and permanent sequelae avoided by instituting the appropriate investigation and treatment as soon as possible after early warning signs develop.

SUBARACHNOID INFECTION

Subarachnoid infection is now an extremely rare complication of regional anesthesia in obstetrics, and the cause may be hard to determine. There is only

Table 24.4
Clinical Criteria for Diagnosing Intraamniotic Infection

Diagnostic Criteria	Percentage Positive Finding[a,b]
Ruptured membranes	100
Fever >37.8°C	100
Maternal tachycardia (>100 bpm)	84
Leukocytosis (>15,000 mm^3)	67
Fetal tachycardia (>160 bpm)	58
Uterine tenderness	25
Foul amniotic fluid	7

[a] Reprinted by permission from Yoder PR, Gibbs RS, Blanco JD, Castaneda YS, St. Clair PJ: A prospective, controlled study of maternal and perinatal outcome after intraamniotic infection at term. Am J Obstet Gynecol 145:695–701, 1983.
[b] Infection confirmed by positive amniotic fluid culture.

one recent report of two cases of puerperal meningitis, but it is a reminder that all possible precautions must be taken to prevent epidural analgesia from becoming a source of CNS infection. In one of the cases, infection appeared to be blood-borne from infected genitalia. However, the second patient showed signs of inflammation around the catheter site, indicating the epidural to be the primary source of the subarachnoid infection (136). Micropore filters were not used in either of these cases, perhaps suggesting that these filters do perform a useful protective function in spite of earlier reports that the incidence of infection is too low to justify their use (137). Cases of chronic adhesive arachnoiditis are probably related to preexisting chronic infection of the spinal canal (138, 139).

In 1980 chloroprocaine came under suspicion as a potential subarachnoid irritant. Some cases of massive subarachnoid injection of 3% chloroprocaine were followed by neurologic complications that varied from delayed recovery to signs of chronic adhesive arachnoiditis (140, 141). The cause was thought to be a combination of factors, including a low pH of 3.1 (142) and the presence of sodium bisulphite as an antioxidant in the formulation of the local anesthetic (143). Sodium bisulphite was excluded from the formulation in 1987, and at the present time general consensus is that chloroprocaine is a safe agent when properly used (144). This topic is discussed at greater length in Chapter 6.

Multidose vials of local anesthetic should not be used for epidural or subarachnoid anesthesia because they contain preservatives such as methylparaben, that are known to be a potential source of delayed arachnoiditis. Moreover, absolute sterility cannot be guaranteed for successive doses once the vial has been broached. One recent report from Italy reviews six cases of arachnoiditis and paralysis following epidural anesthesia with 0.5% bupivacaine plus 1:200,000 epinephrine in which this rule was broken and multiple dose vials were used in five of the six cases. The source of local anesthetic could not be traced in the sixth case. The authors of this report impute the epinephrine as a possible cause of these tragedies, but the real fault would seem to lie in the misuse of multiple-dose vials (145).

VIRAL INFECTIONS

A number of viral infections may cause puerperal paralysis, and if spinal or epidural anesthesia has been used, suspicion is usually cast on the anesthetic as a contributory cause to the adverse outcome rather than as merely associated in time. This section is restricted to the anesthetic implications of two increasingly common viral infections, namely, herpes simplex virus (HSV) and the human immunodeficiency virus (HIV) of the acquired immunodeficiency syndrome (AIDS).

Herpes Simplex Virus (HSV)

Parturients with genital herpes frequently present for cesarean section in the hope of avoiding infection of the child during its passage through a birth canal that may be shedding active virus. Primary HSV infection is associated with viremia, and on rare occasions it may spread widely within the CNS. The severity of the disease is increased during pregnancy, and most cases of disseminated herpetic neurologic sequelae have occurred in pregnant women (146). Therefore it is prudent to avoid major regional anesthesia in such potentially threatening circumstances (147). However, recurrent herpetic lesions in patients with a previous history of genital or oral herpes are limited anatomically to the sacral or trigeminal dermatomes innervated by the sensory ganglia in which the virus is entrenched and from which it migrates centrifugally along their axons to reach cutaneous tissue supplied by them (148, 149).

Generalized dissemination appears to be extremely unlikely during recrudescences in the chronic phases of genital or oral HSV infection. Several reports have reviewed hundreds of cases of cesarean section performed under epidural or spinal anesthesia in patients with secondary genital herpes infection without evidence of neurologic harm (147, 150, 151). Among these reports were five cases of primary infection, and one of these five received a spinal anesthetic. This patient experienced postpartum paresis of one leg, which lasted for a week, and although the deficit was initially attributed to the spinal anesthetic, the precise etiology of the transient palsy could not be clearly defined (151).

The current practice of administering epidural or intrathecal opiates for pain relief in labor and cesarean section has been associated with a greater incidence of reactivation of herpes labialis. However, to date, no reports have appeared of recrudescences of herpes genitalis after intraspinal opiates (152–155).

Human Immunodeficiency Virus (HIV)

Obstetric anesthesiologists should be alert to protect their patients (and themselves) from the possible adverse neurologic (and medicolegal) outcomes arising from occult HIV infection. This section summarizes the relevant context in which appropriate decisions regarding regional anesthesia must be made when faced with HIV-positive patients.

The acquired immunodeficiency syndrome (AIDS) is an inexorably fatal illness: Over 152,000 cases were reported in the United States by November 1, 1990

(156). As with former deadly diseases in the past, such as cholera and tuberculosis, society has been more eager to guard the social susceptibilities of infected individuals rather than to protect the health of the general population. AIDS, the inexorable endpoint of HIV infection, *is* a notifiable disease and must be reported in all states of the United States. However, the median time from HIV infection to development of recognizable AIDS is approximately 10 years; thus, for about a decade, the infected individual remains a potential victim of early AIDS-related sequelae and an occult source of transmissible infection to others. Despite the public health implications of HIV infection, at the time of writing HIV-positive status is not subject to mandatory notification in about one-half of the United States. In the other half it is notifiable, but only under conditions of ensured anonymity. Some individuals with coinfections are at greater risk for harboring HIV virus than others. For example, in one recent survey at a state-funded clinic for sexually transmitted diseases, HIV positivity was found in 21% of African-Americans under treatment for gonorrhea, as opposed to a mean of only 4.7% in the rest of the sample population (156).

It has been said that, currently, all undiagnosed spinal cord lesions should be considered HIV-positive until proven otherwise (157). Approximately 40% of AIDS patients become neurologically symptomatic (158). In autopsies of patients with AIDS, 22% revealed vacuolation of the spinal cord (159), and electron microscopy has shown large fiber losses in 48% of sural nerves (160). In one group of seropositive men, electrophysiologic tests revealed neurologic deficits in 48% whereas 6 to 9 months later the incidence had risen to 67% in the survivors (161).

These harrowing figures in an ever-increasing population of HIV-positive patients have difficult implications for the obstetric anesthesiologist. The informed consent process and preanesthetic interview should take these facts into account, especially if the patient has eluded antenatal care and the possibility of HIV testing.

At the present time there is no evidence that epidural or subarachnoid anesthesia will precipitate spinal pathology in HIV-positive patients; on the other hand, there is no evidence that it will not. In this population, there is a two-thirds chance of neurologic pathology and a two-thirds chance that occult neurologic cases will become overtly symptomatic before they die. A discussion of the risks and benefits of epidural analgesia with HIV-positive patients must therefore try to clarify, as gently and humanely as possible, the gamble that is being offered. Decision making becomes even more poignant for HIV-

positive patients with severe, prolonged, and disabling postdural puncture headache in which the proximate but statistically remote risk of intracranial subdural hematoma (discussed earlier) must be weighed against the statistically higher long-term neurologic risks of the underlying disease (162). It is this author's belief that epidural dextran should be tried as the first line of treatment, as indicated earlier in this chapter. However, epidural blood patch need *not* be withheld under these circumstances, provided proper informed consent has been obtained and witnessed and a second neurologic opinion is placed in the patient's record to support the decision that viremically infected blood will be used with the full knowledge and assent of all concerned.

CHEMICAL CONTAMINANTS OF THE SUBARACHNOID AND EPIDURAL SPACES

The epidural space seems to be remarkably tolerant of some chemical contaminants. For example, epidural injections of 6% aqueous phenol are used by some to relieve terminal cancer pain without any untoward sequelae, and yet the same solution would have disastrous results in the subarachnoid space. Accidental epidural injections of a number of incorrect solutions have been reported, including ephedrine, thiopental (on several occasions), magnesium sulphate (163), potassium chloride, and phenol, and even parenteral nutrition, with results that range from no sequelae to permanent paralysis. The damage caused by epidural potassium chloride appears to be concentration dependent. One observer noted transient effects with 0.2% KCl (164). Another reported intense motor and sensory blockade followed by painful depolarizing spasms with complete recovery after 6.4% KCl (165), whereas a third victim suffered complete paraplegia after 11.25% KCl (166). Interestingly enough, in another case accidental epidural injection of phenol was followed by 9 hr of effective analgesia but no neurologic sequelae after a dose of 30 ml of 0.2% phenol (167). The two cases of accidental epidural parenteral nutrition were equally fortunate. One patient received 300 ml of intralipid with an osmolality of 350 mOsm/kg over a 5-hr period and remained pain free for 24 hr (168). The other patient received 160 ml of hypertonic amino-acid mixture with an osmolality of 2000 mOsm/kg over 2 hr and remained pain free for 27 hr (169). Neither patient experienced any neurologic sequelae: Perhaps the hyperosmolar solution caused enough subliminal damage in the second patient to account for the prolonged analgesia. In one particularly scandalous case which received wide notoriety in Britain, an epidural "top-up" of *paraldehyde* was given to a photographic model during her first labor; permanent and painful tetraplegia followed this piece of negligence (170).

The fault in most of these cases lay in one or more of the following errors:

1. Picking up the wrong ampoule and not reading the label; a fault that can easily occur when drugs with widely different actions are marketed in very similar containers.

2. Not labeling drug-filled syringes, or labeling them incorrectly.

3. Not reading the label on the syringe.

4. Accidentally injecting intravenous medications through an epidural catheter.

All of these seemingly crass errors have been committed by well-trained personnel working under stressful conditions. The only remedy lies in:

1. Constant awareness of the danger.

2. Labeling syringes correctly immediately after they are filled.

3. Identifying all labeled syringes before administering their contents.

4. Never accepting an unlabeled syringe from a third party.

5. Checking the portal of injection to ensure that the right medication is not going into the wrong line, as illustrated by the parenteral nutrition debacles just described.

6. Capping and taping all side ports on epidural infusion lines.

The pia-covered cord and spinal roots in the subarachnoid space are more vulnerable to the effects of chemical contaminants than are the dural-covered elements in the epidural space. A hole in the dura from accidental dural puncture allows epidural solutions to leak into the subarachnoid space, particularly if the injection is made rapidly and under pressure. Thus contaminants that might have been innocuous when excluded by an intact dura become potentially harmful. Craig and Habib (171) reported a case of paraparesis from epidural injection of 1.5% *benzyl alcohol* under these circumstances as follows:

Accidental dural puncture with a 16-gauge needle occurred during induction of epidural analgesia for pain relief in a 24-year-old primiparous woman. After delivery 40 ml of 0.9 per cent saline were injected into the epidural space as a prophylactic measure against a low CSF pressure headache. Unfortunately the saline contained 1.5 per cent benzyl alcohol as a preservative. Paraparesis of the lower limbs followed. Recovery gradually took place over a period of about 16 months.

In this instance the concentration of benzyl alcohol was not high enough to cause damage in the epidural space, and it must be concluded that the saline and preservative leaked into the subarachnoid space through the large needle hole in the dura.

Traces of detergents used for cleaning reusable spinal needles and syringes have been imputed as a possible cause of myelitis if they are accidentally introduced into the subarachnoid space (172). This source of contamination may be considered as a possible explanation for six cases of grave neurologic sequelae reported from Porto Alegre, Brazil (173). Three of the six cases occurred in young women receiving epidural analgesia for childbirth. In all six cases the clinical picture was one of severe adhesive arachnoiditis of a chemical rather than an infective nature, but the cause could not be identified, and detergent contamination is only one of several possibilities.

AVOIDANCE AND DIAGNOSIS OF POSTPARTUM NEUROLOGIC DEFICITS

At the beginning of this chapter it was pointed out that a number of maternal neurologic accidents may attend the process of childbirth, regardless of whether or not a regional anesthetic is given. This section summarizes some of the more common decisions to be made in avoiding the use of regional anesthesia when risks appear to outweigh the benefits, as well as the diagnostic steps to take if an untoward neurologic deficit arises.

Avoidance of Associated Neurologic Deficits

Exhaustive study of the patient's record and elaborate history taking are impossible in the hurried environment of a busy obstetric unit, especially if labor is advanced and the mother is distracted by strong labor pains. If no antenatal anesthesia interview has been documented, an attempt must be made to elicit some salient pieces of information from the patient, her obstetrician, or both.

First, make the history taking as brief and as simple as possible. If a pitocin infusion is running at the time, have it shut off during your preanesthetic exchange of information and the subsequent performance of an epidural block for relief of labor pain. Involve the mother's partner in your interview if he is present. It may be prudent to have him cosign the written history. The history should focus on six major concerns:

1. Is the patient allergic to any drugs you may administer and is she taking any medications or recreational drugs at the present time?

2. Is there reason to suspect any preexisting neurologic compromise (e.g., preexisting sciatica or leg weakness or history of an accident)? If an accident, is it under litigation and did it involve the lumbar spine? If so, general anesthesia may be a preferred choice. On the other hand, if the accident involved both cervical and lumbar areas a lumbar epidural may be the lesser physical and medicolegal risk, provided the patient or husband cosign the preanesthetic notes. In addition, it is prudent to perform a quick check of the lower limb reflexes (these are usually very brisk during active labor), the Babinski sign,

and sensation in the outer border of the foot and calf (i.e., S1 and L5 dermatomes).

3. Has the patient undergone previous back surgery, and are there any cutaneous lesions on the back or signs that suggest underlying spina bifida occulta or a spinal angioma? If the patient has undergone previous surgery for scoliosis, is there a satisfactory interspinous space below the lowest level of fusion? If not, is there a satisfactory sacral hiatus that could be used for caudal anesthesia if outlet forceps are required?

4. Is the patient likely to bleed intraspinally? Is she receiving any medication that may depress platelet function? Does she bruise easily, or has there been an unusual amount of bleeding of the gums after dental hygiene? If so, and if the platelet count is low and only slightly above the cut-off point of 100,000/mm, it is wise to have a bleeding time performed.

5. Is systemic infection present, and if so, is the patient receiving appropriate antibiotics to protect against the risk of metastatic epidural abscess?

6. Finally, the mouth, teeth, and gape should be examined to confirm that endotracheal intubation will be feasible if an unexpected emergency should arise. Be sure to document the findings in the preanesthetic history and confirm that the risks and benefits of the proposed procedure are understood and accepted by the patient.

If epidural analgesia is to be induced in the patient's room, ensure proper sterility precautions. Use disposable manufactured block trays whenever possible. This author believes that all attendants present should be required to wear surgical masks when the tray is opened, since *Staphylococcus aureus* is the most common pathogen in acute epidural abscess, and any person in the room may be harboring it.

Diagnosis

Postpartum neurologic deficits inevitably focus suspicion on whatever regional anesthetic was used during childbirth. Therefore the anesthesiologist should have a clear scheme of investigation in his or her mind so that the necessary diagnostic and therapeutic resources can be deployed. The following questions must be answered:

1. Is the lesion real or imagined?
2. What is the site of the lesion?
3. What is the nature of the lesion?
4. What is the cause?
5. Is there any associated cause, such as diabetes, that requires investigation and treatment?

The following steps are taken in such an investigation.

HISTORY

A careful history is crucial, paying particular attention to the possibility of any antecedent sensory or motor disturbances in the lower limbs.

PHYSICAL EXAMINATION

Careful mapping of sensory and motor deficits, taking note of any sphincter disturbance, will establish whether the lesion is characteristic of a segmental or a peripheral injury. Examination of the back will reveal any local tenderness or cutaneous discoloration that might raise the suspicion of acute spinal infection or underlying arteriovenous anomaly.

SUPPORTING TESTS

According to the results of the history and physical examination, the following tests should be performed:

1. Spinal x-ray examination to ascertain the size and shape of lumbar disc spaces
2. Spinal CT scans at the level of the suspected lesion to help detect small lesions and foreign bodies, such as pieces of sheared epidural catheter
3. Magnetic resonance imaging (MRI) is an extremely helpful but expensive test, and it should be used with cost-benefit ratios in mind
4. Coagulogram to exclude clotting abnormalities
5. Lumbar or cisternal puncture for CSF examination, if indicated by signs and symptoms of epidural abscess
6. Myelography if spinal block is suspected
7. Electromyography of the leg and paraspinous muscles in the event of motor loss. Sequential examinations of limb and paraspinal muscles should be carried out to assess the evolution of denervation patterns and to establish whether the lesion is within the spinal canal and involves both anterior and posterior primary rami, or whether it is distal to the intervertebral foramen and involves only the limb muscles supplied by the anterior primary rami (174–176).

Investigation should also include other systems that may have causal significance. A glucose tolerance test and an examination of urine and feces should be done to exclude diabetes or porphyria as possible underlying causes of neuropathy. If the diagnosis remains obscure, HIV testing should be done in accordance with the dictum that all undiagnosed neurologic deficits should be suspected of HIV-positivity until proven otherwise (157).

Statistically, postpartum neurologic lesions are much more likely to arise from obstetric or natural causes than from the results of concomitant regional anesthesia. In a survey of 780,000 epidural blocks for all types of indications, Usubiaga (121) found an incidence of 1:11,000 neurologic complications. Other smaller populations at specialist centers have had even lower complication rates. Hellman (177) reported on more than 20,000 cesarean sections and vaginal deliveries with epidural anesthesia without a single major neurologic complication. Between 1956 and 1977 approximately 30,000 deliveries were conducted under epidural blockade at the Royal Victoria Hospital, Montreal. During that time several peripheral nerve injuries were attributed to obstetric causes, but no permanent neurologic sequelae were caused by regional anesthesia. The incidence of neurologic complications after well-conducted regional anesthesia is extremely low and far below the naturally occurring incidence of approximately 1 in 3000 that may be expected in a normal obstetric population.

SUMMARY

The neurologic complications of regional anesthesia for obstetrics may be transient or permanent. The transient complications are relatively common and cover a wide range of possibilities. All are trivial if properly managed, but some are potentially lethal if left untreated. Therefore it is of paramount importance that all clinicians using regional anesthesia for obstetrics should be prepared (a) to take all practical steps to avoid technical acts of omission or commission that may lead to neurologic complications and (b) to manage the acute complications that may arise. Permanent complications due to regional anesthesia are extremely rare, with an overall incidence of about 1 in 11,000 and an incidence of less than 1 in 20,000 in specialist centers. Neurologic complications due to natural or obstetric causes occur with an incidence of about 1 in 3000; these are usually trunk or peripheral nerve injuries that tend to resolve in 12 to 16 weeks. Therefore it is very important to be able to distinguish between obstetric and anesthetic causes of neurologic sequelae.

References

1. Turnbull A, Tindall VR, Beard RW, Robson G, Dawson IM, Cloake EP, Ashley JS, Botting B: Maternal deaths associated with anaesthesia. *Report on Confidential Enquiries into Maternal Deaths in England and Wales, 1982–1984.* Her Majesty's Stationery Office, London, 1989, No. 34, pp 96–106.
2. Scott DB, Hibbard BM: Serious nonfatal complications associated with extradural block in obstetric practice. Br J Anaesth 64:537–541, 1990.
3. Donaldson JO: *Neurology of Pregnancy,* 2nd ed. WB Saunders, Philadelphia, 1989.
4. Schreiner EJ, Lipson SF, Bromage PR, Camporesi EM: Neurological complications following general anaesthesia: Three cases of major paralysis. Anaesthesia 38:226–229, 1983.
5. Beatty TE: Second report of the new Lying-in-Hospital, Dublin. Dublin J Med Sci 12:273–313, 1838.
6. Lambrinudi C: Maternal birth palsy. Br J Surg 12:554–557, 1924.
7. Bromage PR: Epidural analgesia for obstetrics. In *Epidural Analgesia.* WB Saunders, Philadelphia, 1978, pp 586–587.
8. La Ban MM, Perrin JCS, Latimer FR: Pregnancy and the herniated disc. Arch Phys Med Rehabil 64:319–321, 1983.
9. Lazorthes G, Poulhes J, Bastide G, Chancolle AR, Azedeh O: La vascularization de la moelle épinière (étude) anatomique et physiologigue). Rev Neurol 106:535–557, 1962.

10. Lazorthes G, Gouazé A, Bastide G, Soutoul JH, Zadeh O, Santini JJ: La vascularization arterielle du rénflement lombaire: Etudes des variations et des suppléances. Rev Neurol 114:109–122, 1966.
11. Bademosi O, Osuntokun BO, Van der Werd HJ, Bademosi AD, Ojo OA: Obstetric neuropraxia in the Nigerian African. Int J Gynaecol Obstet 17:611–614, 1980.
12. Bromage PR: Personal correspondence, 1984.
13. Bromage PR: Anatomy: Arterial supply of the spinal cord. Neurological complications. In *Epidural Analgesia,* WB Saunders, Philadelphia, 1978, pp 54, 680.
14. Rosenblum B, Oldfield EH, Doppman JL, DiChiro G: Spinal arteriovenous malformations: A comparison of dural arteriovenous fistulas and intradural AVMs in 81 patients. J Neurosurg 67:795–802, 1987.
15. Choi IS, Borenstein A: Surgical neuroangiography of the spine and spinal cord. Radiol Clin North Am 26:1131–1141, 1988.
16. Drexler H, Zaroura S, Shapira Y: Transient aphonia and quadriplegia during epidural anesthesia. Anesth Analg 64:365–366, 1985.
17. Hirsch NP, Child CS, Wijetilleka SA: Paraplegia caused by spinal angioma. Possible association with epidural analgesia. Anesth Analg 64:937–940, 1985.
18. Tillman AJB: Traumatic neuritis in the puerperium. Am J Obstet Gynecol 29:660–666, 1935.
19. Hill ED: Maternal obstetric paralysis. Am J Obstet Gynecol 83:1452–1460, 1962.
20. Murray RR: Maternal obstetric paralysis. Am J Obstet Gynecol 88:399–403, 1964.
21. Ong BY, Cohen MM, Esmail A, Cumming M, Kozody R, Palahniuk RJ: Paresthesia and motor dysfunction after labor and delivery. Anesth Analg 66:18–22, 1987.
22. MacArthur C, Lewis M, Knox EG, Crawford JS: Epidural anaesthesia and long-term backache after childbirth. Br Med J 301:9–12, 1990.
23. Vanderick G, Geerinckx K, Van Steenberge AL, DeMuylder E: Bupivacaine 0.125% in epidural block analgesia during childbirth: Clinical evaluation. Br J Anaesth 46:838–844, 1974.
24. Saunders NJ, Spiby H, Gilbert L, Fraser RB, Hall JR, Multon PM, Jackson A, Edmonds DK: Oxytocin infusion during second stage of labor in primiparous women using epidural analgesia: A randomized double-blind placebo controlled trial. Br Med J 299:1423–1426, 1989.
25. Fibuch EF, Opper SE: Back pain following epidurally administered nesacaine-MPF. Anesth Analg 69:113–115, 1989.
26. Stevens RA, Chester WL, Artuso JD, Bray JG, Nellestein JA: Back pain after epidural anesthesia with 2-chloroprocaine in volunteers. Reg Anesth 16:199–203, 1991.
27. Hynson JM, Sessler DI, Glosten B, McGuire J: Back pain following chloroprocaine anesthesia. Anesthesiology 73:A48, 1990.
28. Lee JJ, Roberts RB: Paresis of the fifth cranial nerve following spinal anesthesia. Anesthesiology 49:217–218, 1978.
29. Pavlin DJ, McDonald JS, Child B, Rusch V: Acute subdural hematoma—An unusual sequela to lumbar puncture. Anesthesiology 51:338–340, 1979.
30. Edelman JD, Wingard DW: Subdural hematomas after lumbar dural puncture. Anesthesiology 52:166–167, 1980.
31. Newrick P, Read D: Subdural hematoma as a complication of spinal anesthetic. Br Med J 285:341–342, 1982.
32. Ready LB, Culpin S, Hascke R, Nessby M: Spinal needle determinants of rate of transdural fluid leak. Anesth Analg 69:457–460, 1989.
33. Gielen M: Postdural puncture headache (PDPH): A review. Reg Anesth 14:100–106, 1989.
34. Ravindran RS, Viegas OJ, Tasch MD, Cline PJ, Deaton RL, Brown TR: Bearing down at the time of delivery and the incidence of spinal headache in parturients. Anesth Analg 60:524–526, 1981.
35. Cherala S, Halpern M, Eddi D, Shevade K: Occurrence of headache related to accidental dural puncture effect of bearing down at the time of delivery. Reg Anesth 15:6S, 1990.
36. Franksson C, Gordh T: Headache after spinal anaesthesia and

a technique for lessening its frequency. Acta Chir Scand 94:443–454, 1946.

37. Mihic DN: Postspinal headache and relationship of needle bevel to longitudinal dural fibers. Reg Anesth 10:76–81, 1985.

38. Lybecker H, Moller JT, May O, Nielsen HK: Incidence and prediction of postdural puncture headache: A prospective study of 1021 spinal anesthesias. Anesth Analg 70:389–394, 1990.

39. Norris MC, Leighton BL, DeSimone CA: Needle bevel direction and headache after inadvertent dural puncture. Anesthesiology 70:729–731, 1989.

40. Bromage PR: Identification of the epidural space. In *Epidural Analgesia*. WB Saunders, Philadelphia, 1978, p 195.

41. Lubenow T, Ken-Wong E, Kristof K, Ivankovich O, Ivankovich AD: Inadvertent subdural injection: A complication of an epidural block. Anesth Analg 67:175–179, 1988.

42. Hatfalvi BI: The dynamics of postspinal headache. Headache 17:64–67, 1977.

43. Younker D, Jones MM, Adenwala J, Citrin A, Joyce TH III: Maternal cortical vein thrombosis and the obstetric anesthesiologist. Anesth Analg 68:1007–1012, 1986.

44. Gerwitz EC, Costin M, Marx GF: Cortical vein thrombosis may mimic postdural puncture headache. Reg Anesth 12:188–190, 1987.

45. Ravindran RS, Zandstra G, Viegas OJ: Postpartum headache following regional analgesia: A symptom of cerebral venous thrombosis. Can J Anaesth 36:705–707, 1989.

46. Llewellyn CG, Campbell R, Quartey GR: Intracranial subdural hematoma complicating metrizamide myelography. J Can Assoc Radiol 39:230–231, 1988.

47. Blake DW, Donnan G, Jensen D: Intracranial subdural haematoma following spinal anaesthesia. Anaesth Intensive Care 15:341–342, 1987.

48. Macon ME, Armstrong L, Brown EM: Subdural hematoma following spinal anesthesia. Anesthesiology 72:380–381, 1990.

49. Mantia AM: Clinical report of occurrence of an intracranial hemorrhage following postlumbar puncture headache. Anesthesiology 55:684–685, 1981.

50. Cullen WA, Griffith HR: Postpartum results of spinal anesthesia in obstetrics. Anesth Analg 26:114–121, 1947.

51. Jones RJ: The role of recumbency in the prevention and treatment of postspinal headache. Anesth Analg 53:788–796, 1974.

52. Carbaat PAT, van Grevel H: Lumbar puncture headache: Controlled study on the preventive effect of 24 hour's bed rest. Lancet 2:1133–1135, 1981.

53. Cook PT, Davies MJ, Beavis RE: Bed rest and post lumbar puncture headache: The effectiveness of 24-hour recumbency in reducing the incidence of postlumbar puncture headache. Anaesthesia 44:389–391, 1989.

54. Thornberry EA, Thomas TA: Posture and postspinal headache: A controlled trial in 80 patients. Br J Anaesth 60:195–197, 1988.

55. Miyakawa Y, Meyer JS, Ishihara N, Naritomi H, Nakal K, Hsu MC, Deshmukih MS: Effect of cerebrospinal fluid removal on cerebral blood flow and metabolism in the baboon: Influence of tyrosine infusion and cerebral embolism on cerebrospinal fluid pressure autoregulation. Stroke 8:346–351, 1977.

56. Dodd JE, Efird RC, Rauck RL: Cerebral blood flow changes with caffeine therapy for postdural headaches. Anesthesiology 71:A679, 1989.

57. Camann WR, Murray RS, Mushlin PS, Lambert DH: Effects of oral caffeine on postdural puncture headache: A double blind placebo-controlled trial. Anesth Analg 70:181–184, 1990.

58. Jarvis AP, Greenwalt JW, Fagraeus L: Intravenous caffeine for postdural puncture headache. Anesth Analg 65:316–317, 1986.

59. Ilioff G, Strelec SR, Rothfus W, Teeple E: Does prophylactic ultramuscular caffeine sodium benzoate decrease incidence of postdural puncture headache? Reg Anesth 15:65S, 1990.

60. Crawford JS: The prevention of headache consequent upon dural puncture. Br J Anaesth 44:598–600, 1972.

61. Okell RW, Sprigge JS: Unintentional dural puncture: A survey of recognition and management. Anaesthesia 42:1110–1113, 1987.

62. Barrios-alarcon J, Aldrete JA, Parajas-Topia D: Relief of postlumbar puncture headache with epidural dextran-40: A preliminary report. Reg Anesth 14:78–80, 1989.

63. Gormley JB: Treatment of postspinal headache. Anesthesiology 21:565–566, 1960.

64. Szeinfeld M, Ihmeidan TH, Moser MM, Machado R, Klose KJ, Serafini AN: Epidural blood patch: An evaluation of the volume and spread of blood injected into the epidural space. Anesthesiology 64:820–822, 1986.

65. Carrie LES: Epidural blood patch: Why the rapid response? Anesth Analg 72:129–130, 1991.

66. Ackerman WE, Colclough GW: Prophylactic epidural blood patch: The controversy continues. Anesth Analg 66:913, 1987.

67. Cheek TG, Banner R, Sauter J, Gutsche BB: Prophylactic extradural blood patch is effective. Br J Anaesth 61:340–342, 1988.

68. Trevedi NS, Eddi D, Shevde K: Prevention of headache following inadvertent dural puncture. Reg Anesth 14:51S, 1989.

69. Colonna-Romano P, Shapiro BE: Unintentional dural puncture and proplylactic epidural blood patch in obstetrics. Anesth Analg 69:522–523, 1989.

70. Lievers D: Total spinal anesthesia following proplyactic epidural blood patch. Anesthesiology 73:1287–1289, 1990.

71. Webb PJ, James FM, Wheeler AS: Shivering during epidural analgesia in women in labor. Anesthesiology 55:706–707, 1981.

72. Workhoven MN: Intravenous fluid temperature, shivering and the parturient. Anesth Analg 65:496–498, 1986.

73. Aglio LS, Johnson MD, Datta S, Ostheimer GW: Warm intravenous fluids reduce shivering in parturients receiving epidural analgesia. Anesthesiology 69:A701, 1988.

74. Sevorino FB, Johnson MD, Lema MJ, Datta S, Ostheimer GW, Maulty JS: The effect of epidural sufentanil on shivering and body temperature in the parturient. Anesth Analg 68:530–533, 1989.

75. Browndridge P: Shivering related to epidural blockade with bupivacaine in labour, and the influence of epidural pethidine. Anaesth Intensive Care 14:412–417, 1986.

76. Kepes ER, Martinez LR, Pantuck E, Stark DC: Horner's syndrome following caudal anesthesia. NY State J Med 72:946–947, 1972.

77. Carrie LES, Mohan J: Horner's syndrome following obstetric extradural block. Br J Anaesth 48:611, 1976.

78. Kerr FWL, Alexander S: Descending autonomic pathways in the spinal cord. Arch Neurol 10:249–261, 1964.

79. Fagraeus L, Urban BJ, Bromage PR: Spread of epidural analgesia in early pregnancy. Anesthesiology 58:184–187, 1983.

80. Datta S, Lambert DH, Gregus J, Gissen A, Covino BC: Effect of pregnancy on bupivacaine induced conduction blockade in the isolated rabbit vagus nerve. Anesth Analg 66:123–126, 1987.

81. Flanagan HL, Datta S, Lambert DH, Gissen AJ, Covino BG: Effect of pregnancy on bupivacaine induced conduction blockade in the isolated rabbit vagus nerve. Anesth Analg 66:123–126, 1987.

82. Bromage PR: An evaluation of bupivacaine in epidural analgesia for obstetrics. Can Anaesth Soc 16:46–56, 1969.

83. Pathy GV, Rosen M: Prolonged block with recovery after extradural analgesia for labour. Br J Anaesth 47:520–522, 1975.

84. Cuerden C, Buley R, Downing JW: Delayed recovery after epidural block in labour: A report of four cases. Anaesthesia 32:773–776, 1971.

85. Boys JE, Norman PF: Accidental subdural analgesia. Br J Anaesth 47:1111–1113, 1975.

86. Manchanda VN, Murad SHN, Shilyansky G, Mehringer M: Unusual clinical course of accidental subdural local anaesthetic injection. Anesth Analg 62:1124–1126, 1983.

87. Stevens RA, Stanton-Hicks MD: Subdural injection of local anesthetic: A complication of epidural analgesia. Anesthesiology 63:323–326, 1985.

88. Miller DC, Choi WW, Chestnut DH: Subdural injection of local anesthetics and morphine: A complication of attempted epidural anesthesia. South Med J 82:87–89, 1989.

89. Jones MD, Newton TH: Inadvertent extra-arachnoid injection in myelography. Radiology 80:818–822, 1963.

90. Schultz EH, Brogdon BG: The problem of subdural placement in myelography. Radiology 79:91–96, 1962.

91. Scehzer SH: Subdural space in anesthesia. Anesthesiology 24:869–870, 1963.

92. Lubenow T, Keh-Wong E, Kristof K, Ivankovich O, Ivankovich AD: Inadvertent subdural injection: A complication of an epidural block. Anesth Analg 67:175–179, 1988.

93. Crosby ET, Halpern S: Failure of a lidocaine test dose to identify subdural placement of an epidural catheter. Can J Anaesth 36:445–447, 1989.

94. Hardy PAJ: Can epidural catheters penetrate dura mater? An anatomical study. Anaesthesia 41:1146–1147, 1986.

95. Meiklejohn BH: The effect of rotation of an epidural needle: An in vitro study. Anaesthesia 42:1180–1182, 1987.

96. Phillips DC, MacDonald R: Epidural catheter migration in labour. Anaesthesia 42:661–663, 1987.

97. Kenepp NB, Gutsche BB: Inadvertent intravascular injections during lumbar epidural anesthesia. Anesthesiology 54:172–173, 1981.

98. McGown RG: Accidental marrow sampling during caudal anaesthesia. Br J Anaesth 44:613–615, 1972.

99. Moore DC, Batra MS: The components of an effective test dose prior to epidural block. Anesthesiology 55:693–696, 1981.

100. Leighton BL, Norris MC, Sosis M, Epstein R, Chayen B, Larijani GE: Limitations of epinephrine as a marker of intravascular injection in laboring women. Anesthesiology 66:688–691, 1987.

101. Dain SL, Rolbin SH, Hew EM: The epidural test dose in obstetrics: Is it necessary? Can J Anaesth 34:601–605, 1987.

102. Geerinckx K, Vanderick G, Van Steenberge AL, R Bouche, De Muylder E: Bupivacaine 0.125% in epidural block analgesia during childbirth: Maternal and foetal plasma concentrations. Br J Anaesth 46:937–941, 1974.

103. Prentiss JE: Cardiac arrest following caudal anesthesia. Anesthesiology 50:51–53, 1979.

104. Hurley RJ, Lambert DH: Continuous spinal anesthesia with a microcatheter technique: Preliminary experience. Anesth Analg 70:97–102, 1990.

105. Nagle CJ, McQuay HJ, Glynn CJ: 32-gauge spinal catheters through 26-gauge needles. Anesthesia 45:1052–1054, 1990.

106. Packer NP, Cummins BH: Spontaneous epidural haemorrhage: A surgical emergency. Lancet 1:356–358, 1978.

107. Bromage PR: Neurological complications. In Epidural Analgesia. WB Saunders, Philadelphia, 1978, pp 668–671.

108. Rengachary SS, Murphy D: Subarachnoid hematoma following lumbar puncture causing compression of the cauda equina. J Neurosurg 41:252–254, 1974.

109. Masdeu JC, Breuer AC, Schoene WC: Spinal subarachnoid hematomas: Clue to a source of bleeding in traumatic lumbar puncture. Neurology 29:872–876, 1979.

110. Mayumi T, Dohi S: Spinal subarachnoid hematoma after lumbar puncture in a patient receiving antiplatelet therapy. Anesth Analg 62:777–779, 1983.

111. Edelson RN, Chernik NL, Posner JB: Spinal subdural hematomas complicating lumbar puncture. Arch Neurol 31:134–137, 1974.

112. Guy MJ, Zahra M, Sengupta RP: Spontaneous spinal subdural haematoma during general anaesthesia. Surg Neurol 11:199–200, 1979.

113. Dunn D, Dhopesh V, Mobini J: Spinal subdural hematoma: A possible hazard of lumbar puncture in an alcoholic. JAMA 241:1712–1713, 1979.

114. Greensite FS, Katz J: Spinal subdural hematoma associated with attempted epidural anesthesia and subsequent continuous spinal anesthesia. Anesth Analg 59:72–73, 1980.

115a. Rodgers CRP, Levin J: A critical reappraisal of the bleeding time. Semin Thrombosis Hemostasis 16:1–20, 1990.

115b. Harker LA, Slichter SJ: The bleeding time as a screening test for evaluation of platelet function. N Engl J Med 287:155–159, 1972.

115c. Editorial: The bleeding time. Lancet 337:1447–1448, 1991.

116. Ramanathan J, Sibai BM, Vu T, Chauhan D: Correlation between bleeding times and platelet counts in women with preeclampsia undergoing cesarean section. Anesthesiology 71:188–191, 1989.

117. Kelton JG, Hunter DJS, Neame PB: A platelet function defect in pre-eclampsia. Obstet Gynecol 65:107–109, 1985.

118. Schindler M, Gatt S, Isert P, Morgans D, Cheung A: Thrombocytopenia and platelet functional defects in preeclampsia: Implications for regional anaesthesia. Anaesth Intensive Care 18:169–174, 1990.

119. Hew-Wing P, Rolbin SH, Hew E, Amato D: Epidural anaesthesia and thrombocytopenia. Anaesthesia 44:775–777, 1989.

120a. Harik SI, Raichle ME, Reis DJ: Spontaneous remitting spinal hematoma in a patient on anticoagulants. N Engl J Med 284:1355–1357, 1971.

120b. Messer HD, Forshan VR, Brust JCM, Hughes JEO: Transient paraplegia from hematoma after lumbar puncture: A consequence of anticoagulant therapy. JAMA 235:529–530, 1976.

120c. Ackerman WE, Mushtaque M, Juneja MD, Knapp RK: Maternal paraparesis after anesthesia and cesarean section. South Med J 83:695–697, 1990.

121. Usubiaga JE: Neurological complications following epidural analgesia. Int Anesthesiol Clin 13:19,50, 1975.

122. Katz H, Borden H, Hirscher D: Glass-particles contamination or color-break ampules (letter). Anesthesiology 39:354, 1973.

123. Furgang FA: Glass particles in ampules. Anesthesiology 41:525, 1974.

124. Baker AS, Ojemann RG, Swartz MN, Richardson EP Jr: Spinal epidural abscess. N Engl Med 293:463–468, 1975.

125. Male CG, Martin R: Puerpaeral spinal epidural abscess. Lancet 1:608–609, 1973.

126. Schreiner EJ, Lipson SF, Bromage PR, Camporesi EM: Neurological complications following general anaesthesia. Three cases of major paralysis. Anaesthesia 38:226–229, 1983.

127. Shnider SM, Levinson G: Neurologic complications of regional anesthesia (editorial comment). In Anesthesia for Obstetrics, 2nd ed. SM Shnider, G Levinson, eds. Williams & Wilkins, Baltimore, 1987, p 321.

128. Storniolo FR, Cheek TG, Shelley WC, Gustche BB: The febrile paturient. In The Complicated Patient, 2nd ed. FM James III, AS Wheeler, DM Dewan, eds. FA Davis, Philadelphia, 1988, pp 439–466.

129. Bromage PR: Neurologic complications of regional anesthesia. In Anesthesia for Obstetrics, 2nd ed. SM Shnider, G Levinson, eds. Williams & Wilkins, Baltimore, 1987, pp 320–321.

130. Donaldson JO: Neuropathy. In Neurology of Pregnancy, 2nd ed. WB Saunders, Philadelphia, 1989, p 49.

131. Vaddadi A, Ramanathan J, Angel JJ, Sidai B: Epidural anesthesia in women with chorioamnionitis: A retrospective study. Anesthesiology 73:A863, 1990.

132. Thistlewood JM: Panel summary—Infections and the parturient: Anaesthetic considerations. The febrile parturient. Can J Anaesth 35:270–272, 1988.

133. Carp H, Bailey S: Meningitis after dural puncture in rats. Anesthesiology 73:A862, 1990.

134. Yoder PR, Gibbs RS, Blanco JD, Castaneda YS, St Clair PJ: A prospective, controlled study of maternal and perinatal outcome after intra-amniotic infection at term. Am J Obstet Gynecol 145:695–701, 1983.

135. Gibbs RS, Dinsmoor MJ, Newton ER, Ramamurthy RS: A randomized trial of intrapartum versus immediate postpartum treatment of women with intra-amniotic infection. Obstet Gynecol 72:823–828, 1988.

136. Ready LB, Helfer D: Bacterial meningitis in parturients after epidural anesthesia. Anesthesiology 71:988–990, 1989.

137. Abouleish E, Amortegni AJ, Taylor FH: Are bacterial filters needed in continuous epidural analgesia for obstetrics? Anesthesiology 46:351–356, 1977.

138. Wadia NH, Datsur DK: Spinal meningitides with radioculomyelopathy. I. Clinical features. J Neurol Sci 8:239–260, 1969.
139. Symposium: Lumbar arachnoiditis: Nomenclature, etiology and pathology. Spine 3:21–92, 1978.
140. Ravindran RS, Bond VK, Tasch MD, Gupta CD, Luersson TG: Prolonged neural blockade following regional analgesia with 2-chloroprocaine. Anesth Analg 59:447–451, 1980.
141. Reisner LS, Hochman BN, Plumer MN: Persistent neurologic deficient and adhesive arachnoiditis following intrathecal 2-chloroprocaine injection. Anesth Analg 59:452–454, 1980.
142. Covino BG, Marx GF, Finster M, Zsigmond EK: Prolonged sensory/motor deficits following inadvertent spinal anesthesia. Anesth Analg 59:399–400, 1980.
143. Gissen AJ, Datta S, Lambert D: The chloroprocaine controversy. II. Is chloroprocaine neurotoxic? Reg Anesth 9:135–145, 1984.
144. Abboud TK, Mosaad P, Makar A, Gangolly J, Dror A, Zhu J, Mantilla M, Zaki N, Davis H, Moore J, Swart F, Reyes A: Comparative maternal and neonatal effects of the new and the old formulations of 2-chloroprocaine. Reg Anesth 13:101–106, 1988.
145. Sghirlanzoni A, Marazzi R, Pareyson D, Oliveri A, Bracchi M: Epidural anaesthesia and spinal arachnoiditis. Anaesthesia 44:317–321, 1989.
146. Martens MG: Herpes simplex in pregnancy. In *Infections in Pregnancy*. LC Gilstrap, S Faro, R Alan, eds. Liss Inc, New York, 1990, pp 143–150.
147. Crosby ET, Halpern SH, Rolbin SH: Epidural anaesthesia for caesarean section in patients with active recurrent genital herpes simplex infections: A retrospective review. Can J Anaesth 36:701–704, 1989.
148. Stroop WG, Rock DL, Fraser NW: Localization of herpes simplex virus in the trigeminal and olfactory systems of the mouse central nervous system during acute and latent infections by in situ hybridization. Lab Invest 51:27–38, 1984.
149. Ugolini G, Kuypers HG, Strick PL: Transneuronal transfer of herpes virus from peripheral nerves to cortex and brainstem. Science 243:89–91, 1989.
150. Ramanathan S, Sheth R, Turndorf H: Anesthesia for cesarean section in patients with genital herpes infections: A retrospective study. Anesthesiology 64:807–809, 1986.
151. Bader AM, Camann WR, Datta S: Anesthesia for cesarean delivery in patients with herpes simplex virus type-2 infections. Reg Anesth 15:261–263, 1990.
152. Cardan E: Herpes simplex after spinal morphine. Anaesthesia 39:1031, 1984.
153. Gieraerts R, Navalgund A, Vaes L, Soetens M, Chang J-L, Jahr J: Increased incidence of itching and herpes simplex in patients given epidural morphine after cesarean section. Anesth Analg 66:1321–1324, 1987.
154. Crone L-A A, Conly JM, Clark KM, Crichlow AC, Wardell GC, Zbitnew A, Rea LM, Cronk SL, Anderson CM, Tan LK: Recurrent herpes simplex virus labialis and the use of epidural morphine in obstetric patients. Anesth Analg 67:318–323, 1988.
155. Crone L-A A, Conly JM, Storgard C, Zbitnew A, Cronk SL, Rea LM, Greer K, Berenbaum E, Tan LK, To T: Herpes labialis in parturients receiving epidural morphine following cesarean section. Anesthesiology 73:208–213, 1990.
156. Ward BE, Myers F, Welch JC, Silverman P, Moyer M, Wright L: HIV prevalence survey. Del Med J 63:19–26, 1991.
157. Maki D: AIDS and obstetric anesthesia (personal communication). *Society for Obstetric Anesthesia and Perinatology*, Madison, WI, 1990.
158. Levy RM, Bredesen DE, Rosenblum ML: Neurological manifestations of the acquired immunodeficiency syndrome (AIDS): Experience at UCSF and review of the literature. J Neurosurg 62:475–495, 1985.
159. Petito CK, Navai BA, Cho E-S, Jordan BD, George DC, Price RW: Vacuolar myelopathy pathologically resembling subacute combined degeneration in patients with acquired immunodeficiency syndrome. N Engl J Med 312:874–879, 1985.
160. Mah V, Vartavarian LM, Akers M-S, Vinters HV: Abnormalities of peripheral nerve in patients with human immunodeficiency virus infection. Ann Neurol 24:713–717, 1988.
161. Koralnik IJ, Beaumanoir A, Hausler R, Kohler A, Safran AB, Delacoux R, Vibert D, Mayer E, Burkhard P, Nahory A: A controlled study of early neurologic abnormalities in men with asymptomatic human immunodeficiency virus infection. N Engl J Med 323:864–870, 1990.
162. Frame WA, Lichtmann MW: Blood patch in the HIV-positive patient. Anesthesiology 73:1297, 1990.
163. Dror A, Henriksen E: Accidental epidural magnesium sulphate injection. Anesth Analg 66:1020–1021, 1987.
164. Lin D, Becker K, Shapiro HM: Neurologic changes following epidural injection of potassium chloride and diazepam: A case report with laboratory correlations. Anesthesiology 65:210–212, 1986.
165. Bromage PR: Complications and contraindications. In *Epidural Analgesia*. WB Saunders, Philadelphia, 1978, p 663.
166. Shankar KB, Palkar NV, Nishkala R: Paraplegia following epidural potassium chloride. Anaesthesia 40:45–47, 1985.
167. Guinness JP, Cantees KK: Epidural injection of a phenol-containing ranitidine preparation. Anesthesiology 73:553–555, 1990.
168. Bickler P, Spear R, McKay W: Intralipid solution mistakenly infused into epidural space. Anesth Analg 71:712–713, 1990.
169. Patel PC, Sharif AMY, Fernando PUE: Accidental infusion of total parenteral nutrition solution through an epidural catheter. Anaesthesia 39:383–384, 1984.
170. Brahams D: Record award for personal injuries sustained as a result of negligent administration of epidural anaesthetic. Lancet 1:159, 1982.
171. Craig DB, Habib GG: Flaccid paraparesis following obstetrical anesthesia: Possible role of benzyl alcohol. Anesth Analg 56:219–221, 1977.
172. Winkelman NW: Neurologic symptoms following accidental intraspinal detergent injection. Neurology 2:284–291, 1952.
173. Kliemann FA: Paraplegia and intracranial hypertension following epidural anesthesia: Report of four cases. Arq Neuro-Psiquiatria 33:217–229, 1975.
174. Marinacci AA, Courville CB: Electromyogram in evaluation of neurological complications of spinal anesthesia. JAMA 168:1337–1345, 1958.
175. Marinacci AA: Clinical electromyography: A review. Bull LA Neurol Soc 35:181–200, 1970.
176. Goodgold J, Eberstein A: *Electrodiagnosis of Neuromuscular Diseases*. Williams & Wilkins, Baltimore, 1972.
177. Hellman K: Epidural anaesthesia in obstetrics: A second look at 26,127 cases. Can Anaesth Soc J 12:398–404, 1965.

CHAPTER 25

Anesthesia-Related Maternal Mortality

Gerard M. Bassell, M.B., B.S.

Gertie F. Marx, M.D.

THE SCOPE OF THE PROBLEM

"Reproductive" mortality is usually divided into: pregnancy-related deaths (e.g., from abortion, ectopic pregnancy, and all other gestation-related causes) and contraception-related deaths (e.g., from oral drugs, intrauterine devices, and sterilization) (1). However, the postpartum duration included in this category varies widely. Although most reviews of pregnancy-related mortality limit themselves to 6 weeks after delivery (2, 3), others extend the period to 90 days (4). In New York City, the period extends to 6 months (J. Pakter, personal communication). Because approximately 15% of pregnancy-related fatalities occur more than 6 weeks after parturition (5), extension of the tabulation period past that point should be the aim.

Pregnancy-related deaths have been classified as direct (i.e, due to true obstetric causes, such as uterine hemorrhage); indirect (i.e., due to nonobstetric causes, such as preexisting or incidental medical disease); or unrelated, such as an unplanned accident ("unplanned" because both suicide and homicide may be consequent to the pregnancy, i.e., indirect). In general, deaths from anesthesia have been classified as indirect (6). In 1980 the International Classification of Diseases, 9th Division, Clinical Modification (ICD-9-CM) listed anesthesia as a separate cause of maternal mortality (Table 25.1).

The Maternal Mortality Rate is traditionally defined as the number of maternal deaths divided by the number of live births during the same reporting period. It provides a ratio, not a true rate, because the denominator does not include the entire population at risk for the outcome described by the numerator. In the United States the collection of maternal mortality statistics began in 1915 when mandatory registration of live births was instituted. In the United Kingdom, triennial "Reports on Confidential Enquiries into Maternal Deaths in England and Wales" (CEMD) have been available since 1952.

For international comparisons, England and Wales were chosen as a "standard" population for the following reasons: (a) there was dependable registration; (b) a large population with practically no annual fluctuations in the age-specific rate could be studied; (c) age distribution was nonextreme; and (d) mortality was of the same order as that in the Netherlands and Scandinavia (7). These CEMD reports cover between 1.9 and 2.7 million births per triennium. To date 11 have been published, the first for the years

Table 25.1
The International Classification of Diseases,
9th Revision, Clinical Modification (ICD-9-CM)

668	Complications of the administration of anesthetic or other sedation in labor and delivery
	Includes: Complications arising from the administration of a general or local anesthetic, analgesic, or other sedation in labor and delivery
	Excludes: Reaction to spinal block or lumbar puncture (349.0)
668.0	Pulmonary complications
	Inhalations or aspiration of stomach contents or secretions following anesthesia or sedation in labor and delivery
	Mendelson's syndrome
	Pressure collapse of lung
668.1	Cardiac complications
	Cardiac arrest or failure following anesthesia or other sedation in labor and delivery
668.2	Central nervous system complications
	Cerebral anoxia
668.8	Other complications of anesthesia or other sedation in labor and delivery
668.9	Unspecified complications of anesthesia and other sedation
349	Other and unspecified disorders of the nervous system
349.0	Reaction to spinal or lumbar puncture

1952–1954 (14), and the most recent for the period 1982–1984 (24). In 1991 for the first time the maternal mortality data for the years 1985–1987 for the four countries comprising the United Kingdom (England, Wales, Scotland, Northern Ireland) were combined into a single report (24a). This was made possible, even necessary, by the progressive decline in the number of maternal deaths in Scotland and Northern Ireland, which made maintenance of confidentiality in those countries difficult.

The U.S. maternal mortality was stable, at approximately 60 per 10,000, until the 1930s (6) when a progressive decline began that intensified following World War II. Since then, as in other developed nations, substantial reductions in mortality have been registered in the areas of infection, preeclampsia, and in-hospital hemorrhage so that the current U.S. rate has fallen to about 1 per 10,000 (9.1 per 100,000) (6, 8). However, fatalities related to the administration of anesthesia, rather than undergoing decreases similar to those achieved with other causes of obstetric death, have simply paralleled the overall reduction in pregnancy-related mortality (9–12). To exemplify these trends, maternal deaths over the 20-year period of 1946–1965 were reviewed (11). The total obstetric mortality per 10,000 live births declined from 18.3 during the 5 years from 1946 to 1950, to 13.7 during 1951–1955, 9.6 during 1956–1960, and 7.4 for the years 1961–1965. The corresponding rates for anesthesia-related maternal mortality were reduced from 0.54 per 10,000 live births to 0.41, 0.28, and 0.19. Thus the overall reduction in mortality over the 20-year term of the review was between 35 and 40% for both obstetric and anesthetic causes (Fig. 25.1). Similarly, during the first 36 years of the CEMD reports, pregnancy-related mortality decreased from 68 per 100,000 total births in 1952 to 7.6 in 1985 through 1987 (14–24a). The rate of decline has been maintained at approximately 20% per triennium. Recently, an encouraging trend has been apparent in the statistics from England and Wales. During the period 1970 through 1984, the anesthesia-associated death rate (per million pregnancies) has fallen from 12.8 in the 1970–1972 triennium, to 10.5, 12.1, 8.7, 7.2, and 1.9 during the subsequent triennia (24a) (Table 25.2 and Table 25.3). However, the contribution of anesthesia to the overall number of maternal deaths has remained fairly stable over the same period, ranging from 10.8 to 13%. In the most recent report, deaths associated with anesthesia had declined to 4.4% of direct maternal deaths, but it is not possible to determine if this reduction will continue (24a). Although statistically accurate comparisons between the triennia cannot be made, the decreases in the anesthesia-associated death rate have occurred dur-

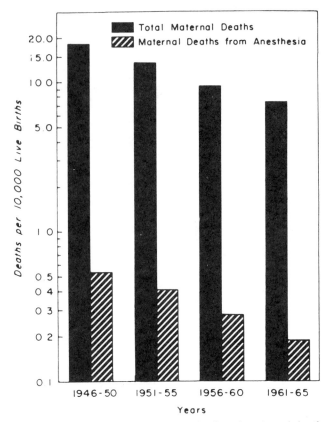

Figure 25.1. Semilogarithmic graph of total maternal death rates (exclusive of nonobstetric deaths) and death rates from anesthetic causes in North Carolina in four 5-year periods: The proportionate decrease in both rates was essentially the same. (Reprinted by permission from Greiss FC Jr, Anderson SG: Elimination of maternal deaths from anesthesia. Obstet Gynecol 29:677–681, 1967.)

ing a period when the number of anesthetics administered to gravidae has increased tremendously. Thus the improvement is probably greater than that suggested by the falling death rate alone. This trend has been maintained in the combined report (24a).

Anesthesia has remained a prominent cause of pregnancy-related mortality. In New York City, it was the third leading factor in the 4-year period of 1973–1976 (Table 25.4) (25), whereas in 1980 it had declined to fifth place, exceeded by ectopic pregnancy, hypertensive disease, pulmonary embolism, and cerebrovascular accident (J. Pakter, personal communication). More recently in New York City, during the period 1981–1983, anesthesia-related deaths (10.83% of the total) had climbed to third place behind ectopic pregnancy and pulmonary embolism (26). Of 95 pregnancy-associated deaths recorded in the state of New York (exclusive of New York City) during 1970–1975, 9.7% were classified as due to anesthesia (27). In the state of Indiana, there were 454 maternal deaths between 1960 and 1980 (mor-

Table 25.2
Direct Deaths by Cause, Rates Per Million Estimated Pregnancies, England and Wales, 1970–1987[a]

	Pulmonary Embolism	Hypertensive Diseases of Pregnancy	Anesthe-sia	Amniotic Fluid Embolism	Abortion	Ectopic Pregnancy	Hemor-rhage	Sepsis, Excluding Abortion	Ruptured Uterus	Other Direct Causes	All Deaths
1970–72	17.6	14.9	12.8	4.8	25.3	11.5	10.4	10.4	3.8	6.9	118.7
1973–75	12.8	13.2	10.5	5.4	10.5	7.4	8.1	7.4	4.3	8.5	88.0
1976–78	18.5	12.5	11.6	4.7	6.0	9.0	10.3	6.5	6.0	8.2	93.4
1979–81[b]	9.0	14.2	8.7	7.1	5.5	7.9	5.5	3.1	1.6	7.5	70.0[c]
1982–84	10.0	10.0	7.2	5.6	4.4	4.0	3.6	1.0	1.2	8.4	55.0
1985–87	9.1	9.4	1.9	3.4	2.3	4.1	3.8	2.3	1.9	7.5	45.6

[a]From Reports on Health and Social Subjects: *Report on Confidential Enquiries into Maternal Deaths in England and Wales*, 1970–1972 through 1985–87. London, Her Brittannic Majesty's Stationery Office, Nos. 11, 14, 26, 29, and 34.
[b]Includes two other direct deaths omitted in the 1976–1978 report.
[c]Rates for the United Kingdom were not available as there was no information on pregnancies for Scotland and Northern Ireland.

Table 25.3
Deaths, Associated with Anesthesia, Estimated Rate Per Million Pregnancies and Percentage of Direct Maternal Deaths, England and Wales, 1970–1987, Compared With United Kingdom, 1985–1987

		Number of Deaths Directly Associated with Anesthesia	Rate Per Million Preg-nancies	% of Direct Maternal Deaths
England & Wales	1970–72	37	12.8	10.8
	1973–75	27	10.5	11.9
	1976–78	27	12.1	12.4
	1979–81	22	8.7	12.4
	1982–84	18	7.2	13.0
	1985–87	5	1.9	4.4
United Kingdom	1985–87	6	N/A	4.3

From Reports on Health and Social Subjects: *Report on Confidential Enquiries into Maternal Deaths in England and Wales*, 1970–1972 through 1985–1987. London, Her Brittanic Majesty's Stationery Office, Nos. 11, 14, 26, 29, and 34.

Table 25.4
The Three Leading Causes of 122 Maternal Mortalities in New York City in the 4-Year Period, 1973–1976[a]

Cause	No.	%
Pulmonary embolism	29	20
Preeclampsia-Eclampsia	20	16
Anesthesia	17	14

[a]Reprinted by permission from Pakter J, Schiffer MA, Nelson F: Maternal and perinatal mortality. In *Clinical Management of Mother and Newborn*. GF Marx, ed. Springer Verlag, New York, 1979, pp 241–264.

tality of 22 per 100,000 live births); anesthesia was the primary cause in 24 of these cases, 16 occurring during 1960–1970 and 8 during 1970–1980 (3). Similarly, in England and Wales, anesthesia accounted for 8.7% of the maternal deaths in the years 1964–1966, 10.9% in 1967–1969, 10.8% in 1970–1972, 11.9% in 1973–1975, 12.4% in both 1976–1978 and 1979–1981, 13.0% in 1982–1984, and 4.4% in 1985–1987 (14–24a). In the 15-year period of 1970–1984, the anesthetic contribution to direct maternal deaths in England and Wales was 11.9%. However, the pattern of anesthetic deaths has changed. Fatalities associated with spinal block have been significantly reduced, whereas deaths related to general anesthesia and epidural block have shown a relative increase (9, 11, 12, 21, 22; J Pakter, personal communication). Thus, of 13 maternal fatalities in New York City between 1979 and 1981, 12 were due to mishaps during general anesthesia (failed intubation being more frequent than pulmonary aspiration of gastric contents) and 1 to a complication of epidural analgesia (accidental intravascular injection of bupivacaine) (J. Pakter, personal communication). In the Indiana report, aspiration of gastric contents was the leading cause of maternal mortality in the 10-year period of 1960–1970, but in the second 10-year period (1970–1980), cardiorespiratory arrest became the more frequent anesthetic problem (3). In England and Wales, during the years 1970–1978 nearly 10 times as many deaths were related to general, as compared with regional, anesthesia: 40 mortalities were caused by inhalation of gastric contents, 28 by intubation problems, and only 7 by complications of regional block (20–22). In the most recent report, of the eight deaths attributable to anesthesia, five were related to a misplaced endotracheal tube, one to pulmonary aspiration of gastric contents, one to a kinked endotracheal tube, and one to cardiovascular collapse fol-

Table 25.5
Maternal Deaths Directly Attributable to Anesthesia[a]

Cause	1973–1975	1976–1978	1985–1988
Inhalation of stomach contents during induction of anesthesia	9	4	1
Inhalation of stomach contents during difficult intubation	4	7	0
Hypoxia due to esophageal/failed intubation/kinked tube	3	9	6
Misuse of drugs	4	3	0
Accidents with apparatus	2	2	0
Subarachnoid injection of anesthetic during attempted epidural block	2	1	0
Miscellaneous causes[b]	7	4	1
TOTAL	31	30	8

[a]Based on data from CEMD Reports 1973–1975, 1976–1978, and 1985–1988 (21, 22, 24a).

[b]Miscellaneous causes included allergic reaction, inadequate reversal of muscle relaxant, intravenous overload, postoperative asphyxial episode, and mismanagement of epidural in a patient with cardiac disease. The 1985–1988 data in this table include two late deaths in which anesthesia was considered to be the main cause of death. These patients were not included in Tables 25.2 and 25.3.

lowing epidural block in a woman with aortic insufficiency (24a). A detailed account of the causes of deaths occurring in 1973–1978 is depicted in Table 25.5.

CAUSES OF ANESTHESIA-RELATED MATERNAL MORTALITY

Deaths Resulting from General Anesthesia

PULMONARY ASPIRATION OF GASTRIC CONTENTS

The anatomic and physiologic changes occurring in the gastrointestinal tract during pregnancy make regurgitation of gastric contents during anesthesia more likely in gravid women than in nonpregnant patients and, should pulmonary aspiration occur, its effects can be more severe. A number of phenomena, of both mechanical and hormonal origin, account for this. First, the rate of gastric emptying is decreased and transit time of bowel contents is increased during pregnancy. These changes are heightened during labor by the effects of pain and anxiety, the recumbent position, and drugs used for the systemic relief of pain (28). Second, the likelihood of regurgitation is enhanced by the progressive pressure of the uterus

and abdominal contents on the stomach, changing its axis from the vertical to the horizontal (29). At the same time, tonus at the gastroesophageal junction is decreased and pressure within the stomach is increased, particularly in the lithotomy position (30). Third, the hormonally induced reduction in gastric tone and motility make nausea and vomiting more likely (31). Finally, although acid and pepsin secretions by the stomach are diminished during the major portion of pregnancy, toward term they tend to increase to above-normal levels (32). Thus, should pulmonary aspiration occur intrapartum, the severity of lung injury could well be greater than it would have been earlier in pregnancy. Therefore parturients must always be considered to have a full stomach, and the gastric contents must be expected to be particularly hazardous.

Pulmonary aspiration of gastric contents can occur following either regurgitation, a passive process, or vomiting, an active one. The quality and volume of aspirate are the major determinants of the type and severity of sequelae. Thus the inhalation of solid foodstuffs has the propensity for producing airway obstruction, varying degrees of pulmonary collapse, mediastinal shift, and reflex bronchospasm. Bronchoscopic removal of aspirated material allows for reinflation of collapsed pulmonary segments and is the appropriate therapeutic maneuver in this situation. Inhalation of liquid gastric juice, particularly with a pH of 2.5 or less, produces the pulmonary acid aspiration (Mendelson's) syndrome. Here, acid injury of the bronchial mucosa is the primary insult and causes bronchiolar spasm, peribronchiolar exudates, focal hemorrhages, and areas of parenchymal necrosis. Therapeutic intervention is aimed at ventilatory support; the role of antibiotics and steroids is still controversial. Complete large airway obstruction or aspiration of a volume of acidic gastric juice sufficient to flood both lungs can result in hypoxic cardiac arrest (33).

Since the recognition of the increased risk of pulmonary aspiration during the peripartum period, significant advances have been made in its prevention. The hazards of aspirating gastric contents should be explained during "preparation for childbirth" classes, and women should be warned to avoid ingestion of all but small amounts of clear liquids once labor is imminent. The incidence of vomiting caused by dehydration and ketosis has been reduced by the widespread use of intravenous hydration with dextrose-containing balanced salt solutions, and vomiting caused by emotional stress or narcotic analgesics has been ameliorated by the employment of small doses of tranquilizers with antiemetic properties when indicated. The probability of regurgitation can also

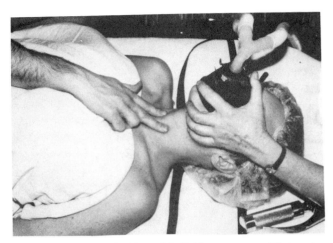

Figure 25.2. Modification of Sellick's maneuver. The assistant places the palmar surface of the hand to the anterior aspect of the patient's chest wall. The palmar aspects of the index and middle fingers, each slightly to either side of the middle of the arch of the cricoid cartilage, are used to press the cricoid posteriorly onto the esophagus.

be decreased by attending to those factors that make it more likely to occur. Thus avoidance of further increases of intragastric pressure, relative to esophageal pressure, is of paramount importance unless the parturient's protective airway reflexes are known to be intact. The use of suprafundal pressure should be restricted to conscious parturients or to those whose airway has been protected by a cuffed endotracheal tube.

Prevention of vomiting or regurgitation is only one of the series of maneuvers that can be expected to reduce the incidence of aspiration pneumonitis in pregnancy. Occlusion of the cervical esophagus with the cricoid cartilage (Sellick's maneuver) deters the passage of regurgitated contents into the nasopharynx and thence into the lower airway. This technique should be a component of all general anesthetics administered to gravidas from the mid-second trimester until 2–3 days postpartum. Pressure on the cricoid cartilage should be applied by a skilled assistant from the time of injection of the drug used for anesthetic induction and should be maintained until the anesthesiologist has inflated the cuff of the endotracheal tube and demonstrated its proper placement. A recent modification of Sellick's maneuver offers two advantages. By placing the palm of the assistant's hand flat against the patient's anterior chest wall under the surgical drapes and using the palmar aspects of the index and middle fingers for the compression (Fig. 25.2), interference with the laryngoscope handle is avoided and large breasts are spread apart by the assistant's forearm (34). If appropriately skilled personnel adhere to these guidelines, "it is certain that

gastric aspiration into the lungs during anaesthesia is preventable" (35).

Forestalling the passage of gastric contents into the airway is obviously the most important factor in avoiding the pulmonary aspiration syndrome. In recent years, however, much work has centered on methods of decreasing the volume and acidity of gastric contents in an attempt to lessen the severity of lung injury should they be inhaled. Oral administration of antacids during labor has been shown to decrease gastric juice acidity, and nonparticulate antacids may be less harmful to the pulmonary parenchyma than particulate ones if aspirated (36–38). Maneuvers such as turning the gravida from side to side to ensure thorough mixing of the antacid with contents of both antral and fundal gastric pouches can further improve acid neutralization (39). Yet, deaths caused by maternal aspiration pneumonitis still occur, even after the routine administration of oral antacids during labor.

Pharmacologic methods of aiding stomach emptying or reducing the volume and acidity of gastric contents have received much recent attention. Metoclopramide, an antiemetic also used to hasten the passage of radiologic contrast medium out of the stomach in nonpregnant patients, has not proved to be consistently effective in term-pregnant women undergoing elective cesarean section (40). Cimetidine, a histamine-2 receptor antagonist, although efficient in reducing gastric volume and acidity (41), may impair hepatic metabolism of hypnotic or narcotic drugs. This may occur in the mother and, since cimetidine crosses the placenta, the newborn. Ranitidine, another histamine-2 receptor antagonist with a structure different from that of cimetidine, does not adversely affect oxidative or conjugative metabolism (42). Despite their popularity the value of histamine-2 receptor antagonists in reducing gastric volume and acidity during labor and their routine use to prevent acid-aspiration pneumonitis remain controversial.

Despite the dissemination of information concerning the pathophysiology of the acid-aspiration syndrome in pregnancy, fatalities continue to occur. More frequent use of regional analgesia during labor, vaginal delivery, and cesarean section can be expected to reduce the incidence of the syndrome. In those clinical situations in which conduction block cannot be used and general anesthesia is required, endotracheal intubation is mandatory with the precautions against regurgitation and aspiration outlined earlier to be used by skilled, knowledgeable operators.

INABILITY TO INTUBATE THE TRACHEA

Passage of an endotracheal tube has become an accepted part of the technique of general anesthesia in obstetrics, but "failure to achieve successful endotracheal intubation is now an important contributor to maternal death" (43). Anatomic abnormalities of the face, neck, or upper airway are the most common causes of difficulty in intubating the trachea. Thus particular care must be taken in assessing the gravida's physiognomy before induction of general anesthesia. If anatomic abnormalities are present, awake endotracheal intubation provides a safer alternative to the usual method (44).

Pregnancy can pose additional problems in achieving safe isolation of the airway. The combination of large breasts and an increased anteroposterior thoracic diameter can severely reduce the room available for manipulation of the laryngoscope handle. These impediments can be ameliorated somewhat by taping large breasts laterally and caudally. Also, a shorter laryngoscope handle has been described for use in obstetrics (45), and this may allow an increased range of movement during difficult airway manipulation. Edema of the laryngeal mucosa occurs in all term-pregnant gravidas to some degree, but it is usually of greater amount and is more often the cause of problems in the preeclamptic woman and, occasionally, in healthy gravidas following prolonged, strenuous bearing-down efforts. If the preeclampsia is severe, swelling of the epiglottis may make visualization of the larynx more difficult than expected, but the more usual problem is a reduction in the caliber of the airway, resulting in an inability to pass an endotracheal tube of anticipated size. Avoidance of any consequent hazard is usually easy. Routine endotracheal intubation in late pregnancy should be accomplished with a tube 0.5 to 1 mm smaller than that used for a similarly sized nonpregnant woman, and preeclamptic gravidas can be expected to require an even smaller tube if the airway is to be secured easily and atraumatically (44).

Despite the above precautions, difficulties with endotracheal intubation have been encountered after anesthesia has been induced (44). The incidence of failed intubation during obstetric anesthesia has been reported to be approximately eight times that encountered in surgical patients (46). Endobronchial intubation is more hazardous in the parturient because of the pregnancy-induced decrease in functional residual capacity (reducing oxygen storage) and increase in metabolic rate (enhancing oxygen use) (47). It is of paramount importance to delay skin incision until successful endotracheal intubation has been confirmed by appropriate auscultation of the upper chest bilaterally, aided by proof of CO_2 exhalation by capnography (48). This allows for discontinuation of the anesthetic and a change in technique should intubation prove impossible. Under such cir-

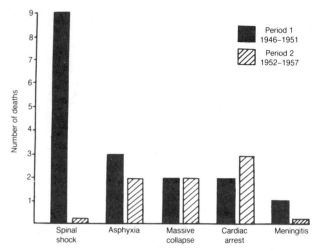

Figure 25.3. Factors in the decline of anesthesia-induced maternal mortality in Bronx County (New York City) comparing two successive 5-year periods: There was no death from "spinal shock" after 1952. (Reprinted by permission from Klein MD, Clahr J: Factor in the decline of maternal mortality. JAMA 168:237–242, 1958.)

cumstances, the parturient should be allowed to regain consciousness so that awake placement of the endotracheal tube can be tried or a regional technique chosen. If surgery has begun before the larynx has been intubated, or if the surgical indication is a maternal life-threatening one (e.g., severe hemorrhage, uterine rupture), an inhalation anesthetic can be continued by mask with maintenance of cricoid pressure and assisted ventilation (but without further muscle relaxant). Safety of the airway must be guaranteed as soon as possible, however, either by passage of an endotracheal tube over a fiberoptic bronchoscope or by cricothyrotomy. Every labor suite should have the instruments required for emergency tracheostomy, and each delivery room should be equipped with a means of providing temporary transtracheal ventilation (44, 49).

Deaths Resulting from Regional Analgesia

SPINAL SHOCK

There have been two reasons for the precipitous decline (Fig. 25.3) in the occurrence of spinal shock (i.e., profound hypotension resulting in cardiopulmonary arrest after spinal anesthesia) in pregnancy. The realization that gravidas require smaller amounts of local anesthetic than do nonpregnant women to produce a similar dermatome level has led to a decrease in the incidence of excessively high levels of spinal block. The occurrence of significant hypotension as a complication of sympathetic blockade has been reduced by the more widespread use of adequate intravenous fluid preloading and prevention of aortocaval compression by uterine displacement.

Decreased Drug Requirement

During pregnancy, a smaller dose of spinally or epidurally administered local anesthetic is required to achieve the desired level of neural blockade. Drug requirement falls to about two-thirds of the usual dose by the third trimester. This phenomenon was first noted clinically but has since been confirmed by three separate studies. When continuous, selective spinal blockade with 0.2% procaine was compared in 10 women prepartum and again postpartum, at least twice the amount of local anesthetic was required to produce sensory analgesia to the fourth cervical dermatome when the measurements were taken approximately 48 hr after delivery (50). Also, when the spread of lumbar epidural analgesia was ascertained in a large number of surgical patients and gravid women after injection of various local anesthetics through wide-bore needles, pregnancy-related discrepancies in the extent of sensory levels were noted (51). For example, a nonpregnant woman of specific age and height in whom blockade to the tenth thoracic dermatome was achieved with 20 ml of 2% lidocaine needed only 14 ml to produce the same extent of denervation when pregnant at term. Finally, in a comparison of the effects of equal doses of spinal anesthetic (hyperbaric tetracaine, 5 mg) administered under identical conditions to obstetric and young gynecologic patients, a significantly more rapid onset, higher level, and longer duration of blockade were produced in the parturients (52).

This altered response appears to be a direct consequence of the physiologic changes induced by gestation. Reduced buffer capacity caused by hyperventilation-induced compensated alkalemia may allow a local anesthetic to remain a salt for a longer time and, therefore, to persist in the compartment of injection for a prolonged period (53). The increased progesterone concentrations of pregnancy can affect smooth muscle behavior and the structure and function of neurons (54). Over the course of gestation, plasma progesterone undergoes a more than 30-fold increase from a nonpregnant level of less than 3 ng/ml to more than 100 ng/ml. At the same time, cerebrospinal fluid concentrations rise from 0.4 to 3.0 ng/ml (55). Epidural venous distension can reduce the capacity of both the epidural and subarachnoid spaces, thus enhancing the spread of local anesthetic solutions, and retarded meningeal capillary circulation may delay drug absorption, thereby prolonging the duration of analgesia (56). The increased degree of lumbar lordosis that occurs during pregnancy may promote an exaggerated cephalad spread of the anesthetic. Inferior vena caval compression plays only an indirect role in that the resultant redistribution of a portion of the venous return to the paravertebral system of veins may produce a further diminution in epidural and subarachnoid space capacities (57). However, reduced drug requirement is unrelated to maternal position and persists despite immediate displacement of the uterus once the anesthetic has been injected. In fact, the decrease in drug requirement for regional block can be demonstrated as early as the latter part of the first trimester before the onset of aortocaval compression and is maintained into the early postpartum period. Thus 23 women receiving epidural analgesia at 8 to 12 weeks of pregnancy had a drug requirement of 21.3 ± 2.1 mg of lidocaine per spinal segment, whereas in 12 nonpregnant controls the corresponding amount was 27.1 ± 2.4 mg ($P < 0.001$) (53). In women undergoing postpartum tubal ligation, analysis of the extent and duration of epidural or spinal blockade revealed a progressive decline in both variables over the first 3 puerperal days (57). It may be significant that the mother's venous distensibility undergoes an almost parallel decrease (58).

Intravenous Fluid Preloading

Sympathetic blockade produces postarteriolar pooling of blood, thereby decreasing effective circulating blood volume. When a large area of the vascular bed is denervated in this manner, venous return to the heart can be reduced. In addition, vascular tone depends more on sympathetic control during pregnancy than it does in the nongravid state. These factors, combined with the effects of the caval component of aortocaval compression, make the pregnant woman more susceptible to the arterial pressure-lowering effects of sympathetic blockade. Thus hypotension is liable to develop at sensory levels of analgesia that would not cause hypotension in nonpregnant women.

Following the demonstration that intravenous fluid administration was effective in reversing the blood pressure fall occurring after spinal anesthesia in pregnant ewes (59), human studies in term-pregnant gravidas were undertaken. In women undergoing elective cesarean section under spinal anesthesia 1 liter of lactated Ringer's solution, as an intravenous preload before injection of the anesthetic, reduced the incidence of significant hypotension (60). Other studies demonstrated that ephedrine was not predictably effective in treating block-induced hypotension unless acute intravenous hydration accompanied its use. This unreliability occurred even when large doses of the drug were administered. However, when concomitant fluid administration was em-

Table 25.6
Incidence of Maternal Hypotension (Decrease in BP >20 mm Hg) In Two Groups of Healthy Parturients of Similar Ages and Weights following Epidural Block with 10 ml of 0.375% Bupivacaine[a]

Group	N	Blood Pressure (mm Hg) before Block (Mean ± SD)	Hypotension after Block	
			N	%
Treatment	51	112.8 ± 11.8	1	2
Control	53	116.6 ± 11.4	15[b]	28[b]

[a]The treatment group was prehydrated with 1 liter of Hartmann's solution within 10 to 15 min before injection of the anesthetic; the control group received no additional intravenous fluid. (Reprinted by permission from Collins KM, Bevan DR, Beard RW: Fluid loading to reduce abnormalities of fetal heart rate and maternal hypotension during epidural analgesia in labour. Br Med J 2:1460–1461, 1978.)
[b]$P < 0.005$.

ployed, ephedrine proved to be effective both prophylactically and therapeutically (61).

Adequate displacement of the uterus from the great vessels is a prerequisite both for the avoidance of block-induced hypotension and for the initiation of therapy if a fall in blood pressure occurs. It should be obvious that the aggressive administration of intravenous fluid and ephedrine will be to no avail unless there is unimpeded return of blood from the lower extremities to the right side of the heart. In the vast majority of gravidas, uterine displacement should be to the left. This can be achieved most efficiently by elevating the right hip with a wedge and tilting the delivery table to the left.

Several investigations have indeed confirmed the efficacy of intravenous prehydration in reducing both the incidence of postblock hypotension and its deleterious effect on the uteroplacental circulation. In one study, maternal blood pressure and fetal heart rate were recorded in 104 parturients who received epidural analgesia during labor. Although all the women were lying on their left sides throughout, only 51 received an intravenous preload of 1 liter of a balanced salt solution just before the local anesthetic was injected. Their incidence of maternal hypotension was significantly lower when compared with that in the nonhydrated gravidas (Table 26.6) (62). Another investigation employed the intravenous radioactive xenon method to assess the effect of epidural block on placental intervillous blood flow (63). Thirty-eight healthy women scheduled for elective cesarean section were studied. Of these, 24 gravidas selected epidural block and were divided into two groups. The first 11 women received 10 ml/kg

intravenously of a plasma expander within 10 min of institution of the block; the other 13 received no fluid preload. The remaining 14 parturients chose general anesthesia and functioned as controls; in them, anesthesia was induced at the conclusion of the blood flow measurements. When the epidural block was administered without a preceding intravenous fluid bolus, maternal mean arterial pressure and intervillous blood flow underwent significant decreases. In contrast, measurements of intervillous blood flow in the preloaded group were comparable to those in the control patients, and arterial pressures declined only to a slight degree. In yet another study, 60 women scheduled for elective cesarean section received 2 liters of a balanced salt solution immediately before institution of an epidural block (64). Systolic blood pressure declined less than 10% from control levels in 78% of the women, and in spite of infusion of a relatively large volume of crystalloid solution, central venous pressure, measured in 20 of the gravidas, rose from an initial mean level of 4.05 ± 0.5 to a mean of 5.72 ± 0.5 cm H_2O after the establishment of the epidural block. This confirms the safety of intravenous fluid preloading in healthy parturients.

CARDIAC ARREST

Since the introduction into clinical practice of the highly lipid-soluble and protein-bound amide local anesthetics, a number of cases of fatal cardiac arrest have occurred in pregnant women exposed to bupivacaine. Typically, cardiovascular collapse, subsequent to a brief grand mal seizure, has followed unintended intravascular injection or rapid absorption from the epidural space of this potent, long-lasting drug during attempted lumbar or caudal epidural block (65). Electrocardiographic patterns have included asystole, ventricular tachycardia, ventricular fibrillation, and complete atrioventricular dissociation, sometimes with only P waves present. Difficult resuscitation has been the norm, with prolonged external cardiac compression and frequent countershock often required (66). All three commercially available concentrations of bupivacaine have been involved, albeit to different extents. The majority of cases have occurred with the 0.75% concentration.

A representative case was described as follows. A healthy gravida chose epidural anesthesia for her elective cesarean section at term.

Sixty seconds after a test-dose of 4 ml of 0.75% bupivacaine, the therapeutic dose of 16 ml was injected. Thirty seconds later, one severe convulsion developed and was followed instantaneously by cardiac asystole. Immediate endotracheal intubation, ventilation with 100% oxygen, and closed cardiac compression were undertaken while the baby was being delivered by section. Normal cardiac rhythm returned after approximately 20 minutes of external massage, two countershocks, intracardiac epinephrine, and intravenous bicarbonate (67).

In managing a catastrophe such as this, two important considerations must be borne in mind. First, external cardiac compression is most effective when performed with the patient in the supine position on an unyielding surface. During late pregnancy, however, this position produces aortocaval compression with a consequent decrease in venous return. This impediment to cardiac filling is detrimental to effective restoration of the circulation; thus delivery of the infant must be considered an important part of the resuscitation attempt. Should immediate delivery be deemed unsafe or impractical, the uterus should be manually displaced at the same time as external cardiac compression is initiated (68). Alternatively, a wooden frame (the Cardiff resuscitation wedge) or similar device that prevents aortocaval compression in pregnant women during cardiopulmonary resuscitation can be used (69). Second, seizures induced by bupivacaine are accompanied by severe acidemia, hypoxemia, and hypercarbia (70). This makes hyperventilation with 100% oxygen and intravenous administration of sodium bicarbonate necessary components of the early management if resuscitation is to have a chance of success.

Bupivacaine-induced seizures and cardiac arrest should be preventable. Careful identification of the epidural space; aspiration of the needle or catheter to identify blood or cerebrospinal fluid; administration of test doses of sufficient magnitude to produce symptoms and signs of toxicity (e.g., tinnitus, agitation, metallic taste, facial paresthesias, sudden drowsiness); and incremental injections of the therapeutic dose allowing sufficient time between aliquots to permit manifestations of either subarachnoid or intravascular placement to become evident are all means by which the technique of epidural block in obstetrics can be made safer.

The use of epinephrine in the anesthetic solution is controversial. When added to the test dose, epinephrine can produce an increase in heart rate if injected into an epidural vein. This tachycardia can be so short lived (20 sec), however, that its recognition may be difficult and, in this regard, use of an electrocardiograph or pulse oximeter during injection of the local anesthetic is suggested. Even with such accurate measurement of the maternal heart rate, however, it is not possible to differentiate between the tachycardia caused by the intravenous injection of a small amount of epinephrine and that associated with uterine contractions (71). Another concern regarding the use of epinephrine as a marker is the

possibility of its producing a decrease in uteroplacental blood flow in situations in which there is already some degree of (recognized or unrecognized) placental insufficiency. As evidence for this risk, epinephrine has been shown to decrease intervillous blood flow in gravid ewes in a dose-related manner (72). In addition, when human parturients received epinephrine (40 µg) as part of an epidural injection, fetal umbilical artery blood velocity systolic/diastolic (S/D) ratios, a measure of vascular resistance, underwent marked change. Those fetuses with normal umbilical arterial resistance before the epidural injection were relatively unaffected. In contrast, when baseline resistance was high, epinephrine-containing epidural injections worsened the situation to the point of producing transient decelerations in the fetal heart rate in two of the six fetuses in this group (73).

At the request of the U.S. Food and Drug Administration in August 1983 the three manufacturers of bupivacaine in North America recommended against the use of the 0.75% concentration in obstetric practice. Consequently, the highest concentration available for use in parturients is 0.5%. Unfortunately, the response of some anesthesiologists has been to increase the volume of the lower concentration to that which will produce an equivalent dose of drug (e.g., 30 ml of 0.5% = 150 mg = 20 ml of 0.75%). Thus the risk to a patient under these circumstances has not been reduced.

UNRECOGNIZED EVENTS DURING REGIONAL BLOCKADE

Recently, a number of maternal deaths attributable to a lack of awareness of the expected symptoms or signs of high spinal or epidural block during cesarean section have occurred. The scenario has tended to follow a predictable pattern: After institution of regional blockade, symptoms of a higher-than-expected level have either been ignored or have engendered an inappropriate response. As might be expected, these incidents have not been reported in the medical literature, but have been represented in the type of closed claims analyses that are occasionally published.

In a case with which one of the authors (Bassell) is familiar, the parturient complained of nausea within the first 5 min following the injection of a tetracaine (15 mg) spinal anesthetic for cesarean section. The anesthesia provider injected droperidol intravenously without measuring a brachial blood pressure or defining the level of sensory blockade. After repeated and progressively weaker patient complaints of dyspnea, diazepam (10 mg) was injected intravenously. Within a few minutes, respiratory arrest had occurred. Late resuscitation complicated by unrecognized esophageal intubation resulted in brain death. Unfortunately, the lack of clinical awareness underlying this event is not unique. Continuing the widespread deployment of sophisticated monitoring devices such as pulse oximeters and capnographs and requiring their use even when regional anesthesia is employed will prevent many maternal deaths. Needless to say, their use during general anesthesia should be mandatory.

CONCLUSION

Elimination of anesthetic-related maternal mortality requires the careful administration of the appropriate anesthetic by well-trained specialists. The inverse relationship between the experience and training of personnel who provide obstetric anesthesia and maternal mortality cannot be overemphasized (74, 75). As hospital services are consolidated, round-the-clock obstetric anesthesia provided by anesthesiologists in well-equipped, fully staffed labor suites should lead to improvements in maternal and fetal safety. The last 25 years have seen the birth of obstetric anesthesia as a recognized subspecialty with its own specialty group, the Society for Obstetric Anesthesia and Perinatology (SOAP). More anesthesiologists-in-training are receiving the type of instruction in obstetric anesthesia principles that allows them to face their responsibilities to parturients with knowledge, experience, and confidence.

References

1. Beral V: Reproductive mortality. Br Med J 2:622–631, 1979.
2. Phillips OC, Hulka JF, Vincent M, Christy WC: Obstetric mortality: A 26-year survey. Obstet Gynecol 25:217–222, 1965.
3. Ravindran RS, Ragan WD: Anesthetic causes of maternal mortality in the state of Indiana from 1960–1980. In *Abstracts of Scientific Papers*, Society for Obstetric Anesthesia and Perinatology, Vancouver, BC, 1983, p 59.
4. Krupp PJ, Barclay DL, Roeling WM, Wegener G: Maternal mortality: A 20-year study of Tulane Department of Obstetrics and Gynecology at Charity Hospital. Obstet Gynecol 35:823–829, 1970.
5. Rubin G, McCarthy B, Shelton J, Rochar RW, Terry J: The risk of childbearing re-evaluated. Am J Publ Health 71:712–716, 1981.
6. Green JR: Changing patterns of maternal mortality. In *Anesthesia for the High-Risk Mother, Fetus and Newborn*. Abstracts of Scientific Papers, San Francisco, 1983, pp 26–34.
7. Bonte JTP, Verbrugge HP: Maternal mortality: An epidemiological approach. Acta Obstet Gynecol Scand 46:445–474, 1967.
8. Atrash HK, Koonin LM, Lawson HW, Franks AL, Smith JC: Maternal mortality in the United States, 1979–1986. Obstet Gynecol 76:1055–1060, 1990.
9. Klein MD, Clahr J: Factors in the decline of maternal mortality. JAMA 168:237–242, 1958.
10. Bjerre B, Astedt B: Maternal mortality in Sweden. Acta Obstet Gynecol Scand 43:1–10, 1964.
11. Greiss FC Jr, Anderson SG: Elimination of maternal deaths from anesthesia. Obstet Gynecol 29:677–681, 1967.
12. Crawford JS: The anaesthestist's contribution to maternal mortality. Br J Anaesth 42:70–73, 1970.
13. Hodgkinson R: Maternal mortality. In *Obstetric Analgesia and Anesthesia.* GF Marx, GM Bassell, eds. Elsevier Scientific, Amsterdam, 1980, pp 375–395.
14. *Report on Confidential Enquiries into Maternal Deaths in England and Wales, 1952–1954.* Her Majesty's Stationery Office, London, 1957, No 97.
15. *Report on Confidential Enquiries into Maternal Deaths in England and Wales, 1955–1957.* Her Majesty's Stationery Office, London, 1960, No 103.
16. *Report on Confidential Enquiries into Maternal Deaths in England and Wales, 1958–1960.* Her Majesty's Stationery Office, London, 1963, No 108.
17. *Report on Confidential Enquiries into Maternal Deaths in England and Wales, 1961–1963.* Her Majesty's Stationery Office, London, 1966, No 115.
18. Arthure H, Tomkinson J, Organe G, Kuck M, Adelstein AM, Weatherall, JAC: *Report on Confidential Enquiries into Maternal Deaths in England and Wales, 1964–1966.* Her Majesty's Stationery Office, London, 1970, No 119.
19. Arthure H, Tomkinson J, Organe G, Bates M, Adelstein AM, Weatherall JAC: *Report on Confidential Enquiries into Maternal Deaths in England and Wales, 1967–1969.* Her Majesty's Stationery Office, London, 1972, No 1.
20. *Report on Confidential Enquiries into Maternal Deaths in England and Wales, 1970–1972.* Her Majesty's Stationery Office, London, 1975, No 11.
21. Tomkinson J, Turnbull A, Robson G, Cloake E, Adelstein AM, Weatherall JAC: *Report on Confidential Enquiries into Maternal Deaths in England and Wales, 1973–1975.* Her Majesty's Stationery Office, London, 1979, No 14.
22. Tompkins J, Turnbull A, Robson G, Dawson I, Cloake E, Adelstein AM, Ashley J: *Report on Confidential Enquiries into Maternal Deaths in England and Wales, 1976–1978.* Her Majesty's Stationery Office, London, 1982, No 26.
23. Turnbull AC, Tindall VR, Robson G, Dawson IMP, Cloake EP, Ashley JSA: *Report on Confidential Enquiries into Maternal Deaths in England and Wales, 1979–1981.* Her Majesty's Stationery Office, London, 1986, No 29.
24. Turnbull A, Tindall VR, Beard RW, Robson G, Dawson IMP, Cloake EP, Ashley JSA, Botting B: *Report on Confidential Enquiries into Maternal Deaths in England and Wales, 1982–1984.* Her Majesty's Stationery Office, London, 1989, No 34.
24a. Tindall VR, Beard RW, Sykes MK, Tighe JR, Hibbard BM, Rosen M, Knight BH, Gordon G, McClure JH, Cameron HM, Pinkerton JHM, Moore J, Toner PG: *Report on Confidential Enquiries into Maternal Deaths in the United Kingdom, 1985–1987.* Her Majesty's Stationery Office, London, 1991.
25. Pakter K, Schiffer A, Nelson F: Maternal and perinatal mortality. In *Clinical Management of Mother and Newborn.* GF Marx, ed. Springer Verlag, New York, 1979, pp 241–264.
26. Dorfman SF: Maternal mortality in New York City, 1981–1983. Obstet Gynecol 76:317–323, 1990.
27. Hughes EC, Cochrane NE, Czyz PL: Maternal mortality study, 1970–1975. NY State J Med 76:2206–2212, 1976.
28. Davison JS, Davison MC, Hay DM: Gastric emptying time in late pregnancy and labour. J Obstet Gynaecol Br Commonw 77:37–41, 1970.
29. Williams NH: Variable significance of heartburn. Am J Obstet Gynecol 42:814–819, 1941.
30. Spence AA, Moir DD, Finlay WEI: Observations on intragastric pressure. Anaesthesia 22:249–256, 1967.
31. Hytten FE, Leitch I: *The Physiology of Human Pregnancy*, 2nd ed. Blackwell Scientific, Oxford, 1971, pp 1–178.
32. Murray FA, Erskine JP, Fielding J: Gastric secretion in pregnancy. J Obstet Gynaecol Br Emp 64:373–381, 1957.
33. Mendelson CL: The aspiration of stomach contents into the lungs during obstetric anesthesia. Am J Obstet Gynecol 52:191–204, 1946.
34. Cowling J: Cricoid pressure: A more comfortable technique. Anaesth Intens Care 10:93–94, 1982.
35. Rosen M: Deaths associated with anaesthesia for obstetrics (editorial). Anaesthesia 36:145–146, 1981.
36. Roberts RB, Shirley MA: Reducing the risk of acid aspiration during cesarean section. Anesth Analg 53:858–868, 1974.

37. Gibbs CP, Spohr L, Schmidt D: The effectiveness of sodium citrate as an antacid. Anesthesiology 57:44–46, 1982.
38. Gibbs CP, Schwartz DJ, Wynne JW, Hood CI, Kuck EJ: Antacid pulmonary aspiration in the dog. Anesthesiology 51:380–385, 1979.
39. Holdsworth JD, Johnson K, Mascall G, Roulston RG, Tomlinson PA: Mixing of antacids with stomach contents: Another approach to the prevention of the acid aspiration (Mendelson's) syndrome. Anaesthesia 35:641–650, 1980.
40. Cohen SE, Barrier G: Efficacy and safety of metoclopramide before cesarean section. In *Abstracts of Scientific Papers*, Society for Obstetric Anesthesia and Perinatology, Vancouver, BC, 1983, p 1.
41. Hodgkinson R, Glassenberg R, Joyce TH III, Coombs DW, Ostheimer GW, Gibbs CP: Comparison of cimetidine with antacid for safety and effectiveness in reducing gastric acidity before elective cesarean section. Anesthesiology 59:86–90, 1983.
42. Abernethy DR, Greenblatt DJ, Eshelman FN, Shader RI: Ranitidine does not impair oxidative or conjugative metabolism: Noninteraction with antipyrine, diazepam and lorazepam. Clin Pharmacol Therapy 35:188–192, 1984.
43. Crawford JS: Difficulty in endotracheal intubation associated with obstetric anesthesia. Anesthesiology 51:475, 1979.
44. Heller PJ, Schneider EP, Marx GF: Pharyngo-laryngeal edema as a presenting symptom in preeclampsia. Obstet Gynecol 162:523–525, 1983.
45. Datta S, Briwa J: Modified laryngoscope for endotracheal intubation of obese patients. Anesth Analg 60:120–121, 1981.
46. Samsoon GLT, Young JRB: Difficult intubation: A retrospective study. Anaesthesia 42:487–490, 1987.
47. Archer GW Jr, Marx GF: Arterial oxygen tension during apnoea in parturient woman. Br J Anaesth 46:358–360, 1974.
48. Bernman JA, Furgiuele JJ, Marx GF: The Einstein carbon dioxide detector. Anesthesiology 60:613–614, 1984.
49. Stinson TW: A simple connector for transtracheal ventilation. Anesthesiology 47:232, 1977.
50. Assali NS, Prystowsky H: Studies on autonomic blockade. I. Comparison between the effects of tetraethylammonium chloride (TEAC) and high selective spinal anesthesia on the blood pressure of normal and toxemic pregnancy. J Clin Invest 29:1354–1360, 1950.
51. Bromage PR: Spread of analgesic solutions in the epidural space and their site of action: A statistical study. Br J Anaesth 34:161–178, 1962.
52. Marx GF, Orkin LR: *Physiology of Obstetric Anesthesia.* Charles C Thomas, Springfield, IL, 1969, pp 97–99.
53. Fagraeus L, Urban BJ, Bromage PR: Spread of epidural analgesia in early pregnancy. Anesthesiology 58:184–187, 1983.
54. Datta S, Lambert DH, Gregus J, Gissen AJ, Covino BJ: Differential sensitivity of mammalian nerve fibers during pregnancy. Anesth Analg 62:1070–1072, 1983.
55. Datta S, Hurley RJ, Naulty JS, Stern P, Lambert DH, Concepcion M, Tulchinsky D, Weiss JB, Ostheimer GW: Plasma and cerebrospinal fluid progesterone concentrations in pregnant and nonpregnant women. Anesth Analg 65:950–954, 1986.
56. Scott DB: Inferior vena cava occlusion in late pregnancy and its importance in anaesthesia. Br J Anaesth 40:120–128, 1968.
57. Marx GF: Regional analgesia in obstetrics. Anaesthesist 20:84–91, 1972.
58. McCausland AM, Hyman C, Winsor T, Trotter AD: Venous distensibility during pregnancy. Am J Obstet Gynecol 81:472–476, 1965.
59. Greiss FC Jr, Crandell DL: Therapy for hypotension induced by spinal anesthesia during pregnancy: Observations on gravid ewes. JAMA 191:793–796, 1965.
60. Wollman SB, Marx GF: Acute hydration for prevention of hypotension of spinal anesthesia in parturients. Anesthesiology 29:374–380, 1968.
61. Marx GF, Cosmi EV, Wollman SB: Biochemical status and clinical condition of mother and infant at cesarean section. Anesth Analg 48:986–993, 1969.
62. Collins KM, Bevan DR, Beard RW: Fluid loading to reduce abnormalities of fetal heart rate and maternal hypotension during epidural analgesia in labour. Br Med J 2:1460–1461, 1978.
63. Huovinen K, Lehtovirta P, Forss M, Kivalo I, Teramo K: Changes in placental intervillous blood flow measured by the Xenon method during lumbar epidural block for elective caesarean section. Acta Anaesthesiol Scand 23:529–533, 1979.
64. Lewis M, Thomas P, Wilkes FG: Hypotension during epidural analgesia for caesarean section: Arterial and central venous pressure changes after acute intravenous loading with two liters of Hartmann's solution. Anaesthesia 38:250–253, 1983.
65. Marx GF: Bupivacaine cardiotoxicity: Concentration or dose? Anesthesiology 65:116, 1986.
66. Albright GA: Cardiac arrest following regional anesthesia with etidocaine or bupivacaine. Anesthesiology 51:285–287, 1979.
67. Marx GF: Maternal complications of regional analgesia. Reg Anesth 6:104–107, 1981.
68. Marx GF: Cardiopulmonary resuscitation of late-pregnant women. Anesthesiology 56:156, 1982.
69. Rees GAD, Willis BA: Resuscitation in late pregnancy. Anaesthesia 43:347–349, 1988.
70. Moore DC, Thompson GE, Crawford RD: Long-acting local anesthetic drugs and convulsions with hypoxia and acidosis. Anesthesiology 56:230–232, 1982.
71. Chestnut DH, Owen CL, Brown CK, Vandewalker GE, Weiner CP: Does labor affect the variability of maternal heart rate during induction of epidural anesthesia? Anesthesiology 68:622–625, 1988.
72. Hood DD, Dewan DM, James FM III: Maternal and fetal effects of epinephrine in gravid ewes. Anesthesiology 64:610–613, 1986.
73. Marx GF, Elstein ID, Schuss M, Anyaegbunam A, Fleischer A: Effects of epidural block with lignocaine and lignocaine-adrenaline on umbilical artery velocity wave ratios. Br J Obstet Gynaecol 97:517–520, 1990.
74. Morgan BM: Maternal death: A review of maternal deaths at one hospital from 1958–1978. Anaesthesia 35:334–338, 1980.
75. Breheny F, McCarthy J: Maternal mortality: A review of maternal deaths over twenty years at the National Maternity Hospital, Dublin. Anaesthesia 37:561–564, 1982.

Obstetric Anesthesia and Lawsuits

Part 1: General Considerations and Recommendations

David Karp, M.A.

Marrs A. Craddick, LLB., J.D.

With some exceptions, malpractice lawsuits against anesthesiologists usually involve catastrophic injuries, including cardiac arrest and death, brain damage, paralysis, and infection. Until recently, anesthesiology was one of the highest risk specialties for liability insurance. In no other medical specialty does the physician render a patient unconscious and insensate (in a physical state still barely understood by medical science), keep the patient suspended and stable while the surgeon or obstetrician performs the operation, then return the patient to consciousness without ill effect. There is an ever-present risk of injury to patients undergoing anesthesia because of the unknown and infinitely variable responses of each patient's body. In obstetric anesthesia, there is an added risk of injury to the fetus or newborn that the anesthesiologist must anticipate and avoid. Actual injury to a patient caused by the mismanagement of anesthesia is infrequent when measured against the total number of local and general anesthetics given each year in the U.S. However, because of the severity of the injuries associated with anesthesia, it is not surprising that many of the highest malpractice damage awards have involved anesthetic complications.

The American Society of Anesthesiologists' (ASA's) adoption in 1986 of anesthesia standards for intraoperative monitoring (1), physician involvement in quality improvement programs, and more effective peer review have contributed to a nationwide decline in the number and severity of anesthesia malpractice claims. Broader anesthesia practice guidelines have been promulgated by the Canadian Anaesthetists' Society (2) and the New Jersey Department of Health (3). The use of formal practice "standards" or "guidelines" not only gives guidance to physicians but strengthens the defense of anesthesiologists in malpractice litigation, except in cases of noncompliance. Before intraoperative monitoring standards were recognized by the specialty, expert anesthesiologists who testified for plaintiffs or defendants frequently expressed only their own individual interpretations of applicable standards of care. Disputes about what constitutes accepted standards and how their validity is to be determined can increase anesthesiologists' liability exposure and can result in unpredictable jury verdicts. In recent years acceptance by anesthesiologists of monitoring guidelines has helped to reduce liability exposure, which in turn has lowered the cost of malpractice liability insurance. Wider adoption of comprehensive practice standards, similar to those in Canada and New Jersey, would tend to ensure more uniform evaluation by jurors, arbitrators, and medical peer reviewers of the appropriateness of anesthesia management in particular cases.

PHYSICIAN-PATIENT RELATIONSHIP

Because of the nature of the specialty, there are two considerable disadvantages with which the anesthesiologist is burdened, as compared with a surgeon or obstetrician, and which increase the chances of being sued. First, the anesthesiologist generally has only relatively short-term personal contact with the patient. Aside from brief conversations during the preanesthesia interview in the operating or delivery room or later conversations in the recovery room, the anesthesiologist's relationship with the patient ordinarily is silent. Second, the anesthesiologist seldom has an opportunity to personally correct a problem that may have resulted from anesthesia. If surgery is unsuccessful, the surgeon may be able to redo the operation and maintain rapport with the patient. The anesthesiologist, on the other hand, seldom is able to treat the patient for injuries related to anesthesia, but must rely on others to do so. As a consequence, the patient may be more critical about a complication from anesthesia than might have been the case had the patient known the anesthesiologist better.

The obstetric anesthesiologist frequently has the opportunity to broaden communication with the patient during labor while administering epidural or caudal anesthesia. The anesthesiologist is more than a consultant to the surgeon or an assistant at delivery or during an operation, and contacts with the patient can be improved if a greater effort is made to establish an independent relationship. Many anesthesiologists now consider it a part of their treatment to make at least one postoperative visit to the patient to learn if any problems resulted from anesthesia, such as damage to teeth secondary to intubation, sore throat, back pain, or other complaints.

In the brief postanesthetic visit, the anesthesiologist can reassure the patient and, when applicable, decide whether specific treatment for a complaint is necessary. The visit should be documented in the chart, and recommendations for treatment should be coordinated with the obstetrician. When problems do exist, a second visit, demonstrating the anesthesiologist's concern, may help to further strengthen rapport with the patient.

"CAPTAIN OF THE SHIP" DOCTRINE IS SOMETIMES INAPPLICABLE

The "captain of the ship" doctrine, under which surgeons or obstetricians could be considered liable for the conduct of all members of the surgical or obstetric team, including the physician-anesthesiologist, does not apply when injury occurs solely as a consequence of the anesthesiologist's professional negligence. The anesthesiologist's independent expertise makes him or her a coequal member of the obstetric team, and the obstetrician is ordinarily responsible only for obstetric decisions. It is anticipated that the obstetrician will consult with the anesthesiologist on matters outside the obstetrician's scope of expertise, and the law recognizes that an obstetrician has to rely on the anesthesiologist to make major decisions concerning the choice of anesthetic agent, the monitoring of vital signs during surgery and delivery, and the administration of perianesthetic drugs. Therefore, because the obstetrician is entitled to rely on the judgment of the anesthesiologist in matters relating to anesthesia, the obstetrician is not liable if it is the judgment of the anesthesiologist that is defective; only the anesthesiologist would be liable in such a case. Nevertheless, some plaintiffs' attorneys believe that they are protecting their clients' interests by suing all persons present during a surgery, even though it is apparent that some may not be liable. For this reason, an obstetrician may sometimes be sued as a defendant in a lawsuit in which an anesthesiologist, a codefendent, is the actual target, and vice versa.

In cases in which the actual cause of injury to the patient is not easily identifiable—such as postoperative infections, adverse reaction to a drug or anesthetic agent, perinatal injuries, or idiopathic complications—the anesthesiologist is likely to be included in the lawsuit along with the obstetrician and virtually all other members of the operating or delivery team. It is often only through the discovery process in litigation that the actual cause of injury can be determined and the person responsible identified.

LITIGATION AGAINST ANESTHESIOLOGISTS

It is a mistake to assume, as many doctors do, that judges and juries are unfavorably disposed toward physicians in malpractice actions. Although everyone has heard or read about large awards in malpractice cases, the overwhelming majority of actions tried in court against doctors and other health care providers end with vindication of the defendant. Defense verdicts are not newsworthy, and are rarely publicized. On the other hand, awards of large sums of money to the plaintiff have news value and are publicized, thus perhaps creating an erroneous impression in the public mind that physicians are losing more often in court than actually is the case. Past experience has shown that doctors prevail in a very large majority of the lawsuits.

RECENT CLAIMS DATA

Recent studies of malpractice claims against anesthesiologists show a decline in the number of such claims and fewer adverse verdicts and settlements.

A 1992 study by the Physician Insurers Association of America (PIAA) analyzed malpractice claims closed between January 1985 and June 1991, as reported by physician-owned insurance carriers (4). Claims against anesthesiologists accounted for less than 5% of all reported claims. Of the 78,712 claims, a total of 3615 claims were made against anesthesiologists. Indemnity payments were made in only 1292 cases, or 36% of the total claims reported against anesthesiologists; 64% of the claims were resolved in the physicians' favor. Claims against anesthesiologists that resulted in payments to claimants comprised less than 1% of paid claims against all physicians.

In the PIAA study, anesthesiologists placed seventh among all specialists in frequency of claims, and tenth in amount of average indemnity payment. The average indemnity payment in an anesthesia-related case was $121,286. (In an earlier study of malpractice claims closed between 1975 and 1978, the National Association of Insurance Commissioners [NAIC] reported that anesthesia claims accounted for 3% of the total claims paid and 11% of the total indemnity dollars paid to litigants. The average indemnity payment for anesthesia claims in the NAIC study was $96,822. Between 1977 and 1978, the size of indemnity payments increased 58% [5, 6].)

The most frequent conditions for which claims were made against anesthesiologists, according to the PIAA, were related to pregnancy and birth. Claims involving central nervous system complications of a procedure were the most expensive (average payment $480,019 on 50 paid claims). (By contrast, the 1980 NAIC study had found that claims involving cardiac or cardiopulmonary arrest were the most expensive, and accounted for one-third of all claims against anesthesiologists.)

An American Society of Anesthesiology Closed Claims Study in 1989 reported that 34% of the cases involved adverse outcomes associated with respiratory events (7). The study noted that 72% of the adverse outcomes could have been prevented with better monitoring. Of interest, professional liability insurers reported a dramatic decline in cases involving cardiopulmonary arrest following the ASA's adoption of monitoring standards of care, which mandate continuous patient monitoring and which restrict anesthesiologists from leaving the operating room while a patient is anesthetized. In the past inadequacy of monitoring or documentation and the failure of anesthesiologists to stay in the operating room while the patient was anesthetized have been serious handicaps in defending anesthesiologists in malpractice cases in which the patient sustained a cardiac arrest, pulmonary arrest, or both. Even before the ASA promulgated its monitoring standards in 1986, a number of California malpractice carriers had already required anesthesiologists to employ similar standards for continuous monitoring and for attending anesthetized patients as a condition of the physicians' liability coverage. But it was the formal adoption of standards that is credited with reducing the frequency of undetected arrest and which has strengthened the defense of anesthesiologists when adverse outcomes occurred despite the use of appropriate monitors.

STANDARDS OF PRACTICE

The success in litigation of defendant-doctors is expected to continue in the future, primarily because it is recognized in the law applicable to physicians that medicine is not an exact science and that human

judgment, which is fallible and also variable, is involved to such an extent that it is difficult to establish clearly in some cases that the judgment exercised by an individual physician was wrong. A trial juror usually is a person who has, in his or her past experience, always been satisfied with and grateful for services rendered to himself or herself and to family members by the medical profession. In addition, the legal representation of members of the medical profession involved with malpractice litigation usually is conducted by experienced trial attorneys who are themselves specialists in litigation of this type and who thoroughly familiarize themselves with medical issues in individual cases and know the applicable law. Moreover, when a jury does impose liability on a member of the medical profession, it is not usually because the jury was confused or because they acted on whim. With rare exceptions, liability has been imposed only where there has been testimony at trial by members of the medical profession that has supported the finding of the jury.

Whatever the reason for which a doctor has been sued, the final determination of culpability, or lack of it, will depend on a determination being made, usually by a jury, as to whether the doctor followed or failed to follow the *standards of practice* for the specialty. Many factors that can affect this determination—for example, the credibility of witnesses, the weight of evidence, the demeanor of the defendant, and the issue of proximate cause (the relationship between the treatment rendered or omitted and the injury). All are considered by the jury (or in arbitration cases by the arbitrator) in reaching a verdict, but it is this determination (i.e., whether the defendant adhered to applicable standards of practice) that is the crux of the case.

The main controversy between the opposing parties in a lawsuit that involves allegations of medical malpractice usually arises from their conflicting efforts to identify and to specify standards (i.e., requirements) of practice that were applicable to the defendant-physician during the period of time that professional services were provided to the patient who subsequently brought the lawsuit. Once the jury has determined what standard actually applied, which is often very difficult for them to do, it is usually a relatively easier task for them to decide whether the conduct of the defendant conformed to the standard. The rules of law that define the duties of the jurors and the methods which they must follow in their efforts to determine the standard that applied have crucial importance and should be fully understood by every member of the medical profession. However, experience suggests that many of them do not understand.

The law itself is generous to physicians; this circumstance has given rise to constant criticism from members of the bar who represent patients who desire to sue their doctors. ***The law recognizes that physicians must make judgments and that all human judgment is fallible.*** Therefore liability is not imposed for mere error in judgment, but rather only for conduct constituting a ***departure from standard practice*** that causes injury to a patient. The law defers to physicians themselves to identify and to define the standards of their profession. The law does not prescribe, much less dictate, to members of the medical profession how injuries and illnesses of patients are to be treated. The ***only*** evidence that may be received in court regarding the existence of an applicable standard of practice in the community in a given set of circumstances involving a physician-patient relationship is the testimony of a knowledgeable physician. The function of the jury is restricted and jurors are not permitted to set up an arbitrary standard of their own to be applied to the conduct of physicians. Their function is limited to weighing and considering the testimony given by members of the medical profession on the issue of what was or was not required of the defendant-physician by applicable standards of practice in the medical community.

It is recognized in law that medicine is not an exact science and that physicians and surgeons can and do differ with each other regarding the choice of treatment for particular problems. There is no limit set in the law regarding the number of different approaches to treatment of any given problem that would be acceptable. The only requirement is that a particular approach to treatment, to be acceptable, must be supported by physicians in good standing in the community.

Neither does the law prescribe the number of physicians who must support a given approach to qualify that approach as one of the methods which is legally acceptable.

The inquiry of a jury in a malpractice case, therefore, is required to be directed toward toward a determination of whether the method or approach selected by the individual defendant-physician under the circumstances of the case presented was one which was accepted at least by some, even if not by all, physicians in good standing in the community. If it was, the inquiry ends and the physician has a complete defense to a charge that he or she departed from standard practice. It is not relevant to continue the inquiry to see what type of result was obtained from treatment selected by the defendant. It may well be that, viewed in the light of later events, a different

method of treatment should have been chosen or that a method other than the one selected by the defendant would have been better suited to bring about the desired result. Hindsight, however, is not the test, and the judgment of the defendant-physician is to be evaluated on the basis of what was presented at the time the judgment was made and not on the basis of how things turned out subsequently.

RES IPSA LOQUITUR

In some malpractice cases, the plaintiff can establish liability against a defendant-physician without having to prove the existence of a specific applicable standard of practice with which the defendant-physician did not comply. That is, the plaintiff may be able to assert the doctrine known as ***res ipsa loquitur***, literally meaning "the thing speaks for itself."

Res ipsa loquitur, a Latin maxim, dates back to a time when proceedings in English courts were conducted in Latin. The doctrine owes its existence to learned judges who were trying to be fair to a plaintiff in a particular case in which the plaintiff had been struck unconscious and was injured by an object that fell from an upper-story window while he was walking by a building occupied by a business owned by the defendant. Until then, English law had required a plaintiff to prove the specific facts constituting the alleged negligence to recover damages for injury caused by negligence. In this case the plaintiff was unconscious, had never been inside the defendant's building, and could not explain how the accident had occurred. Unable to prove negligence in the required way, the plaintiff's case was thrown out in a lower court. The plaintiff appealed to a higher court, which concluded that the decision of the lower court was unfair. In the view of the appellate judges, the situation surrounding the injury to the plaintiff was *res ipsa loquitur*; that is, the situation spoke for itself in that, in the ordinary course of events, objects do not ordinarily fall out of windows and injure innocent passersby unless someone has been careless and negligent. Assessing the conduct of the injured, unconscious, and innocent plaintiff and that of the defendants (who, after all, controlled the instrumentalities that had caused the injury), it seemed unfair to require the plaintiff to prove specifically how the injury had occurred. The defendants were in a much better position to explain. Therefore, it was fair to require them to explain how the accident occurred if it was not due to their negligence.

The court ruled that, where an innocent plaintiff has been injured in a way that ordinarily would not have happened in the absence of negligence, an inference arises that the defendants were negligent res *ipsa loquitur* and the burden then shifts to the defendants to come forth with evidence to rebut the inference of negligence.

In contemporary times, if a plaintiff in a malpractice case can prove that his or her injury was one of a type that does not ordinarily occur in the absence of medical negligence, that his or her attending physicians had exclusive control over the instrumentalities which caused the injury, and that the plaintiff did not contribute to his or her own injury, the plaintiff is not required to produce expert medical testimony that one or more of the defendant physicians failed to comply with an applicable standard of practice. Instead, the plaintiff can, in this situation, rely on the doctrine of *res ipsa loquitur* to avoid what otherwise would result in a failure of required proof. Where *res ipsa loquitur* applies, the main benefit is to relieve the plaintiff of the effort of finding a physician who is willing to testify in support of his or her malpractice claim. When the plaintiff already has or can get an expert witness to testify, the benefit of *res ipsa loquitur* is not needed.

EFFECT OF COMPARATIVE NEGLIGENCE DOCTRINE

Some states have adopted the concept of comparative negligence in adjudicating personal injury lawsuits. This doctrine permits a jury to apportion damages based on the degree of negligence, if any, among all parties (including the plaintiff) who contributed to the injury. Thus, although there is still a risk that the anesthesiologist may be included in a lawsuit based on an injury that is clearly not related to administration of anesthesia, through the concepts of comparative negligence and equitable apportionment of damages, even minimal responsibility for causation of negligent injury likely will be reflected in an assessment of some damages although they might be minimal.

In other states, application of the concept of joint and several liability in malpractice cases can lead to a judgment against both the obstetrician and the anesthesiologist for which each is equally liable, even though the fault of one or the other may be minimal.

PREVENTING THE LAWSUIT

Adhere to Standards of Practice

From the cases in which issues involving the practice of anesthesia have been judicially decided, some basic guidelines have emerged. Some of these minimum practice requirements are:

1. ***Conduct a preanesthetic interview and examination of the patient.*** The extent of the interview and examination depends on how much the doctor

needs to know to be prepared to handle problems that might reasonably be expected to occur in view of the history and findings, and on how much information the patient needs in order to give an informed consent (see below).

2. ***Review the medical chart*** for the current surgery and, when available and relevant, the charts for prior surgeries.

3. ***Record the review of history, findings and proposed anesthetic management in the patient's chart.*** Charting such data is imperative, because studies show that many patients cannot recall preoperative discussions with the anesthesiologist.

4. ***Consult***, as appropriate, with the obstetrician and with other specialists as needed.

5. ***Discuss the risk and hazards of anesthesia with the patient*** so that the patient can freely give consent to be anesthetized.

From the authors' standpoint the required minimums itemized above seem to be nearly universal in the practice of anesthesia. When it comes to evaluating the effort of a physician to fulfill these and other requirements of anesthetic practice, the law is flexible and indulgent. In general, the level of proficiency required of the anesthesiologist is that of other anesthesiologists in the community, or a similar community, who have *average* training and skill. The proficiency of the exceptional or gifted anesthesiologist is not used as a guideline in determining the standard of performance required by law. Although the anesthesiologist personally may not be satisfied to aspire only to the practice of average medicine, the law requires no more; if the anesthesiologist demonstrates proficiency at the level that is average for the community, there is a defense to a charge of negligence. It must be kept in mind, however, that standards of competence change. The anesthesiologist should keep abreast of what is being done by colleagues through educational seminars, continuing education programs, and medical literature.

Monitor the Patient

The types of malpractice suits that, more than any other, have called attention to the anesthesiologist are cardiac arrest cases and cases in which the patient has sustained brain injury secondary to hypoxia or ischemia. It is commonly accepted among anesthesiologists that such complications can occur in the hands of the most proficient and attentive anesthesiologist and that medical science has not yet perfected methods by which the physician can anticipate or even identify all of the reasons why a patient might undergo arrest or become hypoxic during the administration of a "routine" anesthetic. Therefore, the emphasis among anesthesiologists has been to develop methods for detecting these problems so that they can be reversed before injury to the patient occurs.

In view of adoption of monitoring standards by the ASA and other professional organizations, when physicians do not employ the recommended monitoring techniques because of special considerations in individual cases, they should document their reasons for departing from the standards. Except in an emergency, the unavailability of monitoring devices may not be a sufficient reason for proceeding without them.

Obtain an Informed Consent

Few issues in the realm of malpractice litigation have angered and confused physicians as much as the doctrine of "informed consent," which is the product of a series of appellate court decisions. The concept of "informed consent" deals with the questions of how much information a patient needs to be given by a physician to be sufficiently informed before consenting to proposed surgery or anesthesia. At present, the law in several states generally provides that, as an integral part of the physician's overall obligation to the patient, there is a duty of reasonable disclosure of the available options with respect to proposed therapy or surgery and of the dangers inherently and potentially involved in each. A corollary is that it may also be a duty of the physician to discuss risks that will confront the patient if the proposed treatment or procedure is refused.

The purpose of the law can be simply stated. A physician who recommends a particular course of therapy for a patient always has in mind the anticipated benefits that it is hoped will be achieved. In seeking the patient's consent for the treatment, fairness demands that the patient be informed of both the contemplated benefits and potential risks so that the patient personally can make a knowledgeble decision as to whether the benefits outweigh the risks. All information that might reasonably affect this decision should be provided to the patient. The requirement of disclosure has been judicially qualified, however, by acknowledgment that the patient's interest in information does not extend to a lengthy polysyllabic discourse of all possible complications and by recognition that, in electing a procedure, the patient is most concerned with the risk of death or serious bodily injury.

When required to adjudicate a claim by a patient that an informed consent was not obtained, the jury ordinarily is instructed by the judge that a physician must advise the patient of the potential of death or serious harm if it exists, must explain in lay terms the complications that might occur, and must provide any additional information that would be provided by reputable physicians in the community under similar circumstances. The jury is further instructed that the plaintiff must then prove that, had such information been provided, a reasonable person in the same position would have refused the proposed surgery or treatment. In cases in which the sole issue involves informed consent and the evidence indicates that the medical treatment administered to the patient was appropriate, experience has shown that juries generally conclude that a reasonable person, who was adequately informed, would have consented to the proposed procedure.

In anesthesiology, the physician's duty to disclose risks to the patient does not extend to reviewing the choices for anesthetic agents, because the patient is not expected to understand the pharmacologic variations of anesthetic agents. However, a disclosure of the relevant types of anesthesia and the known general risks, including death, paralysis, infection, and idiopathic encephalopathy, cannot be withheld from the patient, except when the patient is in no condition to withstand or understand such disclosure, when the patient requests not to be so advised, or when there is no opportunity for the physician to make the disclosure, such as in emergencies.

The prudent anesthesiologist can probably discharge professional obligations to the patient and comply with the requirements of the law by:

1. *Discussing the choice of anesthetic agent and techniques with the patient and by stating the general reasons for the selection.*
2. *Advising the patient that the administration of any anesthesia involves some risks.*
3. *Inquiring whether the patient wishes to know more specifically about the risks of the anesthesia planned.*

If the patient acknowledges a desire to know the risks, the anesthesiologist should tell the patient the most common complications—such as sore throat, transient backache, hypotension, headache when applicable—as well as rare complications—including death, paralysis, infection, and any other apparent problems that a particular patient may be at risk for—bearing in mind that the purpose is to adequately inform and not frighten the patient.

At the end of the discussion, questions should be invited and answered, and the fact and nature of the conversation should be charted with an entry that indicates that "Major and minor risks discussed; questions answered; patient wants to proceed."

Some patients may prefer not to know the risks of anesthesia; if the patient declines the discussion, the chart should note: "Patient declines discussion of risks." Discussions of risks for incompetent patients should be held with a spouse or next of kin, who probably will be the person who authorizes the surgery or treatment. In those cases in which no next of kin or responsible party is available and the physician believes the patient is not in suitable condition to discuss the risks, the physician may elect to forego such discussion, but should list the reasons for doing so in the patient's chart. Used *judiciously and fairly,* this approach has been held acceptable by the courts.

Although the patient should be enabled to make an informed decision, the patient should not be permitted to dictate medical decisions to the physicians or to force the physician to render or fail to render treatment deemed advisable based on professional judgment. If the patient attempts to dictate a course of treatment contrary to good medical practice, the physician may be well advised to encourage the patient to find another doctor. It is doubtful that the anesthesiologist, who agrees to administer a local anesthetic for a procedure for which a general anesthetic would clearly provide better protection against injury to the patient, will be able later to fashion a successful defense that the type of anesthetic, although contrary to the physician's best medical judgment, was the choice of the patient. Where either method is considered reasonable and acceptable, however, the anesthesiologist should impart to the patient the reasons for the recommendation and should document the reasons if the first choice is not accepted by the patient.

In informed-consent cases, courts consistently have noted that "informed consent" is not the same as "consent form." A consent form signed by a patient before the physician has apparently informed the patient may be invalid. The anesthesiologist should not rely on the obstetrician to explain anesthesia risks to the patient or to obtain informed consent for the administration of anesthesia. Consent forms appearing to have the patient's acknowledgment that anesthesia risks have been discussed can easily be attacked in litigation if the plaintiff can prove that the form was signed before the patient met with the anesthesiologist.

Maintain Equipment and Medical Records

The anesthesiologist has the responsibility for determining that all equipment related to the administration of anesthesia is in proper working order before and during the surgery. Equipment, whether owned by the hospital or by the physician, should be regularly serviced and a service record should be maintained. The selection of equipment is left to the anesthesiologist, and the law does not require that a hospital (or private contractor-physician) select one piece of machinery over another. However, some older equipment may be less helpful to the doctor in de-

tecting anesthetic problems and may impose a greater burden for attentiveness on the doctor. The task of testing all parts of the equipment should not be delegated to a nonphysician, because calibrations for warning devices and gas flow indicators should be attuned to the needs of each particular case in accordance with the physician's judgment.

The medical record has been and always will be one of the firmest foundations on which the defense of a malpractice case is based. In addition to the notes the anesthesiologist makes about preoperative and postoperative visits and examinations, the anesthesia record for labor, delivery, or surgery is an essential part of the medical record. Notations of vital signs, the instillation of drugs, and significant patient response during anesthesia become a permanent record that will help support the actions of the anesthesiologist if a lawsuit occurs many months or years after memories have faded. To prevent subsequent misinterpretation or misunderstanding, the anesthesiologist should try not to chart an inordinate amount of information in abbreviated form in the anesthesia record. Entries should be legible, concise, and properly timed. In cardiac arrest cases the careless or inaccurate charting of the time and nature of resuscitation or medications can mean the difference between a defensible and an indefensible case.

Under no circumstances should the anesthesia record (or any other part of the medical chart, for that matter) be altered after an entry has been made. If there is a need for a correction or amendment, the original, incorrect entry should not be obliterated. It should be simply crossed out with a single line so that the original entry can be read. All changes, additions, or amendments should be initialed, timed, and dated, so that no one can draw the inference that the chart was altered for self-serving purposes. Moreover, the anesthesiologist should never prechart the anesthetic record for personal convenience. Although confident that specific medications will be given or that the flows of anesthetic agents and oxygen will be changed at times, no entries should be made in the chart until after these acts have been accomplished.

Issues in Birth-related Malpractice Suits

The number of birth-related malpractice lawsuits has increased dramatically since 1980. Many multimillion dollar settlements and judgments have involved brain-damaged babies whose perinatal care allegedly was substandard. While most of the cases have focused on the role of the obstetrician (or other physician who delivered the baby) and on the role of nurses in hospital labor and delivery units, anesthesiologists have not been immune from such litigation. One charge that surfaces in these cases is that there was a delay in assembling the medical team, including the anesthesiologist, to perform emergency cesarean section. Hospitals and physicians can defend themselves against such claims by developing a policy for promptly assembling the surgical team in such cases, in accordance with prevailing standards of care, such as those promulgated by The American College of Obstetricians and Gynecologists.

A second issue in birth-related malpractice claims centers on unsuccessful efforts to resuscitate a newborn infant without residual serious mental or physical impairments. The subject of neonatal resuscitation is under scrutiny by medical, religious, and political leaders, and it is unlikely that the questions concerning how and when to abandon resuscitation of an obviously impaired newborn will soon be resolved. Medical staffs are advised to obtain advice from competent medical law attorneys for assistance in formulating policies concerning neonatal resuscitation. "Do not resuscitate" guidelines have been promulgated by several state medical societies and thus far have been acceptable to the courts.

CONCLUSION

It would be understandable if anesthesiologists, and indeed other medical specialists, were disheartened by the liability risks with which they are confronted each time a patient is anesthetized or treated. The malpractice crisis that swept the United States in the spring of 1975 highlighted the complexity of the professional liability problem. The publicity gen-

erated at the time, however, did not accurately reflect the true state of affairs, and it is anticipated that in the future, as in the past, physicians will prevail in the vast majority of lawsuits brought by patients.

It should also be kept in mind that the occurrence of an injury associated with anesthesia or other medical treatment does not in itself establish negligence and, as a consequence, liability. The plaintiff must always prove that the defendant-physician failed to follow standard practice in treating the patient and that it was this failure to do so which caused the injury of which the plaintiff complains. Anesthesiologists who understand their relationship to the patient and to other physicians involved in the treatment and who remain vigilant to the standards in the medical community significantly reduce their exposure to malpractice liability.

References

1. American Society of Anesthesiologists: Standards for Basic Intra-Operative Monitoring, October 21, 1986.
2. Canadian Anaesthetists' Society: *Guidelines to the Practice of Anaesthesia as Recommended by the Canadian Anaesthetists' Society*, 1987.
3. New Jersey Department of Health: Standards of anesthesia care, NJAC 8:43B–18, 1989.
4. Physician Insurers Association of America: *PIAA Data Sharing Reports* (January, 1985 to June, 1991), PIAA, Pennington, NJ, 1989.
5. Sowka, MP: *Malpractice Claims—Final Compilation*. National Association of Insurance Commissionrs, 1980.
6. Brunner, EA: Analysis of anesthesiology mishaps: The National Association of Insurance Commissioners' Closed Claims Study. Int Anesthesiol Clin 22:17–30, 1984.
7. Tinker JH, Dull DL, Caplan RA, Ward RJ, Cheney FW: Role of monitoring devices in prevention of anesthetic mishaps: A closed 780claims analysis. Anesthesiology 71:541–546, 1989.

Obstetric Anesthesia and Lawsuits

Part 2: Review of Obstetric Anesthesia Closed Claims

H.S. Chadwick, M.D.

Since 1985 the Committee on Professional Liability of the American Society of Anesthesiologists (ASA) has been involved in an ongoing project to review malpractice claims against anesthesiologists. The long-term goal of this project is to improve patient safety by devising strategies to prevent anesthetic injuries. Recently a number of studies have been published based on the data collected from this project (1–7). One of these studies focused on the subset of claims resulting from anesthetic care for cesarean section and vaginal delivery (4). The data on obstetric-related claims are of particular interest to those who practice obstetric anesthesia. For the first time reliable data is available regarding the types of injuries that result in claims and the outcomes of such claims (i.e., the proportion of claims that resulted in settlements or awards and the dollar amount of such payments).

Information on anesthetic complications in general and obstetric anesthesia complications in particular is difficult to obtain. One of the best sources of this type of information is maternal mortality data (see Chapter 25). This, however, only provides data about complications that result in maternal death. Information concerning anesthetic-related morbidity is more difficult to obtain. In part, this may be due to a reluctance to publicize adverse outcomes and errors involving anesthetic care. To a large extent, anesthesiologists have operated on the assumption that the same factors that lead to maternal death, result in maternal morbidity in many other instances. Other sources of data about complications of anesthetic care have relied on case reports or research studies designed to determine the incidence of specific complications. These efforts are often limited by difficulty in obtaining reliable data from a large enough sample. Perhaps the current emphasis on quality assurance in medicine will provide new sources of data on anesthetic-related complications. In the meantime the closed claims studies provide a new and relevant source of information about undesired consequences of anesthetic care.

PROBLEMS AND BENEFITS OF CLOSED CLAIMS ANALYSIS

By their nature, closed claims studies have inherent limitations. The cases reviewed in the ASA Closed Claims Project were retrospectively obtained in a nonrandom fashion from participating insurance carriers without control over geographic balance and cover a time period in which anesthetic practices have continued to evolve. Only cases for which there was adequate documentation are included in the study. For any given time period, the total number of claims filed and the total number of anesthetics administered is not known. Not all injuries result in a claim of malpractice, nor is the anesthesiologist necessarily named in an injury that may have been related to anesthetic care. Conversely, anesthesiologists may be named in claims in which there was no anesthetic-related complication. For these reasons it is impossible to determine the incidence of particular complications. Despite these limitations, closed claims analysis can provide specific and valuable information.

The obstetric anesthesia closed claims study (4) allows us to see how those complications that have traditionally been associated with obstetric practice compare with those injuries that actually result in claims. We can compare the obstetric anesthesia claims with other types of anesthesia-related claims to see if different patterns of injury and outcome emerge. Specific questions can be asked: What injuries are most common among filed malpractice claims? In what proportion of claims is newborn injury attributed to anesthetic care? What precipitating events result in the claimed injuries? To what extent does substandard care (as judged by uninvolved anesthesiologists) contribute to the injuries? How is choice of anesthesia related to the claimed injuries? Do more obstetric claims result in payments than nonobstetric claims? Do obstetric claims result in disproportionately large payments? A particular advantage of this closed claims study is that it does not depend on self-reporting by the medical community. Instead, it provides a mechanism by which we can identify problems with anesthetic care based on the consumers' point of view. The study of malpractice claims may allow us to identify areas that require special attention to minimize adverse outcomes and may suggest strategies for limiting liability risk.

THE ASA CLOSED CLAIMS PROJECT

Specially trained, practicing anesthesiologists traveled to the offices of professional liability insurance carriers to review no longer active (closed claims) files of lawsuits against anesthesiologists. A standardized questionnaire consisting of over 140 informational items was completed, according to a set of instructions provided to each reviewer, for claims in which there was enough information to reconstruct the sequence of events and the nature of the injury. Claims for dental damages were not included. In addition to recording specific informational items, reviewers wrote a brief narrative description of each case, summarizing the sequence of events and providing additional details. Typical files reviewed included hospital and anesthesia records, narrative statements by the personnel involved, expert and peer reviews, deposition summaries, outcome reports, and data concerning cost of settlement or award. Each data collection instrument was reviewed by three members of the Closed Claims Project before being entered in a computer database for future analysis.

OBSTETRIC AND NONOBSTETRIC CLAIMS

As of May 1989 a total of 1541 claims were recorded in the ASA Closed Claims Project of which 92% involved cases that occurred between 1975 and 1985. Obstetric claims accounted for 12% (190) and nonobstetric claims 88% (1351) of all cases. The mean maternal age was 28 years in the obstetric claims, compared with a mean patient age of 41 years in the nonobstetric claims. Among the obstetric cases 67% (127) involved cesarean deliveries and 33% (63) involved vaginal deliveries. Of the obstetric claims, 65% (124) were associated with regional anesthesia and 33% (62) with general anesthesia, which is in contrast to the nonobstetric cases in which only 20% had a regional anesthetic and 76% had a general anesthetic. In the study 65% of all the obstetric injuries

and 74% of nonobstetric injuries were considered by the reviewers to be related to anesthetic care.

ANESTHETIC INJURIES

Table 26.1 displays all injuries or complications that had a frequency of 5% or more in the group of obstetric claims, as well as similar injuries in the group of nonobstetric claims. Not surprisingly, maternal or patient death was the leading complication in both obstetric and nonobstetric claims., However, in the group of obstetric claims, newborn brain damage was almost as common as maternal death. Of the 38 cases involving newborn brain injury, 45% (17) were attributed to problems with anesthetic care, 37% (14) to obstetric or congenital problems, and 13% (5) to problems associated with newborn resuscitation. It is interesting that newborn brain damage was one of the most common complications among the obstetric claims, despite the fact that the reviewers considered only 50% (19) of these injuries to have an anesthetic-related cause. Newborn outcome appears to be an important factor in determining if a claim is brought against the anesthesiologist. The anesthesiologist may be co-named in a suit because of the potential for the anesthetic to have contributed to the adverse outcome. Since fewer of the claims involving newborn brain damage appeared to be anesthetic related (50% compared to 76% for all obstetric claims), one might expect that fewer of them would result in payment. However, the payment rate (35%) was not significantly less than that of other obstetric claims (55%). For those claims in which payments were made, the median payment was significantly greater for cases in which the only injury was a damaged infant ($500,000) than for other obstetric claims ($120,000).

To better compare maternal injuries to injuries in the nonobstetric claims, Table 26.2 lists the same injuries as in Table 26.1 but eliminates those claims brought for injuries to the newborn only. By analyzing the data in this way, it can be seen that there are no significant differences between the groups with regard to patient/maternal brain damage and nerve damage. Claims for maternal death, however, constitute a smaller proportion of the obstetric claims than do patient deaths in the nononbstetric group. Claims for less severe injuries were significantly more common in the group of obstetric claims.

One of the most surprising findings of the study was that headache was the third most common complication among the obstetric claims and resulted in payments in over half of the cases. The significantly greater proportion of claims (32%) involving relatively minor injuries such as headache, pain during anesthesia, back pain, and emotional injury among the obstetric cases compared with the nonobstetric cases (4%) is note-

Table 26.1
Most Common Injuries in Obstetric Anesthesia Claims[a,b]

	Non-OB Claims (%) ($n = 1351$)	OB Claims (%) ($n = 190$)	OB Regional (%) ($n = 124$)	OB General (%) ($n = 62$)
Patient/maternal death	39 (524)[c]	22 (41)	12 (15)[c]	42 (26)
Newborn brain damage	NA	20 (38)	19 (23)	24 (15)
Headache	1 (10)[c]	12 (23)	19 (23)[c]	0 (0)
Newborn death	<0.5 (1)[c]	9 (17)	7 (8)	10 (6)
Pain during anesthesia	<0.5 (5)[c]	8 (16)	13 (16)[c]	0 (0)
Patient/maternal nerve damage	16 (209)[c]	8 (16)	10 (12)	7 (4)
Patient/maternal brain damage	13 (174)[c]	7 (14)	7 (9)	8 (5)
Emotional distress	2 (30)	6 (12)	7 (9)	5 (3)
Back pain	1 (8)	5 (9)	7 (9)[c]	0 (0)

[a]The most common injuries for which claims were made in the obstetric group are shown in order of decreasing frequency. Percentages are based on the total claims in each group. Some claims had more than one injury and are represented more than once. Brain damage only includes patients who were alive when the claim was closed. Statistical comparisons are made between obstetric and nonobstetric claims and between obstetric regional and obstetric general anesthetics.
[c]$P \leq 0.01$.
[b]Reprinted by permission from Chadwick HS, Posner K, Caplan RA, Ward RJ, Cheney FW: A comparison of obstetric and nonobstetric anesthesia malpractice claims. Anesthesiology 74:242–249, 1991.

Table 26.2
Most Common Maternal Injuries in Obstetric Anesthesia Claims[a,b]

	Non-OB Claims (%) ($n = 1351$)	Maternal Injury Claims (%) ($n = 151$)
Patient/maternal death	39 (524)[c]	27 (41)
Headache	1 (10)[c]	15 (23)
Pain during anesthesia	<0.5 (5)[c]	11 (16)
Patient/maternal nerve damage	16 (209)	11 (16)
Patient/maternal brain damage	13 (174)	9 (14)
Emotional distress	2 (30)[d]	8 (12)
Back pain	1 (8)[d]	6 (9)

[a]The most common maternal injuries for which claims were made in the obstetric group are shown in order of decreasing frequency. Percentages are based on the total claims in each group. Some claims, especially those with a fatal outcome, had more than one injury and are represented more than once. Cases involving brain damage only include patients who were alive when the claim was closed.
[c]$P \leq 0.01$.
[d]$P \leq 0.05$.
[b]Reprinted by permission from Chadwick HS, Posner K, Caplan RA, Ward RJ, Cheney FW: A comparison of obstetric and nonobstetric anesthesia malpractice claims. Anesthesiology 74:242–249, 1991.

worthy. Obstetric patients may be at greater risk for some of these injuries. For example, the popularity of regional anesthetic techniques in obstetic anesthesia, combined with obstetric patients' greater risk for developing postlumbar puncture headache, may account for the greater number of headache claims in the obstetric group. Almost all claims for pain during anesthesia involved cesarean sections under regional anesthesia. These may have resulted from a reluctance by the anesthesia personnel to convert to a general anesthetic. The high proportion of claims for relatively minor injuries among the obstetric claims may be due to a higher incidence of such problems in that group

of patients. However, other factors such as unrealistic expectations, general dissatisfaction with care provided, and postpartum emotional disturbances may also play a role. Because the true incidence of complications is not known in obstetric and nonobstetric anesthesia, it cannot be concluded that obstetric patients are more litigious, although the quality of anesthetic care was judged similar for both obstetric and nonobstetric claims (Figure 26.1).

CRITICAL EVENTS LEADING TO INJURIES

In the Closed Claims Project an attempt was made to identify those events that precipitated the injuries

STANDARD OF CARE

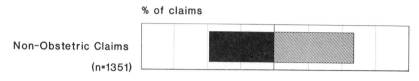

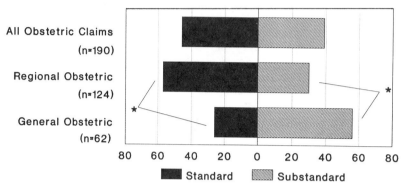

Figure 26.1 The proportion of claims in which the anesthetic care was judged as either standard or substandard. There was no difference between the obstetric and nonobstetric claims. *Indicates $P \le 0.01$ for regional vs. general anes- thesia. (Reprinted by permission from Chadwick HS, Posner K, Caplan RA, Ward RJ, Cheney FW: A comparison of obstetric and nonobstetric anesthesia malpractice claims. Anesthesiology 74:242–249, 1991.)

Table 26.3
Most Common Damaging Events in Obstetric Anesthesia Claims[a,b]

	Non-OB Claims (%) ($n = 1351$)	OB Claims (%) ($n = 190$)	OB Regional (%) ($n = 124$)	OB General (%) ($n = 62$)
Respiratory system	35 (476)[c]	24 (46)	11 (13)[c]	53 (33)
Inadequate ventilation	14 (186)[c]	5 (10)	4 (5)	7 (5)
Difficult intubation	6 (77)	5 (10)	1 (1)[d]	15 (9)
Aspiration	1 (18)[d]	4 (8)	2 (2)	10 (6)
Esophageal intubation	6 (87)	4 (7)	2 (2)	8 (5)
Bronchospasm	2 (27)	3 (5)	1 (1)	7 (4)
Inadequate F_{IO_2}	1 (7)	2 (4)	1 (1)	5 (3)
Airway obstruction	3 (39)	1 (1)	1 (1)	0 (0)
Premature extubation	1 (20)	1 (1)	0 (0)	2 (1)
Convulsion	1 (19)[c]	10 (19)	15 (18)[c]	2 (1)
Equipment problems	4 (56)	6 (11)	6 (7)	6 (4)
Wrong drug/dose	3 (47)	4 (8)	2 (2)	10 (6)
Cardiovascular system	7 (94)[c]	3 (6)	3 (4)	2 (1)
Inappropriate fluid therapy	2 (29)	2 (4)	3 (4)	0 (0)
Excessive blood loss	2 (28)	1 (1)	0 (0)	2 (1)
Wrong blood administered	1 (10)	1 (1)	0 (0)	0 (0)

[a]The most common damaging events in the obstetric claims are illustrated. Percentages are based on the total claims in each group. Specific damaging events were not identified in all cases. Some claims had more than one damaging event, however, for events related to the respiratory system, only the most significant is listed. Statistical comparisons are made between obstetric and nonobstetric claims and between obstetric regional and obstetric general anesthetics.
[c]$P \le 0.01$.
[d]$P \le 0.05$.
[b]Reprinted by permission from Chadwick HS, Posner K, Caplan RA, Ward RJ, Cheney FW: A comparison of obstetric and nonobstetric anesthesia malpractice claims. Anesthesiology 74:242–249, 1991.

for which a claim was filed (Table 26.3). Most of these "damaging" events were related to the respiratory system, both in the group of obstetric and nonobstetric claims. Among the obstetric claims, difficult tracheal intubation, inadequate ventilation, aspiration, and esophageal intubation were the most common events cited, whereas inadequate ventilation was by far the most common damaging event in the nonobstetric group. Those events characterized as "inadequate ventilation" appeared to be due to inadequate gas exchange, although the exact cause of the injury was not always clear. This is understandable when one considers that most of these injuries occurred before the widespread use of pulse oximetry and capnography.

Anesthetic complications are a major cause of maternal mortality (8, 9), and most of these deaths have been related to difficult intubation or pulmonary aspiration (8, 10). Pulmonary aspiration was noted in 8% (16) of the obstetric claims compared to only 2% (29) of nonobstetric claims ($P \leq 0.01$). In the obstetric group, 14 of 16% aspirations occurred with general anesthesia. The two cases of aspiration associated with regional anesthesia occurred during resuscitation efforts following high-spinal blocks.

These data are consistent with reports that difficult intubation and pulmonary aspiration are the leading causes of anesthetic-related maternal mortality, and they support the widely held belief that obstetric patients are at greater risk than nonobstetric patients for having these problems (see Chapter 23). Almost all the cases involving pulmonary aspiration (at least 14 of 16) were associated with either face mask general anesthesia or with difficult or esophageal intubation. A 1981 survey of members of the Society for Obstetric Anesthesia and Perinatology (SOAP) found that, among 21 reported cases of pulmonary aspiration in 1 year, all the patients had undergone general anesthesia. In 19 cases for which tracheal intubation was performed, 14 were reported as difficult intubations (11). The data from the 1981 SOAP survey, as well as the closed claims data, argue for the continued consideration of all obstetric patients as having a full stomach and requiring a protected airway during general anesthesia. The frequency with which adverse outcomes were linked to difficult intubation reinforces the need to have an appropriate protocol and equipment in place at all times for managing patients in whom tracheal intubation proves difficult.

Among the obstetric claims in which regional anesthesia was the primary anesthetic technique, convulsions were the most common critical or damaging event resulting in serious injuries. Convulsions accounted for 10% of all critical events recorded in the obstetric claims, compared with 1% in the nonobstetric claims. Of the 19 convulsions in the obstetric claims, 17 appeared to be due to intravascular injection of local anesthetic during epidural anesthesia. In none of these 17 cases was an epinephrine-containing test dose documented. Bupivacaine was the local anesthetic used in 15 cases, and in 2 cases the anesthetic was not specified. The remaining two convulsions resulting in lawsuits were thought to be eclamptic convulsions. The greater incidence of convulsions among the obstetric claims may be due to the greater popularity of epidural anesthesia in obstetrics. It is also possible, however, that local anesthetic convulsions in pregnant patients are more likely to lead to an adverse outcome in the mother, not to mention the additional risk to the fetus, thereby increasing the likelihood of a claim being filed. It is noteworthy that 83% of the obstetric claims involving convulsions with regional anesthesia resulted in neurologic injury or death to the mother, newborn, or both. Similarly it would appear that a local anesthetic-induced convulsion that does not result in neurologic injury or death is unlikely to result in a lawsuit.

Many of the injuries associated with convulsions occurred before the widespread attention this topic received in the 1980s. The current trends of using effective test doses and fractionating epidural local anesthetic injections and the recommendation to not use bupivacaine 0.75% in obstetrics has probably greatly reduced the occurrence of this untoward event.

Only 6% (11) of the obstetric claims were related to equipment problems. Five of these 11 equipment problems were due to severed epidural catheters. Most of the remainder were due to problems with ventilation equipment and included an expiratory limb of the anesthesia circuit connected to the ventilator, inoperative defibrillator, wrong connector in the circuit, and nitrogen in the oxygen lines during anesthetic administration. Four percent of the obstetric claims involved errors in drug administration. The proportion of claims related to equipment problems or drug errors is relatively low, perhaps because these problems do not often result in serious injury or because the problems were never discovered.

REGIONAL ANESTHESIA VS. GENERAL ANESTHESIA

The greater proportion of claims involving regional anesthesia among the obstetric cases probably relates to the greater popularity of regional anesthesia in obstetrics and not to a greater likelihood of injury associated with regional techniques. However, some injuries (Table 26.1) and damaging events (Table 26.3) showed a significant association with anesthetic technique. Claims for maternal death and events related to the respiratory system were significantly more common in cases involving general anesthetics, whereas claims for headache, pain during anesthesia, backache, and convulsions were significantly more common in cases in which the primary anesthetic was a regional technique. Other injuries such as newborn brain damage, newborn death, and maternal nerve damage were not associated with anesthetic technique. Claims in which a regional anesthetic was used had a significantly lower median severity of injury score than those involving general anesthetics. This was reflected in a lower median payment for obstetric claims involving regional anesthesia (Table 26.4). The significantly higher proportion of maternal deaths among the obstetric claims in which general anesthesia was used is consistent with reports that general anesthesia carries a greater risk of maternal death compared with regional anesthesia (see Chapter 25) (10).

STANDARD OF CARE

For each claim in which sufficient information was available, reviewers were asked to judge the quality of anesthetic care based on the standard of care that a reasonable and prudent anesthesiologist would have exercised at the time the event occurred. The consistency with which appropriateness of care, defined in this way, can be judged by different reviewers has been previously demonstrated (1). The expected standard of care was judged to have been met in 46% of obstetric cases, not met in 39%, and impossible to judge in 15% (Figure 26.1). This is not significantly different from the results seen in the nonobstetric claims, for which the standard of care was judged appropriate in 39% cases and less than appropriate in 47%. In the subset of obstetric claims

that resulted in payments, 30% were identified as having an appropriate standard of care. The standard of care was less than appropriate in 56% of those claims. In both the obstetric and nonobstetric cases the anesthetic care was judged to have been less than appropriate in about half of the cases in which general anesthesia was the primary anesthetic technique and in about one-third of cases in which regional anesthesia was the primary technique.

PAYMENTS

Obstetric claims constitute 12% of the ASA Closed Claims Database, 11% of the total number of payments made, and 13% of the total dollars expended in payments. Payment amounts varied widely but were as high as $6 million in the nonobstetric group and $5.4 million in the obstetric group. Payments were made in 53% of the obstetric claims, which was not significantly different from the 59% payment rate in the nonobstetric claims (Table 26.4). Although, as a group, the obstetric claims were not compensated disproportionately, for those claims in which payments were made, the median payment amount was significantly greater in the obstetric group. Even though there were proportionately more deaths among the nonobstetric claims, there were proportionately more brain injuries (combined maternal and newborn) among the obstetric claims. Because claims for brain injury resulted in higher payments than claims involving death, the higher median payment in the obstetric group may be due to the greater proportion of claims for brain injury, as well as the younger age of obstetric patients and the high costs associated with prolonged care of damaged newborns.

CONCLUSIONS

In conclusion, obstetric anesthesia claims display a medicolegal risk profile that is distinctly different

Table 26.4
Payment Data[a,b]

	Non-OB Claims (%) (n = 1351)	OB Claims (%) (n = 190)	OB Regional (%) (n = 124)	OB General (%) (n = 62)
No payment	32 (431)	38 (72)	43 (53)	27 (17)
Payments made	59 (745)	53 (100)	48 (59)	63 (39)
Median payment	$85,000[c]	$203,000	$91,000[d]	$225,000
Range	$15–6 million	$675–5.4 million	$675–2.5 million	$750–5.4 million

[a]Frequency and amount of payments are illustrated. Percentages are based on the total claims in each group and do not sum to 100% due to missing data. Statistical comparisons are made between payment distributions for obstetric and nonobstetric claims.
[c]$P \leq 0.01$ and for obstetric regional and obstetric general anesthetics.
[d]$P \leq 0.05$. Claims with no payments were excluded from calculations of median payment and range.
[b]Reprinted by permission from Chadwick HS, Posner K, Caplan RA, Ward RJ, Cheney FW: A comparison of obstetric and nonobstetric anesthesia malpractice claims. Anesthesiology 74:242–249, 1991.

from that of nonobstetric claims. Although adverse newborn outcome was judged not to be related to anesthetic care in half of the cases, newborn brain injury was a leading cause of claims against obstetric anesthesiologists. As expected, some damaging events such as pulmonary aspiration and convulsions were more common among the obstetric cases. Unexpectedly, many of the obstetric claims were for relatively minor injuries such as headache, back pain, and emotional injury. Those claims involving general anesthesia had more severe injuries associated with them and resulted in higher payments. Regional anesthetics, however, were also responsible for considerable morbidity and mortality, especially from local anesthetic toxicity. Although there were proportionately more minor injuries and fewer deaths among the obstetric claims (as compared with nonobstetric claims), for those claims resulting in compensation, the median payment was significantly greater in the obstetric claims. This may be related to two factors: the younger age of parturients (as compared with nonobstetric patients) and the high costs associated with lifelong care of brain-damaged mothers or newborns. The data do not provide an answer to the question of whether obstetric patients are more litigious. However, anesthesiologists should be aware that, in the obstetric setting, even minor side effects and complications may result in claims. Obstetric anesthesiologists should become active in prenatal education and make efforts, whenever possible, to establish good rapport with patients. Special care should be taken to provide patients with realistic expectations and knowledge of potential major and minor risks associated with anesthetic procedures.

References

1. Caplan RA, Posner K, Ward RJ, Cheney FW: Peer reviewer agreement for major anesthetic mishaps. QRB 14:363–368. 1988.
2. Caplan RA, Ward RJ, Posner K, Cheney FW: Unexpected cardiac arrest during spinal anesthesia: A closed claims analysis of predisposing factors. Anesthesiology 68:5–11, 1988.
3. Caplan RA, Posner KL, Ward RJ, Cheney FW: Adverse respiratory events in anesthesia: A closed claims analysis. Anesthesiology 72:828–833, 1990.
4. Chadwick HS, Posner K, Caplan RA, Ward RJ, Cheney FW: A comparison of obstetric and nonobstetric anesthesia malpractice claims. Anesthesiology 74:242–249, 1991.
5. Cheney FW, Posner K, Caplan RA, Ward RJ: Standard of care and anesthesia liability. JAMA 261:1599–1603, 1989.
6. Kroll DA, Caplan RA, Posner K, Ward RJ, Cheney FW: Nerve injury associated with anesthesia. Anesthesiology 73:202–207, 1990.
7. Tinker JH, Dull DL, Caplan RA, Ward RJ, Cheney FW: Role of monitoring devices in prevention of anesthetic mishaps: A closed claims analysis. Anesthesiology 71:541–546, 1989.
8. Report on Confidential Enquires into Maternal Deaths in England and Wales, 1982–1983. Her Majesty's Stationery Office, London, 1989, No 34.
9. Kaunitz AM, Hughes JM, Grimes DA, Smith JC, Rochat RW, Kafrissen ME: Causes of maternal mortality in the United States. Obstet Gynecol 65:605–612, 1985.
10. Endler GC, Mariona FG, Sokol RJ, Stevenson LB: Anesthesia-related maternal mortality in Michigan. Am J Obstet Gynecol 159:187–193, 1988.
11. Gibbs CP, Rolbin SH, Norman P: Cause and prevention of maternal aspiration. Anesthesiology 61:112–113, 1984.

NONOBSTETRIC DISORDERS DURING PREGNANCY

CHAPTER 27

Anesthesia for the Pregnant Cardiac Patient

Dennis T. Mangano, Ph.D., M.D.

The pregnant patient with heart disease challenges the anesthesiologist's skills. Pregnancy and labor each impose demands on the circulation, and anesthesia during delivery may compromise an already stressed cardiovascular system. To avoid such a compromise the anesthesiologist must be aware of the nature and progression of heart disease during pregnancy, the normal physiology of labor, delivery and the puerperium, the cardiovascular effects of various anesthetic regimens, and the therapies used to manage acute complications. This chapter discusses the clinical manifestations, pathophysiology, and anesthetic considerations of serious cardiovascular diseases occurring during pregnancy. The first section covers the overall incidence, morbidity and mortality of heart disease. Cardiovascular changes during pregnancy are summarized and anesthetic guidelines are presented. The second, third, and fourth sections describe rheumatic heart disease, congenital heart disease, and several other significant cardiovascular diseases. For each disease the clinical manifestations, pathophysiology, and anesthetic considerations are discussed. The final section reviews the effects of cardiac therapeutics on the fetus. An outline of the chapter is as follows:

I. General Considerations
   A. Cardiovascular Changes During Pregnancy
   B. An Overview of Anesthetic Considerations

II. Rheumatic Heart Disease
   A. Mitral Stenosis
   B. Mitral Insufficiency
   C. Mitral Valve Prolapse
   D. Aortic Insufficiency
   E. Aortic Stenosis

III. Congenital Heart Disease
   A. Ventricular Septal Defect
   B. Atrial Septal Defect

   C. Patent Ductus Arteriosus
   D. Tetralogy of Fallot
   E. Eisenmenger's Syndrome
   F. Coarctation of the Aorta
   G. Congenital Aortic Stenosis

IV. Other Heart Diseases
   A. Primary Pulmonary Hypertension
   B. Hypertensive Disorders
   C. Cardiomyopathy of Pregnancy
   D. Dissecting Aneurysm of the Aorta
   E. Asymmetric Septal Hypertrophy
   F. Coronary Artery Disease
   G. Pericarditis
   H. Pregnancy After Valvular Surgery
   I. Cardiac Transplantation
   J. Open-Heart Surgery During Pregnancy

V. Cardiac Dysrhythmias
   A. Effects of Cardiac Therapeutics on the Fetus
   B. Antiarrhythmics
   C. Vasopressors and Inotropes
   D. Vasodilators
   E. Direct Current Cardioversion

GENERAL CONSIDERATIONS

Over the past 25 years the incidence of heart disease during pregnancy has declined from 3.6% to the present figure of approximately 1.6% (Fig. 27.1) (1–9). Rheumatic heart disease, despite the declining incidence, still accounts for most cases. The incidence of congenital heart disease in pregnant patients has been increasing because a greater number of women with congenital heart lesions now reach the childbearing age due to improvements in medical and surgical therapy (1, 4, 10). Maternal mortality with rheumatic heart disease and pregnancy varies from less than 1% in asymptomatic patients to 17% in patients with mitral stenosis complicated by atrial fibrillation (Table 27.1) (8). Congenital diseases are associated with a large range of mortality; however, several congenital diseases have a high incidence of maternal and fetal mortality regardless of their stage of progression (11). These are primary pulmonary hypertension, dominant right-to-left shunt (Eisenmenger's syndrome, tetralogy of Fallot), severe aortic stenosis, and coarctation of the aorta. These diseases, as well as diseases that have a significant rate of occurrence, are discussed in detail.

Cardiovascular Changes during Pregnancy and Parturition

The cardiovascular changes associated with pregnancy and parturition that were discussed in Chapter 1 are briefly summarized here (12–17). The cardiovascular system is progressively stressed during pregnancy and parturition (Figs. 27.2 to 27.5) (12–17). During labor, pain and apprehension increase and precipitate a progressive increase to stroke volume and cardiac output to 45% over prelabor values (16). Additional stresses are imposed by uterine contraction causing, in effect, an autotransfusion. With each uterine contraction, central blood volume and cardiac output increase by 10 to 25% (17). This acute preload stress is well tolerated by the normal heart but may represent the deciding physiologic stress in a diseased heart that has become increasingly compromised during pregnancy and labor. After delivery the central blood volume increases; obstruction of the vena cava and aorta are relieved and result in a marked increase in stroke volume (up to 80% of prelabor values). Systemic vascular resistance decreases (16). These changes, along with those induced by hemorrhage or the administration of oxytocic drugs, may cause a rapid decompensation in patients with a compromised cardiovascular system.

An Overview of Anesthetic Considerations

Anesthesia for the pregnant patient with heart disease requires an understanding of the type, severity, and progression of the disease in the context of the normal cardiovascular adaptations to pregnancy. The anesthesiologist's assessment of the patient's tolerance to pain during labor and surgery, the autotransfusion of uterine contraction, and the postdelivery changes induced by relief of vena caval obstruction, oxytocic agents, and hemorrhage must each be considered to determine the best anesthetic regimen.

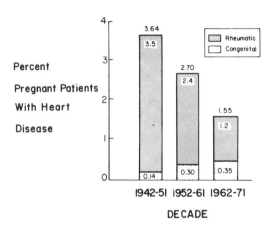

Figure 27.1. Incidence and distribution of heart disease during pregnancy over three decades. (Data were drawn from a review of more than 50,000 cases reported in Szekely P P, Snaith L: *Heart Disease and Pregnancy.* Churchill Livingstone, London, 1974.)

Table 27.1
Incidence and Mortality of Rheumatic and Congenital Heart Disease in Pregnancy

	Distribution (%)	Mortality (%)		References
		Maternal	Fetal	
Rheumatic heart disease (75%)				
Mitral stenosis	90	1–17	3.5	1, 3, 4, 45, 64
Mitral insufficiency	6.5			
Aortic insufficiency	2.5			
Aortic stenosis	1.0			
	100			
Congenital heart disease (25%)				
Ventricular septal defect	7–26	7–40	2–16	10, 58, 61–63, 65
Atrial septal defect	8–38	1–12	1–12	1, 4, 7, 10, 58, 65
Patent ductus arteriosus	6–20	5–6	17	4, 10, 60, 65
Tetralogy of Fallot	2–15	4–12	36–59	1, 4, 7, 10, 65, 70, 71, 73, 74
Eisenmenger's syndrome	2–4	12–33	30–54	1, 2, 4, 62, 63, 67, 71
Coarctation of the aorta	4–18	3–9	10–20	4, 62, 79, 80
Aortic stenosis	2–10		22	1, 4, 64, 65
Pulmonic stenosis	8–16		4	1, 4, 65, 87
Primary pulmonary hypertension	1–2	53	7	1, 4, 59, 62, 66

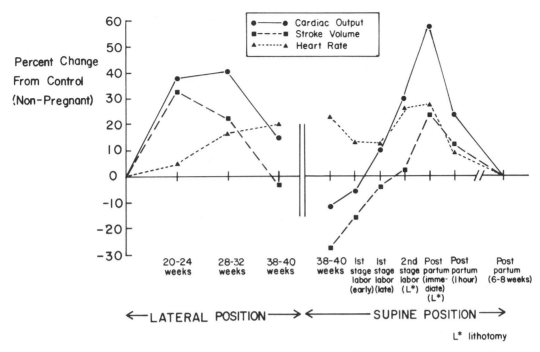

Figure 27.2. Maternal cardiovascular changes during pregnancy and labor from studies on patients in the lateral and supine positions. (Based on data reported by Ueland K, Hansen J: Maternal cardiovascular dynamics. II. Posture and uterine contractions. Am J Obstet Gynecol 103:1–7, 1969; Ueland K, Hansen J: Maternal cardiovascular dynamics. III. Labor and delivery under local and caudal analgesia. Am J Obstet Gynecol 103:8–18, 1969; and Ueland K, Novy M, Peterson E, Metcalf J: Maternal cardiovascular dynamics. IV. The influence of gestational age on the maternal cardiovascular response to posture and exercise. Am J Obstet Gynecol 104:156–164, 1969.)

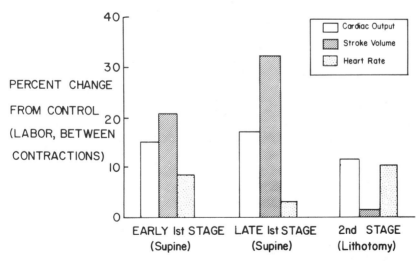

Figure 27.3. Effects of uterine contractions on cardiac output, stroke volume, and heart rate during labor. Values represent percentage increases from control measurements in late pregnancy. (Redrawn from Ueland K, Hansen J: Maternal cardiovascular dynamics. III. Labor and delivery under local and caudal analgesia. Am J Obstet Gynecol 103:8–18, 1969.)

The preanesthetic detection of a symptomatic history either at rest or with exercise is of paramount importance because such a history correlates directly with morbidity and mortality (4, 18, 19). Physical examination plus consultation with the primary physician and cardiologist should also be used to define the severity of the disease. Cardiac medications needed prior to pregnancy should usually be continued throughout pregnancy, labor, and delivery.

For most diseases, no one anesthetic technique is exclusively indicated or contraindicated (20). The primary concern is to avoid and/or treat specific pathophysiologic changes that exacerbate the disease process. These pathophysiologic changes are delineated

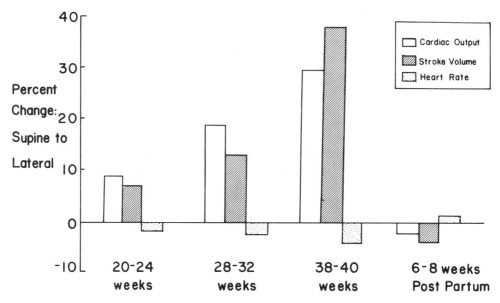

Figure 27.4. Percentage change in cardiac output, stroke volume, and heart rate when the pregnant woman turns from supine to lateral position. (Redrawn from Ueland K, Hansen J: Maternal cardiovascular dynamics. II. Posture and uterine contractions. Am J Obstet Gynecol 103:1–7, 1969.)

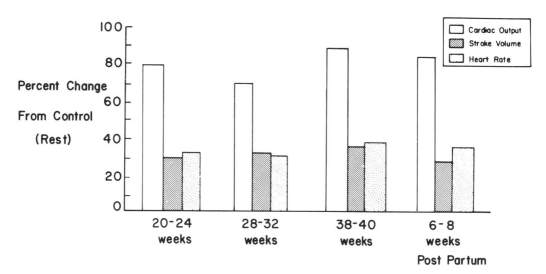

Figure 27.5. Effects of moderate exercise on cardiac output, stroke volume, and heart rate during pregnancy. (Redrawn from Ueland K, Novy M, Peterson E, Metcalf J: Maternal cardiovascular dynamics. IV. The influence of gestational age on the maternal cardiovascular response to posture and exercise. Am J Obstet Gynecol 104:856–864, 1969.)

for each disease, and the recommended anesthetic considerations are discussed.

The decision to use invasive techniques (e.g., a radial arterial line or thermodilution pulmonary artery catheter) depends on the severity and progression of disease. Most asymptomatic patients who have not evidenced disease progression and who have no signs of impaired right or left ventricular performance will have an uneventful course and do not require invasive monitoring. Exceptions are patients, even if asymptomatic, with primary pulmonary hy-

pertension, right-to-left shunt, dissecting aortic aneurysm, severe aortic stenosis, or coarctation of the aorta. In patients with severe heart disease, a full hemodynamic profile—including measurements of cardiac output, vascular resistance, central venous pressure (CVP), and pulmonary capillary wedge (PCW) pressure—is desirable. Based on these measurements a therapeutic plan should be designed for handling each of the acute complications that may occur with that disease. It is well recognized that placement of a pulmonary artery catheter is time consuming, requires expertise, and may have associated morbidity and even mortality. Nonetheless, the author believes that in patients with severe cardiac disease the information derived from pulmonary artery catheterization is worth the risk.

The hemodynamic aberrations seen during labor and delivery may continue after delivery. Thus patients with symptomatic heart disease who have had a complicated labor and delivery period should be monitored in an intensive care unit.

Treatment of complications that occur during an anesthetic course may involve the use of electrocardioversion or pharmacologic agents such as digoxin, propranolol, lidocaine, metaraminol, sodium nitroprusside, and phentolamine. These drugs may have untoward fetal effects. Their use or nonuse depends on the seriousness of maternal impairment and whether that impairment will result in severe fetal morbidity that will outweigh the morbidity associated with the therapy. The author's philosophy is to correct immediately any severe maternal impairment, even though the therapy may cause fetal morbidity.

Finally, it should be clearly understood that there exist few well controlled studies addressing the effects of anesthetics and therapeutics on pregnant patients with heart disease. However, the physiologic changes occurring during pregnancy, the pathophysiology of these disease processes, and the effects of anesthetics on pregnant patients without cardiovascular disease are well documented. The anesthetic and therapeutic considerations and recommendations stated in this chapter have been synthesized from these mostly independent bodies of information and represent the opinions of this author.

RHEUMATIC HEART DISEASE

Rheumatic fever is a diffuse inflammatory disease affecting the heart, joints, and subcutaneous tissues following group A β-hemolytic streptococcal infection. Acute rheumatic fever is evidenced by a history of a streptococcal infection and a subsequent clinical picture that usually includes recurrent migratory polyarthritis with or without carditis. Polyarthritis tends to be self-limited, but the carditis can progressively and permanently damage valves or heart muscle. Although the prophylactic administration of antibiotics generally prevents the sequelae of rheumatic fever, rheumatic heart disease continues to commonly cause death in the United States and in many other countries (18, 19, 21–23). Left or right ventricular failure, atrial dysrhythmias, systemic or pulmonary embolism, and infective endocarditis may complicate rheumatic heart disease during pregnancy (Table 27.2). Although the incidence of these

Table 27.2
Pregnant Patients with Rheumatic Heart Disease[a]

Major Complications	Incidence (%)
Left or right ventricular failure	8.5
Atrial dysrhythmias	6.5
Systemic or pulmonary embolism	1.6
Infective endocarditis	0.4

[a]Data adapted from Szekely P, Snaith L: *Heart Disease and Pregnancy*. Churchill Livingstone, London, 1974.

complications during pregnancy has progressively decreased, they still occur in 15% of patients.

Mitral Stenosis

Rheumatic fever usually first occurs in 6- to 15-year-old children. If carditis occurs, mitral insufficiency ensues followed in about 5 years by mitral stenosis. Symptoms usually do not appear for another 15 years. Pulmonary congestion, pulmonary hypertension, and right ventricular failure develop 5 to 10 years after the occurrence of symptoms (24, 25). On average, symptoms appear at 31 years and proceed in 7 years to total incapacity (26). Without surgical correction 20% of totally incapacitated patients die in 6 months, 50% in 5 years, 75% in 10 years, and 90% in 15 years (26–29).

CLINICAL MANIFESTATIONS

The initial symptoms are fatigue and dyspnea on exertion with progression to paroxysmal nocturnal dyspnea, orthopnea, and dyspnea at rest. Hemoptysis with rupture of bronchopulmonary varices and pulmonary or systemic arterial embolization occur infrequently. When mitral stenosis is severe, supraimposition of stresses such as atrial fibrillation, pulmonary embolism, infection, or pregnancy may precipitate rapid decompensation.

Physical examination may reveal a presystolic or middiastolic murmur that, if faint, will only be heard when the patient lies on her left side. The intensity of the murmur correlates poorly with the degree of stenosis, perhaps because other hemodynamic effects (e.g., depressed cardiac output) reduce flow through the valve. In addition to this murmur an opening snap may be heard at the base of the heart along the left sternal border. Atrial fibrillation occurs in approximately one-third of patients with severe mitral stenosis.

Radiologic studies are normal early in the course of mitral stenosis, but left atrial and right ventricular enlargement occur as the disease progresses. Severe mitral stenosis may produce generalized pulmonary edema.

The electrocardiogram shows a broadened P wave in lead V_1, signifying left atrial enlargement. Right axis deviation signifies right ventricular enlargement. Cardiac catheterization commonly shows capillary wedge pressures of 25 to 30 mm Hg (normal is 0 to 12 mm Hg) occurring when the mitral valve orifice area is less than 2 cm². There is an associated increase in pulmonary vascular resistance. Severe mitral stenosis is consistent with valvular diastolic pressure gradients in excess of 25 mm Hg (normal is 5 mm Hg or less) (19).

PATHOPHYSIOLOGY

The decrease in mitral valve orifice area impairs left ventricular filling (Fig. 27.6). Although the left atrium initially may overcome this obstruction, ventricular filling is eventually decreased; left atrial volume and pressure, pulmonary venous pressure, and PCW pressure then rise. Transudation of fluid into the pulmonary interstitial space occurs, pulmonary compliance decreases, and the work of breathing rises, producing progressive dyspnea on exertion. With

pulmonary hypertension, pulmonary artery medial thickening and fibrosis result, and pulmonary vascular resistance becomes permanently elevated. Right ventricular hypertrophy, dilation, and failure then occur, leading to tricuspid insufficiency with hepatic and peripheral congestion. Atrial fibrillation, tachycardia, or increased metabolic demands (e.g., pregnancy and labor) may exacerbate the above processes (30–32). With pregnancy an anatomically moderate stenosis can become functionally severe (7). Pregnant patients with mitral stenosis have an increased incidence of pulmonary congestion (25%), atrial fibrillation (7%), and paroxysmal atrial tachycardia (3%) (4). Left ventricular dysfunction is uncommon (15%) with pure mitral stenosis (19), and its presence suggests an associated element of mitral or aortic insufficiency.

ANESTHETIC CONSIDERATIONS

Asymptomatic patients without evidence of pulmonary congestion have minimally increased risk and do not require additional invasive monitoring but should be attended with caution. On the other hand, patients with marked symptoms may be at significant risk, and radial artery and pulmonary artery monitoring is recommended (Fig. 27.7). The following considerations should be noted (Table 27.3).

1. *Neither sinus tachycardia nor atrial fibrillation with a rapid ventricular response is tolerated well.* Digoxin therapy used to control atrial fibrillation prior to pregnancy should be continued (with readjustment of dose, if necessary) to maintain ventricular rates below 110 beats per min (bpm). Development of atrial fibrillation with a rapid ventricular response may dramatically decrease cardiac output and produce pulmonary edema (29). The treatment is cardioversion starting with 25 watt-sec of energy. The fetal safety of cardioversion has been documented (34, 35). If cardioversion is unavailable, or if time (minutes) allows, propranolol (0.2 to 0.5 mg intravenously every 3 min) may be used to lower

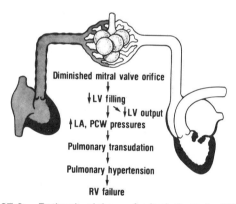

Figure 27.6. Pathophysiology of mitral stenosis. LV = left ventricle; LA = left atrial; PCW = pulmonary capillary wedge; RV = right ventricle.

Figure 27.7. Intrapartum alterations in pulmonary capillary wedge pressure (*PCWP*) in eight patients with mitral stenosis. (Reprinted by permission from Clark SL, Phelan JP, Greenspoon J, Aldahl D, Horenstein J: Labor and delivery in the presence of mitral stenosis: Central hemodynamic observations. Am J Obstet Gynecol 152:984–988, 1985.)

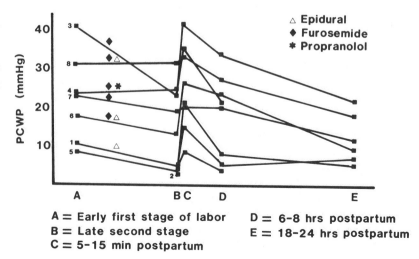

Table 27.3
Mitral Stenosis: Anesthetic Considerations

1. Prevent rapid ventricular rates.
2. Minimize increases in central blood volume.
3. Avoid marked decreases in systemic vascular resistance.
4. Prevent increases in pulmonary artery pressure.

the rate below 110 bpm. Propranolol administration should be discontinued when a total dose of 0.1 mg/kg is given or evidence of heart failure occurs (increasing PCW). Digitalization is used in stable situations where prolonged but not immediate (seconds to minutes) ventricular rate control is necessary. Digoxin 0.50 mg intravenously is given over 10 min followed by 0.25 mg intravenously every 2 hr to achieve a full digitalizing dose. Each dose has an effect in 15 min with a full effect in 1 to 2 hr.

Sinus tachycardia in excess of 140 bpm or causing decreased cardiac output or increased PCW should be corrected immediately by reversing a precipitating event (pain, light general anesthesia, hypercarbia, acidosis) or by administering propranolol as described above.

2. *Marked increases in central blood volume are poorly tolerated.* Overtransfusion, Trendelenburg position, or autotransfusion via uterine contraction can precipitate right ventricular failure, pulmonary hypertension, pulmonary edema, or atrial fibrillation. Increases in CVP or PCW may be used to assess increases in central blood volume.

3. *Marked decreases in systemic vascular resistance may not be tolerated.* With severe stenosis, decreases in systemic vascular resistance are compensated by increases in heart rate (stroke volume is fixed). This response is limited and marked increases in heart rate may lead to decompensation. The author recommends that, if necessary, systemic vascular resistance be maintained with an intravenous infusion of metaraminol (10 mg in 250 ml of saline). Because ephedrine may increase heart rate, it is not recommended.

4. *Exacerbation of pulmonary hypertension and right ventricular failure can be precipitated by multiple factors.* Any degree of hypercarbia, hypoxia, acidosis, lung hyperinflation, or increased lung water can elevate pulmonary vascular resistance. Prostaglandins used to treat uterine atony should be used with caution since they may have effects on the pulmonary vasculature.

If pulmonary hypertension and right ventricular compromise persist, inotropic support with dopamine (3 to 8 μg/kg/min) and pulmonary vasodilation with low dose sodium nitroprusside (0.1 to 0.5μg/kg/min) are recommended. Higher doses of nitroprusside may produce undesirable vasodilation and elevated maternal and fetal cyanide levels (see final section). Prolonged mechanical ventilation may be required if hemodynamic or pulmonary complications occur.

ANESTHESIA FOR VAGINAL DELIVERY AND CESAREAN SECTION

The author recommends segmental lumbar epidural anesthesia for labor and vaginal delivery (36, 37). This eliminates the pain and tachycardia that attend uterine contractions. Perineal analgesia blocks the urge to push and thereby prevents exertion, fatigue, and the deleterious effect of a Valsalva maneuver. Fetal descent is accomplished by the uterine contractions per se, and delivery is facilitated with vacuum extraction or outlet forceps. Hypotension may be prevented by continuous left uterine displacement and judicious fluid infusion. Prophylactic ephedrine and rapid hydration should be avoided. If hypotension occurs metaraminol is the preferred vasopressor.

Either regional or general anesthesia may be used for cesarean section. A continuous lumbar epidural block is preferred to spinal anesthesia because epidural anesthesia produces more controllable hemodynamic changes. The anesthetic level should be established slowly by titration of local anesthetic through the epidural catheter. Epinephrine is omitted from the local anesthetic because of the potential for tachycardia and peripheral vasodilation.

As with regional anesthesia for vaginal delivery, a blood pressure reduction associated with decreased PCW pressure may be cautiously treated with fluid infusion to reestablish normal filling pressures. If PCW pressure remains normal or if pulmonary artery monitoring is not possible, hypotension should be corrected by infusion of metaraminol.

If general anesthesia is used, drugs that produce tachycardia, such as atropine, pancuronium, meperidine, and ketamine, should be avoided. Patients with mild disease may be managed with an intravenous thiopental induction, intubation, and light general anesthesia. Those with moderate or severe stenosis may be unduly stressed by this regimen, and a slow induction with halothane or intravenous fentanyl is recommended. If significant right or left ventricular compromise exists, fentanyl is preferred to halothane. With either technique tachycardia may follow endotracheal intubation or surgical incision; it should be treated by increasing the anesthetic depth or with propranolol. A halothane or fentanyl induction increases the risk of maternal aspiration or neonatal depression, but the author believes that the benefits outweigh these hazards.

Mitral stenosis may produce pulmonary dysfunction. The usual assessment of respiratory adequacy (arterial blood gases, pulmonary mechanics, chest roentgenogram) must be made on weaning from con-

trolled ventilation. Intensive care unit monitoring in
the postoperative period may be necessary.

Mitral Insufficiency

Mitral insufficiency is the second most common
valvular defect in pregnancy (4, 24). Left ventricular
volume work is chronically increased. This is usually
tolerated well, and patients with insufficiency may
remain asymptomatic for 30 to 40 years. However,
congestive heart failure follows, and with symptoms,
a rapid downhill course occurs with a 5-year mortality of 50%. Other complications occurring during
the fourth or fifth decade are atrial fibrillation, systemic embolization, and bacterial endocarditis (24,
38, 39).

Because complications usually occur late in life—
after the childbearing age—most patients with mitral
regurgitation tolerate pregnancy well. However,
Szekely and Snaith (4) reported a 5.5% incidence of
pulmonary congestion during pregnancy. In addition, they reported a 4.3% incidence of atrial tachycardia, a 2.8% incidence of pulmonary embolism,
and an 8.5% incidence of infective endocarditis.

CLINICAL MANIFESTATIONS

The principal symptoms of advanced mitral insufficiency are those of left ventricular failure. The
cardinal sign is a pansystolic murmur of blowing
quality, loudest at the cardiac apex, referred to the
left axilla or the infrascapular area. Atrial fibrillation
occurs in approximately one-third of patients. With
mild mitral insufficiency the electrocardiogram is
normal, but advanced mitral insufficiency produces
signs of left ventricular hypertrophy and, at times,
right ventricular hypertrophy. Roentgenographic
findings in mild mitral insufficiency are normal.
However, severe mitral insufficiency causes left ventricular and especially left atrial enlargement. Late
sequellae associated with mitral insufficiency include pulmonary congestion, pulmonary hypertension, and right ventricular enlargement (18, 22).

PATHOPHYSIOLOGY

With mitral insufficiency there is regurgitation of
blood from the left ventricle through the incompetent
mitral valve into the left atrium (Fig. 27.8). With
chronic mitral insufficiency, the left atrium adapts
to this increased blood volume by dilating and increasing its compliance. When left atrial pressure
rises, pulmonary venous and PCW pressures also rise,
causing pulmonary congestion and edema. With progressive left ventricular failure, pulmonary hypertension and right ventricular compromise will occur.
Left atrial pressure does not increase until late in the
course of the disease; thus the left atrium protects
the pulmonary venous, capillary, and arterial beds

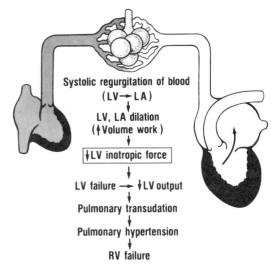

Figure 27.8. Pathophysiology of mitral insufficiency. *LV* =
left ventricle; *LA* = left atrium; *RV* = right ventricle.

from pressure overload. Left ventricular dilation occurs as well because of the increase in preload afforded by the hypervolemic left atrium. Forward
ejection of blood through the aortic valve can be impaired by as much as 50 to 60% and depends on the
ratio of resistance through the aortic valve to that
through the insufficient mitral valve. Reduction of
left ventricular afterload can then play an important
role in decreasing the amount of regurgitant blood
flow and increasing forward cardiac output.

The chronically compromised left ventricle may
not tolerate the increase in intravascular volume associated with pregnancy, and pulmonary congestion
may occur (40). Changes in systemic resistance may
play an important role. The decreased peripheral resistance of pregnancy may improve forward flow at
the expense of regurgitant flow (41). In contrast, pain,
apprehension, uterine contractions, or surgical stimulation associated with labor and delivery may increase systemic vascular resistance by augmenting
sympathetic activity. The resultant decrease in forward flow and increase in regurgitant flow may precipitate acute left ventricular failure and pulmonary
congestion (40). It should be noted that the murmurs
of mitral and aortic insufficiency may decrease during pregnancy (41).

ANESTHETIC CONSIDERATIONS

Asymptomatic patients with mild mitral insufficiency and an unchanging murmur throughout pregnancy may be approached in a routine but cautious
fashion. In symptomatic patients radial artery and
pulmonary artery monitoring is desirable. Table 27.4
gives the principal anesthetic considerations.

Table 27.4
Mitral Insufficiency: Anesthetic Considerations

1. Prevent peripheral vasoconstriction.
2. Avoid myocardial depressants.
3. Treat acute atrial fibrillation immediately.
4. Maintain a normal or slightly elevated heart rate.
5. Monitor PCW pressure and intensity of murmur.

1. *Large increases in systemic vascular resistance can cause acute decompensation of the left ventricle.* Treatment consists of left ventricular afterload reduction with low doses of sodium nitroprusside (0.1–0.5 μg/kg/min) or phentolamine (0.1 to 1 μg/kg/min).

2. *Myocardial depressants are not well tolerated.* Because left ventricular impairment usually accompanies mitral insufficiency, even minimal myocardial depression may result in significant compromise.

3. *Atrial fibrillation can cause left ventricular decompensation.* The preferred treatment is direct current countershock as outlined in the section on mitral stenosis.

4. *Bradycardia is not tolerated well.* Forward stroke volume may be limited, and cardiac output will principally depend on heart rate. Maintenance of normal to slightly elevated heart rates is advocated.

5. *The amount of regurgitant flow correlates with:* (a) *the intensity of the insufficiency murmur and* (b) *the size of the v wave in the PCW pressure tracing.* Both can be useful parameters in assessing the amount of ventricular failure with chronic insufficiency. PCW pressure is a poor measure of left atrial volume or left ventricular end-diastolic volume since the left atrium is very compliant. However, minor changes in pressure indicate changes in left ventricular end-diastolic volume. On the other hand, with acute mitral insufficiency, the left atrium will be less compliant, and changes in the PCW pressures correlate with changes in left atrial and left ventricular end-diastolic pressures. The anesthetic considerations in regard to pulmonary hypertension and right ventricular compromise are delineated in the section on mitral stenosis and apply here as well.

6. *Afterload reduction may be useful therapy.* Left ventricular failure may benefit from afterload reduction with small amounts of sodium nitroprusside or phentolamine, combined with dopamine to give left ventricular inotropic support.

ANESTHESIA FOR VAGINAL DELIVERY AND CESAREAN SECTION

For labor and vaginal delivery, lumbar epidural analgesia is recommended. This technique will prevent the peripheral vasoconstriction associated with the pain of labor and will increase the forward flow of blood. This latter advantage also applies to regional versus general anesthesia for cesarean section. However, regional anesthesia will increase venous capacitance and may require administration of intravenous fluids to maintain the filling volume of the enlarged left ventricle. Constant left uterine displacement and a 10-degree Trendelenburg position should be used to maintain venous return. The positive inotropic and chronotropic effects of ephedrine are especially useful in preventing and treating hypotension.

Nitrous oxide–relaxant anesthesia may be dangerous because of the associated peripheral vasoconstriction. However, when combined with sodium nitroprusside to prevent peripheral vasoconstriction, this technique may be useful in patients with compromised ventricular function because this approach avoids myocardial depression and maintains an elevated heart rate. However, in patients without severe ventricular compromise, halothane or isoflurane may be added to the nitrous oxide.

Mitral Valve Prolapse

Mitral valve prolapse (MVP) is the most common congenital valvular lesion, occurring in 5 to 10% of the general population. Because of the large spectrum of pathologic changes in the mitral valve apparatus that occur with this syndrome, it has been referred to by a variety of names, including the following syndromes: the systolic click-murmur, Barlow's, billowing mitral valve, mitral cusp, sloppy mitral valve, and redundant cusp. MVP is most prevalent in younger females, commonly during the childbearing years. In over 85% of patients with MVP, the disease is asymptomatic and benign. In the remaining 15%, mitral regurgitation develops over a 10- to 15-year period and requires alteration of medical management.

The majority of patients with MVP during pregnancy do not have mitral insufficiency and tolerate pregnancy and delivery well (43). Only with mitral insufficiency or with other coexisting diseases, such as toxemia, have complications been reported.

CLINICAL MANIFESTATIONS

Although the majority of patients with MVP are asymptomatic, a number of diverse clinical manifestations have been associated with the syndrome. Among these symptoms are anxiety, palpitations, dyspnea, chest discomfort, light-headedness, emotional disturbances, and symptoms associated with autonomic nervous dysfunction, such as orthostatic hypotension. Patients are sometimes marfanoid or have thoracic skeletal abnormalities. The cardinal sign of MVP is a mid- to late systolic click, occurring after the beginning of the upstroke of the carotid pulse. In addition, the click is often accompanied by a mid- to late crescendo systolic murmur, with the duration of the murmur reflecting the severity of the mitral regurgitation. With severe MVP, the click occurs early and the murmur becomes holosystolic. The electrocardiogram is usually normal in asymptomatic patients, but occasionally has inverted or biphasic T waves and nonspecific ST changes in the inferior leads. Arrythmias are common, particularly paroxysmal supraventricular tachycardia due to presence of atrioventricular bypass tracts. Other supraventricular and ventricular tachyarrhythmias, bradyarrhythmias, and conduction blocks have been reported with this condition. The echocardiographic findings are significant and often diagnostic for MVP. M-mode echocardiography demonstrates sudden posterior movement of the posterior leaflet during midsystole resulting in a "question mark" sign as well as "hammocking" of the posterior leaflet into the left atrium. Two-dimensional echocardiography may be the most definitive test, demonstrating mitral valve leaflets in the left atrium during ventricular systole.

With mitral insufficiency, the clinical manifestations as described in the previous section will occur.

PATHOPHYSIOLOGY

With MVP, the cordae tendineae are elongated, causing the mitral leaflets to prolapse into the left atrium when ventricular volume decreases during mid- to late systole. The systolic click is produced by a sudden tensing of the elongated cordae and the prolapsing leaflets. The crescendo systolic murmur represents retrograde flow during systole from the left ventricle to the left atrium. Conditions that decrease left ventricular volume, such as hypovolemia, venodilation, increased airway pressure, or tachycardia, cause an earlier prolapsing of the mitral leaflets during systole and an earlier and louder crescendo murmur with increased regurgitation. Conditions that increase ventricular volume, on the other hand, such as bradycardia, afterload augmentation, hypervolemia, or negative inotropic agents, cause a delayed click and murmur, and at times may mask these signs of MVP. Generally, when the click and murmur occur earlier in the cycle the degree of regurgitation is greater. However, certain conditions such as infusion of venodilators (nitrates) or augmentation of afterload (phenylephrine) cause paradoxical changes. With nitrates, ventricular volume decreases and produces an earlier systolic click and murmur; however, because of the lower left ventricular systolic pressure, the regurgitant fraction decreases as does the intensity of the murmur. With increases in systemic vascular resistance, such as with administration of phenylephrine, the click and onset of the murmur are delayed, but ventricular volume and systolic pressure

increase, causing increased regurgitation and intensity of the murmur. Thus, when mitral insufficiency occurs with MVP, the anesthetic considerations are similar to those with mitral insufficiency alone.

In pregnant patients with MVP, the physiologic changes occurring with pregnancy appear to have little effect when no other cardiovascular abnormalities exist. The incidence of antepartum and intrapartum complications, as well as signs of fetal distress, are not increased when compared with pregnant patients without cardiac disorders. However, in patients with coexisting cardiovascular disorders such as toxemia, complications such as congestive heart failure have been reported.

ANESTHETIC CONSIDERATIONS

Asymptomatic patients without mitral insufficiency with an unchanging murmur throughout pregnancy should be approached in a routine but cautious fashion. Otherwise, in patients who manifest symptoms of mitral insufficiency, or in those with crescendo murmurs that are increased in intensity during pregnancy, special consideration is warranted. Table 27.5 gives the principal anesthetic considerations. Decreases in left ventricular volume generally cause increased prolapse, and are not tolerated well. Treatment consists of reversing these effects (such as decreasing airway pressure) and administration of intravenous fluids. Maintenance of intravascular and intraventricular volume and acute treatment of blood loss is necessary. Antiarrhythmics should be continued pre-, intra-, and postoperatively. Treatment of paroxysmal supraventricular tachycardia, especially when decreased peripheral perfusion occurs, should be aggressive (see dysrhythmias section). In patients with moderate to severe mitral insufficiency, the anesthetic considerations for mitral insufficiency apply. Prevention of peripheral vasoconstriction, avoidance of myocardial depressants, and maintenance of a normal to slightly elevated heart rate will decrease the regurgitant fraction and enhance forward flow.

For patients without mitral insufficiency or with mild mitral insufficiency, maneuvers or drugs that increase ventricular volume will decrease the degree of prolapse. Generally, no special considerations or

---

Table 27.5
Mitral Valve Prolapse: Anesthetic Considerations

1. Avoid decreases in preload.
2. Continue antiarrhythmic therapy.
3. With MVP and moderate to severe mitral insufficiency the same considerations as listed for mitral insufficiency alone apply.

treatment modalities are necessary in these patients. Maintenance of ventricular volume, afterload, and normal or even depressed contractility should be beneficial.

ANESTHESIA FOR VAGINAL DELIVERY AND CESAREAN SECTION

In patients without mitral insufficiency or with mild insufficiency, no particular anesthetic technique appears to be superior. In patients with moderate to severe mitral insufficiency, lumbar epidural analgesia for labor and vaginal delivery is recommended (44). This technique prevents the peripheral vasoconstriction associated with the pain of labor and will increase the forward flow of blood. This advantage also applies to regional versus general anesthesia for cesarean section. With regional anesthesia, the increase in venous capacitance will require the administration of intravenous fluid to maintain the filling volume of the enlarged left ventricle, and minimize the degree of prolapse. Left uterine displacement and Trendelenburg positioning should be used to maintain venous return.

Nitrous oxide-relaxant anesthesia, when accompanied by tachycardia and peripheral vasoconstriction, may be detrimental for several reasons. Tachycardia may reduce intraventricular volume and increase the degree of prolapse. Peripheral vasoconstriction will increase left ventricular systolic pressure and regurgitant flow. However, in patients with marked ventricular dysfunction, a nitrous oxide–relaxant technique may be beneficial because of its lack of associated myocardial depression. In these circumstances, maintenance of a normal to low-normal systemic vascular resistance using, for example, sodium nitroprusside appears to be effective. In patients without severe ventricular dysfunction the inhalational agents can be used effectively.

Aortic Insufficiency

A 7- to 10-year latent period after an acute attack of rheumatic fever usually precedes the development of aortic regurgitation with associated widened pulse pressure, decreased systemic diastolic pressure, and bounding peripheral pulses (19, 24). The disease usually remains asymptomatic for another 7–10 years. Patients presenting with (a) left ventricular enlargement, (b) electrocardiographic evidence of ventricular hypertrophy, and (c) a large peripheral pulse pressure have a 33% chance of developing heart failure, angina, or death within 1 year, 50% within 2 years, 65% within 3 years, and 87% within 6 years (24). Patients with one or two of these signs have a 10% chance of developing heart failure, angina, or death over a 10-year period, and patients with none

of these signs have uneventful courses over the same period (18, 19, 22).

Because symptoms usually develop during the fourth or fifth decades of life, most patients with dominant aortic insufficiency have uneventful pregnancies. However, heart failure complicates 3–9% of such patients during pregnancy (1, 4, 7, 40).

CLINICAL MANIFESTATIONS

The symptoms of aortic insufficiency relate to left ventricular failure. Moderately severe insufficiency produces a widened pulse pressure with diastolic blood pressures below 60 mm Hg (18, 19, 24). Systolic pressure is commonly less than 160 mm Hg. An early blowing diastolic murmur is usually heard along the left sternal border in the second, third, or fourth intercostal space. Duration of the diastolic murmur depends on the severity of aortic insufficiency. The electrocardiogram in severe insufficiency displays increased QRS amplitude, depressed ST segments, inverted T waves, and a horizontal axis. Atrial fibrillation suggests concomitant mitral valve disease or myocardial failure with moderately severe aortic insufficiency. Chest roentgenogram will reveal left ventricular dilation.

PATHOPHYSIOLOGY

With aortic insufficiency left ventricular volume overload occurs (Fig. 27.9). This volume depends on the area of the regurgitation orifice, the diastolic pressure gradient between aorta and left ventricle, and the duration of diastole (46). With chronic volume overload, the left ventricle becomes eccentrically distended and compliance increases. Left ventricular end-diastolic pressure remains normal for several years. The left ventricle usually tolerates this chronic increase in left ventricular volume work and can be-

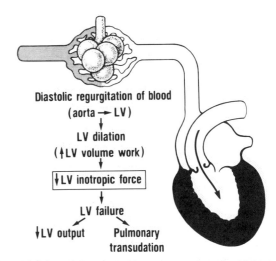

Figure 27.9. Pathophysiology of aortic insufficiency. *LV* = left ventricle.

come markedly distended without evidencing cardiac failure. However, once failure begins, forward stroke volume decreases, end-diastolic volume precipitously increases, and left ventricular end-diastolic pressure rises above normal. Pulmonary capillary congestion and signs of pulmonary edema follow (19, 47).

The decrease in systemic vascular resistance and the increase in heart rate during pregnancy may reduce both the regurgitant flow and the intensity of the murmur of insufficiency (42, 48). On the other hand, the increase in intravascular volume seen throughout pregnancy and the increases in systemic vascular resistance with the stress of labor and delivery can lead to left ventricular dysfunction.

ANESTHETIC CONSIDERATIONS

Asymptomatic patients without signs of pulmonary congestion have minimally increased risk. Symptomatic patients with an increased murmur intensity, decreased diastolic blood pressure, increased peripheral pulse pressure, or signs of pulmonary congestion are at increased risk and may benefit from radial artery and pulmonary artery catheterization. The following points should be considered (Table 27.6).

1. *Systemic vascular resistance increases can precipitate left ventricular failure.* This should be corrected by titration with a vasodilator such as sodium nitroprusside or phentolamine. Usually, less than 0.5 µg/kg/min of nitroprusside is necessary.

2. *Bradycardia is poorly tolerated.* Bradycardia increases the duration of ventricular diastole and, consequently, the amount of blood regurgitated across the aortic valve. Heart rates should be maintained between 80 and 100 bpm.

3. *Myocardial depressants exacerbate left ventricular failure.* Aortic insufficiency usually produces left ventricular impairment. If myocardial reserve is small, minimal myocardial depression may result in failure.

4. *Decreasing diastolic blood pressure, increasing arterial pulse pressure, or increasing intensity or duration of the aortic murmur indicate left ventricular compromise.* PCW pressure elevation is a late sign, and even small elevations may suggest significant left ventricular failure.

5. *Afterload reduction may be useful therapy.*

Table 27.6
Aortic Insufficiency: Anesthetic Considerations

1. Avoid marked increases in systemic vascular resistance.
2. Maintain a normal or slightly elevated heart rate.
3. Avoid myocardial depressants.
4. Monitor arterial diastolic pressure, PCW pressure, and intensity of murmur.

Left ventricular failure may benefit from afterload reduction with small amounts of sodium nitroprusside or phentolamine, combined with dopamine to give left ventricular inotropic support.

ANESTHESIA FOR VAGINAL DELIVERY AND CESAREAN SECTION

For aortic insufficiency the anesthetic management is comparable to that of mitral insufficiency (see previous section). Continuous lumbar epidural analgesia will prevent peripheral vasoconstriction and is recommended for vaginal delivery. For cesarean section regional or general anesthesia, as previously described, may be used.

Aortic Stenosis

Aortic stenosis appears as the dominant valve lesion in 0.5 to 3% of parturients (1, 4, 7, 45). This relative rarity results from the 35- to 40-year latent period between acute rheumatic fever and symptoms of severe stenosis: congestive failure, syncope, and angina. Most patients become symptomatic in their fifth or sixth decade (49). Progressive decompensation follows the appearance of symptoms, with a 50% mortality within 5 years. Sudden death occurs in 3 to 10% of these patients (18, 19, 24, 50). Asymptomatic pregnant patients with aortic stenosis are not at increased risk (4), although they have reduced hemodynamic responses to the demands of pregnancy and exercise (51). Symptomatic aortic stenosis markedly increases maternal and fetal morbidity and mortality (1, 4, 7, 52).

CLINICAL MANIFESTATIONS

The cross-sectional area of the aortic valve orifice in normal adults is 2.6 to 3.5 cm^2 (53). A 25 to 50% decrease in area results in a loud aortic systolic murmur. Narrowing to less than 1 cm^2 markedly increases left ventricular end-diastolic pressures (Fig. 27.10). Areas below 0.75 cm^2 produce exertional dyspnea, angina pectoris, and syncope (19, 53, 54, 55). The principal physical finding is a systolic ejection murmur loudest in the second right intercostal space adjacent to the sternum and radiating into the neck. Intensity of the murmur may not correlate with the degree of stenosis. A low cardiac output or decreased velocity of ejection decreases the intensity of the murmur. The electrocardiogram in severe aortic stenosis shows left ventricular hypertrophy and occasionally a left bundle branch block. Radiographs may show left ventricular enlargement, post-stenotic dilation of the aorta, and, in older adults, calcification of the aortic valve. Catheterization findings are usually normal when the aortic valve orifice area exceeds 1 cm^2. Smaller areas usually produce a systolic pressure gradient between the aorta and left ventricle. A gradient of 50 mm Hg or more indicates severe ste-

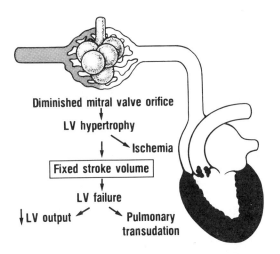

Figure 27.10. Pathophysiology of aortic stenosis. *LV* = left ventricle.

nosis, except in patients with congestive heart failure, where reduced left ventricular stroke volume may produce only 30-mm Hg gradients even with severe aortic stenosis (17, 18).

ANESTHETIC CONSIDERATIONS

The appearance of symptoms, evidence of left ventricular failure, or progression of stenosis suggest monitoring via radial artery and pulmonary artery catheters (56). The following considerations should be noted (Table 27.7).

1. *Decreases in systemic vascular resistance are poorly tolerated.* In normal patients increases in stroke volume and heart rate usually compensate for a decrease in systemic vascular resistance. Aortic stenosis relatively fixes stroke volume, and patients with stenosis must rely on elevation of heart rate to maintain blood pressure. However, elevations of heart rate above 140 bpm will decrease diastolic filling and cardiac output. Vascular resistance should be maintained during anesthesia by using light levels or by using a vasoconstrictor (e.g., metaraminol).

2. *Bradycardia is poorly tolerated for the reasons outlined above.*

3. *Decreases in venous return and left ventricular filling are poorly tolerated.* Because of the increased and fixed afterload, left ventricular stroke volume will be maintained only if the end-diastolic volume is adequate. Marked decreases in ventricular filling will decrease stroke volume and cardiac output (Fig. 27.11). Additionally, since the ventricle is noncompliant, small changes in fluid loading will result in large changes in filling pressure (Fig. 27.12).

ANESTHESIA FOR VAGINAL DELIVERY AND CESAREAN SECTION

These patients usually tolerate the hemodynamic effects of pain and stress. When possible, avoid sympathetic blockade; if regional anesthesia is necessary,

Table 27.7
Aortic Stenosis: Anesthetic Considerations

1. Avoid decreases in systemic vascular resistance.
2. Avoid bradycardia.
3. Maintain venous return and left ventricular filling.

a gradually administered continuous epidural technique is indicated. Because hypotension is poorly tolerated, maternal blood pressure should be sustained with left uterine displacement, fluids, and metaraminol or ephedrine. For labor and vaginal delivery, systemic medication, inhalation analgesia, and pudendal nerve block anesthesia are suggested. For cesarean section, general anesthesia with the standard nitrous oxide–relaxant technique is recommended (57). Halogenated anesthetics, with their potential for undue myocardial depression, should be avoided when evidence of severe left ventricular compromise exists. Signs or symptoms of ventricular ischemia associated with hypotension indicate the need to elevate or maintain systemic vascular resistance with metaraminol.

CONGENITAL HEART DISEASE

The major categories of congenital heart disease are: left-to-right shunt (ventricular septal defect, atrial septal defect, patent ductus arteriosus), right-to-left shunt (tetralogy of Fallot, Eisenmenger's syndrome), and congenital valvular and vascular lesions (coarctation of the aorta, aortic stenosis, pulmonary stenosis).

In women with congenital heart disease, pregnancy may be affected by (a) the cardiac status; (b) the anatomic diagnosis; (c) pulmonary hypertension; and (d) the type of operative repair, if any, and the degree of residual impairment.

Left-to-Right Shunt

VENTRICULAR SEPTAL DEFECT

Ventricular septal defect (VSD) occurs in 7% of adults with congenital heart disease. The size of the VSD and the degree of pulmonary hypertension determine the course of patients with VSD (10, 19, 58). The VSD in most adult patients is small, with a minimal left-to-right shunt, insignificant pulmonary hypertension, and no symptoms. Pregnancy is usually uneventful (10), but rarely may be complicated by bacterial endocarditis or congestive heart failure (10, 45, 59).

The few patients with uncorrected large VSDs usually display growth retardation, recurrent respiratory infection, pulmonary hypertension, and left and right ventricular compromise (60). Their mortality during pregnancy is between 7 and 40% (4, 7, 61–63). Severe right ventricular failure with shunt reversal (Eisen-

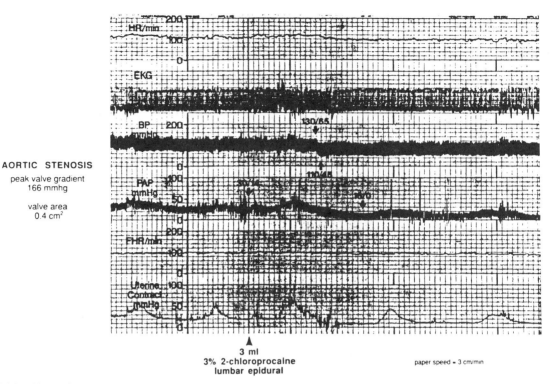

Figure 27.11. Hemodynamic responses to an epidural test dose of a rapid-acting anesthetic in a patient with severe aortic stenosis. *HR* = heart rate; *ECG* = electrocardiogram; *BP* = blood pressure; *PAP* = pulmonary artery pressure; *FHR* = fetal heart rate. Shortly after injection of 3 ml of 3% 2-chloroprocaine, there was a dramatic fall in PAP and BP, likely resulting from a small but rapid increase in vascular capacitance. (Reprinted by permission from Easterling TR, Chadwick HS, Otto CM, Benedetti TJ: Aortic stenosis in pregnancy. Obstet Gynecol 72:113–118, 1988.)

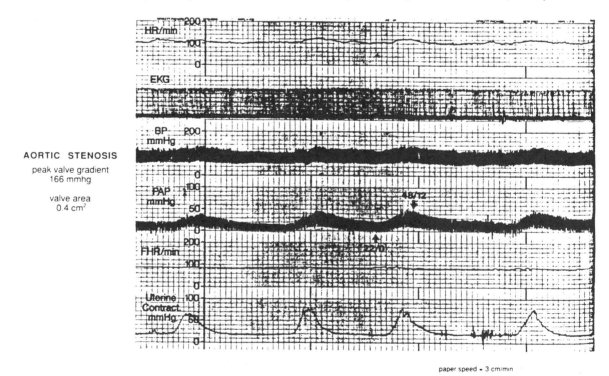

Figure 27.12. Hemodynamic responses of a patient with severe aortic stenosis to increased vascular return associated with uterine contractions. *HR* = heart rate; *ECG* = electrocardiogram; *BP* = blood pressure; *PAP* = pulmonary artery pressure; *FHR* = fetal heart rate. (Reprinted by permission from Easterling TR, Chadwick HS, Otto CM, Benedetti TJ: Aortic stenosis in pregnancy. Obstet Gynecol 72:113–118, 1988.)

menger's syndrome) is the major complication. Operative correction of the VSD before pregnancy does not increase maternal or fetal morbidity or mortality during pregnancy (4, 10, 64).

Clinical Manifestations

A small VSD produces a mild pansystolic murmur in the fourth or fifth left intercostal space, a normal chest roentgenogram, and a right bundle branch pattern on the electrocardiogram. Intracardiac pressures are normal with minimal left-to-right shunting. A moderate to large VSD produces loud pansystolic murmurs with expiratory splitting of the second heart sound and evidence of left ventricular enlargement. Eventually, right ventricular enlargement occurs. Right ventricle oxygen saturation is increased as a result of the left-to-right shunt. Right ventricular end-diastolic pressure, pulmonary artery pressure, and left ventricular end-diastolic pressure are increased. A moderate VSD usually decreases pulmonary vascular resistance; a large VSD usually increases it. Prolonged elevation of pulmonary vascular resistance causes bidirectional and eventually right-to-left shunting with concomitant cyanosis and clubbing.

Pathophysiology

The left-to-right shunt associated with a small VSD initially increases pulmonary blood flow and secondarily decreases pulmonary vascular resistance, thus preserving normal pulmonary artery pressures. The increase in left ventricular volume work is well tolerated. With a larger VSD, the greater left-to-right shunt markedly increases pulmonary blood flow, but pulmonary vascular resistance cannot compensate for this increased flow and pulmonary hypertension develops. The increase in left ventricular volume work leads to left ventricular dysfunction, elevation of PCW pressure, and exacerbation of the pulmonary hypertension. Right ventricular failure follows, with eventual equalization of right and left ventricular pressures, and bidirectional or reverse shunting with peripheral cyanosis follows (62, 63).

With pregnancy, elevations in heart rate, cardiac output, and intravascular volume may increase the left-to-right shunt, exacerbate pulmonary hypertension, and cause left and right ventricular failure. Elevation of vascular resistance with stress associated with labor and surgical stimulus increases right and left ventricular dysfunction. Bidirectional shunting or right-to-left shunting may result. If right ventricular afterload is increased as much as left afterload is increased, then there may be no increase in shunting.

Anesthetic Considerations

A small VSD in an asymptomatic patient with normal ventricular function does not require specialized monitoring. Symptoms, abnormal ventricular function, or a large VSD indicate monitoring via radial and pulmonary artery catheters. The following points should be considered (Table 27.8).

1. *Systemic vascular resistance increases may not be tolerated.*
2. *Marked increases in heart rate are poorly tolerated.* An increased systemic vascular resistance or heart rate may increase the left-to-right shunt. Pulmonary hypertension and ventricular failure may follow. Therefore adequate anesthesia is essential to prevent the sympathetic response that attends pain during labor and delivery, endotracheal intubation, and surgical stimulation. Vasodilation with low doses of sodium nitroprusside or phentolamine (0.1 to 0.5 μg/kg/min) may be needed to reduce shunting and improve cardiac output.
3. *With pulmonary hypertension and right ventricular compromise, marked decreases in systemic vascular resistance may not be well tolerated.* With a marked decrease in systemic vascular resistance, a right-to-left shunt and hypoxia will occur. Pressure decreases consequent to regional anesthesia should be corrected.
4. *Factors that increase pulmonary vascular resistance should be avoided in patients with pulmonary hypertension and evidence of right ventricular compromise.* These factors are discussed in the sections on mitral stenosis and primary pulmonary hypertension.

Anesthesia for Vaginal Delivery and Cesarean Section

For labor and vaginal delivery continuous lumbar epidural anesthesia permits control of systemic resistance and painful stimuli. For cesarean section, either regional or general anesthesia may be used. If regional anesthesia is selected, a continuous lumbar epidural technique will ensure slower changes in systemic resistance and allow more time for correction of pressure changes. General anesthesia that combines inhalation and narcotic techniques may

---

Table 27.8
Anesthetic Considerations: Ventricular Septal Defect

1. Avoid marked increases in systemic vascular resistance.
2. Avoid marked increases in heart rate.
3. With pulmonary hypertension, avoid marked decreases in systemic vascular resistance.
4. With pulmonary hypertension, avoid marked increases in pulmonary vascular resistance.

best minimize increases in systemic vascular resistance and myocardial depression. Addition of a vasodilator may be necessary.

Peripheral cyanosis in the presence of an elevated cardiac output indicates an imbalance between the pulmonary and systemic resistances with right-to-left shunt as the most probable cause. One hundred percent oxygen should be delivered. The systemic vascular resistance should be increased by lightening anesthesia or by administering small amounts of metaraminol. Peripheral cyanosis associated with a depressed cardiac output indicates right and/or left ventricular failure. Therapy includes an increase in oxygen delivery, withdrawal of anesthesia, and use of an inotrope such as dopamine.

ATRIAL SEPTIC DEFECT

Atrial septal defect (ASD) occurs in 17.5% of adults with congenital heart disease and is the most common congenital heart lesion (4, 10, 60, 65). Atrial septal defect is consistent with prolonged longevity (8, 59). Cardiac dysrhythmia, pulmonary hypertension, right ventricular failure, and left ventricular failure are commonly not seen until the fourth or fifth decades. Most women with uncorrected ASD tolerate pregnancy well, even when pulmonary blood flow is increased (4, 10). However, the risk of left ventricular failure during pregnancy is increased (1, 7, 66). Maternal and fetal mortality range between 1 and 12% (1, 4, 7, 66, 67).

Clinical Manifestations

Physical examination reveals fixed expiratory splitting of the second heart sound and a systolic ejection murmur at the upper left sternal border whose intensity varies with the degree of left-to-right shunt (19). The electrocardiogram usually exhibits right axis deviation with an osteum secundum defect. Chest roentgenogram may show right ventricular enlargement, pulmonary artery prominence, and increased pulmonary vascular markings. Cardiac catheterization of the parturient usually reveals normal pulmonary artery, right ventricular, and right atrial pressures even with moderate right ventricular dilation.

Pathophysiology

The left-to-right shunting increases right ventricular preload, right ventricular volume work, and pulmonary blood flow. However, a compensatory decrease in pulmonary vascular resistance keeps pulmonary artery pressures normal until the fourth or fifth decade. The increase in right and left atrial blood volume eventually causes right and left atrial distension and associated supraventricular dysrhythmias, particularly atrial fibrillation. The chronically elevated pulmonary blood flow causes pulmonary vascular changes, leading to increased pulmonary vas-

cular resistance, and pulmonary hypertension. Right ventricular failure may occur with prolonged increase in volume work, particularly when pressure work increases secondary to pulmonary hypertension.

Pregnancy accelerates these changes by increasing blood volume and cardiac output with consequent increases in left-to-right shunt, right ventricular volume work, pulmonary blood flow, and left ventricular volume work. Pulmonary hypertension and right and left ventricular dysfunction may follow. Left atrial distension may precipitate supraventricular dysrhythmias. Supraventricular dysrhythmias are particularly hazardous because incomplete emptying of the left atrium occurs and left atrial volume and pressure increase and exacerbate the left-to-right shunt.

Anesthetic Considerations

Most asymptomatic patients without evidence of pulmonary hypertension or right ventricular compromise do not require unusual care. Symptoms, pulmonary hypertension, or right ventricular failure indicate radial artery, pulmonary artery, and right atrial pressure monitoring. The following considerations should be noted (Table 27.9).

1. *Supraventricular dysrhythmias are poorly tolerated and may increase left-to-right shunt.* Medications (digoxin, quinidine, etc.) given to control chronic supraventricular dysrhythmias should be continued and adjusted throughout pregnancy and the puerperium. The acute onset of supraventricular dysrhythmias should be treated with direct current cardioversion or propranolol if right ventricular failure or systemic hypotension occur. Digitalization is recommended if these complications are absent.

2. *Increased systemic vascular resistance may not be tolerated.*

3. *Marked decreases in pulmonary vascular resistance are poorly tolerated.* An increase in peripheral resistance or a decrease in pulmonary resistance may increase the left-to-right shunt and cause systemic hypotension.

4. *Increases in pulmonary vascular resistance exacerbate preexisting pulmonary hypertension, and right ventricular failure may occur.*

Table 27.9
Anesthetic Considerations: Atrial Septal Defect

1. Prevent or immediately treat supraventricular dysrhythmias.
2. Avoid increases in systemic vascular resistance.
3. Avoid decreases in pulmonary vascular resistance.
4. With pulmonary hypertension, avoid further increases in pulmonary vascular resistance.

Anesthesia for Vaginal Delivery and Cesarean Section

For labor, vaginal delivery, and cesarean section segmental continuous lumbar epidural anesthesia avoids the hazard of increases in systemic vascular resistance. General anesthesia may be used if the above considerations are borne in mind.

PATENT DUCTUS ARTERIOSUS

Patent ductus arteriosus (PDA) constitutes 15% of all congenital heart disease (4). Early surgical intervention presently makes this a rarely significant finding during pregnancy. Patients with a small ductus usually have a benign clinical course until the fourth or fifth decade of life, when left or right ventricular failure may occur. However, a ductus of large internal diameter (greater than 1 cm) may produce growth retardation, respiratory infection, congestive heart failure, and pulmonary hypertension during childhood and early adult life. Even without congestive heart failure prior to pregnancy, maternal mortality from ventricular failure is 5 to 6% in unoperated pregnancy patients (4, 10).

Clinical Manifestations

A PDA produces a continuous murmur, enveloping the second heart sound with late systolic accentuation, terminating in late or middiastole, and radiating to the first left intercostal space. A large ductus enlarges the left ventricle and widens the arterial pulse pressure. The electrocardiogram can be normal (with a small ductus) or demonstrate left or right ventricular hypertrophy (with a large ductus). The chest roentgenogram can appear normal (with a small ductus) or can demonstrate left ventricular, left atrial, or pulmonary artery enlargement. Right ventricular enlargement is seen with severe pulmonary hypertension.

Pathophysiology

The left-to-right shunt of aortic blood via the ductus to the pulmonary artery increases central circulatory flow at the expense of peripheral flow. Both length and cross-section of the ductus determine resistance to flow and hence the amount of left-to-right shunt. A small internal diameter (less than 1 cm) generally permits a small left-to-right flow. A secondary decrease in pulmonary vascular resistance prevents the increase in pulmonary artery flow from producing pulmonary hypertension. Both the left and right ventricles tolerate this small increase in flow.

A ductus with a moderate internal diameter (1 to 2 cm) permits a significant increase in pulmonary blood flow. Pulmonary hypertension ultimately results from the inability of the pulmonary vasculature to compensate for the increased flow. Left ventricular volume work is increased, and left ventricular failure

eventually ensues. With failure, elevation of left ventricular end-diastolic pressure further exacerbates the pulmonary hypertension. Progressive medial hypertrophy and intimal fibrosis increase pulmonary resistance, and right ventricular failure follows.

A large internal diameter (greater than 2 cm) telescopes the temporal development of the above changes. Severe pulmonary hypertension with right ventricular failure may eventually produce a right-to-left shunt and peripheral cyanosis (Eisenmenger's syndrome).

The increased intravascular volume associated with pregnancy can increase shunting, pulmonary hypertension, and left ventricular volume work. In addition, the increased heart rate and stroke volume will increase myocardial oxygen demand and may compromise left ventricular function during stressful periods, such as uterine contractions. The decrease in systemic vascular resistance, seen throughout pregnancy and particularly during the postpartum period, can lead to shunt reversal and cyanosis, particularly in patients with a large ductus.

Anesthetic Considerations

Asymptomatic patients with normal hemodynamics and no evidence of ventricular dysfunction do not require unusual care. Evidence of left ventricular failure, pulmonary hypertension, right ventricular failure, or reversal of the left-to-right shunt indicates monitoring via an arterial line and a pulmonary artery catheter with the following considerations noted (Table 27.10).

1. *Increases in systemic vascular resistance may not be tolerated.* Proportionate increases in pulmonary vascular resistance may not occur and left-to-right shunt may increase.

2. *Marked increases in blood volume may be poorly tolerated.* Acute hypervolemia may precipitate failure by increasing left ventricular volume work and oxygen consumption.

3. *Marked decreases in systemic vascular resistance or increases in pulmonary resistance may lead to reverse shunting in patients with preexisting pulmonary hypertension and right ventricular compromise* (see the section on Eisenmenger's syndrome).

Table 27.10
Anesthetic Considerations: Patent Ductus Arteriosus

1. Avoid increases in systemic vascular resistance.
2. Avoid marked increases in blood volume.
3. With pulmonary hypertension, avoid marked decreases in systemic vascular resistance or increases in pulmonary vascular resistance.
4. With left ventricular failure, avoid myocardial depressants.

4. *Patients with left ventricular failure may not tolerate additional myocardial depression.*

Anesthesia for Vaginal Delivery and Cesarean Section

Use of a continuous epidural technique for labor, vaginal delivery, and cesarean section prevents increases in systemic vascular resistance associated with pain. In addition, decreases in systemic vascular resistance may reduce left-to-right shunt. If general anesthesia is selected for cesarean section, increases in systemic vascular resistance should be rapidly treated by deepening anesthesia or use of a vasodilating agent such as sodium nitroprusside or phentolamine.

The use of simultaneous pulse oximetry of the right hand and foot as a monitor of both pulmonary function and shunt fraction has been shown to be useful (68). Blood flow to the right arm is predominantly preductal; thus SaO_2 in the right arm is determined by FIO_2, pulmonary function, and cardiac output, as well as the degree and direction through the PDA. When the SaO_2 of the right arm is constant, the SaO_2 of the foot changes inversely with the amount of right-to-left shunting through the PDA.

Right-to-Left Shunt

TETRALOGY OF FALLOT

Tetralogy of Fallot constitutes 15% of all congenital heart disease and is the most common cyanotic congenital heart disease (19, 65, 69). This anomaly is characterized by right ventricular outflow obstruction, VSD, right ventricular hypertrophy, and overriding aorta. In the past, few women demonstrated tetralogy of Fallot during pregnancy because most died before the childbearing age. However, antibiotic therapy and palliative or corrective surgery have increased the number of parturients presenting with corrected or uncorrected tetralogy of Fallot (10, 60, 65).

Pregnancy increases the morbidity and mortality of uncorrected tetralogy of Fallot, particularly in patients with a history of syncope, polycythemia, decreased arterial oxygen saturation (less than 80%), and right ventricular hypertension (1, 5, 7, 62, 70–72). Left ventricular failure, bacterial endocarditis, and cerebral thrombosis are increased. Most complications develop immediately postpartum when systemic vascular resistance is lowest, thereby exacerbating the right-to-left shunt. In parturients with uncorrected tetralogy of Fallot, 40% suffer from heart failure and 12% die (1). The fetal death rate is 36%. Patients undergoing pulmonary valvulotomy during pregnancy are not at increased risk, but fetal mortality approaches 50% (73, 74). Maternal mortality is not increased in patients with a corrected tetralogy

of Fallot, but fetal mortality can be as high as 25% (1, 64, 70).

Clinical Manifestations

Uncorrected tetralogy of Fallot causes cyanosis, clubbing, and a systolic thrill at the left sternal border near the second or third intercostal space. The degree of pulmonary hypertension and pulmonary blood flow determine the loudness of the thrill. The electrocardiogram suggests right ventricular hypertrophy. Chest roentgenogram demonstrates an enlarged heart but sparse peripheral pulmonary vasculature. Catheterization reveals decreased pulmonary artery pressure and significant right-to-left shunt.

Pathophysiology

The increased resistance to right ventricular outflow promotes right-to-left shunting via the ventricular septal defect. Shunting and, therefore, cyanosis depend on the size of the VSD, the obstruction to outflow from the right ventricle, and the ability of the right ventricle to overcome that obstruction. The obstruction may result from a fixed pulmonic stenosis or dynamic infundibular hypertrophy. If infundibular hypertrophy exists, increases in myocardial contractility or decreases in right ventricular volume may increase outflow obstruction (see the section on asymmetric septal hypertrophy). If significant hypertrophy does not exist, maintenance of right ventricular contractility is important for preservation of pulmonary blood flow and peripheral oxygenation. Regardless of the type of right ventricular outflow obstruction, decreases in systemic vascular resistance may exacerbate shunting and produce cyanosis.

Labor and postpartum changes may compromise these patients. The stress of labor may increase pulmonary vascular resistance and consequently increase the right-to-left shunt. Decreases in systemic vascular resistance noted throughout pregnancy and after delivery may increase the right-to-left shunt and produce cyanosis. Finally, patients with infundibular obstruction may be particularly at risk during labor, when increases in contractility may be highest.

Anesthetic Considerations

If the tetralogy has not been corrected, then special considerations are warranted, including radial artery and CVP monitoring. Patients with corrected tetralogy of Fallot may suffer from residual right ventricular failure and also require special considerations (see the section on primary pulmonary hypertension). In the absence of symptoms or right ventricular compromise, the usual anesthetic considerations can be applied. The following considerations should be noted (Table 27.11).

1. *Decreases in systemic vascular resistance, blood volume or venous return are not well toler-*

Table 27.11
Anesthetic Considerations: Tetralogy of Fallot

1. Avoid decreases in systemic vascular resistance.
2. Avoid decreases in blood volume.
3. Avoid decreases in venous return.
4. Avoid myocardial depressants.

ated. A fall in systemic vascular resistance increases the right-to-left shunt. A fall in blood volume or a decrease in venous return will decrease the ability of the right ventricle to perfuse the lungs. With right ventricular compromise high central blood volumes are necessary for maintenance of right ventricular output.

2. *Myocardial depressants may not be well tolerated.* In patients with right ventricular compromise, even small amounts of myocardial depression may not be tolerated, and inotropic support with dopamine may be necessary.

Maternal and fetal prognoses depend on the severity of pulmonary hypertension (2, 58, 68). Maternal mortality has been reported to be between 12 and 33% and fetal mortality between 30 and 54% (62, 63, 67, 71).

Anesthesia for Vaginal Delivery and Cesarean Section

For labor and vaginal delivery these patients are likely to be most safely managed with systemic medication, inhalation analgesia, or paracervical or pudendal block anesthesia. Epidural or spinal anesthesia should be used with extreme caution. To avoid decreases in systemic vascular resistance and venous return, volume infusion and continuous left uterine displacement are recommended. Ephedrine should be administered cautiously, because it may produce a marked increase in pulmonary vascular resistance.

For cesarean section a general anesthetic technique is preferred. If the patient does not present with infundibular obstruction, light planes of anesthesia should be well tolerated, and nitrous oxide–relaxant (and narcotic after the delivery) may be most efficacious. However, if the patient does present with infundibular stenosis, increases in myocardial contractility or heart rate and decreases in ventricular volume will not be well tolerated, and an inhalation anesthetic, such as halothane or isoflurane, might be most efficacious. Maintenance of normal or slightly elevated right ventricular filling pressure and systemic vascular resistance is advocated (see the section on asymmetric septal hypertrophy).

Increasing peripheral cyanosis occurring in patients without infundibular obstruction usually indicates a decrease in systemic vascular resistance or increased right ventricular compromise. Treatment consists of delivering the maximum concentration of oxygen and decreasing the anesthetic depth. Increasing peripheral cyanosis in patients with a history of significant infundibular obstruction is usually precipitated by tachycardia, increased myocardial contractility, or decreased right ventricular volume. Treatment consists of increasing the depth of halothane or isoflurane anesthesia, increasing venous return and central blood volume, and decreasing contractility and heart rate by titration of propranolol.

EISENMENGER'S SYNDROME

Eisenmenger's syndrome consists of pulmonary hypertension and a right-to-left or bidirectional shunt with peripheral cyanosis (10, 19). The shunt may be atrial, ventricular, or aortopulmonary. The incidence of Eisenmenger's syndrome has been reported to be approximately 3% of all patients with congenital heart disease; it is commonly found with left-to-right shunt reversal during the end stages of patent ductus arteriosus, ventricular septal defect, and atrial septal defect (65). Most patients with Eisenmenger's syndrome have a particularly poor prognosis, and survival beyond the age of 40 is uncommon. This condition is not amenable to surgical correction; high pulmonary artery pressures with fixed vascular resistance are not reversed by surgical intervention (10, 58, 65).

Maternal and fetal prognoses depend on the severity of pulmonary hypertension (2, 58). Maternal mortality has been reported to be between 12 and 33% and fetal mortality between 30 and 54% (62, 63, 67, 71).

Clinical Manifestations

Clinical manifestations of Eisenmenger's syndrome are dependent on the degree of pulmonary hypertension and right-to-left shunt (2, 19). The type of murmur detected is a function of the specific right-to-left defect (e.g., a systolic ejection murmur with ASD, or a holosystolic murmur with VSD). The electrocardiogram usually demonstrates right ventricular hypertrophy with right axis deviation, and the chest roentgenogram usually demonstrates increased pulmonary artery markings with a prominent right ventricle.

Pathophysiology

The degree of right-to-left shunt depends on the severity of pulmonary hypertension and the size of the right-to-left circulatory communication (Fig. 27.13). In addition, the relationship between the pulmonic and systemic vascular resistance plays an important role. Increases in pulmonary vascular resistance or decreases in systemic vascular resistance exacerbate the right-to-left shunt and produce peripheral cyanosis. The third factor that affects the

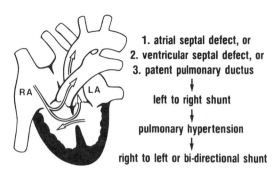

1. atrial septal defect, or
2. ventricular septal defect, or
3. patent pulmonary ductus

↓

left to right shunt

↓

pulmonary hypertension

↓

right to left or bi-directional shunt

Figure 27.13. Pathophysiology of Eisenmenger's syndrome. *RA* = right atrium; *LA* = left atrium.

degree of shunt is the contractile state of the right ventricle. Progressive right ventricular dysfunction will decrease pulmonary blood flow and increase shunt.

Pregnancy is not tolerated well. In patients with Eisenmenger's syndrome the typical fall in pulmonary vascular resistance during pregnancy is not seen since the resistance is fixed. However, the decrease in systemic vascular resistance does occur, and, consequently, the right-to-left shunt markedly increases (7, 62, 75). Increases in heart rate and stroke volume will increase right ventricular oxygen consumption and, in the presence of relatively desaturated blood, may produce right ventricular compromise with increased right-to-left shunt (19, 75).

Diuresis is usually seen in the postdelivery period and may increase hematocrit and thus decrease blood viscosity and pulmonary blood flow. Adequate crystalloid replacement and maintenance of hematocrit below 55% are advocated.

Anesthetic Considerations

All patients with Eisenmenger's syndrome are at markedly increased risk and should be monitored with radial arterial and central venous catheters. The following considerations should be noted (Table 27.12).

1. *Decreases in systemic vascular resistance or venous return are not well tolerated* (see section on tetralogy of Fallot).

2. *Elevations of pulmonary vascular resistance are not well tolerated.* Even minimal hypercarbia, acidosis, or hypoxia should be avoided; if they do occur, they should be treated aggressively (see the section on primary pulmonary hypertension).

Anesthesia for Vaginal Delivery and Cesarean Section

The anesthetic management of patients with Eisenmenger's syndrome is essentially identical to that previously outlined for patients with tetralogy of Fallot (76–78).

Table 27.12
Anesthetic Considerations: Eisenmenger's Syndrome

1. Avoid decreases in systemic vascular resistance.
2. Avoid decreases in venous return.
3. Avoid increases in pulmonary vascular resistance (e.g., hypercarbia, acidosis, hypoxia).

Other Congenital Heart Diseases

COARCTATION OF THE AORTA

Coarctation of the aorta represents approximately 8% of all cases of congenital heart disease in adults (65). The incidence of this disease in the pregnant population has been steadily decreasing because most cases are surgically corrected in early childhood. With corrected lesions maternal and fetal morbidity and mortality are not increased (7, 79, 80). The maternal mortality for patients with uncorrected coarctation of the aorta has been reported to be between 3 and 9%, and fetal mortality may be as high as 20% (4, 7, 79, 80). The incidence of congenital heart disease in the offspring is also elevated and is between 3 and 5% (4, 10). The principal risks to the mother with coarctation of the aorta are left ventricular failure, aortic rupture, and infective endocarditis.

Clinical Manifestations

Physical examination usually reveals a significant difference in blood pressures obtained in the upper and lower extremities or in the right and left upper extremities. Other findings with significant stenosis include an increase in intensity of the aortic component of the second heart sound, a medium-pitched systolic blowing murmur (heard best between the scapulae), a ventricular heave, and a laterally displaced point of maximal impulse. Late in the course, the electrocardiogram will demonstrate signs of left ventricular hypertrophy, and the chest roentgenogram will demonstrate left ventricular enlargement and a characteristic "three" sign in the aortic knob. Cardiac catheterization is indicated in complicated cases and is useful in assessing the severity of the disease.

Pathophysiology

Coarctation, like aortic stenosis, represents a fixed obstruction to left ventricular ejection. Thus, stroke volume tends to be limited, and increases in cardiac output are achieved primarily through increases in heart rate. Because of increased left ventricular afterload, ventricular pressure work increases and concentric hypertrophy occurs. Patients with mild coarctation tolerate this well and progression to ventricular dilation and failure occurs late in the course. With severe coarctation these complications will be precipitated much earlier. In addition to these ventricular changes, pathologic changes in the arterial wall at the site of coarctation will occur and serve as the nidus for dissection and rupture.

Both left ventricular compromise and vascular wall damage can be exacerbated by pregnancy. Because stroke volume is limited, the increased intravascular volume and increased metabolic demand seen in pregnancy can be accommodated only by increases in heart rate. During periods of high demand (labor) or acute increases in intravascular volume (uterine contraction), supranormal heart rates may not be able to compensate for limited stroke volume, and left ventricular failure will occur. With respect to vascular wall damage, there is evidence that anatomic changes in the aortic intima and media can be precipitated by pregnancy (79, 80). With increased heart rate and contractility seen with stress, the rate of ejection of blood from the left ventricle will increase and may cause aortic dissection and rupture. Finally, systemic arterial dilation seen during pregnancy and immediately after delivery may not be tolerated because stroke volume is fixed.

Anesthetic Considerations

Asymptomatic patients without left ventricular enlargement or dysfunction can be approached in the usual fashion. Other patients may be at markedly increased risk and should be monitored with radial artery and pulmonary artery catheters. The following considerations should be noted (Table 27.13).

1. *Decreases in systemic vascular resistance are not well tolerated.* Because stroke volume is fixed, compensation for decreases in systemic vascular resistance is limited, and hypotension may result. Maintenance of systemic vascular resistance in a normal to slightly elevated range with either metaraminol or "light" anesthesia is recommended. Particular caution should be given to the period immediately after delivery.

2. *Decreases in heart rate are not well tolerated.* In the presence of a fixed stroke volume, cardiac output is primarily determined by heart rate. Vagal stimulants, medications, or anesthetics that either decrease the heart rate or depress the sinus node should be avoided. Bradycardia should be treated by removing the precipitant cause and, if necessary, administering atropine or isoproterenol.

3. *Decreases in left ventricular filling are not well tolerated.* In the presence of a fixed obstruction to left ventricular emptying, adequate stroke volume

Table 27.13
Anesthetic Considerations: Coarctation of the Aorta

1. Avoid decreases in systemic vascular resistance.
2. Avoid bradycardia.
3. Maintain left ventricular filling.

will require high end-diastolic volumes. Venous return must be maintained, hypovolemia avoided, and atrial dysrhythmias promptly treated.

Anesthesia for Vaginal Delivery and Cesarean Section

The anesthetic management of these patients is similar to those with rheumatic aortic stenosis as previously described. For vaginal delivery, systemic medication, inhalation analgesia, or pudendal nerve block are recommended. For cesarean section, light general anesthesia using a nitrous oxide–relaxant technique is advocated. Increased levels of heart rate, contractility, and vascular resistance can be maintained with this technique. In addition, if the possibility of aortic dissection exists, the anesthetic considerations listed in the section on dissecting aneurysm of the aorta should be noted.

CONGENITAL AORTIC STENOSIS

Congenital aortic stenosis can be supravalvular, valvular, or subvalvular (81, 83). The supravalvular lesion has been described in the maternal rubella syndrome (84), and the narrowing occurs just distal to the coronary artery orifices. The subvalvular lesion may be diaphragmatic or muscular (such as asymmetric septal hypertrophy). However, the most common valvular form, as well as the most common congenital malformation of the heart, is the bicuspid aortic valve occurring in 1 to 2% of the general population (85). Unlike the supravalvular and subvalvular forms, the bicuspid form may not become clinically apparent until late in adult life. Studies by Bacon and Matthews (86) suggested that 20 to 30% of patients with a congenitally bicuspid aortic valve eventually develop aortic stenosis, secondary to blood turbulence and fibrin deposition.

Mendelson (1), Ueland (64), and Szekely and Snaith (4) reported on 14 patients with congenital aortic stenosis complicating pregnancy. Ten of fourteen pregnancies were uncomplicated. In the other four pregnancies one was terminated because of intractable heart failure, and three required aortic valvulotomy during pregnancy. Of these three patients, one had an uncomplicated postoperative course and an uneventful delivery, one had a miscarriage 10 days after operation, and the third patient delivered a child with congenital abnormalities who died at the age of 4 months. Thus, with congenital aortic stenosis, as with rheumatic aortic stenosis, the maternal morbidity and fetal mortality seem to be increased.

Aside from asymmetric septal hypertrophy (which is discussed later in this chapter), the pathophysiology and anesthetic considerations of congenital aortic stenosis are similar to those already described for rheumatic aortic stenosis (Table 27.7).

CONGENITAL PULMONIC STENOSIS

Isolated pulmonic stenosis constitutes approximately 13% of all congenital heart disease (65). The lesion may be valvular or subvalvular (infundibular stenosis) (87). The valvular lesion is usually non-progressive until late in adult life (19). However, the subvalvular lesion, which has a different pathophysiology, can be progressive. The considerations for patients with subvalvular stenosis are discussed in the section on asymmetric septal hypertrophy. Only valvular stenosis is discussed here.

Mendelson (1) and Szekely and Snaith (4) reviewed a total of 71 patients with isolated pulmonic stenosis during pregnancy. There were no maternal deaths; however, 5 of the 71 pregnancies were complicated by right ventricular failure, and there were 3 fetal deaths.

Clinical Manifestations

In patients with severe right ventricular failure, decreased left ventricular output occurs and the symptoms of fatigue and syncope result. Auscultation reveals a pulmonic ejection click following the first heart sound and a systolic ejection murmur in the second left intercostal space. With increasing severity of pulmonic stenosis, the murmur has an increased duration and a late systolic accentuation; in addition, the pulmonic component of the second heart sound is delayed, with an expiratory splitting of the second heart sound. In mild pulmonic stenosis the electrocardiogram usually reveals a right bundle branch block. With severe stenosis, a predominant R wave is seen in lead V_1 that usually exceeds 20 mm in height (88); it is usually correlated with a right ventricular systolic pressure of at least 80 mm Hg (89). Right ventricular strain manifested by negative T waves in the right precordial leads may occur as well. The characteristic radiologic finding is prominence of the left pulmonary artery. With severe stenosis right ventricular and atrial enlargement are usually seen.

Pathophysiology

With progressive stenosis of the right ventricular outflow tract, pressure work increases and concentric hypertrophy occurs. The right ventricle seems to adapt readily to this situation. Right ventricular output is maintained until late in the course of the disease, notably when right ventricular systolic pressure exceeds approximately 80 mm Hg (90). As right ventricular output decreases so does left ventricular preload and, therefore, cardiac output. Systemic vascular resistance increases in an effort to compensate for the decreased left ventricular output. However, as right ventricular failure progresses, further decreases in cardiac output are uncompensated, and

symptoms of low cardiac output—such as fatigue and syncope—occur with exercise and later at rest.

Although patients with isolated pulmonary valvular stenosis have uneventful courses until late in life (19)—that is, after the childbearing years—their course may become complicated during the stressful periods of pregnancy, labor, and delivery (1, 4). Right ventricular failure can be precipitated during pregnancy by both the increase in intravascular volume (increasing right ventricular preload, stroke work, and oxygen consumption) and the increase in heart rate (increasing oxygen consumption). Furthermore, the decrease in systemic vascular resistance, which is usually seen during pregnancy, and especially after delivery, may counteract an important compensatory mechanism needed during low right ventricular output states.

Anesthetic Considerations

Patients who are asymptomatic without progression of right ventricular compromise may be approached in the usual manner. Otherwise, radial artery and CVP monitoring is advocated. The first sign of impending right ventricular failure may be a subtle but progressive rise in end-diastolic pressure or CVP. In providing anesthesia the following considerations should be noted (Table 27.14).

1. *Marked increases or decreases in right ventricular filling pressure are not well tolerated.* Maintenance of the patient's right ventricular filling pressure in its usual range is necessary for effective contraction of the ventricle against the increased pulmonic resistance. Excessive volume transfusion may overdistend the right ventricle and produce further right ventricular failure. On the other hand, sudden drops in venous return, such as obstruction of the vena cava or acute hemorrhage, will decrease the effectiveness of right ventricular contraction.

2. *Decreases in heart rate are not well tolerated.* Right ventricular output will depend primarily on heart rate because stroke volume is limited. Maintenance of at least normal (90 to 110 bpm) heart rates, by choosing drugs with a positive chronotropic effect and using light anesthesia, is recommended.

3. *Marked decreases in systemic vascular resistance may not be tolerated.* With a low output state, systemic pressure is preserved by increases in vas-

Table 27.14
Anesthetic Considerations: Congenital Pulmonic Stenosis

1. Avoid marked increases in intravascular volume.
2. Avoid marked decreases in venous return.
3. Avoid bradycardia.
4. Avoid marked decreases in systemic vascular resistance.
5. Avoid myocardial depressants.

cular resistance. Maintenance of a normal to high systemic vascular resistance by light levels of general anesthesia or by the addition of a vasoconstrictor, such as ephedrine or metaraminol, is advocated.

4. *Negative inotropes may not be well tolerated.* The contractile state of the right ventricle may be compromised, and further myocardial depression may result from negative inotropes such as halothane or enflurane. Likewise, use of medications or techniques with positive inotropic action is efficacious.

Anesthesia for Vaginal Delivery and Cesarean Section

For labor and vaginal delivery, techniques that reduce systemic vascular resistance and venous return should be used with extreme caution. These patients are probably best managed with systemic or inhalation analgesics and pudendal blocks.

If epidural, caudal, or spinal anesthesia is chosen, prophylactic administration of intravenous fluids and ephedrine is recommended. Maintenance of a normal CVP is necessary. Decreases in systemic vascular resistance should be anticipated and immediately corrected with left uterine displacement and ephedrine or metaraminol.

For cesarean section general anesthesia using a nitrous oxide–relaxant technique is recommended. Maintenance of vascular resistance, heart rate, and contractility is the goal. If signs of right ventricular failure develop (elevation of filling pressure), treatment consists of lightening the anesthetic level and administering an inotrope such as dopamine.

In addition to these congenital diseases, a number of others exist but are certainly more rare. Recently, case reports have appeared which suggest that such conditions can be approached safely despite their inherent difficulties (91, 95). The anesthetic considerations will vary depending on the disease itself and its progression.

OTHER HEART DISEASES

Primary Pulmonary Hypertension

Primary pulmonary hypertension is a disease that particularly affects young women (96, 98). Maternal mortality is more than 50% (62, 99). Most deaths occur during the periods of labor and the puerperium, and the pattern is similar to that described in Eisenmenger's syndrome (7, 10, 62, 66, 100). There is speculation that amniotic fluid embolism might be a possible precipitating factor in the fulminant course of this disease during labor and the puerperium (4).

CLINICAL MANIFESTATIONS

The principal symptoms of this disease, exertional dyspnea and fatigue, characteristically occur late in its natural course as differentiated from other causes of pulmonary hypertension. These symptoms are due to a low fixed cardiac output. The signs of this disease are dependent on the degree of pulmonary hypertension and right ventricular compromise. Usually, patients are acyanotic, have cool extremities with poor peripheral pulses, and have a quiet precordium. Prominent A waves in the deep jugular veins can be noted. Late in the disease, a systolic ejection murmur is heard over the pulmonary valve. In addition, evidence of tricuspid insufficiency can be detected. The electrocardiogram usually reveals right ventricular hypertrophy and right atrial enlargement. Chest roentgenogram shows a prominent main pulmonary artery and a slightly enlarged heart with a right atrial and right ventricular configuration. Late in the course of this disease the heart size may increase considerably. Cardiac catheterization demonstrates isolated pulmonary hypertension in the face of a normal PCW pressure.

PATHOPHYSIOLOGY

Pulmonary hypertension is present when the pulmonary artery pressure exceeds 30/15 mm Hg or the mean pulmonary artery pressure exceeds 25 mm Hg (83). With elevation of pulmonary pressure, morphologic changes occur in the pulmonary vasculature producing medial hypertrophy and intimal fibrosis. A large spectrum of changes can occur in this vasculature, and the reactivity of these vessels can be quite variable. With increasing pulmonary hypertension, right ventricular afterload and, therefore, right ventricular pressure work increase. The right ventricle hypertrophies and eventually fails, causing an elevated right ventricular end-diastolic pressure and a decreased cardiac output. This elevation of end-diastolic pressure is reflected by an elevation of CVP, producing passive congestion of the liver and peripheral edema. With progression of the disease, the right ventricle will become dilated, and tricuspid insufficiency will occur. Characteristically, throughout this course, the PCW or left ventricular preload is not elevated. The left ventricle usually functions well; however, left ventricular output falls because of the failing right ventricle.

ANESTHETIC CONSIDERATIONS

It is imperative that the degree of pulmonary hypertension and right ventricular failure be assessed before proceeding with an anesthetic plan. If possible, the reactivity of the pulmonary vasculature should be determined, for it may be responsive to pharmacologic vasodilation. Monitoring of radial artery and pulmonary artery pressure is recommended in all patients (102, 103). The following considerations should be noted (Table 27.15).

Table 27.15
Anesthetic Considerations: Primary Pulmonary Hypertension

1. Avoid increases in pulmonary vascular resistance.
2. Avoid marked decreases in venous return.
3. Avoid marked decreases in systemic vascular resistance.
4. Avoid myocardial depressants.

1. *Increases in pulmonary vascular resistance are not well tolerated.* Hypercarbia, hypoxia, acidosis, lung hyperinflation, pharmacologic vasoconstrictors, and stress can markedly elevate pulmonary vascular resistance and should be avoided.

2. *Marked decreases in right ventricular volume are not well tolerated.* Early correction of fluid and blood loss and avoidance of inferior vena caval obstruction are important for the maintenance of normal to slightly elevated CVP.

3. *Marked decreases in systemic vascular resistance may not be well tolerated.* Cardiac output is limited by a fixed right ventricular output. The patient may be unable to compensate for decreases in systemic vascular resistance.

4. *Right ventricular contractility may be compromised, and negative inotropes may result in marked depression of ventricular function.*

ANESTHESIA FOR VAGINAL DELIVERY AND CESAREAN SECTION

In these patients pain, anxiety, and stress are especially detrimental, because pulmonary vascular resistance may increase markedly. Adequate psychologic support and analgesia are mandatory. For labor and vaginal delivery, intravenous narcotics, inhalation analgesia, intrathecal morphine (101), and paracervical and pudendal nerve blocks are recommended. It is recognized that neonatal depression from the narcotics may result, and use of neonatal naloxone should be anticipated. In addition, opioids may cause maternal hypercapnia, potentially increasing the pulmonary vascular resistance. Nevertheless, these techniques are preferred to major conduction anesthesia because they are not associated with marked peripheral vasodilation and reduction in venous return. However, conduction anesthesia can be performed safely if attention to detail is meticulous, as demonstrated by several recent case reports (102, 103). These patients are frequently ideal candidates for subarachnoid and/or epidural narcotics, as described in Chapters 9 and 10.

If a continuous epidural technique is used, a dermatome-by-dermatome titration of local anesthetic is recommended. Meticulous attention must be given to changes in venous capacitance and vascular resistance. Continuous intravenous titration of fluids is necessary. Correction of small decreases in

systemic vascular resistance is not advocated, because the treatment might have a marked effect on the pulmonary vascular resistance. Only marked decreases in systemic vascular resistance should be corrected by titration of ephedrine.

For cesarean section general anesthesia is preferred. The conventional rapid induction with thiopental, succinylcholine, and endotracheal intubation may precipitate marked pulmonary hypertension and right ventricular failure. One suggested approach is an inhalation induction with halothane and oxygen. There is some evidence that use of an inhalation agent, such as halothane or isoflurane may decrease pulmonary vascular resistance (105). Intubation should not be performed until an adequate depth of anesthesia is achieved. To avoid possible hypoventilation and hypercarbia during induction, it is suggested that the patient by paralyzed with pancuronium immediately after loss of consciousness; ventilation can then be controlled. Hyperinflation of the lungs should be avoided, and a tidal volume of 5 to 10 ml/kg is recommended.

It is recognized that there is an increased risk of aspiration with this technique. Antacids should be administered prior to induction, and cricoid pressure should be applied continuously until intubation is performed.

The most serious complication is right ventricular decompensation resulting from increases in pulmonary hypertension. An early sign is a subtle but progressive elevation of CVP even though other parameters are stable and normal. If this should occur, hypercarbia, hypoxia, acidosis, and light anesthesia should be ruled out or corrected. If the situation persists, inotropes such as dopamine or isoproterenol should be titrated slowly. If these measures fail, pulmonary vasodilation with low dose sodium nitroprusside or phentolamine (0.1 to 0.5 μg/kg/min) should be attempted.

Hypertensive Disorders

The incidence of hypertension during pregnancy from all causes is approximately 6%, a quarter of these patients having preexistent hypertension (106–109). In addition to essential hypertension, the principal causes of hypertension are toxemia, renal disease, and, more rarely, coarctation of the aorta and pheochromocytoma. Both maternal and fetal morbidity and mortality seem to be affected by the occurrence, degree, pattern, and treatment of hypertension during pregnancy (4, 106–114). With essential hypertension, patients whose blood pressure does not exceed 160/100 mm Hg before and during the first 20 weeks of pregnancy have, as a rule, an excellent prognosis (106). In addition, those who demonstrate the characteristic fall in systolic blood pressure during the second trimester seem to have much lower fetal mortality (4.6%) as compared with those who show no fall (16%). Patients with essential hypertension who receive antihypertensive drugs during pregnancy had a lower incidence of toxemia (6% versus 18%) and fetal mortality (9% versus 24%) in comparison with a similar group of patients who did not receive antihypertensive therapy but were managed with rest, sedation, and salt restriction (106).

The cardiovascular changes seen in patients with preeclampsia–eclampsia and essential hypertension have been studied and contrasted with those changes seen in normal pregnancy. Recent data seem to indicate that patients with preeclampsia or essential hypertension have a lower cardiac index and smaller increase in blood volume than patients with hypertension during pregnancy. Patients with toxemia have been shown to have increased sensitivity to the effects of catecholamines (115), vasopressin (116), and angiotensin II (117). As in normal pregnancy, patients with essential hypertension seem to have a marked increase in sensitivity to ganglionic blocking drugs, which may precipitate severe hypotension. However, in patients with toxemia this sensitivity has not been demonstrated (118, 119). A complete discussion of preeclampsia–eclampsia is found in Chapter 17.

CLINICAL MANIFESTATIONS

The clinical manifestations of hypertension will depend on its etiologic factors. In general, symptoms of serious end organ involvement—such as transient cerebral ischemic attacks, left ventricular failure, angina, or renal insufficiency—are indicative of long-standing or malignant hypertension and warrant special consideration. Especially noteworthy are signs of left ventricular hypertrophy or dilation, which indicate more severe myocardial damage. These signs are a displaced point of maximal impulse, left ventricular heave on physical examination, left ventricular strain pattern (in addition to an excessive left ventricular voltage pattern) on electrocardiogram, and an enlarged and "boot-shaped" heart on chest roentgenogram.

PATHOPHYSIOLOGY

Hypertension affects nearly all organs of the body. Two pathophysiologic changes are noteworthy. First, with long-standing or severe hypertension arterial damage may occur and alter both the distribution of organ blood flow and its autoregulatory processes. There is evidence that these tissues may require higher perfusion pressures than normal to maintain tissue blood flow (19, 120). Second, with increased systemic pressure, left ventricular pressure work pro-

gressively increases, and the ventricle concentrically hypertrophies. Ventricular dilation and cardiomegaly occur later in the disease process when significant myocardial compromise and failure occur (18, 19).

Pregnancy can complicate the course of preexisting hypertension, can uncover essential hypertension, or can precipitate new forms of hypertension, such as toxemia (4, 106–113). The mechanisms by which these changes occur are increases in intravascular volume, increases in cardiac demand (heart rate, stroke volume), acute increases in systemic vascular resistance with stress, and changes in renal or endocrine function. The final result is left ventricular ischemia and failure with decreased cardiac output and decreased organ (including uterine) perfusion.

ANESTHETIC CONSIDERATIONS

The continuation of antihypertensive medications is recommended. In patients with severe or malignant hypertension prior to delivery, blood pressure should be reduced to reasonable levels (160 to 180/100 to 110 mm Hg) with intravenous vasodilators such as hydralazine. These patients may be very sensitive to vasodilators, and slow titration is recommended. With left ventricular failure radial artery and pulmonary artery monitoring is recommended.

ANESTHESIA FOR VAGINAL DELIVERY AND CESAREAN SECTION

For labor and vaginal delivery, regional anesthesia is recommended and is discussed fully in Chapter 17. Because labor pains can exacerbate hypertension and its sequelae, a continuous lumbar epidural technique is advocated. Intravascular volume may be relatively decreased in these patients and sympathectomy may lead to severe hypotension. Hydration prior to administration of a block and correction of hypotension with left uterine displacement and small amounts of ephedrine (2.5 mg intravenously) are suggested.

For cesarean section either regional or general anesthesia is acceptable. With regional anesthesia, administration of at least 1000 ml of crystalloid prior to the regional block is recommended. With general anesthesia, addition of a halogenated agent should prevent the acute rise in blood pressure associated with light planes of anesthesia. With severe or malignant hypertension associated with left ventricular dysfunction, radial artery and PCW pressure monitoring is advocated. Sodium nitroprusside or phentolamine may be necessary to treat an acute hypertensive crisis.

Cardiomyopathy of Pregnancy

The occurrence of left ventricular failure late in the course of pregnancy or during the first 6 months of the postpartum period without known causes has been termed cardiomyopathy of pregnancy, peripartum cardiomyopathy, puerperal cardiomyopathy, and postpartal heart disease (4, 72, 121–126). It is not clear whether this condition is closely related to pregnancy or whether pregnancy exacerbates a preexisting, latent myocardial disorder. The incidence of this disorder is increased in older multiparous women; in the presence of twins, toxemia, viral infection, poor nutrition, and genetic disorders; and in members of the black race (127). The long-term prognosis is highly variable. Mortality is between 15 and 60% (4, 107, 125). The occurrence of heart failure during subsequent pregnancies and the long-term survival seems to depend on the return of heart size to normal 6 months after the first episode of cardiomyopathy. Demakis and Rahimtoola (122) studied the clinical course of this disease in 27 women. All patients presented with left ventricular failure during the last month of pregnancy or within the first 5 months of the postpartum period. In 14 of the 27 patients, heart size returned to normal within 6 months. However, in 13 patients cardiomegaly persisted beyond 6 months. Eleven of these thirteen patients had chronic congestive heart failure and died after an average of 4.7 years.

CLINICAL MANIFESTATIONS

The clinical manifestations associated with this disorder are signs and symptoms of left or right ventricular failure (4, 19). Pulmonary embolism or infarction may also occur (128). The electrocardiogram demonstrates left ventricular hypertrophy, diffuse ST-T wave abnormalities, or left ventricular conduction defects. The chest roentgenogram is consistent with either left, right, or biventricular failure.

PATHOPHYSIOLOGY

Either left or right myocardial damage may be significant while the patient remains asymptomatic until a physiologic stress such as pregnancy occurs. With pregnancy a deleterious effect may be produced by several normal physiologic changes: the increase in preload associated with the stresses of uterine contraction or surgery and the increase in cardiac demand (heart rate, stroke volume, contractility). With progressive ventricular failure, end-diastolic volume increases (decreasing subendocardial blood flow), cardiac output decreases (decreasing coronary perfusion), and myocardial oxygen demand increases. Thus a myocardial oxygen supply–demand imbalance occurs, leading to further ventricular compromise.

ANESTHETIC CONSIDERATIONS

Patients presenting with ventricular failure (left or right) prior to delivery should be treated with bed rest, salt restriction, diuresis, digitalization, and preload–afterload reduction as necessary. If ventricular failure persists at the time of delivery, monitoring with a radial arterial line and a pulmonary artery catheter is recommended. Acute increases in afterload occurring with endotracheal intubation or surgical incision can precipitate left ventricular failure and should be anticipated and controlled with a vasodilator.

ANESTHESIA FOR VAGINAL DELIVERY AND CESAREAN SECTION

For labor and vaginal delivery regional anesthesia is recommended. With a continuous epidural technique, deleterious increases in afterload secondary to stress can be avoided. In addition, the resultant preload and afterload reduction may be efficacious in patients with ventricular compromise. A slow titration of the local anesthetic is suggested. Prehydration and prophylactic ephedrine should not be routinely used. Continuous fetal heart rate monitoring will help determine when the fall in blood pressure should be treated.

For cesarean section either regional or general anesthesia may be used. If general anesthesia is chosen, a nitrous oxide–relaxant technique is recommended in patients with marked ventricular failure. Afterload reduction with either sodium nitroprusside or phentolamine may be necessary. If regional anesthesia is chosen, a continuous epidural technique is recommended, because significant changes in systemic vascular resistance and venous capacitance will occur more slowly and are more easily corrected.

Dissecting Aneurysm of the Aorta

Although dissecting aneurysm of the aorta is more commonly found in men over 50 years of age, there has been a well-recognized association between pregnancy and dissecting aneurysm of the aorta (129). Up to 50% of dissecting aneurysms in women less than 40 years old occurred in association with pregnancy (129–131). Possible etiologic factors are syphilis, sepsis, Erdheim's medial necrosis, arteriosclerosis, and coarctation of the aorta. The effect of pregnancy per se on the histologic changes in the aorta is controversial (7, 130). However, pathologic changes occurring with pregnancy, such as hypertension, are known to influence the course of aortic dissection. The maternal mortality of patients with acute dissection of the aorta is similar to that of nonpregnant patients and depends on the extent of the process and the location of the intimal tear (4). During pregnancy, maternal mortality ranging from 19 to 91% has been reported (2).

CLINICAL MANIFESTATIONS

An abrupt, excruciating pain is the most characteristic feature. Most commonly the pain begins in the thorax or abdomen and migrates posteriorly to the interscapular or lumbar areas (18, 19). However, pain can also originate in the neck, extremities, or jaw. Painless dissection is most commonly seen in patients with Marfan's syndrome. Physical examination usually demonstrates hypertension and tachycardia; however, with dissection, hypotension may occur. If the ascending aorta is involved, a murmur of aortic insufficiency may be found; if the abdominal aorta is involved, a palpable tender aneurysm may be detected. Other findings include asymmetric pulses in the major vessels, focal neurologic signs, or evidence of myocardial ischemia.

PATHOPHYSIOLOGY

With aortic medial degeneration and the hydraulic stresses of pulsatile flow, dissection will occur. In approximately 70% of patients the dissection originates in the ascending aorta; in the remainder it usually originates distal to the left subclavian artery (19). Dissection may be localized or extend throughout the aorta. Proximal extension may involve the aortic valve (producing aortic insufficiency), the pericardium, or the left pleural space. Distal extension may involve the femoral vessels. In addition, dissection may occur primarily in the anterior or posterior regions of the aorta. With posterior dissection, tamponade may occur and slow the dissection process; with anterior dissection, acute rupture with hemorrhage into a body cavity may occur.

ANESTHETIC CONSIDERATIONS

The Nonemergent Situation

Patients with a history of aortic dissection that has been well controlled medically should continue to receive their medications throughout pregnancy, labor, and delivery. Regional anesthesia for labor and delivery (vaginal or cesarean section) is recommended. Maintenance of both a pain-free state and normal to slightly decreased blood pressure (a systolic pressure between 90 and 110 mm Hg) is necessary. Continuous fetal heart rate monitoring should be employed to determine the acceptable degree of hypotension. If general anesthesia is selected for cesarean section, an inhalation technique with halothane is suggested because hypertension and tachycardia will be less likely and the force of ventricular ejection of blood may be decreased.

Trimethaphan and propranolol are useful for control of hypertension and tachycardia. These drugs are recommended if hemodynamic control cannot be achieved by a quiet environment, reassurance, pain control with a regional anesthetic, and mild sedation.

Rupture with severe hemorrhage should always be anticipated. Two large-bore intravenous catheters should be placed; at least 8 units of whole blood should be available; and preparation for rapid intubation and resuscitation should be made.

The Emergent Situation

In patients presenting with progressive dissection requiring emergency surgical correction, all efforts should be made to expedite surgery. However, the induction of anesthesia is critical.

In patients who are normotensive to hypertensive, an inhalation induction with halothane is recommended. Control of blood pressure and minimization of the response to endotracheal intubation will help prevent hemodynamic decompensation prior to surgical control of the aorta. Immediately prior to induction, the surgical field should be prepped and draped, and the surgeon should be prepared to make an incision and cross-clamp the aorta if severe hypotension should occur with induction or intubation. Patients who are mildly to severely hypotensive may not be able to tolerate an inhalation agent, a barbiturate, or even a narcotic prior to intubation. Rapid induction with succinylcholine with or without ketamine is recommended. Even with marked sympathetic stimulation, blood pressure elevation may not occur because of severe intravascular volume depletion. Immediate surgical control of the aorta is the only treatment.

After control of the aortic dissection classic cesarean section should be performed.

Asymmetric Septal Hypertrophy

Asymmetric septal hypertrophy (ASH), also known as idiopathic hypertrophic subvalvular stenosis, is a cardiomyopathy characterized by a marked hypertrophy of the ventricle involving the interventricular septum and the outflow tract (83, 132–135). During ventricular systole constriction of the outflow tract occurs, producing obstruction to ventricular ejection. Typically, ASH is a disease of young adults, with the majority of patients being in their third and fourth decades.

Several authors have reported that pregnant patients with ASH have an increased risk for left ventricular failure and supraventricular dysrhythmias (4, 136–139). Brown et al. (134) reported on 12 patients; 1 developed left ventricular failure in her last month of pregnancy, and 2 developed atrial dysrhythmias in late pregnancy. Of the 12 patients, 3 died during the first postpartum year. On the other hand, Turner et al. (137) and Szekely and Snaith (4) reported on 13 patients with ASH during pregnancy and found that only 1 patient had a complicated pregnancy marked by episodes of supraventricular tachycardia without evidence of left ventricular failure. All patients had normal deliveries, and there was no evidence of an increased morbidity or mortality during the postpartum period. Thus the course of patients with ASH during pregnancy is quite variable.

CLINICAL MANIFESTATIONS

The most frequent symptoms of patients with ASH are exertional dyspnea, angina pectoris, and syncope (140). Late in the course of the disease, symptoms of left ventricular failure occur as well. On physical examination the heart is usually enlarged with a left ventricular lift, a double apical impulse, and a systolic murmur commencing late after the first heart sound and best heard at the apex (19). The electrocardiogram is usually abnormal with evidence of left ventricular hypertrophy; in addition, a Wolff-Parkinson-White syndrome or abnormal Q waves in the inferior or left precordial leads may be seen (140). Chest roentgenogram usually displays an enlarged left ventricle.

PATHOPHYSIOLOGY

Patients with ASH involving the left ventricle exhibit a marked hypertrophy of the entire left ventricle with a bulging of the ventricular myocardium in the septal region several centimeters below the aortic valve. The ventricular cavity is relatively small. With each systolic contraction the muscle about the outflow tract constricts and left ventricular ejection is obstructed. Progression of left ventricular hypertrophy eventually leads to ventricular failure.

Agents or events that increase myocardial contractility will exacerbate the left ventricular outflow obstruction and precipitate failure (19). Decreases in systemic vascular resistance may also cause an increase in left ventricular ejection force and increase obstruction (18, 19). Decreases in left ventricular preload will decrease the size of the left ventricle cavity during systole and increase obstruction (141). Thus rapid atrial rates or loss of atrial kick is not well tolerated (142).

During pregnancy the increase in intravascular volume is helpful in these patients because it will cause left ventricular distension and decrease the amount of outflow obstruction. However, the decrease in systemic vascular resistance and the increase in heart rate and myocardial contractility seen throughout pregnancy may be deleterious and may precipitate left ventricular failure.

ANESTHETIC CONSIDERATIONS

In patients who are symptomatic or present with a hemodynamically significant atrial dysrhythmia, monitoring with an arterial line and a pulmonary artery catheter may be especially helpful. In addition, the following points should be noted (Table 27.16).

Table 27.16
Anesthetic Considerations: Asymmetric Septal Hypertrophy

1. Avoid decreases in blood volume and venous return.
2. Avoid or correct supraventricular tachycardia, atrial fibrillation, and atrial flutter.
3. Avoid decreases in systemic vascular resistance.
4. Avoid increases in myocardial contractility.
5. Treat ventricular compromise with phenylephrine, intravenous fluids, and propranolol.

1. *Decreases in preload are not well tolerated.* Maintenance of slight hypervolemia is recommended because the increase in ventricular volume tends to decrease the amount of outflow obstruction.

2. *Supraventricular tachycardia, atrial fibrillation, or atrial flutter are not well tolerated.* With these dysrhythmias ventricular filling will be decreased. Immediate treatment with direct current cardioversion or propranolol is advocated.

3. *Decreases in systemic vascular resistance are not well tolerated.* Maintenance of a normal to a slightly elevated systemic resistance is advocated because the degree of outflow obstruction will be minimized.

4. *Increases in contractility may not be well tolerated.* Increases in myocardial contractility may markedly increase outflow obstruction.

5. *The treatment of ventricular failure with ASH is markedly different from the usual treatment of failure.* Increasing afterload (metaraminol) and preload (intravenous fluids) and decreasing heart rate (propranolol) and contractility (propranolol and halothane) are efficacious.

ANESTHESIA FOR VAGINAL DELIVERY AND CESAREAN SECTION

Anesthesia for labor and vaginal delivery is best provided with systemic or inhalation analgesics and paracervical and pudendal blocks. Major regional anesthetic techniques may reduce systemic vascular resistance and venous return, thereby increasing outflow obstruction. However, such regional techniques can be used if the attention to detail is meticulous, as recently reported (138). If these techniques are used, prophylactic administration of intravenous fluids, continuous left uterine displacement, and, if necessary, metaraminol infusion may be used to maintain blood pressure. For cesarean section a general anesthetic with an inhalation agent, such as halothane, is recommended because the degree of outflow obstruction may be reduced by the negative inotropic and chronotropic effects of halothane (139).

Coronary Artery Disease

Coronary artery disease occurring prior to or during pregnancy is uncommon and has been reported in approximately 1 in 10,000 pregnancies (4). In 108 cases of acute myocardial infarction during pregnancy the maternal and fetal mortalities were 35 and 37%, respectively (4, 7, 143–148). Seventy percent of the patients who did succumb had a myocardial infarction during the last trimester. The clinical manifestations and pathophysiology are similar to those in the nonpregnant patient (18, 19).

ANESTHETIC CONSIDERATIONS

Patients with a history of crescendo angina, recent (6 weeks) myocardial infarction, or congestive heart failure should be monitored with an arterial line and a pulmonary artery catheter. Patients maintained on nitrates or propranolol for treatment of angina should have their medications continued throughout pregnancy, labor, delivery, and the puerperium.

ANESTHESIA FOR VAGINAL DELIVERY AND CESAREAN SECTION

For labor and vaginal delivery, regional anesthesia is recommended. Regional anesthesia will minimize pain and stress, which could precipitate angina, and may decrease afterload and preload, which will be beneficial. However, severe decreases in afterload (producing systemic diastolic pressures below 50 mm Hg) or large increase in heart rate (greater than 120 bpm) can precipitate decreased diastolic filling of the coronary arteries and angina. Correction with metaraminol or propranolol, respectively, is advocated. Administration of nitroglycerin to treat angina in the presence of a sympathetic block may cause a further decrease in preload and cardiac output and may produce more ischemia.

For cesarean section either regional or general anesthesia may be used. The considerations for regional anesthesia are discussed above. For general anesthesia the most important consideration is to minimize the stress of intubation and surgery. If there is no evidence of congestive failure, an inhalation technique is recommended. If congestive failure is present and general anesthesia is selected, a nitrous oxide–relaxant technique with narcotic supplementation is suggested. Evidence of myocardial ischemia on the electrocardiogram (lead V_5 preferably) should be approached by first "normalizing" blood pressure and heart rate, changing the anesthetic level, or administering therapeutics (sodium nitroprusside, propranolol). With normalized vital signs but persistent evidence of ischemia, administration of sublingual nitroglycerine is suggested.

The rapid hemodynamic changes during the postpartum period can precipitate ischemia. An uneventful delivery does not ensure that the patient will have an uncomplicated course. Because of the marked changes in systemic vascular resistance and blood volume occurring during the postpartum period, the patient should be closely monitored, preferably in an intensive care unit.

Finally, a recent study using continuous Holter monitoring in 25 patients undergoing elective cesarean section under either spinal or epidural anesthesia demonstrated that the occurrence of ST-segment depression is common (150). ST-segment depression suggestive of myocardial ischemia occurred in 16 patients. Eight of these patients had entirely normal regional wall motion on two-dimensional precordial echocardiography. It was interesting that patients in whom ST depression developed had significantly more tachycardia at delivery than those who did not have ST depression. Thus these authors concluded that ST-segment depression is a nonspecific finding in this population group. Although they could not identify the cause of the echocardiographic changes, the relationship between ST depression and heart rate suggests that it may be, at least in part, a rate-related phenomenon.

Pericarditis

Pericarditis is an uncommon complication during pregnancy with few cases reported (150–152). Tamponade is even a less common complication. The anesthetic considerations are similar to those cited for the nonpregnant patient. Most important, however, is a clear understanding of the physiologic significance of the pericarditis. In that regard, precordial (or even transesophogeal) echocardiography can be performed safely, and is invaluable (152).

Pregnancy after Valvular Surgery

There have been more than 700 cases of pregnancy after mitral valvulotomy and more than 150 cases after mitral and aortic valve replacement (4, 153–160).

MITRAL VALVULOTOMY

Patients with a previous mitral valvulotomy have increased maternal and fetal mortality, pulmonary embolization, and atrial fibrillation (Table 27.17) (4, 153–155). These complications can be seen to be related to residual right and left ventricular dysfunction, residual pulmonary hypertension, and a dilated, compliant left atrium. Although these statistics are not as foreboding as those for patients with prosthetic valves (especially mitral valves), they are significantly higher than those for patients without heart disease and warrant special anesthetic considerations.

Anesthetic Considerations

1. *Assessment of the status of the valvulotomy should be made throughout pregnancy and prior to delivery.* Changes in signs or symptoms with preg-

Table 27.17
Maternal and Fetal Complications in Patients with Previous Valvular Surgery

Surgical Procedure	Mortality (%)		Maternal Morbidity (Emboli, Hemorrhage) (%)	Incidence of Fetal Malformations (%)	References
	Maternal	Fetal			
Mitral valvulotomy	2.4–5.5	5.5–16.5	6.6–8.0	1	4, 153–155
Mitral valve replacement	1.2	41	36	20	4, 156–160
Mitral and aortic valve replacement	0	87	Unknown	Unknown	4, 156–160
Aortic valve replacement	0	14	21	2	4, 156–160

nancy and exercise are particularly important. Residual or new mitral stenosis or insufficiency may be present. If so, the previously discussed anesthetic considerations for these lesions should be applied (Tables 27.3 and 27.4).

2. *Residual pulmonary hypertension may exist despite correction of the valvular lesion.* Pulmonary hypertension may be subtle, and symptoms of associated low cardiac output may be precipitated only with exercise or stress. If symptoms or signs exist, the considerations listed under primary pulmonary hypertension also apply here (Table 27.15).

3. *Residual right or left ventricular dysfunction may exist.* Patients with corrected mitral valvular lesions have been shown to have decreased cardiac output and a decreased response of cardiac output with exercise. The considerations are those described under mitral stenosis and insufficiency (Tables 27.3 and 27.4).

4. *Atrial fibrillation is associated with a marked increase in morbidity.* The incidence of systemic embolization and left atrial failure (pulmonary edema with a depressed cardiac output) is increased. Maintenance and adjustment of medications such as digoxin or quinidine throughout pregnancy, labor, and delivery are necessary. Treatment of acute atrial fibrillation is outlined in the sections on mitral stenosis and dysrhythmias.

5. *The choice of anesthetic is dependent on the type and severity of residual disease involving the mitral valve, pulmonary artery, and left and right ventricles.* For a discussion of these considerations, see the sections on mitral stenosis and insufficiency.

MITRAL VALVE REPLACEMENT

More than 100 cases of pregnancy after mitral valve replacement have been reported (4, 7, 156–160). Although maternal mortality is not significantly different from that associated with valvulotomy, maternal morbidity, fetal mortality, and fetal malformations are significantly increased (Table 27.17).

In the nonpregnant population, mitral valve replacement is associated with a number of chronic, postoperative complications: thromboembolism, paravalvular regurgitation, ball or disc variance,

hemolysis, and endocarditis. In addition, these patients typically have a low resting cardiac output, a subnormal increase in cardiac output with exercise, residual pulmonary vascular disease, and some degree of right or left ventricular dysfunction (161–165). Pregnancy aggravates these complications further because of increased intravascular volume, increased myocardial oxygen demand and increased risk of thromboembolism.

Anesthetic Considerations

1. *All patients should be assumed to have some degree of residual myocardial dysfunction and pulmonary hypertension.* Occurrence or progression of any signs or symptoms during pregnancy, especially with exercise or stress, indicate that a considerable amount of residual myocardial damage exists. The anesthetic considerations listed in the previous section and in the sections on mitral valve disease will then apply here as well.

2. *Pulmonary artery monitoring is recommended with symptomatic disease or with evidence of ventricular compromise, or pulmonary hypertension.* Because the risk of endocarditis is increased in these patients, a strictly sterile technique must be used in the placement and maintenance of this catheter.

3. *These patients are invariably anticoagulated.* Usually coumarin anticoagulants are replaced with heparin during pregnancy (166–173). One anesthetic approach is to continue the patient on heparin therapy throughout labor and delivery, avoiding all forms of regional anesthesia, and using systemic medication, inhalation analgesia, and general anesthesia if necessary. The second approach is to discontinue heparin immediately prior to labor and administer protamine until coagulation tests become normal. Regional anesthesia can then be conducted and heparin resumed 24 hr after removal of the epidural catheter (170). Because experience with the latter technique is limited, the morbidity associated with this technique cannot truly be assessed at this time.

AORTIC VALVE REPLACEMENT

Patients with an aortic valve prosthesis have a lower incidence of complications than those with a mitral prosthesis (Table 27.17) (4, 156–160). The reasons for this difference can be attributed to the difference in myocardial function and the more restricted use of anticoagulants in patients with aortic valve prostheses (171–173). Cardiac output at rest and in response to exercise is generally normal in patients with aortic valve prostheses, and ventricular function in general seems to be better (174–176). However, abnormalities do exist and depend principally on the preoperative myocardial status and the quality of valve function. The complications in nonpregnant patients include ball and disc variance, paravalvular regurgitation, hemolysis, endocarditis, and thromboembolism. Compared to patients with mitral valve prostheses, however, the risk of thromboembolism, residual pulmonary hypertension, or right ventricular compromise is not as great.

Anesthetic Considerations

1. *All patients should be assumed to have some degree of residual myocardial dysfunction.* Symptoms or signs of left ventricular compromise, especially with stress or exercise, are indicative of increased risk, and the anesthetic considerations delineated under the sections on aortic insufficiency and stenosis should be applied (Tables 27.6 and 27.7).

2. *Pulmonary artery monitoring is recommended with symptomatic disease or with evidence of left ventricular compromise.*

3. *If the patient is anticoagulated the anesthetic management should be modified as previously discussed.*

Cardiac Transplantation

Cardiac transplantation is an accepted procedure. Little is known about the physiologic changes that occur during pregnancy in the patient who has undergone an orthotopic heart transplantation. The first case has only recently been reported (152). Further study is necessary given the expected increase in this population.

Open-Heart Surgery During Pregnancy

Approximately 200 cases of cardiac surgery during pregnancy have been reported (4, 5, 179–191). From these cases it seems that maternal mortality is no different from nonpregnant patients having open-heart surgery. However, the fetal mortality is very high (33 to 50%). Zitnik et al. (184) reviewed 21 cases and found no correlation of pump time, ischemic time, or type of perfusate with maternal or fetal mortality. Consideration should, therefore, be given to less invasive procedures, such as closed valvulotomy. Recently the feasibility of performing closed mitral and aortic valvulotomy (percutaneous balloon techniques) have been demonstrated (177, 178).

ANESTHETIC CONSIDERATIONS

Basic considerations for anesthetic management of pregnant patients undergoing nonobstetric operations are discussed in Chapter 14. A detailed delineation of the anesthetic considerations for open-heart surgery is beyond the scope of this chapter. However, the following basic considerations should be noted.

1. *The anesthetic consideration for the various cardiac lesions are particularly applicable for patients undergoing open-heart surgery.*

2. *The fetus should be monitored as fully as possible during the operation and postoperative periods* (Chapter 35).

3. *Monitoring systemic vascular resistance as well as systemic blood pressure is recommended throughout the perioperative period, and particularly during cardiopulmonary bypass.* Uterine blood flow depends on both uterine perfusion pressure and vascular resistance. Agents that increase systemic vascular resistance probably increase uterine vascular resistance as well and may result in decreased uterine blood flow in the face of an elevated systemic pressure. If continuous fetal heart rate monitoring indicates fetal distress during cardiopulmonary bypass and arterial pressure is low, perfusion pressure should be increased by increasing flow rate. If fetal distress occurs and vascular resistance is high, small doses of hydralazine are recommended.

Cardiac Dysrhythmias

Cardiac dysrhythmias are common during pregnancy even in patients without detectable organic heart disease. Most normal pregnant patients manifest some type of cardiac dysrhythmia during pregnancy, labor, and delivery (4, 7, 192–200). Fortunately, most of these dysrhythmias are benign. The more serious dysrhythmias are usually found in association with rheumatic heart disease and are considered here.

ATRIAL FIBRILLATION

Atrial fibrillation occurring during pregnancy is usually associated with advanced rheumatic mitral valve disease, primarily dominant mitral stenosis (4, 7). Patients with recent onset of atrial fibrillation during pregnancy have an increased mortality and an increased incidence of heart failure and embolization. Mendelson (1) reported on 117 pregnancies in which atrial fibrillation had occurred and found that the maternal mortality was 17% and fetal mortality was 50%; heart failure developed in 52% of the cases. Szekely and Snaith (4) found that 62% of the patients who developed atrial fibrillation during pregnancy had associated heart failure. In approximately half the cases heart failure developed before the onset of atrial fibrillation, and in the remaining half it developed 1 week to 6 months after the onset of atrial fibrillation. In addition, they found a high incidence of systemic (13%) and pulmonary (18%) emboliza-tion. These authors also reported that the incidence of atrial fibrillation after mitral valvulotomy was higher in pregnant (31%) than in nonpregnant (16.5%) pa-tients (194).

Treatment

Patients who have had a history of atrial fibrilla-tion and who have responded well to treatment should be maintained on this therapy (digitalis, propranolol, quinidine) throughout pregnancy; the doses of these drugs should be adjusted to achieve ventricular rates between 90 and 110 bpm. The effects of these drugs on the fetus are discussed in the following section. Patients without underlying heart disease who de-velop new atrial fibrillation during pregnancy, labor, and delivery should be treated immediately if evi-dence of hypotension, left ventricular failure, or my-ocardial ischemia exists. If these changes are pro-found, direct current cardioversion, starting with 100 watt-sec, should be performed immediately. If elec-trocardioversion is unavailable or if more time per-mits (minutes), administration of propranolol should be instituted. Rapid digitalization will also slow the ventricular response but will take a minimum of 15 to 30 min before significant slowing occurs, and is not recommended for the acute life-threatening sit-uation. However, if time does permit (hours), digi-talization is the treatment of choice. When the patient is fully digitalized, restoration of a sinus rhythm can then be accomplished with quinidine or procain-amide. In patients with advanced rheumatic heart disease who develop atrial fibrillation, rapid decom-pensation can occur, and immediate direct current cardioversion or propranolol administration is rec-ommended.

ATRIAL FLUTTER

Atrial flutter is rarely seen in normal patients and is less commonly found than atrial fibrillation. The atrial rate is usually between 280 and 320 bpm and a 2:1 block usually exists, resulting in a ventricular rate of about 150 bpm.

Treatment

There are few reports of atrial flutter during preg-nancy (1, 4). The clinical implications and the gen-eral guidelines of therapy are similar to those of atrial fibrillation. However, several differences do exist. Treatment with direct current cardioversion usually requires less energy; 20 watt-sec are often successful. Approximately 30% of the patients will convert to atrial fibrillation, usually with a slower ventricular response. Atrial fibrillation is then treated as dis-cussed above.

PAROXYSMAL ATRIAL TACHYCARDIA

Paroxysmal atrial tachycardia (PAT) can occur during pregnancy with or without underlying or-ganic heart disease (1, 4). Szekely and Snaith (196) reported no increased incidence of morbidity when PAT was associated with structurally normal hearts. Mendelson (1) reported a 14% incidence of heart fail-ure and a 5.5% mortality when PAT was associated with mitral stenosis. Szekely and Snaith (4) reported on pregnant patients with rheumatic heart disease who developed PAT. Eight-five percent of the PAT occurred during pregnancy, labor, and delivery and 15% occurred postpartum. Peak incidence occurred during the third trimester of pregnancy. Moderate to severe mitral stenosis was present in 90% of the pa-tients and mitral regurgitation in 10% of the patients. All patients manifested cardiac enlargement. Eighty-eight percent of the paroxysms lasting for more than 6 hr were associated with left ventricular failure, whereas paroxysms lasting less than 2 hr were not associated with ventricular failure.

Treatment of choice for life-threatening PAT dur-ing pregnancy is direct current countershock. If more time permits, any of the following treatment modal-ities can be instituted: edrophonium (5 to 10 mg in-travenously), carotid sinus stimulation, propranolol, or digoxin. Neosynephrine, sometimes used to slow the heart reflexly, should not be used in the pregnant patient.

OTHER DYSRHYTHMIAS

Other dysrhythmias occurring during pregnancy, such as heart block, bundle branch block, Wolff-Parkinson-White syndrome, and ventricular dys-rhythmias are uncommon but can precipitate signif-icant complications, especially in the patient with underlying organic heart disease (1, 4, 45, 197–199). Treatment of these dysrhythmias is identical to that in the nonpregnant patient (18, 19).

EFFECTS OF CARDIAC THERAPEUTICS ON THE FETUS

A variety of medications (antiarrhythmics, vaso-pressors, and vasodilators) as well as electrocardio-version are used to treat maternal cardiac disorders (200, 201). The effects of these therapeutics on the fetus and uterine blood flow and contractility must be considered. Many of the drugs are discussed in more detail in the chapters on obstetric anesthesia and uterine blood flow (Chapter 3), effects of anes-thesia on uterine activity and labor (Chapter 4), per-inatal pharmacology (Chapter 5), and choice of local anesthetics in obstetrics (Chapter 6).

Antiarrhythmics

LIDOCAINE

High maternal blood levels of lidocaine (greater than 5 µg/ml) are associated with neonatal depression. The usual therapeutic level for suppression of ventricular dysrhythmias is 2 to 5 µg/ml (18), which is comparable to that found with conventional obstetric anesthesia. Very high blood levels of lidocaine—greater than 200 µg/ml in pregnant ewes—were found to cause a dose-related transient (2 to 3-min) decrease in uterine blood flow and a simultaneous increase in intrauterine pressure (175). However, constant intravenous infusion (plasma level of 2 to 4 µg/ml) did not significantly change maternal or fetal hemodynamics or blood gases or uterine blood flow or tone (203, 204).

QUINIDINE

Few studies have investigated the safety of quinidine use during pregnancy. However, because pregnancy is associated with a decrease in plasma pseudocholinesterase activity, quinidine may exacerbate the effects of esters such as succinylcholine. In fact, quinidine has recently been shown to have an inhibitory effect on plasma pseudocholinesterase, which may explain these effects (205). It should, thus, be used cautiously.

PROPRANOLOL

Propranolol crosses the placenta (206). Interference with autonomic responses during labor (207) and depressant effects on the neonate have been reported (208). Fetal bradycardia and hypoglycemia resolving over a prolonged period (3 days) have been associated with the administration of propranolol (209). Decreased fetal hepatic metabolism may prolong the half-life of propranolol. In pregnant ewes, propranolol causes an impairment of the fetal response to anoxia (210, 211).

ESMOLOL

Esmolol hydrochloride, a β_1-adrenergic selective antagonist with an elimination half-life of 9 min, has been gaining increasing use recently to control perioperative hypertension or tachyarrhythmias because of its ease of titratability. Recent investigations have shown that esmolol crosses the placental membrane of gravid ewes rapidly (213), and production of an equivalent degree of β-blockade is slow following prolonged infusion. However, another study demonstrated that the metabolism of esmolol is rapid in the fetus, as it is in the mother (214). Fetal heart rate and blood pressure decreased 12 and 7%, respectively, but fetal acid-base status remained un-

altered. Its safety thus remains to be further determined in a larger study.

LABETOLOL

Labetolol hydrochloride, a nonselective β-andrenergic and selective α_1-adrenergic blocking agent, is widely used in treating intraoperative and postoperative hypertension. It has been demonstrated to be safe for both the mother and the fetus for treatment of both acute and chronic hypertension (214–216).

VERAPAMIL

Verapamil has been shown to decrease uterine blood flow in awake pregnant ewes (218). These changes may not be physiologically important to the fetus, but may be consequential in patients with cardiovascular dysfunction. Placental transfer of verapamil hydrochloride is limited in the pregnant ewe, but prolongation of the PR-interval in the fetal heart occurs without changes in the acid-base status (219).

AMIODARONE

Amiodarone has been shown to produce both coronary and peripheral vasodilation, probably by interfering with vascular smooth muscle excitation contracture coupling. Its use during pregnancy has not been investigated. However, a recent case report described the use of epidural anesthesia in a patient receiving amiodarone therapy for recurrent atrial and ventricular dysrhythmias (218). Attention to anesthetic interaction was emphasized.

NICARDIPINE

Nifedipine and nicardipine have been shown to have substantial tocolytic effects in vitro and in vivo. However, their safety during pregnancy remains unknown. Recently, in the pregnant rabbit, nicardipine was found to be associated with an increase in heart rate and cardiac output and a fall in uteroplacental blood flow (219). Nifedipine effectively lowers maternal blood pressure and heart rates but does not decrease uterine blood flow in awake pygmy goats (220). Thus further studies are necessary to document the safety of such agents.

Vasopressors and Inotropes

NOREPINEPHRINE

In pregnant ewes during sympatholytic hypotension, norepinephrine restores maternal blood pressure to normal without increasing uterine blood flow (222). In normotensive ewes uterine blood flow decreases despite a marked increase in maternal blood pressure (223). Norepinephrine also produces an increase in uterine tonus and intensity and frequency of contraction (224).

METARAMINOL

In pregnant ewes with spinal hypotension, metaraminol will restore maternal blood pressure to normal and, on the average, will increase uterine blood flow to 70 to 80% of normal (225). Some reports indicate that maternal blood pressure and uterine blood flow are returned to normal, but fetal acidosis and hypoxia are not necessarily corrected (226).

PHENYLEPHRINE, METHOXAMINE, AND ANGIOTENSIN II

In pregnant ewes with spinal hypotension, these drugs restore maternal blood pressure to normal but without increasing reduced uterine blood flow (227). In normotensive ewes they also produce uterine vasoconstriction and decreased uterine blood flow.

EPHEDRINE

In hypotensive pregnant ewes, ephedrine was found to restore maternal blood pressure to normal, increase uterine blood flow to 85% of normal, and correct fetal hypoxia and acidosis (223, 225, 226). Comparison with metaraminol revealed that ephedrine caused less maternal bradycardia and a greater increase in uterine blood flow (187).

Recently, it has been demonstrated that ephedrine may increase fetal atrial natriuretic peptide (227), which may be expected because ephedrine crosses the placenta freely. Such findings, although potentially important, have unknown implications at present.

EPINEPHRINE

Despite increases in systemic blood pressure, epinephrine markedly decreases uterine blood flow (221). In low doses epinephrine decreases uterine contractility, and in high doses it increases uterine contractility (228).

ISOPROTERENOL

Isoproterenol causes a decrease in mean blood pressure and uterine blood flow. No direct vasodilation of gravid uterine vessels has been demonstrated (229). Uterine contractions are inhibited by approximately 50% when doses of 2 to 8 μg/min are administered (230).

DOPAMINE

Differing effects of dopamine on uterine blood flow have been reported (231–234). In normotensive sheep dopamine increased uterine blood flow despite an increase in uterine vascular resistance (231). However, in pregnant ewes high does of dopamine increased maternal cardiac output and blood pressure but decreased uterine blood flow and did not change renal blood flow (232). Doses less than 10 μg/kg/min produced no significant change in maternal hemo-

dynamics. In pregnant ewes with spinal hypotension and decreased uterine blood flow, dopamine in doses sufficient to maintain blood pressure at control values (20 to 40 μg/kg/min) further decreased uterine blood flow and increased uterine vascular resistance (233). In hypotensive patients undergoing cesarean section, dopamine (2 to 10 μg/kg/min) restored systolic pressure to 100 mm Hg without depression of Apgar scores. However, depression of maternal arterial Po_2 was found when compared to controls. Infants also had a significantly lower Po_2 in umbilical arterial and venous blood than control (234).

DIGOXIN

Digoxin crosses the placental barrier in both the exteriorized and the intrauterine fetal lamb preparations, and the half-life is significantly longer in the ewe (235, 236). The amount that crossed the placenta was found to be small but could preserve cardiac function in these preparations. In this study (198) no toxicity was found. Observations on three women during their 11th and 12th weeks of pregnancy showed that less than 1% of the administered digitoxin was detectable in the fetus (239). On the other hand, one case report revealed that digitoxin may profoundly affect the fetus. A mother who ingested 8.9 mg of digitoxin during her eighth month of pregnancy gave birth to an infant with digitalis intoxication who died shortly after birth (240).

AMRINONE AND MILRINONE

Few studies are available on amrinone and milrinone use during pregnancy. However, a recent report demonstrated that milrinone was associated with maternal tachycardia and an increase in uterine blood flow, whereas the fetal condition was unchanged (241). Further investigation is necessary.

Vasodilators

SODIUM NITROPRUSSIDE

In pregnant ewes with phenylephrine-induced hypertension, sodium nitroprusside restores blood pressure to normal values, but uterine blood flow remains depressed (242). Furthermore, in ewes, prolonged administration may produce fetal death from cyanide toxicity (243).

HYDRALAZINE

In pregnant ewes hydralazine lowers blood pressure to control values during phenylephrine-induced hypertension and increases uterine blood flow by 15% (242). In comparison with sodium nitroprusside, hydralazine is slower in onset but produces a greater increase in cardiac output and heart rate and a greater decrease in systemic vascular resistance at the same systemic pressure (243).

Direct Current Cardioversion

Use of direct current cardioversion during pregnancy has been reported by Vogel et al. (34), Sussman et al. (199), and Schroeder and Harrison (35). Energies as high as 100 watt-sec were used. Gestation and delivery were normal in all cases. Monitoring of fetal heart rate revealed no apparent effect on the fetus.

References

1. Mendelson CL: *Cardiac Disease in Pregnancy*. Davis, Philadelphia, 1960.
2. Mendelson CL: Acute cor pulmonale and pregnancy. Clin Obstet Gynecol 11:992–1009, 1968.
3. Barnes CG: *Medical Disorders in Obstetrics Practice* 3rd ed. Blackwell, Oxford, 1970.
4. Szekely P, Snaith L: *Heart Disease and Pregnancy*. Churchill Livingstone, London, 1974.
5. Ueland K: Cardiovascular diseases complicating pregnancy. Clin Obstet Gynecol 21:429–442, 1978.
6. Niswander K, Berendes H, Deutschberger J, Lipko N, Westphal MC: Fetal mortality following potentially anoxigenic conditions. Am J Obstet Gynecol 98:871–876, 1967.
7. Burwell CS, Metcalfe J: *Heart Disease and Pregnancy*. Little, Brown, Boston, 1958, pp 210, 217, 220.
8. Szekely P, Snaith L: Atrial fibrillation and pregnancy. Br Med J 1:1407–1410, 1961.
9. Sugrue D, Blake S, MacDonald D: Pregnancy complicated by maternal heart disease at the National Maternity Hospital, Dublin, Ireland, 1969 to 1978. Am J Obstet Gynecol 139:1–6, 1981.
10. Cannell DE, Vernon CP: Congenital heart disease and pregnancy. Am J Obstet Gynecol 85:744–753, 1961.
11. Shime J, Mocarski EJM, Hastings D, Webb GD, McLaughlin PR: Congenital heart disease in pregnancy: Short- and long-term implications. Am J Obstet Gynecol 156:313–322, 1987.
12. Kerr M: Cardiovascular dynamics in pregnancy and labor. Br Med Bull 24:19–24, 1968.
13. Liley AW: Clinical and laboratory significance of variations in maternal and plasma volume in pregnancy. Int J Gynecol Obstet 8:358–362, 1970.
14. Metcalfe J, Ueland K: Maternal cardiovascular adjustments to pregnancy. Prog Cardiovascular Dis 16:363, 1974.
15. Ueland K, Novy M, Peterson E, Metcalfe J: Maternal cardiovascular dynamics. IV. The influence of gestational age on the maternal cardiovascular response to posture and exercise. Am J Obstet Gynecol 104:856–864, 1969.
16. Ueland K, Hansen J: Maternal cardiovascular dynamics. III. Labor and delivery under local and caudal analgesia. Am J Obstet Gynecol 103:8–18, 1969.
17. Ueland K, Hansen J: Maternal cardiovascular dynamics. II. Posture and uterine contractions. Am J Obstet Gynecol 103:1–7, 1969.
18. Hurse JW: *The Heart*. McGraw-Hill, New York, 1978.
19. Fowler NO: *Cardiac Diagnosis and Treatment*. Harper & Row, New York, 1976.
20. Milsom I, Forssman L, Biber B, Dottori O, Rydgren B, Sivertsson R: Maternal haemodynamic changes during caesarean section: A comparison of epidural and general anaesthesia. Acta Anaesth Scand 29:161–167, 1985.
21. Sonnenblick E, Lesch M: *Valvular Heart Disease*. Grune & Stratton, New York, 1974.
22. Spagnuolo M, Pasternack B, Taranta A: Risk of rheumatic fever recurrences after streptococcal infections. N Engl J Med 285:641–647, 1971.
23. Jones TD: The diagnosis of rheumatic fever. JAMA 126:481, 1944.
24. Rapaport E: Natural history of aortic and mitral valve disease. Am J Cardiol 35:221–227, 1975.
25. Selzer A, Cohn E: Natural history of mitral stenosis: A review. Circulation 45:878–890, 1972.
26. Wood P: An appreciation of mitral stenosis. Br Med J 1:1051–1063, 1954.
27. Keith TA, Fowler NO, Helmsworth JA, Gralnick H: The course of surgically modified mitral stenosis. Am J Med 34:308–319, 1963.
28. Hultgren H, Hubis H, Shumway N: Cardiac function following mitral valve replacement. Am Heart J 75:302–312, 1968.
29. Braunwald E, Braunwald NS, Ross J Jr, Morrow AG: Effects of mitral valve replacement on the pulmonary vascular dynamics of patients with pulmonary hypertension. N Engl J Med 273:509–514, 1965.
30. Stott DK, Marpole DGF, Bristow JD, Kloster FE, Griswold HE: The role of left atrial transport in aortic and mitral stenosis. Circulation 41:1031–1041, 1970.
31. Hildner FJ, Javier RP, Cohen LS, Samet P, Nathan MJ, Yahr WZ, Greenberg JJ: Myocardial dysfunction associated with valvular heart disease. Am J Cardiol 30:319–326, 1972.
32. Arani DT, Carleton RA: The deleterious role of tachycardia in mitral stenosis. Circulation 36:511–516, 1967.
33. Hemmings GT, Whalley DG, O'Connor PJ, Benjamin A, Dunn C: Invasive monitoring and anaesthetic management of a parturient with mitral stenosis. Can J Anaesth 34:182–185, 1987.
34. Vogel JHK, Pryor R, Blount SG Jr: Direct-current defibrillation during pregnancy. JAMA 193:970–971, 1965.
35. Schroeder JS, Harrison DC: Repeated cardioversion during pregnancy: Treatment of refractory paroxysmal atrial tachycardia during three successive pregnancies. Am J Cardiol 27:445–446, 1971.
36. Lynch C III, Rizor RF: Anesthetic management and monitoring of a parturient with mitral and aortic valvular disease. Anesth Analg 61:788–792, 1982.
37. Clark SL, Phelan JP, Greenspoon J, Aldahl D, Horenstein J: Labor and delivery in the presence of mitral stenosis: Central hemodynamic observations. Am J Obstet Gynecol 152:984–988, 1985.
38. Perloff JK, Roberts WC: The mitral apparatus: Functional anatomy of mitral regurgitation. Circulation 46:227–239, 1972.
39. Braunwald E: Mitral regurgitation, physiological, clinical and surgical considerations. N Engl J Med 281:425–33, 1969.
40. Baxley WA, Kennedy JW, Feild B, Dodge HT: Hemodynamics in ruptured chordae tendineae and chronic rheumatic mitral regurgitation. Circulation 48:1288–1294, 1973.
41. Goodman DJ, Rossen RM, Holloway EL, Alderman EL, Harrison DC: Effect of nitroprusside on left ventricular dynamics in mitral regurgitation. Circulation 50:1025–1032, 1974.
42. Marcus FI, Ewy GA, O'Rourke RA, Walsh B, Belich AC: The effect of pregnancy on the murmurs of mitral and aortic regurgitation. Circulation 41:795–805, 1970.
43. Alcantara LG, Marx GF: Cesarean section under epidural analgesia in a parturient with mitral valve prolapse. Anesth Analg 66:902–903, 1987.
44. Alderson JD: Cardiovascular collapse following epidural anaesthesia for caesarean section in a patient with aortic incompetence. Anaesthesia 42:643–645, 1987.
45. Dack S, Bader ME, Bader RA, Gelb IJ: Heart disease. In *Medical, Surgical and Gynecologic Complications of Pregnancy*, 2nd ed. JJ Rovinsky, AF Guttmacher, eds. Williams & Wilkins, Baltimore, 1965, p 1.
46. Brawley RK, Morrow AG: Direct determinations of aortic blood flow in patients with aortic regurgitation. Circulation 35:32–45, 1967.
47. Schlant RC, Nutter DO: Heart failure in valvular heart disease. Medicine 50:421–451, 1971.
48. Judge TP, Kennedy JW, Bennett LJ, Wills RE, Murray JA, Blackmon JR: Quantitative hemodynamic effects of heart rate in aortic regurgitation. Circulation 44:355–367, 1971.
49. Finegan RE, Gianelly RE, Harrison DC: Aortic stenosis in the elderly. N Engl J Med 281:1261–1264, 1969.
50. Frank S, Johnson A, Ross J Jr: Natural history of aortic valvular stenosis. Br Heart J 35:41–46, 1973.

51. Ueland K, Novy MJ, Metcalfe J: Hemodynamic responses of patients with heart disease to pregnancy and exercise. Am J Obstet Gynecol 113:47–59, 1972.

52. Arias F, Pineda J: Aortic stenosis and pregnancy. J Reprod Med 20:229–232, 1978.

53. Frank S, Ross J Jr: The natural history of severe acquired valvular aortic stenosis. Am J Cardiol 19:128–129, 1967.

54. Liedtke AJ, Gentzler RD II, Babb JD, Hunter AS, Gault JH: Determinants of cardiac performance in severe aortic stenosis. Chest 69:192–200, 1976.

55. Lee SJK, Jonsson B, Bevegard S, Karlof I, Astrom H: Hemodynamic changes at rest and during exercise in patients with aortic stenosis of varying severity. Am Heart J 79:318–331, 1970.

56. Easterling TR, Chadwick HS, Otto CM, Benedetti TJ: Aortic stenosis in pregnancy. Obstet Gynecol 72:113–118, 1988.

57. Redfern N, Bower S, Bullock RE, Hull CJ: Alfentanil for caesarean section complicated by severe aortic stenosis. Br J Anaesth 59:1309–1312, 1987.

58. Bloomfield DK: The natural history of ventricular septal defect in patients surviving infancy. Circulation 29:914–955, 1964.

59. Snaith L, Szekely P: Cardiovascular surgery in relation to pregnancy. In *Advances in Obstetrics and Gynecology.* SL Marcus, CC Marcus, eds. Williams & Wilkins, Baltimore, 1967, p 220.

60. Rudolph AM: *Congenital Diseases of the Heart.* Year Book Medical Publishers. Chicago, 1974.

61. Ullery JC: The management of pregnancy complicated by heart disease. Am J Obstet Gynecol 67:834–866, 1954.

62. Jones AM, Howitt G: Eisenmenger syndrome in pregnancy. Br Med J 1:1627–1631, 1965.

63. Neilson G, Galea EG, Blunt A: Eisenmenger's syndrome and pregnancy. Med J Aust 1:431–434, 1971.

64. Ueland K: Cardiac surgery and pregnancy. Am J Obstet Gynecol 92:148–162, 1965.

65. Campbell M: The incidence and later distribution of malformations of the heart. In *Paediatric Cardiology.* H Watson, ed. Lloyd-Luke, London, 1968, p 71.

66. Jewett JF, Ober WB: Primary pulmonary hypertension as a cause of maternal death. Am J Obstet Gynecol 71:1335–1341, 1956.

67. Copeland WE, Wooley CF, Ryan JM, Runco V, Levin HS: Pregnancy and congenital heart disease. Am J Obstet Gynecol 86:107–110, 1963.

68. Pollack KL, Chestnut DH, Wenstrom KD: Anesthetic management of a parturient with Eisenmenger's syndrome. Anesth Analg 70:212–215, 1990.

69. Sellers JD, Block FE, McDonald JS: Anesthetic management of labor in a patient with dextrocardia, congenitally corrected transposition, Wolff-Parkinson-White syndrome, and congestive heart failure. Am J Obstet Gynecol 161:1001–1003, 1989.

70. Meyer EC, Tulsky AS, Sigmann P, Silber EN: Pregnancy in the presence of tetralogy of Fallot. Am J Cardiol 14:874–879, 1964.

71. Jacoby WJ: Pregnancy with tetralogy and pentalogy of Fallot. Am J Cardiol 14:866–873, 1964.

72. Kirklin JW, Karp RB: *The Tetralogy of Fallot.* Saunders, Philadelphia, 1970.

73. Dunborg G, Brouset P, Bricaud H, Fontan F, Trarieux M, Fontanille P: Correction complete d'une triade de Fallott en circulation extracorporelle chez une femme enceinte. Arch Mal Coeur 52:1389–1391, 1959.

74. Baker JL, Russell CS, Grainger RG, Taylor DG, Thornton JA, Verel D: Closed pulmonary valvotomy in the management of Fallot's tetralogy complicated by pregnancy. J Obstet Gynaecol Br Commonw 70:154–157, 1963.

75. Cutforth R, Catchlove B, Knight LW, Dudgeon G: The Eisenmenger syndrome and pregnancy. Aust N Z J Obstet Gynaecol 8:202–210, 1968.

76. Spinnato JA, Kraynack BJ, Cooper MW: Eisenmenger's syndrome in pregnancy: Epidural anesthesia for elective cesarean section. N Engl J Med 304:1215–1217, 1981.

77. Robinson S: Pulmonary artery catheters in Eisenmenger's syndrome: Many risks, few benefits. Anesthesiology 58:588–589, 1983.

78. Muller BJ, Steude G: General anesthesia administered to a patient with Eisenmenger's syndrome undergoing cesarean section. Anesthesiol Rev 9:32–35, 1982.

79. Goodwin JF: Pregnancy and coarctation of the aorta. Clin Obstet Gynecol 4:645–664, 1961.

80. Deal K, Wooley CF: Coarctation of the aorta and pregnancy. Ann Intern Med 78:706–713, 1973.

81. Cohen LS, Friedman WF, Braunwald E: Natural history of mild congenital aortic stenosis elucidated by serial hemodynamic studies. Am J Cardiol 30:1–5, 1972.

82. Pansegrau DG, Kioshos JM, Durnin RE, Kroetz FW: Supravalvular aortic stenosis in adults. Am J Cardiol 31:635–641, 1973.

83. Parker B: The course in idiopathic hypertrophic muscular subaortic stenosis. Ann Intern Med 70:903–911, 1969.

84. Varghese PH, Izukawa T, Rowe RD: Supravalvular aortic stenosis as part of rubella syndrome with discussion of pathogenesis. Br Heart J 31:59–62, 1969.

85. Roberts WC: The congenitally bicuspid aortic valve: A study of 85 autopsy cases. Am J Cardiol 26:72–83, 1970.

86. Bacon APC, Matthews MB: Congenital bicuspid aortic valves and the etiology of isolated aortic valvular stenosis. Q J Med 28:545–560, 1959.

87. Kirklin JW, Connolly DC, Ellis FH Jr, Burchell HB, Edwards JE, Wood EH: Problems in the diagnosis and surgical treatment of pulmonic stenosis with intact ventricular septum. Circulation 8:849–863, 1953.

88. Bentivoglio LG, Maranhao V, Downing DF: Electrocardiogram in pulmonary stenosis with intact septa. Am Heart J 59:347–357, 1960.

89. Cayler GG, Ongley P, Nadas AS: Relation of systolic pressure in the right ventricle to the electrocardiogram: A study of patients with pulmonary stenosis and intact ventricular septum. N Engl J Med 258:979–982, 1958.

90. Moller I, Wennevold A, Lyngborg KE: The natural history of pulmonary stenosis: Long-term follow-up with serial heart catheterizations. Cardiology 58:193–202, 1973.

91. Wilton NCT, Traber KB, Deschner LS: Anaesthetic management for caesarean section in a patient with uncorrected truncus arteriosus. Br J Anaesth 62:434–438, 1989.

92. Copel JA, Harrison D, Whittemore R, Hobbins JC: Intrathecal morphine analgesia for vaginal delivery in a woman with a single ventricle: A case report. J Reprod Med 31:274–276, 1986.

93. Baumann H, Schneider H, Drack G, Alon E, Huch A: Pregnancy and delivery by caesarean section in a patient with transposition of the great arteries and single ventricle: Case report. Br J Obstet Gynaecol 94:704–708, 1987.

94. Sellers JD, Block FE Jr, McDonald JS: Anesthetic management of labor in a patient with dextrocardia, congenitally corrected transposition, Wolff-Parkinson-White syndrome, and congestive heart failure. Am J Obstet Gynecol 161:1001–1003, 1989.

95. Strickland RA, Oliver WC Jr, Chantigian RG, Ney JA, Danielson GK: Anesthesia, cardiopulmonary bypass, and the pregnant patient. Mayo Clin Proc 66:411–429, 1991.

96. Kaufman JM, Ruble PE: The current status of the pregnant cardiac patient. Ann Intern Med 48:1157–1170, 1958.

97. Avido DM: *The Lung Circulation.* Pergamon Press, Oxford, 1965.

98. Wagenvoort CA, Wagenvoort N: *Pathology of Pulmonary Hypertension.* Wiley, New York, 1977.

99. Coleman PN, Edmunds AWB, Tregillus J: Primary pulmonary hypertension in three sibs. Br Heart J 21:81–88, 1959.

100. Nelson DM, Main E, Crafford W, Ahumada GG: Peripartum heart failure due to primary pulmonary hypertension. Obstet Gynecol 62:58S–63S, 1983.

101. Abboud TK, Raya J, Noueihid R, Daniel J: Intrathecal morphine for relief of labor pain in a parturient with severe pulmonary hypertension. Anesthesiology 59:477–479, 1983.
102. Power KJ, Avery AF: Extradural analgesia in the intrapartum management of a patient with pulmonary hypertension. Br J Anaesth 63:116–120, 1989.
103. Robinson DE, Leicht CH: Epidural analgesia with low-dose bupivacaine and fentanyl for labor and delivery in a parturient with severe pulmonary hypertension. Anesthesiology 68:285–288, 1988.
104. Cheng DCH, Edelist G: Isoflurane and primary pulmonary hypertension. Anaesthesia 43:22–24, 1988.
105. Stoelting RK, Reis RR, Longnecker DE: Hemodynamic responses to nitrous oxide-halothane and halothane in patients with valvular heart disease. Anesthesiology 37:430–435, 1972.
106. Sullivan JM: Blood pressure elevation in pregnancy. Prog Cardiovasc Dis 16:375, 1974.
107. Barnes CG: *Medical Disorders in Obstetric Practice.* 3rd ed. Blackwell, Oxford, 1970. pp 50–52, 54–56, 58, 60.
108. Browne FJ: Chronic hypertension and pregnancy. Br Med J 2:283, 1947.
109. Wallen I: The infant mortality in specific hypertensive disease of pregnancy and in essential hypertension. Am J Obstet Gynecol 66:36–45, 1953.
110. Kincaid-Smith P, Bullen M, Mills J: Prolonged use of methyldopa in severe hypertension in pregnancy. Br Med J 1:274–276, 1966.
111. Leather HM, Humphreys DM, Baker P, Chad MA: A controlled trial of hypotensive agents in hypertension in pregnancy. Lancet 2:488–490, 1968.
112. Ross JH, Wright JA: Successful twin pregnancy after treatment of malignant essential hypertension. Br Med J 2:545, 1958.
113. Hamilton M: Presymptomatic diagnosis of hypertension. In *Proceedings of the 5th International Congress of Hygiene and Preventive Medicine. Vol. 1.* Rome. 1968, p 132.
114. Smith SL, Douglas BH, Langford HG: A model of preeclampsia. Johns Hopkins Med J 120:220–224, 1967.
115. Chesley LC, Talledo E, Bohler CS, Zuspan FP: Vascular reactivity to angiotensin II and norepinephrine in pregnant and nonpregnant women. Am J Obstet Gynecol 91:837–842, 1965.
116. Dieckmann WJ, Michel HL: Vascular effects of posterior pituitary extracts in pregnant women. Am J Obstet Gynecol 33:131, 1937.
117. Talledo OE, Chesley LC, Zuspan FP: Renin-angiotensin system in normal and toxemic pregnancies. Am J Obstet Gynecol 100:218–221, 1968.
118. Brust AA, Assali NS, Ferris EB: Evaluation of neurogenic and humoral factors in blood pressure maintenance in normal and toxemic pregnancy using tetraethylammonium chloride. J Clin Invest 27:717, 1948.
119. Assali NS, Prystowsky H: Studies on autonomic blockade. J Clin Invest 29:1354–1366, 1950.
120. Koch-Weser J: Correlation of pathophysiology and pharmacotherapy in primary hypertension. Am J Cardiol 32:499–510, 1973.
121. Walsh JJ, Burch GE: Postpartal heart disease. Arch Intern Med 108:817–822, 1961.
122. Demakis JG, Rahimtoola SH: Peripartum cardiomyopathy. Circulation 44:964–968, 1971.
123. Demakis JG, Rahimtoola SH, Sutton GC, Meadows R, Szanto PB, Tobin JR, Gunnar RM: Natural course of peripartum cardiomyopathy. Circulation 44:1053–1061, 1971.
124. Veille JC: Peripartum cardiomyopathies: A review. Am J Obstet Gynecol 148:805–818, 1984.
125. Homans DC: Peripartum cardiomyopathy. N Engl J Med 312:1432–1437, 1985.
126. Gambling DR, Flanagan ML, Huckell VF, Lucas SB, Kim JHK: Anaesthetic management and non-invasive monitoring for caesarean section in a patient with cardiomyopathy. Can J Anaesth 34:505–508, 1987.
127. Goodwin JF, Oakley CM: The cardiomyopathies. Br Heart J 34:545–552, 1972.
128. Stuart KL: Cardiomyopathy of pregnancy and the puerperium. Q J Med 37:463–478, 1968.
129. Kitchen DH: Dissecting aneurysm of the aorta in pregnancy. J Obstet Gynaecol Br Commonw 81:410–413, 1974.
130. Schnitker MA, Bayer CA: Dissecting aneurysm of the aorta in young individuals, particularly in association with pregnancy: With report of a case. Ann Intern Med 20:486, 1944.
131. McGeachy TE, Paullin JE: Dissecting aneurysm of the aorta. JAMA 108:1690, 1937.
132. Frank S, Braunwald E: Idiopathic hypertrophic subaortic stenosis: Clinical analysis of 126 patients with emphasis on the natural history. Circulation 37:759–788, 1968.
133. Powell JW Jr, Whiting RB, Dinsmore RE, Sanders CA: Symptomatic prognosis in patients with idiopathic hypertrophic subaortic stenosis (IHSS). Am J Med 55:15–24, 1973.
134. Reis RL, Peterson LM, Mason DT, Simon AL, Morrow AG: Congenital fixed subvalvular aortic stenosis: An anatomical classification and correlations with operative results. Circulation 43 (suppl I):I-11–I-18, 1971.
135. Swan DA, Bell B, Oakley CM, Goodwin J: Analysis of symptomatic course and prognosis and treatment of hypertrophic obstructive cardiomyopathy. Br Heart J 33:671–685, 1971.
136. Brown AK, Doukas N, Riding WD, Jones WE: Cardiomyopathy and pregnancy. Br Heart J 29:387–393, 1967.
137. Turner GM, Oakley CM, Dixon HG: Management of pregnancy complicated by hypertrophic obstructive cardiomyopathy. Br Med J 11:281–284, 1968.
138. Minnich ME, Quirk JG, Clark RB: Epidural anesthesia for vaginal delivery in a patient with idiopathic hypertrophic subaortic stenosis. Anesthesiology 67:590–592, 1987.
139. Boccio RV, Chung JH, Harrison DM: Anesthetic management of cesarean section in a patient with idiopathic hypertrophic subaortic stenosis. Anesthesiology 65:663–665, 1986.
140. Braunwald E, Lambrew CT, Rockoff SD, Ross J Jr, Morrow AG: Idiopathic hypertrophic subaortic stenosis. I. A description of the disease based upon an analysis of 64 patients. Circulation 30 (suppl IV):IV-3–IV-213, 1964.
141. Mason DT, Braunwald E, Ross J Jr: Effects of changes in body position on the severity of obstruction to left ventricular outflow in idiopathic hypertrophic subaortic stenosis. Circulation 33:374–382, 1966.
142. Glancy DL, Shepherd RL, Beiser GD, Epstein SE: The dynamic nature of left ventricular outflow obstruction in idiopathic hypertrophic subaortic stenosis. Ann Intern Med 75:589–592, 1971.
143. Watson H, Emslie-Smith D, Herring J, Hill IGW: Myocardial infarction during pregnancy and the puerperium. Lancet 2:523–525, 1960.
144. Fletcher E, Knox EW, Morton P: Acute myocardial infarction in pregnancy. Br Med J 11:586–590, 1967.
145. Ginz B: Myocardial infarction in pregnancy. J Obstet Gynaecol Br Commonw 77:610–615, 1970.
146. Husaini MH: Myocardial infarction during pregnancy: Report of two cases with a review of the literature. Postgrad Med J 47:660–665, 1971.
147. Curry JJ, Quintana FJ: Myocardial infarction with ventricular fibrillation during pregnancy treated by direct current defibrillation with fetal survival. Chest 58:82–88, 1970.
148. Canning B St J, Green AT, Mulcahy R: Coronary heart disease in the puerperium. J Obstet Gynaecol Br Commonw 76:1018–1020, 1969.
149. McLintic AJ, Pringle SD, Lilley S, Houston AB, Thorburn J: Electrocardiographic changes during cesarean section under regional anesthesia. Anesth Analg 74:51–56, 1992.
150. Simpson WG, DePriest PD, Conover WB: Acute pericarditis complicated by cardiac tamponade during pregnancy. Am J Obstet Gynecol 160:415–416, 1989.
151. Sachs BP, Lorell BH, Mehrez M, Damien N: Constrictive pericarditis and pregnancy. Am J Obstet Gynecol 154:156–157, 1986.
152. Moustafa E, Zina AAA, Kassem M, El-Tabbakh G: Echocardiography of the pericardium in pregnancy. Obstet Gynecol 69:851–853, 1987.

153. Schenker JG, Polishuk WZ: Pregnancy following mitral valvotomy: A survey of 182 patients. Obstet Gynecol 32:214–220, 1968.
154. Wallace WA, Ellis LB: Pregnancy following closed mitral valvuloplasty: Long-term follow-up. Circulation 40 (suppl III):III-211, 1969.
155. Wallace WA, Harken DE, Ellis LB: Pregnancy following closed mitral valvuloplasty: Long-term study with remarks concerning necessity for cardiac management. JAMA 217:297–304, 1971.
156. Harrison RC, Roschke EJ: Pregnancy in patients with cardiac valve prostheses. Clin Obstet Gynecol 18:107–123, 1975.
157. Villoria FE: Montoya L, Recasens E: Protesis valvulares y'embarazo. Rev Clin Esp 140:537, 1976.
158. Lutz DJ, Noller KL, Spittell J Jr, Danielson GK, Fish CR: Pregnancy and its complications following cardiac valve prosthesis. Am J Obstet Gynecol 131:460–468, 1978.
159. Ibera-Perez C, Arevalo-Toledo N, Alvarez-De la Cadena O, Noreiga-Guerra L: The course of pregnancy in patients with artificial heart valves. Am J Med 61:504–512, 1976.
160. Buxbaum A, Aygen MM, Shahin W, Levy MJ, Ekerling B: Pregnancy in patients with prosthetic heart values. Chest 59:639–642, 1971.
161. Braunwald E, Braunwald N, Ross J, Morrow AG: Effects of mitral valve replacement on the pulmonary vascular dynamics of patients with pulmonary hypertension. N Engl J Med 273:509–514, 1965.
162. Kloster F, Bristow D, Starr A, McCord CW, Griswold HE: Serial cardiac output and blood volume studies following cardiac valve replacement. Circulation 33:528–539, 1966.
163. Austen W, Corning H, Moran J, Sanders CA, Scannell JG: Cardiac hemodynamics immediately following mitral valve surgery. J Thorac Cardiovasc Surg 51:468–473, 1966.
164. Hultgren H, Hubis H, Shumway N: Cardiac function following mitral valve replacement. Am Heart J 75:302–312, 1968.
165. Gilbert CS, Sullivan GJ, McLaughlin JJ: Heart disease in pregnancy: Ten year report from the Lewis Memorial Maternal Hospital. Obstet Gynecol 9:58–63, 1957.
166. Tejani N: Anticoagulant therapy with cardiac valve prosthesis during pregnancy. Obstet Gynecol 42:785–793, 1973.
167. Varkey GP, Brindle GF: Peripheral anesthesia and anticoagulant therapy. Can Anaesth Soc J 21:106–109, 1974.
168. Shaul WL, Hall JG: Multiple congenital anomalies associated with oral anticoagulants. Am J Obstet Gynecol 127:191–198, 1977.
169. Bloomfield DK: Fetal deaths and malformations associated with the use of coumarin derivatives in pregnancy: A critical review. Am J Obstet Gynecol 107:883–888, 1970.
170. Saks DM, Marx GF: Management of a parturient with cardiac valve prosthesis. Anesth Analg 55:214–216, 1976.
171. Stevenson RE, Burton OM, Ferlanto GJ, Taylor HA: Hazards of oral anticoagulants during pregnancy. JAMA 243:1549–1551, 1980.
172. Hall JG, Pauli RM, Wilson KM: Maternal and fetal sequelae of anticoagulation during pregnancy. Am J Med 68:122–140, 1980.
173. Nageotte MP, Freeman RK, Garite TJ, Block RA: Anticoagulation in pregnancy. Am J Obstet Gynecol 141:472, 1981.
174. Bristow JD, McCord CW, Starr A, Ritzman LW, Griswold HE: Clinical and hemodynamic results of aortic valvular replacement with a ball-valve prosthesis. Circulation 29 (suppl I):I-36–I-46, 1964.
175. McHenry MM, Smeloff EA, Davey TB, Kaufman B, Fong WY: Hemodynamic results with full-flow orifice prosthetic valves. Circulation 35 (suppl I):I-24–I-37, 1967.
176. Ross J Jr, Morrow AG, Mason DT, Braunwald E: Left ventricular function following replacement of the aortic valve: Hemodynamic response to muscular exercise. Circulation 33:507–516, 1966.
177. Vosloo S, Reichart B: The feasibility of closed mitral valvotomy in pregnancy. J Thorac Cardiovasc Surg 93:675–679, 1987.
178. Angel JL, Chapman C, Knuppel RA, Morales WJ, Sims CJ: Percutaneous balloon aortic valvuloplasty in pregnancy. Obstet Gynecol 72:438–440, 1988.
179. Kay C, Smith K: Surgery of the pregnant cardiac patient. Am J Cardiol 12:293–295, 1963.
180. Zuhdi N, Carey JL, Schmidt A, Greer A: Total body perfusion and pregnancy. J Int Coll Surg 43:43–46, 1965.
181. Lee WH Jr, Pate JW: Surgical aspects of heart disease in pregnancy. GP 28:78, 1963.
182. Jacobs WM, Cooley D, Goen GP: Cardiac surgery with extracorporeal circulation during pregnancy. Obstet Gynecol 25:167–169, 1965.
183. Harthorne JW, Buckley MJ, Grover JW, Austen WG: Valve replacement during pregnancy. Ann Intern Med 67:1032–1034, 1967.
184. Zitnik RS, Brandenburg RO, Sheldon R, Wallace RB: Pregnancy and open-heart surgery. Circulation 39 and 40(suppl I):I-257–I-262, 1969.
185. Eilen B, Kaiser IH, Becker RM, Cohen MN: Aortic valve replacement in the third trimester of pregnancy: Case report and review of the literature. Obstet Gynecol 57:119–121, 1981.
186. El-Maraghy M, Senna IA, El-Tehewy F, Bassiouni M, Ayoub A, El-Sayed H: Mitral valvotomy in pregnancy. Am J Obstet Gynecol 145:708–710, 1983.
187. Cavalieri RL, Watkins Jr L, Abraham RA, Berkay HS, Niebyl JR: Acute bacterial endocarditis with postpartum aortic valve replacement. Obstet Gynecol 59:124–125, 1982.
188. Nagorney DM, Field CS: Successful pregnancy 10 years after triple cardiac valve replacement. Obstet Gynecol 57:386–388, 1981.
189. Levy DL, Warriner III RA, Burgess GE: Fetal response to cardiopulmonary bypass. Obstet Gynecol 56:112–115, 1980.
190. Trimakas AP, Maxwell KD, Berkay S, Gardner TJ, Achutt SC: Fetal monitoring during cardiopulmonary bypass for removal of a left atrial myxoma during pregnancy. Johns Hopkins Med J 144:156–160, 1979.
191. Martin MC, Pernoll ML, Boruszak AN, Jones JW, LoCicero J III: Cesarean section while on cardiac bypass: Report of a case. Obstet Gynecol 57:41S–45S, 1981.
192. Upshaw CB: A study of maternal electrocardiograms recorded during labor and delivery. Am J Obstet Gynecol 107:17–27, 1970.
193. Spritzer RC, Seldon M, Mattes LM, Donoso E, Friedberg CK: Serious arrhythmias during labor and delivery in women with heart disease. JAMA 211:1005–1007, 1970.
194. Szekely P, Snaith L: Atrial fibrillation and pregnancy. Br Med J 1:1407–1410, 1961.
195. Pine HL, Fox L, Shook D McK: Paroxysmal ventricular tachycardia complicating pregnancy. Am J Cardiol 15:732–734, 1965.
196. Szekely P, Snaith L: Paroxysmal tachycardia in pregnancy. Br Heart J 15:195–198, 1953.
197. Mendelson CL: Disorders of the heart beat in pregnancy. Am J Obstet Gynecol 72:1268–1299, 1956.
198. Mowbray R: Heart block and pregnancy: A review. J Obstet Gynaecol Br Emp 55:432, 1948.
199. Sussman HF, Duque D, Lesser ME: Atrial flutter with 1:1 A-V conduction. Dis Chest 49:99–102, 1966.
200. Dicke JM: Cardiac arrhythmias in pregnant women. Contemporary Ob/Gyn. July 1983, pp 159–184.
201. Dicke JM: Which therapeutic agents for cardiac arrhythmias? Contemporary Ob/Gyn. July 1983, pp 187–197.
202. Greiss FC Jr, Still JG, Anderson S: Effects of local anesthetic agents on the uterine vasculatures and myometrium. Am J Obstet Gynecol 124:889–899, 1976.
203. Biehl D, Shnider SM, Levinson G, Callender K: The direct effects of circulating lidocaine on uterine blood flow and foetal well being in the pregnant ewe. Can Anaesth Soc J 24:445–451, 1977.
204. Biehl D, Shnider SM, Levinson G, Callender K: Placental transfer of lidocaine. Anesthesiology 48:409–412, 1978.
205. Kambam JR, Franks JJ, Smith BE: Inhibitory effect of quin-

idine on plasma pseudocholinesterase activity in pregnant women. Am J Obstet Gynecol 157:897–899, 1987.

206. Joelsson I, Barton MD, Daniel S, James S, Adamsons K: The response of the unanesthetized sheep fetus to sympathomimetic amines and adrenergic agents. Am J Obstet Gynecol 114:43–50, 1972.

207. Joelsson I, Barton MD: The effect of blockade on the receptors of the sympathetic nervous system of the fetus. Acta Obstet Gynecol Scand 48 (suppl 3):75–79, 1969.

208. Barnes AG: Chronic propranolol administration during pregnancy. J Reprod Med 5:179–180, 1970.

209. Renou P, Newman W, Wood C: Autonomic control of fetal heart rate. Am J Obstet Gynecol 105:949–953, 1969.

210. Tunstall ME: The effect of propranolol on the onset of breathing at birth. Br J Anaesth 41:792, 1969.

211. Reed RL, Cheney CB, Fearon RE, Hook R, Hehre FW: Propranolol therapy throughout pregnancy: A case report. Anaesth Analg 53:214–218, 1974.

212. Castro MI, Eisenach JC: Maternally administered esmolol produces fetal β-blockade and hypoxemia. Anesthesiology 69:A708, 1988.

213. Ostman PL, Chestnut DH, Robillard JE, Weiner CP, Hdez MJ: Transplacental passage and hemodynamic effects of esmolol in the gravid ewe. Anesthesiology 69:738–741, 1988.

214. Frishman WH, Chesner M: Beta-adrenergic blockers in pregnancy. Am Heart J 115:147–152, 1988.

215. MacPherson M, Broughton PF, Rutter N: The effect of maternal labetalol on the newborn infant. Br J Obstet Gynaecol 93:539–542, 1986.

216. Michael CA: Intravenous labetalol and intravenous diazoxide in severe hypertension complicating pregnancy. Aust N Z J Obstet Gynaecol 26:26–29, 1986.

217. Murad SHN, Tabsh KMA, Shilyanski G, Kapur PA, Ma C, Lee C, Conklin KA: Effects of verapamil on uterine blood flow and maternal cardiovascular function in the awake pregnant ewe. Anesth Analg 64:7–10, 1985.

218. Murad SHN, Tabsh KMA, Conklin KA, Shilyanski G, Ziadlourad F, Kapur PA, Flacke WE: Verapamil: Placental transfer and effects on maternal and fetal hemodynamics and atrioventricular conduction in the pregnant ewe. Anesthesiology 62:49–53, 1985.

219. Koblin DD, Romanoff ME, Martin DE, Hensley FA Jr., Larach DR, Stauffer RA, Luck JC: Anesthetic management of the parturient receiving amiodarone. Anesthesiology 66:551–553, 1987.

220. Lirette M, Holbrook RH, Katz M: Cardiovascular and uterine blood flow changes during nicardipine HCl tocolysis in the rabbit. Obstet Gynecol 69:79–82, 1987.

221. Veille JC, Bissonnette JM, Hohimer AR: The effect of a calcium channel blocker (nifedipine) on uterine blood flow in the pregnant goat. Am J Obstet Gynecol 154:1160–1163, 1986.

222. Greiss FC Jr, Crandell DL: Therapy for hypotension induced by spinal anesthesia during pregnancy. JAMA 191:793–796, 1965.

223. Greiss FC Jr, Pick JR: The uterine vascular bed: Adrenergic receptors. Obstet Gynecol 23:209–213, 1964.

224. Cibils LA, Pose SV, Zuspan FP: Effect of 1-norepinephrine infusion of uterine contractility and the cardiovascular system. Am J Obstet Gynecol 84:307–317, 1962.

225. James FM III, Greiss FC, Kemp RA: An evaluation of vaso-

pressor therapy for maternal hypotension during spinal anesthesia. Anesthesiology 33:25–34, 1970.

226. Lucas W, Kirschbaum T, Assali NS: Spinal shock and fetal oxygenation. Am J Obstet Gynecol 93:583–587, 1965.

227. Levinson G, Shnider SM: Vasopressors in obstetrics. In *Clinical Anesthesia*. HL Zauder, ed. Davis, Philadelphia, 1973, p 77.

228. Shnider SM, deLorimier AA, Holl JW, Chapler FK, Morishima HO: Vasopressors in obstetrics. I. Correction of fetal acidosis with ephedrine during spinal hypotension. Am J Obstet Gynecol 102:911–919, 1968.

229. Johnson MD, Datta S, Murphy M, Carr D, Ostheimer GW: Atrial natriuretic peptide in maternal and umbilical cord blood during elective cesarean section. Anesthesiology 69:A703, 1988.

230. Kaiser IH, Harris JS: The effect of adrenalin on the pregnant human uterus. Am J Obstet Gynecol 59:775–784, 1950.

231. Kresnow N, Rolett EL, Yurchak PM, Hood WB Jr, Gorlin R: Isoproterenol and cardiovascular performance. Am J Med 37:514–525, 1964.

232. Mahon WA. Reid DWJ, Day RA: The in vivo effects of beta adrenergic stimulation and blockade on the human uterus at term. J Pharmacol Exp Ther 156:178–185, 1967.

233. Blanchard K, Dandavino A, Nuwayhid B, Brinkman CR III, Assali NS: Systemic and uterine hemodynamic responses to dopamine in pregnant and nonpregnant sheep. Am J Obstet Gynecol 130:669–673, 1978.

234. Callender K, Levinson G, Shnider SM, Feduska NJ, Biehl DR, Ring G: Dopamine administration in the normotensive pregnant ewe. Obstet Gynecol 51:586–589, 1978.

235. Rolbin SH, Levinson G, Shnider SM, Biehl DR, Wright RG: Dopamine treatment of spinal hypotension decreases uterine blood flow in the pregnant ewe. Anesthesiology 51:36–40, 1979.

236. Clark RB, Brunner JA: Dopamine as a vasopressor for the treatment of spinal hypotension during cesarean section. Anesthesiology 53:514–517, 1980.

237. Hernandez A, Burton RM, Goldring D, Klint R: The effects of maternally administered digoxin upon the cardiovascular hemodynamics of the fetal lamb. Am Heart J 85:511–517, 1973.

238. Berman W, Ravenscroft PJ, Sheiner LB, Heymann MA, Melmon KL, Rudolph AM: Differential effects of digoxin at comparable concentrations in tissues of fetal and adult sheep. Circ Res 41:635–642, 1977.

239. Okita GT, Plotz EJ, Davis ME: Placental transfer of radioactive digitoxin in pregnant women and its fetal distribution. Circ Res 4:376–380, 1956.

240. Sherman JL, Locke RV: Transplacental neonatal digitalis intoxication. Am J Cardiol 6:834–837, 1960.

241. Baumann AL, Santos AC, Wlody D, Pedersen H, Morishima HO, Finster M: Maternal and fetal effects of milrinone and dopamine. Anesthesiology 71:A855, 1989.

242. Ring G, Krames E, Shnider SM, Wallis KL, Levinson G: Comparison of nitroprusside and hydralazine in hypertensive pregnant ewes. Obstet Gynecol 51:598–602, 1977.

243. Naulty J, Cefalo RC, Lewis PE: Fetal toxicity of nitroprusside in the pregnant ewe. Am J Obstet Gynecol 139:708–711, 1981.

CHAPTER 28

Anesthesia for the Pregnant Patient with Asthma

Edward A. Eisler, M.D.

Although the respiratory system usually adapts well to the physiologic stresses of pregnancy (1, 2), changes in minute ventilation, oxygen consumption, and lung volumes can lead to dyspnea in parturients without respiratory disease (3, 4). When these stresses are superimposed on preexisting lung disease, aggressive management may be required to prevent fetal distress or maternal complications. Asthma is the most common respiratory disorder in women of childbearing age. Management of the asthmatic patient through pregnancy, labor, and delivery is detailed below. Other diseases of the respiratory system, including bronchiectasis, sarcoidosis, tuberculosis, and cystic fibrosis, can also complicate pregnancy and are reviewed elsewhere (1, 3, 5, 6).

CLASSIFICATION AND PATHOPHYSIOLOGY

As defined by the American Thoracic Society and the American College of Chest Physicians, asthma is a disease characterized by increased responsiveness of the airways to various stimuli, manifested by widespread airway narrowing, which changes in severity either spontaneously or as a result of therapy (7). Episodic wheezing and dyspnea due to spasm and hypertrophy of bronchial smooth muscle, inflammation, mucosal congestion, and inspissation of thick secretions are the most common features (Fig. 28.1). Two major clinical subgroups have been identified: extrinsic (or allergic) and intrinsic (or idiopathic). Patients with extrinsic asthma usually have onset of symptoms in childhood and a positive family history of allergic disease. Acute attacks in these patients are often seasonal and can be precipitated by specific antigens. Blood and sputum eosinophilia, elevated serum immunoglobulin (IgE), and positive reactions to skin testing with environmental antigens are common findings. In contrast, patients with intrinsic asthma, the more common type of asthma, have negative family histories for allergic diseases, normal serum IgE, no blood eosinophilia, and negative skin testing. Acute attacks in these patients may be pre-

cipitated by viral illness or irritant exposure. Also included in the intrinsic group are patients whose symptoms are induced by cold air, exercise, or aspirin (8).

Although airway narrowing is the common feature of both subgroups, the precise pathophysiology of asthma has yet to be clearly elucidated. Imbalances in neural control of airway tone, alterations in mucosal permeability and microvascular leakage, immunologic components, inflammatory processes, and biochemical mediators may all have important roles in the initiation and propagation of an acute asthma attack. Previously, attention was focused on primary bronchoconstrictor mechanisms, possibly due to an abnormality of smooth muscle (9), which led to an emphasis on bronchodilator therapy. However, recently a characteristic inflammatory response has been recognized in chronic asthma (10). This finding, in conjunction with recent clinical studies demonstrating the efficacy of inhaled corticosteroids (11), has led many clinicians to view asthma as a primary inflammatory process with bronchoconstriction as a response to the inflammation (12). Although the precise link between symptoms, airway inflammation, and bronchial hyperresponsiveness is still uncertain (10), there is compelling evidence based on animal experiments that the degree of this exaggerated response is related to the extent of inflammation of the airway (12).

Mast cells, macrophages, eosinophils, neutrophils, and lymphocytes are all present in the airways of patients with asthma. Release of histamine from mast cell granules can produce bronchial smooth muscle contraction and an increase in vascular permeability. Although mast cells are probably important in the acute bronchoconstrictor response to an allergen, clinical experiences indicate that degranulation of mast cells is not the initial stimulus to produce bronchial muscle hyperactivity. For example, drugs that stabilize mast cells are less effective than corticosteroids (13); antihistamines are not

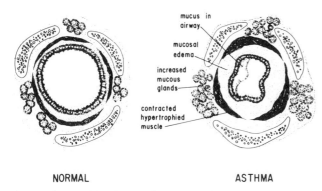

NORMAL   ASTHMA

Figure 28.1. Bronchial wall in asthma (diagrammatic). Note the hypertrophied, contracted smooth muscle, edema, mucous gland hypertrophy, and secretion in the lumen. (Reprinted by permission from West JB: *Pulmonary Pathophysiology—the Essentials*. Williams & Wilkins, Baltimore, 1977, p 81.)

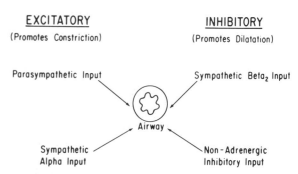

Figure 28.2. Neurohumoral control of airways. (Reprinted by permission from Hirshman CA: Airway reactivity in humans. Anesthesiology 58:171–177, 1983.)

effective in preventing acute bronchospasm; and blood histamine levels are not elevated during asthma attacks. Eosinophils are the inflammatory cells most characteristic of asthma. Eosinophils are perhaps attracted to the airways by the release of eosinophilic chemotactic factor of anaphylaxis (ECF-A) (14). Although little is known about the pharmacology of eosinophils, they appear to release proteins that are toxic to epithelial cells in the airway (15). T lymphocytes are also common in the airways of patients with asthma. Interleukin-5 released from these cells may be important in retaining and priming eosinophils in the airway (12). Macrophages may also be important in the continued propagation of the inflammatory response. Neutrophil infiltration is not a prominent feature of asthma.

Inflammatory mediators also include slow-reacting substance of anaphylaxis (SRS-A) (16), prostaglandins, leukotrienes, and platelet-activating factor. Platelet-activating factor induces many features of asthma (17) and may be the most important signal that recruits and activates eosinophils in the airways of patients with asthma (18).

Neural control of airway tone is complex and involves parasympathetic, sympathetic, and nonadrenergic systems (Fig. 28.2). Stimulation of the parasympathetic system, which predominates in large, central airways, leads to bronchoconstriction. Endotracheal tube-induced bronchospasm appears to be mediated through these fibers (19). Stimulation of α-adrenergic receptors also leads to bronchoconstriction, but this is of less importance because there are few α-receptors in the lung. Relaxation of bronchial smooth muscle occurs by stimulation of β_2-adrenergic receptors. Acquired and congenital deficiencies of β_2-receptors have been described in some asth-

matic patients (9). A nonadrenergic, noncholinergic system may also be involved (20). Neuropeptides released from these sensory nerves include substance P (a potent inducer of microvascular permeability and mucus secretion), neurokinin A (a potent bronchoconstrictor), and calcitonin gene-related peptide (an effective and long-lasting dilator of bronchial vessels) (12). Bradykinin may be the trigger that leads to the release of these peptides from exposed nerve endings, which would then amplify and spread the inflammatory response (21). Thus airway hyperreactivity can result from cholinergic dominance, β-adrenergic blockade, or imbalances in the poorly characterized nonadrenergic, noncholinergic system.

The intracellular cyclic nucleotides, particularly cyclic adenosine monophosphate (cAMP) and cyclic guanosine monophosphate (cGMP), may control bronchomotor tone. After cholinergic stimulation, cGMP increases and causes smooth muscle contraction. Increases in cGMP also promote mast cell degranulation and cause increases in local release of histamine and other biochemical mediators. Through a series of intermediary reactions, increases in intracellular cAMP lead to bronchial smooth muscle relaxation by interfering with actinmyosin coupling of smooth muscle fibers. Intracellular cAMP also regulates release of histamine and other mediators of capillary permeability from mast cells and basophils. Although the exact pathophysiology remains unclear, the capacity of adrenergic and cholinergic agents to influence mediator release and alter bronchial smooth muscle contractility through cyclic nucleotides suggests that imbalances or defects in the autonomic nervous system might predispose to asthma (8).

EFFECTS OF PREGNANCY ON ASTHMA

Asthma occurs in approximately 1% of pregnant women, with a reported range from 0.4 to 1.3% (22–26). Ten to 15% of these women will require hospitalization for acute severe attacks of asthma during their pregnancy (26, 27). The effect of pregnancy on asthma varies widely. Several studies have shown that more than 40% of patients had a deterioration in their condition during pregnancy (28, 29). In contrast, Schaefer and Silverman (22) found that 93% of the patients they studied had no change in severity of symptoms. Turner et al. (23) summarized the results of nine clinical studies involving over 1000 asthmatic patients and noted that symptoms remained unchanged in half of the patients, worsened in approximately one-fourth of the patients, and improved in the remaining patients.

Adolescent asthmatics are particularly at risk for exacerbations of their asthma during pregnancy. In a study of 28 pregnancies in patients between 14 and 19 years of age, nearly two-thirds required hospitalization for status asthmaticus (30).

Several physiologic changes of pregnancy may influence the course of asthma during pregnancy. Increases in plasma cortisol, progesterone, cAMP, and maternal histaminase occur during pregnancy and may help alleviate symptoms. The increases in cortisol and progesterone may be responsible for the 50% decrease in bronchomotor tone and airway resistance observed in normal pregnancy (31). There is a decrease in cell-mediated immunity, particularly a decrease in T-cell lymphocyte function. This may help decrease the maternal response to antigen challenge. However, this decrease in cell-mediated immunity may make the parturient more susceptible to viral upper respiratory infections that can precipitate asthma attacks. Other changes that could worsen asthma include increases in bronchoconstricting prostaglandins, congestion of inferior nasal turbinates with resulting increases in upper airway congestion (32), and increased antigen exposure from the developing fetus. Maternal hyperventilation and the subjective feeling of dyspnea mentioned earlier may lead to maternal anxiety and apprehension, and precipitate an asthma attack. Decreases in pulmonary reserve coupled with an increase in oxygen consumption may make it more difficult for the patient to tolerate mild exacerbations.

It is difficult to predict the course of asthma for an individual pregnancy, although it appears that patients with more severe disease are more likely to have a deterioration during pregnancy (33). Women whose asthma worsened in a previous pregnancy should expect similar decompensation with subsequent pregnancies (28, 34). Worsening of symptoms usually occurs between the 29th and 36th weeks of gestation (35). However, in one study of severe asthmatics, 50% of patients had respiratory difficulties during the intrapartum or immediate postpartum pe-

riods (36). Unlike preeclampsia, it is rare for dramatic improvements in asthma symptoms to occur after delivery of the fetus. However, Topilsky et al. (37) reported the case of a patient whose asthma worsened progressively until the 18th week of pregnancy. Despite increasing doses of steroids, the patient required mechanical ventilation and maximum bronchodilator therapy. Within 12 hr after removal of the fetus by hysterotomy, she improved dramatically, was extubated, and her medical regimen quickly weaned. Gluck and Gluck (28) have suggested that parturients with increases in serum IgE levels during pregnancy are the patients most likely to experience exacerbations of asthma.

EFFECTS OF ASTHMA ON PREGNANCY

A large Norwegian study found significant increases in labor complications among asthmatic patients when compared to patients without respiratory disease (38). Hemorrhage, hyperemesis, toxemia, and induced labor were the most common abnormalities noted. Another study that included 16 patients classified as "severe asthmatics" reported two maternal deaths attributed to asthma in the peripartum period (25). A more recent prospective study involving nearly 200 pregnancies focused on careful prenatal management of respiratory disease (39). In this study, preeclampsia occurred more often in asthmatic patients, especially in patients with severe asthma. Cesarean delivery was also more common in asthmatic patients, but no other maternal morbidity was noted (39). In several studies in which corticosteroids were frequently used to treat severe maternal asthma, complications were infrequent and no maternal deaths occurred (40–42).

Deaths from asthma in the population at large have risen over the past decade (43). In a study of patients who had an asthma-induced respiratory arrest, this near fatal result was caused by exacerbations of severe asthma and not treatment-induced cardiac dysrhythmias. Although it had been previously proposed that deaths were frequently due to drugs used to treat asthma (44), results from this study suggest that undertreatment rather than overtreatment is the major contributor to the observed increase in mortality from asthma (43). It also appears that better treatment of maternal asthma leads to less perinatal maternal complications (39, 42).

Several studies have shown that preterm delivery, low–birth-weight infants, and perinatal death occur more frequently in pregnancies complicated by asthma (22, 25, 38). Low–birth-weight infants were more common even in studies in which maternal asthma was well controlled (42, 45). Hypoglycemia occurs more often in infants of mothers with severe asthma than in infants of mothers with less severe disease (39). It is not known whether these adverse outcomes are due to fetal effects of maternal medicines or fetal hypoxia secondary to maternal asthmatic attacks. However, a better outcome is more likely in patients in whom asthma is well controlled.

TREATMENT OF ASTHMA DURING PREGNANCY

Treatment plans for the pregnant asthmatic need to be individualized, carefully monitored, and altered appropriately to control episodic attacks. The main goals in therapy are to prevent maternal and fetal hypoxia while limiting exposure of the fetus to potentially harmful drugs. Few clinical studies of drug teratogenicity are available to guide the clinician in choice of therapeutic options. Often the study group size is too small to permit a high degree of statistical confidence that a drug is safe (46). The physician should attempt to minimize drug usage, particularly during the first trimester, but not at the risk of attack of severe uncontrolled asthma. The fetus is at much greater jeopardy from repeated bouts of maternal hypoxia than from exposure to small amounts of antiasthmatic drugs (47). Even though some drugs have been implicated as potential teratogens, it is important to remember that "maternal disease which necessitates the initiation of therapeutic intervention makes it difficult, if not impossible, to extricate the effects of the treatment from those of the maternal complaint" (48).

The asthmatic patient should be advised to avoid potential precipitating environmental factors such as strenuous exercise, smoke, strong perfume, fresh paint, and other irritants (27). Proper nutrition, appropriate hydration, moderate physical activity, and adequate rest and sleep are important in controlling the disease process. Infections should be treated vigorously.

When antiasthma therapy is needed, treatment traditionally has begun with an inhaled β-adrenergic agent and/or a theophylline preparation. However, the wisdom of this therapeutic approach has now been questioned. Because asthma appears to be a primary inflammatory process with reactive bronchospasm, antiinflammatory therapy is now the first line of therapy used by many clinicians (12). Indeed, one study has shown that inhalation corticosteroids are more effective than inhalation β_2-agonists for patients with newly detected mild asthma (49). Inhaled beclomethasone appears to be both a safe and effective therapy for pregnant asthmatics (50).

A large retrospective Canadian study has demonstrated an increased risk of death or near death when β_2-agonists were used on a regular and frequent basis (51). Although it is possible that this observed effect simply identified those patients with more severe disease, these authors reviewed evidence that suggests that regular, frequent use of inhaled β_2-agonists may make asthma worse, perhaps by increasing airway hyperresponsiveness (51). Other authors have suggested that inhaled β-agonists not be prescribed on a regular schedule, but be reserved for acute attacks (52). For patients whose asthma is severe enough to require daily treatment, inhaled antiinflammatory agents are preferred (12, 51).

To decrease systemic side effects and decrease fetal exposure, the inhaled route of administration of either β_2-agonists or corticosteroids should be employed first (53). If this initial therapy fails, oral aminophylline is added because its bronchodilating abilities may have a synergistic effect (12). Some authors suggest that cromolyn sodium can also be used safely in pregnancy (26).

Although there is some evidence of congenital malformations when laboratory animals are given large doses of aminophylline (3), most authors agree that aminophylline therapy is safe during pregnancy (54–57). Sustained-release preparations of epinephine are associated with an increase in fetal malformations when used in the first trimester (1). One large study has shown that inhaled β-agonist bronchodilator therapy is not associated with any increased maternal or fetal morbidity (58). However, there is little available data about the safety of more specific β_2-adrenergic agents such as terbutaline, metaproterenol, or albuterol in very early pregnancy (57).

Two studies have indicated that oral corticosteroids can be used safely in severe asthmatics (40, 59). In particular, prednisone and prednisolone are well suited for long-term oral use in pregnancy because they cross the placenta poorly (maternal to fetal concentration is 10:1).

However, the use of large doses of steroids has been associated with intrauterine growth retardation in humans (48) and congenital abnormalities, particularly cleft palate, in laboratory animals (60). Steroids should be used sparingly at the lowest effective dose. Every-other-day therapy is preferable.

Sedatives should be avoided because many produce congenital anomalies in animals (61). A list of drugs to be avoided in the treatment of asthma and asthmatic-related infections is given in Table 28.1. Prostaglandin $F_{2\alpha}$ is used intraamniotically for second-trimester abortions. However, patients with a history of asthma are very susceptible to bronchoconstriction with this drug (23, 62). Because significant airway constriction has been demonstrated when this drug was given to asthmatic patients, alternate means for terminating pregnancy should be considered in these patients (62, 63).

Table 28.1
Drugs to Avoid in Pregnancy Complicated by Asthma

Aspirin
Tartrazine dyes
Iodine-containing preparations
Tetracycline
Hydroxyzine
Prostaglandin $F_{2\alpha}$
Brompheniramine maleate
β-Blockers

Table 28.2
Pulmonary Function Changes during an Acute Asthma Attack

Total airway resistance	↑
Forced vital capacity	↓
Forced expiratory volume (1 sec)	↓
Total lung capacity	↑
Functional residual capacity	↑
Residual volume	↑
Expiratory reserve volume	↓
Inspiratory reserve volume	↓
Maximum midexpiratory flow rate	↓

ACUTE ASTHMA ATTACKS DURING PREGNANCY

An acute asthmatic attack can be life threatening to the pregnant patient. Chest tightness, shortness of breath, wheezing, and cough are common presenting symptoms. Patients are generally quite aware of their disease process and are able to give a subjective appraisal of the severity of an acute asthma attack and their response to treatment (64). Use of accessory muscles of respiration and the presence of both inspiratory and expiratory wheezes are indicative of severe airway obstruction. Additional signs of potentially life-threatening disease include heart rate greater than 120, respiratory rate greater than 30, forced expiratory volume (FEV_1) less than 1 liter, and pulsus paradoxus more than 18 mm Hg. A "silent chest" with little air movement is an ominous sign of impending respiratory failure. Changes in pulmonary function during an acute attack are shown in Table 28.2.

Because upper respiratory infections are the most common precipitants of acute asthma attacks in pregnancy (23), evidence of a precipitating infection or irritant exposure should be sought by history and physical examination. A chest x-ray is unlikely to add useful information if no indication of infection is found by history or examination (65). However, a chest x-ray may be necessary when the patient's symptoms do not respond well to treatment. The radiation dose from posteroanterior and lateral films is about 50 mrad to the chest and only 2 to 5 mrad to the gonads. The minimal dose for fetal teratogenic concern is much greater, at a level of 1 to 5 rad (3). Serial measurements of parameters such as FEV_1 and arterial blood gases are useful for monitoring the patient's condition, but treatment should not be unduly delayed for the purpose of diagnostic procedures.

Prompt treatment is essential. An outline for therapy is given in Table 28.3. Appropriate antibiotic therapy should be given if there is clinical suspicion of an infectious process. Other important considerations are as follows.

1. *The importance of early institution of oxygen therapy can not be overemphasized.* The precarious oxygenation status of the fetus was demonstrated in a series of studies utilizing induced mild hypoxemia in mothers at term (66). When maternal inspired oxygen was lowered from 21 to 15%, the maternal Po_2 fell from 91 mm Hg to 65 mm Hg with little change in arterial oxygen content. In contrast, fetal umbilical vein Po_2 fell from 32 mm Hg to 26 mm Hg, resulting in a substantial reduction in oxygen content because of the steep slope of the hemoglobin-oxygen dissociation curve. Oxygen delivery to the fetus may be further impaired by alkalosis induced by maternal hyperventilation (67), which commonly occurs during an acute asthma attack.

2. *Inhaled β_2-agonists provide excellent relief of acute bronchoconstrictive symptoms* (52). For subcutaneous administration, epinephrine and terbutaline appear to be equally effective. In early pregnancy terbutaline may be preferred because of the potential for fetal malformations with repeated doses of epinephrine (1). However, terbutaline should be used very cautiously in late pregnancy because of the risk of maternal complications, particularly pulmonary edema (69).

3. *The pregnant patient's requirement for theophylline may increase during the second and third trimester* (55). This is due to an increased volume of distribution with an unchanged clearance. Since the parturient's weight also changes, dosages given on a milligram-per-kilogram basis may only need to be altered slightly. Intravenous theophylline therapy should be monitored by blood levels. Levels should be drawn after 10 hr of therapy and more frequently if toxic reactions such as nausea, tremors, and dysrhythmias occur.

4. *Since steroids take several hours to be effective, they should be given early if symptoms do not rapidly improve.* A "wait and see" attitude about institution of steroid therapy may expose the mother and fetus to serious risk.

5. *Arterial blood gases should be monitored frequently in the unstable patient.* A mild asthma attack is characterized by a pH of 7.38 or higher, a Pco_2

Table 28.3
Management of Acute Asthmatic Attack during Pregnancy

Initial Therapy	If No Improvement, Add	If No Improvement, Add

1. Supplemental oxygen
2. Inhaled bronchodilator (e.g., isoetharine 0.5 ml in 2.5 ml saline or metaproterenol 0.3 ml in 2.5 ml saline)
or
Subcutaneous injection of β-agonist (e.g., 0.3 ml of 1:1000 epinephrine or 0.25 mg terbutaline sulfate) Repeat, if needed
	1. Intravenous hydration
	2. Intravenous aminophylline
	  a. Loading dose:
	    • No prior theophylline—5.6 mg/kg lean body weight over 20 min (400 mg max)
	    • Previous inadequate theophylline—2.5 mg/kg lean body weight over 20 min (400 mg max)
	    • Previous adequate theophylline—no loading dose
	  b. Then, continuous infusion
	    • 0.5 mg/kg/hr—normal
	    • 0.7 mg/kg/hr—smokers, teenagers
	    • 0.3 mg/kg/hr—coexisting heart disease, liver disease, or cimetidine therapy
		1. Hospital admission
		2. Serial ABG and spirometry

3. Initial laboratory examinations (e.g., ABG, CBC, spirometry as therapy is begun)		3. Intravenous corticosteroid therapy: Cortisol sodium succinate (Solu-Cortef) 100 to 200 mg q 2 to 6 hr *or* Methyl prednisolone sodium succinate (Solu-Medrol) 40 mg q 2 to 6 hr

of 30 mm Hg or less, and a low normal Po_2. The combination of low arterial Po_2, normal pH, and normal Pco_2 indicates a moderate attack and possible danger because the patient may be too tired to hyperventilate in an attempt to increase oxygenation. A Pco_2 greater than 35 mm Hg or a pH less than 7.35 indicates a severe attack, and the patient should be transferred to an intensive care setting (26).

6. *The fetal heart rate should be continually monitored.*

When maximal medical management is ineffective and arterial blood gases continue to deteriorate, endotracheal intubation may be required. Woo (70) recommended tracheal intubation when (a) total vital capacity is less than 10 ml/kg, (b) dead space–tidal volume ratio (V_D/V_T) is greater than 0.6, or (c) the alveolar–arterial oxygen tension gradient (A-a gradient) is greater than 300 torr while breathing 100% oxygen. If mechanical ventilation is instituted patients should be adequately sedated to decrease the risk of barotrauma. Muscle relaxants may also be required in some cases. Humidification of inhaled gases, slow respiratory rates, and adequate expiratory times will also facilitate mechanical ventilation. There are several reports in which bronchoalveolar lavage or warm metaproterenol solution irrigation and suction

was used to successfully treat severe asthma-induced respiratory failure during the third trimester (71, 72).

MANAGEMENT OF LABOR AND VAGINAL DELIVERY

It is important for the anesthesiologist to obtain an appropriate history and perform a physical exam as soon as possible after the pregnant asthmatic patient is admitted to the labor suite. Essential areas of assessment include medications currently taken (especially whether or not steroids have been used recently), predisposing factors in acute attacks, known allergies, previous anesthetic history, and presence of recent respiratory infections. A history of a persistent cough may be the sole manifestation of reactive airway disease in pregnant women (73). Physical examination should focus on the cardiac and respiratory systems. Chest auscultation while the patient performs a forced expiration maneuver may elicit wheezing not audible during normal tidal volume ventilation. In patients with a history of severe asthma, arterial blood gases, electrocardiogram, complete blood count, and pulmonary function tests, particularly forced vital capacity (FVC) and FEV_1, will provide useful baseline information. If there is an indication of current respiratory infection, sputum should be sent for culture and a chest x-ray obtained.

The patient should continue receiving previous medications throughout her hospital admission and additional therapies should be added as needed to optimize respiratory status. Intermittent positive pressure breathing (IPPB) with bronchodilators is not recommended because it is of questionable benefit and has been associated with barotrauma when used in the third trimester (74).

Aminophylline, β-sympathomimetics (i.e., terbutaline), and epinephrine have all been shown to slow labor (75, 76). The progress of labor should be carefully monitored when these drugs are given for asthma. Pitocin, not prostaglandins, should be used if necessary to augment labor.

Similarly, prostaglandin $F_{2\alpha}$ and ergonovine should be avoided as therapy for postpartum hemorrhage because both have been reported to exacerbate asthma when used in this setting (53). Particular caution should be exercised when using terbutaline because of the risk of maternal pulmonary edema (69) and with intravenous aminophylline because of the risk of fetal toxicity (77–79). Fetal side effects including irritability, tachycardia, jitteriness, vomiting, and opisthotonus have been observed even with therapeutic theophylline levels (79). The preterm infant is particularly at risk because of the prolonged half-life of theophylline secondary to immature enzyme systems (78). Theophylline should be monitored by maternal serum levels and levels kept between 10 and 14 μg/ml (low therapeutic range).

If the patient has recently needed corticosteroids, it is recommended that hydrocortisone (100 mg intramuscularly) be given upon admission and then every 8 hr for 24 hr (57). This recommendation is made even though several studies have shown that much lower doses are effective in steroid-treated patients undergoing major surgery (80, 81). The important advantages of supplemental corticosteroids in these laboring parturients include providing adequate exogenous corticosteroids for the physiologic stress of labor (82), preventing exacerbations of asthma, and preventing the possibility of adrenal insufficiency in patients who have been steroid dependent (57).

Minute ventilation increases progressively throughout labor and may equal 20 liters/min (57). Because hyperventilation is a known precipitant of acute asthmatic attacks, the importance of optimal respiratory status before the onset of labor cannot be overemphasized. Adequate maternal hydration during labor may help overcome additional fluid losses caused by hyperventilation and minimize inspissation of thickened secretions. Because fetuses of asthmatic mothers may be at increased risk for perinatal complications, oxygen supplementation during labor is recommended. Continuous fetal heart tracings and uterine activity monitoring are advantageous. More invasive monitoring, such as an intraarterial catheter, may be indicated should an acute asthmatic attack occur during labor.

Small amounts of narcotics can be used for pain relief during the first stage of labor. "Although large doses of morphine and meperidine produce constriction of the bronchi, this effect is rarely seen after therapeutic doses in man" (83). Meperidine and fentanyl are preferred over morphine because of the latter's greater propensity for histamine release (84). Narcotics should not be given if there is evidence of respiratory compromise. Other sedatives are best avoided, particularly in combination with narcotics.

Epidural analgesia is the ideal method of pain relief for labor. Advantages include lack of maternal sedation, decreases in maternal stress and anxiety, and elimination of maternal hyperventilation in response to painful uterine contractions. Epidural analgesia has been used to effectively treat an acute asthma attack during labor after specific bronchodilator therapy had become ineffective (85). The epidural anesthetic must be carefully titrated to avoid an excessively high block and respiratory compromise. Low concentrations of local anesthetics (i.e., lidocaine 1% or bupivacaine 0.25%) should be used to avoid excessive motor blockade. Some authors advise using epinephrine-containing local anesthetic solutions (1:200,000 dilution) because low-dose absorption of the epinephrine will aid bronchial dilatation (86) without adversely affecting neonatal outcome. Large amounts of local anesthetic containing epinephrine may slow the progress of labor, but this effect can easily be ameliorated by pitocin (87). The continuous infusion technique described in Chapter 9 is recommended because it offers the advantages of a continuous stable anesthetic level and steady pain relief. The addition of fentanyl to the local anesthetic appears to produce profound analgesia with minimal effect on maternal respiratory effort or fetal well-being (85).

Regional anesthesia is also useful for vaginal delivery. A preexisting epidural can be extended or a low spinal or saddle block placed to provide perineal analgesia and pain-free delivery. A pudendal block can also be used either by itself or in combination with inhalation or intravenous analgesia with patients for whom a spinal or epidural anesthetic is contraindicated or otherwise not possible. Low concentrations of enflurane have been used to provide effective pain relief during delivery (88). This technique offers the advantages of concomitant administration of high concentrations of oxygen and the bronchodilating actions of the inhaled agent. This technique should be used with extreme caution to avoid loss of protective upper airway reflexes. Intravenous sedation using low doses of ketamine, a bronchodilator, has been described in Chapter 8. Low-dose ketamine has the advantage of providing analgesia while maintaining appropriate protective upper airway reflexes (89). There can be an increase in oral secretions with this technique that may necessitate the use of a drying agent such as glycopyrrolate.

REGIONAL ANESTHESIA FOR CESAREAN DELIVERY

Regional anesthesia offers many advantages for the pregnant asthmatic patient undergoing cesarean delivery during nonemergency conditions. The foremost reason is that this technique obviates the need for airway instrumentation and irritation. Regional anesthesia reliably blocks the maternal stress response to delivery, while general anesthesia does not (90). Epidural anesthesia does not block the fetal stress response that may be necessary for adaptation to extrauterine life (90). Regional anesthesia provides a smoother transition from the operation to recovery and allows for careful titration of analgesics without additional sedation and respiratory depression from residual anesthetic gases.

Epidural anesthesia provides several additional benefits. A catheter technique can be used and the catheter reinjected with local anesthetic or narcotics to provide postoperative pain relief. Epinephrine-containing local anesthetic solutions may have additional bronchodilating effects as discussed earlier. There is a greater difference between sensory level and level of motor blockade with epidural anesthesia than with spinal anesthesia. Freund et al. (91) found the level of motor blockade to be 2.8 dermatomal segments lower than sensory level with spinals and 4.6 segments lower with epidurals. Thus respiratory function may be better preserved with epidural anesthesia.

Respiratory compromise is a major potential hazard with regional anesthesia. The maternal position may limit respiration (6). Blockade of thoracic muscles of respiration may lead to difficulty in coughing and clearing secretions. Thoracic muscle blockade may lead to an abnormal sensation of respiration from the change to a diaphragmatic pattern of breathing. However, by carefully controlling the level of anesthesia these complications can be minimized. Freund and co-workers (91) found that mean inspiratory capacity fell only 3% with epidural anesthesia and mean expiratory reserve volume fell only 21%. With a sensory level of T4 (approximate motor block to T8 with

epidural anesthesia) there are only minimal changes in ventilatory parameters (Fig. 28.3).

Because bronchospasm can occur during regional anesthesia (92–94), the patient should bring her inhaler (if she is accustomed to using one) into the delivery room. An intraoperative asthmatic attack should be managed as outlined in Table 28.3.

Adequate prehydration, early treatment of hypotension, and supplemental oxygen may help decrease the incidence of nausea and vomiting. Emotional support and distraction techniques such as shoulder massage or focusing attention on the baby should be used in preference to intravenous sedation to relieve maternal fear and anxiety. Supplemental narcotics can be used in small doses after delivery of the newborn. The use of minimal traction by a gentle surgeon may greatly reduce the discomfort associated with manipulation of the peritoneum during surgical repair. In particular, the surgeon should avoid exteriorizing the uterus, if possible, to decrease discomfort and lower the risk of air embolism.

GENERAL ANESTHESIA FOR CESAREAN DELIVERY

A general anesthetic technique for the pregnant asthmatic must attempt to eliminate complications from two potential medical problems: (a) reactive airways disease and (b) increased risk of aspiration. Because the pregnant patient is presumed to have a full stomach, the anesthetic technique of rapid-se-

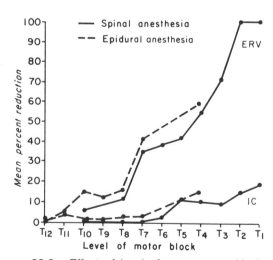

Figure 28.3. Effect of level of motor nerve block during spinal and epidural anesthesia on inspiratory capacity (IC) and expiratory reserve volume (ERV). Changes in ventilatory parameters are plotted as percentage reduction from control. (Reprinted by permission from Freund FG, Bonica JJ, Ward RJ, Akamatsu TJ, Kennedy WF: Ventilatory reserve and level of motor block during high spinal and epidural anesthesia. Anesthesiology 28:834–837, 1967.)

quence induction and endotracheal intubation with subsequent awake extubation is used. However, the most common single factor that precipitates an attack of wheezing during general anesthesia is the presence of an endotracheal tube (93). Furthermore, reflex bronchospasm is most likely to occur when the endotracheal tube is placed or manipulated in the presence of light anesthesia (95)—exactly the conditions frequently seen with a rapid induction and awake extubation technique. However, general anesthesia is indicated for emergency surgery or when regional anesthesia is not possible.

The patient should be given a clear antacid to decrease gastric pH. H_2-receptor blockers such as cimetidine or ranitidine should not be used because they may provoke bronchospasm (96). Histamine mediates bronchospasm via H_1 receptors, whereas bronchodilation is mediated by H_2 receptors; thus selective blockade of H_2 receptors could unmask unopposed bronchoconstriction.

A rapid intravenous induction is performed after a full 3 min of preoxygenation. Thiopental is best avoided because it does not reliably protect against reflex-induced bronchospasm in doses used clinically for induction of anesthesia (97). Ketamine is the agent of choice for rapid induction in patients with reactive airways disease (89). Ketamine has been shown to decrease airway resistance in patients with pulmonary dysfunction (98, 99). Ketamine has also been shown to prevent bronchospasm in previously sensitized laboratory animals challenged with antigen (100). This effect appears to be mediated through the sympathetic nervous system (100). Ketamine is not arrhythmogenic in the presence of aminophylline (101). Although ketamine was not associated with any higher incidence of maternal or fetal complications when compared to thiopental (102, 103), emergence reactions and psychic disturbances have been reported following its use (89). Small doses of diazepam can attenuate these reactions (89). Succinylcholine has been used safely for intubation in asthmatics (92, 93, 98). Application of 4% lidocaine to the larynx is not recommended because this practice delays intubation and can lead to reflex bronchoconstriction in asthmatics (104, 105).

Inhalational agents should be used for maintenance of anesthesia. Halothane has been considered the anesthetic agent of choice for the asthmatic patient (92, 93). Isoflurane, halothane, and (presumably) enflurane prevent bronchoconstriction by direct effects on airway smooth muscle and depression of reflex pathways (106). Because of these bronchodilating properties, isoflurane and enflurane are acceptable alternatives to halothane. The combination of intravenous aminophylline and halothane has been

associated with ventricular dysrhythmias in laboratory animals (107) and patients (76). This effect is more pronounced with high levels of aminophyline (107). Because of this interaction, enflurane or isoflurane should be used in the patient receiving intravenous aminophylline, or whenever there is a possibility of potentially toxic theophylline levels.

Controlled ventilation with high concentrations of humidified oxygen is recommended. Large tidal volumes and slow respiratory rates should be used. Allowing ample time for expiration will help prevent air trapping. If additional muscle relaxation is needed during surgery, vecuronium and pancuronium are preferred over the relaxants associated with histamine release (curare, metocurine, atracurium). Residual muscle blockade should be reversed with neostigmine or edrophonium prior to extubation. Because muscarinic actions of these drugs can precipitate asthma, a sufficient dose of intravenous atropine should precede their use (6).

Intraoperative asthmatic attacks can be successfully treated by temporarily deepening halothane anesthesia (92, 93), while a search for other causes of intraoperative wheezing is undertaken. Table 28.4 lists an appropriate differential diagnosis. If there is any question of airway patency, a suction catheter should be passed to rule out obstruction and to clear thick secretions.

Because exposure to high concentrations of halothane will lead to uterine relaxation, narcotics and small doses of benzodiazepines should be given intravenously after the baby is delivered to maintain increased anesthetic depth. Should asthmatic bronchospasm persist in the presence of adequate anesthesia depth, inhaled β_2-agonists should be given directly through the breathing circuit (97). T-piece adapters and connectors are available for many commonly used aerosolized bronchodilators or a jet nebulizer can be placed into the inspiratory limb of the anesthetic circuit (Figs. 28.4 to 28.6).

Table 28.4
Causes of Wheezing during General Anesthesia

Bronchial asthma
Mechanical obstruction of the endotracheal tube
Inadequate anesthesia for the surgical stimulation resulting in active expiratory efforts
Inadequate neuromuscular blockade
Endobronchial intubation
Overinflation of the endotracheal tube cuff
Pulmonary edema
Aspiration of gastric contents
Anaphylactic or anaphylactoid reaction
Amniotic fluid embolism
Pneumothorax

Figure 28.4. A fluorocarbon propellant generator with T-piece and connectors. (Reprinted by permission from Kingston HGG, Hirshman CA: Perioperative management of the patient with asthma. Anesth Analg 68:844–855, 1984.)

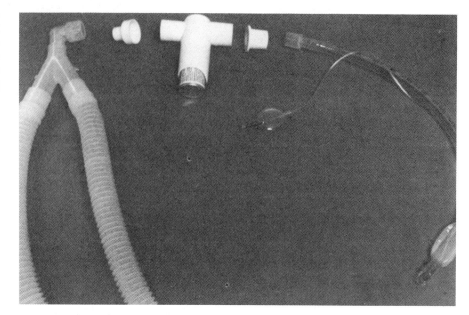

Figure 28.5. A jet nebulizer connected to an oxygen source. (Reprinted by permission from Kingston HGG, Hirshman CA: Perioperative management of the patient with asthma. Anesth Analg 68:844–855, 1984.)

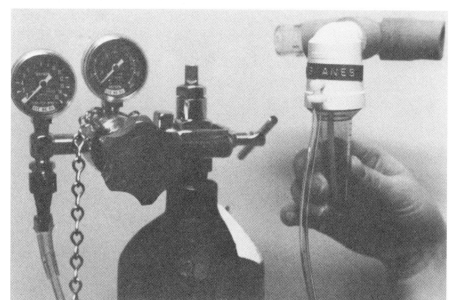

Figure 28.6. A jet nebulizer placed in the inspiratory limb of an anesthesia circuit. (Reprinted by permission from Kingston HGG, Hirshman CA: Perioperative management of the patient with asthma. Anesth Analg 68:844–855, 1984.)

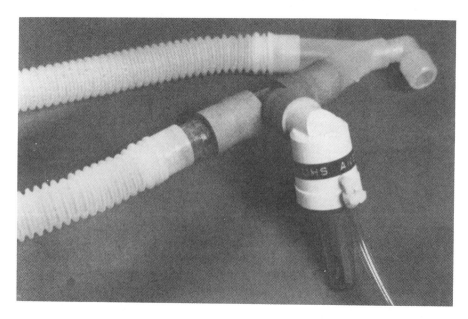

At the end of surgery the patient is extubated awake after complete reversal of muscle relaxants. Delaying extubation until the patient is awake enough to protect against aspiration can lead to bronchospasm, but this technique is necessary because aspiration can be disastrous in a patient with bronchospastic disease. Small doses of narcotics will help decrease coughing and bucking on the endotracheal tube during awakening. Intravenous lidocaine has been shown to block reflex bronchoconstriction of the kind caused by endotracheal tubes (105, 108). Administration of a 75 to 100-mg intravenous bolus of lidocaine followed by an infusion of 1 to 4 mg/min may be a useful adjuvant. If there is any question of adequacy of ventilation, the patient should be ventilated postoperatively until her bronchospastic disease is better controlled. Humidifed oxygen and inhaled bronchodilators can be important therapies in the immediate postoperative period.

SUMMARY

Pregnancy can exacerbate bronchospasm, particularly in patients with severe asthma. Treatment is aimed at preventing maternal and fetal hypoxia. A better fetal outcome is anticipated when maternal asthma is well controlled. Inhaled corticosteroids appear to be a safe and effective first-line treatment for chronic asthma. Oxygen, inhaled bronchodilators, and intravenous aminophylline are used to treat acute attacks. Systemic corticosteroids should be used in severe cases. Maternal pain and hyperventilation can be alleviated by epidural analgesia during labor and delivery. A well-controlled epidural anesthetic provides excellent conditions for cesarean delivery. General anesthesia techniques include induction with ketamine and maintenance of anesthesia with inhaled agents, particularly halothane.

References

1. Niederman MS, Matthay RA: Asthma and other severe respiratory diseases during pregnancy. In *Critical Care of the Obstetric Patient*. RL Berkowitz, ed. Churchill Livingston, New York, 1983, pp 335–366.
2. DeSwiet M: Respiratory disease in pregnancy. Postgrad Med J 55:325–328, 1979.
3. Weinberger SE, Weiss ST, Cohen WR, Weiss JW, Johnson TS: Pregnancy and the lung. Am Rev Resp Dis 121:559–581, 1980.
4. Milne JA, Howie AD, Pack AI: Dyspnoea during normal pregnancy. Br J Obstet Gynaecol 85:260–263, 1978.
5. Novy MJ, Edwards MJ: Respiratory problems in pregnancy. Am J Obstet Gynecol 99:1024–1045, 1967.
6. Brown WU: Respiratory Problems. In *Obstetric Anesthesia: The Complicated Patient*. FM James III, AS Wheeler, eds. Davis, Philadelphia, 1982, pp 103–121.
7. Samet J: Epidemiological approaches for the identification of asthma. Chest 91:745–785, 1987.
8. Don HF, Koopman W, Mathieu A: Asthma and other allergic disorders: Current immunologic concepts and anesthetic considerations. In *Immunologic Aspects of Anesthetic and Surgical Practices*. A Mathieu, BD Kahan, eds. Grune & Stratton, New York, 1975, pp 289–313.
9. Szentivanji A: The beta adrenergic theory of atopic abnormality in bronchial asthma. J Allergy 42:203–232, 1968.
10. Barnes PJ: New concepts in the pathogenesis of bronchial hyperresponsivenss and asthma. J Allergy Clin Immunol 83:1013–1026, 1989.
11. Greenberger PA, Patterson R: The outcome of pregnancy complicated by severe asthma. Allergy Proc 9:539–543, 1988.
12. Barnes PJ: A new approach to the treatment of asthma. N Engl J Med 321:1517–1527, 1989.
13. Svendsen UG, Frølund L, Madsen F, Nielsen NH, Holstein-Rathlou NH, Weeke B: A comparison of the effects of sodium cromoglycate and beclomethasone dipropionate on pulmonary function and bronchial hyperreactivity in subjects with asthma. J Allergy Clin Immunol 80:68–74, 1987.
14. Kay AB, Austen KF: IgE mediated release of an eosinophil leukocyte chemotactic factor from human lung. J Immunol 107:899, 1971.
15. Frigas E, Gleich GJ: The eosinophil and the pathophysiology of asthma. J Allergy Clin Immunol 77:527–537, 1986.
16. Orange RP, Austen WG, Austen KF: Immunologic release of histamine and SRS-A from human lung. I. Modulation by agents influencing cellular levels of cyclic 3'5' adenosine monophosphate. J Exp Med 134(suppl):136, 1971.
17. Barnes PJ, Chung KF, Page CD: Platelet-activating factor as a mediator of allergic disease. J Allergy Clin Immunol 81:919–934, 1988.
18. Beasley R, Roche WR, Roberts JA, Holgate ST: Cellular events in the bronchi in mild asthma and after bronchial provocation. Am Rev Respir Dis 139:806–817, 1989.
19. Boushey HA, Holtzman MJ, Shelley JM, Nadel JA: Bronchial hyperactivity. Am Rev Resp Dis 121:389–413, 1980.
20. Hirshman CA: Airway reactivity in humans. Anesthesiology 58:170–177, 1983.
21. Barnes PJ: Asthma as an axon reflex. Lancet 1:242–245, 1986.
22. Schaefer G, Silverman F: Pregnancy complicated by asthma. Am J Obstet Gynecol 82:182–191, 1961.
23. Turner ES, Greenberger PA, Patterson R: Management of the pregnant asthmatic patient. Ann Intern Med 93:905–918, 1980.
24. Friedman A, Solomons E: Asthma in pregnancy. Am J Obstet Gynecol 74:318–323, 1957.
25. Gordon M, Niswander KR, Berendes H, Kantor AG: Fetal morbidity following potentially anoxigenic obstetric conditions. VII. Bronchial asthma. Am J Obstet Gynecol 106:421–429, 1970.
26. Hernandez E, Angell CS, Johnson JWC: Asthma in pregnancy: Current concepts. Obstet Gynecol 55:739–743, 1980.
27. Holbreich M: Asthma and other allergic disorders in pregnancy. Am Fam Pract 25:187–192, 1982.
28. Gluck JC, Gluck PA: The effects of pregnancy on asthma: A prospective study. Ann Allergy 37:164–168, 1976.
29. Jensen K: Pregnancy and allergic disease. Acta Allergol (Kbh) 6:44–53, 1953.
30. Apter AJ, Greenberger PA, Patterson R: Outcomes of pregnancy in adolescents with severe asthma. Arch Intern Med 149:2571–2575, 1989.
31. Gee JBL, Pacher BS, Miller JE, Robin ED: Pulmonary mechanics during pregnancy. J Clin Invest 46:945–952, 1967.
32. Fishburne JI: Physiology and disease of the respiratory system in pregnancy. J Reprod Med 22:177–189, 1979.
33. Williams DA: Asthma and pregnancy. Acta Allerg 22:311–323, 1967.
34. Weinstein AM, Dubin BD, Podleski WK, Spector SL, Fair RS: Asthma and pregnancy. JAMA 241:1161–1165, 1979.
35. Schatz M, Harden K, Forsyth A, Chilingar L, Hoffman C, Sperling W, Zeiger RS: The course of asthma during pregnancy, postpartum and with successive pregnancies: A prospective analysis. J Allergy Clin Immunol 81:509–517, 1988.
36. Kochenour NK, Lavey JP: Managing asthma in the pregnant patient. Contemp Obstet Gynecol 7:27–35, 1976.

37. Topilsky M, Levo Y, Spitzer SA, Levinski U, Atsmon A: Status asthmaticus in pregnancy: A case report. Ann Allergy 32:151–153, 1974.

38. Bahna SL, Bjerkedal T: The course and outcome of pregnancy in women with bronchial asthma. Acta Allergy 27:397–406, 1972.

39. Stenius-Aarniala B, Pirala P, Teramo K: Asthma and pregnancy: A prospective study of 198 pregnancies. Thorax 43:12–18, 1988.

40. Schatz M, Patterson R, Zeitz S, O'Rourke J, Melam H: Corticosteroid therapy for the pregnant asthmatic patient. JAMA 233:804–807, 1975.

41. Fitzimmons R, Greenberger PA, Patterson R: Outcome of pregnancy in women requiring corticosteroids for severe asthma. J Allergy Clin Immunol 78:349–353, 1986.

42. Greenberger PA, Patterson R: The outcome of pregnancy complicated by severe asthma. Allergy Proc 9:539–543, 1988.

43. Barger LW, Vollmer WM, Felt RW, Buist AS: Further investigation into the recent increase in asthma death rates: A review of 41 asthma deaths in Oregon in 1982. Ann Allergy 60:31–39, 1988.

44. Robin ED: Death from bronchial asthma. Chest 93:614–618, 1988.

45. Lao TT, Huengsburg M: Labour and delivery in mothers with asthma. Eur J Obstet Gynaecol Reprod Biol 35:183–190, 1990.

46. Pratt WR: Allergic disease in pregnancy and breast feeding. Ann Allergy 47:355–360, 1981.

47. Sinaiko RJ, German DF: Perspective on asthma in pregnancy. West J Med 131:315–316, 1979.

48. Reinisch JM, Simon NG, Karow WG, Gandelman R: Prenatal exposure to prednisone in humans and animals retards intrauterine growth. Science 202:436–438, 1978.

49. Haahtela T, Järvinen M, Kaua T: Comparison of a beta-2 agonist, terbutaline with an inhaled corticosteroid, budesonide, in newly detected asthma. N Engl J Med 325:388–392, 1991.

50. Greenberger PA, Patterson R: Beclomethasone diproprionate for severe asthma during pregnancy. Ann Intern Med 98:478–480, 1983.

51. Spitzer WO, Suissa S, Ernst P, Horwitz RI, Habbick B, Lockcroft D, Boivin J-F, McNutt M, Buist AS, Rebuck AS: The use of beta agonists and the risk of death and near death from asthma. N Engl J Med 326:501–506, 1992.

52. Burrows B, Lebowitz MD: The beta agonist dilemma. N Engl J Med 326:560–561, 1992.

53. D'Alonzo GE: The pregnant asthmatic patient. Semin Perinatol 14:119–129, 1990.

54. Marx CM, Fraser DG: Treatment of asthma in pregnancy. Obstet Gynecol 57:766–767, 1981.

55. Pollowitz JA: Theophylline therapy during pregnancy. JAMA 243:651–652, 1980.

56. Greenberger P, Patterson R: Safety of therapy for allergic symptoms during pregnancy. Ann Intern Med 89:234–237, 1978.

57. Greenberger PA, Patterson R: Management of asthma during pregnancy. N Engl J Med 312:897–902, 1985.

58. Schatz M, Reiger RS, Harden KM, Hoffman CD, Forsythe AB, Chilingar LM, Porreco RP, Benenson AS, Sperling WL, Saunders BS: The safety of inhaled bronchodilators during pregnancy. J Allergy Clin Immunol 82:686–695, 1988.

59. Snyder RD, Snyder D: Corticosteroid for asthma during pregnancy. Ann Allergy 41:340–341, 1978.

60. Warrell DW, Taylor R: Outcome for the fetus of mothers receiving prednisolone during pregnancy. Lancet 1:117–118, 1968.

61. Walker B, Patterson A: Induction of cleft palate in mice by tranquilizers and barbiturates. Teratology 10:159–163, 1974.

62. Kreisman H, Van de Wiel W, Mithel CA: Respiratory function during prostaglandin-induced labor. Am Rev Resp Dis 111:564–566, 1975.

63. Fishburne JJ, Brenner WE, Braaksma JT, Hendricks CH: Bronchospasm complicating intravenous prostaglandin $F_{2\alpha}$ for therapeutic abortion. Obstet Gynecol 39:892–896, 1972.

64. Huff RW: Asthma in pregnancy. Med Clin North Am 73:653–660, 1989.

65. Findley LJ, Sohn SA: The value of chest roentgenograms in acute asthma in adults. Chest 80:535–540, 1981.

66. Wulf KH, Kung LW, Lehman V: Clinical aspects of placental gas exchange. In Respiratory Gas Exchange and Blood Flow in the Placenta. LD Long, H Barkels, eds. National Institutes of Health, Bethesda, MD, 1972, pp 505–521.

67. Levinson G, Shnider SM, deLorimier AA, Steffenson JL: Effects of maternal hyperventilation on uterine blood flow and fetal oxygenation and acid-base status. Anesthesiology 40:340–347, 1974.

68. Wilson AF: Drug treatment of acute asthma. JAMA 237:1141–1143, 1977.

69. Benedetti TJ: Maternal complications of parenteral β-sympathomimetic therapy for premature labor. Am J Obstet Gynecol 145:1–7, 1983.

70. Woo SW: Anesthetic considerations. In Bronchial Asthma: Mechanisms and Therapeutics. EB Weiss, MS Segol, eds. Little, Brown, Boston, 1976.

71. Schreier L, Cutler RM, Saigal V: Respiratory failure in asthma during the third trimester: Report of two cases. Am J Obstet Gynecol 160:80–81, 1989.

72. Munakota M, Shosaka A, Fujimoto S: Bronchoalveolar lavage during third trimester pregnancy in patients with status asthmaticus: A case report. Respiration 51:252–255, 1987.

73. Geller M, Coslovsky S: Persistent cough as the sole manifestation of asthma in pregnancy. Ann Allergy 43:310, 1979.

74. Hague WM: Mediastinal and subcutaneous emphysema in a pregnant patient with asthma. Br J Obstet Gynaecol 87:440–443, 1980.

75. Caritis SN, Edelstone DI, Mueller-Heubach E: Pharmacologic inhibition of preterm labor. Am J Obstet Gynecol 133:557–577, 1979.

76. Stirt JA, Sullivan SF: Aminophylline. Anesth Analg 60:587–602, 1981.

77. Arwood LL, Dasta JF, Friedman C: Placental transfer of theophylline: Two case reports. Pediatrics 63:844–846, 1979.

78. Labovitz E, Spector S: Placental theophylline transfer in pregnant asthmatics. JAMA 247:786–788, 1982.

79. Yeh TF, Pildes RS: Transplacental aminophylline toxicity in a neonate. Lancet 1:910, 1977.

80. Symreng T, Karlberg BE, Kagedal B, Schildt B: Physiological cortisol substitution of long-term steroid-treated patients undergoing major surgery. Br J Anaesth 53:949–953, 1981.

81. Gran L, Pahle JA: Rational substitution therapy for steroid-treated patients. Anaesthesia 33:59–61, 1978.

82. Jolivet A, Blanchier H, Gautray JP, Dhem N: Blood cortisol variations during late pregnancy and labor. Am J Obstet Gynecol 119:775–783, 1974.

83. Jaffe JH, Martin WR: Opioid analgesics and antagonists. In The Pharmacologic Basis of Therapeutics, 8th ed. AG Gilman, TW Rall, AS Nies, P Taylor, eds. Macmillan, New York, 1980, pp 494–534.

84. Aviado DM: Regulation of bronchomotor tone during anesthesia. Anesthesiology 42:68–80, 1975.

85. Younker M, Clark T, Tessem J, Joyce TH III, Kubicek M: Bupivacaine-fentanyl epidural analgesia for a parturient in status asthmaticus. Can J Anaesth 34:609–612, 1987.

86. Marx GF: Obstetric anesthesia in the presence of medical complications. Clin Obstet Gynecol 17:165–180, 1974.

87. Craft JB Jr, Epstein BS, Coakley CS: Effect of lidocaine with epinephrine versus lidocaine (plain) on induced labor. Anesth Analg 51:243–246, 1972.

88. Abboud TK, Shnider SM, Wright RG, Rolbin SH, Craft JB, Henriksen EH, Johnson J, Jones MJ, Hughes SC, Levinson G: Enflurane analgesia in obstetrics. Anesth Analg 60:133–137, 1981.

89. White PF, Way WL, Trevor AJ: Ketamine—its pharmacology and therapeutic uses. Anesthesiology 56:119–136, 1982.

90. Namba Y, Smith JB, Fox GS, Challis JRG: Plasma cortisol concentrations during caesarean section. Br J Anaesth 52:1027–1031, 1980.

91. Freund FG, Bonica JJ, Ward RJ, Akamatsu TJ, Kennedy WF: Ventilatory reserve and level of motor block during high spinal and epidural anesthesia. Anesthesiology 28:834–837, 1967.
92. Gold MI, Helrich M: A study of the complications related to anesthesia in asthmatic patients. Anesth Analg 42:283–293, 1963.
93. Shnider SM, Papper EM: Anesthesia for the asthmatic patient. Anesthesiology 22:886–892, 1961.
94. Mallampati SR: Bronchospasm during spinal anesthesia. Anesth Analg 60:839–840, 1981.
95. Benatar SR: Anesthesia for the asthmatic. S Afr Med J 59:409–412, 1981.
96. Manchikanti L, Kraus JW, Edds SP: Cimetidine and related drugs in anesthesia. Anesth Analg 61:595–602, 1982.
97. Kingston HGG, Hirshman CA: Perioperative management of the patient with asthma. Anesth Analg 63:844–855, 1984.
98. Huber FC, Reves JG, Gutierrez J, Corssen G: Ketamine: Its effect on airway resistance in man. South Med J 65:1176–1180, 1972.
99. Corssen G, Gutierrez J, Reves JG, Huber FC: Ketamine in the anesthetic management of asthmatic patients. Anesth Analg 51:588–596, 1972.
100. Hirshman CA, Downes H, Farbood A, Bergman NA: Ketamine block of bronchospasm in experimental canine asthma. Br J Anaesth 51:713–717, 1979.
101. Stirt JA, Berger JM, Roe SD, Ricker SM, Sullivan SF: Cardiovascular effects of ketamine following administration of aminophylline in dogs. Anesth Analg 61:685–688, 1982.
102. Peltz B, Sinclair DM: Induction agents for caesarean section. Anaesthesia 28:37–42, 1973.
103. Jones MM, Joyce TH III, Adenwala J, Mawji F: Comparison of thiopental-nitrous oxide-halothane with ketamine-oxygen-halothane as anesthetic agents for cesarean section. Anesth Analg 64:S233, 1985.
104. Fish JE, Peterman VI: Effects of inhaled lidocaine on airway function in asthmatic subjects. Respiration 37:201–207, 1979.
105. Downes H, Hirshman CA: Lidocaine aerosols do not prevent allergic bronchoconstriction. Anesth Analg 60:28—32, 1981.
106. Hirshman CA, Edelstein G, Peetz S, Wayne R, Downes H: Mechanisms of action of inhalational anesthesia on airways. Anesthesiology 56:107–111, 1982.
107. Stirt JA, Berger JM, Ricker SM, Sullivan SF: Arrhythmogenic effects of aminophylline during halothane anestheisa in experimental animals. Anesth Analg 59:410–416, 1980.
108. Downes H, Hirshman CA, Leon DA: Comparison of local anesthetics as bronchodilator aerosols. Anesthesiology 58:216–220, 1983.

CHAPTER 29

Anesthesia for the Pregnant Diabetic Patient

Sanjay Datta, M.D.

Diabetes is the most common medical problem of pregnancy, occurring once in every 700 to 1000 gestations (1). However, advances in the obstetric and anesthetic management of diabetic parturients have considerably decreased perinatal mortality for insulin-dependent diabetic mothers (2). This chapter reviews the metabolic and hormonal adjustments in normal and diabetic pregnancy; the maternal, fetal, and neonatal complications of diabetes during pregnancy; and modern modes of treatment.

FUEL-HORMONE BALANCE DURING PREGNANCY

Pregnancy is associated with hyperplasia of the β cells of the maternal islets of Langerhans. Islets from pregnant animals secrete more insulin and are more sensitive to a lower dose of glucose than are islets from nonpregnant animals (3). These morphologic and secretory changes can be induced by treating animals with gestational hormones such as estrogen, progesterone, and human placental lactogen. Compared with nonpregnant controls, humans in the second half of pregnancy have higher basal plasma concentrations of immunoreactive insulin; therefore any glucose load produces a faster increase in insulin to higher peak plasma concentrations.

Pregnancy produces major changes in the homeostasis of all metabolic fuels. Plasma concentrations of glucose in the postabsorptive state decline as pregnancy advances, owing to increasing placental uptake of glucose and a probable limitation on hepatic output of glucose. Gluconeogenesis could be limited by a relative lack of the major substrate alanine.

Although fat deposition is accentuated in early pregnancy, later in gestation lipolysis is enhanced, and in the postabsorptive state more glycerol and free fatty acids (FFAs) are released. The lipolytic effects of human placental lactogen override the antilipolytic influence of insulin. Ketogenesis is also accentuated in the postabsorptive state during pregnancy.

During pregnancy the balance of metabolic fuels also differs for the fed state. Despite associated hyperinsulinism, the disposal of glucose is impaired, producing somewhat higher maternal blood levels, perhaps to ensure maximal "feeding" of the conceptus. The antiinsulin effects of gestation have been attributed to interference of human placental lactogen, progesterone, and cortisol (4). The decay of administered insulin in plasma is not greater during pregnancy, despite the presence of placental insulin receptors and degrading enzymes. Glucagon is well suppressed by glucose during pregnancy, and the secretory response of glucagon to amino acids is not higher than levels during nonpregnancy.

METABOLIC DISORDERS IN PARTURIENTS

Deficient secretion of insulin in type I insulin-dependent parturients increases glucose concentrations in the blood after meals. In the postabsorptive state, the liver manufactures more glucose by breakdown of glycogen secondary to lack of inhibition by insulin. Concentrations of insulin-sensitive branched-chain amino acids such as leucine, isoleucine, and valine are higher in diabetic subjects having fasting hyperglycemia (i.e., having glucose levels higher than 105 mg/dl during fasting) (5). Gluconeogenesis mainly takes place from the mobilization of amino acids and glycerol from the muscle and fat stores, respectively. Some of the FFAs released from adipose cells can be converted in the liver to triglycerides, cholesterol, and phospholipids (6). Knopp and colleagues (5) found elevated plasma triglyceride levels in obese pregnant women having gestational or adult-onset diabetes. In contrast, when compared with normal parturients, patients having juvenile-onset diabetes did not differ in plasma triglyceride levels. Because of a lack of insulin in diabetic patients, increased amounts of FFAs are converted to ketone bodies, acetoacetate, and β-hydroxybutyric acid. During pregnancy the physiologic changes of insulin resistance, increased lipolysis, and ketogenesis increase metabolic disturbances in diabetic women.

DIABETIC KETOACIDOSIS

Diabetic ketoacidosis is a major cause of perinatal morbidity. The fetal death rate can reach as high as 90%. Without careful and rigorous treatment, diabetic pregnant women are at increased risk of severe hyperglycemia and ketoacidosis (7). Four factors are mainly responsible for ketoacidosis in diabetics: a relative insulin deficiency, an excess of stress hormone, a lack of food, and dehydration. Glucose accumulates in extracellular fluid because of relative insulin deficiency and excessive stress hormone. Because of a lack of effect of insulin on adipose cells and because of elevated catecholamine and glucagon levels, excessive amounts of FFA are released. These increased FFAs provide increased substrate for hepatic ketogenesis. Water loss from osmotic diuresis secondary to glucosuria is excessive. Despite dehydration and hyperosmolarity, most patients with ketoacidosis can be hyponatremic. Insulin deficiency and glucagon excess exacerbate the loss of sodium in urine. Another major factor in hyponatremia is the shift of intracellular water to the extracellular space—because, without adequate insulin, cells are impermeable to glucose. Urinary and gastrointestinal losses produce a marked deficit in total body potassium. The potential for hyponatremia and hypokalemia must be a major consideration when treatment is formulated.

Hypertension

The incidence of hypertension and preeclampsia is higher in diabetic parturients than in the normal population (Table 29.1). Diabetic pregnant patients with associated nephropathy (class F) and hypertension may be more prone to pulmonary edema; this is related to both low colloidal oncotic pressure and left ventricular dysfunction (8).

Stiff Joint Syndrome (SJS)

Stiff joint syndrome is a rare condition seen in juvenile-onset diabetic patients and consists of rapidly progressive microangiopathy, nonfamilial short stature, tight waxy skin, and limited joint mobility or joint contractures. SJS frequently first involves the small joints of the digits and hands, and therefore, the failure to approximate the palmar surfaces of the interphalangeal joints ("prayer sign") is highly correlated with SJS (Fig. 29.1). Involvement of the atlanto-occipital joint may prohibit proper extension of the neck, and one might encounter difficult intubation in such a patient (9).

Table 29.1

Incidence of Prematurity, Hypertensive Complications, and Prematurity Caused by Preeclampsia in Gravidas with Insulin Requiring Diabetes, Antedating Pregnancy[a,b]

White's Class	Prematurity (%) (<37 weeks)	Hypertensive Complications (%)	Premature Deliveries due to Preeclampsia (%)
B	20.4	17.5	23.8
C	17.4	23.1	28.6
D	25.7	30.7	26.9
F	52.5	66.1	45.2
R	30.5	25.0	36.8
All classes combined	26.2	29.8	32.7

[a] Modified from Greene MF, Hare JW, Krache M, Phillippe M, Barss VA, Saltzman DH, Nadel A, Younger MD, Heffner L, Scherl JE: Prematurity among insulin-requiring diabetic gravid women. Am J Obstet Gynecol 161:106–111, 1989.
[b] Subjects grouped in White's classes. N = 420.

WHITE'S CLASSIFICATION OF PREGNANT DIABETIC WOMEN

White (10) classified diabetic pregnant women on the basis of the duration and severity of diabetes (Table 29.2). This system, which was used worldwide, was originally designed to predict perinatal outcome and to define arbitrary management goals. Because perinatal mortality has declined dramatically in all of White's classes, this system is no longer used to describe and compare populations of pregnant diabetic women. However, certain characteristics of patients in the different White classes are still pertinent. The risk of complications is minimal in gestational diabetic patients (glucose intolerance of pregnancy) or in class A patients whose diabetes is well controlled by diet alone; such patients may be otherwise managed as normal pregnant women. If insulin is required to keep fasting plasma glucose levels at less than 105 mg/dl or postprandial plasma glucose levels at less than 120 mg/dl, the patient should be managed as in class B. Class B women whose insulin dependence is of recent onset will probably have residual islet β cell function; although control of hyperglycemia may be easier than in class C or D patients, fetal and neonatal risk are generally equivalent. Finally, the most complicated and difficult pregnancies occur in women with renal, retinal, or coronary vascular disease.

PERINATAL MORBIDITY

Even with substantial advances in the treatment of diabetes, maternal mortality is slightly higher in diabetic parturients (11). Associated vascular disease

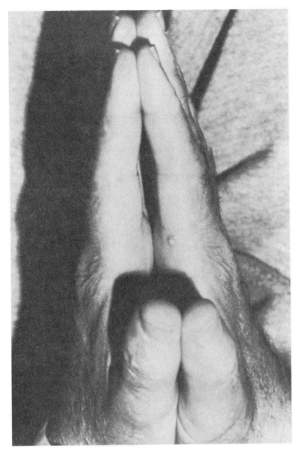

Figure 29.1. The patient is unable to approximate the palmar surfaces of the phalangeal joints despite maximal effort (a "prayer sign") because of diabetic stiff joint syndrome, which may also involve the atlanto-occipital joint (Reprinted by permission from Hogan K, Russy D, Springman SR: Difficult laryngoscopy and diabetes mellitus. Anesth Analg 67: 1162–1165, 1988.)

such as myocardial infarction, hypertension, and preeclampsia or renal disease can bring about major complications. Polyhydramnios is still common in diabetic parturients. Maternal convulsions following hypoglycemia can occur in early pregnancy in insulin-treated patients. Ketoacidosis may develop during the second and third trimesters.

The leading causes of morbidity in neonates of diabetic mothers are major congenital anomalies, intrauterine fetal distress, prematurity, respiratory distress syndrome (RDS), macrosomia, birth trauma, and neonatal hypoglycemia (12). At present congenital anomalies are the most frequent cause of perinatal mortality and morbidity in diabetic parturients. The incidence of congenital anomalies is as high as three times greater in infants of diabetic mothers. Poor metabolic control during the period from 4 to 8 weeks of pregnancy appears to be related to a higher incidence of such anomalies (14). In addition to in-

creased perinatal mortality, morbidity is also greater among these infants: hypoglycemia, hyperbilirubinemia, and hyperglycemia occur much more frequently in infants of diabetic mothers.

MANAGEMENT

Diet and Insulin Therapy

The diet of a diabetic parturient should consist of 30 to 35 cal/kg of ideal body weight. Carbohydrates should comprise 40 to 50% of the total calories, the remaining calories being divided between fat and protein. Lewis et al. (15) suggested that more protein be included in the diet to keep glucose concentrations at a constant level.

The ultimate goal of insulin therapy during pregnancy should be to avoid not only hyperglycemia, but also hypoglycemic reactions. The percentage of hemoglobin A_{Ic} (Hb A_{Ic}), a minor variant of hemoglobin A, increases with the severity of the disease (Fig. 29.2). Hemoglobin A_{Ic} also correlates well with mean daily capillary blood glucose levels over a few weeks during pregnancy (12). A sequential measurement of Hb A_{Ic} (range 5 to 10%) will provide the physician with another indicator of long-term control (Fig. 29.3). However, because insulin dosage must be frequently adjusted during the metabolically dynamic state of pregnancy, glucose levels (in capillary blood or urine) must be ascertained several times each day. Self-monitoring of capillary blood glucose levels at home with glucose oxidase strips and portable reflectance colorimeters has proved reliable in almost all patients and provides excellent end-points of therapy (16). At Brigham and Women's Hospital, the obstetrician's goal is to keep the average capillary blood glucose level at 100 mg/dl or less during fasting and at less than 140 mg/dl at 2 hr after eating.

Most insulin-dependent parturients require at least two injections of a 1:2 mixture of regular and intermediate-acting insulin each day to prevent fasting and postprandial hyperglycemia. Usually, two-thirds of the insulin is given before breakfast and one-third before supper. Occasionally, to manage patients whose blood glucose level is difficult to control, regular insulin is given three or four times each day with one or two injections of intermediate-acting insulin. Small portable pumps for continuous infusions of regular insulin are used at a few perinatal centers.

Monitoring of the Fetus

In the past decade the incidence of sudden intrauterine death in the third trimester of pregnancies complicated by diabetes was about 5 to 10%. Poor control of diabetes accompanied by ketoacidosis, preeclampsia, and diabetes-induced nephropathy were the major causes. Other factors included a combi-

Table 29.2
A Summary of White's (8) Classification of Diabetic Pregnant Women

Class	Characteristics	Implications
Gestational diabetes	Glucose intolerance diagnosed during pregnancy	Diagnosis before 30 weeks gestation is important to prevent macrosomia; treatment with diabetic pregnancy diet of adequate calories to prevent maternal weight loss; goal is fasting plasma glucose <105 mg/dl, 2-hr postprandial plasma glucose <120 mg/dl; if insulin is necessary, manage as in classes B, C, D.
A	Chemical diabetes diagnosed before pregnancy; managed by diet alone; any age of onset	Management same as gestational diabetes.
B	Insulin treatment necessary before pregnancy; onset ≥ age 20 years; duration < 10 years	Some endogenous insulin secretion may persist; insulin resistance at the cellular level in obese women; fetal and neonatal risks equivalent to class C and D, as in management.
C	Onset age 10–20 years, or duration 10–20 years	Insulin-deficient diabetes of juvenile onset.
D	Onset < age 10 years, or duration > 20 years, or chronic hypertension (not preeclampsia) or benign retinopathy (tiny hemorrhages)	Fetal macrosomia or intrauterine growth retardation possible; so-called retinal microaneurysms may progress during pregnancy, then regress after delivery.
F	Diabetic nephropathy with proteinuria	Anemia and hypertension common; proteinuria increases in third trimester, declines after pregnancy; fetal intrauterine growth retardation common; perinatal survival about 85% under optimal conditions; bed rest necessary (class T [postrenal transplant] outlook is good).
R	Malignant proliferative retinopathy	Neovascularization; risk of vitreous hemorrhage or retinal detachment; laser photocoagulation is useful; abortion usually not necessary; route of delivery is controversial.
H	Coronary artery disease	Grave maternal risk.

nation of relative fetal hypoxia and hyperglycemia, severe hypoglycemia, or fetal myocardial dysfunction.

Recent technologic advances have allowed for the earlier detection of fetal distress and have facilitated prevention of stillbirth. For example, ultrasound quantitates fetal activity patterns. Also, measurement of estriol levels in maternal urine and serum is an important diagnostic tool because estriol is produced by the placenta from aromatization of dehydroepiandrosterone sulfate, manufactured by the fetal adrenals and further hydroxylated in the fetal liver. Hence, most estriol in the maternal compartment is a product of fetal placental function. Chronically low maternal levels (below 95% confidence limits for the stage of gestation) or a rapid fall below 40% from the mean estriol level of the previous 3 days may indicate fetal distress. Estriol assays must be performed daily to be of value in preventing stillbirths in high-risk pregnancies. However, more recently, ultrasound ex-

aminations of fetal well-being are rapidly replacing the importance of estriol determinations.

In such pregnancies, the fetal heart rate should also be monitored routinely. The oxytocin challenge test (OCT) was the first test to be used to establish the adequacy of placental perfusion. Deceleration of the fetal heart rate after uterine contractions signifies transient fetal hypoxia and deranged uteroplacental function. Recently, nonstress tests have become popular for the same purpose. With good long-term variability of the fetal heart rate and accelerations greater than 15 beats per minute (bpm) with fetal movements, fetal well-being can be predicted. If the fetus is nonreactive even with stimulation, a full OCT is performed. Diabetic parturients should be hospitalized early if control of diabetes is poor, if hypertension is significant, or if fetal well-being is suspected of being in jeopardy. In the hospital, estriol levels should be measured daily and nonstress tests performed at least twice a week. If results of the estriol

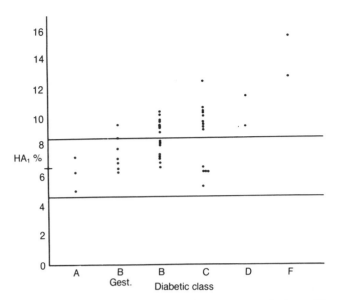

Figure 29.2. Hemoglobin A₁ (*HA₁*) measurements (*n* = 43) in 21 pregnant diabetic patients by diabetic class. Gestational class B includes gestational diabetics who require insulin to keep fasting blood sugar less than 100 mg/100 ml. Normal range for pregnancy is indicated (4.7–8.7%). Stepwise increase in hemoglobin A₁ by class related to increases in mean blood sugar, which also increased by class. (Reprinted by permission from O'Shaughnessy R, Russ J, Zuspan FP: Glycosylated hemoglobins and diabetes mellitus in pregnancy. Am J Obstet Gynecol 135:783–790, 1979.)

and fetal heart rate tests remain normal, the pregnancies should continue until term. Diagnostic specificity is increased by using both tests.

Experience at Brigham and Women's Hospital indicates that diabetic gravidas in whom capillary blood glucose levels can be extremely well controlled in the third trimester are at very low risk of antepartum fetal distress. Therefore such patients are not admitted to the hospital until the 38th or 39th week of gestation. After 36 week's gestation they are seen biweekly to assess the results of home blood glucose monitoring and nonstress tests.

Timing and Route of Delivery

Unless risks to the mother and fetus make it impossible, pregnancy should not be terminated until the 38th week of gestation to reduce neonatal morbidity from preterm deliveries. Before delivery the lecithin-sphingomyelin (L-S) ratio should be obtained by amniocentesis. According to the experience at Brigham and Women's Hospital, the incidence of severe RDS is 12% when the L-S ratio is 2:3. Therefore fetal lung is considered mature when the L-S ratio is 3.5 or greater (Fig. 29.4). Other amniotic fluid assays such as desaturated phosphatidylcholine, phosphatidylglycerol (PG), or the so-called

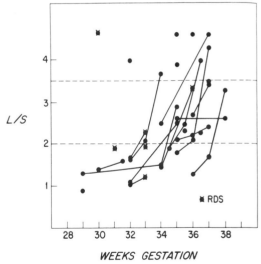

Figure 29.4. Lecithin-sphinogomyelin (*L/S*) values obtained at amniocentesis in pregnant women with diabetic nephropathy. Values representing sequential samples in the same patient are connected with *solid lines. Dotted line at 2* indicates usual level of predicted fetal lung maturity for infants of nondiabetic mothers. *Dotted line at 3.5* indicates levels used to predict low risk of severe respiratory distress syndrome in insulin-dependent diabetes mellitus. Amniotic fluid sample with an L/S value of 4.5 at 30 weeks was obtained after treatment of gravida with dexamethasone. (Reprinted by permission of Kitzmiller JL, Aiello LM, Kaldany A, Younger MD: Diabetic vascular disease complicating pregnancy. Clin Obstet Gynecol 24:112, 1981.)

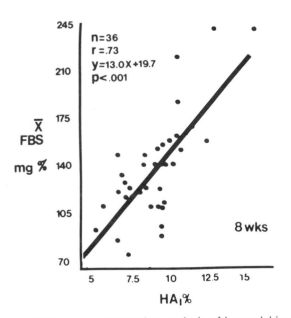

Figure 29.3. Linear regression analysis of hemoglobin A₁ (*HA₁*) from pregnant diabetic patients on mean of fasting blood sugar (*FBS*) values from prior 8 weeks. Standard error of the estimate = 26.9 mg/100 ml. (Reprinted by permission from O'Shaughnessy R, Russ J, Zuspan FP: Glycosylated hemoglobins and diabetes mellitus in pregnancy. Am J Obstet Gynecol 135:783–790, 1979.)

foam test are being evaluated for greater diagnostic specificity. The presence of PG in quantities greater than 1000 ng/ml is an extremely reliable indicator of fetal lung maturity. However, only 50% of fetuses will have fetal lung immaturity when the phosphatidylglycerol amount is less than 1000 ng/ml. Thus at Brigham and Women's Hospital, both L-S and PG are used for observation of fetal lung maturity.

The route of delivery is determined by several factors. If the ultrasonic examination confirms that the fetus is large (4300 g, 9.5 lb) cesarean section should be performed because of the possibility of shoulder dystocia. Otherwise, provided that the cervix and pelvis are favorably positioned, labor should be induced because fewer risks are associated with vaginal delivery. If the cervix is unfavorable for induction of labor, an attempt is made to "ripen" the cervix by inserting laminaria overnight. Continuous monitoring of the fetal heart rate and scalp pH values should be used routinely during labor because the incidence of intrapartum fetal distress (i.e., persistent late decelerations and scalp pH of less than 7.25) is high in pregnancies complicated by diabetes. At the author's institution, if progress of cervical effacement and dilatation is minimal on the first day, a "staged induction" is performed.

β-Adrenergic drugs such as salbutamol (17), terbutaline, and ritodrine (18) are used to arrest premature labor. These drugs can cause hyperglycemia and, subsequently, metabolic acidosis as a result of increased lactate and ketones. Corticosteroids are also used to accelerate lung maturation in premature babies. In diabetic subjects, these drugs also possess a potent hyperglycemic effect (19). As a result, severely uncontrolled diabetes can occur within a few hours of starting treatment, leading to a substantial increase in insulin requirement. Such an increase is best prevented by continuously infusing low doses of regular insulin intravenously.

Glucose and Insulin Therapy during Labor or Before Cesarean Section

Tight control of diabetes in the intrapartum period is essential. Maternal hypoglycemia may interfere with the progress of labor, whereas hyperglycemia may increase fetal distress.

Glucose crosses the placenta by facilitated diffusion. Oakley et al. (20) reported that, when maternal blood glucose levels were within the physiologic range, the difference in maternal and fetal blood glucose levels was approximately 20 mg/dl or less. In hyperglycemia, when the maternal level was over 300 mg/dl, the fetal blood glucose level plateaued at 150-200 mg/dl. At the author's institution, glucose levels in umbilical cord blood at delivery correlated well

with the somewhat higher maternal levels. Also, there did not seem to be an upper limit on placental transfer of glucose. Umbilical vein glucose concentrations were very high (over 300 mg/dl) after acute maternal volume expansion with solutions containing dextrose.

Disturbed glucose homeostasis during labor can result in neonatal hypoglycemia. Light et al. (21) observed a direct correlation between the rate of disappearance of glucose in infants of diabetic mothers (and ultimate neonatal hypoglycemia) and the concentration of glucose in umbilical cord blood. This relationship has been attributed to maternal hyperglycemia, producing fetal hyperglycemia and consequently fetal hyperinsulinemia.

Lactate concentrations increase in the plasma of the fetus when glucose or fructose levels are high in human (22) or animal (23) mothers. Shelley (24) observed an increased accumulation of lactate in fetal lambs during hyperglycemia and hypoxia. Bassett and Madill (25) confirmed these results. However, hyperglycemia did not appear to be harmful to well-oxygenated fetuses. Robillard et al. (26) compared fetal blood gases, pH, and plasma lactate concentrations at different levels of hyperglycemia in well-oxygenated sheep fetuses. Plasma lactate concentration increased, pH decreased (from 7.38 to 7.32), and blood gases were stable in the fetus when fetal plasma glucose concentrations were over 150 mg/dl. However, severe metabolic acidosis and concomitant decreases in blood gases and pH (from 7.38 to 7.18) occurred when fetal plasma glucose concentrations were over 300 mg/dl. Preliminary studies in primates by this author and others (27) showed that acute hyperglycemia accentuated metabolic acidosis secondary to acute hypoxia.

A well-recognized plan for insulin management for labor and delivery consists of administering one-third to one-half the pregnancy dose in the morning. Because the diabetic parturient is sensitive to insulin after delivery, insulin shock is possible if delivery is earlier than anticipated. West and Lowy (28) described low-dose intravenous infusion of insulin and glucose during labor. Patients were given a normal dose of insulin the day before delivery; thereafter food was withheld after 10 PM. The next morning the patients were given 1 liter of 5% dextrose every 6 hr together with Actrapid insulin, usually 1 to 2 units/hour. The insulin infusion was adjusted to keep the blood glucose concentrations between 90 and 125 mg/dl. None of the neonates became hypoglycemic.

On the other hand, Soler and Malins (29) also achieved good metabolic control of diabetic mothers and their babies by administering a standard dose of intermediate-acting insulin (i.e., 24 units for those requiring more than 60 units/day in the third trimester, and 16 units for those requiring less). During labor Soler and Malins infused 200 ml of 5% dextrose (10 g of glucose) hourly. This regimen was very successful if the blood glucose level during fasting on the day of induction of labor was less than 100 mg/dl. If the blood glucose level was higher, they recommended an intravenous infusion of insulin during labor.

Brudenell (30) reported a higher incidence of fetal distress when mothers were given a subcutaneous injection of insulin instead of an intravenous infusion of insulin (21% vs. 4%). Jovanovic and co-workers (31) studied glucose and insulin requirements during induction of labor in 10 insulin-dependent women with previously well-controlled diabetes. All patients received their usual subcutaneous dose of insulin in the morning (26 units PZI and 40 units NPH before breakfast) and before supper (10 units PZI). All had small amounts of food at 9 PM and no food after midnight. In the morning, the patients were transferred to the labor and delivery floor, where they had an external fetal monitor placed and connected to a Biostator to keep blood glucose concentrations between 70 and 90 mg/dl. (This machine maintains a constant glucose blood level using a continuous sensing device.) Glucose (5% dextrose with lactated Ringer's solution) was infused at a rate of 150 ml/hr. Blood glucose levels were kept normal during the administration of 7.5 mg of dextrose/hr, despite the fact that none of these patients required insulin in the intrapartum period.

The author's protocol for administering insulin during labor varies according to the fasting blood glucose level. If such levels are less than 120 mg/dl, intermediate-acting insulin is administered in one-third the daily dose given during pregnancy, and capillary blood glucose levels are measured every 1 to 2 hr during labor. If capillary blood glucose levels exceed 120 mg/dl during labor, an intravenous infusion of 0.5 to 2 units of regular insulin per hour is added. If the original fasting blood glucose levels are higher than 120 mg/dl, an intravenous infusion of insulin is used from the very beginning. In diabetic parturients, surprisingly little insulin is required to keep blood glucose levels almost normal during labor. If cesarean section is scheduled early in the morning, no insulin is given until after surgery. However, if abdominal delivery is planned later in the day, this author follows the same protocol for labor.

Anesthetic Considerations

Optimal anesthetic management of diabetic parturients requires an understanding of a few special pathophysiologic changes that occur in such patients.

DERANGED UTEROPLACENTAL BLOOD FLOW

Placental abnormalities are associated with even mild, well-controlled gestational diabetes in the mother (32). Nylund et al. (33) compared the uteroplacental blood flow index in the last trimester of pregnancy for 26 women with diabetes mellitus with that for 41 healthy control parturients. After injecting indium-113m intravenously, these investigators recorded the radiation over the placenta with a computer-linked gamma camera. Uteroplacental blood flow decreased 35 to 45% in diabetic parturients. Also, the index tended to be further impaired in those patients with higher blood glucose values. However, the reduction in the blood flow index in gestational diabetes did not differ statistically from that in severe diabetes. This result substantiated the ultrastructural study of the placenta by Jones and Fox (32), who observed identical placental abnormalities in women with well-controlled diabetes and in parturients with long-standing, moderately controlled disease. Bjork and Persson (34) observed that the placenta of diabetic patients was denser because the villi were enlarged. These enlarged villi can reduce the uteroplacental blood flow by reducing the intervillous space. Such changes in placental perfusion cause the infants of diabetic parturients to be more vulnerable to reduced placental blood flow.

IMPAIRMENT OF OXYGEN TRANSPORT

Hemoglobin A_{Ic} is two to three times higher in insulin-treated diabetes than in control subjects (35). In Hb A_{Ic}, glucose has entered the internal cavity of hemoglobin, and as glucose becomes convalently bound to two β-chains, the approximation of the H helices to each other is prevented. This movement is a normal allosteric response of the hemoglobin molecule for oxygen loading. In contrast to hemoglobin A, the oxygen affinity of Hb A_{Ic} is little affected by the in vitro addition of 2,3-diphosphoglycerate (2,3 DPG). No effect occurs because the binding of 2,3-DPG to hemoglobin is impaired by the presence of a hexose on the NH_2-terminal residues of HB A_{Ic} (36). Madsen and Ditzel (37) observed that red blood cell oxygen transport, saturation, and oxygen tension are impaired in insulin-dependent diabetic subjects (Figs. 29.5 and 29.6). In poorly regulated patients, in whom concentrations of Hb A_{Ic} are higher and concentrations of 2,3-DPG tend to be lower, oxygen release at the tissue level may be more impaired.

Another disadvantage of poor control of maternal diabetes is a chronic fluctuation of fetal blood glucose. Maternal hyperglycemia will be associated with

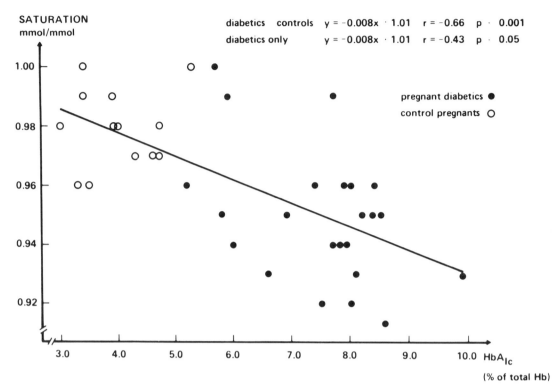

Figure 29.5. Correlation between hemoglobin A$_{lc}$ and arterial oxygen saturation in the diabetic women and in the total material. (Reprinted by permission of Madsen H, Ditzel J: Changes in red blood cell oxygen transport in diabetic pregnancy. Am J Obstet Gynecol 143:421–424, 1982.)

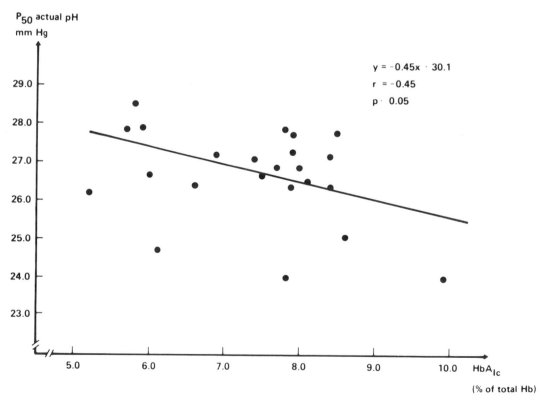

Figure 29.6. Correlation between hemoglobin A$_{lc}$ and P$_{50}$ (the partial pressure of oxygen at a hemoglobin saturation of 50%) at actual pH in diabetic women. (Reprinted by permission from Madsen H, Ditzel J: Changes in red blood cell oxygen transport in diabetic pregnancy. Am J Obstet Gynecol 143:421–424, 1982.)

fetal hyperglycemia and subsequently may lead to fetal hypoxemia and acidosis (38).

DERANGED BUFFERING CAPACITY IN INFANTS OF DIABETIC MOTHERS

In 1981 Brouillard et al. (39) observed that the infants of diabetic mothers may have a decreased buffering capacity and a different response to an increased acid load. In these infants, the affinity of hemoglobin to oxygen increased. Values for the partial pressure of oxygen at a hemoglobin saturation of 50% (P_{50}) were significantly lower in infants of diabetic mothers than in control infants (17.9 vs 22.6 torr). Normally as CO_2 or fixed acid increases in the blood, oxyhemoglobin affinity decreases and O_2 is released, thereby increasing the amount of reduced hemoglobin. This reduced hemoglobin is thus available for buffering. This principle is the "Bohr effect." When CO_2 or fixed acid is decreased in the blood, oxyhemoglobin affinity increases. Thus more hemoglobin is available for binding with O_2 because of its release of hydrogen ion. This is called the "Haldane effect." The higher intracellular pH values in infants of diabetic mothers is consistent with the fact that oxyhemoglobin affinity was also higher.

This multiplicity of problems makes the infants of diabetic mothers more vulnerable to hypoxia; hence, careful anesthetic management is mandatory.

Anesthetic Management

For labor and vaginal delivery, moderate pain relief can be obtained by administering small doses of narcotics in the early part of the first stage of labor. Lumbar epidural block can provide excellent pain relief for both labor and delivery. Pearson (40) noted that the fetus commenced the second stage in a less acidotic state when mothers were given epidural anesthesia than when mothers were given no anesthesia. Acidosis was metabolic in origin and was related to high lactate concentration. In 1980 Shnider et al. (41) showed that epidural anesthesia reduced the maternal endogenous catecholamines during labor, a reduction that might benefit placental perfusion. Such a benefit might be more important in diabetic parturients.

Spinal anesthesia can also be used if required at the time of delivery. If rapid infusion of a dextrose-free solution is necessary to treat hypotension while avoiding hyperglycemia, a separate intravenous catheter should be used. Also, it is important to realize that the fetus of a diabetic mother might be quite susceptible to hypoxia secondary to maternal hypotension.

Anesthesia for cesarean section requires special attention for diabetic parturients. The incidence of cardiovascular depression is higher during regional

anesthesia for cesarean section and is related to higher sympathetic blockade accentuated by compression of the inferior vena cava and aorta by the uterus.

In 1977 Datta and Brown (42) compared spinal and general anesthesia for abdominal delivery in healthy mothers and diabetic parturients. Infants of diabetic mothers given spinal anesthesia were more acidotic than infants of diabetic mothers given general anesthesia. Acidosis appeared to be related to both maternal diabetes and maternal hypotension. Subsequently, maternal and neonatal acid-base values were also examined after epidural anesthesia was administered in this special group of parturients (43). The incidence of neonatal acidosis (i.e., an umbilical artery pH value of 7.20 or less) during epidural anesthesia was 60%. Fetal acidosis was related to both the degree of maternal diabetes and to the presence of maternal hypotension. The umbilical artery pH value was always greater than 7.20 when the mother was not hypotensive. In both studies 5% dextrose with lactated Ringer's solution was used for acute volume expansion.

The genesis of fetal acidosis in diabetic parturients appears to be complex. The human placenta produces lactate in vitro, especially during hypoxia (44) or increased glycogen deposition, as occurs in maternal diabetes (10). The placenta of the ewe can also produce lactic acid (45). In sheep, such lactate accounts for 25% of fetal oxygen consumption, compared with 50% attributable to glucose use. Glycogen-rich placentas of diabetic parturients might contribute lactate to fetal blood during conditions of relative hypoxia, such as decreased uterine blood flow, which may happen during hypotension.

In human pregnancies, elevated fetal blood glucose levels have been associated with acidosis at birth. Swanstrom and Bratteby (46) observed a significant correlation between blood glucose concentrations and base deficits in infants with low 1-min Apgar scores. In a randomized controlled study of maternal intravenous fluid administration (with or without dextrose) in healthy patients undergoing cesarean delivery, Kenepp et al. (47) found significantly lower umbilical artery pH values in glucose-loaded infants. Fetal lactic acidemia might occur as a result of hypoxia (secondary to maternal hypotension) in the presence of hyperglycemia after acute volume loading with solutions containing dextrose. To test this hypothesis, Kitzmiller and co-workers (27) noticed the effect of acute hyperglycemia in monkey fetuses in response to acute maternal hypoxia. Hyperglycemic fetuses had (a) a greater reduction in arterial oxygen tension and content than did normoglycemic controls, despite similar values for maternal arterial oxygen partial pressure in each group, and (b) severe metabolic acidosis, compared with a modest reduction of arterial pH in normoglycemic fetuses. However, hyperglycemic monkey fetuses exposed to moderate maternal hypoxia did not have greater increases in blood lactate levels than did normoglycemic fetuses. Further investigation is necessary to determine the full nature of the interrelationship between blood glucose levels, oxygen content, and pH in pregnancies complicated by hyperglycemia. An additional risk of maternal and fetal hyperglycemia that accompanies acute volume expansion with dextrose-containing solutions before cesarean section in diabetic parturients is the occurrence of neonatal hypoglycemia. Soler and Mallins (29) reported an incidence of over 40% in their series when the mean maternal blood glucose level at delivery was more than 130 mg/dl.

Finally, Carson et al. (48) observed that chronic infusion of insulin directly into the sheep fetus increased fetal glucose uptake and oxidative use of glucose by the fetus and, surprisingly, reduced fetal arterial oxygen content. They speculated that hyperinsulinemia may increase oxygen consumption and that fetal hyperglycemia and hyperinsulinemia might result in reduced fetal oxygenation in pregnancies complicated by uncontrolled diabetes (38).

This author and others (49) recently reevaluated acid-base status in 10 rigidly controlled insulin-dependent diabetic mothers and 10 healthy nondiabetic controls undergoing spinal anesthesia for cesarean section. Dextrose-free intravenous solutions were used for volume expansion before induction of anesthesia, and hypotension was prevented in all cases by prompt treatment with ephedrine. No significant differences occurred in acid-base values between diabetic and nondiabetic mothers and between infants of diabetic mothers and infants of control subjects. Therefore, if maternal diabetes is well controlled, if dextrose-containing solutions are not used for maternal intravascular volume expansion before delivery, and if maternal hypotension is avoided, spinal anesthesia appears to be a safe technique for diabetic mothers undergoing cesarean section (Table 29.3).

In summary, the following criteria should be considered in the use of anesthesia for cesarean section in diabetic parturients.

1. *Acute hydration should be provided by administration of a dextrose-free solution before induction of anesthesia.* A separate intravenous catheter should be used. Solutions containing dextrose should be administered by constant infusion pump at the rate of 7.5 g/hr.

2. *Routine left uterine displacement should be*

Table 29.3
Comparison of Acid–Base and Blood Gas Data in Two Studies on Spinal Anesthesia for Cesarean Section for Diabetic and Nondiabetic Patients[a,b]

	1977		1982[c]	
	Healthy (n = 15)	Diabetic (n =15)	Healthy (n =10)	Diabetic (n =10)
Maternal artery				
pH	7.43 ± 0.02[d]	7.43 ± 0.01	7.42 ± 0.01	7.40 ± 0.006
Po$_2$ (torr)	218 ± 9	209 ± 7	200 ± 9	205 ± 8
Pco$_2$ (torr)	34 ± 4	33 ± 1	33 ± 2	33 ± 1
BD (mEq/liter)	0.67 ± 0.68	0.86 ± 0.56	1.3 ± 0.6	2.7 ± 0.5
Umbilical vein				
pH	7.34 ± 0.01	7.29 ± 0.02	7.35 ± 0.01	7.33 ± 0.01
Po$_2$ (torr)	37 ± 3	30 ± 2	30 ± 1	32 ± 3
Pco$_2$ (torr)	48 ± 2	52 ± 2	45 ± 2	48 ± 2
Umbilical artery				
pH	7.28 ± 0.01	7.20 ± 0.02	7.30 ± 0.01	7.27 ± 0.01
Po$_2$ (torr)	18 ± 1	18 ± 2	22 ± 2	20 ± 2
Pco$_2$ (torr)	63 ± 2	67 ± 2	50 ± 2.5	56 ± 2
BD (mEq/liter)	1.87 ± 0.73	5.67 ± 0.98	3 ± 0.7	4 ± 1
ΔBase deficit[d]	0.58 ± 0.25	4.14 ± 1.01	1.7 ± 0.3	1.4 ± 1

[a] Data taken from Datta S, Brown WU Jr: Acid-base status in diabetic mothers and their infants following general or spinal anesthesia for cesarean section. Anesthesiology 47:272–276, 1977; and Datta S, Kitzmiller JL, Naulty JS, Ostheimer GW, Weiss JB: Acid-base status of diabetic mothers and their infants following spinal anesthesia for cesarean section. Anesth Analg 61:662–665, 1982.
[b] Values are mean ± SE. Po$_2$ = oxygen partial pressure; Pco$_2$ = carbon dioxide partial pressure; BD = base deficit.
[c] In the 1982 study, prehydration was accomplished with dextrose-free solution and developing hypotension was treated immediately with ephedrine.
[d] Maternal artery base deficit − umbilical artery base deficit.

provided from the beginning of induction of anesthesia until delivery.

3. Hypotension should be treated promptly with intravenous injection of 10 to 30 mg of ephedrine.

4. An ester-type local anesthetic such as 2-chloroprocaine, which is rapidly hydrolyzed in both maternal and fetal plasma by pseudocholinesterase, might be considered.

5. Amide local anesthetics having a long half-life, such as mepivacaine, should be avoided.

6. Well-conducted general anesthesia can be used, if necessary, with good neonatal outcome. One should be aware of SJS and the possibility of difficult intubation in such patients.

After the procedure, regular insulin can be administered as needed in small doses. Lev-Ran (50) noted a drop in the insulin requirement to zero for 1 or 2 days in 11 of 12 patients undergoing cesarean section; in 3 of these 11 patients, hypoglycemia appeared. This temporary drop in the insulin requirement was followed by a steep rise in blood glucose levels. Thus judicious use of insulin is essential at this stage.

References

1. White P: Pregnancy and diabetes: Medical aspects. Med Clin North Am 49:1015, 1965.
2. Kitzmiller JL, Cloherty JP, Younger MD, Tabatabaii A, Rothchild SB, Sosenko I, Epstein MF, Singh S, Neff RK: Diabetic pregnancy and perinatal morbidity. Am J Obstet Gynecol 1312:560–580, 1978.
3. Kitzmiller JL: The endocrine pancreas and maternal metabolism. In *Maternal-Fetal Endocrinology.* DT Tulchinski, RJ Ryan, eds. WB Saunders, Philadelphia, 1980, pp. 58–83.
4. Malaisse WJ, Malaisse-Lagae F, Picard C, Flament-Durand J: Effects of pregnancy and chorionic growth hormone upon insulin secretion. Endocrinology 84:41–44, 1969.
5. Knopp RH, Montes A, Childs M, Li JR, Mabuchi H: Metabolic adjustments in normal and diabetic pregnancy. Clin Obstet Gynecol 24:21–49, 1981.
6. Kalkhoff RK, Jacobson M, Lemper D: Relative effects of progesterone, pregnancy and the augmented insulin response. J Clin Endocrinol 31:24–28, 1970.
7. Kitzmiller JL: Diabetic ketoacidosis. Contemp Obstet Gynecol 20:141–168, 1982.
8. Datta S, Greene MF: The diabetic parturient. In *Anesthetic and Obstetric Management of High Risk Pregnancy.* S Datta, ed. Mosby Year Book, St Louis, pp 407–422.
9. Hogan K, Rusy D, Springman SR: Difficult laryngoscopy and diabetes mellitus. Anesth Analg 67:1162–1165, 1988.
10. White P: Diabetes mellitus in pregnancy. Clin Perinatol 1:331–347, 1974.
11. Gabbe SG, Mestman JG, Freeman RK, Goebelsmann UT, Lowensohn RI, Nochimson D, Cetrulo C, Quilligan EJ: Management and outcome of pregnancy in diabetes mellitus, classes B to R. Am J Obstet Gynecol 129:723–732, 1977.
12. Datta S, Kitzmiller JL: Anesthetic and obstetric management of diabetic pregnant women. Clin Perinatol 9:153–166, 1982.
13. Robert MF, Neff NK, Hubbell JP, Taeusch HW, Avery ME: Maternal diabetes and the respiratory distress syndrome. N Engl J Med 294:354–360, 1976.
14. Gabbe SG: Congenital malformations in infants of diabetic mothers. Obstet Gynecol Surv 32:125–132, 1977.
15. Lewis SB, Murray WK. Wallin JD, Coustan DR, Daane TA,

Tredway DR, Navins JP: Improved glucose control in non-hospitalized pregnant diabetic patients. Obstet Gynecol 48:260–267, 1976.
16. Counstan DR: Recent advances in the management of diabetic pregnant women. Clin Perinatol 7:299–311, 1980.
17. Fredholm BB, Lunell NO, Persson B, Wager J: Actions of salbutamol in late pregnancy: Plasma cyclic AMP, insulin and C-peptide, carbohydrate and lipid metabolites in diabetic and nondiabetic women. Diabetologia 14:235–242, 1978.
18. Steel JM, Parboosingh J: Insulin requirements in pregnant diabetics with premature labour controlled by ritodrine. Br Med J 1:880, 1977.
19. Watkins PJ: Diabetic control in pregnancy and labour. J R Soc Med 71:202–204, 1978.
20. Oakley NW, Beard RW, Turner RC: Effect of sustained maternal hyperglycemia in normal and diabetic pregnancies. Br Med J 1:466–469, 1972.
21. Light IJ, Keenan WJ, Sutherland JM: Maternal intravenous glucose administration as a cause of hypoglycemia in the infant of the diabetic mother. Am J Obstet Gynecol 113:345–350, 1972.
22. Pearson JF, Shuttleworth R: The metabolic effects of a hypertonic fructose infusion on the mother and fetus during labor. Am J Obstet Gynecol 111:259–265, 1971.
23. Ames AC, Cobbolds Maddock J: Lactic acidosis complicating treatment of ketosis in labour. Br Med J 4:611–613, 1975.
24. Shelley HJ: The use of chronically catheterized foetal lambs for the foetal metabolism in combine. In *Foetal and Neonatal Physiology.* RS Gross, KW Dawes, PW Nathanielsz, eds. Cambridge University Press, London, 1973, pp 360–381.
25. Bassett JM, Madill D: Influence of prolonged glucose infusions on plasma insulin and growth hormone concentrations of foetal lambs. J Endocrinol 62:299–309, 1974.
26. Robillard JE, Sessions C, Kennedy RL, Smith FG Jr: Metabolic effects of constant hypertonic glucose infusion in well-oxygenated fetuses. Am J Obstet Gynecol 130:199–203, 1978.
27. Kitzmiller JL, Phillipe M, VonOeyen P, Datta S, Brouillard E: Hyperglycemia, hypoxia and fetal acidosis in rhesus monkeys. *Abstracts of Scientific Papers,* Society for Gynecologic Investigation, St. Louis, 1981, p 98.
28. West TET, Lowy C: Control of blood glucose during labor in diabetic women with combined glucose and low dose insulin infusion. Br Med J 1:1252–1254, 1977.
29. Soler NG, Malins JM: Diabetic pregnancy: Management of diabetes on the day of delivery. Diabetologica 15:441–446, 1978.
30. Brudenell JM: Delivering the baby of the diabetic mother. J R Soc Med 71:207–211, 1978.
31. Jovanovic L, Peterson CM, Saxena BB, Dawood MY, Saudek CD: Feasibility of maintaining normal glucose profiles in insulin-dependent pregnant diabetic women. Am J Med 68:105–112, 1980.
32. Jones CJP, Fox H: Placental changes in gestational diabetes. An ultrastructural study. Obstet Gynecol 48:274–280, 1976.
33. Nylund L, Lunell N-O, Lewander R, Persson B, Sarby B: Uteroplacental blood flow in diabetic pregnancy: Measurements with indium 113m and a computer-linked gamma camera. Am J Obstet Gynecol 144:298–302, 1976.
34. Bjork O, Persson B: Placental changes in relation to the degree of metabolic control in diabetes mellitus. Placenta 3:367–378, 1983.
35. Trivelli LA, Ranney HM, Lai H-T: Hemoglobin components in patients with diabetes mellitus. N Engl J Med 284:353–357, 1971.
36. Bunn HF, Briehl RW: The interaction of 2, 3-diphosphoglycerate with various human hemoglobin. J Clin Invest 49:1088–1095, 1970.
37. Madsen H, Ditzel J: Changes in red blood cell oxygen transport in diabetic pregnancy. Am J Obstet Gynecol 143:421–424, 1982.
38. Milley JR, Rosenberg AA, Phillipps AF, Molteni RA, Jones MD Jr, Simmons MA: The effect of insulin on ovine fetal oxygen extraction. Am J Obstet Gynecol 149:673–680, 1984.
39. Brouillard RG, Kitzmiller JL, Datta S: Buffering capacity and

oxyhemoglobin affinity in infants of diabetic mothers. Anesthesiology 55:A318, 1981.

40. Pearson JF: The effect of continuous lumbar epidural block on maternal and fetal acid-base balance during labor and at delivery. In *Proceedings of the Symposium on Epidural Analgesia in Obstetrics.* A Doughty, ed. Lewis, London, 1972, pp. 16–30.

41. Shnider SM, Abboud T, Artal R, Henriksen EH, Stefani SJ, Levinson G: Maternal endogenous catecholamines decrease during labor after lumbar epidural anesthesia. Am J Obstet Gynecol 147:13–15, 1983.

42. Datta S, Brown WU Jr,: Acid-base status in diabetic mothers and their infants following general or spinal anesthesia for cesarean section. Anesthesiology 47:272–276, 1977.

43. Datta S, Brown WU Jr. Ostheimer GW, Weiss JB, Alper MH: Epidural anesthesia for cesarean section in diabetic parturients: Maternal and neonatal acid base status and bupivacaine concentration. Anesth Analg 60:574–580, 1981.

44. Gabbe SG, Demer SLM, Greep RO, Villee AC: The effects of hypoxia on placental glycogen metabolism. Am J Obstet Gynecol 114:540–545, 1972.

45. Shelley JH, Bassett JM, Milner RDG: Control of carbohydrate metabolism in the fetus and newborn. Br Med Bull 31: 37–43, 1975.

46. Swanstrom S, Bratteby LE: Metabolic effects of obstetric regional analgesia and of asphyxia in the newborn infant during the first two hours after birth. Acta Paediatr Scand 70:791–800, 1981.

47. Kenepp NB, Shelley WC, Kuman S, Gutsche BB, Gabbe S, Delivoria-Papadopoulos M: Effects on newborn of hydration with glucose in patients undergoing cesarean section with regional anaesthesia. Lancet 1:645, 1980.

48. Carson BS, Phillips AF, Simmon MA, Battaglia FC, Meschia G: Effects of a sustained insulin infusion upon glucose uptake and oxygenation of the ovine fetus. Pediatr Res 13:147–152, 1980.

49. Datta S, Kitzmiller JL, Naulty JS, Ostheimer GW, Weiss JB: Acid-base status of diabetic mothers and their infants following spinal anesthesia for cesarean section. Anesth Analg 61:662–665, 1982.

50. Lev-Ran A: Sharp temporary drop in insulin requirement after cesarean section in diabetic patients. Am J Obstet Gynecol 120:905-908, 1974.

CHAPTER 30

Anesthesia for Neurosurgery during Pregnancy

Mark A. Rosen, M.D.

Over the past four decades, maternal mortality has progressively declined because of improved management of the major obstetric problems of hemorrhage, infection, and toxemia. As a result, the relative incidence of deaths resulting from nonobstetric causes during pregnancy has increased. Chief among nonobstetric causes are neurologic disorders. Those most common during pregnancy are intracranial tumors or subarachnoid hemorrhage (SAH) resulting from rupture of either a saccular aneurysm (1–9) or an arteriovenous malformation (AVM) (10–14). According to angiographic, surgical, and autopsy findings, SAH is the reported cause of 5 to 24% of maternal deaths (7, 8, 15). Primary and metastatic intracranial tumors are less common during the childbearing years, but their clinical course may be aggravated by pregnancy and make surgery a prerequisite for delivery of a viable infant.

This chapter reviews the pathophysiology of SAH, intracranial tumors, and benign intracranial hypertension during pregnancy and discusses an approach to the anesthetic management of these clinical situations. Although other neurosurgical disorders such as cerebral cysts or abscesses, sinus thrombosis, hydrocephalus (16–18), and spinal cord diseases (19, 20) are not specifically discussed, the principles of anesthetic management reviewed in this chapter may apply to them as well.

The objectives of neuroanesthetic management during pregnancy are the same as those for other nonobstetric surgery during gestation: to ensure maternal safety, to avoid teratogenic drugs, to prevent fetal asphyxia, and to avoid inducing preterm delivery. The goal of anesthesia for labor and delivery is to provide analgesia without endangering the fetus or aggravating the maternal neurologic disorder.

INTRACRANIAL TUMORS DURING PREGNANCY

Except for the neurologic complications of choriocarcinoma (21, 22), the relationship between preg-

nancy and a wide variety of intracranial tumors that present with symptoms during pregnancy is probably fortuitous (23). Although the incidence of brain tumors is no greater in pregnant than nonpregnant women, the clinical symptoms of tumors such as meningiomas (24), angiomas, neurofibromas, and pituitary adenomas (25, 26) are often precipitated or exacerbated by pregnancy. The mechanism of exacerbation is uncertain, but it is probably either tumor swelling caused by the generalized water retention characteristic of pregnancy (27, 28) or the engorgement of blood vessels feeding the tumor. There is no evidence that pregnancy itself increases mitotic activity. Pregnancy also does not alter the clinical signs, symptoms, indicators for diagnostic testing, or decisions to use corticosteroid treatment for cerebral edema or radiation treatment for tumors (with appropriate fetal shielding) when neurologic symptoms are mistaken for symptoms occurring in normal or complicated pregnancy. For example, vomiting may be interpreted as a normal occurrence in early pregnancy; headache or visual disturbance may be interpreted as preeclampsia; and convulsions may be mistakenly attributed to eclampsia (29–31). Consideration should be given to postponing elective surgical resection until after delivery when the maternal physiologic functions affected by pregnancy have returned to normal and the risk of adversely affecting the fetus is nonexistent. If a patient's clinical condition deteriorates during pregnancy, a craniotomy may be necessary.

SUBARACHNOID HEMORRHAGE DURING PREGNANCY

Subarachnoid hemorrhage (SAH) during pregnancy is typically related to either congenital saccular (berry) aneurysms or cerebral AVMs (with approximately equal frequency). Estimates of the incidence of SAH vary from less than 1 per 10,000 to 1 per 2500 pregnancies (1, 32). Precise incidence is difficult to determine because of the frequency of incorrect diagnosis (2).

Pathology

Saccular aneurysms are caused by congenital defects of the muscularis of arterial walls that occur at bifurcation or branching sites at or near the circle of Willis (Fig. 30.1). With continued stress by the forces of blood pressure, the internal elastica of the muscularis undergoes degeneration. The resulting aneurysms are usually less than 1 cm in diameter but can be as large as 5 cm. Autopsy specimens from women of reproductive age reveal a 0.5 to 1% incidence of unruptured saccular aneurysms.

An *AVM* is a network of tangled, interconnected thin-walled vessels in which arterial blood passes directly to venous drainage without intervening capillaries. Most AVMs are high-flow, low-resistance shunts with mean pressures of about half of systemic mean arterial pressures. The network is usually supplied by more than one artery and ranges in size from microscopic to massive. An AVM commonly extends from the surface of the brain into the parenchyma and may also occur in the spinal cord.

Etiology

Although distension leading to rupture of an AVM or saccular aneurysm often occurs when the patient is at rest, the most frequent precipitating factor for aneurysm rupture appears to be an episode of increased blood pressure, which may occur with coughing, straining, coitus, defecation, lifting, or emotional stress. There appears to be no correlation between hypertension and bleeding from an AVM (33).

No clear correlation between pregnancy and rupture of saccular aneurysms or AVMs has been established. Although some studies conclude that the association is merely coincidental (1, 2, 4, 5, 34), other studies suggest the incidence of saccular aneurysm rupture increases during the 30th to 40th gestational week, whereas the incidence of AVM rupture increases during the second trimester, shortly before labor, during delivery, and in the early puerperium (35). However, rupture of either may occur at any time during gestation, labor, or delivery. Physiologic factors that may contribute to rupture during pregnancy include the cardiovascular stresses of increased cardiac output and increased blood volume and the hormonal changes that affect the connective tissue integrity of vessel walls. The direct role of either of these factors remains unknown.

Pathophysiology

When an AVM or aneurysm ruptures, the sudden high-pressure leakage of blood raises intracranial pressure (ICP) and can cause reactions ranging from headache and drowsiness to coma, rapid brain dis-

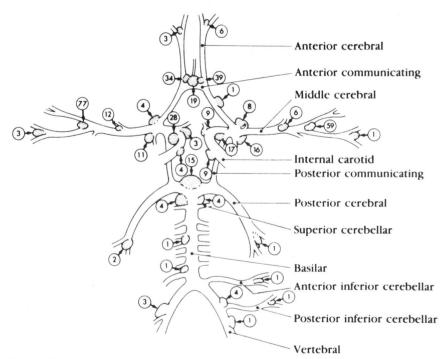

Figure 30.1. Location of 407 aneurysms in 300 consecutive patients. Numbers in circles represent the incidence. (Reprinted by permission from Peerless SJ: Intracranial aneu- rysms, neurosurgery. In *Handbook of Neuroanesthesia: Clinical and Physiologic Essentials*, 2nd ed. P Newfield, JE Cottrell, eds. Little, Brown, Boston, 1991.)

placement, and death, depending on the severity of the hemorrhage. The hemorrhage may remain subarachnoid or blood may dissect into brain parenchyma, resulting in focal neurologic deficits. An AVM involves brain parenchyma more often than does an aneurysm. The blood and its breakdown products irritate the meninges, parenchyma, and blood vessels. Meningeal irritation causes headache and sterile meningitis, which can lead to subacute or chronic communicating hydrocephalus. Brain irritation can evoke adverse descending autonomic discharges, causing hypertension, cardiac arrhythmias, and electrolyte and water disturbances. Vasospasm, caused in part by the breakdown products of extravasated blood, can lead to ischemia or infarction, resulting in neurologic deficits 5 to 7 days after the initial hemorrhage.

Prognosis

The prognosis for pregnant and nonpregnant patients is similar following rupture of a saccular aneurysm or an AVM. Frequently, hemorrhage recurs during the first few weeks following rupture (12, 36). With a saccular aneurysm, the overall mortality is higher. With an AVM, survivors sustain increased neurologic disability because of hemorrhage location and the tendency to bleed into brain tissue.

Diagnosis

An AVM (more often than an aneurysm) can sometimes be diagnosed before rupture via a history of severe headaches, seizures, bruits, cranial nerve palsies, or focal neurologic deficits. Typically, however, the presentation is SAH. The initial symptoms are the abrupt onset of severe headache (usually described as bursting or explosive); photophobia; nuchal rigidity; diplopia; nausea; vomiting; vertigo; disturbances of consciousness ranging from drowsiness or confusion to coma; seizures; migraines; bruits; and possibly focal or lateralizing neurologic signs such as hemiparesis.

Subarachnoid hemorrhage is diagnosed by a history and physical examination and confirmed by magnetic resonance imaging (MRI) or computed tomographic (CT) scanning and the appearance at lumbar puncture of grossly bloody or xanthochromic cerebrospinal fluid (CSF), with the latter occurring if the blood has hemolyzed since rupture. If there are lateralizing neurologic deficits or a suspicion of increased ICP, lumbar puncture should be deferred (37) and noninvasive MRI or CT scanning used. Although AVMs and aneurysms of less than 1 cm may not be visible, the site of the bleeding can be located. Angiography will confirm the specific cause and is safe for the fetus, provided the mother is in a stable con-

dition at the time (38, 39) and the fetus is protected by radiographic shielding.

DIFFERENTIAL DIAGNOSIS

The principal differential diagnosis of a ruptured saccular aneurysm or an AVM is either fulminant toxemia of pregnancy (with or without intracerebral hemorrhage) or a cerebrovascular accident secondary to chronic hypertension. An accurate diagnosis also includes the elimination of other neurologic conditions, such as meningitis or brain abscess, venous thrombosis, brain tumor, or intracranial vascular complications of choriocarcinoma.

Distinguishing toxemia of pregnancy from SAH is difficult, and errors in diagnosis and treatment have been made. The symptoms of hypertension, proteinuria, and either convulsions or coma can occur with both conditions. When hypertension and proteinuria are severe and edema generalized, the diagnosis is usually toxemia. Although both symptomatologies include headache, the toxemic headache is typically frontal and boring (or throbbing), whereas that of SAH is explosive or bursting. In addition, epigastric pain occasionally accompanies toxemia, but not SAH. Unusually high blood pressure also occurs more frequently with toxemia, but the hemorrhage of a ruptured aneurysm or AVM may raise ICP and cause a reflex increase in blood pressure. Because these profiles are similar, early neurologic consultation is advised whenever the diagnosis is uncertain or toxemic patients present with unusual findings.

MANAGEMENT OF SUBARACHNOID HEMORRHAGE: CONCERNS AND TREATMENT

Successful outcome of SAH requires aggressive and prompt investigation and treatment. The neurologic management of SAH is the same for pregnant and nonpregnant patients. The goals of treatment are to preserve life, reduce disability, prevent recurrent hemorrhage, and (for the pregnant patient) preserve fetal life. If an aneurysm remains untreated during a pregnancy, massive hemorrhage may recur and kill both mother and fetus.

Medical Management

The initial treatment of SAH is conservative. Traditional management includes (a) antihypertensive therapy to avoid increases in blood pressure caused by hypertension secondary to preexisting disease or irritation from subarachnoid blood; (b) absolute bed rest in a dark, quiet room; and (c) the cautious use of sedatives and analgesics to avoid emotional excitement. Stool softeners are recommended to avoid straining and the Valsalva maneuver. Steroids are administered to reduce cerebral edema and anticonvulsants are administered to prevent seizures. Some medical centers use antifibrinolytic agents such as ϵ-aminocaproic acid to inhibit lysis of the clot formed at the bleeding site and to prevent recurrent bleeding. Vasospasm is treated by increasing the intravascular volume and applying various regimens that increase blood pressure, including aminophylline and isoproterenol, and agents to counteract vasospasm, such as calcium channel-blocking drugs.

Abortion or cesarean section are performed only if obstetrically indicated. Exceptions arise when fetal maturity is adequate and the size, location, and surgical assessment of the lesion suggest urgent neurosurgical repair (40) or when massive hemorrhage occurs late in pregnancy and the mother is in deep coma and moribund (41). Cesarean section may be necessary to save a viable fetus, and the staff must be prepared to perform an agonal cesarean section.

Surgical Management

The decision and time for surgery are determined by the site and surgical accessibility of a lesion, a patient's clinical condition (particularly the clinical grade of consciousness), and the presence of vasospasm. These decisions should rarely, if ever, be influenced by pregnancy. If SAH occurs after fetal lung maturity is possible, consideration should be given to elective cesarean delivery followed by repair of the aneurysm or AVM. Factors contributing to the successful decline in the morbidity and mortality of intracranial aneurysm surgery include early clipping of the aneurysm after the initial bleed (< 1 to 2 weeks) to decrease the risk of re-bleed (about 20% in the first 2 weeks); the use of antifibrinolytic agents; better control of cerebral edema; and improved preoperative and postoperative intensive care, particularly postoperative hypervolemic and hypertensive therapy. Improvements in surgical and anesthetic techniques include the use of magnification and illumination, self-retaining retraction, use of temporary proximal clips, adjuncts to decrease ICP and produce brain relaxation, anesthetic techniques to maximize cerebral perfusion during temporary cerebral artery occlusion, deliberate hypotension, and intravascular volume expansion and hypertension after permanent clip application (42). Surgical clipping, trapping, ligation, or reinforcement of saccular aneurysms has greatly reduced the incidence of and mortality from recurrent hemorrhage. The advantages of surgical resection and ligation of the feeding arteries of an AVM depend on its size and location. Alternative interventional therapies include particulate embolization, obliteration with intravascular glue, and proton-beam irradiation.

Anesthetic Management

The particular hazards of anesthesia during pregnancy stem from physiologic changes in the mother and potential adverse effects on the fetus. Hormonal secretions from the corpus luteum and the placenta and the mechanical effects of the gravid uterus induce major changes in practically every organ system. It is important to understand these changes and their implications for anesthetic management to ensure the safest possible administration of anesthesia during pregnancy. These concerns are the subject of Chapters 1 and 14.

AVOIDANCE OF FETAL ASPHYXIA

Fetal oxygenation depends on maternal arterial oxygen content and placental blood flow. Although hypotension and hypocarbia are commonly induced during neurosurgery, these techniques may place a fetus at risk for intrauterine asphyxia. This can be avoided by maintaining normal maternal PaO_2, $PaCO_2$, and uterine blood flow.

The causes and treatment of maternal hypoxia during general anesthesia do not differ from those for any ventilated patient. The hyperoxia that commonly occurs during anesthesia presents no risk to the fetus. Maternal PaO_2 may rise to 600 mm Hg without producing a fetal PaO_2 above 45 to 60 mm Hg. Thus the fetus is never at risk in utero for premature closure of the ductus arteriosus or retrolental fibroplasia.

Maternal $PaCO_2$ directly affects fetal $PaCO_2$. Maternal hypercapnia causes fetal respiratory acidosis. Hypocapnia produced by excessive positive pressure ventilation may increase mean intrathoracic pressure, decrease venous return, and decrease cardiac output, causing a decrease in uterine blood flow that can harm the fetus. Maternal alkalosis will reduce the umbilical blood flow by direct vasoconstriction, increasing the affinity of maternal hemoglobin for oxygen and thereby decreasing the release of oxygen to the fetus at the placenta. Fetal hypoxia and acidosis may result.

Maternal blood pressure directly affects uterine arterial blood flow. A decrease in blood pressure leading to hypotension causes a decrease in uterine blood flow that may lead to fetal asphyxia. During light anesthesia induced with halothane, the decrease in blood pressure is slight and does not significantly reduce uterine blood flow because uterine vascular resistance also decreases. However, deep halothane anesthesia producing maternal hypotension (30% decrease from control) impairs uterine blood flow and results in fetal asphyxia. Therefore significant maternal hypotension should be avoided or treated promptly by administering fluids, reducing anesthetic concentration, or administering an appropriate vasopressor such as ephedrine if necessary.

AVOIDANCE OF TERATOGENIC DRUGS

Each organ and system during gestation undergoes a critical stage of differentiation during which vulnerability to teratogens is greatest and specific malformations may occur. In humans, the first trimester of pregnancy appears to be the most vulnerable period.

Teratogenicity may be induced by exogenous agents at different stages of gestation, yet it remains undetected until birth or later. To produce a defect requires that (a) a teratogen be introduced at the dose that causes defect; (b) the embryo or fetus be at a species-specific developmental stage; and (c) the embryo or fetus be genetically susceptible to the teratogen.

Almost all commonly used anesthetic and premedicant drugs are known to be teratogenic in some animal species. Hyperbaric oxygenation, hypoxia, and hypercapnia may also be teratogenic in animals. In surveys of women anesthetized for surgery during pregnancy (first trimester included), no specific drug was found safer than another, and no specific agent was found to be teratogenic (43–49). However, too few cases have been reported to support a conclusion that anesthetic drugs are nonteratogenic. Nevertheless, the choice of anesthesia for obstetric patients undergoing neurosurgery is not currently influenced by a concern for teratogenic effects. (For a more detailed discussion of anesthetic agent teratogenesis, see Chapter 14.)

PREVENTION OF PRETERM LABOR

It has been suggested that abdominal operations during pregnancy may cause preterm labor during the postoperative period, and that anesthesia and surgery during pregnancy may increase the risk of first and second trimester spontaneous abortions. Although the influence of anesthetics on preterm labor is unknown, the likelihood that anesthetics may stimulate preterm labor during a neurosurgical procedure is small. In fact, no direct correlation of neurosurgical procedures with preterm labor exists. Nevertheless, patients should be monitored intraoperatively and postoperatively (for at least 24 hr) for uterine contractions. Early detection of preterm labor is critical for early treatment with labor-inhibiting drugs that may avoid premature delivery. During a neurosurgical procedure, the use of drugs that increase uterine tone, such as α-adrenergic vasopressors, should be avoided, as should the rapid intravenous administration of anticholinesterase drugs.

Complications of Adjuvants to Lower Intracranial Pressure

During neurosurgery, osmotic diuresis, controlled hypotension, hypothermia, and hypocarbia are com-

monly induced to lower ICP. In the pregnant patient, however, these adjuvants may adversely affect the fetus. The decision to use them should depend on the gravity of the maternal impairment and the determination that the risk of maternal or fetal morbidity from the impairment is greater than that posed by the use of the adjuvant. A recent trend has been towards an increased use of temporary clips instead of deliberate hypotension to reduce pressure in an aneurysm during dissection before permanent clip application.

OSMOTIC DIURETICS

Osmotic diuretics such as mannitol and urea are used to reduce cerebral water content. They have been shown to traverse the placenta, raise the fetal plasma osmotic pressure, and cause a net flow of water from the fetus to the mother (50, 51). This fluid exchange decreases fetal blood volume, total body water, and extracellular fluid volume and can cause severe fetal dehydration. However, low doses of osmotic diuretic agents have been used without adverse fetal outcome (41). Consequently, these drugs should be used only when absolutely necessary during pregnancy and should be given in low doses, recognizing potential adverse fetal effects.

CONTROLLED HYPOTENSION

Inducing controlled hypotension in a pregnant patient undergoing craniotomy for vascular lesions will reduce the likelihood of maternal cerebral hemorrhage but may cause fetal asphyxia. Although hypotensive techniques have been successfully used in some cases (1, 8, 52), fetal death or distress (based on fetal heart rate monitoring) has resulted from their use in others (6, 53, 54). The "success" reported is often measured by a living fetus or live birth with no assessment of fetal neurologic status or pediatric follow-up.

The hazard to the fetus depends on the severity and duration of the maternal hypotension. Fetal risk is directly related to uterine blood flow, which varies directly with maternal blood pressure. When uterine blood flow is reduced sufficiently, fetal asphyxia results, damaging the fetal central nervous system, heart, and lungs. In fetal monkeys who sustained asphyxia of intermediate severity and duration with consequent acidosis, permanent brain injury occurred, producing lesions similar to those of human cerebral palsy (55). Severe asphyxia produced fetal death from myocardial failure.

The drugs commonly used to induce hypotension are halogenated anesthetic agents, sodium nitroprusside, nitroglycerin, and trimethaphan. Light *halothane or isoflurane* anesthesia is not associated with significant reductions in uterine blood flow because of concomitant decreases in uterine vascular resistance. However, high concentrations of these agents, which depress myocardial contractility and produce significant hypotension, cause decreased uterine blood flow and consequent fetal asphyxia.

Sodium nitroprusside (SNP), the drug most widely used for inducing hypotension, rapidly penetrates the placenta. SNP is degraded to cyanogen, then transformed to thiocyanate (by the liver enzyme rhodonase). Cyanogen is potentially toxic to the fetus (56, 57). In pregnant animals given SNP, peak arterial cyanide levels appearing in the fetus are significantly higher than those in the mother. This may be due to a more rapid fetal formation of cyanide or to a slower fetal rate of detoxification and excretion. In hypertensive pregnant sheep given SNP, the hemodynamic effects of the drug compromise uterine blood flow (58, 59). Although SNP has been used to treat systemic and pulmonary hypertension and to induce intraoperative hypotension without harm to the fetus (60, 61), its administration to pregnant patients should be limited to small doses for short periods of time. If tachyphylaxis or metabolic acidosis develop or if more than 0.5 mg/kg/h is infused, SNP should be promptly discontinued.

To date, the use of *nitroglycerin* (NTG) during pregnancy has demonstrated no adverse fetal or neonatal effects. NTG has been shown to be effective in reducing norepinephrine-induced hypertension in gravid ewes (62), and has been used successfully in humans (63, 64). It is essentially nontoxic and metabolizes the glyceryl dinitrate and nitrite in the presence of glutathione. Onset is slower than that of SNP, and more patients are resistant to its hypotensive effect. Since NTG is absorbed on many plastics, it should be infused using glass bottles and polyethylene tubing.

The use of *trimethaphan* to induce hypotension via ganglionic blockade has greater effect on pregnant than nonpregnant women. In supine pregnant women, the hypotensive effect of autonomic blockade depends primarily on venous pooling of blood, which decreases the return of blood to the heart and diminishes cardiac output. Autonomic blockade also prevents the increase in neurogenic tone of the capacitance vessels that ordinarily compensates for the venous obstruction resulting when the uterus of the supine patient compresses the inferior vena cava. Trimethaphan-induced blockade also prolongs the action of succinylcholine by inhibiting plasma pseudocholinesterase and may impair neurologic assessment in the postoperative period by causing dilation of the pupils.

When it is necessary to induce hypotension in pregnant patients, blood pressure reduction should be limited in depth and duration to the minimum required, based on clinical judgment. The fetal heart rate should be closely monitored because fetal tolerance will depend on fetoplacental reserve. Maternal arterial pH should be measured frequently to avoid risks of severe fetal or maternal compromise.

HYPOCAPNIA/HYPERVENTILATION

Extreme maternal hyperventilation may result in a reduction of uterine blood flow, a decrease in placental oxygen transfer, a decrease in fetal P_{O_2}, anaerobic metabolism, and fetal metabolic acidosis. Thus in theory, the use of hyperventilation should be avoided. Mild hyperventilation is probably safe, although the fetal heart rate must be monitored for adverse effects. Fetuses with good reserves will not become acidotic in response to moderate maternal hyperventilation, but those in precarious or borderline situations may react adversely to even mild degrees of maternal hyperventilation. Normal maternal Pa_{CO_2} is 32 mm Hg, with a pH of 7.40 to 7.45. Hyperventilation that decreases Pa_{CO_2} by 5 to 10 torr is probably safe and easily reversible if fetal tachycardia or bradycardia indicate fetal intolerance. As with induced hypotension, the use of hyperventilation should be limited in extent and duration to the minimum required, based on clinical judgment. During periods of arterial occlusion with a temporary clip application, anesthetic techniques should be employed to maximize cerebral perfusion, including maintenance of blood pressure in the high normal range, and Pa_{CO_2} in the low normal range.

HYPOTHERMIA

Moderate hypothermia (temperatures of 28 to 32° C), properly used, decreases cerebral metabolic requirements for oxygen and reduces blood flow to the brain. Although uterine vascular resistance increases and uteroplacental blood flow decreases during hypothermia, oxygen transfer is unaffected. If maternal respiratory acidosis is prevented, the gas and acid-base contents of fetal blood will parallel those of the mother (65). The fetus will also become hypothermic, and its metabolic needs will proportionately decrease (66). For example, the fetal heart rate parallels the decrease in maternal heart rate during cooling, increasing again during rewarming (67, 68). The response of the fetus during hypothermia does not appear to increase the risk of fetal morbidity (1, 3, 6, 10, 11, 13, 52, 53, 68–71).

Monitoring of the Mother and Fetus during Craniotomy

In addition to the monitors used during major neurosurgical procedures (e.g., intraarterial catheter,

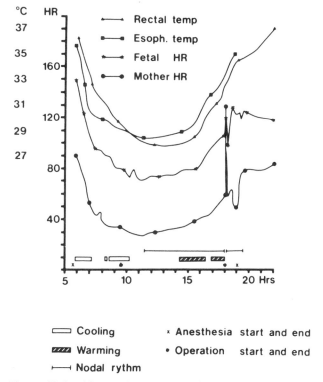

Figure 30.2. Maternal temperature (esophageal and rectal) and heart rate (maternal and fetal) during anesthesia with hypothermia. The times when cooling and warming of the mother were performed and the time during which the mother had modal rhythm are indicated. The hours indicate the time of the day. (Reprinted by permission from Stange K, Hallidin M: Hypothermia in pregnancy. Anesthesiology 58:460–461, 1983.)

Doppler air-embolism monitor, and right atrial catheter), monitors of the fetus and uterus should be used if possible. If the uterine fundus is above the level of the umbilicus, an external tocodynamometer is usually effective for monitoring uterine activity. An external Doppler fetal heart rate monitor will usually detect fetal heart rate after the 16th week of pregnancy. Doppler monitoring is particularly useful because changes in heart rate may signal an abnormality in maternal ventilation, uterine perfusion, or fetal well-being. Close observation of maternal blood pressure and prompt treatment of hypotension and hypoxia are essential if the fetus is to have the best chance of surviving with an intact nervous system.

The responses of the mother and fetus to anesthesia are also important monitors of the well-being of both. For example, anesthetics that readily traverse the placenta diminish the normal beat-to-beat variability of the fetal heart rate. The drop in fetal heart rate during induced hypothermia parallels a decrease in the maternal heart rate (Fig. 30.2). However, when patterns of bradycardia emerge, they may indicate a fetal response to maternal hypotension or hypoxia.

Maternal systolic blood pressure of less than 100 torr may be associated with pathologic fetal bradycardia, which can begin a few minutes after the onset of maternal hypotension and may be preceded by mild tachycardia. Thus fetal tachycardia may also be an indicator of both maternal hypoxia and fetal distress.

THE ANESTHETIC COURSE FOR NEUROSURGERY

The Preanesthetic Visit

The preanesthetic visit is an essential part of each patient's preparation and assessment before surgery. The visit should include a physical examination, history taking, and an analysis of laboratory findings and consultants' reports. The patient's clinical grade should be assessed according to the Hunt system (72): Higher grades in this system are often associated with vasospasm, increased ICP, and increased surgical mortality. Any neurologic deterioration associated with preoperative decreases in blood pressure should be noted to avoid intraoperative systemic blood pressures that fall below critical levels of cerebral perfusion pressure. Before surgery, the patient's state of hydration and electrolyte balance should also be evaluated and corrected if necessary. Abnormalities in electrocardiogram data are common after SAH, including T wave inversion or flattening, S-T segment depression or elevation, U waves, and prolonged Q-T intervals. Sinus bradycardia and premature ventricular contractions are also common.

Special efforts should be made to decrease the patient's apprehension by providing reassurance and emotional support. Maternal stress and anxiety are associated with an increased release of endogenous catecholamines that decreases uterine blood flow, potentially harming the fetus. The patient is concerned not only for her own welfare, but for that of her unborn child. The anesthesiologist should convey optimism about both the maternal and fetal prognosis and reassure the mother that the welfare of the baby will be considered at all times.

Preoperative Medication

Heavy sedation is contraindicated because of the potential for respiratory depression, potential exacerbation of depressed consciousness, and delayed postoperative recovery of consciousness. Preoperative sedation may be omitted in many cases, with increased safety for the patient. If some sedation is necessary, pentobarbital (50 to 100 mg intramuscularly) may be preferable to benzodiazepines, phenothiazines, or narcotics. If possible, patients should be given medication to reduce gastric acidity.

Transport and Positioning of the Patient

Ideally, after the beginning of the second trimester, patients should not be placed in the supine or prone positions when transported to surgery or positioned on the surgical table. They should be placed in either a sitting or lateral decubitus position. If placed supine, left uterine displacement should be used. Proper positioning will minimize the risk of obstruction of the vena cava by removing the weight of the gravid uterus from the great vessels. The patient's legs should be wrapped in elastic bandages and placed level to her heart to facilitate venous return from the lower extremities. Her eyes should be protected with a small amount of protective eye ointment, tape, and patches.

Induction and Intubation

To establish an airway and protect the patient from possible regurgitation and aspiration, induction of anesthesia with intravenous drugs should be followed immediately by intubation of the trachea using a cuffed endotracheal tube and a rapid-sequence technique. This is important for pregnant women at more than 20 weeks of gestation and for all women with a history of gastric reflux.

The rapid-sequence technique of intravenous induction and endotracheal intubation, commonly performed for women undergoing cesarean delivery, is acceptable for neurosurgical patients provided they are adequately anesthetized before laryngoscopy. Pretreatment with a nondepolarizing drug can be followed by administration of succinylcholine without risk of increasing ICP. Alternatively, either a low or priming dose of a short-acting nondepolarizing drug can be given before the intubating dose (73–75). For example, 0.01 mg/kg of vecuronium can be given 4 min before a rapid-sequence induction using 0.1 mg/kg of vecuronium as the intubating dose for neuromuscular blockade. The conscious patient can be asked to voluntarily hyperventilate immediately before induction.

In a lightly anesthetized patient, rapid-sequence laryngoscopy and intubation may cause hypertension. This will raise the transmural pressure across the wall of an aneurysm and possibly cause rupture (Fig. 30.3). Administering a large dose of thiopental in combination with intravenous lidocaine or pretreatment with intravenous fentanyl can ameliorate this response. The use of nitroprusside (76), nitroglycerin (63), or short-acting β-blocking agents such as esmolol or labetalol to achieve a stable, modest blood pressure reduction (15 to 25%) immediately before induction will also blunt the hypertensive response.

Maintenance of Anesthesia

Light general anesthesia is usually adequate for positioning the patient. Additional thiopental (1 to

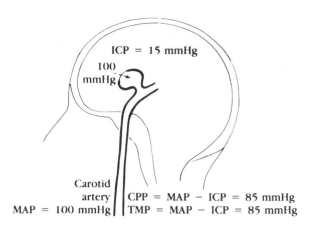

Figure 30.3. The transmural pressure (*TMP*) of the aneurysm is the same as the cerebral perfusion pressure (*CPP*) and equal to the difference between arterial pressure (*MAP*) and intracranial pressure (*ICP*). (Reprinted by permission from Colley PS: Intracranial aneurysms, anesthesia. In *Handbook of Neuroanesthesia: Clinical and Physiologic Essentials*, 2nd ed. P Newfield, JE Cottrell, eds. Little, Brown, Boston, 1991.)

2 mg/kg) is given 30 to 60 sec before placement of the pin headholder. Once adequate controlled ventilation has been established, inhalation anesthesia can be used to supplement the intravenous agents used for induction. Isoflurane may be preferable to halothane or enflurane because it has less effect on cerebral blood volume and thus helps to maintain cerebral perfusion and because it reduces cerebral metabolic oxygen requirements. In addition, isoflurane's low blood gas solubility permits more rapid elimination of the anesthetic at the conclusion of the surgical procedure.

Postoperative Management

The postoperative management of pregnant patients after craniotomy differs only slightly from that of nonpregnant patients. Although smooth emergence and extubation are ideal, extubation should be delayed until the patient is sufficiently awake to protect her airway from regurgitation and aspiration of gastric contents. Maintaining left uterine displacement is important to avoid hypotension from the supine compression of the great vessels by the gravid uterus. The patient should be placed in a lateral position with her head slightly elevated during the entire postoperative period, including during transport from the operating room to the recovery area. The fetal heart rate and uterine tone should be monitored for at least 24 hr or until the mother's condition is stable. Maternal hypotension, hypertension, or respiratory depression could adversely affect both the mother and fetus. If these occur, they must be promptly and aggressively treated. Delayed ischemia (vasospasm) is a major cause of morbidity in the postoperative period. Treatment is directed at increasing cerebral perfusion pressure by increasing systemic arterial pressure with inotropic agents, such as dopamine or phenylephrine, to maximize cerebral perfusion in areas with dysfunctional autoregulation, which are passively dependent on systemic arterial pressure. However, the beneficial effects of these maneuvers must be weighed against the potential risks of reducing uterine blood flow, resulting in fetal asphyxia.

ANESTHETIC MANAGEMENT OF DELIVERY IN PATIENTS WITH AN ANEURYSM, AVM OR BRAIN TUMOR

Preventing hypertension and increased ICP is crucial to managing labor and delivery successfully in women with documented unclipped aneurysms, nonexcised AVMs, or intracranial tumors (especially tumors that have not been surgically treated). Obstetric indications should be used for decisions about the method of delivery. Vaginal delivery is acceptable for patients with increased intracranial pressure. However, the second stage of labor must be shortened and maternal straining with the Valsalva maneuver avoided because it raises both intracranial and CSF pressures (7, 77, 78). Immediately following the Valsalva maneuver, there is a reduction in CSF pressure accompanied by an increase in cardiac output and blood pressure, which is the result of increased venous return to the heart. The net effect on transmural pressure of cerebral vessels is not precisely known. Until cerebral hemodynamics during labor are better understood, it is best to avoid Valsalva maneuvers in women with cerebrovascular disease, thus reducing the possibility of rupturing tenuous cerebral vessels.

To shorten the second stage of labor and avoid maternal straining, the administration of segmental lumbar epidural or caudal anesthesia and the use of outlet forceps are recommended. For the first stage of labor, a properly administered epidural block will decrease pain and the increased blood pressure and cardiac output resulting from painful contractions. It will also prevent the Valsalva maneuver by blocking the reflex urge to bear down. Epidural and caudal anesthesia may be contraindicated in patients with increased ICP because of the risk of dural puncture or of increasing ICP further by injecting local anesthetic into the epidural space and elevating CSF pressure. Dural puncture may cause a sudden leakage of CSF that decreases CSF pressure and produces cerebellar herniation. Although the likelihood of dural puncture and elevated CSF pressure is somewhat re-duced with the caudal approach to the epidural space, caudal anesthesia has been associated with neurologic sequelae in patients with increased ICP (79).

Alternate forms of analgesia, although less effective than epidural or caudal anesthesia, include paracervical and pudendal blocks, inhalation analgesics, and systemic narcotics. Paracervical blocks have been associated with fetal compromise, but they may be a satisfactory alternative for women with increased ICP. Pudendal blocks are safe and useful for the second stage of labor. However, administration of narcotics and inhalation agents during spontaneous ventilation may raise $PaCO_2$, induce maternal respiratory acidosis, increase cerebral blood flow, and raise ICP. If general anesthesia is necessary either for vaginal delivery or for manual removal of the placenta, the rapid-sequence intravenous induction technique described earlier should be used.

Low-spinal anesthesia is another alternative. This approach may be contraindicated in patients who have intracranial hypertension in the presence of an aneurysm or AVM. A reduction in CSF pressure may increase the transmural pressure (MAP-ICP) in the aneurysm, increasing the potential for rupture.

When cesarean delivery is required, epidural anesthesia with a sensory level of T4 is recommended. If general anesthesia is necessary, the concerns and techniques discussed earlier apply. Although elective cesarean delivery has been recommended for patients with untreated AVMs (6), most authorities advocate this procedure only for accepted obstetric or fetal indications. For patients with a documented saccular aneurysm or AVM—whether ruptured or unruptured, or surgically or conservatively treated—cesarean delivery provides no definite advantage over vaginal delivery in protecting against intracerebral hemorrhage (2, 3, 5–8, 80, 81); aneurysm rupture has occurred during elective cesarean delivery (2, 77).

If labor supervenes after SAH, a procedure combining cesarean section and neurosurgery may be used, although vaginal and cesarean delivery should be considered before neurosurgical intervention (6, 9). The choice of procedure in this situation is guided by the severity of the maternal clinical condition, the feasibility of terminating preterm labor, and the maturity of and potential hazard to the fetus.

After successful surgical occlusion of an aneurysm or AVM, there appears to be no need for specialized management of labor and delivery. Even induction of labor with an oxytocic agent is not contraindicated. Considering that the incidence of unruptured aneurysms in women is reportedly 0.5 to 1%, many pregnant women with this vascular anomaly apparently undergo labor and deliver without incident.

BENIGN INTRACRANIAL HYPERTENSION

Pseudotumor cerebri, or benign intracranial hypertension, is a syndrome characterized by increased intracranial pressure without a focal lesion or hydrocephalus. The syndrome involves elevated ICP, normal CSF composition, normal mental status, and no focal intracranial lesions. Treatment of this syndrome involves control of the intracranial pressure to protect vision by repetitive lumbar punctures to drain CSF, steroids to reduce brain swelling, acetazolamide to reduce CSF production, or surgery to create a shunt of CSF to the peritoneal cavity.

Pregnancy may exacerbate the symptoms of this syndrome: headaches and visual disturbances (82–84). However, the increased ICP is not a contraindication to labor and delivery. Labor analgesia may be provided by an epidural technique (85). Spinal anesthesia has been advocated as the method of choice for cesarean section because it is safe and technically easy and a postdural puncture CSF leak would be beneficial (86). Before performing a spinal anesthetic for patients with lumboperitoneal shunts, localization of the site of entry of the shunt into the subarachnoid space is important.

References

1. Cannell DE, Botterell EH: Subarachnoid hemorrhage and pregnancy. Am J Obstet Gynecol 72:844–855, 1956.
2. Pedowitz P, Perell A: Aneurysms complicated by pregnancy. Part II. Aneurysms of the cerebral vessels. Am J Obstet Gynecol 73:736–749, 1957.
3. Pool JL: Treatment of intracranial aneurysms during pregnancy. JAMA 192:209–214, 1965.
4. Fliegner JRH, Hooper RS, Kloss M: Subarachnoid haemorrhage and pregnancy. J Obstet Gynaecol Br Commonw 76:912–917, 1969.
5. Amias AG: Cerebral vascular disease in pregnancy. I. Haemorrhage. J Obstet Gynaecol Br Commonw 77:100–120, 1970.
6. Robinson JL, Chir B, Hall CJ, Sedzimir CB: Subarachnoid hemorrhage in pregnancy. J Neurosurg 37:27–33, 1972.
7. Hunt HB, Schifrin BS, Suzuki K: Ruptured berry aneurysms and pregnancy. Obstet Gynecol 43:827–837, 1974.
8. Minielly R, Yuzpe AA, Drake CG: Subarachnoid hemorrhage secondary to ruptured cerebral aneurysm in pregnancy. Obstet Gynecol 53:64–70, 1979.
9. Young DC, Leveno KJ, Whalley PJ: Induced delivery prior to surgery for ruptured cerebral aneurysm. Obstet Gynecol 61:749–752, 1983.
10. Smolik EA, Nash FP, Clawson JW: Neurological and neurosurgical complications associated with pregnancy and the puerperium. South Med J 50:561–572, 1957.
11. Boba A: Hypothermia: Appraisal of risk in 110 consecutive patients. J Neurosurg 19:924–933, 1962.
12. Locksley HB: Report on the cooperative study of intracranial aneurysms and subarachnoid hemorrhage. Section V, Part II. Natural history of subarachnoid hemorrhage, intracranial aneurysms and arteriovenous malformations: Based on 6368 cases in the cooperative study. J Neurosurg 25:321–368, 1966.
13. Dunn JM, Raskind R: Rupture of a cerebral arteriovenous malformation during pregnancy. Obstet Gynecol 30:423–426, 1967.
14. Dunn JM, Weiss SR, Raskind R: Rupture of intracranial arteriovenous malformation in pregnancy. Int Surg 49:241–247, 1968.
15. Barno A, Freeman DW: Maternal deaths due to spontaneous subarachnoid hemorrhage. Am J Obstet Gynecol 125:384–392, 1976.
16. Monfared AH, Koh KS, Apuzzo MLJ, Collea JV: Obstetric management of pregnant women with extracranial shunts. Can Med Assoc J 120:562–563, 1979.
17. Howard TE, Herrick CN: Pregnancy in patients with ventriculoperitoneal shunts: Report of two cases. Am J Obstet Gynecol 141:99–101, 1981.
18. Cast MJ, Grubb RL, Strickler RC: Maternal hydrocephalus and pregnancy. Obstet Gynecol 62(Suppl):29–31, 1983.
19. Mealey J, Carter JE: Spinal cord tumor during pregnancy. Obstet Gynecol 32:204–209, 1968.
20. Apuzzio J, Pelosi MA, Ganesh VV, Caterini H, Iffy L: Spinal cord tumors during pregnancy. Int J Gynaecol Obstet 17:608–610, 1980.
21. Jones WB: Gestational trophoblastic neoplasms: The role of chemotherapy and surgery. Surg Clin North Am 58:167–179, 1978.
22. Weed JC, Woodward KT, Hammond CB: Choriocarcinoma metastatic to the brain: Therapy and prognosis. Semin Oncol 9:208–212, 1982.
23. Aminoff MJ: Neurological disorders and pregnancy. Am J Obstet Gynecol 132:325–335, 1978.
24. Ehlers N, Malmros R: The suprasellar meningiomas. Acta Ophthalmol 121(Suppl):1, 1973.
25. Magyar DM, Marshall JR: Pituitary tumors and pregnancy. Am J Obstet Gynecol 132:739–751, 1978.
26. Mills RP, Harris AB, Heinrichs L, Burry KA: Pituitary tumor made symptomatic during hormone therapy and induced pregnancy. Ann Ophthalmol 11:1672–1676, 1979.
27. Weyand RD, MacCarty C, Wilson RB: The effect of pregnancy on intracranial meningiomas occurring about the optic chiasm. Surg Clin North Am 31:1225–1233, 1951.
28. Donaldson JO: Tumours. In Neurology of Pregnancy. Saunders, Philadelphia, 1978, p 158.
29. O'Connell JEA: Neurological problems in pregnancy. Proc R Soc Med 55:577–582, 1962.
30. Chaudhuri P, Wallenburg HCS: Brain tumors and pregnancy: Presentation of a case and a review of the literature. Eur J Obstet Gynecol Reprod Biol 11:109–114, 1980.
31. Graham JG: Neurological complications of pregnancy and anaesthesia. Clin Obstet Gynaecol 9:333–350, 1982.
32. Miller HJ, Hinkley CM: Berry aneurysms in pregnancy: A ten year report. South Med J 63:279–285, 1970.
33. Szabo MD, Crosby GM, Sundaram P, Dodson BA, Kjellberg RN: Does hypertension cause spontaneous hemorrhage of intracranial arteriovenous malformations? Anesthesiology 70:761–763, 1989.
34. Horton JC, Chambers WA, Lyons SL, Adams RD, Kjellberg RN: Pregnancy and the risk of hemorrhage from cerebral arteriovenous malformations. Neurosurgery 27:867–872, 1990.
35. Rish BL: Treatment of intracranial aneurysms associated with other entities. South Med J 71:553–557, 1978.
36. Graf CJ: Prognosis for patients with nonsurgically treated aneurysms: Analysis of the cooperative study of intracranial aneurysms and subarachnoid hemorrhage. J Neurosurg 35:438–443, 1971.
37. Samson DS, Clark K, Hodosh RM: Treatment of subarachnoid hemorrhage. In The Treatment of Neurological Diseases. RN Rosenberg, ed. Spectrum, New York, 1979, pp 117–142.
38. Mathew NT, Meyer JS, Hartmann A: Diagnosis and treatment of factors complicating subarachnoid hemorrhage. Neuroradiology 6:237–245, 1974.
39. Tuttelman RM, Gleicher N: Central nervous system hemorrhage complicating pregnancy. Obstet Gynecol 58:651–656, 1981.
40. Lennon RL, Sundt TM Jr, Gronert GA: Combined cesarean section and clipping of intracerebral aneurysm. Anesthesiology 60:240–242, 1984.
41. Kofke WA, Wuest HP, Mc Ginnis LA: Cesarean section following ruptured cerebral aneurysm and neuroresuscitation. Anesthesiology 60:242–245, 1984.
42. Solomon RA, Fink ME, Lennihan L: Early aneurysm surgery

and prophylactic hypervolemic hypertensive therapy for the treatment of aneurysmal subarachnoic hemorrhage. Neurosurgery 23:699–704, 1988.

43. Smith BE: Fetal prognosis after anesthesia during gestation. Anesth Analg Curr Res 42:521–526, 1963.

44. Shnider SM, Webster GM: Maternal and fetal hazards of surgery during pregnancy. Am J Obstet Gynecol 92:891–900, 1965.

45. Brodsky JB, Cohen EN, Brown BW, Wu ML, Witcher C: Surgery during pregnancy and fetal outcome. Am J Obstet Gynecol 138:1165–1167, 1980.

46. Duncan PG, Pope WDB, Cohen M, Greer N: The safety of anesthesia and surgery during pregnancy. Anesthesiology 64:790–794, 1986.

47. Crawford JS, Lewis M: Nitrous oxide in early human pregnancy. Anaesthesia 41:900–905, 1986.

48. Aldridge LM, Turnstall ME: Nitrous oxide and the fetus. Br J Anaesth 58:1348–1356, 1986.

49. Mazze RI, Kallen B: Reproductive outcome following anesthesia and operation during pregnancy: A registry of 5,405 cases. Am J Obstet Gynecol 161:1178–1185, 1989.

50. Battaglia F, Prystowsky H, Smisson C, Hellegers A, Bruns P: Fetal blood studies. XIII. The effect of the administration of fluids intravenously to mothers upon the concentrations of water and electrolytes in plasma of human fetuses. Pediatrics 25:2–10, 1960.

51. Bruns PD, Linder RO, Drose VE, Battaglia F: The placental transfer of water from fetus to mother following the intravenous infusion of hypertonic mannitol to the maternal rabbit. Am J Obstet Gynecol 86:160–167, 1963.

52. Wilson F, Sedzimir CB: Hypothermia and hypotension during craniotomy in a pregnant woman. Lancet 2:947–949, 1959.

53. Pevehouse BC, Boldrey E: Hypothermia and hypotension for intracranial surgery during pregnancy. Am J Surg 100:633–634, 1960.

54. Aitken RR, Drake CG: A technique of anesthesia with induced hypotension for surgical correction of intracranial hemorrhages. Clin Neurosurg 21:107–114, 1974.

55. Brann AW Jr, Myers RE: Central nervous system findings in the newborn monkey following severe in utero partial asphyxia. Neurology 25:327–338, 1975.

56. Lewis PE, Cefalo RC, Naulty JS, Rodkey FL: Placental transfer and fetal toxicity of sodium nitroprusside. Gynecol Invest 8:A58, 1977.

57. Naulty J, Cephalo RC, Lewis PE: Fetal toxicity of nitroprusside in the pregnant ewe. Am J Obstet Gynecol 139:708–711, 1981.

58. Ring G, Krames E, Shnider SM, Wallis KL, Levinson G: Comparison of nitroprusside and hydralazine in hypertensive pregnant ewes. Obstet Gynecol 50:598–602, 1977.

59. Lieb SM, Zugaib M, Nuwayhid B, Tabsh K, Erkkola R, Ushioda E, Brinkman CR III, Assali NS: Nitroprusside-induced hemodynamic alterations in normotensive and hypertensive pregnant sheep. Am J Obstet Gynecol 139:925–931, 1981.

60. Donchin Y, Amirav B, Sahar A, Yarkoni S: Sodium nitroprusside for aneurysm surgery in pregnancy. Br J Anaesth 50:849–851, 1978.

61. Rigg D, McDonogh A: Use of sodium nitroprusside for deliberate hypotension during pregnancy. Br J Anaesth 53:985–987, 1981.

62. Wheeler AS, James FM III, Meis PJ, Rose JC, Fishburne II, Dewan DM, Urban RB, Greiss FC Jr: Effects of nitroglycerin and nitroprusside on the uterine vasculature of gravid ewes. Anesthesiology 52:390–394, 1980.

63. Snyder SW, Wheeler AS, James FM III: The use of nitroglycerin to control severe hypertension of pregnancy during cesarean section. Anesthesiology 51:563–564, 1979.

64. Hood DD, Dewan DM, James FM III, Bogard TD, Floyd HM: The use of nitroglycerin in preventing the hypertensive response to tracheal intubation on severe preeclamptics. Anesthesiology 59:A423, 1983.

65. Vandewater SL, Paul WM: Observations on the foetus during experimental hypothermia. Can Anaesth Soc J 7:44–51, 1960.

66. Assali NS, Westin B: Effects of hypothermia on uterine circulation and on the fetus. Proc Soc Exp Biol Med 109:485–488, 1962.

67. Hess OW, Davis CD: Electronic evaluation of the fetal and maternal heart rate during hypothermia in a pregnant woman. Am J Obstet Gynecol 89:801–807, 1964.

68. Stange K, Halldin M: Hypothermia in pregnancy. Anesthesiology 58:460–461, 1983.

69. Kamrin RP, Masland W: Intracranial surgery under hypothermia during pregnancy. Arch Neurol 13:70–76, 1965.

70. Hehre FW: Hypothermia for operations during pregnancy. Anesth Analg Curr Res 44:424–428, 1965.

71. Matsuki A, Oyama T: Operation under hypothermia in a pregnant woman with an intracranial arteriovenous malformation. Can Anaesth Soc J 19:184–191, 1972.

72. Hunt WE, Hess RM: Surgical risk as related to time of intervention in the repair of intracranial aneurysms. J Neurosurg 28:14–20, 1968.

73. Schwarz S, Ilias W, Lackner F, Mayrhofer O, Foldes FF: Rapid tracheal intubation with vecuronium: The priming principle. Anesthesiology 62:388–391, 1985.

74. Mehta MP, Choi WW, Gergis SD, Sokoll MD, Adolphson AJ: Facilitation of rapid endotracheal intubations with divided doses of nondepolarizing neuromuscular blocking drugs. Anesthesiology 62:392–395, 1985.

75. Taboada JA, Rupp SM, Miller RD: Redefining the priming principle for vecuronium during rapid sequence induction of anesthesia. Anesthesiology 63:A573, 1985.

76. Ellis SC, Wheeler AS, James FM III, Rose JC, Meis PJ, Greiss FC Jr, Urban RB, Shihabi Z: Sodium niroprusside for hypertension in gravid ewes. Anesthesiology 55:A302, 1981.

77. McCausland AM, Holmes F: Spinal fluid pressures during labor: Preliminary report. West J Surg Obstet Gynecol 65:220–233, 1957.

78. Marx GF, Zemaitis MT, Orkin LR: Cerebrospinal fluid pressures during labor and obstetrical anesthesia. Anesthesiology 22:348–354, 1961.

79. Abouleish E: Caudal analgesia. In *Pain Control in Obstetrics*. E Abouleish, ed. Lippincott, Philadelphia, 1977, pp 225–256.

80. Daane TA, Tandy RW: Rupture of congenital intracranial aneurysms in pregnancy. Obstet Gynecol 15:305–314, 1960.

81. Baker JW: Subarachnoid haemorrhage associated with pregnancy. Aust N Z J Obstet Gynaecol 9:12–17, 1969.

82. Elian M, Ben-Tovim N, Bechar M, Bornstein B: Recurrent benign intracranial hypertension (pseudotumor cerebri) during pregnancy. Obstet Gynecol 31:685–688, 1968.

83. Kassam SH, Hadi HA, Fadel HE, Sims W, Jay WM: Benign intracranial hypertension in pregnancy: Current diagnostic and therapeutic approach. Obstet Gynecol Surv 38:314–321, 1983.

84. Koontz WL, Herbert WNP, Cefalo RC: Pseudomotor cerebri in pregnancy. Obstet Gynecol 62:324–327, 1983.

85. Palop R, Choed-Amphai E, Miller R: Epidural anesthesia for delivery complicated by benign intracranial hypertension. Anesthesiology 50:159–160, 1979.

86. Abouleish E, Ali V, Tang RA: Benign intracranial hypertension and anesthesia for cesarean section. Anesthesiology 63:705–707, 1985.

CHAPTER 31

Anesthesia for the Pregnant Patient with Neuromuscular Disorders

Samuel C. Hughes, M.D.

Neuromuscular diseases are not common during the childbearing years but, when they occur, have important implications for the obstetrician and the anesthesiologist. This group of diseases may markedly affect the management of a patient and the administration of drugs during labor and delivery (1, 2). This chapter reviews the more common anesthetic problems encountered and those that might serve as guides to managing similar or related problems. All of these conditions require highly individualized care to balance complex medical conditions and their specific presentations during pregnancy.

MYOTONIC SYNDROMES

The myotonic syndromes are a group of autosomal dominant degenerative diseases including *myotonia congenita, myotonic dystrophy*, and *paramyotonia congenita*. The latter is the rarest of these syndromes and appears only on exposure to cold (1). A case of cold-induced abortion in a woman with paramyotonia congenita has been reported (3). In all three syndromes, the skeletal muscle is especially affected and generally characterized by weakness and wasting. Myotonia is characterized by difficulty in initiating muscle movement with delayed muscle relaxation following contraction and is present to some degree in all three manifestations. The basic defect may be in membrane chloride permeability (4).

Myotonia congenita is rare and consists of myotonia and pseudohypertrophy of some voluntary muscles. Dystrophic changes do not occur. The myotonia is said to be most severe following rest but improved with exercise. The disease is most often autosomal dominant, appearing in childhood and rarely progressing in severity. In its purest form, myotonia congenita does not affect the cardiac and smooth muscles. Unlike myotonic dystrophy, there is no mental deterioration, infertility, or decrease in life expectancy. This disease often responds to oral therapy with phenytoin, quinine sulfate, or procainamide, which may diminish muscle stiffness and

cramping. In one reported case, the disease increased in severity during pregnancy and improved after delivery with no obstetric complications (5).

Myotonic dystrophy (also called *myotonia atrophica*) is the most common and most severe of these syndromes. Onset is often in the second decade of life, but it may present without myotonia in neonates in a severe form characterized by thin, weak muscles. When onset is neonatal, death often results within a few months from respiratory weakness. For some individuals bearing the gene, the only manifestation may be cataracts in old age. Electromyographic changes occur early in the disease (before myotonia) and can be demonstrated clinically (6). Death usually occurs during the sixth decade of life from bulbar involvement, cardiac defects, or aspiration pneumonia.

Typically, patients with myotonic dystrophy demonstrate myotonia and wasting of skeletal muscles including facial, cervical, and proximal limb muscles. Often, they exhibit an early frontal baldness, gonadal atrophy, and endocrine failure. Other manifestations of particular importance to the anesthesiologist are cardiac conduction defects with a prolonged P-R interval and heart block that may cause benign arrhythmias or sudden death. Respiratory involvement is related to impaired mechanical ability. There may be weakness of both the diaphragm and intercostal muscles accompanied by chronic hypoventilation, hypercapnia, and decreased arterial oxygen saturation. During the perioperative period, decreased pharyngeal muscle strength and repeated aspiration can cause further respiratory problems.

Although smooth muscle involvement can occur, too few obstetric cases have been reported to study the effect of myotonic dystrophy on labor (7, 8). The disease is associated with ovarian insufficiency, amenorrhea, infertility, and, among women who become pregnant, a high incidence of spontaneous abortion (5, 9). The small number of patients studied makes it unwise to relate the effects of the disease to the course of labor and delivery. Increased muscle weakness during pregnancy has been related to the effects of progesterone (10). Involvement of the adrenal glands may result in adrenocortical insufficiency. Polyhydramnios is reportedly associated with the disease, including generalized weakness, hypotonia, and multiple contractures.

In one review of 15 obstetric patients with myotonic dystrophy, 8 had spontaneous vaginal deliveries, 5 required low forceps delivery or vacuum extraction, and 2 required cesarean delivery (8). Other investigators have reported an increased severity of symptoms at about the seventh month of pregnancy, and the increased muscle weakness may make it difficult for the patient to fully cooperate in the delivery (10). Tocolysis with ritodrine, a β-mimetic used to delay premature labor, reportedly provoked the symptoms of myotonic dystrophy (12).

Anesthetic Management of Patients with Myotonic Syndromes

The anesthesiologist managing a patient with myotonic dystrophy should evaluate the extent of the disease, the potential for untoward responses to otherwise routine anesthetic agents, and the obstetric course of the patient. The initial evaluation should include an estimation of pulmonary function and an electrocardiogram (ECG) to determine the potential for restrictive lung disease and cardiac arrhythmias. If analgesia for labor pain is required, narcotics and sedatives should be used with caution. All central nervous system depressants, including thiopental, diazepam, and inhalation agents, have been associated with apnea in these patients (13, 14). Imposing a central respiratory depression on an already atrophic respiratory musculature would most likely cause respiratory difficulty in these patients. Regional anesthesia including epidural, spinal, or pudendal block provides satisfactory anesthesia and avoids the risk of respiratory depression. Consequently, the anesthetic technique suggested for patients with myotonic disorders is local or conduction anesthesia (15-20).

If general anesthesia is required, a cautious approach is suggested. The use of depolarizing muscle relaxants in a patient with myotonic dystrophy is considered extremely hazardous and should be avoided. Marked, generalized skeletal muscle contracture proportional to the dose will develop, leading to difficulty in ventilating the patient (13) (Fig. 31.1). A review of the literature on succinylcholine, however, reveals that both relaxation of the myotonic state and general myotonia have been reported following the use of the drug, suggesting that the response of myotonic patients to this drug is unpredictable (Table 31.1) (21).

The response of these patients to nondepolarizing

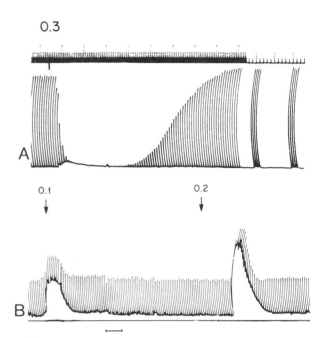

Figure 31.1. The response of a patient with myotonia to succinylcholine, demonstrated by evoked thumb adduction in response to stimulation of the ulnar nerve at 0.15 Hz. Time scale = 1 min. *A* represents the normal response and *B* the abnormal contracture seen when succinylcholine is administered to a patient with myotonia. (Adapted from Mitchell MM, Ali HH, Savarese JJ: Myotonia and neuromuscular blocking agents. Anesthesiology 49:44–48, 1978.)

muscle relaxants appears normal, although a prolonged response to curare has been reported (22). Rapid-sequence endotracheal intubation can be accomplished with a sufficient dose of a nondepolarizing agent, and anesthesia can be maintained with nitrous oxide, oxygen, and a potent inhalation agent. Narcotics should be used sparingly following delivery of the infant. Extubation should be performed only when a patient is fully alert and able to maintain good ventilation. Despite an earlier report of myotonic crisis (generalized contractures) precipitated by the drug (16), reversal of muscle relaxants with neostigmine appears to be safe (13), although this remains controversial (21).

Generalized contractures may result from mechanical, as well as electrical, stimulation. Neither regional anesthesia nor nondepolarizing muscle relaxants prevent myotonic spasms. The effects of volatile anesthetic agents are uncertain but appear to be minimal. However, muscles in myotonic spasm will become flaccid when injected with a local anesthetic. There is no agreement on the treatment of generalized sustained muscle contraction if it occurs during surgery, but intravenous administration of quinine (300 to 600 mg) has been used, as have large doses of steroids (23). Dantrolene has also been suggested (1).

Table 31.1.
Neuromuscular Disorder and Their Response to Muscle Relaxants[a]

Neuromuscular Disorder	Response to Succinylcholine	Response to Nondepolarizing Muscle Relaxants
Upper motor neuron lesion	Hyperkalemia, monitor unaffected side	Resistant
Lower motor neuron lesion	Hyperkalemia, monitor unaffected side	Sensitive
Neurofibromatosis	Contractures, resistant to Sch	Sensitive
Myasthenia gravis	Resistant/sensitive if an anti-cholinesterase	Sensitive
Myasthenic syndrome	Sensitive	Sensitive
Muscular dystrophy	nl/hyperkalemia	nl/sensitive
Myotonia	Contractures/hyperkalemia	Resistant
Peripheral neuropathy	Resistant	Sensitive

[a]Adapted from Azar I: The response of patients with neuromuscular disorders to muscle relaxants: A review. Anesthesiology 61:173–187, 1984.

Table 31.2
Causes of Seizures during Pregnancy[a]

Eclampsia
Idiopathic epilepsy
Trauma
Drug, alcohol withdrawal
Arteriovenous malformation
Brain tumor
Metabolic disorder: uremia, hypoglycemia, electrolyte abnormality, hepatic failure

[a]Adapted from Dichter MA: The epilepsies and convulsive disorders. In *Harrison's Principles of Internal Medicine*, 10th ed. RG Petersdorf, RD Adams, E Braunwald, KJ Isselbacher, JB Martin, JD Wilson, eds. McGraw-Hill, New York, 1983, pp 2018–2028.

In summary, patients having myotonic syndromes often present with significant multisystem disease having variable effects of pregnancy. For labor and delivery, regional anesthesia may avoid many of the risks of general anesthesia while providing adequate analgesia or anesthesia.

EPILEPSY

Epilepsy is a chronic seizure disorder affecting approximately 0.5 to 2% of the population (24). Seizures may be caused by intracranial birth injury, metabolic disturbances, trauma, acute infection, brain tumors, or alcoholism; they may also be of idiopathic origin (Table 31.2). The latter is perhaps the most common and may occur at any age, but usually appears before age 20 years. In obstetric patients, the typical presentation is idiopathic epilepsy with drug therapy in progress.

A review of the Norwegian Medical Birth Registry compared 371 epileptic women with over 100,000 nonepileptic women and found that epileptic women had an increased incidence of hemorrhage, toxemia, and obstetric intervention (including forceps and cesarean delivery) (Table 31.3) (25). In addition, neonatal mortality was approximately fourfold higher.

The authors concluded that women with epilepsy should be considered a high-risk group. Although there is controversy about the extent of the problem (26), these patients deserve careful consideration.

Interaction of Pregnancy and Epilepsy

True idiopathic epilepsy may be first diagnosed during pregnancy. The incidence of epilepsy for women in the childbearing years has been reported to be 50 per 100,000 (27). However, there is no evidence that pregnancy causes epilepsy or is in itself epileptogenic. In one review of 59 epileptic mothers studied through 153 pregnancies, 45% had more frequent seizures, 50% showed no change, and 5% had fewer seizures (28). The patients having more frequent seizures before pregnancy are likely to have an increased frequency of seizures during pregnancy.

Pregnancy produces several physiologic and metabolic changes that may affect the course of epilepsy. Arterial CO_2 tension decreases during pregnancy, but arterial pH usually changes little because of adequate metabolic compensation. During labor, severe pain producing hyperventilation may produce alkalosis and vomiting and potentiate pH changes, thereby inducing seizures. During pregnancy, fluid retention may be epileptogenic and patients should avoid rapid weight gains. In addition, renal plasma flow and glomerular filtration rate increase markedly. In one study phenobarbitone clearance did not show any significant changes, whereas the clearance of phenytoin increased, often by as much as 100% (29). The resulting decrease in serum phenytoin could lead to an increased frequency of seizures; serum levels should therefore be monitored frequently during pregnancy (Fig. 31.2) (30). Because the clearance of phenytoin returns to normal within a few months of delivery, drug dosage must be carefully adjusted postpartum to avoid drug intoxication.

Obstetric epilepsy cases may also become more complex because of patients' variable compliance to

Table 31.3
Epilepsy and Pregnancy: Maternal and Neonatal Complications and Outcome[a,b]

	Epilepsy (n = 371)	Control (n = 125,423)	Significance (P)
Obstetric/maternal complications			
Vaginal hemorrhage	5.1%	2.2%	<0.001
Toxemia	7.5%	4.7%	<0.01
Cesarean delivery	3.2%	1.1%	<0.001
Forceps delivery	6.3%	2.4%	<0.001
Intervention in labor (e.g., induction, rupture of membranes, surgical delivery)	17.3%	7.7%	<0.001
Neonatal outcome			
Gestation<37 weeks	8.9%	5.0%	<0.01
Birth weight<2500 g	7.4%	3.7%	<0.001
Congenital malformation	4.5%	2.2%	
Neonatal death rate	29.3/1000 births	8.0/1000 births	<0.001

[a]Frequency of complications during pregnancy in epileptic women and neonatal outcome from the Norwegian Medical Birth Registry and Central Bureau of Statistics, 1967–1968.
[b]Adapted from Bjerkedal T, Bahna SL: The course and outcome of pregnancy in women with epilepsy. Acta Obstet Gynecol Scand 52:245–248, 1973.

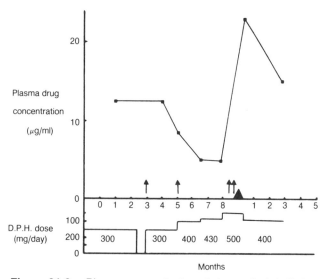

Figure 31.2. Plasma concentration of phenytoin (μ/ml) during pregnancy with the doses administered. The time of childbirth is shown by the *solid triangle*; the *arrows* indicate the occurrence of seizures. Therapeutic range for phenytoin is 10–20 μg/ml. (Adapted from Lander CM, Edwards VE, Eadie MJ, Tyrer JH: Plasma anticonvulsant concentrations during pregnancy. Neurology 27:128–131, 1977.)

drug therapy during pregnancy. For example, patients may be more conscientious about taking medication during pregnancy or may decrease medication because of concern for teratogenicity. It has been suggested that in some cases, the emotional factors and stress surrounding pregnancy also may influence epilepsy.

Gestational Epilepsy

Some authors refer to a true gestational epilepsy (31, 32). By strict definition, this is a seizure or con-

vulsion that occurs only with pregnancy. It may occur at any time during pregnancy or immediately postpartum. These patients have no evidence of toxemia or previous history of epilepsy and appear to recover completely. While Knight and Rhind (28) referred to 14 such patients, 6 of their patients had abnormal electroencephalogram responses or other potential causes for seizure, including previous skull fracture and intracerebral vascular malformation. Pregnancy may have only revealed a previously existing problem. However, there may be the rare pregnant patient with no obvious pathologic condition or seizure history who presents with an apparent epilepsy that resolves with delivery. Treatment in this case is symptomatic, but other, more common pathologic states must first be excluded.

Teratogenic Effects of Anticonvulsant Therapy

The incidence of fetal malformations in the offspring of epileptic women is about two and one-half times that for the general population (33). This is most likely due to anticonvulsant medication, but a genetic predisposition cannot be ruled out. One of the problems reported is the fetal hydantoin syndrome, which presents with altered growth and development and the potential for cleft lip and palate, cardiac lesions, and hypoplasia of nails and digits. Because treatment of epilepsy often consists of more than one drug, it is difficult to assign blame to a particular drug, but hydantoins and barbiturates have been incriminated. Ideally, the epileptic woman contemplating pregnancy should have her anticonvulsant medication tapered to the minimum effective dosage or discontinued (if possible) before becoming pregnant. For many women, discontinuing drug therapy is not possible and major manipulation of drug therapy should clearly be avoided during pregnancy. However, most women with epilepsy, even those taking anticonvulsant medications, will have uneventful pregnancies and can expect to deliver healthy babies.

When barbiturates are used to control seizures, the placental transfer of the drug is rapid. The ratio of umbilical cord vein to maternal artery phenobarbital concentration is 0.95 (34). Neonates may suffer from a drug-induced depression of vitamin K-dependent clotting factors (35). Because phenobarbital, primidone, or phenytoin may produce a transient depression of prothrombin and factors V and VII, vitamin K should be administered to neonates of mothers receiving anticonvulsant therapy. In addition, neonates may demonstrate the clinical signs of barbiturate withdrawal, including hyperexcitability, tremulousness, and decreased sucking. The newborn should be carefully observed for these signs for several days in the nursery.

Status Epilepticus during Pregnancy

Status epilepticus can occur with pregnancy, triggered by physiologic changes or alterations in drug level and therapy. It should be treated vigorously with standard anticonvulsant therapy and routine airway management with special attention to the potential for aspiration. Intubation, paralysis with muscle relaxants, and controlled ventilation with oxygen protect the patient from aspirating, decrease respiratory and metabolic acidosis, and ensure adequate oxygenation of mother and fetus. Phenytoin (Dilantin) as a slow intravenous drip (13 to 18 mg/kg) is the drug of choice for terminating status epilepticus, although it may cause a drop in blood pressure and mild atrioventricular block. Diazepam (Valium) in incremental doses or phenobarbital (Luminal) at a dose of 10 to 20 mg/kg may be given intravenously but may cause respiratory depression. Even with therapy, the mortality for status epilepticus may be as high as 10% (24). However, if the condition is properly managed in obstetric patients, the outcome has been reported to be good, with the pregnancy continuing to term (28).

Anesthetic Management of Patients with Epilepsy

The anesthesiologist managing a pregnant epileptic patient must consider the cause of the epilepsy and the treatment in progress, as well as the obstetric course. Anticonvulsant drugs being taken should be identified. The availability of serum levels, drawn late in the pregnancy or in early labor, would make it possible to optimize dosage. The therapeutic range for phenytoin is 10 to 20 μg/ml, which is usually achieved by taking 3 to 5 mg/kg/day. The therapeutic range for phenobarbital is 10 to 50 μg/ml, achieved with a dose of 1 to 5 mg/kg/day (Table 31.4).

Drug interactions may be complex with epileptic patients. For example, the addition of phenobarbital to the therapeutic regimen of a patient receiving phenytoin may decrease the phenytoin serum level by enzyme induction. On the other hand, drugs that compete with phenytoin for a common metabolic pathway (e.g., dicumarol, isoniazid, sulfonamides, diazepam, and chloramphenicol) may increase the phenytoin serum levels. In addition, phenobarbital enzyme induction speeds metabolism of methoxyflurane (36). Consequently, another less readily metabolized potent agent should be used when inhalation analgesia is required for labor and delivery.

Fortunately, local anesthetics do not appear to interact significantly with anticonvulsant medications; in fact, lidocaine has been used to terminate epileptic seizure (37). Regional anesthesia is therefore a safe and appropriate choice for the typical epileptic patient. During labor and delivery, regional anesthetics prevent the hyperventilation and respiratory alkalosis that could provoke seizure. Preliminary data noted an increased incidence of seizures postpartum in patients who had received spinal anesthesia (38). However, these findings have not been confirmed.

If general anesthesia is indicated, the routine technique as described elsewhere in this text is satisfactory. In animals, d-tubocurarine interacts with both phenytoin and lidocaine, causing a greater than usual depression of twitch height in epileptic patients, and prolonged neuromuscular blockade (39). Monitoring the neuromuscular function should avoid any potential problems. Some investigators advise against using any drugs with the potential for causing convulsion or seizure-like activity, including ketamine, althesin, and enflurane (40). However, enflurane, the most common of these agents, does not appear to increase seizure activity in patients with a history of convulsive disorders (41, 42). Using the low levels of enflurane suggested for general anesthesia before delivery or for enflurane analgesia is acceptable, provided $PaCO_2$ is maintained in the near-normal range. A narcotic and diazepam combination may be used to supplement nitrous oxide and oxygen following delivery.

NEUROFIBROMATOSIS

Neurofibromatosis was first described by Von Recklinghausen in 1882. The disease is inherited as an autosomal dominant disorder and occurs in 1 in 3000 births (43). The defective gene causing the dis-

Table 31.4
Commonly Used Antiepileptic Drugs[a]

Generic Name	Trade Name	Dosage (Adult p.o.)	Half-life	Therapeutic Range
Phenytoin	Dilantin	3–5 mg/kg/day	24 hr (variable)	10–20 μg/ml
Phenobarbital	Luminal	1–5 mg/kg/day	90 hr	10–50 μg/ml
Primidone	Mysoline	10–25 mg/kg/day	8 hr	2–10 μg/ml

[a]Adapted from Dichter MA: The epilepsies and convulsive disorders. In *Harrison's Principles of Internal Medicine*, 10th ed. Petersdorf RG, RD Adams, E Braunwald, KJ Isselbacher, JB Martin, JD Wilson, eds. McGraw-Hill, New York, 1983, pp 2018–2028.

order has now been identified. The classic manifestations include café au lait spots or increased skin pigmentation and neurofibromas involving the skin. In the 19th century, an Englishman named John Merrick suffered such bizarre and deforming tumors that he was called the "Elephant Man." The neurofibromas arise from the neurilemma sheath (Schwann cells) and the fibroblasts of peripheral nerves. The tumors may involve nerve roots or blood vessels and arise in or around most organs and body cavities. They are often totally benign and only a cosmetic problem. Occasionally, they produce serious problems, such as intracranial tumors (in 5 to 10% of patients) or a compromised airway, the latter developing particularly if they occur in the mediastinum or cervical regions (44). In most patients, neurofibromatosis is a multifaceted syndrome associated with some osseous changes and (in rare cases) endocrine disorders such as pheochromocytoma and hyperthyroidism (45). The association with pheochromocytoma is probably overestimated, and some authors indicate that the frequency with which they coincide is only 1% (44). In 5 to 10% of cases of neurofibromatosis, one of the tumors will become sarcomatous (43).

Pregnancy and Neurofibromatosis

The pregnant patient with neurofibromatosis may have particular problems caused by the increase in neurofibroma size associated with pregnancy and the potential for hemorrhaging into the lesions themselves (45). Tumor growth regresses after pregnancy. It is difficult to judge how common these problems are, but because paravertebral and spinal neurofibromas are often present, the pregnant patient should be observed for any change in neurologic function (Fig. 31.3). Spontaneous hemothorax has also been reported in the parturient with neurofibromatosis (46).

Vascular changes have also been associated with the disease and, in advanced form, may be characterized by fibrous transformation of the intima (47). Renovascular hypertension associated with neurofibromatosis is often diagnosed before age 20 years and may be present in the obstetric patient. Swapp and Main (45) reviewed 11 patients with 24 preg-

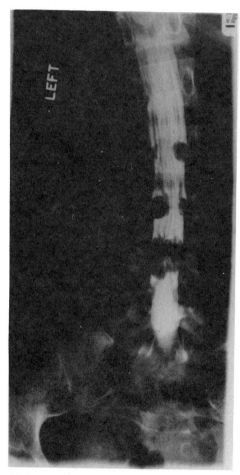

Figure 31.3. Lumbar spine and pelvis showing neurofibromas encroaching on the spine of a 25-year-old female with neurofibromatosis. This patient had only mild upper extremity symptomatology at the time of this radiographic study.

nancies. Ten of these patients were already hypertensive or developed hypertension with pregnancy. While the blood pressure elevations of these patients is mild, renovascular hypertension must be considered in the differential diagnosis of hypertension during pregnancy or at delivery.

Finally, there are several reports of abnormal responses to muscle relaxants in patients with neurofibromatosis (48-50). It is suggested that these patients have a prolonged response to nondepolarizing muscle relaxants. Furthermore, some patients with neurofibromatosis are reported to be resistant to succinylcholine, whereas others have a prolonged response. An abnormal response to muscle relaxants might be attributed to a denervation phenomenon produced by generalized neurofibromatosis, but there is no good evidence that this occurs (1, 50). This author has used both succinylcholine and nondepolarizing agents in these patients with the standard, expected results. However, given the diversity of the clinical features of this disease, using the minimal effective dose and monitoring neuromuscular function carefully are recommended when relaxants are required.

Anesthetic Management of Patients with Neurofibromatosis

The initial evaluation of the patient should include a particularly careful history to elicit signs and symptoms indicative of significant disease. That is, simple café au lait spots and cutaneous neurofibromas are probably not cause for alarm. However, intracranial neurofibromas or lesions near the spine might alter the management of pregnancy significantly. A history of labile hypertension might be indicative of pheochromocytoma or of renal vascular disease. Such cardiac lesions as pulmonary stenosis and coarctation of the aorta have also been reported in these patients.

In most cases the patient can be managed in a routine manner and according to her wishes as the obstetric course requires. There are no unique considerations for selecting drugs or techniques unless there is more extensive disease present (as suggested in the preceding section). The possibility of cystic lung lesions leading to pneumothorax should be considered if intubation is required. The anesthesiologist must also examine the airway for evidence of laryngeal or neck involvement, which would make intubation difficult. Muscle relaxants should be carefully monitored. Regional anesthesia is perfectly acceptable, but before administering a conduction block, an attempt should be made to elicit symptomatology and document the presence of paraspinous tumors.

Since one-third of these patients are diagnosed only by chance on routine physical examination and one-third are referred because of cosmetic problems, it is likely that the outcome in pregnant patients with neurofibromatosis will be good.

ACUTE IDIOPATHIC POLYNEURITIS: LANDRY-GUILLAIN-BARRÉ SYNDROME

The Landry-Guillain-Barré-Strohl syndrome (LGBS) was first described by Landry in 1859 as a neurologic disorder with ascending paralysis and later modified by specific cerebrospinal fluid (CSF) findings by Guillain, Barré, and Strohl in 1916 (51). The cause of LGBS remains unknown, although the clinical profile has been well documented and the prognosis has improved. The diagnosis is based on typical clinical findings supported by the demonstration of increased protein in the CSF with a normal cell count. The rise in protein probably results from inflammation of nerve roots in the subarachnoid space. There is segmental demyelination throughout the peripheral nervous system.

The syndrome of iodiopathic polyneuritis is characterized by the sudden onset of weakness and paralysis. It is usually symmetric and ascending in nature, spreading cephalad from simple paresis and impaired tendon reflexes of the lower extremities to possible bulbar symptoms with respiratory depression over a 2-week course. The patient recovers in approximately 6 months, but residual findings occur in perhaps 5 to 10% of these patients. A review of 10 series including 425 nonobstetric patients with LGBS revealed a 21% mortality (52). At least three maternal deaths have been reported, although improved medical management of the disease during pregnancy should make this uncommon (53, 54).

When considering a diagnosis of LGBS during pregnancy, it is important to rule out disorders with similar symptomatology, such as vitamin-B complex deficiency associated with hyperemesis gravidarum, porphyria, or poisoning with lead or other heavy materials. There are no preventive measures for LGBS nor is there any cure, so treatment is symptomatic. The onset of dyspnea, cyanosis, and bronchial congestion is symptomatic of respiratory failure and possible pulmonary infection, both leading causes of maternal death in this syndrome. Improved medical support, including early diagnosis of impending respiratory failure and aggressive intervention in the more serious cases, has undoubtedly improved the outlook for these patients. A recent case report demonstrating the joint efforts of the obstetric and intensive care teams is an example of successful patient management (Fig. 31.4).

Pregnancy and LGBS

The onset of LGBS does not occur at any particular point during the pregnancy. There appears to be no direct relationship between LGBS onset or severity and pregnancy, and there is no reason to terminate a pregnancy because of the disease. The maternal and perinatal mortality (>10%), however, indicates that patients require expert care (56). Infants born to mothers with LGBS are normal, and there is no evidence that the disease is teratogenic. Infant survival

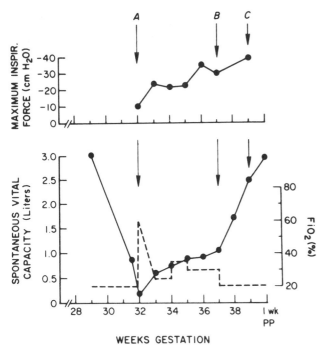

Figure 31.4. Respiratory function during late pregnancy in a patient with LGBS. The *top figure* represents maximum inspiratory force and the vital capacity (*solid line*) is shown in the *lower figure*. The FiO₂ is shown by the broken line. *A* represents initiation of mechanical ventilation; *B*, the cessation of mechanical ventilation; *C*, the delivery; and *PP*, the postpartum period. The rapid fall in vital capacity and decreased maximum inspiratory force (normal > −40 cm H₂O) necessitated ventilatory support at 32 weeks' gestation. A tracheotomy was performed and the patient was ventilated until 37 weeks' gestation with delivery of a healthy infant 2 weeks later. (Reprinted by permission from Bravo RH, Katz M, Inturrisi M, Cohen NH: Obstetric management of Landry-Guillian-Barré syndrome: A case report. Am J Obstet Gynecol 142:714–715, 1982.)

is at least 88% (51). The higher incidence of prematurity is probably related to the severity of the disease and the necessity for respiratory intervention, but with careful support maternal recovery and delivery of a healthy baby can be expected in most cases.

Anesthetic Management of Patients with LGBS

Anesthesia for patients with LGBS is controversial. If general anesthesia is required, these patients are like any patients with generalized weakness and disability. Succinylcholine should not be administered because an excessive release of potassium could result. These patients may also be more sensitive to nondepolarizing muscle relaxants. Controlled ventilation should be used, and the need to support ventilation postoperatively should be anticipated. If intravenous analgesia is considered, narcotics should

be used with care in LGBS patients with bulbar involvement. Autonomic nervous system dysfunction may occur, with wide fluctuations in blood pressure and heart rate (57). Repeated blood gas analysis and evaluation of respiratory sufficiency may be necessary during labor and delivery when a combination of increased respiratory demands, patient position, and poor respiratory function may seriously compromise the patient.

The use of regional anesthesia is controversial. In general, regional anesthesia is avoided in patients with neurologic dysfunction, and psychoprophylaxis and local anesthesia are recommended by some (55). However, several anesthesiologists from major centers have stated that regional analgesia exerted no influence on the course of chronic neurologic diseases (58). They reported on two LGBS patients given regional anesthesia without resulting problems. This review has been criticized, however, because of the absence of detailed information on agents, dosages, and the length of follow-up (59). The use of epidural anesthesia may be acceptable for analgesia during labor and perhaps delivery (when expulsive forces are decreased and vacuum or forceps extraction may be required), especially because the use of narcotics in LGBS patients introduces the potential for respiratory depression. The use of regional anesthesia may also be possible for cesarean delivery in patients with adequate pulmonary function. However, if cesarean delivery is indicated in patients with significant bulbar involvement, a general anesthetic is more appropriate because of the potential for respiratory compromise.

For LGBS patients particularly, pulmonary function should be carefully monitored with respiratory support at hand. The close cooperation of the obstetrician and the anesthesiologist, and appropriate intensive care support as needed, should enable the mother to deliver a healthy baby.

MULTIPLE SCLEROSIS

Multiple sclerosis (MS) is a demyelinating disease of the central nervous system characterized by multiple, random sites of demyelination in the brain and spinal cord. It is a remittent disease of young adults with exacerbation and remissions occurring over the years. The diagnosis depends on physical findings, neurologic history, and the exclusion of other neuromuscular diseases. There is no known cure for the disease; treatment includes physical therapy and symptomatic care. Steroids may shorten the length of an acute attack.

MS is not a hereditary disorder, although it is more common in some families. Few cases have been reported among the obstetric population. While the historical literature suggests that women with MS neither marry nor have children, more recent analysis indicates otherwise and fails to demonstrate definite adverse effects of pregnancy on the course of the disease.

The etiology of MS is unknown, but it is interesting to note the close relationship between geographic latitude and the risk of developing the disease. There is a lower incidence of the disease at the equator, for example, when compared to the northern temperate zones of North America and Europe. It is generally believed that there is a viral agent that initiates an altered immune reaction in a genetically susceptible individual.

The course of the disease is characterized by exacerbations and remissions with symptoms (depending on site of demyelination) developing over 2 to 3 days, stabilizing for several weeks, then clearing. The interval between exacerbations may be several years but is unpredictable. Eventually, residual symptoms lead to profound disability. However, the young obstetric patient is often without significant permanent disability and may be in a period of remission.

Pregnancy and MS

The effect of pregnancy on the course of multiple sclerosis is ill defined. Relapses or exacerbations may be caused by infection, fever, excessive fatigue, and emotional trauma or stress. During pregnancy, all of these conditions may occur and produce a relapse of the disease or an exacerbation in symptomatology. However, a direct relationship between pregnancy and changes in the course of the disease has not been demonstrated. It has been said that rest during the puerperium is helpful.

The time of onset of MS relapse during pregnancy in patients previously diagnosed as having MS is similar to the time of onset of the disease during pregnancy. That is, about one-half of MS relapses occur before pregnancy, and the remainder during the first 3 months postpartum; exhaustion, stress, and child care may contribute to the latter (Table 31.5) (60). One study found that the overall relapse rate in women with MS is 0.16 per year, whereas during pregnancy, it is 0.25 per pregnancy year (61). Others suggest that the relapse rate is equivalent when comparing pregnant with nonpregnant patients (62, 63).

In summary, the patient with MS appears to be at some risk for a relapse of the disease during pregnancy, although this assumption is controversial and not well documented. If a relapse occurs, it happens with equal frequency during the 9 months of pregnancy and 3 months postpartum. It is unclear whether physical, emotional, or the many physiologic and hormonal changes of pregnancy are responsible for any change in the disease status. Furthermore, one must keep in mind that the incidence of MS and pregnancy is higher during the third decade of life.

Anesthetic Management of Patients with MS

Although surgery and anesthesia have been implicated in the exacerbation of MS, there is little evidence to support any intrinsic relationship (64). The method of delivery chosen for the pregnant MS patient should be based on obstetric considerations. General anesthesia using drugs such as succinylcholine, barbiturates, narcotics, and various volatile agents has been successful. In one review, in which 42 MS patients were given 88 general anesthetics, only one patient experienced an attack of the disease during the postoperative period. As a result, the rate of relapse was only 0.14 relapse per patient year (Table 31.6) (65). This compared favorably with an expected rate of approximately 0.27 relapse per patient year at that center.

Regional anesthesia has been associated with a relapse of MS, although the evidence is not strong. The study just mentioned reviewed seven patients given nine spinal anesthetics. One relapse occurred, and the authors suggested that spinal anesthesia might be best avoided in pregnant MS patients. The same authors concluded that local anesthesia (e.g., peripheral blocks) was completely safe. However, the blood-brain barrier may be impaired in these pa-

Table 31.5
Multiple Sclerosis and Relapses during Pregnancy[a]

	New Onset (First Attack)	Previously Diagnosed (Relapse)
Number of pregnancies	15	133
Number of episodes	15	29
Time of relapse		
During pregnancy	6	13
Postpartum (3 months)	9	16

[a]Modified from Müller R: Pregnancy in disseminated sclerosis. Acta Psychiatr Neurol Scand 26:397–409, 1951.

Table 31.6
Multiple Sclerosis and Anesthesia[a]

Number of Patients	Anesthetics	Number of MS Exacerbations
42	88 general	1
7	9 spinal	1
1	3 caudal	0
98	1000 local	14

[a]Modified from Bamford C, Sibley W. Laguna J: Anesthesia in multiple sclerosis. Can J Neurol Sci 5:41–44, 1978.

tients, resulting in a toxic response to local anesthetic at lower than expected doses (66).

There is no strong evidence that spinal or lumbar epidural anesthesia exacerbates MS, and there have been no controlled studies. Most reports are anecdotal in nature because of the small number of patients studied. In one of the few large studies, Schapira demonstrated that spinal puncture alone did not exacerbate the disease (67). In his review of 250 diagnostic spinal taps, 231 patients reported no change in their disease, 14 reported *improvement*, and only 5 reported deterioration of their condition. Myelography was undertaken in 5 of these patients with no apparent adverse effects. However, the possibility of a relapse or exacerbated symptoms resulting from the effects of spinal or epidural anesthesia cannot be ignored. The controversy over 2-chloroprocaine suggests that a local anesthetic could be neurotoxic, perhaps especially on a demyelinated nerve in an MS patient.

Epidural anesthesia has been used successfully for labor and delivery (58, 68). In one clinical report, the patient experienced mild MS exacerbations in the form of hypoesthesia on the inner thigh following delivery (68). Although this response lasted for several weeks, the authors concluded that the use of epidural anesthesia should not be prohibited in pregnant MS patients. Warren and co-workers suggested that epidural anesthesia might be less risky than spinal anesthesia because the concentration of local anesthetic in the white matter of the spinal cord is lower—1.37 mg/kg (spinal) vs. 0.4 mg/kg (epidural) (68). A clinical review from the same institution and representing 32 pregnancies in 20 women suggested that higher concentrations of local anesthetics may increase the relapse rate (69). However, the obstetric course that leads to the need for higher concentrations of local anesthetics seems the most likely cause of any increase in the incidence of relapse. Although the relationship between the use of regional anesthesia and potential problems for MS patients is unclear, using as dilute a solution of local anesthetic as possible for lumbar epidural administration seems prudent.

When a general anesthetic is required, the routine sequence of thiopental, succinylcholine, $N_2O:O_2$, and halothane or isoflurane is suggested; narcotics, diazepam, and other standard agents have also been used successfully. The suggestion that sodium thiopental may have a deleterious effect on the course of MS or may cause a relapse (70) has not been substantiated (71, 65). The potential of succinylcholine-induced increased release of potassium from muscle tissue is unlikely unless there is severe neurologic deficit with muscle wasting. In the otherwise healthy

Table 31.7
Pathogenesis of Myasthenia Gravis:
An Autoimmune Disorder

A 70–90% decrease in number of acetylcholine receptors.
Acetylcholine receptor IgG antibodies in 70% or more of patients.
Abnormality in T-cell function responsible for abnormal autoimmune response
Postsynaptic membrane abnormalities.
Wider clefts between nerve and muscle.

patient with MS in remission, the use of succinylcholine is acceptable (21). There has been some concern about the effects of the volatile agents on the immune response and postoperative infection, but there is no evidence that immune status following surgery is affected significantly by the choice of anesthetic agent or technique.

Perhaps as important as the choice of anesthetic agent or technique is the practice of dealing openly with the pregnant MS patient, providing choice, support, and as much information as the patient can assimilate. The effects of regional anesthetic, for example, should be explained ahead of time because this resulting muscle weakness could easily be confused with exacerbation of the disease.

MYASTHENIA GRAVIS

First described in 1672, myasthenia gravis is a chronic disease characterized by weakness and easy fatigability. It most often affects the oculomotor, facial, laryngeal, pharyngeal, and respiratory muscles, and the latter are of particular concern to the anesthesiologist. Patients generally recover somewhat with the rest and improve with anticholinesterase therapy. Myasthenia can occur at all ages and is twice as common in females. Onset is usually in the third decade of life for women, with an overall incidence of approximately 1 in 19,000 to 1 in 40,000 (72). The disease may be totally benign or life threatening. The pathogenesis includes findings of specific abnormalities at the neuromuscular junction of striated muscle while the myometrium remains unaffected (Table 31.7), and its contractile force is unimpaired. The disease may be aggravated to variable extents by several factors, including infection, excitement, fatigue, loss of sleep, diet, and alcohol use. Furthermore, menstruation or pregnancy may cause an exacerbation of myasthenia gravis in many patients.

Pregnancy and Myasthenia Gravis

In a review of 202 myasthenia gravis patients with 292 pregnancies, it was noted that 30% experienced remissions, 45% deterioration of their condition, and 25% no change in the disease pattern during pregnancy (73). Other studies have also reported similar changes in symptomatology (74). In addition, the experience of previous pregnancy was not found helpful in predicting the course of subsequent pregnancies. It has been suggested that altered hormonal relationships during pregnancy may cause a relapse of the disease (75). However, neither the administration of birth control pills nor estrogen therapy appears to benefit the myasthenic patient. In addition, the incidence of exacerbations is high (30%) in the postpartum period when hormonal changes are normalizing (73). In summary, the course of the disease during pregnancy, labor, and delivery is highly variable and unpredictable, and requires the careful attention of the obstetric team because the patient's presentation may vary from benign to full-blown myasthenic crisis (too little anticholinesterase) or cholinergic crisis (too much anticholinesterase). A cholinergic crisis may be associated with excessive tearing, hypersalivation, bradycardia, sweating, abdominal cramping, and diarrhea. A "nonreactive crisis" has been reported and results from the sudden development of refractoriness to antiacetylcholinesterase medications. This may have been related to the administration of betamethasone (76). The correct diagnosis is imperative for acute management.

EDROPHONIUM TEST

Edrophonium chloride (Tensilon) is very similar in action to neostigmine but shorter acting. Both are anticholinesterases and are quarternary ammonium compounds that do not cross the blood-brain barrier. Consequently, there is minimal placental transfer of these compounds (77). When given intravenously, edrophonium chloride can rapidly demonstrate the presence of myasthenia gravis. Even if it exacerbates the condition (cholinergic crisis), this effect is short lasting (78). The patient's muscle strength should first be assessed by vital capacity, grip strength, or other objective methods so that changes may be noted. Next, 2 mg of edrophonium chloride should be administered intravenously, and if there is no deterioration in symptoms, a further dose of 8 mg should be given. If inadequately treated, the patient will have a rapid increase in muscle strength.

Intravenous neostigmine methylsulfate has also been used as a test, but it is slower in onset and longer in duration. This test must be performed with equipment for respiratory intervention at hand because fatalities have occurred. It has been suggested that uterine cholinergic receptors may be affected by intravenous anticholinesterase therapy, resulting in increased uterine tone and an increased incidence of abortions and possibly premature labor. Although reported results vary, intravenous drug therapy should

Table 31.8
Suggested Preoperative Assessment in Myasthenia Gravis

Assess extent of respiratory or bulbar involvement.
Determine frequency and severity of myasthenic attacks.
Note type and dosage of anticholinesterase and other drugs.
Consider pulmonary function tests.
Conduct laboratory studies: CBC, electrolytes, serum protein, ECG, and chest radiographic series.

nevertheless be considered thoughtfully during pregnancy.

Labor and Delivery

The factors previously mentioned that affect the course of myasthenia gravis may be present during labor. They include emotional stress, physical exertion, minor infections, and fatigue. However, the disease does not affect labor itself and the use of outlet forceps may shorten the second stage of labor and avoid fatigue. The cesarean section rate is not increased in these patients. However, problems may result from pharmacologic intervention during labor and delivery. For example, aminoglycosides, kanamycin, and gentamicin reportedly exacerbate the symptoms of myasthenia gravis (79). Magnesium sulfate, commonly used in the treatment of preeclampsia, may produce a neuromuscular block in the myasthenic patient, resulting in respiratory insufficiency (80). The use of magnesium sulfate is therefore best avoided in these patients.

Anesthetic Management of Patients with Myasthenia Gravis

Preanesthetic assessment of a patient with myasthenia gravis ideally begins with a visit by the anesthesiologist before labor. A formal consultation when the patient is near term might be appropriate to evaluate the patient and the extent of her illness. The laboratory work required to evaluate these patients is more extensive than that usually performed, as is the history taking and physical examination for myasthenic symptoms (Table 31.8). Bulbar weakness, for example, may lead to nutritional compromise and abnormalities of hemoglobin, serum electrolytes, or protein. Because focal necrosis of the myocardium has been reported, an ECG is recommended (81, 82). Recently performed pulmonary function tests help to determine the extent of the disease and efficacy of therapy and provide information valuable for managing possible respiratory insufficiency. Clearly, the anesthetic management of patients with myasthenia gravis must be based on careful preanesthetic assessment and tailored to the particular obstetric situation.

Anticholinesterase therapy is the mainstay of treatment for myasthenic patients and should be adjusted to provide optimal symptomatic relief before labor. Other therapeutic modalities are often helpful in more difficult cases (Table 31.9). Anticholinesterase therapy must be maintained during labor and constantly reevaluated. Because gastric uptake is unreliable during labor and delivery, it is recommended that the patient's routine oral dose be converted to the equivalent intramuscular dose (Table 31.10).

The postpartum period may also be hazardous. Plauche reported that 30% of pregnant myasthenic patients have exacerbated symptoms during this period (73). Thus the patient should be monitored for at least 10 days postpartum, preferably in the hospital, with adjustment of anticholinesterase therapy as needed (83). Breastfeeding is probably not a risk to the mother, provided she is well rested because anticholinesterase drugs are not transmitted in detectable amounts in breast milk (84).

ANESTHESIA FOR VAGINAL DELIVERY

Traditional intravenous analgesia and sedation with narcotics and tranquilizers must be used cautiously in myasthenic patients, particularly if there is respiratory or bulbar involvement. It is recommended that these drugs be administered in less than the usual doses to avoid retention of secretions and respiratory depression. Many clinicians recommend the use of regional anesthesia for vaginal delivery of myasthenic patients (78, 83–85).

Table 31.9
Treatment of Myasthenia Gravis

Anticholinesterase therapy
Thymectomy in younger patients (improvement in 57–86% of patients)
Corticosteroids for immunosuppressive actions (improvement in 70–100% of patients)
Plasmapheresis and thoracic duct drainage (useful in some patients)
Immunosuppressive drugs (reserved for patients who are resistant to standard therapies)

Table 31.10
Commonly Used Anticholinesterase Drugs and Equivalent Doses

Drug	IV Dose (mg)	IM Dose (mg)	Oral Dose (mg)
Neostigmine (Prostigmine)	0.5	0.7–1.0	15.0
Pyridostigmine (Mestinon)	2.0	3.0–4.0	60.0

Whether administered as a low spinal or continuous epidural, regional anesthesia provides pain relief with minimal or no systemic medication, prevents fatigue, and allows for the use of outlet forceps (when necessary) to shorten the second stage of labor. Although high blood levels of local anesthetics may interfere with neuromuscular transmission, this is unlikely to be a clinical problem. The levels required to alter neuromuscular transmission (in animal models) are toxic, and despite the pathology of the myasthenic patient's neuromuscular junction, there is no evidence of an altered response to local anesthetics in these patients (86).

On theoretical grounds, 2-chloroprocaine, an ester-type local anesthetic metabolized by plasma cholinesterase, is not recommended for epidural anesthesia in a myasthenic patient (83). For patients receiving anticholinesterase therapy, plasma cholinesterase activity is significantly decreased, which increases the risk of anesthetic overdose or toxicity (87). The reality of this danger is unclear, but amide local anesthetics may be more appropriate because their metabolism is unaltered by the disease. Another alternative is the use of intrathecal morphine for the first stage of labor, although further anesthetic intervention is required if the use of outlet forceps is necessary to shorten the second stage of labor. The use of epidural sufentanil might be another alternative (see Chapter 10).

When general anesthesia is required for vaginal delivery, the anesthesiologist must perform a rapid-sequence induction with immediate intubation because of the possibility of a full stomach. In a severely compromised myasthenic patient, intubation may be accomplished with thiopental alone, although a muscle relaxant is often also required. Because these patients are especially sensitive to nondepolarizing agents, the onset of muscle relaxation is rapid and can be obtained with 2 to 3 mg of curare (88). Because the redistribution and excretion of curare is unaltered by the disease, the duration of effect is the same as that in normal patients.

Intubation can be equally well accomplished using succinylcholine (30 to 50 mg), but anticholinesterase therapy prolongs the duration of succinylcholine effects for as much as 90 min. According to some experts, the response to succinylcholine is unpredictable, and it is claimed that some patients may be resistant to succinylcholine (21).

Once intubation is complete, ventilation should be controlled and any of the volatile inhalation agents may be used (if necessary) to relax the uterus or to supplement N_2O and O_2 until delivery is accomplished.

ANESTHESIA FOR CESAREAN DELIVERY

Either regional or general anesthesia can be used for cesarean delivery, provided careful attention is given to the extent of respiratory involvement. If the patient presents with only ocular myasthenia or minimal disease with no anticholinesterase therapy, anesthetic management is relatively routine. However, if there is bulbar or respiratory muscle movement, general anesthesia with endotracheal intubation is more appropriate, unless the disease is well controlled with anticholinesterase therapy. Even then, careful consideration should be given to the combined effects of a high motor block and preexisting respiratory problems in these patients.

During general anesthesia, the use of muscle relaxants in the myasthenic patient is usually unnecessary and best avoided. If a small dose of curare or succinylcholine is used to facilitate endotracheal intubation, it will probably suffice for the surgery as well. If further relaxation is needed, 0.5 to 1 mg of curare in incremental doses is recommended, with careful monitoring of the response (83). In myasthenic patients undergoing thymectomy, Baraka and Dajani (89) used atracurium (0.09 to 0.21 mg/kg) and achieved 75 to 90% neuromuscular block. The newer nondepolarizing short-acting drugs have proved very useful. Reversal of nondepolarizing muscle relaxants can be accomplished with incremental doses of neostigmine (0.5 mg) or pyridostigmine (1 mg) with the response monitored by a nerve stimulator. If the patient's disease was well controlled before surgery, extubation should be expected without complications.

The postoperative course, however, must be monitored very carefully for 48 hr. The anticholinesterase requirements may vary, and repeated evaluation (including measurements of vital capacity) is suggested. Adequate ventilatory support, endotracheal suctioning, and chest physical therapy must be *readily* available. If a regional anesthetic has been used, postoperative administration of epidural morphine may provide pain relief uncomplicated by the significant sedation and respiratory depression that might result from larger doses of intramuscular or intravenous narcotics. The catheter could be left in place for 24 hr to facilitate pain management.

Neonatal Myasthenia Gravis

Neonatal myasthenia gravis is a transient disease occurring in approximately 12% of the infants born to mothers with myasthenia gravis (90). It usually presents with generalized muscle weakness, weak reflexes, and respiratory distress and is probably caused by placental transfer of maternal antibodies (91). Although 80% of these cases appear within the first 24 hr of life, neonatal myasthenia can occur up

Table 31.11
Anticholinesterase Drugs in Neonatal Myasthenia Gravis[a,b]

Drug	Dosage
Diagnosis	
Edrophonium (Tensilon)— for rapid diagnosis	1 mg IV
Treatment	
Pyridostigmine bromide (Mestinon)	1 mg/kg orally q 3–4 hr with feeding
Neostigmine bromide (Prostigmin)	0.3 mg/kg orally q 4 hr with feeding
Neostigmine methylsulfate (Prostigmin)	0.05 to 0.25 mg IM q 2–3 hr

[a]Therapy for neonatal myasthenia gravis must be titrated to the symptomatic response of the newborn once the diagnosis is made.
[b]Adapted from Rudolph AM, Hoffman JIE, Rudolph CD, eds: *Pediatrics*, 17th ed. Appleton-Century-Crofts, Norwalk, CT, 1982, p 1688.

to 4 days after birth (2). The delayed onset may be explained by placental transfer of maternal anticholinesterases. The infant who has not become symptomatic by the fourth day postpartum may be allowed to leave the hospital. If the condition is suspected, it can be diagnosed by rapid improvement in movement and crying following an intramuscular injection of 0.5 to 1 mg of edrophonium.

The anesthesiologist must be prepared to intervene in the delivery room if the respiratory status of the infant is inadequate. The previous delivery of a healthy infant by a myasthenic mother does not preclude the birth of an infant with neonatal myasthenia gravis on a subsequent delivery. The obstetric team must always be prepared to diagnose and treat the problem. Approximately 80% of infants with neonatal myasthenia gravis require anticholinesterase therapy, but the disease spontaneously clears within 2 to 4 weeks (Table 31.11) (90, 92). The goal in treating these infants is to allow feeding and breathing without producing a vigorous cry or strong, active movement, for fear of invoking cholinergic weakness requiring further intervention with atropine. As the infant's strength improves, anticholinesterase therapy should be tapered off and the length of the interval between treatments increased. Complete recovery can be expected.

SPINAL CORD INJURY: PARAPLEGIA AND QUADRIPLEGIA

Spinal cord transection is most commonly caused by trauma and results in either paralysis of the lower extremities (paraplegia) or of all four extremities (quadriplegia). Extensive cord damage from infection, tumors, or vascular lesions may also cause permanent spinal cord damage and create similar chronic problems (94). Better medical care of the young patient with spinal cord injury has opened the way for paraplegic and quadriplegic women to become successful mothers, and the anesthesiologist must consider the special problems of pregnancy, labor, and delivery in these women (94).

Acute transection of the spinal cord produces a flaccid paralysis and loss of sensation below the lesion. The initial phase, characterized by hypotension, bradycardia, and the potential ECG abnormalities indicative of myocardial damage, lasts for 2 to 3 weeks and requires careful medical attention. Amenorrhea lasting for 2 to 3 months following spinal cord injury is common. The chronic state that follows the injury is characterized by potential muscle rigidity and spasm, as well as anemia and recurrent urinary infections, especially during pregnancy. The risk of a stillbirth or fetal abnormality appears to be increased for the women who suffer spinal cord injury during pregnancy (95).

Autonomic Hyperreflexia: Mass Reflex

This reflex was first described in 1917 by Head and Riddoch and consists of pilomotor erection, excessive sweating, facial flushing, dilated pupils, severe headache, bradycardia, and severe paroxysmal hypertension (96). Increased blood pressure can result in loss of consciousness and convulsions if the stimulus is not removed, and retinal as well as fatal cerebral or subarachnoid hemorrhages have been reported (97). The syndrome appears not to occur if the lesion is below T7 but occurs in over 85% of patients with a cord injury above this level (98, 99).

Autonomic hyperreflexia is the result of afferent impulses entering the isolated cord and initiating focal segmental reflexes that are neither modulated nor inhibited by higher centers (100, 101). Stimulation of the skin below the cord lesion, bladder distension, fecal impaction, rectal examination, genital stimulation, or contraction of a hollow viscus including the gut and uterus may bring about a massive stimulation of the sympathetic nervous system. The isolated adrenal glands receive their sympathetic nerve supply from the greater splanchnic nerve (T5–T9) and may be partially responsible for the response. However, Debarge and co-workers (102) concluded that the response was more likely caused by norepinephrine from the adrenergic sympathetic nerve endings than by any direct outflow from the adrenal glands. They also suggest that the pressor response to similar doses of catecholamines was greater in quadriplegic patients than in normal control subjects, which helps to explain the severe hypertension resulting from relatively minimal stimulation in some

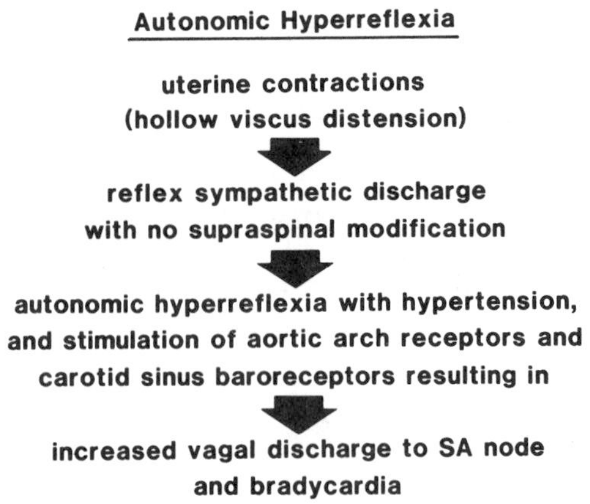

Autonomic Hyperreflexia

uterine contractions
(hollow viscus distension)

reflex sympathetic discharge
with no supraspinal modification

autonomic hyperreflexia with hypertension,
and stimulation of aortic arch receptors and
carotid sinus baroreceptors resulting in

increased vagal discharge to SA node
and bradycardia

Figure 31.5. Etiology and signs of an autonomic hyperreflexic response.

Table 31.12
Hyperkalemia after Administration of Succinylcholine (60 mg IV)[a,b]

Time (min)	K+	ECG
1	3.88	NSR
3	8.93	↑ ↑ T waves and
5	9.05	wide QRS

[a]Electrocardiographic and plasma potassium changes following 60 mg IV of succinylcholine in a patient with recent onset of hemiparesis.
[b]Adapted from Cooperman LH, Strobel GE, Kennel EM: Massive hyperkalemia after administration of succinylcholine. Anesthesiology 32:161–164, 1970.

cases. Regardless of the cause, the body's only defense mechanism for uncontrolled paroxysmal hypertension is vagally mediated bradycardia resulting from stimulation of carotid sinus baroreceptors and aortic arch receptors (Fig. 31.5) (103). During uterine contractions, premature ventricular beats, ventricular bigeminy, atrioventricular nodal block, and prominent U waves have been observed (2).

A further concern for the anesthesiologist is the risk of hyperkalemia resulting from the administration of succinylcholine in these patients. The hyperkalemic response may occur with many neuromuscular diseases, as well as with massive trauma or crush or burn injuries (104). The risk is not great during the first few hours following cord damage, but the administration of a depolarizing muscle relaxant may be hazardous for up to 6 months or more following the injury, and it is best to avoid succinylcholine if there is any question. The short-acting nondepolarizing agents, vecuronium and atracurium, may obviate the problem. The degree of hyperkalemia resulting from the administration of succinylcholine to a patient with recent central nervous system damage can be catastrophic (Table 31.12)

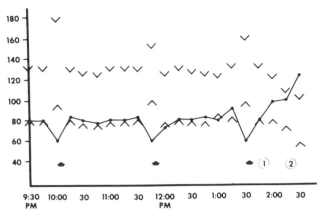

Figure 31.6. Epidural anesthesia and autonomic hyperreflexia: The vital signs of a 24-year-old paraplegic (T4 level) woman in labor showing the response to bupivacaine 0.25% via an epidural catheter. Δ = diastolic pressure; ▽ = systolic pressure; ● = pulse rate; ↑ = epidural injection of 0.25% bupivacaine; *1* = first twin delivered; and *2* = second twin delivered. (Adapted from Watson DW, Downey GO: Epidural anesthesia for labor and delivery of twins of a paraplegic mother. Anesthesiology 52:259–261, 1980.)

Labor and Delivery

In 1872, Sir James Simpson demonstrated normal parturition in swine after removal of the thoracic and lumbar cord (93). Cord damage per se is not an indication for cesarean delivery, and a vaginal delivery can be expected unless there is an obstetric reason to indicate otherwise. In a review of 39 deliveries of 26 paraplegic women, 21 had normal vaginal deliveries, 15 forceps deliveries, and only 3 cesarean deliveries (93). The relatively high rate of forceps deliveries was undoubtedly due to the paralysis of musculature responsible for the expulsive forces.

With complete cord transection above the T10 level, a painless labor can be expected. However, if cord damage is incomplete or below this level, painful labor may result. If cord damage is above the T10 level, there is also an increased incidence of premature labor that may not be appreciated by the patient. Weekly examination in the third trimester of pregnancy is recommended (especially in multigravidas) to detect cervical changes indicative of the onset of labor (105).

Anesthetic Management of Patients with Spinal Cord Transection

Depending on the level of the cord lesion, analgesia for labor and delivery per se is probably rarely required for these patients. The general medical condition of the patient and the extent of cord damage must first be evaluated. A history of increased blood pressure with urinary retention, for example, should alert the health care team to the possible presence of autonomic hyperreflexia.

For control of autonomic hyperreflexia in any patient with a T7 level injury or higher, epidural anesthesia should be considered. The ability of epidural analgesia to block autonomic hyperreflexia is well established but seems to be regularly overlooked by some (106–109). Although spinal anesthetics provide adequate anesthesia, administering a continuous epidural anesthetic offers more flexibility. Stirt and co-workers (101) reported effective control of autonomic hyperreflexia during labor using epidural anesthesia in a quadriplegic patient. Eight hours after the onset of labor, the patient experienced facial flushing, apprehension, and diaphoresis, and her blood pressure increased to 220/110 with a contraction. An epidural anesthetic was administered to modify or block this response and a healthy newborn was later delivered with forceps.

A similar course was undertaken in the delivery of twins from a paraplegic mother; in this case, 0.25% bupivacaine was effective in blocking autonomic hyperreflexia (Fig. 31.6)(103). In another case, in which the use of sodium nitroprusside to control blood pressure during evacuation of a dead fetus was attempted, it became necessary to administer a continuous epidural block to control wide swings in the patient's blood pressure (109). Clearly, when considering the use of sodium nitroprusside in these patients, placental transfer of the drug, as well as difficulty in titrating the dose and potential toxicity, must be carefully evaluated (110). The success of regional anesthesia in controlling autonomic hyperreflexia and providing extended anesthesia for pregnant cord-injured patients makes it the clear choice (101, 103, 107–109). A case report suggested that epidural meperidine may be useful as well (Fig. 31.7) (111). However, epidural fentanyl was not entirely successful in blocking autonomic hyperreflexia in another case report (112). Meperidine's success may be related to its local anesthetic properties.

A regional anesthetic (either spinal or epidural) is also appropriate for cesarean delivery. One author has suggested that general anesthesia can be used to control blood pressure in cord-injured patients during general surgery (113). However, the depth of anesthesia required to achieve this, the uterine atony induced by the use of volatile inhalation agents, and the requisite use of significant intravenous agents that profoundly affect the newborn make general anesthesia a less desirable choice for these patients (Table 31.13). Nevertheless, if general anesthesia is to be used for a cesarean delivery, a rapid-sequence intubation with cricoid pressure can be accomplished using a nondepolarizing agent to facilitate intubation. The latter is nec-

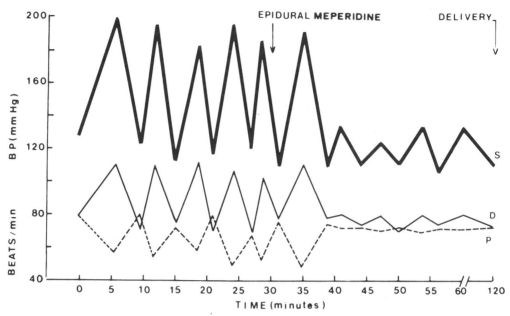

Figure 31.7.   Epidural meperidine and autonomic hyperreflexia. A graphic recording of blood pressure and heart rate changes before and after administration of epidural meperidine. S = systolic blood pressure; D = diastolic blood pressure; P = heart rate. (Reprinted by permission from Baraka A: Epidural meperidine for control of autonomic hyperreflexia in a paraplegic paturient. Anesthesiology 62:688–690, 1985.)

Table 31.13
Anesthesia and the Control of Blood Pressure in Patients with Spinal Cord injury[a,b]

Group (N)	Anesthetic Technique	Preanesthesia Systolic Blood Pressure (Torr)[c]	Intraoperative Systolic Blood Pressure (Torr)[c]	P
A (19)	Topical anesthesia, sedation, or no anesthesia	135 ± 20	172 ± 44	<0.005
B (13)	General anesthesia	110 ± 13	107 ± 34	<0.8
C (46)	Spinal anesthesia	117 ± 19	103 ± 21	<0.001

[a]Both general anesthesia and spinal anesthesia effectively controlled blood pressure changes in patients at risk for autonomic hyperreflexia.
[b]Reprinted with permission from Lambert DH, Deane RS, Mazuzan JE: Anesthesia and the control of blood pressure in patients with spinal cord injury. Anesth Analg 61:344–348, 1982.
[c]Values are means $\pm$ SD. Preanesthesic systolic blood pressures: A vs. B, $P < 0.001$; A vs. C, $P < 0.005$; B vs. C, $P < 0.3$. Intraoperative systolic blood pressures: A vs. B, $P < 0.001$; A vs. C, $P < 0.001$; B vs. C, $P < 0.7$.

essary if the cord injury is more recent than 6 months to 1 year. Although the general anesthetic will provide unconsciousness and amnesia, a regional anesthetic should also be used to block autonomic hyperreflexia.

References

1. Abouleish E: Neurologic disease. In *Obstetric Anesthesia: The Complicated Patient.* FM James, AS Wheeler, eds. Davis, Philadelphia, 1982, pp 57–86.
2. Donaldson JO: *Neurology of Pregnancy.* Saunders, Philadelphia, 1978.
3. Chitayat D, Etchell M, Wilson D: Cold-induced abortion in paramyotonia congenita. Am J Obstet Gynecol 158:435–436, 1988.
4. Barchi RL: Myotonia. An evaluation of the chloride hypothesis. Arch Neurol 32:175–180, 1975.
5. Hakim A, Thomlinson J: Myotonia congenita in pregnancy. J Obstet Gynaecol Br Commonw 76:561–562, 1969.
6. Chutorian AB, Koenigsberger R: The muscular dystrophies. In *Brenneman's Practice of Pediatrics*, UC Kelley, ed. Harper & Row, Hagerstown, MD, 1971, pp 6–10.
7. Harvey JC, Sherbourne DH, Siegel CI: Smooth muscle involvement in myotonic dystrophy. Am J Med 39:81–90, 1965.
8. Sarnat HB, O'Connor T, Byrne PA: Clinical effects of myotonic dystrophy on pregnancy and the neonate. Arch Neurol 33:459–465, 1976.
9. Gardy HH: Dystrophia myotonica in pregnancy: Report of a case. Obstet Gynecol 21:441–445, 1963.

10. Hopkins A, Wray S: The effect of pregnancy on dystrophia myotonica. Neurology 17:166–168, 1967.
11. Dunn LJ, Dierker LJ: Recurrent hydramnios in association with myotonia dystrophica. Obstet Gyencol 42:104–106, 1973.
12. Sholl JS, Hughey MJ, Hirschmann RA: Myotonic muscular dystrophy associated with ritodrine tocolysis. Am J Obstet Gynecol 151:83–86, 1985.
13. Mitchell MM, Ali HH, Savarese JJ: Myotonia and neuromuscular blocking agents. Anesthesiology 49:44–48, 1978.
14. Dundee JW: Thiopentone in dystrophica myotonica. Anesth Analg Curr Res 31:257–262, 1952.
15. Wheeler AS, James FM: Local anesthesia for laparoscopy in a case of myotonia dystrophia (letter). Anesthesiology 50:169, 1979.
16. Kaufman L: Anaesthesia in dystrophia myotonica (abridged): A review of the hazards of anaesthesia. Proc R Soc Med 53:183–188, 1960.
17. Harris MN: Extradural anesthesia and dystrophia myotonia. Anaesthesia 39:1032–1033, 1984.
18. Cope DK, Miller JN: Local and spinal anesthesia for cesarean section in a patient with myotonic dystrophy. Anesth Analg 65:687–690, 1986.
19. Patterson RA, Tousignant M, Skene DS: Cesarean section for twins in a patient with myotonic dystrophy. Can Anaesth Soc J 32:418–421, 1985.
20. Camann WR, Johnson MD: Anesthesia management of a parturient with myotonia dystrophia: A case report. Reg Anesth 15:41–43, 1990.
21. Azar I: The response of patients with neuromuscular disorders to the muscle relaxants: A review. Anesthesiology 61:173–187, 1984.
22. Mudge BJ, Taylor PB, Vanderspek AFL: Perioperative hazards in myotonic dystrophy. Anaesthesia 35:492–495, 1980.
23. Hook R, Anderson EF, Noto P: Anesthetic management of a parturient with myotonia atrophica. Anesthesiology 43:689–692, 1975.
24. Dichter MA: The epilepsies and convulsive disorders. In Harrison's Principles of Internal Medicine, 10th ed., RG Petersdorf, RD Adams, E Braunwald, KJ Isselbacher, JB Martin, JD Wilson, eds. McGraw-Hill, New York, 1983, pp 2018–2028.
25. Bjerkedal T, Bahna SL: The course and outcome of pregnancy in women with epilepsy. Acta Obstet Gynecol Scand 52:245–248, 1973.
26. Hiilsmaa VK, Bardy A, Teramo K: Obstetric outcome in women with epilepsy. Am J Obstet Gynecol 152:499–504, 1985.
27. Hopkins A: Neurological disorders. Clin Obstet Gynecol 4:419–433, 1977.
28. Knight AH, Rhind EG: Epilepsy and pregnancy: A study of 153 pregnancies in 59 patients. Epilepsia 16:99–110, 1975.
29. Mygind KI, Mogens D, Christiansen J: Phenytoin and phenobarbitone plasma clearance during pregnancy. Acta Neurol Scand 54:160–166, 1976.
30. Lander CM, Edwards VE, Eadie MJ, Tyrer JH: Plasma anticonvulsant concentrations during pregnancy. Neurology 27:128–131, 1977.
31. Maroni E, Markoff R: Epilepsie und schwangerschaft. Gynaecologia 168:418–421, 1969.
32. Dimsdale H: The epileptic in relation to pregnancy. Br Med J 2:1147–1150, 1959.
33. Laidlaw JL, Richens A: A Textbook of Epilepsy. Churchill Livingstone, London, 1976, p. 227.
34. Melchior JC, Svensmark O, Trolle D: Placental transfer of phenobarbitone in epileptic women and elimination in newborns. Lancet 2:860–861, 1967.
35. Solomon GE, Hilgartner MW, Kutt H: Coagulation defects caused by phenobarbitol and primidone. Neurology 23:445–451, 1973.
36. Van Dyke RA: Metabolism of volatile anesthetics. III. Induction of microsomal dechlorinating and ether-cleaving enzymes. J Pharmacol Exp Ther 154:364–369, 1966.
37. Bohm E, Flodmark S, Ptersen I: Effect of lidocaine (Xylo-
caine®) on seizure and interseizure electroencephalograms in epileptics. Arch Neurol Psychiatry 81:550–556, 1959.
38. Aravapalli R, Abouleish E, Aldrete JA: Anesthetic implications in the parturient epileptic patient. Anesth Analg 67:S3, 1988.
39. Harrah HD, Way WL, Katzung BG: The interaction of d-tubocurarine with antiarrhythmic drugs. Anesthesiology 33:406–410, 1970.
40. Evans DEN: Anesthesia and the epileptic patient: A review. Anaesthesia 30:34–45, 1975.
41. Roizen MF: Anesthetic implications of concurrent diseases. In Anesthesia, 3rd ed. RD Miller, ed. Churchill Livingstone, New York, 1990, p 846.
42. Oshima E, Urabe N, Shingu K, Mori K: Anticonvulsant actions of enflurane on epilepsy models in cats. Anesthesiology 63:29–40, 1985.
43. Adams RP, DeLong GR: Developmental and other congenital abnormalities of the nervous system. In Harrison's Principles of Internal Medicine, 10th ed. RG Petersdorf, RD Adams, E Braunwald, KJ Isselbacher, JB Martin, JD Wilson, eds. McGraw-Hill, New York, 1983, pp 2133–2142.
44. DeFalque RJ, Musunuru VS: Diseases of the nervous system. In Anesthesia and Co-Existing Disease, AK Stoelting, SF Dierdorf, eds. Churchill Livingstone, New York, 1983, pp 314–316.
45. Swapp GH, Main RA: Neurofibromatosis in pregnancy. Br J Dermatol 88:431–435, 1973.
46. Brady DB, Bolan JC: Neurofibromatosis and spontaneous hemothorax in pregnancy: Two case reports. Obstet Gynecol 63:35S, 1984.
47. Bourke E, Gatenby PBB: Renal artery dysplasia with hypertension in neurofibromatosis. Br J Med 3:681–682, 1971.
48. Manser J: Abnormal responses in Von Recklinghausen's disease (letter). Br J Anaesth 42:183, 1970.
49. Magbagbeola JAO: Abnormal responses to muscle relaxants in a patient with Von Recklinghausen's disease (multiple neurofibromatosis) (letter). Br J Anaesth 42:710, 1970.
50. Baraka A: Myasthenic response to muscle relaxants in Von Recklinghausen's disease. Br J Anaesth 46;701–703, 1974.
51. Ahlberg G, Ahlmark G: The Landry-Guillain-Barré syndrome and pregnancy. Acta Obstet Gynecol Scand 57:377–380, 1978.
52. Ravn H: The Landry-Guillain-Barré syndrome: A survey and a clinical report of 127 cases. Acta Neurol Scand 43 (Suppl):1–64, 1967.
53. Osler LD, Sidell AD: The Guillain-Barré syndrome: The need for exact diagnosis criteria. N Engl J Med 262:964–969, 1960.
54. Rudolph JH, Norris FH Jr, Garvey PH, Friederich MA: The Landry-Guillain-Barré syndrome in pregnancy: A review. Obstet Gynecol 26:265–271, 1965.
55. Elstein M, Legg NJ, Murphy M, Park DM, Sutcliffe ML: Guillain-Barré syndrome in pregnancy. Anaesthesia 26:216–224, 1971.
56. Bravo RH, Katz M, Inturrisi M, Cohen NH: Obstetric management of Landry-Guillain-Barré syndrome: A case report. Am J Obstet Gynecol 142:714–715, 1982.
57. Greenland P, Griggs RC: Arrhythmic complications in Guillain-Barré syndrome. Arch Intern Med 140:1053–1055, 1980.
58. Crawford JS, James FM III, Nolte H, Van Steenberge A, Shah JL: Regional anesthesia for patients with chronic neurological disease and similar conditions (letter). Anaesthesia 36:821, 1981.
59. Jones RM, Healy TEJ: A reply (letter). Anaesthesia 36:821–822, 1981.
60. Muller R: Pregnancy in disseminated sclerosis. Acta Psychiatr Neurol Scand 26:397–409, 1951.
61. Schapira K, Poskanzer DC, Newell DJ, Miller H: Marriage, pregnancy and multiple sclerosis. Brain 89:419–428, 1966.
62. McAlpine D, Compston N: Some aspects of the natural history of disseminated sclerosis. Q J Med 21:135–167, 1952.
63. Tillman AJB: The effect of pregnancy on multiple sclerosis and its management. In Multiple Sclerosis and the Demyelinating Diseases. Research Publications of the Association

for Research in Nervous and Mental Disease, No. 28, 1950, pp 548–582.

64. Ridley A, Schapira K: Influence of surgical procedures on the course of multiple sclerosis. Neurology 11:81–82, 1961.

65. Bamford C, Sibley W, Laguna J: Anesthesia in multiple sclerosis. Can J Neurol Sci 5:41–44, 1978.

66. Eickhoff K, Wikstrom J, Poser S, Bauer H: Protein profile of cerebrospinal fluid in multiple sclerosis with special reference to the function of the blood brain barrier. J Neurol 214:207–215, 1977.

67. Schapira K: Is lumbar puncture harmful in multiple sclerosis? J Neurol Neurosurg Psychiatry 22:238, 1959.

68. Warren TM, Datta S, Ostheimer GW: Lumbar epidural anesthesia in a patient with multiple sclerosis. Anesth Analg 61:1022–1023, 1982.

69. Bader AM, Hunt CO, Data S, Naulty JS, Ostheimer GW: Anesthesia for the obstetric patient with multiple sclerosis. J Clin Anesth 1:21–24, 1988.

70. Baskett PJF, Armstrong R: Anaesthetic problems in multiple sclerosis. Are certain agents contraindicated? Anaesthesia 31:1211–1216, 1976.

71. Siemkowicz E: Multiple sclerosis and surgery. Anaesthesia 31:1211–1216, 1976.

72. Foldes FF, McNall PG: Myasthenia gravis: A guide for anesthesiologists. Anesthesiology 23:837–872, 1962.

73. Plausche WC: Myasthenia gravis in pregnancy. Am J Obstet Gynecol 29:691, 1979.

74. Osserman KE: Obstetrics. In *Myasthenia Gravis*. KE Osserman, ed. Grune & Stratton, New York, 1958, pp 239–242.

75. Frenkel M, Ehrlich EN: The influence of progesterone and mineralocorticoids upon myasthenia gravis. Ann Intern Med 60:971–981, 1964.

76. Catanzarite VA, Mittargue AM, Sandberg EC, Dyson DC: Respiratory arrest during therapy for premature labor in a patient with myasthenia gravis. Obstet Gynecol 64:819–822, 1984.

77. Edery H, Porath G, Zahavy J: Passage of 2-hydroxyaminomethyl-N-methylpyridinium methanesulfonate to the fetus and cerebral spaces. Toxicol Appl Pharmacol 9:341–346, 1966.

78. Foldes FF: Myasthenia gravis. Monogr Anesthesiol 3:345–393, 1975.

79. Hokkanen E: The aggravating effect of some antibiotics on the neuromuscular blockade in myasthenia gravis. Acta Neurol Scand 40:346–352, 1964.

80. Cohen BA, London RS, Goldstein PG: Myasthenia gravis and preeclampsia. Obstet Gynecol 48:355, 1976.

81. Genkins G, Mendelow H, Sobel HJ, Osserman KE: Myasthenia gravis: Analysis of thirty-one consecutive postmortem examinations. In *Myasthenia Gravis*, HR Viets, ed. Charles C Thomas, Springfield, IL, 1961, pp 519–530.

82. Mendelow H: Pathology. In *Myasthenia Gravis*, KE Osserman, ed. Grune & Stratton, New York, 1958, pp. 10–43.

83. Rolbin SH, Levinson G, Shnider SM, Wright RG: Anesthetic considerations for myasthenia gravis and pregnancy. Anesth Analg Curr Res 57:441–447, 1978.

84. McNall PG, Jafarnia MR: Management of myasthenia gravis in the obstetrical patient. Am J Obstet Gynecol 92:518–525, 1965.

85. Coaldrake LA, Livingstone PA: Myasthenia gravis in pregnancy. Anaesth Intens Care 11:254–257, 1983.

86. Usubiaga JE, Wikinski JA, Morales RL, Usubiaga LEJ: Interaction of intravenously administered procaine, lidocaine and succinylcholine in anesthetized subjects. Anesth Analg Curr Res 46:39–45, 1967.

87. Foldes FF, Smith JC: The interaction of human cholinesterases with anticholinesterases used in the therapy of myasthenia gravis. Ann NY Acad Sci 135:287–301, 1966.

88. Mulder DG, Braitman H, Wei-i L, Herrmann C Jr: Surgical management in myasthenia gravis. J Thorac Cardiovasc Surg 63:105–113, 1972.

89. Baraka A, Dajani A: Atracurium in myasthenics undergoing thymectomy. Anesth Analg 63:1127–1130, 1984.

90. Namba T, Brown SB, Grob D: Neonatal myasthenia gravis: Report of two cases and review of the literature. Pediatrics 45:488–504, 1970.

91. Keesey J, Lindstrom J, Cokely H, Herrmann C Jr: Antiacetylcholine receptor antibody in neonatal myasthenia gravis (letter). N Engl J Med 296:55, 1977.

92. Penn AS: Diseases of the neuromuscular junction. In *Pediatrics*, 19th ed. AM Rudolph, JIE Hoffman, CD Rudolph, eds. Appleton & Lange, Norwalk, CT, 1991, p 1801.

93. Robertson DNS: Pregnancy and labour in the paraplegic. Paraplegia 10:209–212, 1972.

94. Guttmann L: *Spinal Cord Injuries: Comprehensive Management and Research.* Blackwell Scientific, Oxford, 1973.

95. Goller H, Paeslack V: Our experiences about pregnancy and delivery of the paraplegic women. Paraplegia 8:161–166, 1970.

96. Head H, Riddoch G: The automatic bladder, excessive sweating and some other reflex conditions in gross injuries of the spinal cord. Brain 40:188–263, 1917.

97. Kurnick NB: Autonomic hyperreflexia and its control in patients with spinal cord lesions. Ann Intern Med 44:678–686, 1956.

98. Kendrick WW, Scott JW, Jousse AT, Botterell EH: Reflex sweating and hypertension in traumatic transverse myelitis. Treatment Servs Bull Can (Ottawa) 8:437–448, 1953.

99. Ciliberti BJ, Goldfein J, Rovenstine EA: Hypertension during anesthesia in patients with spinal cord injuries. Anesthesiology 15:273–279, 1953.

100. Quimby CW Jr, Williams RN, Greifenstein FE: Anesthetic problems of the acute quadriplegic patient. Anesth Analg Curr Res 52:333–340, 1973.

101. Stirt JA, Marco A, Conklin KA: Obstetric anesthesia for a quadriplegic patient with autonomic hyperreflexia. Anesthesiology 51:560–562, 1979.

102. Debarge O, Christensen NJ, Corbett JL, Eidelman BH, Frankel HL, Mathias CJ: Plasma catecholamines in tetraplegics. Paraplegia 12:44–49, 1974.

103. Watson DW, Downey GO: Epidural anesthesia for labor and delivery of twins of a paraplegic mother. Anesthesiology 52:259–261, 1980.

104. Cooperman LH, Strobel GE, Kennell EM: Massive hyperkalemia after administration of succinycholine. Anesthesiology 32:161–164, 1970.

105. Rossier AB, Ruffieux M, Ziegler WH: Pregnancy and labour in high traumatic spinal cord lesions. Paraplegia 7:210–216, 1969.

106. Young BK, Katz M, Klein SA: Pregnancy after spinal cord injury: Altered maternal and fetal response to labor. Obstet Gynecol 62:59–63, 1983.

107. Marx GF: Editorial comment. Obstet Anesth Digest 4:6, 1984.

108. Katz VL, Thorp JM, Cefolo RC: Epidural analgesia and autonomic hyperreflexia: A case report. Am J Obstet Gynecol 162:471–472, 1990.

109. Ravindran RS, Cummins DF, Smith IE: Experience with the use of nitroprusside and subsequent epidural analgesia in a pregnant quadriplegic patient. Anesth Analg 60:61–63, 1981.

110. Lewis PE, Cefalo RC, Naulty JS, Rodkey FL: Placental transfer and fetal toxicity of sodium nitroprusside. Gynecol Invest 8:46, 1977.

111. Baraka A: Epidural meperidine for control of autonomic hyperreflexia in a paraplegic parturient. Anesthesiology 62:688–690, 1985.

112. Abouleish E, Hanley ES, Palmer SM: Can epidural fentanyl control autonomic hyperreflexia in a quadriplegic parturient? Anesth Analg 68:523–526, 1989.

113. Lambert DH, Deane RS, Mazuzan JE: Anesthesia and the control of blood pressure in patients with spinal cord injury. Anesth Analg 61:344–348, 1982.

CHAPTER 32

Anesthesia for the Morbidly Obese Pregnant Patient

Sheila E. Cohen, M.B., Ch.B., F.F.A.R.C.S.

DEFINITIONS

Obesity is a disease of modern civilization that afflicts more than 20% of the United States population. It is more than a social or cosmetic problem to the pregnant patient, as evidenced by accumulating data that point to significantly increased maternal and fetal risk with this condition (1–4). In a recent report of maternal mortality in Michigan, obesity was a risk factor in 80% of anesthetic deaths (2). Because of the prevalence of obesity in our society, the obese parturient may be the most common high-risk patient encountered by the obstetric anesthesiologist. Although obesity usually results from excessive caloric intake and not abnormal metabolism, the cause is often obscure. Hereditary, environmental, social economic, and psychologic factors all seem to be important (5). The tendency to obesity begins early in life, with an increased number of fat cells being present in the first year. Familial eating patterns tend to result in obese mothers overfeeding their children, so that they similarly become overweight.

Obesity is defined as an excess of body fat. In nonobese young men approximately 15 to 18% of body weight is composed of fat; in females this figure is 20 to 25% (5). In both groups the proportion of body fat tends to increase with age. Although sophisticated measurements of body fat are necessary to accurately define and quantitate obesity, in most instances the diagnosis is readily apparent. Obesity can be classified in a variety of ways. Individuals less than 20% in excess of ideal weight have been described as **overweight**, and those more than 20% as **obese**. **Morbid obesity** is said to be present when body weight is more than twice normal, or when it exceeds by more than 100 lbs the ideal weight for age and height. Ideal weight can be taken from Metropolitan Life Insurance tables (6) or can be calculated using the **Broca Index**:

Ideal weight (kg) = height (cm) − 100

Techniques used to quantitate adiposity more accurately have included complex measurements of body density and determinations of fat or water content by isotopic or chemical dilution. Simple γ methods include measurement of skinfold thickness, indices such as weight/height, or the **ponderal index** (height/$\sqrt[3]{}$ weight). The most useful of these simple measurements of obesity is the **body mass index** (BMI), which affords the best correlation with the degree of adiposity and is least affected by variations in height (7):

$$\text{BMI} = \frac{\text{weight (kg)}}{\text{height (m}^2)}$$

A BMI of less than 25 is normal, 25 to 29 connotes overweight, and over 30 frank obesity.

Among obese individuals there are two subgroups: those with simple obesity and a small minority, comprising 5 to 10%, who exhibit the obesity hypoventilation syndrome (OHS), also referred to as the "Pickwickian syndrome" (8). Patients in the latter category are extremely obese and suffer from hypoventilation (hypoxemia and hypercarbia), somnolence, edema, polycythemia, and cardiomegaly. It is fortunate that most obese parturients do not suffer from this syndrome, as it carries with it significant risk of morbidity and mortality.

RISKS OF THE OBESE PARTURIENT

Obesity induces changes in anatomy, physiology, psychopathology, and biotransformation of anesthetic agents. Similarly, pregnancy is associated with significant deviations from the normal state. When these two conditions coexist, the resultant effect is unpredictable and potentially hazardous. In addition, obese individuals frequently suffer from other medical problems, including cardiovascular disease (particularly hypertension and coronary artery disease), diabetes, cirrhosis, and cholelithiasis (6). Fatty infiltration of the liver can occur, and abnormal liver function tests have been reported (9). These conditions and obstetric factors render the obese parturient and her newborn particularly prone to developing complications during pregnancy (3, 4, 10–18).

The complications reported in association with obesity in pregnancy are listed in Table 32.1. Because the definitions of obesity vary markedly among investigators, comparisons among studies are difficult. Most of the literature is not confined to morbidly obese parturients (who comprise about 6 to 10% of pregnant women in the United States [4]) but includes those with lesser degrees of obesity. Chronic or pregnancy-induced hypertension has been reported in from 23 to 41% and diabetes in 4 to 18% of obese parturients (3, 4, 10–12, 14). Among obese gravidas presenting for anesthesia in one institution, 47% had antenatal medical disease (17). These rates, which are 5 to 10 times those in normal weight mothers, explain much of the maternal and fetal morbidity. The newborns of obese parturients are large for gestational age (3, 4, 14, 15), with obesity and diabetes both positively influencing fetal weight. The degree of macrosomia is surprising in view of the lower than normal pregnancy weight gain and the increased incidence of hypertension and multiple gestation (4, 15). Prolonged gestation is common in obesity and results in frequent induction of labor (14, 15). Some studies also have reported increased incidences of dysfunctional labor, failed induction, and prolongation of the second stage (12, 14).

The larger babies born to obese mothers may be more at risk for birth trauma and asphyxia, often as a consequence of shoulder dystocia (4, 14). This, along with a higher incidence of malpresentations and twins and a tendency to dysfunctional labors, may explain

the high rate of operative delivery quoted in a number of studies (3, 11, 12). In contrast, Gross et al. (15) found no significant differences in abnormalities of labor or the rate of either operative vaginal or primary cesarean deliveries in a series of women weighing more than 90 kg. However, the rate of repeat cesarean sections was increased in these moderately overweight women (15). In a larger study involving 10,000 mothers of various weights, Garbaciak et al. (3) reported an increased incidence of primary cesarean sections in obese and morbidly obese parturients. When antepartum complications were present, the incidence increased from 18% in normal weight women to 23% in both obese and morbidly obese mothers. When antepartum complications were absent, the cesarean section rates were 10%, 12%, and 20% in normal weight, obese, and morbidly obese mothers, respectively. The marked increase in the latter group may relate to the more frequent occurrence of fetal umbilical cord accidents, meconium staining, and late decelerations noted in these patients (3). These complications did not affect perinatal mortality, however, which was increased only in the infants of mothers with antepartum complications such as diabetes or hypertension. In a recent analysis of almost 57,000 pregnancies, Naeye (16) challenged the hypothesis that adverse neonatal outcome in obesity is related only to maternal complications and fetal macrosomia. Data from this study revealed a progressive increase in perinatal mortality with increasing pregravid maternal weight. Although factors inherently related to obesity, such as maternal diabetes, advanced maternal age, and an increased incidence of dizygous twinning, were associated with greater mortality, acute chorioamnionitis with consequent preterm labor made the biggest contribution to adverse perinatal outcome. It is not known how chorioamnionitis might be related to increased maternal weight.

Many of the above complicating conditions are associated with the need for operative vaginal delivery or cesarean section, thereby necessitating anesthesia. Hood et al. (17) reported a 62% cesarean section rate in 117 women weighing over 300 lbs, whereas Wolfe and colleagues (18) found that 58% of 107 women weighing from 200 to 504 lbs underwent primary cesarean section. Although few studies relate specifically to pregnant patients, anesthesia and surgery in nonpregnant obese patients have been associated with increased morbidity and mortality (19–23). Following surgery for duodenal ulcer, perioperative mortality in obese patients was two and one-half to three times that of nonobese patients (19). Sudden death, not apparently due to myocardial infarction, has been reported during anesthesia in these

Table 32.1
Pregnancy-Related Complications in the Obese Parturient

Maternal Complications	Obstetric/Neonatal Complications
Gestational diabetes	Increased perinatal mortality
Hypertension (chronic and PIH)	Inadequate weight gain
	Prolonged gestation
Urinary tract infection	Macrosomia
Increased cesarean section rate	Twins/breech/ malpresentation
Anesthesia complications	Dysfunctional labor patterns
Blood loss > 1000 ml at cesarean	Shoulder dystocia
	Birth asphyxia
Prolonged surgery	Birth trauma
Postpartum hemorrhage	Neonatal hypoglycemia
Thrombophlebitis	
Wound infections/ dehiscence	

patients. In a critical review of the literature, Pasulka et al. (24) concluded that the risks to the obese patient of *elective* surgery performed in specialized centers by experienced personnel may not be significantly increased. Unfortunately, this is seldom the situation faced by most obstetric patients. Maternal mortality statistics provide convincing evidence that obesity is a significant hazard to the pregnant patient. Obesity was a risk factor in 12 of 15 anesthesia-related maternal deaths in Michigan between 1972 and 1984 (2), with inability to accomplish endotracheal intubation the principal cause of death in recent years. An earlier report from the Chicago Maternity Center found that 4 of 7 maternal deaths occurred in women weighing more than 200 lbs (25). Similar data from Minnesota between 1963 and 1972 revealed that 12% of all maternal deaths occurred in obese women; pulmonary embolus was the leading cause of death in this series (13). Although mortality data do not classify obesity as a cause of death, it seems clear that anesthesia, surgery, and pregnancy pose significant risks to the obese woman. Perioperative morbidity also is increased in obese individuals (26). Complications during cesarean section include prolonged surgery and blood loss exceeding 1000 ml, whereas in the postoperative period, wound infections and thrombophlebitis occur with greatly increased frequency (14, 18, 24, 26).

PHYSIOLOGIC DISTURBANCES

The physiologic changes that accompany both pregnancy (27) (see also Chapter 1) and obesity (24, 28, 29) have been extensively studied. However, few data relate specifically to obese parturients. During pregnancy, the most major changes result from hormonal influences and the mechanical effects of the enlarging uterus. The metabolic demands of the fetus, placenta, and breasts also are responsible for some changes, but these exert a relatively minor influence compared with the other causes. In the obese state, most of the deviations from normal result from the added metabolic and mechanical burden of excess fat. Although many of the physiologic changes in obesity and pregnancy are in the same direction, the magnitude of the resultant abnormality frequently is not known. In view of the wide variation in the degree of physiologic derangement that can exist, evaluation of each patient is mandatory.

Respiratory Changes

LUNG VOLUMES

Both pregnancy and obesity result in an exaggerated lumbar lordosis. In very obese patients a thoracic kyphosis may also be present (27–29). The normal parturient has a widened transverse diameter of the chest due to cephalad pressure by the gravid uterus. Diaphragmatic excursion also is greater than usual. In obesity, the chest wall tends to be splinted in a position of inspiration by abdominal fat, which elevates the ribs. Although diaphragmatic movement again is greater than normal, chest wall adiposity significantly hinders respiratory excursion. Chest wall compliance is decreased in pregnancy and, to a much greater extent, in obesity. In the latter condition compliance relates directly to the weight of adiposity in this region, rather than to total body weight. Inspiratory capacity is therefore abnormal in obesity, but not in normal pregnancy. In addition, in very obese individuals respiratory muscle efficiency is frequently reduced (28). In a study of healthy young adults with moderate to severe obesity, Ray et al. (30) found that respiratory changes were of two types: those which changed in proportion to the degree of obesity, such as expiratory reserve volume (ERV) and diffusing capacity for carbon monoxide, and those which changed only in extreme obesity, such as vital capacity, total lung capacity, and maximum voluntary ventilation.

Individually, pregnancy and obesity are associated with a decrease in ERV and, hence, functional residual capacity (FRC). This results from cephalad pressure by the gravid uterus in pregnancy, and intraabdominal fat and added weight on the chest wall in obesity (27–29). In obese nonpregnant individuals, ERV may be reduced to 20% of its predicted value in the sitting position and may be totally obliterated in the Trendelenburg position (Fig. 32.1). The net

EFFECT OF POSITION ON LUNG VOLUMES

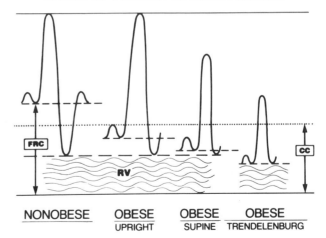

NONOBESE   OBESE UPRIGHT   OBESE SUPINE   OBESE TRENDELENBURG

Figure 32.1. Effect of position change on lung volumes in nonobese compared with markedly obese subjects. *FRC* = functional residual capacity; *RV* = residual volume; *CC* = closing capacity. (Reprinted by permission from Vaughan RW: Pulmonary and cardiovascular derangements in the obese patient. In *Anesthesia and the Obese Patient*, BR Brown Jr, ed. Davis, Philadelphia, 1982, pp 19–39.)

effect is that FRC may be smaller than closing capacity (the lung volume at which terminal airways close during expiration), leading to closure of dependent airways during tidal ventilation. This results in shunting of deoxygenated blood through nonventilated alveoli, with consequent arterial hypoxemia. Shunt fractions of 10 to 25% of cardiac output have been reported in obesity (31). Although in pregnancy FRC is reduced by 30%, airway closure in the sitting position has variously been reported not to occur (32), or conversely to be present in about 25% of women, the majority of whom, however, are smokers (33). Assumption of the supine, lithotomy, or Trendelenburg position (Fig. 32.1), induction of general anesthesia, and the insertion of abdominal packs during surgery all result in additional decreases in FRC in both pregnancy and obesity. In these situations there is the potential for significant deterioration in oxygen saturation (28). Damia et al. (34) recently demonstrated decreases in FRC of 51% following induction of general anesthesia and muscle paralysis in a group of morbidly obese surgical patients. This decrease, which was considerably greater than that seen in normal weight patients, resulted in lung volumes less than baseline residual volumes. FRC returned toward preanesthesia values after laparotomy incision, only to decrease again with skin closure (34). Extrapolation of these findings to obese parturients undergoing cesarean section suggests that pulmonary function might improve significantly after abdominal incision and delivery of the fetus.

It is fortunate that the effects of obesity and pregnancy on lung volumes do not appear to be additive. When the obese gravida reaches the second half of pregnancy, subdiaphragmatic uterine compression would be expected to lead to further encroachment on FRC, with increased airway closure and ventilation perfusion mismatching. In one of the few investigations of respiratory function in obese parturients, Eng and associates (35) studied women weighing 50 to 140% above normal (Table 32.2). Measurements were made during the last trimester of pregnancy and 2 months postpartum, at which stage it was assumed that normalcy had resumed. Although the usual respiratory changes of pregnancy occurred, they were not exaggerated, and FRC decreased to a slightly lesser extent than normal. Surprisingly, FRC was larger than had previously been reported for both pregnant and obese individuals. The authors suggested that their results were due to measurements having been made with subjects in the sitting rather than the supine position, as had been the case in other studies. In spite of the fact that FRC was greater than anticipated, moderate hypoxemia was present with mean PaO_2 values of 85 and 86 for

Table 32.2
Respiratory Function during Pregnancy[a,b]

	Third Trimester (Pregnant)	Postpartum (Nonpregnant)
Lung volumes[c]		
VC (liters)	3.76	3.92
ERV	0.79	0.94[d]
FRC	2.06	2.14
FEV 1.0	3.2	3.3
Arterial blood gases		
pH (torr)	7.44	7.44
PO_2 (torr)	85	86
PCO_2 (torr)	30	36[d]
Base excess (mEq/liter)	−4.2	+0.03[d]

[a] Data from Eng M, Butler J, Bonica J: Respiratory function in pregnant obese women. Am J Obstet Gynecol 123:241–245, 1975.
[b] Respiratory function in 12 obese women during the last trimester of pregnancy and 2 months postpartum (nonpregnant). The change in FRC is not statistically significant and represents a decrease during pregnancy of only 3%. Ventilatory changes are similar to those found in nonobese parturients.
[c] VC = vital capacity; ERV = expiratory reserve volume; FRC = functional residual capacity; FEV 1.0 = forced expiratory volume in 1 sec.
[d] $P < 0.001$ compared to the pregnant state.

pregnant and nonpregnant states, respectively. These data indicate that obesity has a significant deleterious effect on ventilation–perfusion mismatching, which is not further worsened by the pregnant state. It should be noted that only half of the patients in this study could be classified as morbidly obese.

Blass (36) studied a group of women who were considerably more obese and similarly found that pregnancy did not have a detrimental effect on oxygenation. Arterial PO_2 was higher in 27 gravidas between 250 and 500 lbs presenting for cesarean section than it was in women of similar weights who had undergone gastrojejunal bypass. However, these groups are not strictly comparable, because patients undergoing remedial surgery may have been more severely incapacitated by their obesity. The authors suggest that the hyperventilation and flaring of the chest wall that occur during pregnancy exert a beneficial effect in obese women.

VENTILATION

Pregnancy is associated with small (10 to 20%) increases in oxygen consumption and metabolic rate and a large (70%) increase in alveolar ventilation (27). These appear to be hormonally induced (progesterone and estrogen effect) rather than a response to increased metabolism. In obesity, hyperventilation at rest is usual as the excess fat "organ" requires oxygen and generates carbon dioxide; additional cardiorespiratory work is necessary just to mechanically transport the additional weight (28). In patients with simple morbid obesity the mechanical cost of breathing is increased by 30% and with OHS it is increased by as much as 300% above that of normal individuals (37). Eng et al. (35) reported ventilatory changes in obese parturients similar to those in their normal counterparts. Nevertheless, this added burden results in the obese parturient expending significant amounts of energy on ventilatory work, particularly during an unmedicated labor when hyperventilation is often extreme.

Cardiovascular Changes

Similar changes in cardiovascular function are induced by both pregnancy and obesity (27–29, 31). The increases in cardiac output and blood volume in pregnancy are predominantly a function of hormonal influences, with the added effect of the low-resistance placental circulation acting as an arteriovenous shunt. Whereas in pregnancy cardiac output increases by 35 to 45%, in obesity it may double. In the latter condition, blood volume and cardiac output expand in proportion to the increased mass of fat tissue that must be perfused. Also, the additional work of breathing and hypoxemia (if present) stimulate cardiac output. In obesity, resting left ventricular end-diastolic pressure is at the upper limit of normal, explaining the increase in stroke volume that is present. In contrast to the normal pregnant state, when blood pressure decreases somewhat because of lowered vascular resistance, in obesity systolic and diastolic pressures are often elevated, while systemic vascular resistance remains normal. Abnormal mean pulmonary artery and pulmonary capillary pressures have been reported in some extremely obese subjects at rest, with excessive increases following exercise (38). The obese individual is thus subjected to considerable added stresses when she becomes pregnant. Cardiac work and myocardial oxygen consumption already are increased, yet must respond to additional demands imposed by elevations in cardiac output of 45% in labor and 80% in the immediate postpartum period. This is clearly a period of great risk to mothers with hypertension or coronary artery disease. During the second half of pregnancy, aortocaval compression by the uterus in the supine position can severely reduce cardiac output and placental perfusion. This problem is greatly exacerbated in the obese parturient if a large fat panniculus adds to compression of the great vessels.

Gastrointestinal Changes

The problems in the normal pregnant woman of delayed gastric emptying, diminished lower esophageal sphincter tone, and hyperacidity are compounded in the obese mother by a high incidence of hiatus hernia and greatly elevated intragastric pressure. The latter results from compression of intraabdominal structures by omental fat and the weight of the panniculus. Vaughan et al. (39) found 75% of obese surgical patients to be at risk for developing aspiration pneumonitis, having both a gastric pH of less than 2.5 and a volume in excess of 25 ml (Fig. 32.2). In Roberts and Shirley's study of pregnant patients (40), obesity also conferred added risk. Among women in labor weighing over 160 lbs, mean gastric volume was 131 ml, compared with only 22 ml in women of normal weight (28).

Pathophysiology of OHS

In some massively obese patients, hyperventilation gives way to hypoventilation, with consequent hypercapnia, hypoxemia, polycythemia, and somnolence (41). Pulmonary artery pressure is often high and cardiac failure can result. Fortunately, this syndrome usually develops later in life and these patients seldom become pregnant.

EVALUATION OF THE PATIENT

An anesthetic consultation during pregnancy is highly desirable in view of the potential pathophysiologic changes described above. If this has not been accomplished, it should be performed on admission to the labor suite. At this examination the respiratory and cardiovascular systems must be carefully eval-

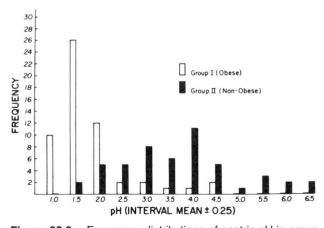

Figure 32.2. Frequency distributions of gastric pH in group I (obese) and group II (nonobese) surgical patients. The distribution curve for group I patients is skewed to the left. (Reprinted by permission from Vaughan RW, Bauer S, Wise L: Volume and pH of gastric juice in obese patients. Anesthesiology 43:686–689, 1975.)

uated, inquiring for symptoms of dyspnea, edema, dizziness in the supine position (indicating severe aortocaval compression), and exercise tolerance. The blood pressure should be checked with an adequately sized cuff, bearing in mind that, while a cuff that is too small will give falsely high pressures, an overly large cuff also will give erroneous results. The chest should be examined for signs of left ventricular hypertrophy and pulmonary congestion. Severe "heartburn" indicates that significant gastroesophageal reflux is present.

It is most important at this time to carefully evaluate the airway, because failed intubation, currently the leading cause of maternal anesthetic mortality, is a particular hazard in the obese parturient. Difficulty relates to the degree of adiposity of the face, shoulders, neck, and breasts. The usual atlantooccipital gap is frequently nonexistent in the obese patient (Fig. 32.3), with the result that extension of the head is either impossible or results in bowing of the cervical spine and forward displacement of the larynx (42). Insertion of the laryngoscope may be hindered by grossly enlarged breasts (Fig. 32.3), particularly when the patient is in a position of left lateral tilt. A history of easy intubation with prior

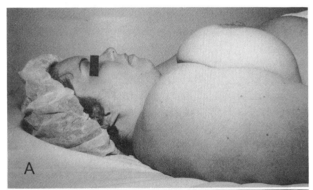
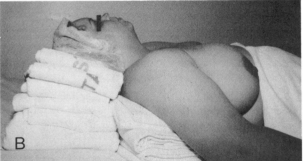

Figure 32.3. *A,* Obese pregnant woman in the supine position. The atlantooccipital gap is obliterated by fat and access with a laryngoscope is hindered by large breasts. *B,* The same patient positioned with the shoulders elevated and the occiput further elevated so that the head assumes the "sniffing" position. Access to the airway is greatly facilitated.

anesthetics is no guarantee that problems will not be encountered, because weight usually has increased significantly during pregnancy. Inspection of the distribution of body fat, with evaluation of the lumbar area for ease of palpation of bony landmarks and degree of lordosis, is important with respect to performance of regional anesthesia. The arms should be examined to predict potential difficulty with insertion of intravenous and intraarterial catheters.

In addition to the usual laboratory investigations, an electrocardiogram, liver function tests, and a glucose tolerance test should be ordered. Measurement of oxyhemoglobin saturation in the sitting, supine, and Trendelenburg positions using a pulse oximeter provides an easy way to assess the present degree of airway closure and the potential for deterioration with further decreases in FRC. In patients demonstrating desaturation with these maneuvers or in those with extreme obesity, pulmonary function tests and arterial blood gas analysis should be performed. Finally, the predelivery visit affords an ideal opportunity to explain to the patient the problems engendered by her condition and to appraise her of the risks and benefits of alternative analgesic management plans. Although apparently cheerful, many morbidly obese individuals are in fact intensely embarrassed and depressed by their appearance. If the anesthesiologist is to secure the patient's cooperation, disparaging remarks about her weight and the difficulties that it will cause must be avoided.

ANESTHETIC CONSIDERATIONS

Drug Metabolism and Toxicity in the Obese Individual

Abnormal biotransformation of volatile anesthetic agents, with increased formation of reactive intermediates or toxic end products, has been reported in morbidly obese patients (43, 44). This appears to result from increased retention of lipid-soluble agents in the abnormally large depot of body fat, with subsequent prolonged biodegradation. This is most significant with methoxyflurane, which is extremely lipid soluble. Young et al. (43) reported higher peak inorganic fluoride levels following methoxyflurane anesthesia in obese surgical patients than in normal controls; mean peak serum inorganic fluoride levels of 56 μmol in obese patients were in the range associated with subclinical nephrotoxicity, and four individuals had peak levels in the toxic range. Similarly, fluoride production following enflurane administration to obese patients occurs at a rate twice that of nonobese patients exposed to comparable dosages (44). Maximum serum fluoride levels in obese individuals were 60% higher than in normal patients (28 vs. 17 μmol) but were insufficiently high to result in abnormal renal function. Isoflurane is metabolized to a much lesser extent than is enflurane and results in considerably lower fluoride levels in obese patients (Fig. 32.4) (45). Unlike enflurane, fluoride levels after isoflurane are similar in obese and normal weight patients. Halothane is usually not metabolized to form inorganic fluoride. However, in morbidly obese patients elevated inorganic fluoride levels follow halothane administration, indicating that reductive metabolism has taken place (46). This is of concern, because this abnormal metabolic pathway has been associated with halothane hepatotoxicity in animals. To date there is no evidence that halothane administration to obese individuals routinely results in hepatic dysfunction. Although serum bromide levels following halothane anesthesia are higher in obese patients than in normal individuals, sedative levels are not attained (46). From the point of view of toxicity, isoflurane is currently the agent of choice for obese patients. Enflurane and halothane are probably acceptable, provided dosage is not excessive. Methoxyflurane should not be used in this population.

Although delayed recovery from inhalation anesthesia in obesity might be expected because of retention of volatile agents in body fat, this does not appear to be the case. Cork et al. (47) found no difference between the recovery time of obese individuals who had received fentanyl and those who had received halothane or enflurane. Obese patients often require large doses of intravenous anesthetic agents because their volume of drug distribution is greatly expanded. Dose requirements of succinylcholine (48) are increased in obesity in proportion to body weight, BMI, and surface area, rather than relating to lean body mass, as might be expected. This is due to the increases in blood and extracellular fluid volumes, which are proportionate to the enlarged body surface area (5) as well as to an increase in pseudocholinesterase levels in obesity (48).

Studies in which pancuronium was administered to obese patients have yielded controversial results. Tsueda et al. (49) found that larger dose requirements for pancuronium in obese patients were related to body surface area, whereas Söderberg et al. (31) suggest that dosage for this agent should be based on ideal body weight. Varin and colleagues (50) studied atracurium in obese patients and recommended dosing on the basis of body weight. Although the volume of distribution for atracurium was not increased in these obese patients, a higher drug concentration was required to obtain a degree of blockade comparable to that of nonobese patients (50). However, the duration of neuromuscular blockade was not prolonged even when large doses of atracurium were given (Fig. 32.5, A), (50, 51) probably because drug disposition does not depend on hepatic or renal clearance. In contrast, prolonged recovery from vecuronium has been reported in obesity (Fig. 32.5, B) and has been attributed to delayed hepatic elimination, possibly resulting from fatty infiltration of the liver or a relative reduction in hepatic blood flow (51). The prolonged action and elimination of metocurine that occurs in obese patients has been explained by decreased urinary clearance resulting from exaggerated effects of anesthesia on renal function (52). Overdosage with relaxants other than atracurium can be minimized by reducing maintenance doses and increasing the interval between supplements. Regardless of which anesthetic drugs are used, careful postanesthetic surveillance is essential to detect residual muscle paralysis or respiratory depression caused by large doses of intravenous agents.

Monitoring

The sophistication of monitoring techniques employed should depend on the degree of obesity (and consequent cardiopulmonary impairment) and whether other conditions such as preeclampsia or diabetes are present. A correctly sized blood pressure cuff is adequate for the moderately obese mother having an uncomplicated labor. In more complex situ-

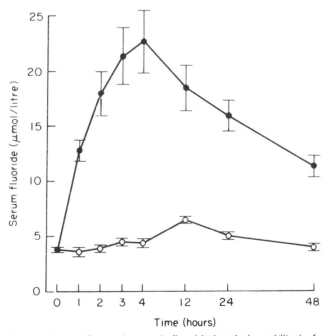

Figure 32.4. Serum inorganic fluoride levels (μmol/liter) after enflurane anesthesia (●) and isoflurane anesthesia (○) in obese surgical patients (mean ± SEM). (Reprinted by permission from Strube PJ, Hulands GH, Halsey MJ: Serum fluoride levels in morbidly obese patients: Enflurane compared with isoflurane anaesthesia. Anaesthesia 42:685–689, 1987.)

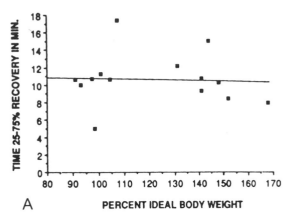

A   **PERCENT IDEAL BODY WEIGHT**

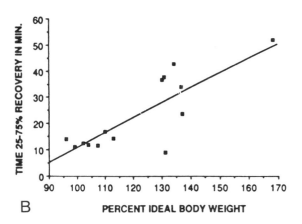

B   **PERCENT IDEAL BODY WEIGHT**

Figure 32.5. Regression lines relating time for 25 to 75% recovery of twitch response and body weight in surgical patients following: *A*, atracurium, 0.5 mg/kg ($r = 0.06$); and *B*, vecuronium, 0.1 mg/kg, ($r = 0.81$). (Reprinted by permission

from Weinstein JA, Matteo RS, Ornstein E, Schwartz AE, Goldstoff M, Thal G: Pharmacodynamics of vecuronium and atracurium in the obese surgical patient. Anesth Analg 67:1149–1153, 1988.)

ations an automated device, or an intraarterial catheter that facilitates repeated blood gas analyses, is preferable. Central venous and pulmonary artery catheters are indicated in special situations such as preeclampsia or cardiac or respiratory failure. Percutaneous placement of these monitors and even an intravenous catheter can prove very difficult and occasionally a cutdown is necessary. Noninvasive monitoring of oxygenation with pulse oximetry is mandatory during general or regional anesthesia for cesarean section and is helpful during labor in the morbidly obese parturient. End-tidal carbon dioxide monitoring also should be used during general anesthesia to confirm correct placement of the endotracheal tube and permit appropriate adjustment of ventilation. The electrocardiogram must be monitored during major anesthesia and a nerve stimulator used whenever muscle relaxants are employed. During labor, monitoring of contractions and fetal heart rate is often hindered by the thickness of the abdominal wall. Direct internal monitoring of these parameters with a scalp electrode and an intrauterine pressure catheter is usually necessary.

Anesthesia for Vaginal Delivery

During labor the mother should remain in the lateral sitting or semirecumbent position to minimize closure of dependent airways and aortocaval compression. Intravenous access is best secured early in labor. Oxygen should be administered throughout labor to prevent hypoxemia, which may result from ventilation perfusion abnormalities and from the enormously increased metabolic and cardiorespiratory activity. Epidural analgesia decreases respiratory work and oxygen consumption, improves oxygenation, and prevents the increase in cardiac output

that results from catecholamine secretion during labor. It also is advantageous in view of the frequent need for operative vaginal or cesarean delivery. Major technical difficulties may present when instituting regional anesthesia in obese mothers, although the distribution of fat is sometimes such that the procedure is easier than would have been predicted from weight alone.

As might be expected, the depth at which the epidural space is located correlates strongly with patient weight and the degree of obesity (53, 54). Hood and associates (17) found that, whereas 94% of morbidly obese parturients ultimately obtained successful epidural anesthesia, the catheter had to be replaced once in 46% of patients and two or more times in 21% of patients. Increasing patient weight significantly decreased the likelihood of successful epidural placement by residents, but not by attending anesthesiologists (17). Insertion of an epidural catheter early in labor is desirable to allow time for placement and confirmation that the block is functional. Experienced personnel must be available to perform these challenging procedures, and special long needles (15 or 20 cm) are sometimes required. When a normal length needle is used, it may be submerged up the hilt, thereby indenting the subcutaneous tissue. In this circumstance, an assistant may be needed to prevent displacement of the needle by securing it with a hemostat (55). A loss-of-resistance technique is preferable to the "hanging drop" method, because epidural pressure in obesity cannot be relied upon to be subatmospheric. The sitting position is most comfortable for the patient and provides the easiest identification of the midline. If no bony landmarks can be located, extensive infiltration of the area with local anesthetic enables exploration with a fine needle to localize a vertebral spinous process or lamina.

Once the epidural space has been located, insertion of the catheter for 5 cm rather than the usual 3 to 4 cm has been recommended to discourage displacement of the catheter due to mobility of the layer of subcutaneous fat (56). For the same reason, secure taping of the catheter also is essential. The volume of local anesthetic needed to provide adequate epidural analgesia is less in the obese individual (see below) (57, 58), probably because adipose tissue and increased venous distension from severe aortocaval compression decrease the capacity of the epidural space. A block that is too high or too dense will further weaken respiratory muscle function and impair the ability to push in the second stage of labor. Infusions of dilute solutions of local anesthetics combined with opioids provide excellent analgesia for labor, with minimal motor blockade. Although these mixtures have not specifically been studied in obese parturients, they appear ideal because they allow the patient to move herself and facilitate maternal expulsive efforts during the second stage of labor. Conservative doses of opioids are recommended, however, as experience with use of intraspinal opioids for postcesarean analgesia suggests that the obese parturient is at greater risk of respiratory depression (59, 60).

If epidural analgesia proves technically impossible, first-stage pain can be managed with small doses of intravenous narcotics. Spinal block is often easier to perform than epidural and is appropriate for the second stage of labor, particularly when operative vaginal delivery is planned. Several investigators have reported higher than expected levels of spinal blockade in obese nonpregnant patients (61–63), attributing this to increased cerebrospinal fluid pressure caused by epidural venous congestion or excessive extradural fat. An additional factor may be the large buttocks effectively placing the patient in a Trendelenburg position relative to the true horizontal of the operating table (64). When epidural placement for labor analgesia proves technically difficult, we sometimes administer a single spinal injection of opioid (usually sufentanil, 7.5 to 10 μg [65]) with the goal of establishing analgesia while efforts to insert the epidural catheter proceed. Continuous spinal anesthesia also can be considered in this situation. However, the recent occurrence of several cases of cauda equina syndrome in surgical patients who received larger than usual doses of local anesthetic via very small gauge spinal catheters has raised concern about this technique (66).

Inhalation analgesia with nitrous oxide can be administered for the latter part of the first and all of the second stage of labor, provided that consciousness and active laryngeal reflexes are maintained and oxygen saturation is closely monitored. Anesthesia can be induced particularly rapidly, because of the degree of hyperventilation present in the obese woman in labor. Methoxyflurane should not be used for reasons already discussed. General anesthesia should rarely be necessary for vaginal delivery, but if unavoidable, it should be performed as described in the following for cesarean section. It must be remembered that the Trendelenburg and lithotomy positions, which often are employed during vaginal delivery, have a deleterious effect on oxygenation. In these situations, positive pressure ventilation should be used to prevent airway closure.

Anesthesia for Cesarean Section

Obese parturients presenting for cesarean section have a high incidence of complications such as diabetes or preeclampsia, with the coexisting medical condition often directly or indirectly being the cause for the procedure. As previously discussed, perioperative morbidity and mortality are high in this group. Reviews of anesthesia for obese patients (1, 14, 21–23, 56, 67–70) describe problems with both regional and general anesthesia. In recent years general anesthesia has been implicated more often than regional in causing maternal deaths (1). For elective cesarean section regional anesthesia appears to be advantageous because it results in a lower incidence of intraoperative hypertension and postoperative respiratory complications (55, 67–69). The major goals of anesthetic management are prevention of aspiration, careful management of the airway and of ventilation, and avoidance of additional cardiovascular stress. Technical difficulties relate to transporting the patient to the operating room, securing her on a narrow operating table, and displacing the uterus adequately to avoid aortocaval compression.

Much discussion has centered on the ideal surgical approach to the uterus (70, 71). Caudad retraction of the panniculus to permit a midline incision traditionally has been favored because abdominal access is facilitated and operating time until delivery minimized. However, Ahern and Goodlin (71) preferred cephalad retraction to enable a Pfannenstiel incision, which has less potential for wound dehiscence and for causing hypoxemia in the postoperative period. In a study of morbidity following cesarean section in obese women, Wolfe et al. (18) found that choice of skin incision did not influence the postoperative course. If a transverse incision is considered desirable, an attempt should be made to retract the panniculus vertically, thus removing its weight from the great vessels (Fig. 32.6). Severe aortocaval compression caused by cephalad retraction of a 70-kg panniculus has resulted in death of the

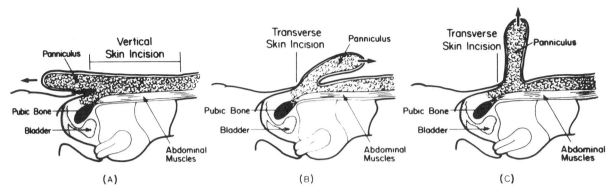

Figure 32.6. The panniculus is shown (*A*) retracted caudad to permit a vertical incision above; (*B*) retracted cephalad to permit a transverse Pfannenstiel incision; and (*C*) retracted vertically. Direction of retraction is shown by arrows. (Reprinted by permission from Hodgkinson R, Husain FJ: Caesarean section associated with gross obesity. Br J Anaesth 52:919–923, 1980.)

fetus in one extremely obese woman (70). Cephalad retraction of a large panniculus also decreases chest wall compliance, causing dyspnea in patients who are awake and necessitating higher inflation pressures in those undergoing general anesthesia. Whenever possible, fetal heart rate should be monitored during the surgical procedure. The induction-delivery interval is often prolonged, and fetal deterioration can result from decreases in uterine perfusion due to excessive retraction or abnormalities in maternal ventilation.

GENERAL ANESTHESIA

General endotracheal anesthesia is necessary for some emergency cesarean deliveries or for elective cases when regional anesthesia is contraindicated or not feasible for technical reasons.

Prevention of Aspiration Pneumonitis

To decrease the risk of pneumonitis should aspiration occur, measures should be taken to increase gastric pH and decrease gastric volume. In elective cases, histamine H_2-receptor antagonists such as cimetidine or ranitidine should be administered the night before and the morning of operation. In a study in nonpregnant obese surgical patients, only 13% of those who had received cimetidine had a gastric pH of less than 2.5, compared with 65% of patients who had been premedicated with atropine or glycopyrrolate (72). Using the same criteria, Lam et al. (73) found only 10% of morbidly obese patients at risk from aspiration following intravenous injection of 300 mg of cimetidine at least 60 min before induction of anesthesia, compared with 77% in the control group. Prophylactic administration of oral or intravenous ranitidine is recommended for morbidly obese parturients in labor as a precaution should general anesthesia become necessary. Metoclopramide, a dopamine antagonist that increases lower esophageal

sphincter tone in gravid patients (74), should be particularly beneficial in obese mothers. A 10- to 20-mg dose administered intravenously 30 min or more before induction of anesthesia may also accelerate gastric motility and, hence, decrease the volume of gastric contents (75). When an obese patient is admitted to the labor ward for urgent cesarean section, an H_2 blocker and metoclopramide should be administered immediately to inhibit gastric acid secretion and facilitate emptying of food that may be in the stomach. In addition, all patients should receive 15 to 30 ml of a nonparticulate antacid, such as 0.3 molar sodium citrate, immediately before induction of anesthesia to neutralize gastric pH.

Airway Management

Endotracheal intubation can present major difficulties in the obese parturient because of fat deposits in the neck, shoulders, and breasts. Failed intubation, often in association with pulmonary aspiration, is one of the most common causes of anesthetic deaths in obese parturients (2). Difficulties should be anticipated beforehand, rather than discovering after induction of anesthesia that the patient can neither be intubated nor ventilated. Careful positioning as shown in Figure 32.3 can greatly facilitate access to the airway. The shoulders are elevated, allowing the breasts to fall away from the neck and chin, while folded towels are used to support the occiput and place the head in the sniffing position. This opens up an area that is often submerged in rolls of fat, allowing insertion of the laryngoscope. The short-handled laryngoscope (76) and the adjustable-angle blade (77) can be helpful in the obese parturient (Fig. 32.7). An added hazard in these patients is laryngeal edema, which can accompany grossly excessive weight gain in pregnancy (78) or generalized edema in preeclampsia (79). A small-diameter endotracheal tube

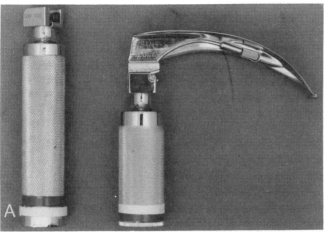 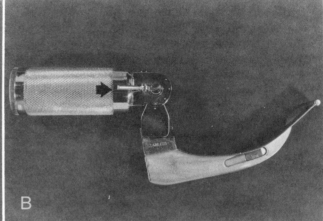

Figure 32.7. *A,* Short handle (*right*) for laryngoscope compared with conventional length handle (*left*). *B,* Adjustable-angle laryngoscope. A blade lock (*arrow*) allows positioning of the blade at 180, 135, 90, or 45 degrees to the handle. The blade can be inserted parallel to the handle and the angle then decreased to 135 or 90 degrees to allow tongue retraction and exposure of the larynx. (Reprinted by permission from Patil VU, Stehling LC, Zauder HL: An adjustable laryngoscope handle for difficult intubations. Anesthesiology 60:609, 1984.)

should therefore always be prepared. The anesthesiologist also should have immediately available some means of ventilating the patient should attempts at intubation fail. A 12- or 14-gauge intravenous cannula or a specially designed cricothyrotomy needle with which the anesthesiologist is familiar can be introduced through the cricothyroid membrane into the trachea and connected to a high pressure source of ventilation (80, 81). However, technical difficulties should be anticipated because of adiposity of the neck and low compliance of the chest wall. If airway obstruction or failed intubation does occur, hypoxia and acidosis develop with alarming rapidity. The decreased FRC stores less oxygen, and oxygen consumption and carbon dioxide production are greatly increased in the obese parturient. An oximeter and a capnograph thus are extremely helpful when airway complications arise in the obese parturient. If difficulty with the airway is anticipated before induction of anesthesia, awake intubation can be performed (6, 7) either blindly or with the aid of a fiberoptic laryngoscope. Fiberoptic laryngoscopy is not to be recommended in the emergency situation to practitioners unskilled in this technique.

Anesthetic Technique

Rapid induction of anesthesia with thiopental (3 to 4 mg/kg) and succinylcholine (1 to 1.5 mg/kg) is usually performed in the emergency situation and in elective cases if the airway appears favorable. Concurrent with injection of the induction agents, cricoid pressure must be applied by a skilled assistant. The optimal method of preoxygenation before induction in the obese parturient is controversial. In obese surgical patients (82) and nonobese pregnant patients (83), 3 min of preoxygenation and four vital capacity breaths proved equally effective at increasing arterial oxygen tension. However, the former technique resulted in slight retention of carbon dioxide in morbidly obese patients (82). Of most importance in the obese parturient, in whom intubation difficulties are common, is the safe duration of apnea. In a study of normal healthy patients, Gambee et al. (84) demonstrated longer times to desaturation during apnea following 3 min of preoxygenation than following four vital capacity breaths. Because oxygen saturation during apnea decreases much more quickly in both morbidly obese patients (85) and pregnant women (86), a 3- to 5-min period of denitrogenation is recommended in the obese parturient.

Anesthesia can be maintained with nitrous oxide 50% and low concentrations of a volatile anesthetic until delivery, after which the latter may be discontinued and a short-acting narcotic administered. Paralysis with a neuromuscular blocking agent is usually necessary to facilitate surgical access. Positive pressure ventilation with large tidal volumes minimizes airway closure (29, 87), although positive end-expiratory pressure does not appear to improve oxygenation, probably because it also decreases cardiac output (87, 88). Catecholamine release during endotracheal intubation can be hazardous in the hypertensive obese gravida, who is particularly prone to developing pulmonary edema because of her expanded blood volume. Treatment of severe hypertension with vasodilators or short-acting β-adrenergic blockers may be indicated; the choice of drug therapy will depend on the presence or absence of invasive monitoring. The obese mother must be fully awake before extubation, and postoperative ventilation must be continued if adequate arousal and respiratory and neuromuscular function cannot be demonstrated. Because hypoxemia is common in obese patients in the immediate postoperative period, oxygen saturation should be monitored and supplemental oxygen administered in the postanesthetic care unit (89).

REGIONAL ANESTHESIA

Regional blockade avoids intubation difficulties and, provided hypotension does not develop, is associated with greater cardiovascular stability than is general anesthesia in the hypertensive parturient (90). Also, aspiration should be less of a hazard. However, this risk does exist with regional anesthesia, and the precautions recommended for general anesthesia should be employed. Postoperative respiratory complications have been reported to occur less frequently with regional than with general anesthesia (67).

Epidural anesthesia is preferable to spinal anesthesia for cesarean section because of its greater controllability and the ability to titrate the block to the desired level and extend it for prolonged procedures. Spinal anesthesia is often technically easier to perform and is useful in the moderately obese gravida in whom markedly prolonged surgery is not anticipated. Long-acting local anesthetics such as bupivacaine should be used, with the addition of opioids and perhaps epinephrine to ensure a dense block of adequate duration. Continuous spinal anesthesia offers an alternative approach in cases in which the surgical procedure is likely to be long and difficult. In normal weight individuals, some anesthesiologists use very small-gauge spinal catheters with the goal of minimizing the risk of postdural puncture headache. However, because technical difficulties with insertion and subsequent kinking may cause problems in the obese parturient, use of a larger catheter may be preferable.

Hypotension with regional anesthesia must be prevented by preloading the circulation with fluids, adequate displacement of the uterus and the panniculus from the inferior vena cava and aorta, and prompt treatment of any decrease in blood pressure with additional fluids and ephedrine. When all these precautions were taken, the incidence of hypotension (<100 mm Hg systolic blood pressure) was only 12% in one series of obese patients receiving epidural anesthesia for cesarean section (57). Several studies have demonstrated that higher levels of anesthetic block result in obese patients (57, 58, 67). Hodgkinson and Husain (57) found the extent of analgesia to be positively correlated with BMI and body weight.

These authors also found that, in obesity, cephalad spread of epidural block was limited when the patient was in the sitting position, in contrast to patients of normal weight in whom gravity did not affect the block (58). They recommended using a reduced dosage of local anesthetic and performing the block with the patient sitting to minimize unwanted autonomic blockade and maintain respiratory muscle tone. Spinal anesthesia is also performed most easily with the patient in the sitting position. Despite the fact that the level of spinal block tends to be higher in obese patients (see preceding), this author does not recommend decreasing the local anesthetic dosage. An inadequate spinal block may necessitate emergency induction of general anesthesia after the operation has started, presenting a hazardous situation for the obese gravida. Control of the level of spinal blockade can be accomplished by using routine doses of hyperbaric solutions, with careful positioning of the patient in a slight head-up position as soon as an adequate level of anesthesia has been obtained.

Embarrassment of ventilation by large breasts, the fat panniculus, and insertion of packs in the abdomen must be guarded against. Sedation following delivery should be kept to a minimum to avoid hypoventilation. If respiratory inadequacy does occur, general anesthesia with endotracheal intubation and positive pressure ventilation must be undertaken. A major advantage of regional anesthesia is that it permits the use of intraspinal opioid analgesia, postoperatively. Leaving the epidural catheter in situ allows for continuation of analgesia for several days if necessary.

POSTOPERATIVE MANAGEMENT

The obese parturient continues to be at risk after delivery, particularly if surgical intervention was necessary. Wound dehiscences and infections are more frequent in these individuals, and hospitalization is often prolonged. Postoperatively, respiratory complications are frequent (25) and hypoxemia can persist for several days (Fig. 32.8) (91, 92). Vertical abdominal incisions result in more severe hypoxemia on the second to fifth postoperative day than do transverse incisions (Fig. 32.8) (92). Supplemental oxygen should be administered and the patient placed in the sitting position, as this minimizes airway closure and improves oxygenation (93). Intensive chest physiotherapy is helpful to aid the clearing of secretions. Severely obese patients in whom cardiac or respiratory dysfunction was present preoperatively should recover in the intensive care unit, at least for the first 24 to 48 hr.

Adequate postoperative analgesia is essential if deep

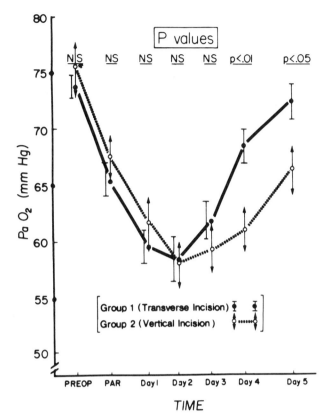

Figure 32.8. Decrease in Pa_{O_2} (torr) with time postoperatively in group I (transverse incision) and group II (vertical incision) patients. (Reproduced by permission from Vaughan RW, Wise L: Choice of abdominal operative incision in the obese patient: A study using blood gas measurements. Ann Surg 181:829–835, 1975.)

breathing is to be encouraged and atelectasis avoided. Parenteral, epidural, or spinal opioids (94–99) or epidurally administered local anesthetics (67, 69) can be employed, but care must be taken to avoid central respiratory depression or respiratory muscle weakness. The analgesia that results from intraspinal opioids encourages better ventilation, earlier mobility (thus guarding against deep vein thrombosis), and earlier restoration of bowel function, and it facilitates nursing care (94, 95, 98). However, because respiratory depression is a greater risk in the obese parturient (59, 60), it is mandatory that ventilation be continuously monitored for the first 24 hr, either on the postpartum ward or in the intensive care unit. Prophylaxis against deep vein thrombosis with low-dose heparin is advocated by many for obese surgical patients (100, 101) because thrombophlebitis and pulmonary embolus are a major cause of mortality, particularly in the postpartum period (13). Some experts consider heparin prophylaxis to be a contraindication to the use of regional anesthesia because of the risk of epidural hematoma. However, reports of

the safe use of epidural anesthesia in anticoagulated patients suggest that this risk is minimal, if appropriate precautions are taken (102, 103).

SUMMARY

In the obese parturient, morbidity and mortality are high because of abnormal anatomy, physiology, and responses to anesthesia. Hypertension, hypotension, hypoxia, and acidosis can develop with great rapidity when complications occur; the margin of safety in these circumstances is very much reduced. The anesthesiologist must be aware of the particular problems of the morbidly obese mother and ensure that an appropriate level of expertise is available for her care. All too often, the attitude of the health care team mirrors the negative view that society holds of these people, with the result that they are not afforded the attention warranted by their medical condition.

References

1. Endler GC: The risk of anesthesia in obese parturients. J Perinatol 10:175–179, 1990.
2. Endler GC, Mariona FG, Sokol RJ, Stevenson LB: Anesthesia-related maternal mortality in Michigan. Am J Obstet Gynecol 159:187–193, 1988.
3. Garbaciak JA, Richter M, Miller MS, Barton JJ: Maternal weight and pregnancy complications. Am J Obstet Gynecol 152:238–245, 1985.
4. Kliegman RM, Gross T: Perinatal problems of the obese mother and her infant. Obstet Gynecol 66:299–306, 1985.
5. Bray GA: *The Obese Patient, Vol 9.* Saunders, Philadelphia, 1976, pp 2–93.
6. Metropolitan Life Insurance Company: New weight standards for men and woman. Stat Bull Metrop Insur Co 40:3–6, 1959.
7. Keys A, Fidanze F, Karvonen MJ, Kimura N, Taylor HL: Indices of relative weight and obesity. J Chronic Dis 25:329–343, 1972.
8. Burwell CS, Robin ED, Whaley RD, Bickelmann AG: Extreme obesity associated with alveolar hypoventilation: A Pickwickian syndrome. Am J Med 21:811–818, 1956.
9. Bentley JB: The liver in obesity. In *Anesthesia and the Obese Patient.* BR Brown Jr, ed. Davis, Philadelphia, 1982, pp 41–53.
10. Roopnarinesingh SS, Pathak UN: Obesity in the Jamaican parturient. J Obstet Gynaecol Br Commonw 77:895–899, 1970.
11. Tracy TA, Miller GL: Obstetric problems of the massively obese. Obstet Gynecol 33:204–208, 1969.
12. Freedman MA, Wilds PL, George WM: Grotesque obesity: A serious complication of labor and delivery. South Med J 65:732–736, 1972.
13. Maeder EC, Barno A, Mecklenburg F: Obesity: A maternal high-risk factor. Obstet Gynecol 45:669–671, 1975.
14. Johnson SR, Kolberg BH, Varner MW, Railsback LD: Maternal obesity and pregnancy. Surg Gynecol Obstet 164:431–437, 1987.
15. Gross T, Sokol RJ, King KC. Obesity in pregnancy: Risks and outcome. Obstet Gynecol 56:446–450, 1980.
16. Naeye RL: Maternal body weight and pregnancy outcome. Am J Clin Nutr 52:273–279, 1990.
17. Hood DD, Dewan DM, Kashtan K: Anesthesia outcome in the morbidly obese parturient. Anesthesiology 73:A952, 1990.
18. Wolfe HM, Gross TL, Sokol RJ, Bottoms SF, Thompson KL: Determinants of morbidity in obese women delivered by cesarean. Obstet Gynecol 71:691–696, 1988.

19. Postlethwait RW, Johnson WD: Complications following surgery for duodenal ulcer in obese patients. Arch Surg 105:438–440, 1972.

20. Fisher A, Waterhouse TD, Adams AP: Obesity: Its relation to anaesthesia. Anaesthesia 30:633–647, 1975.

21. Catenacci AJ, Anderson JD, Boersma D: Anesthetic hazards of obesity. JAMA 175:657–665, 1973.

22. Fox GS: Anesthesia for intestinal short circuiting in the morbidly obese with reference to the pathophysiology of gross obesity. Can Anaesth Soc J 22:307–315, 1975.

23. Gould AB: Effect of obesity on respiratory complications following general anesthesia. Anesth Analg 41:448–452, 1962.

24. Pasulka PS, Bistrian BR, Benotti PN, Blackburn GL: The risks in obese patients. Ann Intern Med 104:540–546, 1986.

25. Benaron HBW, Tucker BE: The effect of obstetric management and factors beyond clinical control on maternal mortality rates at the Chicago Maternity Center from 1959–1963. Am J Obstet Gynecol 110:1113–1118, 1971.

26. Nielsen TK, Hökegård KH: Postoperative cesarean section morbidity: A prospective study. Am J Obstet Gynecol 146:911–916, 1983.

27. Cohen SE: Why is the pregnant patient different? Semin Anesth 1:73–82, 1982.

28. Vaughan RW: Pulmonary and cardiovascular derangements in the obese patient. In Anesthesia and the Obese Patient. BR Brown Jr, ed. Davis, Philadelphia, 1982, pp 19–39.

29. Bendixen HH: Morbid obesity. In Refresher Courses in Anesthesiology, Vol 6. SG Hershey, ed. Lippincott, Philadelphia, 1978, pp 1–14.

30. Ray CS, Sue DY, Bray G, Hansen JE, Wasserman K: Effects of obesity on respiratory function. Am Rev Resp Dis 128:501–506, 1983.

31. Söderberg M, Thomson D, White T: Respiration, circulation and anesthetic management in obesity: Investigation before and after jejuno-ileal bypass. Acta Anaesthesiol Scand 21:55–61, 1977.

32. Templeton A, Kelman GR: Maternal blood gases (PAO$_2$-PaO$_2$), physiological shunt and VD/VT in normal pregnancy. Br J Anaesth 48:1001–1104, 1976.

33. Holdcroft A, Bevan DR, O'Sullivan JC, Sykes MK: Airway closure and pregnancy. Anaesthesia 32:517–523, 1977.

34. Damia G, Mascheroni D, Croci M, Tarenzi L: Perioperative changes in functional residual capacity in morbidly obese patients. Br J Anaesth 60:574–578, 1988.

35. Eng M, Butler J, Bonica J: Respiratory function in pregnant obese women. Am J Obstet Gynecol 123:241–245, 1975.

36. Blass NH: Regional anesthesia in the morbidly obese. Reg Anesth 4:20–22, 1979.

37. Sharp JT, Henry JP, Sweany SK, Meadows WR, Pietras RJ: The total work of breathing in normal and obese men. J Clin Invest 43:728–738, 1964.

38. Backman L, Freyschuss V, Holbug D, Melcher A: Cardiovascular function in extreme obesity. Acta Med Scand 193:437–446, 1973.

39. Vaughan RW, Bauer S, Wise L: Volume and pH of gastric juice in obese patients. Anesthesiology 43:686–689, 1975.

40. Roberts RB, Shirley MA: Reducing the risk of acid aspiration during cesarean section. Anesth Analg 53:859–868, 1974.

41. Rochester DF, Enson Y: Current concepts in the pathogenesis of the obesity-hypoventilation syndrome. Am J Med 57:402–420, 1974.

42. Nichol HC, Zuck D: Difficult laryngoscopy. The "anterior" larynx and the atlantooccipital gap. Br J Anaesth 55:141–144, 1983.

43. Young SR, Stoelting RK, Peterson C, Madura JA: Anesthetic biotransformation and renal function in obese patients during and after methoxyflurane or halothane anesthesia. Anesthesiology 42:451–457, 1975.

44. Bentley JB, Vaughan RW, Miller MS, Calkins JM, Gandolfi AJ: Serum inorganic fluoride levels in obese patients during and after enflurane anesthesia. Anesth Analg 58:409–412, 1979.

45. Strube PJ, Hulands GH, Halsey MJ: Serum fluoride levels in morbidly obese patients: Enflurane compared with isoflurane anaesthesia. Anaesthesia 42:685–689, 1987.

46. Bentley JB, Vaughan RM, Gandolfi AJ, Cork RC: Halothane biotransformation in obese and nonobese patients. Anesthesiology 57:94–97, 1982.

47. Cork RC, Vaughan RW, Bentley JB: Best general anesthetic agent for morbidly obese patient. Anesthesiology 53:A258, 1980.

48. Bentley JB, Borel JD, Vaughan RW, Gandolfi AJ: Weight, pseudocholinesterase activity and succinylcholine requirement. Anesthesiology 57:48–49, 1982.

49. Tsueda K, Warren JE, McCafferty LA, Nagle JP: Pancuronium bromide requirements during anesthesia for the morbidly obese. Anesthesiology 48:436–439, 1978.

50. Varin F, Ducharme J, Théorêt Y, Besner JG, Bevan DR, Donati F: Influence of extreme obesity on the body disposition and neuromuscular blocking effect of atracurium. Clin Pharmacol Ther 48:18–25, 1990.

51. Weinstein JA, Matteo RS, Ornstein E, Schwartz AE, Goldstoff M, Thal G: Pharmacodynamics of vecuronium and atracurium in the obese surgical patient. Anesth Analg 67:1149–1153, 1988.

52. Schwartz AE, Matteo RS, Ornstein E, Chow FT, Diaz J: Pharmacokinetics and dynamics of metocurine in the obese. Anesthesiology 65:A295, 1986.

53. Palmer SK, Abram SE, Maitra AM, von Colditz JH: Distance from the skin to the lumbar epidural space in an obstetric population. Anesth Analg 62:944–946, 1983.

54. Maiklejohn BH: Distance from the skin to the lumbar epidural space in an obstetric population. Reg Anesth 15:134–136, 1990.

55. Maitra AM, Palmer SK, Bachhuber SR, Abram SE: Continuous epidural analgesia for cesarean section in a patient with morbid obesity. Anesth Analg 58:348–349, 1979.

56. Dewan DD: Anesthesia for the morbidly obese parturient. In Problems in Anesthesia, Vol 3. DD Hood, ed. JB Lippincott, Philadelphia, 1989, pp 56–68.

57. Hodgkinson R, Husain FJ: Obesity and the cephalad spread of analgesia following epidural administration of bupivacaine for cesarean section. Anesth Analg 59:89–92, 1980.

58. Hodgkinson R, Husain FJ: Obesity and spread of epidural anesthesia. Anesth Analg 60:421–424, 1981.

59. Brockway MS, Noble DW, Sharwood-Smith GH, McClure JH: Profound respiratory depression after extradural fentanyl. Br J Anaesth 64:243–245, 1990.

60. Abouleish E, Rawal N, Rashad MN: The addition of 0.2 mg subarachnoid morphine to hyperbaric bupivacaine for cesarean delivery: A prospective study of 856 cases. Reg Anesth 16:137–140, 1991.

61. Pitkänen MT: Body mass and spread of spinal anesthesia with bupivacaine. Anesth Analg 66:127–131, 1987.

62. Taivainen T, Tuominen M, Rosenberg PH: Influence of obesity on the spread of spinal analgesia after injection of plain 0.5% bupivacaine at the L3-4 or L4-5 interspace. Br J Anaesth 64:542–546, 1990.

63. McCulloch WJD, Littlewood DG: Influence of obesity on spinal analgesia with isobaric 0.5% bupivacaine. Br J Anaesth 58:610–614, 1986.

64. Greene N: Physiology of Spinal Anesthesia, 3rd ed. Williams & Wilkins, Baltimore, 1981, p 6.

65. Leicht CH, Evans DE, Durkan WJ: Intrathecal sufentanil for labor analgesia: Results of a pilot study. Anesthesiology 73:A981, 1990.

66. Rigler ML, Drasner K, Krejcie TC, Yelich SJ, Scholnick FT, DeFontes J, Bohner D: Cauda equina syndrome after continuous spinal anesthesia. Anesth Analg 72:275–281, 1991.

67. Buckley FP, Robinson NB, Simonowitz DA, Dellinger EP: Anaesthesia in the morbidly obese. Anaesthesia 38:840–851, 1983.

68. Bromage PR, Fox GS: Obesity: Its relation to anaesthesia. Anaesthesia 31:557–558, 1976.

69. Gelman S, Laws HL, Potzick J, Strong S, Smith L, Erdemir H: Thoracic epidural vs. balanced anesthesia in morbid obes-

ity: An intraoperative and postoperative hemodynamic study. Anesth Analg 59:902–908, 1980.
70. Hodgkinson R, Husain FJ: Caesarean section associated with gross obesity. Br J Anaesth 52:919–923, 1980.
71. Ahern JK, Goodlin RC: Cesarean section in the massively obese. Obstet Gynecol 51:509–510, 1978.
72. Wilson SL, Mantena NR, Halverson JD: Effects of atropine, glycopyrrolate, and cimetidine on gastric secretions in morbidly obese patients. Anesth Analg 60:37–40, 1981.
73. Lam AM, Grace DM, Penny FJ, Vezina WC: Prophylactic intravenous cimetidine reduces the risk of acid aspiration in morbidly obese patients. Anesthesiology 65:684–687, 1986.
74. Brock-Utne JG, Dow TGB, Welman S, Dimopoulos GE, Moshal MG: The effect of metoclopramide on the lower esophageal spincter in late pregnancy. Anaesth Intens Care 6:26–29, 1978.
75. Bylsma-Howell M, Riggs KW, McMorland GH, Rurak DW, McErlane B, Price JDE, Axelson JE: Placental transport of metoclopramide: Assessment of maternal and neonatal effects. Can Anaesth Soc J 30:487–492, 1983.
76. Datta S, Briwa J: Modified laryngoscope for endotracheal intubation of obese patients. Anesth Analg 60:120–121, 1981.
77. Patil VU, Stehling LC, Zauder HL: An adjustable laryngoscope handle for difficult intubations. Anesthesiology 60:609, 1984.
78. Spotoft H, Christensen P: Laryngeal oedema accompanying weight gain in pregnancy. Anaesthesia 36:71, 1981.
79. Seager SJ, Macdonald R: Laryngeal oedema and preeclampsia. Anaesthesia 35:360–362, 1980.
80. Millar WL: Management of a difficult airway in obstetrics. Anesthesiology 52:523–524, 1980.
81. Benumof JL, Scheller MS: The importance of transtracheal ventilation in the management of the difficult airway. Anesthesiology 71:769–778, 1989.
82. Goldberg ME, Norris MC, Larijani GE, Marr AT, Seltzer JL: Preoxygenation in the morbidly obese: A comparison of two techniques. Anesth Analg 68:520–522, 1989.
83. Norris MC, Dewan DM: Preoxygenation for cesarean section: A comparison of two techniques. Anesthesiology 62:827–829, 1985.
84. Gambee AM, Hertzka RE, Fisher DM: Preoxygenation techniques: Comparison of three minutes and four breaths. Anesth Analg 66:468–470, 1987.
85. Jense HG, Dubin SA, Silverstein PI, O'Leary-Escolas U: Effect of obesity on safe duration of apnea in anesthetized humans. Anesth Analg 72:89–93, 1991.
86. Archer GW, Marx GF: Arterial oxygen tension during apnoea in parturient women. Br J Anaesth 46:358–360, 1974.
87. Eriksen J, Anderson J, Rasmussen JP, Sorensen B: Effects of ventilation with large tidal volumes or positive end-expiratory pressure on cardiorespiratory function in anaesthetized obese patients. Acta Anaesth Scand 22:241–248, 1978.

88. Salem MR, Dalal FY, Zygmunt MP, Mathrubhutham M, Jacobs HK: Does PEEP improve intraoperative arterial oxygenation in grossly obese patients? Anesthesiology 48:280–281, 1978.
89. Morris RW, Buschman A, Warren DL, Philip JH, Raemer DB: The prevalence of hypoxemia detected by pulse oximetry during recovery from anesthesia. J Clin Monit 4:16–20, 1988.
90. Hodgkinson R, Husain FJ, Hayashi RH: Systemic and pulmonary blood pressure during caesarean section in parturients with gestational hypertension. Can Anaesth Soc J 27:389–394, 1980.
91. Vaughan RW, Engelhardt RC, Wise L: Postoperative hypoxemia in obese patients. Ann Surg 180:877–882, 1974.
92. Vaughan RW, Wise L: Choice of abdominal operative incision in the obese patient: A study using blood gas measurements. Ann Surg 181:829–835, 1975.
93. Vaughan RW, Wise L: Postoperative arterial blood gas measurements in obese patients: Effect of position on gas exchange. Ann Surg 182:705–707, 1975.
94. Rawal N, Sjöstrand UH, Dahlström B, Nydahl P, Ostelius J: Epidural morphine for postoperative pain relief: A comparative study with intramuscular narcotic and intercostal nerve block. Anesth Analg 61:93–98, 1982.
95. Rawal BM, Sjöstrand U, Christoffersson E, Dahlström B, Arvill A, Rydman H: Comparison of intramuscular and epidural morphine for postoperative analgesia in the grossly obese: Influence on postoperative ambulation and pulmonary function. Anesth Analg 63:583–592, 1984.
96. Bromage PR, Camporesi E, Chestnut D: Epidural narcotics for postoperative analgesia. Anesth Analg 59:473–480, 1980.
97. Rawal N, Sjöstrand U, Dahlström B: Postoperative pain relief by epidural morphine. Anesth Analg 60:726–731, 1981.
98. Cohen SE, Woods WA: The role of epidural morphine in the postcesarean patient: Efficacy and effects of bonding. Anesthesiology 58:500–504, 1983.
99. Rosen MA, Hughs SC, Shnider SM, Abboud TK, Norton M, Dailey PA, Curtis JD: Epidural morphine for the relief of postoperative pain after cesarean delivery. Anesth Analg 62:666–672, 1983.
100. Kakkar VV: Prevention of fatal postoperative thromboembolism by low dose heparin: An international multicenter trial. Lancet 2:45–51, 1975.
101. Gallus AS, Hirsh J, O'Brien SE, McBride JA, Tuttle RJ, Gent M: Prevention of venous thrombosis with small subcutaneous doses of heparin. JAMA 235:1980–1982, 1976.
102. Rao TLK, Adel AE: Anticoagulation following placement of epidural and subarachnoid catheters: An evaluation of neurologic sequelae. Anesthesiology 55:618–620, 1981.
103. Odoom JA, Sih IL: Epidural analgesia and anticoagulant therapy. Anaesthesia 38:254–259, 1983.

CHAPTER 33

Anesthesia for the Pregnant Patient with Immunologic Disorders

Stephen Halpern, M.D., F.R.C.P.C.

Immunologic mechanisms play a role in a wide variety of pathologic states. These may be acute and life threatening, such as severe anaphylaxis, or they may be subacute or chronic, as in such diseases as rheumatoid arthritis and renal allograft rejection. None of these preclude pregnancy. Acute events can occur at any time but are most common during labor and delivery, when parenteral drugs are administered most frequently. Chronic diseases cause a decrease in fertility and an increase in first trimester abortions, but a significant number of patients with such disorders are now able to deliver viable fetuses. Recently, human immunodeficiency virus (HIV) infection and the resultant compromise of the immune system has become prevalent in women of childbearing age. This chapter reviews the pathophysiology of immune-mediated tissue injury, the effects of immunodeficiency, and the anesthetic management appropriate for parturients with these disorders.

THE IMMUNE SYSTEM

The immune system is composed of cellular elements (lymphocytes, plasma cells, and macrophages), their humoral products (e.g., immunoglobulins), and complement. Normally these interact in an organized fashion to rid the body of foreign material (i.e., antigens) that may cause harm. However, in the process they may cause inflammation and tissue damage. Destruction of normal tissue may also occur in autoimmune disorders in which the immune response is directed against autoantigens. Patients with acquired immunodeficiency syndrome (AIDS) have a defect in cellular immunity caused by the destruction of helper T lymphocytes by the HIV virus (1). The pivotal role of this cell in the immune system is shown in Figure 33.1. The clinical manifestations are outlined at the end of this and the following chapter.

There are four classic mechanisms by which the immune system causes injury: anaphylaxis (type 1), cytotoxic reactions (type II), circulating immune complexes (type III), and delayed hypersensitivity reactions (type IV). These are shown in Table 33.1.

ANAPHYLAXIS (TYPE I)

Anaphylaxis is a sudden, unexpected, detrimental reaction to a second exposure of antigen in which histamine, slow-reacting substance of anaphylaxis (SRS-A), and other mediators are released by the reaction of the antigen with immunoglobulin (IgE) in the surface of mast cells (2). The term *anaphylactoid* defines the clinical manifestations of anaphylaxis and mediator release without implying an immunologic basis (3). The two phenomena are indistinguishable by observation alone, and therefore the term *anaphylaxis* is usually reserved for situations in which specific IgE mediation has been proven.

Many of the signs and symptoms of an anaphylactic reaction are caused by the release of histamine into the general circulation. This has a profound effect on the smooth muscle in many organ systems. Histamine causes vasodilatation in capacitance vessels and arteries. Small venules dilate and endothelial cells constrict, causing an increase in permeability to plasma proteins and edema formation. Histamine causes an increase in heart rate and contractility and predisposes the heart to arrhythmias by slowing atrioventricular conduction. Blood pressure usually falls when histamine is given parenterally. All these effects are caused by activation of both H_1 and H_2 receptors (4).

Histamine constricts most extravascular smooth muscle. For instance, bronchial muscle constricts when exposed to histamine, particularly in asthmatic patients. In normal subjects, this effect is less marked, implying that another substance (probably slow-reacting substance of anaphylaxis [SRS-A]) is responsible for the severe bronchoconstriction sometimes seen. Histamine has no effect on the smooth muscle of the pregnant uterus (4).

Clinically, during an anaphylactic reaction the patient may suffer from respiratory, cardiovascular, skin, or gastrointestinal symptoms. Laryngeal edema and bronchospasm may cause severe respiratory distress leading to cyanosis and death. Cardiovascular symptoms include hypotension or cardiac arrhythmia, which may lead to ventricular fibrillation or asystole. The electrocardiogram (ECG) may show sinus tachycardia, sinus bradycardia, nonspecific ST segment changes, atrial fibrillation, or ventricular tachycardia (5). Nausea, vomiting, and diarrhea may be prominent. Finally, urticaria and angioedema may be present (Table 33.2).

If anaphylaxis occurs in the pregnant patient, the treatment must be modified to take into account the

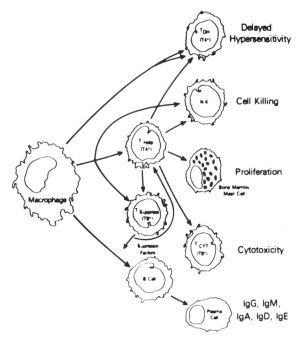

Figure 33.1. Cell-mediated responses. The central role of T4 (helper) lymphocytes. (From Sever JL: HIV: Biology and immunology. Clin Obstet Gynecol 32:423–428, 1989.)

physiologic status of the mother and fetus. The aim of treatment is to maintain maternal and fetal oxygenation. Hypotension may be prominent, and this must be treated immediately with left uterine displacement, colloid solutions (6) through a large-bore intravenous cannula, and vasopressors. Epinephrine is considered the drug of choice for severe anaphylaxis (3, 5, 7); however, because it is a potent uterine artery constrictor, it should be used in the minimum effective dose to correct hypotension and bronchospasm. This usually is accomplished by giving small intravenous boluses (50 to 100 μg) at 30- to 45-sec intervals until the desired effect is achieved. ECG monitoring should be used because cardiac dysrhythmias may result from both the anaphylactic response and epinephrine therapy (8–10).

If severe upper airway obstruction with stridor and cyanosis occurs, endotracheal intubation or cricothyroidotomy may be performed. Epinephrine, together with an H_1 receptor-blocking agent, is the treatment of choice in this situation.

Both epinephrine and aminophylline are indicated to relieve bronchospasm (5, 11). These drugs cause uterine relaxation and may increase bleeding if delivery occurs immediately after their use. Aminophylline crosses the placenta and may cause neonatal toxicity (12).

Neither steroids nor H_1 receptor-blocking drugs are useful as the sole treatment of immediate life-threatening anaphylaxis (3). The latter may play a role in the reduction of itching resulting from urticaria and swelling caused by angioedema. All antihistamines cross the placenta and may cause newborn depression. Diphenhydramine or promethazine effectively treats these symptoms and causes minimal adverse response in the neonate.

The pregnant patient near term is exposed to a number of drugs that have been implicated in ana-

Table 33.1
Immune Mechanisms of Tissue Injury

Mechanism	Mediators	Examples
Type I: Anaphylaxis	IgE; histamine; slow-reacting substance of anaphylaxis (SRS-A); eosinophil chemotactic factor	Anaphylactic shock; urticaria; atopy; angioedema
Type II: Cytotoxic reaction	IgG; IgM; complement Erythroblastosis fetalis; immune thrombocytopenia	Hemolytic transfusion reaction Goodpasture's syndrome
Type III: Immune complex	Immune complexes; complement; phagocytes; lysosomal enzymes	Systemic lupus erythematosus; rheumatoid arthritis; progressive systemic sclerosis
Type IV: Delayed hypersensitivity	T lymphocytes; lymphokines; macrophages; complement[a]; antibodies[a]	Allograft rejection; tuberculin test

[a] Not required for the reaction to take place.

Table 33.2
Signs and Symptoms of Anaphylaxis

System	Symptom	Sign
Cardiovascular	Lightheadedness Palpitations	Hypotension Cardiac arrhythmia; cardiovascular collapse
Respiratory	Dyspnea	Stridor; laryngeal edema; wheezing; pulmonary edema
Skin	Itching; swelling	Urticaria; angioedema
Gastrointestinal	Nausea; vomiting; diarrhea	Dehydration

phylactic reactions (13–14). In particular, many patients claim to be allergic to the "——caines" (i.e., local anesthetics). Hypersensitivity reactions to both ester (15) and amide (16) local anesthetics have been reported. When an allergic reaction occurs, ester-type derivatives of paraaminobenzoic acid such as procaine, tetracaine, and chloroprocaine are usually the group implicated (17). Documented cases of allergic reactions to amide-type local anesthetics are extremely rare. In most instances either preservatives in the local anesthetics, such as paraben (18–20), or other drugs concomitantly administered are at fault.

Ideally, the pregnant patient who has experienced an adverse response to local anesthetics in the past should be seen in consultation by an anesthesiologist before her expected date of delivery. A detailed history should be taken about her symptoms at the time she received the offending drug. Often, the classic symptoms of anaphylaxis are not elicited and another diagnosis is suggested. Reactions to local anesthetics are most commonly caused by relative overdose, intravascular injection, or the effect of vasoconstrictors in the solution. However, the history may not exclude allergic reaction in some cases.

It is best to avoid the offending agent if it is known. If the offending agent is unknown, intradermal testing and progressive subcutaneous challenge with an amide anesthetic may be useful. This topic has been reviewed (15, 20–23). The procedure should be done in a facility with resuscitation equipment available. Paraben-containing local anesthetics should also be tested because paraben has been reported to cause anaphylaxis (20). The skin tests should be compared with negative (saline) and positive (histamine) controls. A positive test result is present if, after 20 min, a wheal or erythema is noted to be greater in size than the histamine control or if increasing the concentration of local anesthetic produces an increasing skin reaction. Patients who have no symptoms after

the challenge test can be told that their risk of an allergic reaction to the local anesthetic tested is the same as that of the general population (20).

In addition to local anesthetics, intravenous anesthetics, narcotics, and antibiotics also cause anaphylactic or anaphylactoid reactions. These are often used in combination with other drugs, making the offending agent difficult to identify. However, a safe, efficacious system of intradermal drug testing has been devised for these agents (22, 23).

CYTOTOXIC REACTIONS (TYPE II)

The cytotoxic immune response is initiated in the circulation by the combination of IgM or IgG antibodies with antigens in cell membranes. These antibodies either act as opsonins and cause cell destruction in the reticuloendothelial system, primarily by splenic trapping, or they bind to complement and cause lysis of the cell in the circulation.

Antibodies can be directed against the red blood cells, platelets, or other antigens. If the immune response is directed toward red blood cells, life-threatening hemolysis can occur, either when red blood cells are destroyed by complement or in the spleen. Blood transfusion with ABO-incompatible blood usually leads to immediate destruction of red blood cells in the circulation by IgM antibodies. Complement activation, in addition to causing cell lysis, releases activated coagulation enzymes, fibrinolysins, and kinins that account for the severe hemodynamic and renal manifestations, as well as the accompanying disseminated intravascular coagulation. Autoimmune hemolytic anemia, whether or not it is associated with collagen vascular disease, is often caused by IgG antibodies that cause less dramatic cell destruction in the spleen. However, severe anemia, refractory to blood transfusion, may result.

Immune thrombocytopenic purpura is a condition in which platelets are destroyed by antibodies. These antibodies are often of the IgG class, leading to platelet sequestration in the spleen, liver, and bone marrow (24). This condition is more fully discussed in Chapter 19. A cytotoxic mechanism of injury also is postulated in Goodpasture's syndrome. The target antigens in this condition are glomerular basement membrane and pulmonary blood vessels. Complement is fixed, releasing chemotactic factors that attract neutrophils and macrophages to the site of inflammation. Lysosomal enzymes are released, causing damage to the kidney (glomerulonephritis) and lung (pulmonary hemorrhage). Erythroblastosis fetalis is an example of a pathologic cytotoxic immune response that occurs only in pregnancy. This condition is considered in detail.

Erythroblastosis Fetalis

Teleologically, maternal antibodies of the IgG class are actively transported to the fetus in utero to protect it from infection during the first months of postnatal life. Whereas the placenta forms an effective barrier against other classes of antibody such as IgM, IgA, and IgE, it cannot discriminate between beneficial and pathologic IgG antibodies. As a result, irregular anti-Rh antibodies that were formed during a previous exposure to Rh antigen can gain access to the fetus. These antibodies bind to fetal red blood cells if they contain the Rh antigen. Usually anti-Rh is not complement fixing and therefore red blood cell destruction takes place extravascularly in the fetal spleen. This results in fetal anemia, the severity of which will depend on the maternal antibody titer and the time of onset. Both the rate of rise of maternal antibody titer and the amount of bilirubin found in the amniotic fluid as a result of red blood cell destruction help the obstetrician to evaluate the fetus early in gestation and determine whether or not a course of intrauterine blood transfusions would be beneficial (25).

About 50% of fetuses with erythroblastosis are mildly affected. Slight anemia with polychromasia and evidence of red blood cell destruction on blood smear is present at birth. Mild jaundice may also occur but no treatment is required. About 25% of neonates with erythroblastosis are moderately affected and have unconjugated hyperbilirubinemia in addition to moderately severe anemia. This occurs because of continuing hemolysis after birth. Phototherapy or (in more severe cases) exchange transfusion is required to prevent kernicterus and permanent brain damage. The remaining 25% of neonates are severely affected and hydrops fetalis develops before term if left untreated. Subcutaneous edema, effusions, severe anemia, and hepatosplenomegaly are seen clinically. Edema and effusions can appear before cardiac decompensation because of hypoalbuminemia (26). In addition, portal hypertension may account for ascites (27). Because of liver involvement, vitamin K-dependent clotting factors may be greatly reduced. Coagulation may also be impaired by thrombocytopenia secondary to splenomegaly. Human studies show that umbilical vein blood flow is inversely proportional to the fetal hemoglobin and is decreased toward normal by intrauterine blood transfusion (28). The fetal heart rate can be normal in spite of increased flow, indicating that other mechanisms such as a decrease in blood viscosity are important in maintaining fetal cardiac output. Hepatosplenomegaly occurs on the basis of extramedullary erythropoiesis in an attempt to increase red cell production. The liver also shows fatty degeneration and hemosiderin deposits. Organomegaly, especially if associated with tense ascites, may cause dystocia during delivery.

The placenta becomes grossly edematous, sometimes weighing as much as the fetus itself. The edema may cause the placenta to become a barrier to nutrients, leading to chronic fetal malnutrition (26).

The fetal heart rate tracing often reflects the severity of the anemia. Although a sinusoidal pattern is associated with severe anemia, it may be transient and difficult to interpret or even absent (29). As the fetal condition worsens, the tracing progresses from nonreactive to a persistent tachycardia to decelerations.

Once it has been established that the fetus is likely to be severely affected, intrauterine transfusions with Rh-negative blood are used to maintain the fetal hematocrit at an acceptable level until fetal lung maturity is achieved. In spite of transfusion, however, the fetus may suffer significant asphyxia at birth due to anemia and the neonate may suffer hypoxia because of pulmonary edema secondary to heart failure.

During labor the fetus must be stressed as little as possible and fetal oxygenation must be maintained. In the severely affected fetus, a cesarean delivery may be indicated if it is thought that labor would be deleterious. For an abdominal delivery, either regional or general anesthesia may be used as described in Chapter 12.

If vaginal delivery is planned, continuous segmental epidural analgesia is safe and effective for the relief of pain in the first stage of labor. Catecholamine release and hyperventilation due to labor pain are diminished when pain is relieved. Furthermore, if hypotension is prevented, it has been shown that uterine intervillous blood flow may be increased by this technique (30). The block can be extended at the time of delivery to include the perineum. Because many of these patients deliver preterm fetuses, pelvic muscle relaxation may be useful at delivery and can be supplied by the perineal dose of local anesthetic.

IMMUNE COMPLEX DISEASES (TYPE III)

Immune complex diseases occur when antigen-antibody complexes are deposited in various tissues. These cause complement activation and release of vasoactive and chemotactic factors. Acutely, the immune complexes are phagocytized by neutrophils that in turn release lysosomal enzymes, causing cell damage. Monocytes and T lymphocytes are responsible for continuing cell destruction.

Immune complexes can be detected normally in the circulation in the third trimester of pregnancy (31), but these are usually removed by the reticuloendothelial system. In patients with immune complex diseases, soluble antigen and antibody form multimolecular complexes that bind complement, causing cellular damage (32). As their concentration increases, they precipitate and are deposited in vascular beds, glomerular basement membranes, and serous cavities. These deposits cause the vasculitis, glomerulonephritis, and polyserositis typical of this group of diseases. Circulating immune complexes or the antibody component of these can be detected in cord blood after delivery (31).

Although immune complex diseases may have a number of causes (Table 33.3), the collagen vascular diseases are of particular interest because they are the most common of the group that coexists with pregnancy. Rheumatoid arthritis, systemic lupus erythematosis, and progressive systemic sclerosis (scleroderma) are considered in detail.

Rheumatoid Arthritis

Rheumatoid arthritis is a chronic inflammatory disease of diarthrodial joints that is frequently combined with the dysfunction of other organ systems (33). It is more common in females and can occur in any age group. The etiologic factors of the disease are unknown, but there is strong evidence that tissue damage is caused by immune complexes, complement, and lysosomal enzymes. Juvenile rheumatoid arthritis is a similar disease with an onset before age 16 years. This condition can result in crippling sequelae by childbearing age.

The primary manifestations of rheumatoid arthritis occur in the joints. Initially, there is a mild inflammation that may progress to thickening of the synovium, articular cartilage destruction, and ankylosis, causing an almost total lack of mobility of the joint. The tendons and ligaments of other joints may be weakened, resulting in instability and subluxation. The small joints of the hands and feet are usually affected first, but any diarthrodial joint can be involved. Of particular interest to the anesthesiologist are the temporomandibular, cricoarytenoid, and atlantoaxial joints because of disease in these areas (34).

Table 33.3
Conditions Associated with Immune Complexes

Etiology	Examples
Exogenous antigen	Serum sickness
Postinfectious	Poststreptococcal glomerulonephritis
Collagen vascular diseases	Rheumatoid arthritis; systemic lupus erythematosus; progressive systemic sclerosis
Pregnancy	Preeclampsia-eclampsia

The temporomandibular joint may become severely ankylosed. As a result, it becomes impossible to open the mouth sufficiently to permit oral intubation. The ability to intubate the trachea may be further diminished in patients with juvenile rheumatoid arthritis because of micrognathia from mandibular disease in childhood. Cricoarytenoid arthritis causes constriction of the glottic opening in about one-third of patients (35). Finally, involvement of the cervical spine is common. Clinical manifestations include neck pain and stiffness. Radiologic evidence of involvement is common and includes generalized osteoporosis and bone erosion. With time the cartilage is destroyed and the ligaments become lax, producing atlantoaxial instability. If the patient suffers from posterior subluxation, neck extension may be hazardous (Fig. 33.2) (36).

If possible, the patient should be seen by an anesthesiologist before she is in labor to identify potential

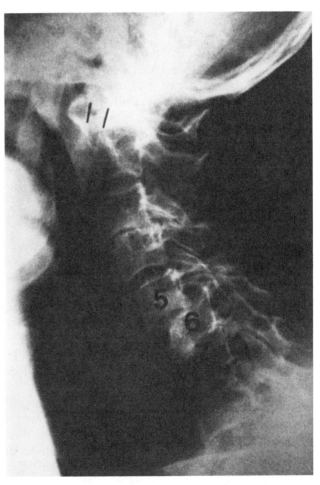

Figure 33.2. Lateral cervical spine radiograph demonstrating generalized osteoporosis, atlantoaxial subluxation, serial subaxial subluxations, and vertebral endplate erosions (vertebrae 6 and 7). (From Crosby ET, Lui A: The adult cervical spine. Can J Anaesth 37:77–93, 1990.)

airway problems. The temporomandibular joint can be tested by asking the patient to open her mouth. At least a 4-cm opening is required to admit a laryngoscope and endotracheal tube orally. The patient should be viewed from the side to note micrognathia and flexion of the cervical spine. She should be asked to flex and extend her neck. Limitations should be noted, and atlantoaxial instability can be demonstrated if sensory or motors symptoms are produced by this maneuver. Lateral radiographs of the cervical spine in the neutral position and in voluntary flexion and extension are also helpful in diagnosing instability (36). Hoarseness, stridor, and shortness of breath suggest cricoarytenoid arthritis. Indirect or direct fiberoptic laryngoscopy can be used to identify the extent of laryngeal stenosis and vocal cord immobility.

Other skeletal abnormalities due to rheumatoid or juvenile rheumatoid arthritis include deformities of the hips that limit flexion and abduction (37) and bony pelvis abnormalities that may lead to cephalopelvic disproportion. The intervertebral facet joints of the lumbar vertebral column may be involved with arthritis. Examination of the back and radiographs of the lumbosacral spines (taken before pregnancy) may be helpful in showing which facets are least affected.

In addition to skeletal manifestations, rheumatoid arthritis affects other organ systems. Visceral involvement is more common in those patients with high serum rheumatoid factor titers (38). Of prime importance are the respiratory and cardiovascular effects. Patients with severe disease may suffer from restrictive lung disease. This may be due to pleural effusions, spinal disease leading to kyphosis, and (to a lesser extent) fixation of the ribs by arthritis. As the gravid uterus becomes larger during pregnancy, this restriction may become more severe because of impaired diaphragmatic excursion. The heart may also function abnormally because pericardial effusion, cardiomyopathy, conduction defects, and valvular heart disease may occur. Cardiac reserve may be taxed as pregnancy reaches the middle of the third trimester and cardiac output and blood volume become maximal. Labor also causes an increased demand for cardiac output.

Of the medications often prescribed for rheumatoid arthritis, only aspirin and corticosteroids are recommended for use during pregnancy (39). Large doses of aspirin near the time of delivery predispose the patient to delayed onset of labor, prolonged labor, and increased blood loss during delivery (38). Anemia is common because of iron deficiency secondary to gastrointestinal loss. Aspirin also interferes with platelet function for several days after discontinuation of the drug. Prolonged use of steroids, particu-

larly in high doses for a prolonged period of time, causes numerous metabolic derangements (Table 33.4). Adrenal suppression may also occur in the mother and, rarely, in the neonate.

For patients with mild disease who have no joint deformities and who require no medication to control the symptoms of rheumatoid arthritis, the methods of administering pain relief during labor and delivery are the same as those in normal pregnancy. Patients who have received any aspirin within 3 to 5 days should have their bleeding time measured before a major conduction block is instituted. An abnormal bleeding time may preclude a block. In addition a large-bore intravenous catheter should be placed and blood should be available for transfusion not because of the increased risk of postpartum hemorrhage.

Patients who have joint deformities require special attention if a major conduction block or general anesthesia is used. Severe contractures of the large joints may be present and the range of motion of each of these joints should be determined before anesthesia is commenced so that overextension and dislocation do not occur under anesthesia. It is particularly important to test the hip joints by maximally abducting and flexing them before placing the patients into stirrups. Some patients have osteoporosis secondary to steroid treatment or immobility and care must be taken with positioning to avoid fractures. Finally, peripheral neuropathy may occur secondary to rheumatoid arthritis. Although this is not an absolute con-

Table 33.4
Toxicity of Adrenocorticosteroids

Maternal
  Hypokalemia
  Sodium retention and edema
  Hyperglycemia
  Increased susceptibility to infection
  Peptic ulceration
  Osteoporosis
  Avascular necrosis of hip
  Proximal muscle weakness
  Psychosis
  Cataracts
  Adrenal insufficiency
  Cushingoid habitus
  Striae
  Acne
Fetal
  Adrenal insufficiency
  Leukopenia
  Infections
  (?) Congenital malformations
Other
  Suppression of estriol secretion

traindication to spinal or epidural anesthesia, it should be documented before commencement of the block.

Anesthesia for vaginal delivery can be managed in the usual fashion with the following special considerations. If the patient has severe airway abnormalities, ensure that the patient remains conscious at all times because loss of muscle tone may result in upper airway obstruction that may not be safely overcome because of abnormal anatomy. Patients with flexion deformities of the cervical spine and micrognathia are most prone to obstruction under anesthesia (34). In addition, as in all laboring patients, a full stomach may be present and unconsciousness may lead to aspiration pneumonitis. Conduction analgesia may be used if coagulation is normal, although this may be technically difficult. A large dose of anesthetic accidentally administered intravenously would be catastrophic; seizures causing cervical subluxation and quadriplegia may result. This caveat also applies to paracervical or pudendal blocks. Spinal anesthesia using a small dose of lidocaine, bupivacaine, or tetracaine could be used for a saddle block to facilitate forceps delivery. The use of subarachnoid or epidural narcotics, as described in Chapter 10, may be particularly useful in these patients.

Patients with long-standing, crippling rheumatoid arthritis are more likely to require a cesarean section because of hip joint or pelvic bony involvement. Regardless of the anesthetic technique used, a large-bore intravenous catheter should be placed preoperatively and blood should be available in anticipation of increased blood loss secondary to aspirin ingestion. For elective cesarean section, lumbar epidural, spinal, or general anesthesia can be used. If there are upper airway deformities or cervical spine abnormalities, conduction anesthesia may be preferred. Special care must be taken to avoid intravascular injection of local anesthetics or an excessively high block. If epidural anesthesia is chosen, an appropriate test dose should be used and the level should be increased slowly by giving small volumes through the catheter. Spinal anesthesia has the advantage of requiring far less local anesthetic, thus making the possibility of a systemic reaction remote. The level of the block can be controlled by positioning the patient and by the dose of drug. If general anesthesia is used in patients with severe airway deformities, the airway must be secured while the patient is awake. This can be done by a blind nasal or (preferably) a fiberoptic technique. Topical anesthesia of the upper airway is required, but little or no sedation should be used to maintain consciousness and to minimize drug transfer to the fetus. A vasoconstrictor should be applied to the nasal mucosa to avoid epistaxis.

The neck should be manipulated very gently to avoid cervical subluxation. The awake patient may complain of pain or paresthesia if subluxation occurs before permanent neurologic damage has occurred. A tracheostomy under local anesthesia may be necessary if intubation is impossible.

After induction, the patient should be carefully positioned. The head should be supported by several pillows if there is a severe flexion deformity of the neck. The arms may have to be placed at the sides if there is restriction of shoulder movement. Some patients require hip flexion, which can be accomplished by placing pillows under the knees. Left uterine displacement should be used. If general anesthesia is used, the patient must be wide awake before extubation. If glottic narrowing is severe, she should be observed for several hours postextubation in an area where reintubation or tracheostomy can be performed.

If an emergency cesarean section must be performed in a patient with a severely deformed upper airway and the fetus must be delivered in the shortest possible time, the experience of the anesthesiologist and the operating team determines the conduct of anesthesia. After the airway has been secured, spinal anesthesia or, if there is a contraindication to this, general anesthesia can be done as previously described. If the operating team has had experience using local anesthesia, an abdominal wall field block with local infiltration using 1% procaine or 0.5% lidocaine is an alternative. Supplemental sedation is usually required but loss of consciousness should be avoided.

In summary, rheumatoid arthritis is an immunologic disease involving the musculoskeletal, cardiovascular, respiratory, and hematologic systems. In particular, joint disease in the head and neck may limit the anesthesiologist's access to the patient's airway. Because management of the pregnant patient requires airway control to prevent aspiration of gastric contents, a careful assessment of these factors is mandatory and the problems must be recognized by all members of the surgical team. By carefully planning the obstetric and anesthetic management, the appropriate equipment and personnel can be available at the time of delivery to ensure a successful outcome.

Systemic Lupus Erythematosus

Systemic lupus erythematosus (SLE) is a chronic inflammatory disease thought to be caused by a disturbance in immunoregulatory mechanisms resulting from the interaction of genetic, hormonal, and environmental factors (40). Most patients with the disorder have hypergammaglobulinemia and a reduction in serum complement. In addition, immune deposits have been found in the glomerular basement membrane on renal biopsy and at the dermal-epidermal junction in biopsies of involved areas of skin. However, unlike rheumatoid arthritis, the joint symptoms are usually mild and severe deformities are rare. There is a high incidence of the disease in females (female/male ratio, 9:1) (41), many of whom are of childbearing age.

The manifestations of SLE may be mild and confined to one organ system or fulminating, leading rapidly to death. Fever, weight loss, and fatigue may be the first signs of the disease. The skin may be affected, causing the classic malar "butterfly rash." Involvement of mucous membranes with painful ulcerations in the pharynx, mouth, or vagina may also occur. Polyserositis is relatively common, with pleurisy occurring in 50% of cases. The polyarthralgia or arthritis associated with SLE follows the same distribution as rheumatoid arthritis but is usually milder. Avascular necrosis of the head of the femur may result from either chronic steroid therapy or vasculitis. Other manifestations such as pulmonary hemorrhage and cerebrovascular accidents may also be caused by vasculitis.

The heart may be affected in a number of ways. Pericarditis occurs in over 50% of patients with SLE. Cardiac tamponade is uncommon, but the patient may experience chest pain. Myocarditis can also be present and cause congestive heart failure. Del Rio and co-workers (42) have demonstrated that patients with SLE have a decreased myocardial reserve. This may be caused by coronary arteritis, focal or generalized myocarditis, or focal necrosis and atrophy of the myocardium. Some patients have cardiac valvular lesions (Libman-Sacks endocarditis) that are usually asymptomatic. However, prophylactic antibiotics against bacterial endocarditis are indicated for labor and delivery.

Lupus nephritis is common and accounts for the majority of fatalities due to SLE. Renal impairment may be mild, moderate, or severe, although patients with a creatinine clearance of less than 50 ml/min rarely become pregnant (43). In addition, hypertension commonly occurs with lupus nephritis. Proteinuria and the nephrotic syndrome often accompany lupus nephritis, and if this occurs in the third trimester, it may be clinically impossible to distinguish worsening of the renal disease from toxemia of pregnancy (44).

Many of the neurologic complications of SLE may be due to the vasculitis or to steroid treatment. Up to 25% of deaths in SLE patients occur because of intracerebral bleeding or status epilepticus (40). Other manifestations include psychosis, transverse mye-lopathy, cranial nerve palsies, and peripheral neuropathy.

There may be several coagulation defects in patients with SLE. The platelet count may be low in active disease because of antiplatelet antibodies and splenomegaly. In addition, circulating anticoagulants may be present. The lupus anticoagulant (LA) is a nonspecific antibody directed towards phospholipids and therefore causes an abnormality in the phospholipid-dependent coagulation factors. It is usually suspected if the activated thromboplastin time is prolonged and confirmed with tests proving factor nonspecificity and phospholipid dependency (45). LA is an in vitro phenomenon, and patients do not exhibit abnormal bleeding. In fact, many develop both arterial and venous thrombosis. The presence of LA indicates a high risk for premature delivery and fetal loss. Because there is a high incidence of thrombosis, care must be taken to ensure that the patient is not taking anticoagulants or drugs that inhibit platelet function. Finally, other conditions such as pre-eclampsia must be ruled out because coagulopathies related to this condition may contraindicate regional anesthesia.

In contrast to LA, specific anticoagulants are associated with SLE and other collagen vascular diseases. These are diagnosed by demonstration of factor specificity and are associated with abnormal bleeding. Factor VIII inhibitors are the most common (46), but antibodies to other clotting factors have been found. Their presence contraindicates the use of regional block.

During pregnancy, many patients with moderate or severe symptoms of SLE receive corticosteroids. These medications may result in a number of side effects in the mother and newborn (Table 33.4).

The infant may be affected by maternal SLE. Transient skin rashes, leukopenia, hemolytic anemia, and thrombocytopenia (41, 47) may occur because of transplacental passage of antibodies. Congenital heart block due to circulating antiribonucleoprotein antibody has been reported in the offspring of patients with SLE (48). The diagnosis must be considered if fetal bradycardia is detected in a patient with autoimmune disease.

The conduct of anesthesia for pregnant patients with SLE depends on the severity of the disease, the organ systems involved, and the medications the patients are receiving. Of major importance is the evaluation of the renal, cardiovascular, respiratory, and coagulation systems. A urinalysis and blood urea nitrogen, serum creatinine, serum electrolytes, and blood sugar studies should be performed on all patients with SLE when they are admitted in labor. With these, an assessment of renal impairment and proteinuria can be made. Casts in the urine sediment indicate active nephritis. Hypokalemia and glucose intolerance are common in patients receiving corticosteroids. The cardiovascular system is best evaluated by physical examination. Heart rate, arterial blood pressure, and central venous pressure should be assessed. The heart should be auscultated for murmurs (suggestive of valvular heart disease), extra sounds (suggestive of heart failure), and friction rubs. Auscultation of the chest may reveal basilar rales if heart failure is present. An ECG may be useful to assess rhythm abnormalities and ischemic changes. A history of hemoptysis and shortness of breath accompanied by a pleural rub on physical examination suggests pulmonary vasculitis and possible pulmonary infarct. Pleural effusions are common and may be large enough to cause respiratory embarrassment. If dyspnea is present, arterial blood gases should be drawn and hypoxemia treated with supplemental oxygen. Finally, a prothrombin time, activated thromboplastin time, platelet count, and possibly bleeding time measurements should be done.

Analgesia for vaginal delivery can be given using narcotics, inhalational analgesia, or if coagulation is normal, continuous lumbar epidural analgesia. Meperidine or fentanyl can be used for the first stage of labor because they have a relatively short half-life and, like most narcotic analgesics, are metabolized in the liver. Methoxyflurane and enflurane are avoided in patients with SLE because the vast majority of them have some renal involvement. For inhalational analgesia, self-administered nitrous oxide in oxygen provides satisfactory analgesia. Finally, intrathecal or epidural opiates, with or without local anesthetics, may be useful. A neurologic examination should be done before initiating a conduction block. Although a fixed neurologic deficit is not an absolute contraindication to regional block, it should be documented. If raised intracranial pressure is suspected, subarachnoid block should be avoided and epidural anesthesia performed most cautiously because of the possibility of accidentally puncturing the dura. In patients with LA, regional anesthesia may be used if the diagnosis of LA is certain, if the patient has not recently taken any drugs to interfere with coagulation, and if there are no serious coagulation defects. The risks and benefits of the procedure should be thoroughly discussed with the patient. Patients on long-term corticosteroid therapy require steroid coverage.

Cesarean section may be performed safely under regional or general anesthesia. All patients with SLE should have 2 units of compatible blood prepared in advance because cross-matching problems can arise as the result of irregular antibodies in the serum.

Similar to vaginal delivery, steroid coverage is indicated for those patients receiving long-term steroid therapy. Regional anesthesia is the technique of choice if coagulation is normal. If severe renal disease is present, a central venous or pulmonary artery catheter may be required to assess cardiac filling and optimize cardiac output. Hourly urine output using a Foley catheter should be assessed. An arterial line may be placed to monitor blood pressure if hypertension is difficult to control or if continuing hypoxia requires repeated arterial blood gas analyses. These monitors are especially helpful in preventing pulmonary edema when giving the patient crystalloid while performing an epidural block and when replacing blood volume after uterine incision. Supplemental oxygen should be given to the patient throughout the procedure.

If general anesthesia is indicated for maternal or fetal reasons, a rapid-sequence induction using preoxygenation, thiopental, succinylcholine, cricoid pressure, and endotracheal intubation with a cuffed endotracheal tube should be used. This sequence may have to be modified for extremely ill patients with severe cardiac disease. If myocardial function is poor, oxygen is administered, appropriate monitoring is initiated, and anesthesia induced with a reduced dose of thiopental combined with a narcotic such as fentanyl. This technique should result in less myocardial depression. Succinylcholine is still used as a muscle relaxant to facilitate endotracheal intubation unless the patient has recently suffered paralysis from a recent cerebrovascular accident. Succinylcholine is then contraindicated because of the possibility of causing massive hyperkalemia. An intubating dose of a short-acting nondepolarizing muscle relaxant may be used. Agents that require renal excretion to terminate their action, such as gallamine, metocurine, and (to a certain extent) pancuronium, should be avoided if renal failure is present. Blood volume should be meticulously maintained to ensure optimum uterine and renal blood flow, and transfusion with packed red blood cells should be started early if the patient is severely anemic before surgery. Extubation should take place when the patient's laryngeal reflexes have fully recovered. Finally, the delivery should take place in a facility that is prepared to take care of the infant should it be affected with neonatal SLE.

Progressive Systemic Sclerosis (Scleroderma)

Progressive systemic sclerosis (PSS) is a generalized disorder of connective tissue characterized by inflammatory, fibrotic, and vascular lesions in the skin and viscera. Although the cause is unknown, it has been classified as an autoimmune disorder because autoimmune hemolytic anemia, hypergammaglobulinemia, rheumatoid factor, and numerous autoantibodies have been found in patients with this disease. In addition to skin involvement, PSS causes impairment of kidney, heart, lung, and gastrointestinal tract function (49).

Involved areas of the skin show sclerosis and massive thickening of the dermis and subcutaneous tissue (50). The skin of the extremities is often bound down to the digits, with the condition later extending proximally and sometimes including the trunk. It may be impossible to clinically assess the position of the fetus if the induration of the skin over the abdomen is severe (51). The skin of the face may become tightly adherent to underlying structures, limiting the ability to open the mouth. Thus orotracheal intubation may be difficult. Nasotracheal intubation may also be difficult and hazardous because of decreased size of the external nares and mucosal telangectasias that may bleed if traumatized, although they rarely hemorrhage spontaneously (52). Because of these deformities an anesthetic mask may fit poorly, causing difficulty when preoxygenation or intermittent positive pressure ventilation by mask are necessary.

The kidneys are involved in almost half of patients with PSS. Proteinuria, hypertension, and azotemia are the usual manifestations (53). The nephrotic syndrome associated with pregnancy has been reported (54).

One of the hallmarks of PSS is an increase in vascular reactivity to cold. Raynaud's phenomenon is common and is associated with a decrease in renal blood flow in some patients (53). In addition, coronary vascular spasm may occur, causing arrhythmias and angina in patients with anatomically normal coronary arteries (55). The myocardium may show focal or generalized fibrosis leading to congestive heart failure.

The entire gastrointestinal tract can be involved with PSS, causing malnutrition secondary to malabsorption. This may also cause a prolongation of the prothrombin time due to malabsorption of vitamin K. There is abnormal esophageal motility, leading to incomplete emptying, lower esophageal sphincter incompetence, and peptic strictures (52). There may also be difficulty in swallowing due to tongue and palate abnormalities. These changes make the aspiration of both lower esophageal and gastric contents a hazard.

Pulmonary function is often impaired. Interstitial fibrosis leading to a restrictive pattern and a decrease in diffusing capacity are the usual defects (49). Pulmonary hypertension may also be present (56). In

pregnancy, hypoxemia may be aggravated because of the abdominal mass (causing a decrease in the already compromised functional residual capacity) and because of the increased metabolic rate. Hypoxia may further increase pulmonary artery pressures, leading to cor pulmonale.

As in both rheumatoid arthritis and SLE, peripheral joints are often arthritic. This can lead to severe deformities, particularly of the small joints of the hands and feet.

Pregnancies complicated by PSS put both the mother and fetus at high risk for morbidity and mortality (50). In one review of 17 case reports, 42% of patients experienced a worsening of their PSS during pregnancy. In addition, there were three maternal deaths. There is an increased incidence of preeclampsia-eclampsia in patients with PSS (57). Although it is rare for the autoantibodies associated with PSS to cause disease in the fetus or neonate (58), organ compromise and hypertension in the mother may lead to stress in utero. Prematurity and a high incidence of perinatal deaths occur, particularly in patients with renal disease (59).

A number of treatments have been used in an attempt to halt the progression of the disease. Antiinflammatory agents, corticosteroids, antimetabolites, and plasmapheresis have been tried with little success. However, the patient may be taking a number of medications for symptomatic relief. During pregnancy, aspirin and antihypertensive agents are the most frequent drugs prescribed.

The pregnant patient with severe PSS poses several difficult anesthetic management problems. Often there is a lack of suitable peripheral veins for intravenous therapy. If the small veins on the hand or wrist are used for injection of drugs or infusion of cold fluids, painful venospasm or Raynaud's phenomenon may be provoked. Therefore it is desirable to use a large forearm or central vein for these purposes. To keep vascular spasms to a minimum, the delivery suite and all intravenous fluids should be warmed. Blood pressure may have to be measured with an ultrasound device because decreased arterial blood flow may make Korotkoff sounds difficult to hear. Indwelling arterial catheters should be avoided if possible because these may provoke distal vasospasm and gangrene.

Epidural anesthesia may be indicated for relief of labor pain or operative delivery. Technically this may be difficult because of changes in the overlying skin or arthritis in the lumbar spine. Local anesthetics appear to have a prolonged duration of action in patients with PSS (60); therefore it has been suggested that short-acting ester anesthetics can be used (61). After an appropriate test dose, these can be given in small increments through an epidural catheter. Vasopressors should be used in small doses intravenously to avoid severe hypertension and vasospasm. For the same reasons, ergot preparations should be used with caution.

General anesthesia may be required for fetal distress. The problems associated with this technique depend on the patient's pathophysiologic condition. Before induction, an attempt should be made to empty the lower esophagus of secretions with an orogastric tube. Next, a nonparticulate antacid should be given. Since the patient often has decreased esophageal motility and distal strictures, oral antacids may not neutralize gastric acid, although it is helpful to neutralize the residual contents in the esophagus. Ranitidine may be useful to reduce gastric acid secretion. Metoclopramide is used to accelerate gastric emptying, but its efficacy in PSS has not been proven. If a difficult intubation is suspected because of restricted mouth opening, awake oral intubation under local anesthesia using a fiberoptic laryngoscope may be the safest way to secure the airway before induction of anesthesia. Nasotracheal intubation may cause severe bleeding from the nose. If intubation is impossible, a tracheostomy may be required.

Intraoperative monitoring is often difficult in patients with PSS, and the benefits of using each monitoring device must be weighed against the risks. A Foley catheter should be used and hourly urine output should be recorded. Arterial blood pressure should be monitored noninvasively. A central venous catheter is helpful to monitor pressure and infuse fluids. If severe lung disease is present, arterial blood for blood gas measurement should be obtained percutaneously using a 25-gauge needle. An indwelling arterial catheter should be avoided. Noninvasive measurement of oxygen saturation and end-tidal carbon dioxide reduces the need for obtaining arterial blood. Unfortunately, pulse oximetry may be of limited use in patients with severe vasospastic disease since all sites (fingers, ears, nose) may be affected.

A pulmonary artery catheter is helpful if congestive heart failure or severe pulmonary hypertension is present. Unfortunately, it is technically difficult to correctly position the catheter if the heart is severely dilated and pulmonary artery pressures are high. In addition, cardiac arrhythmias are common.

Hypotension may occur with peripheral vasodilation. This must be treated promptly by decreasing the concentration of any volatile anesthetic agents used, administering fluids, and giving small doses of vasopressor if necessary. During the course of the anesthetic, high concentrations of oxygen should be used; these should be continued in the recovery period if respiratory symptoms or hypoxemia were detected preoperatively.

DELAYED HYPERSENSITIVITY REACTIONS (TYPE IV)

Delayed hypersensitivity, as exemplified by allograft rejection and by the tuberculin test in the skin, is mediated by T lymphocytes. Unlike reactions caused by histamine release, which occur immediately, the signs of inflammation begin to occur approximately 12 hr after the antigen is introduced, with a peak severity at 24 to 48 hr. During this time, previously sensitized T lymphocytes release soluble mediators that attract macrophages and other T lymphocytes to the site of antigen production. These are activated by other soluble mediators to become cytotoxic or "killer" cells. Although antibodies and complement are not necessary for this type of reaction, they are often involved.

In addition to being the chief reaction against allografted tissue, delayed hypersensitivity is the immune response commonly directed against many viruses, fungi, protozoa, and bacteria. It is thought that there are deficiencies in T lymphocyte function during pregnancy that may account for the observed increase in some types of infection and for the fact that the fetus, which is antigenically distinct from the mother, is not rejected (62).

Recently, through the manipulation of this portion of the immune system, a number of different major organs have been successfully transplanted in humans, resulting in increased longevity and quality of life. The kidney is by far the most commonly transplanted organ and, although there are isolated reports of pregnancy in patients who have received bone marrow (63) and liver (64) transplants, there are many patients who have had kidney transplants who have delivered viable newborns. The physiology and anesthetic management of these patients are now considered in detail.

Normally, renal blood flow and glomerular filtration rate (GFR) increase during the first trimester of pregnancy, reaching a peak at the end of the second trimester. Although the transplanted kidney is ectopic and denervated, the GFR often increases early in pregnancy (Fig. 33.3) (65). During the third trimester, GFR declines slightly as in normal pregnant patients. Proteinuria may also appear in the third trimester, but in the absence of hypertension it is not significant and often resolves postpartum (65).

The most common problems that occur in the pregnant patient with a renal transplant are related to a decrease in renal function during gestation and the immunosuppressive medication they are taking. Both of these may also affect the fetus adversely.

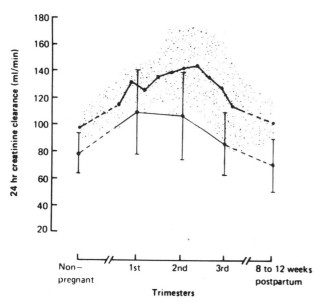

Figure 33.3. Serial 24-hr creatinine clearance (mean ± SD) during 10 pregnancies in 8 women with renal transplants. Measurements from 10 healthy women (mean ± SD) are shown by the *upper line* and *dotted area*. (Reprinted by permission from Davidson JM, Lindheimer MD: Pregnancy in renal transplant recipients. J Reprod Med 27:613–621, 1982.)

Some patients have systemic disease such as diabetes, systemic lupus, and others that necessitated the renal transplant. These may adversely affect maternal and fetal outcome.

Renal function can be assessed by measuring blood urea nitrogen and serum creatinine. Both of these are inversely proportional to the GFR, although the serum creatinine is a more specific test. When the serum creatinine is higher than 1.6 mg/dl, maternal morbidity and fetal morbidity and mortality increase (66). Other tests of renal function are warranted in the pregnant patient with a renal transplant. These include serum electrolytes and glucose, routine and microscopic urinalysis, and 24-hr urine collections for protein and creatinine studies.

Pregnant patients with renal allografts continue to take their immunosuppressive medications throughout pregnancy. These medications include corticosteroids, azathioprine, and recently, cyclosporine. Pharmacologic doses of corticosteroids, in addition to affecting lymphocyte function, cause a number of side effects, some of which are life threatening (Table 33.4). Azathioprine may cause an increased incidence of congenital anomalies (64), toxic hepatitis, and bone marrow suppression (67). Cyclosporine, a peptide antirejection agent, is both hepatotoxic and nephrotoxic (68, 69). In addition, there may be an association between cyclosporine and intrauterine growth retardation (70).

Because all renal transplant patients take one or

more of these drugs, they are at high risk for infection. Therefore strict aseptic technique should be used before any invasive procedure. In addition, those patients that were treated with hemodialysis before transplantation are at high risk for carrying hepatitis B antigen.

Serious rejection episodes occur in 9% of renal transplant patients during pregnancy (64). A rise in serum creatinine with oliguria, proteinuria, hypertension, fever, and tenderness over the graft are the most common signs and symptoms. In addition, casts often appear in the urine. This must be distinguished from toxemia of pregnancy because toxemia occurs in 27% of pregnant patients with renal transplants (64) and the treatment of the two conditions is radically different. The definitive diagnosis can be made by biopsying the transplanted kidney.

If acute rejection has been diagnosed a short time before delivery, the patient may have severe renal failure and require dialysis. The anesthetic care of these patients must include a careful assessment of their cardiovascular status. In addition to the usual monitors, the severely hypertensive patient with poor renal function may require invasive hemodynamic monitoring. Cardiac output should be optimized to maintain both uterine blood flow and blood flow to the transplanted kidney. Low urine output and a rising serum creatinine are indications for frequent determinations of the serum potassium. If hyperkalemia occurs, it can be treated acutely with intravenous calcium to reverse the myocardial depressant effect of potassium. Potassium may also be shifted into cells using glucose, insulin, and bicarbonate. Ion exchange resins or dialysis may be necessary to remove excess potassium from the body if anuria is present.

High doses of immunosuppressants are usually given to treat rejection episodes. If large doses of corticosteroids have been used, the serum glucose level may be elevated, necessitating insulin therapy. Hyperglycemia should be avoided at the time of birth because this may result in hyperinsulinemia and hypoglycemia in the neonate. Patients on immunosuppressant drugs may also acquire unusual infections, particularly in the lungs. Supplemental oxygen should be given to maintain arterial oxygen content as near normal as possible.

If dialysis is required because of rejection before delivery, hemodialysis is usually the treatment modality used (66). Although care is taken to ensure that all the heparin used during the dialysis is neutralized after treatment, a partial thromboplastin time should be done before any regional block is administered.

Preeclampsia frequently occurs during pregnancy in patients with renal transplant. This may necessitate preterm delivery of the fetus. Magnesium must be used with great caution if the creatinine is elevated, and frequent blood samples should be drawn and the levels tested.

There is significant perinatal morbidity in infants born to mothers who have received a renal transplant. In one series, 45% were delivered prematurely and 25% were small for gestational age. Respiratory distress syndrome, hyperviscosity, congenital anomalies, adrenocortical insufficiency, and sepsis also occurred in the newborn (64). Therefore the neonate should be born in a center equipped to treat these problems.

The choice of anesthetic management for labor and delivery depends primarily on graft function. Most patients who conceive and are able to carry viable fetuses have good renal function and therefore their fluid, electrolyte, and acid-base statuses are normal. However, they may be at risk for such problems as uterine rupture (71) because of steroid treatment and therefore a large-bore intravenous cannula should be placed. In addition, steroid cover is indicated. Parenteral narcotics, inhalational analgesia with nitrous oxide, or (if there are no contraindications) epidural analgesia can be used for pain relief for vaginal delivery. Methoxyflurane should not be used for inhalation analgesia.

Cesarean section is required in 25 to 100% of pregnancies (64, 71, 72), necessitated by avascular necrosis of the hip, pelvic bony abnormalities, toxemia, or deteriorating renal function. The transplanted kidney is located in the false pelvis and rarely causes obstruction to vaginal delivery. Steroid cover is indicated preoperatively. When positioning the patient, care must be taken to protect any functioning shunts or fistulas that had been used as vascular access for hemodialysis.

Blood loss may be increased because of the previous surgery in the bladder area. While blood transfusion before renal transplant significantly increases the chance of a successful graft (73), transfusion after the graft is in place does not have this effect and may be detrimental. If a blood transfusion is required, washed or frozen red blood cells should be used to avoid introducing an excessive amount of white blood cells and platelet antigens into the circulation.

Either regional or general anesthesia may be used. If regional anesthesia is chosen, hypotension must be avoided before and after delivery of the infant to ensure good renal perfusion. Fluid infusions should be tailored to the patient and depend on her preoperative intravascular volume, renal function, and expected blood loss. Central venous or pulmonary artery pressure should be monitored in patients with severe oliguria, and fluid should be restricted if in-

travascular hypervolemia is present. If an epidural is performed, large doses of bupivacaine should be avoided in patients with severe graft compromise (74). Ephedrine can be used to raise the blood pressure if hypotension occurs in spite of normal cardiac filling pressures. After the delivery of the infant, an oxytocin infusion should be started to contract the uterus and promote hemostasis. Ergot preparations should be avoided if possible because, in large doses, these may cause generalized arteriolar constriction and may decrease graft blood flow.

If general anesthesia is chosen, many of the same considerations for regional anesthesia apply. In addition such nephrotoxic agents as methoxyflurane and muscle relaxants that depend on renal elimination, such as gallamine, metocurine, and pancuronium, should be avoided. Succinylcholine can be used, but it may cause an increase in potassium of 0.5 to 1 mEq/liter (75). This is not dangerous unless the serum potassium is already abnormally high.

In summary, the number of pregnancies with good outcomes is increasing in renal transplant patients. Their anesthetic management depends on their degree of renal impairment and the resulting hemodynamic and metabolic changes. Since all transplant patients take a number of antirejection and possibly other drugs, the interaction of these with the stress of labor and anesthesia must be recognized. If renal function is normal, the anesthetic management is similar to that in normal pregnant patients. Patients with severe renal impairment require intensive hemodynamic monitoring and frequent electrolyte determinations to ensure a successful outcome for both mother and fetus.

IMMUNE DEFICIENCY SYNDROMES

Immune deficiency syndromes can be either congenital or acquired and may involve abnormalities in T lymphocytes, B lymphocytes, or both. In addition, complement deficiencies may result in autoimmune phenomena and increased infections. The more severe congenital syndromes are fatal in early childhood, but others are compatible with a normal life span.

Regardless of how immunodeficiency begins, all are characterized by an unusual susceptibility to infection. Patients with abnormalities in humoral immunity have recurrent pyogenic infections with staphylococci, *Haemophilus influenzae*, and *Streptococcus pneumoniae*. Abnormalities in T-cell function result in disseminated viral and fungal infections (76).

The most common types of immunodeficiencies are caused by specific immunosuppressive drugs or HIV infection. The latter is becoming an increasingly widespread problem and will be discussed in detail below and in the following chapter.

Acquired Immunodeficiency Syndrome (AIDS)

AIDS is a defect in cell-mediated immunity caused by the human immunodeficiency virus (HIV). In North America, it has been primarily a male to male sexually transmitted disease but the number of women of childbearing age contracting the disease is increasing. Between 1989 and 1991, women accounted for 12% of the reported cases of AIDS, compared with 9% from 1981 to 1988 (77, 77a). Underreporting makes this number an underestimate of the actual incidence. The risk factors for exposure are shown in Table 33.5.

The clinical course and natural history of HIV infection have been described according to the Walter Reed (WR) classification system (Table 33.6). The observation of patients at various stages of the illness show that virtually all patients progress over time. Although the course of the disease is usually slowly progressive, it can be very rapid with about 1% of patients progressing from stage 1 to 6 in less than 14 months and 10% within 36 months. Over 90% of patients advance at least 1 stage during 36 months of observation (78). The diagnosis of AIDS requires

Table 33.5
Risk Factors for Exposure to the HIV Virus in Women[a]

Exposure Category	Percent Affected
Intravenous (IV) drug use	57.2
Sex with an IV drug user	20.2
Receipt of a blood transfusion or tissue from an infected donor	4.8
Sex with a man born in a pattern II country[b]	
Women born in a pattern II country	4.6
Women born elsewhere	0.3
Sex with a bisexual male	3.3
Sex with an HIV-positive male of undetermined mode of exposure	2.9
Sex with a man with hemophilia	0.4
Hemophilia or coagulation disorder	0.3
Sex with a transfusion recipient with HIV infection	0.2
Undetermined exposure	5.7

[a] Reprinted by permission from Gayle JA, Selik RM, Chu SY: Surveillance for AIDS and HIV infection among Black and Hispanic children of childbearing age 1981–1989. MMWR 39:23–30, 1990.
[b] Pattern II countries are those where heterosexual contact is the primary mode of transmission of HIV.

documentation of HIV infection and the following clinical criteria: severe immunosuppression without obvious cause; specified opportunistic infections (Table 33.6); severe, involuntary weight loss; or dementia.

Clinically, pregnant patients with HIV infection present three main problems: (a) the effect of HIV infection on themselves; (b) the potential effect of HIV infection on the infant, including perinatal transmission; and (c) possible spread of the disease among health care workers.

The vast majority of pregnant patients with HIV infection are asymptomatic. Normally during pregnancy, the number of T-helper cells drops until the seventh month when they stabilize and increase until delivery. Patients with HIV infection follow the same pattern, but their levels tend to be 10 to 20% below those of controls. Patients who have a T-helper cell count of less than 300 cells per μL have a high incidence of opportunistic infections, pneumonia, and postpartum abscess (79).

The effect of pregnancy on HIV infection is controversial. Because pregnancy impairs T-cell responses to other viral illnesses such as cytomegalovirus and rubella, it was thought that HIV infection may follow a more fulminant course. There are no data to support this contention, and progression from an asymptomatic to symptomatic state does not occur commonly. In a series of 20 patients who died of AIDS within 1 year of termination of pregnancy, most died of *Pneumocystis carinii* pneumonia. With advances in the treatment and prophylaxis of this disease, it may become less common in the future. Others died of candidiasis, tuberculosis, and central nervous system lymphoma (80).

Pregnancy may mask some of the symptoms of HIV infection. Symptoms such as anorexia, weight loss, and fatigue are common in early pregnancy and must be distinguished from progression of HIV or opportunistic infection (81). Some therapy such as azidothymidine (AZT) may be relatively contraindicated (82). This drug is known to cross the placenta in significant concentrations in the rodent (83) and ovine (84) models. Interestingly, the use of antiviral agents is currently under study in an effort to prevent transmission of HIV to the fetus (84).

The incidence of transmission of the HIV virus to offspring is between 13 and 73% (Table 34.4). Transmission of the virus to the fetus is known to occur early in pregnancy but the frequency of intrapartum transmission to the infant is unknown. Cesarean section does not reduce the transmission rate (82). However, it may be wise to take precautions during labor and delivery to reduce the chance of transmission. These precautions may include avoiding scalp clips,

Table 33.6
Walter Reed Classification for the Clinical Course of AIDS

Stage	Laboratory	Symptoms
0	None	Exposure to known carrier but no symptoms
1	Antibodies, virions	Flu-like illness appearing for weeks to months
2	Decreasing T-helper cell count	Generalized lymphadenopathy for months to 5 years
3	T-helper cell count of less than 400	Subclinical immune dysfunction
4	Partial cutaneous anergy	
5	Total cutaneous anergy	Superficial fungal infections (e.g., thrush)
6	Definitional opportunistic infections—pneumocystosis, crptoccocosis, etc.	

clearing blood and secretions from the infant atraumatically as soon as possible after delivery, and avoiding venipuncture and vitamin-K inoculation before thoroughly cleaning the infant (85). Patients with clinical AIDS are at high risk for complicated pregnancies. Preterm deliveries and stillbirths are common (80). Infection of the fetus with opportunistic organisms such as cytomegalovirus or toxoplasma can have devastating effects.

Health care workers are concerned with the potential for transmission of HIV to themselves by exposure to body fluids. In 1985 the Centers for Disease Control (CDC) proposed that, because many patients may be carriers of both HIV and hepatitis B virus although their status at the time of treatment is unknown, universal precautions for the prevention of exposure should be exercised. This is especially true when blood, amniotic fluid, or other body fluids contaminated with blood are encountered. Although the risk of contracting HIV infection in this manner is small, the exact risk depends on several factors. These include the incidence of HIV infection in the population, the transmission rate after a single needle stick or other exposure, and the number of exposures experienced by each health care worker. The incidence of seroconversion after a single needle stick is about 0.5%. By 1988 17 cases of occupational transmission by needle stick had been documented (86). Table 33.7 contains some practical suggestions for the protection of health care workers on the labor unit (87).

Other patients must also be protected from the transmission of HIV. The virus is rapidly killed outside the body. Reusable equipment that comes into contact with mucous membranes such as laryngoscope blades should be sterilized via high-level sterilization—that is, hot water pasteurization or accepted chemical sterilization (87).

The anesthetic management of the parturient with HIV infection must take several factors into consid-

Table 33.7
Universal Precautions and Prevention of Spread of HIV to Health Care Workers on the Labor Unit

1. Vinyl or latex gloves should be worn when handling material contaminated with body fluids at risk (amniotic fluid, blood, pericardial fluid, pleural fluid, peritoneal fluid, synovial fluid, cerebrospinal fluid, semen, and vaginal secretions). These should be disposed of after use and not washed.
2. Care should be taken when handling sharp contaminated objects. Needles should not be recapped or manipulated by hand. All sharp objects should be placed in a puncture-resistant container.
3. Hands should be washed thoroughly after any procedure for which exposure to above mentioned fluids occurred, whether gloves have been used or not.
4. Eye protection or face guards and gowns should be used when there is a potential for splashes of blood or amniotic fluid.
5. The neonate should be handled with gloves immediately after delivery. The oropharynx should not be suctioned with direct mouth suction, rather a suction bulb or wall suction should be used.

eration. A thorough history and physical examination must be performed to determine what, if any, clinical impact the disease has made. Anemia, thrombocytopenia, and circulating anticoagulants may be present (82). A neurologic examination must be performed because HIV infection is associated with progressive neurologic deficits. Pneumonitis caused by opportunistic infection may be present and account for severe hypoxemia. Other systemic or central nervous system infections may contraindicate the use of regional block.

A 1989 survey conducted by the Society for Obstetric Anesthesia and Perinatology of its members showed that anesthesiologists have some reservations concerning regional block in the patient with clinical AIDS because of the possibility that progressive neurologic deficit may be blamed on the procedure (88). Pain relief in labor may be achieved by other means such as narcotics or nitrous oxide, although these may be less than satisfactory in some cases. Consultation with the anesthesiologist for patient assessment and to explain the risks of the procedure before labor starts may avoid the unnecessary denial of regional anesthesia to these patients.

The effect of general anesthesia on T-cell function is controversial. Early studies did not show depression in T-cell numbers when halothane or enflurane was given to volunteers. Other studies have shown greater T-cell suppression after general anesthesia for surgery when compared with epidural anesthesia, possibly as a result of the reduction of the cortisol response to trauma (89). The clinical implications of these observations are not clear. It should be noted that the immunosuppression associated with the trauma and endocrine changes of surgery probably is more important than the type of anesthetic.

In summary, the anesthesiologist will encounter the patient with HIV infection and AIDS more frequently. Asymptomatic patients may be treated as any other because universal precautions should be taken to avoid exposure to potentially contaminated body fluids from both the mother and newborn. When formulating an anesthetic plan for patients with clinical AIDS, their respiratory, cardiovascular, and neurologic status must be assessed. In addition, the needs of the fetus and plans for delivery must be known. Ideally, the anesthesiologist will see the patient before labor begins to discuss anesthetic techniques. A detailed discussion of the anesthetic considerations for HIV-infected patients is presented in Chapter 34.

References

1. Sever JL: HIV: Biology and Immunology. Clin Obstet Gynecol 132:423–428, 1989.
2. Barrett JT: *Textbook of Immunology: An Introduction to Immunochemistry and Immunobiology*, 4th ed. CV Mosby, St. Louis, 1983.
3. Watkins J, Clark RSJ: Report of a symposium: Adverse responses to intravenous agents. Br J Anaesth 50:1159–1164, 1978.
4. Garrison GC: Histamine, bradykinin and 5-hydroxytryptamine and their antagonists. In *The Pharmacological Basis of Therapeutics*, 8th ed, AG Gilman, TW Rall, AS Nies, P Taylor, eds. Pergamon Press, New York, 1990, pp 575–599.
5. Kelly JF, Patterson R: Anaphylaxis: Course, mechanism and treatment. JAMA 227:1431–1436, 1974.
6. Fisher MM: Blood volume replacement in acute anaphylactic cardiovascular collapse related to anesthesia. Br J Anaesth 49:1023–1026, 1977.
7. Ford RM: The management of acute allergic disease including anaphylaxis. Med J Aust 1:222–223, 1977.
8. Cheng TC, Pouget JM: Electrocardiographic changes in oral penicillin anaphylaxis. IL Med J 160:172–174, 1981.
9. Sullivan T: Cardiac disorders in penicillin-induced anaphylaxis. JAMA 248:2161–2162, 1982.
10. Zavecz JH, Levi R: Separation of primary and secondary cardiovascular events in anaphylaxis. Circ Res 40:15–19, 1977.
11. Fisher MM: The management of anaphylaxis. Med J Aust 1:793, 1977.
12. Labovitz E, Spector S: Placental theophyllin transfer in pregnant asthmatics. JAMA 247:786–789, 1982.
13. Levy JH, Rockoff MA: Anaphylaxis to meperidine. Anesth Analg 61:301–303, 1982.
14. Etter MS, Herlich M, Mac Kenzie MS: Immunoglobulin E fluctuation in thiopental anaphylaxis. Anesthesiology 52:181–183, 1980.
15. Incaudo G, Shatz M, Patterson R, Rosenberg M, Yamamoto F, Hamberger R: Administration of local anesthetics to patients with prior history of adverse reactions. J Allergy Clin Immunol 61:339–345, 1978.
16. Brown DT, Beamish D, Wildsmith JAW: Allergic reaction to an amide local anesthetic. Br J Anaesth 53:435–437, 1981.
17. Aldrete JA, Johnson DA: Allergy to local anesthetics. JAMA 207:356–357, 1969.
18. Shatz M: Skin testing and incremental challenge in the evaluation of adverse reactions to local anesthetics. J Allergy Clin Immunol 74:606–616, 1984.
19. Assem ESK, Punnia-Moorthy A: Allergy to local anesthetics: An approach to definitive diagnosis. Br Dent J 164:44–47, 1988.
20. Nagel JE, Fuscaldo JT, Fireman P: Paraben allergy. JAMA 237:1594–1595, 1977.
21. de Shazo RD, Nelson HS: An approach to the patient with a history of local anesthetic hypersensitivity: Experience with 90 patients. J Allergy Clin Immunol 63:387–394, 1979.
22. Sage D: Intradermal testing following anaphylactoid reaction during anaesthesia. Anaesth Intensive Care 9:381–386, 1981.
23. Fisher MM: Intradermal testing in the diagnosis of acute anaphylaxis during anaesthesia: Results of five years experience. Anaesth Intensive Care 7:58–61, 1979.
24. Kagan R, Laros RK: Immune thrombocytopenia. Clin Obstet Gynecol 26:537–546, 1983.
25. Bowman JM: Rh erythorblastosis fetalis 1975. Semin Hematol 12:189–207, 1975.
26. Rote NS: Pathophysiology of Rh immunization. Clin Obstet Gynecol 25:243–253, 1982.
27. Pritchard JA, MacDonald PC, Gant N: Other diseases of the fetus and newborn infant. In *Williams Obstetrics*, 17th ed. JA Pritchard, PC MacDonald, NF Gant, eds. Appleton-Century–Crofts, Norwalk CT, 1985, pp 769–792.
28. Kirkinen P, Jouppila P, Eik-Nes S: Umbilical vein blood flow in rhesus-isoimmunization. Br J Obstet Gynaecol 90:640–643, 1983.
29. Haines CJ, Read MD: Characteristic fetal heart rate changes in severe rhesus isoimmunization. Aust N Z J Obstet Gynaecol 23:114–116, 1983.
30. Hollmén AL, Jouppila R, Jouppila P, Koivula A, Vierola H: Effect of extradural analgesia using bupivacaine and 2-chloroprocaine on intervillous blood flow during normal labor. Br J Anaesth 54:837–842, 1982.
31. Gleicher N, Adelsberg BR, Lui TL, Cederqvist LL, Phillips RN, Siegel I: Immune complexes in pregnancy. III. Immune complexes in immune-complex associated conditions. Am J Obstet Gynecol 142:1011–1015, 1982.
32. Eisenberg RA, Cohen PL: The role of immunologic mechanisms in the pathogenesis of rheumatic diseases. In *Primer on Rheumatic Diseases*, 9th ed. HR Schumacher Jr, ed. The Arthritis Foundation, Atlanta, GA, 1988, pp 36–44.
33. Hess EV: Rheumatoid arthritis: Epidemiology, etiology, rheumatoid factor, pathology, pathogenesis. In *Primer on Rheumatic Diseases*, 9th ed. HR Schumacher Jr, ed. The Arthritis Foundation, Atlanta, GA, 1988, pp 83–96.
34. Edelist G: Principles of anesthetic management in rheumatoid arthritic patients. Anesth Analg 43:227–231, 1964.
35. Phelps JA: Laryngeal obstruction due to cricoarytenoid arthritis. Anesthesiology 27:518–522, 1966.
36. Crosby ET, Lui A: The adult cervical spine: Implications for airway management. Can J Anaesth 37:77–93, 1990.
37. Hodgekinson R: Anesthetic management of a parturient with severe rheumatoid arthritis. Anesth Analg 60:611–612, 1981.
38. Bulmash JM: Rheumatoid arthritis in pregnancy. Obstet Gynecol Ann 8:223–276, 1979.

39. Klipple GL, Cercere FA: Rheumatoid arthritis and pregnancy. Rheum Dis Clin North Am 15:213–240, 1989.
40. Alacorn-Segovia D: Systemic lupus erythematosus: Pathology and pathogenesis. In *Primer on Rheumatic Diseases*, 9th ed. HR Schumacher Jr, ed. The Arthritis Foundation, Atlanta, GA, 1988, pp 96–98.
41. Scott JS: Systemic lupus erythematosus and allied disorders in pregnancy. Clin Obstet Gynecol 6:461–471, 1979.
42. del Rio A, Vazquez JJ, Sobrino, JA, Gil A, Barbado J, Mate I, Ortiz-Vazquez J: Myocardial involvement in systemic lupus erythematosus: A non-invasive study of left ventricular function. Chest 74:414–417, 1978.
43. Fine LG (Moderator): Systemic lupus erythematosus in pregnancy. Ann Intern Med 94:667–677, 1981.
44. Zulman JI, Talal N, Hoffman GS, Epstein WV: Problems associated with the management of pregnancies in patients with systemic lupus erythematosus. J Hematol 7:37–49, 1980.
45. Triplett DA, Brandt J: Laboratory identification of the lupus anticoagulant. Br J Haematol 73:139–142, 1989.
46. Reece EA, Romero R, Hobbins J: Coagulopathy associated with Factor VIII Inhibitor: A literature review. J Reprod Med 29:53–58, 1984.
47. Vetter VL, Rashkind WJ: Congenital complete heart block and connective tissue disease (editorial). N Engl J Med 309:236–238, 1983.
48. Scott JS, Maddison PJ, Taylor PV, Esacher E, Scott O, Skinner RP: Connective-tissue disease, antibodies to ribonucleoprotein, and congenital heart block. N Engl J Med 309:209–212, 1983.
49. Medsger TA: Systemic sclerosis and localized scleroderma. In *Primer on Rheumatic Diseases*, 9th ed. HR Schumacher Jr, ed. The Arthritis Foundation, Atlanta, GA, 1988, pp 111–117.
50. Johnson TR, Banner EA, Winklemann RK: Scleroderma in pregnancy. Obstet Gynecol 23:467–469, 1964.
51. Swanesaratnam V, Chong HL: Scleroderma and pregnancy. Aust N Z J Obstet Gynaecol 22:123–124, 1982.
52. Weisman RA, Calceterra TC: Head and neck manifestations of scleroderma. Ann Otol Rhinol Laryngol 87:332–339, 1978.
53. Cannon PJ, Hassar M, Case DB, Casserella WJ, Sommers SC, LeRoy EC: The relationship between hypertension and renal failure in scleroderma (progressive systemic sclerosis) to structural and functional abnormalities of the renal cortical circulation. Medicine 53:1–46, 1974.
54. Palma A, Sanchez-Palencia A, Armas JR: Progressive systemic sclerosis and the nephrotic syndrome. Arch Intern Med 141:520– 521, 1981.
55. Bulkley BH, Ridolfi RL, Salyer WR, Hutchins GM: Myocardial lesions of progressive systemic sclerosis: A cause of cardiac dysfunction. Circulation 53:483–490, 1976.
56. Young RH, Mark GJ: Pulmonary vascular changes in scleroderma. Am J Med 64:998–1004, 1978.
57. Karlen JR, Cooke WA: Renal scleroderma in pregnancy. Obstet Gynecol 44:349–354, 1974.
58. Levy DL: Fetal-neonatal involvement in maternal autoimmune disease. Obstet Gynecol Surv 37(suppl):122–127, 1982.
59. Maymon R, Fegin M: Scleroderma in pregnancy. Obstet Gynecol Surv 44:530–534, 1989.
60. Eisele JH, Reitan JA: Scleroderma, Raynaud's phenomenon, and local anesthetics. Anesthesiology 34:386–387, 1971.
61. Thompson J, Conklin K: Anesthetic management of a pregnant patient with scleroderma. Anesthesiology 59:69–71, 1983.
62. Gall SA: Maternal adjustments in the immune system in normal pregnancy. Clin Obstet Gynecol 26:521–536, 1983.
63. Deeg HJ, Kennedy MS, Sanders JE, Thomas ED, Storb B: Successful pregnancy after marrow transplantation for severe aplastic anemia and immunosuppression with cyclosporine. JAMA 250:647, 1983.
64. Penn J, Makowski EL, Harris P: Parenthood following renal transplantation. Kidney Int 18:221–233, 1980.
65. Davison JM, Lindheimer MD: Pregnancy in renal transplant recipients. J Reprod Med 27:613–621, 1982.
66. MacCarthy P, Pollack VE: Maternal renal disease: Effect on the fetus. Clin Perinatol 8:307–319, 1981.
67. Calabresi P, Parks RE: Antiproliferative agents and drugs used for immunosuppression. in *The Pharmacologic Basis of Therapeutics*, 8th ed. AG Gilman, TW Rall, AS Nies, P Taylor, eds. Macmillan, New York, 1990, pp 1209–1263.
68. Morris PJ: Cyclosporin A: Transplantation 32:349–354, 1981.
69. Ryffel B, Donatsch P, Madorin M, Matter BE, Ruttimann G, Schon H, Stoll R, Wilson J: Toxicological evaluation of cyclosporin A. Arch Toxicol 53:107–141, 1983.
70. Hou S: Pregnancy in organ transplant recipients. Med Clin North Am 73:667–683, 1989.
71. Farber M: Pregnancy and renal transplantation. Clin Obstet Gynecol 21:931–935, 1978.
72. Whetham JCG, Cardella C, Harding M: Effect of pregnancy on graft function and graft survival in renal cadaver transplant patients. Am J Obstet Gynecol 145:193–197, 1983.
73. Gutterman RD: Selection and preparation of donors and recipients for renal transplantation. In *Textbook of Nephrology*. SG Massry, RJ Glassock, eds. Williams & Wilkins, Baltimore, 1983, pp 9.13–9.17.
74. Gould DB, Aldrete JA: Bupivacaine cardiotoxicity in a patient with renal failure. Acta Anaesthesiol Scand 27:18–21, 1983.
75. Hilgrenberg JC: Renal disease. In *Anesthesia and Co-existing Disease*. RK Stoelting, SF Dierdorf, eds. Churchill Livingston, New York, 1983, p 394.
76. Cooper MD, Lawton III AR: Immune deficiency diseases. In *Harrison's Principles of Internal Medicine*, 11th ed. E Braunwald, KJ Isselbacher, RG Petersdorf, J Wilson, JB Martin, AS Fauci, eds. McGraw-Hill, New York, 1987, pp 1385–1392.
77. Gayle JA, Selik RM, Chu SY: Surveillance for AIDS and HIV infection among Black and Hispanic children and women of childbearing age 1981–1989. MMWR 39:23–30, 1990.
77a. Centers For Disease Control: The second 100,000 cases of acquired immune deficiency syndrome: United States, June, 1981–December, 1991. MMWR 41:28–29, 1992.
78. Settlage RH: AIDS in obstetrics: Diagnosis, course, and prognosis. Clin Obstet Gynecol 32:437–444, 1989.
79. Landesman SH: Human immunodeficiency virus infection in women: An overview. Semin Perinatol 13:2–6, 1989.
80. Koonin LM, Ellerbrock TV, Atrash HK, Rogers MF, Smith JC, Hogue CRJ, Harris MD, Chavkin W, Parker AL, Halpin GJ: Pregnancy-associated deaths due to AIDS in the United States. JAMA 261:1306–1309, 1989.
81. Rich K: Maternal AIDS: Effects on mother and infant. Ann NY Acad Sci 562:241–247, 1989.
82. Finekind L, Minkoff HL: HIV in pregnancy. Clin Perinatol 15:189–202, 1988.
83. Little BB, Bawdon RE, Christmas JT, Sobhi S, Gilstrap LC III: Pharmacokinetics of azidothymidine during late pregnancy in Long-Evans rats. Am J Obstet Gynecol 161:732–734, 1989.
84. Hughes SC, Thirion AV, Messer C, Hazzanzadeh K, Gambertoglio JG, Rosen MA, Shnider SM: Placental transfer and acute maternal and fetal effects of AZT in the pregnant ewe. In *Society of Perinatal Obstetricians*. New Orleans, 1989. A393.
85. Connon E, Bardeguez A, Apuzzio J: The intrapartum management of the HIV-infected mother and her infant. Clin Perinatol 16:899–908, 1989.
86. Mead PB: AIDS: Risk to the health profession. Clin Obstet Gynecol 32:485–496, 1989.
87. Guidelines for the prevention of transmission of human immuno-deficiency virus to health–care and public safety workers. MMWR 38:1–37, 1989.
88. Douglas JM: AIDS and obstetric anesthesia. SOAP Newslett 21:9, 1989.
89. Stevenson GW, Hall SC, Rudnick S, Seleny FL, Stevenson HC: The effect of anesthetic agents on the human immune response. Anesthesiology 72:542–552, 1990.

FETUS AND NEWBORN

CHAPTER 34

Human Immunodeficiency Virus in the Delivery Suite

Patricia A. Dailey, M.D.

Infection with the human immunodeficiency virus (HIV) and subsequent acquired immunodeficiency syndrome (AIDS) is occurring with increasing frequency in women of childbearing age and their children. Many women do not realize they are at risk for HIV infection and may not realize they are infected with HIV until they develop AIDS or bear a child who is infected. Accordingly, health care workers must assume that every patient we care for has a blood-borne pathogen (whether it is HIV, hepatitis B [HBV], or the next unknown virus) and must take appropriate precautions to prevent transmission between mother and fetus/neonate, patient and health care worker, and patient and patient.

EPIDEMIOLOGY

The number of women with AIDS has been steadily increasing, with women accounting for an increasing proportion of all AIDS cases in the United States. From November 1989 through October 1990, women accounted for 11% of all reported cases in adults (1). Among all cases of AIDS in women, 85% occurred among women of childbearing age (15–44 years) (1). Most women with AIDS were young, black or Hispanic, and residents of urban areas on the Atlantic coast (Fig. 34.1). Overall, 51% of women with AIDS were infected through intravenous drug use and 29% through heterosexual contact (2). HIV/AIDS is among the 10 leading causes of death in women of reproductive age, and if current mortality trends continue, HIV/AIDS will be one of the 5 leading causes of death by 1991 (Fig. 34.2) (3).

By the end of 1990 over 15,000 cases of AIDS in women were reported to the Centers for Disease Control (1). However, this is a gross underestimate of the seroprevalence of HIV infection. It has been predicted that at least 100,000 women in the United States are infected with HIV (4). The prevalence of seropositivity for HIV antibody in women ranges from a low of 0.004% among female blood donors in Massachusetts to a high of 57% among New Jersey prostitutes (5). Table 34.1 presents seroprevalence studies of women receiving prenatal care.

HIV-infected women often remain undiagnosed until the onset of AIDS or until a perinatally infected child becomes ill. One approach to assessing the prevalence of HIV infection in childbearing women is to test the blood of their newborn infants for HIV antibody. Antibodies to HIV are transferred transplacentally from mother to fetus and can persist in the infant beyond 10 months of age (6, 7). The presence of antibody in the newborn does not necessarily indicate HIV infection of the newborn, but it does represent HIV infection of the mother. Several studies have screened umbilical cord blood or neonatal heel-stick specimens for the presence of HIV antibody (5). They are summarized in Table 34.2. The prevalence rates range from 0 to 4.3% (5). In 1987 one in fifty-seven women who delivered at Boston City Hospital was HIV-positive (8).

Diagnosis of maternal HIV infection may be delayed during pregnancy due to the nonspecific symptoms of infection such as fatigue, anorexia, and weight loss. All patients should be offered counseling and *voluntary* HIV testing. Controversy surrounds the issue of *mandatory* testing for HIV of all patients.

HIV has a long incubation period between infection and overt illness; the estimated median incubation period is at least 7 years in homosexual men (9). In general, women have a shorter mean length of survival between the diagnosis of AIDS and death than do men; 298 days for women vs 347 days for men (10). It has been suggested that there may be an accelerated progression of HIV infection with pregnancy. The effects of pregnancy on HIV are unknown. Cell-mediated immunity is depressed during pregnancy, especially during the second and third trimesters of gestation (11, 12). Within 28 to 30 months postpartum, 45 to 75% of asymptomatic pregnant women, identified because their children developed HIV disease, developed symptoms themselves (13).

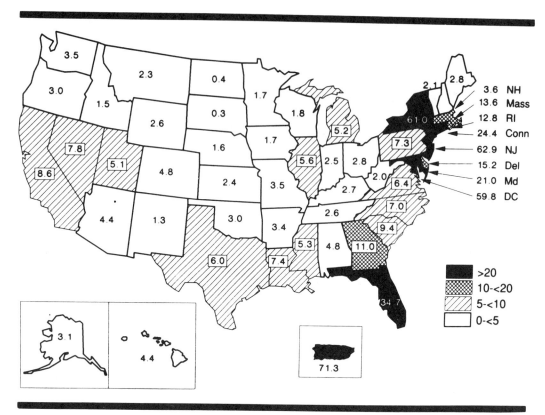

Figure 34.1. Cumulative incidence rates of cases of acquired immunodeficiency syndrome in women by state of residence per 100,000 women, United States, through December 31, 1990. (Reprinted with permission from Ellerbrock TV, Bush TJ, Chamberland ME, Oxtoby MJ: Epidemiology of women with AIDS in the United States, 1981 through 1990: A comparison with heterosexual men with AIDS. JAMA 265:2971–2975, 1991.)

This is a higher rate of symptoms than the 13 to 34% reported for antibody-positive homosexual men, intravenous drug users, and hemophiliacs who were followed for up to 6 years. At least 26 maternal deaths attributable to HIV disease have been reported in the medical literature in the United States (Table 34.3) (14–18). Most women died of *Pneumocystis carinii* pneumonia. The interval between termination of pregnancy and death ranged from 3½ hr to 19 weeks. Overall, the interval between AIDS diagnosis and death ranged from 1 day to 15 months (14).

TRANSMISSION OF HIV IN THE HEALTH CARE SETTING

There is a significant potential for transmission of HIV in the labor and delivery setting. With the "humanization" of obstetric practice to create a more natural and home-like setting, health care workers have often stopped using the physical and protective barriers of drapes, gowns, and gloves. However, patients infected with HIV or other blood-borne infections such as hepatitis B cannot always be identified. It has been difficult to convince obstetric staff of the need to protect themselves and their patients by us-

ing the universal precautions recommended by the Centers for Disease Control (CDC) to minimize body fluid contact (19). Before discussing more specific suggestions related to the prevention of transmission of HIV infection in the labor and delivery setting, the universal precautions guidelines will be reviewed.

HIV has been isolated from blood and body fluids and tissues including semen, vaginal secretions, saliva, breast milk, tears, urine, cerebrospinal fluid (CSF) alveolar fluid, and amniotic fluid. However, epidemiologic evidence has implicated only blood, semen, vaginal secretions, and possibly breast milk in transmission (20). The rate of isolation of the virus varies with the fluid. For example, of 71 men with HIV infection, the virus was detected in 28 of 50 blood samples but in only 1 of 83 saliva samples (21).

Universal blood and body fluid precautions are recommended for all patients–not just patients with known or suspected infection. The CDC's recommendations (20) provide that:

1. All health care workers should routinely use appropriate barrier precautions to prevent skin and mucous membrane exposure when contact with blood or other body fluids of any patient is anticipated. Gloves should be worn for touching blood and body

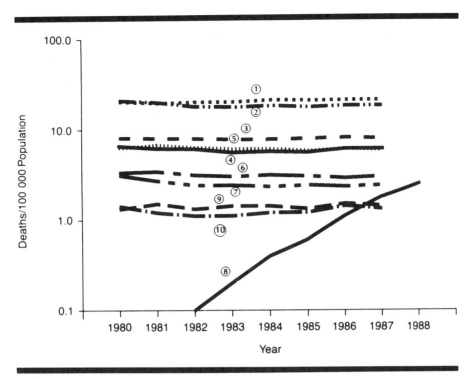

Figure 34.2. Death rates for HIV/AIDS and other leading causes in women 15 to 44 years of age, 1980 through 1988. 1 = neoplasm; 2 = unintentional injuries; 3 = heart disease; 4 = homicide; 5 = suicide; 6 = cerebrovascular disease; 7 = chronic liver disease and cirrhosis; 8 = human immunodeficiency virus/acquired immunodeficiency syndrome; 9 = diabetes mellitus; and 10 = pneumonia and influenza. (Reprinted with permission from Chu Sy, Buehler JW, Berkelman RL: Impact of the human immunodeficiency virus epidemic on mortality in women of reproductive age, United States. JAMA 264: 225–229, 1990.)

fluids, mucous membranes, or nonintact skin of all patients, for handling items or surfaces soiled with blood or body fluids, and for performing venipuncture and other vascular access procedures. Gloves should be changed after contact with each patient. Masks and protective eyewear or face shields should be worn during procedures that are likely to generate droplets of blood or other body fluids to prevent exposure of mucous membranes of the mouth, nose, and eyes. Gowns or aprons should be worn during procedures that are likely to generate splashes of blood or other body fluids.

2. Hands and other skin surfaces should be washed immediately and thoroughly if contaminated with blood or other body fluids. Hands should be washed immediately after gloves are removed.

3. All health care workers should take precautions to prevent injuries caused by needles, scalpels, and other sharp instruments or devices during procedures, when cleaning used instruments, during disposal of used needles, and when handling sharp instruments after procedures. To prevent needle stick injuries, needles should not be recapped, purposely bent or broken by hand, removed from disposable syringes, or otherwise manipulated by hand. After they are used, disposable syringes and needles, scalpel blades, and other sharp items should be placed in puncture-resistant containers for disposal; the puncture-resistant containers should be located as close as practical to the use area. Large-bore reusable needles should be placed in a puncture-resistant container for transport to the reprocessing area.

4. Although saliva has not been implicated in HIV transmission, to minimize the need for emergency mouth-to-mouth resuscitation, mouthpieces, resuscitation bags, or other ventilation devices should be available for use in areas in which the need for resuscitation is predictable.

5. Health care workers who have exudative lesions or weeping dermatitis should refrain from all direct patient care and from handling patient care equipment until the condition resolves.

The CDC has clarified their recommendations to say that universal precautions do not apply to feces, nasal secretions, sputum, sweat, tears, urine, and vomitus unless they contain visible blood (22). While the CDC says universal precautions do not apply to saliva (i.e., gloves are not necessary when feeding patients or wiping saliva from skin), they do recommend the use of gloves as a general infection control practice when suctioning endotracheal tubes, during digital examination of mucous membranes, and during dental procedures. Blood is frequently in the mouth following endotracheal intubation. Forty-one persons had their oral se-

Table 34.1
Human Immunodeficiency Virus Antibody Studies in Women Receiving Prenatal Care[a]

Region	Location	Year	% Positive	No. Positive/ No. Tested	Remarks
Entire clinic population tested					
Northeast	Brooklyn, NY	1986–1987	5.9	15/255	Haitians
	New York City, NY	1986–1987	1.5	22/1497	
Midwest	Central Illinois	1987	0	0/97	
	Central Wisconsin	1986	0	0/1000	
South	North Carolina	1987	0	0/200	
	South Carolina	1988	0.1	1/1268	
	Jacksonville, FL	1986–1987	0.7	2/299	
	Baltimore, MD	1986–1987	1.3	16/1245	
West	Long Beach, CA	1986–1987	0	0/227	
	Alameda County, CA	1987	0	0/342	
	San Francisco, CA	1988	0.9	3/327	
Puerto Rico	San Juan	1987	1.2	42/3603	
Women at high risk for HIV infection targeted					
Midwest	Chicago, IL	1986–1987	25.0	15/60	IVDU
			1.1	1/90	Non-IVDU
	Chicago, IL	1986–1987	9.8	10/102	Mainly IVDU
	Detroit, MI	1986–1987	9.4	16/170	IVDU
South	Baltimore, MD	1986–1987	29.6	34/115	
	Baltimore, MD	1986–1987	21.6	19/88	

[a] Reprinted with permission from Shapiro CN, Schulz SL, Lee NC, Dondero TJ: Review of human immunodeficiency virus in the United States. Obstet Gynecol 74:800–808, 1989.
HIV = human immunodeficiency virus; IVDU = intravenous drug user.

cretions tested for occult blood to assess the incidence of blood in the mouth after routine endotracheal intubation. Twenty of the 41 were not intubated and served as controls. Only 1 of these 20 tested positive for occult blood. Twenty-one patients underwent general anesthesia with oral endotracheal intubation. Secretions were suctioned from the pharynx at the time of extubation. Of the 21 specimens, 13 tested positive for blood (23). The CDC also comments that the use of gloves for oral examinations and treatment in the dental setting may also protect the patient from exposure to the dental worker's blood (22).

Although gloves should reduce the incidence of contamination of hands, they cannot prevent penetrating injuries due to needles or other sharp instruments. Several studies have shown that double gloving may prevent perforations of the inner glove and cutaneous exposure of the hand (24, 25). Surgical or examination gloves should not be washed or disinfected for reuse. Washing may enhance the penetration of liquids through undetected holes in the glove and disinfectants may cause deterioration (22).

Universal precautions cost at least $336 million in the United States in fiscal year 1989. However, it is estimated that testing all hospital-admitted patients for HIV and HBV would cost $2.6 billion annually nationwide (26). Compared with the testing of all patients, the relative costs of isolation materials used for universal precautions seem beneficial. The author and editors do not recommend HIV testing of all patients for several reasons: (a) serologic results may not be available for patients treated on an emergency basis; (b) it may take 6 to 12 weeks for a patient infected with HIV to develop antibodies detectable by currently used screening tests; (c) universal precautions are effective in preventing other blood-borne infections such as HBV (27); and (d) there is no evidence to suggest that preoperative testing for HIV infection would reduce the frequency of accidental exposures to blood (25).

TRANSMISSION FROM MOTHER TO FETUS AND NEONATE

The transplacental route is the major mode of infection among infants, accounting for about 75 to 80% of all pediatric AIDS cases (28). HIV infection may be transmitted to the fetus in utero via the maternal circulation, to the infant during labor and delivery by inoculation or ingestion of blood and other infected fluids, and to the infant after birth through infected breast milk. Based on current epidemiologic evidence, it is believed that the risk of perinatal transmission of HIV by the transplacental route is between 13% and 73% (Table 34.4) (29–38). Seropositive women with more advanced HIV-related disease or T4-cell counts of less than 400 per cubic millimeter were more likely to transmit HIV infection to their babies (38).

The timing of perinatal transmission has been

Table 34.2
Human Immunodeficiency Virus Antibody Studies of Cord Blood Specimens[a]

Region	Location	Year	% Positive	No. Positive/ No. Tested
Northeast	Boston, MA	1987	1.6	16/1000
	Statewide, MA[b]	1987	0.3	81/30,708
	Newark, NJ	1987	4.3	26/604
	Brooklyn, NY	1986–1987	2.0	12/602
	Manhattan, NY	1986–1987	2.3	28/1192
	Manhattan, NY	1987	2.7	6/224
	New York City, NY	1987	1.3	26/1934
	Manhattan	1987	2.8	9/320
	Bronx	1987	1.6	5/312
	Brooklyn	1987	1.6	11/674
	Queens	1987	0.3	1/312
	Staten Island	1987	0	0/107
	Other/unknown	1987	0	0/209
	Upstate New York[b]	1987–1988	0.2	110/70,684
	New York City, NY[b]	1987–1988	1.3	786/60,866
	Manhattan[b]	1987–1988	1.7	182/10,798
	Bronx[b]	1987–1988	1.9	225/11,910
	Brooklyn[b]	1987–1988	1.2	266/21,286
	Queens[b]	1987–1988	0.7	96/14,086
	Staten Island[b]	1987–1988	0.6	17/2786
	Other/unknown[b]	1987–1988	0.1	2/2231
	Philadelphia, PA	1987	0	0/366
South	Miami, FL[c]	1986–1988	4.2	105/2475
	Baltimore, MD	1985	0.7	5/673
Puerto Rico	San Juan	1986–1987	1.2	11/909

[a] Reprinted with permission from Shapiro CN, Schulz SL, Lee NC, Dondero TJ: Review of human immunodeficiency virus in the United States. Obstet Gynecol 74:800–808, 1989.
[b] Filter-paper testing of neonatal heel-stick specimens.
[c] Haitian women.

difficult to determine. A characteristic facial malformation (microcephaly, ocular hypertelorism, prominent box-like forehead, flat nasal bridge, and a prominent philtrum) has been described in an uncontrolled study of 20 infected infants, suggesting that infection may occur between the 12th and 16th week of gestation (Fig. 34.3) (39). However, a controlled study found no supporting evidence of an AIDS embryopathy (40).

At present, there is no direct evidence that HIV can be acquired by the infant during its passage through the birth canal (46). However, in a study of twins born to HIV-infected mothers, the first child delivered was twice as likely to be infected with HIV than the second (Table 34.5) (83). Cesarean section does not prevent infection in the child (28, 31, 41–43). Precautions by health care workers to possibly lessen the risk of transmission of the virus from mothers who are HIV positive to the infant in the perinatal period include (29, 44, 45):

1. Avoidance of percutaneous umbilical cord sampling (PUBS). It is possible that the fetus would be infected by "sharing a needle" with the mother.
2. Avoidance of fetal scalp clips and fetal scalp sampling in labor unless absolutely necessary. Puncture sites in the fetal scalp could serve as a portal of entry for the virus.
3. Avoidance of delivery techniques (vacuum, forceps) that could produce abrasions and breaks in the infant's skin.
4. Removal of all maternal blood and fluids as thoroughly as possible immediately after delivery and before venipuncture or injections.
5. Until more is known about the transmission of virus in breast milk, counsel mothers known to be infected to not breastfeed their infants.

Some surveys have reported on dozens of babies who have not contracted HIV infection despite being breast fed by infected mothers. However, in one study 83% of infants who were breastfed became infected, as compared with 25% of those who were bottlefed (37). In addition, there are reports of mothers who were infected postpartum by blood transfusions whose breastfed babies then seroconverted (46).

In the postpartum period, regular hospital infection control guidelines should be followed. Isolation of asymptomatic seropositive women is not recommended. Mothers should be given full access

Table 34.3
Selected Characteristics of Women who Died of AIDS during or within One Year after Pregnancy Termination, United States 1983–1988[a]

Case	Year of Death	Age (yr)	Race/ Ethnicity	Transmission Categories	Pregnancy Outcome	EGA[b]	Interval Between Pregnancy Termination and Death	Major Opportunistic Disease	Interval Between AIDS Diagnosis and Death
1	1983	23	Black	IVDA[c]	PLB[d]	29	137	Kaposi's sarcoma	156
2	1984	22	Hispanic	Partner IVDA	NA[e]	NA	96	PCP[f]	27
3	1984	29	Black	Heterosexual (foreign born)	PLB	35	138	Candidiasis	225
4	1984	33	White	IVDA	Undel[g]	26	Undel	PCP	11
5	1984	24	Hispanic	IVDA	NA	NA	44	PCP	51
6	1985	27	Black	IVDA and foreign born	Undel	14	Undel	PCP	1
7	1985	22	Black	Undetermined	PLB	28	4	PCP	NA
8	1985	27	White	IVDA	PLB	33	30	PCP	95
9	1985	38	White	IVDA	Stillbirth	29	1	PCP	127
10	1986	35	White	IVDA	NA	NA	NA	PCP	79
11	1986	23	Hispanic	Partner IVDA	PLB	35	38	Central nervous system lymphoma	423
12	1986	30	Hispanic	IVDA	PLB (twins)	28	20	PCP	74
13	1986	36	Black	Partner IVDA	PLB	27	64	Disseminated tuberculosis	198
14	1987	26	Black	IVDA	Stillbirth	25	5	PCP	89
15	1987	26	Hispanic	Partner IVDA	PLB	25	3	PCP	66
16	1987	19	Black	Undetermined	PLB	26	3	PCP	6
17	1987	33	White	IVDA	PLB	24	2	PCP	7
18	1987	27	Black	Partner IVDA	Undel	NA	Undel	PCP	48
19	1987	22	Black	Partner IVDA	NA	NA	89	PCP	461
20	1988	27	Black	Heterosexual (foreign born)	Undel	22	Undel	PCP	4

[a] Reprinted from Koonin LM, Ellerbrock TV, Atrash HK, Rogers MF, Smith JC, Hogue CJR, Harris MA, Chavkin W, Parker AL, Halpin GJ: Pregnancy-associated deaths due to AIDS in the United States. JAMA 261:1306–1309, 1989.
[b] EGA = estimated gestational age (weeks).
[c] IVDA = intravenous drug abuser.
[d] PLB = premature live birth.
[e] NA = information not available.
[f] PCP = *Pneumocystis carinii* pneumonia.
[g] Undel = died during pregnancy, undelivered.

to their infants unless they have untreated pulmonary tuberculosis. Women infected with HIV should be medically evaluated (ideally antenatally) to rule out any incipient opportunistic infection or malignancy including *Mycobacterium tuberculosis*, hepatitis B virus, cytomegalovirus, toxoplasmosis, chlamydia, and herpes simplex, as well as gonorrhea and syphilis.

PREVENTION OF HIV TRANSMISSION BETWEEN PATIENT AND HEALTH CARE WORKER

As the number of pregnant women with HIV infection increases, perinatal health care workers become more at risk for occupational exposure to HIV. Historically, it has been difficult to convince obstetric staff to protect themselves by using blood and body fluid precautions with all patients. The following recommendations have been made when caring for all patients:

1. Thorough handwashing is one of the most important methods of preventing infection. Handwashing is mandatory before and after any and all procedures, after caring for a woman or infant, and between touching infants in the nursery. This includes handwashing after diaper, sanitary napkin, or linen changes.

2. Personnel with direct contact with the mother or newborn during delivery should wear gown and gloves.

3. Those exposed to the possibility of a splash of fluid (such as blood or amniotic fluid) should wear a mask and protective eyewear during the delivery.

4. Secretions in the neonate's oropharynx may be infected with HIV. Although no cases of virus transmission have been documented when using mouth to

Table 34.4
Risk of Transplacental Infection[a]

Reference	Number of Patients	Method of Diagnosis	Length of Follow-Up (Mos)	Transmission Rate (%)
30	372	HIV ab/culture/clin dis[b]	18+	13
31	20	HIV ab/clin dis	30	65
32	64	HIV ab/clin dis	14	37
33A	248	HIV IgM/culture	12	73
33B	46	HIV IgM/culture	12	33
34	6	Tissue culture (abortus)	NA	33
35	71	HIV ab/clin dis	36	30
36	37	HIV ab/clin dis	12	50
37	117	HIV ab/culture/clin dis	18	27
38	92	HIV ab/culture/clin dis	12	39

[a]Based on Nanada D, Minkoff HL: HIV in pregnancy: Transmission and immune effects. Clin Obstet Gynecol 32:456–466, 1989.
[b]*HIV ab* = HIV antibody; *clin dis* = clinical disease, and NA = not applicable.

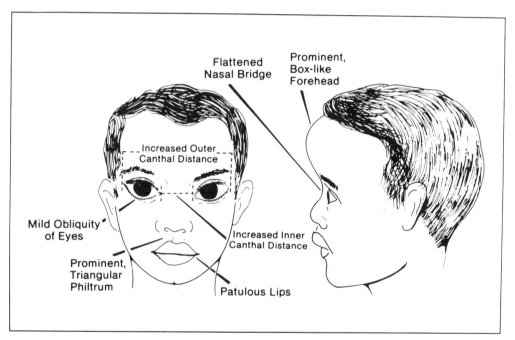

Figure 34.3. The existence of an HIV embryopathy is controversial. This is an illustration of major facial features ascribed to human T-cell lymphotrophic virus type III embryopathy. (Reprinted with permission from Marion RW, Wiznia AA, Hutcheon G, Rubinstein A: Human T cell lymphotrophic virus type III (HTLV-III) embryopathy: A new dysmorphia syndrome. Am J Dis Child 140:638–640, 1986.)

tube or DeLee trap, it is prudent to use devices connected to a wall or bulb suction. An example is shown in Figure 34.4. No data exist defining the optimum vacuum level necessary for safe and effective tracheal suction of meconium in infants. Some have arbitrarily used 100 to 130 mm Hg negative pressure; others have found that 80 mm Hg is adequate (47–49).

5. Contaminated linens and disposables, as well as blood and amniotic fluid specimens, should be handled following hospital infection control procedures.

6. It has been suggested that obstetricians avoid par-

acervical blocks and pudendal blocks for pain relief as these are procedures performed by guidance of a needle to certain landmarks by palpation. These blocks are not performed under direct visualization (45).

PREVENTION OF HIV TRANSMISSION TO HEALTH CARE WORKERS

Both HIV and the hepatitis B virus (HBV) are blood-borne pathogens. The HBV epidemiology model represents a "worst case" model in regard to transmission of HIV in health care settings. The risk of acquiring HBV infection after a needle stick from a HBV carrier ranges from 8 to 20%; the risk of HIV infection after a needle stick from an HIV-positive patient is less than 1%. Annually, 18,000 health care workers become infected with occupationally acquired HBV, and 200 to 300 healthcare workers die as a result of the HBV infection or its complications (50, 51). The apparent differences in transmissibility between HBV and HIV may be explained by the relative concentrations of each virus in the blood of carriers. HBV carriers positive for HBeAg may have 100 million to 1 billion active particles per ml of blood, whereas HIV carriers may have 10,000 virus particles per ml of blood (52).

Several factors that affect the risk for occupational transmission of HIV infection have been suggested. They include the type of exposure (percutaneous, mucosal, or cutaneous), the type of fluid involved, the concentration of HIV in the fluid, the severity of the exposure (depth, extent, and tissue involved), physical factors (temperature, pH, and humidity), and possibly the time between the withdrawal of the specimen from the source patient and the exposure (53). Most seroconversions follow deep intramuscular exposure or deep cuts. One of six (16.6%) subjects with cuts from sharp instruments became HIV seropositive after exposure to blood or blood-containing body fluids from HIV-infected patients (53).

The amount of infectious HIV has been quantitated in the blood of infected persons (Fig. 34.5) (52). HIV-infected asymptomatic patients had 1 in 50,000 peripheral blood mononuclear cells (PBMCs) harboring the virus or 20 tissue culture-infective doses (TCIDs) per 10^6 cells; plasma had 30 TCIDs per milliliter. When such a patient's condition progressed to AIDS-related complex or AIDS, the viral titer increased to approximately 1 in 400 PBMCs or 2200 to 2700 TCIDs per 10^6 cells; the plasma had 3200 to 3500 TCIDs per milliliter. The total titer of HIV in whole blood can be determined. If 1 ml of blood is assumed to contain an average of 0.65 ml of plasma and 2×10^6 PBMCs, the blood of asymptomatic HIV seropositive patients contains approximately 60 TCIDs per milliliter and that of patients with AIDS or AIDS-related complex contains about 7000 TCIDs per milliliter. This has important implications with regard to the transmission of HIV in the health care setting. During needle stick accidents in health care settings, the amount of blood involved is typically about 1 μl (54). This would represent 0.06 TCIDs if the blood were from an asymptomatic seropositive patient or 7 TCIDs if from a symptomatic patient (Fig. 34.6). However, a 250-ml unit of blood from an asymptomatic seropositive patient could contain 15,000 TCIDs or 1,750,000 TCIDs from a symptomatic patient. This is why the transfusion of HIV-infected blood results in an extremely high rate of HIV infection among recipients in comparison with a low rate of infection after a needle stick. In one study 111 of 124 (89.5%) patients became HIV positive after being transfused with HIV-contaminated blood components (55).

As of March 1988, 5.4% of adults with AIDS were classified as health care workers (51). Of these, 5% had no known risk factors other than occupational exposure. Several prospective studies are ongoing to assess the risk of nosocomial acquisition of HIV infection among health care workers in the United States. These studies indicate the risk of seroconversion following percutaneous exposure to blood from HIV-infected patients is less than 1% (53, 56–58). The level of risk associated with the exposure of nonintact skin or mucous membranes is likely to be far

Table 34.5
Prevalence of HIV Infection in Twins Born to Women Infected with HIV[a]

Delivery Method	Prevalence of HIV Infection	
	First Born (%)	Second Born (%)
Vaginal	50	19
Cesarean Section	38	19

[a]Data from Goedert JJ, Duliege AM, Amos CI, Felton S, Biggar RJ and The International Registry of HIV-Exposed Twins: Lancet 38:1471–1475, 1991.

ADAPTER (15 mm. O.D.)   MECONIUM ASPIRATOR   SUCTION LINE

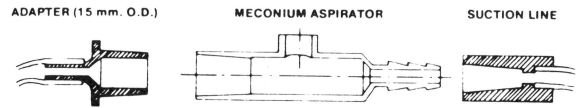

Figure 34.4. One commonly used device for meconium aspiration. The small end with the barbed fitting is connected to the suction line (suction set at 80 mm Hg or less). Following intubation of the patient, the larger end of the meconium aspirator is connected to the endotracheal tube adapter. The manufacturer recommends that suction be applied for no more than 2 sec at a time and that the suctioning be done while the endotracheal tube is being withdrawn. (Meconium Aspirator. Neotech Products, Inc. 9614-F Cozycroft Avenue, Chatsworth, CA 91311.)

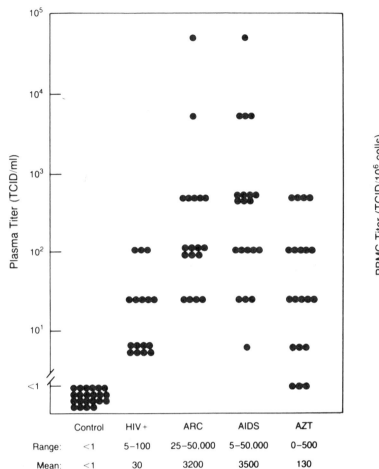

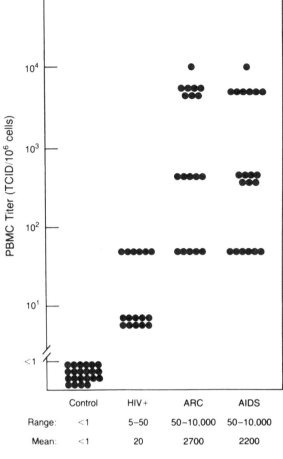

Figure 34.5. Titers of infectious HIV-1 in plasma and peripheral blood mononuclear cells (PBMC; i.e., lymphocytes and monocytes) in 22 control subjects and 54 patients in different stages of HIV-1 infection. *HIV+* = asymptomatic seropositive patients; *ARC* = patients with AIDS-related complex; *AZT* = patients receiving long-term zidovudine treatment; and *TCID* = tissue-culture infective doses. (Reprinted with permission from Ho DD, Moudgil T, Alam M: Quantitation of human immunodeficiency virus type 1 in the blood of infected persons. N Engl J Med 321:1621–1625, 1989.)

less than that associated with needle stick exposures (51). The chance of HIV infection from HIV-contaminated blood or fluids on one's skin is less than 0.5%.

NEEDLE STICK PRECAUTIONS

Strategies to prevent accidental needle stick were discussed in the section on universal precautions. Unfortunately, health care workers are often faced with two competing hazards—of recapping and not recapping the needle. It has yet to be determined whether recapping poses a greater risk than not recapping when a competing hazard is present (59). Four common reasons for recapping needles are: (*a*) to protect oneself during disassembly of a device with an exposed needle; (*b*) to protect oneself from exposed needles when several items are to be carried to a disposal box in a single trip, (*c*) to store a syringe safely between uses if its contents are to be administered in two or more doses at different times; and

(*d*) to protect others who are passed on the way to the disposal box. The optimal solution is to reduce the use of needles. At a minimum, a fixed barrier should be provided between the hands and the needle after use.

Needles used to access intravenous lines are a leading cause of needle stick injury. In a study of needle stick injury caused by various devices in a university hospital, of 326 injuries studied, disposable syringes accounted for 35%, intravenous tubing and needle assemblies for 26%, prefilled cartridge syringes for 7%, phlebotomy needles for 5%, intravenous catheter stylets for 2%, and other devices for 13% (59). However, when the data were corrected for the number of each device purchased, disposable syringes had the lowest rate of needle sticks (6.9 per 100,000 purchased) and intravenous tubing and needle assemblies had the highest (36.7 per 100,000 purchased) (Fig. 34.7).

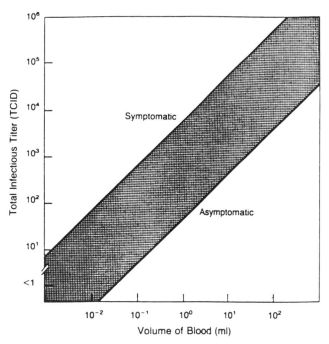

Figure 34.6. Total HIV-1 titer in relation to volume of blood from asymptomatic patients (*bottom line*) and symptomatic patients (*top line*). The two lines were derived with the use of the data shown in Figure 34.5. (Reprinted with permission from Ho DD, Moudgil T, Alam M: Quantitation of human immunodeficiency virus type 1 in the blood of infected persons. N Engl J Med 321:1621–1625, 1989.)

The needles used to access intravenous lines may place health care workers and patients at risk of contracting HIV, hepatitis, and other blood-borne diseases because these needles may become contaminated with blood while in the intravenous port. When intravenous fluid was aspirated from the injection ports of 100 consecutive recovery room patients at Parkland Memorial Hospital, blood was present in samples from 14 patients. In 8 of the 14 patients blood was not visible but was detected by guiac testing. Three of these patients had not received a blood transfusion, their intravenous line was not started before they came to the operating room, nor did they have their blood pressure cuff on the same arm (60). Administration of drugs via in-line stopcocks or one-way injection valves instead of needles is one method of decreasing the risk of puncture wounds from needles accessing intravenous ports.

Management of Exposures

If a health care worker has parenteral (e.g., needle stick or cut) exposure to blood or other body fluids, bleed the wound, and pour 70% isopropyl alcohol directly on the wound or clean with soap and water. If blood or body fluids containing blood contaminate intact skin, the area should be immediately washed with soap and water (61). In the case of mucous mem-

brane exposure (e.g., splash to the eye or mouth), the site should be copiously irrigated. ***Immediately report the incident to the facility's occupational and/or infection control health department.*** The source patient should be informed of the incident and tested for serologic evidence of infection after consent is obtained. If the source patient has a positive test result or refuses testing, the health care worker involved should be counseled regarding the risk of infection and evaluated as soon as possible to determine if they are HIV positive. The health care worker should be retested at 6 weeks, 12 weeks, and at periodic intervals thereafter (i.e., 3 months, 6 months, and 1 year) if he or she was found to be seronegative (20). Most infected persons are expected to seroconvert 6 to 12 weeks after exposure. The health care worker should report and seek medical evaluation for any acute febrile illness that occurs within 12 weeks after the exposure. An illness characterized by fever, rash, or lymphadenopathy may be indicative of recent HIV infection (20).

The efficacy of zidovudine (AZT) prophylaxis to prevent HIV infection following needle stick exposure to HIV has not been proved and its use for this purpose is controversial (62). There are documented failures of zidovudine prophylaxis (63). However, if used, zidovudine therapy should be started within 1 hr after the needle stick or penetration if it is to have much chance of effectiveness. A short course would last between 2 to 6 weeks at the advice of an infectious disease consultant.

PREVENTION OF HIV TRANSMISSION BY HEALTH CARE WORKERS

Standard sterilization and disinfection procedures for patient care equipment currently recommended for use are adequate to sterilize or disinfect items contaminated with blood or other body fluids from persons infected with HIV (Table 34.6) (20). Techniques that will kill the common viruses will also kill HIV. Techniques that produce high-level disinfection should be routinely used for processing equipment that contact mucous membranes (i.e., laryngoscope blades and breathing circuits) but do not penetrate sterile body cavities or enter the bloodstream. High-level disinfection is a procedure that kills vegetative organisms and viruses but not necessarily large numbers of bacterial spores. Items should be thoroughly cleaned before exposure to sterilization or disinfection. Activated 2% glutaraldehyde is an efficient viricidal and bactericidal cold sterilizing agent (65, 84). It is of relatively low toxicity; is not corrosive to lensed and metal instruments; has a short sterilization period; and is effective for 2 weeks, during which time it can be reused.

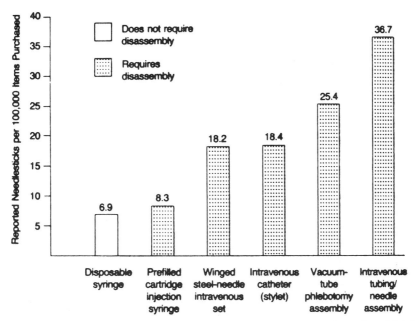

Figure 34.7. Reported needle stick injury rates per 100,000 items purchased for six devices with needles. (Reprinted with permission from Jagger J, Hunt EH, Brand-Elnaggar J, Pearson, RD: Rates of needle-stick injury caused by various devices in a university hospital. N Engl J Med 319:284–288, 1988.)

Table 34.6
Some Common Disinfectants with Their Use Dilutions and Properties[a]

Disinfectants	Use dilution (active)	Level of disinfection	Inactivates[b] Bacteria	Lipophilic viruses	Hydrophilic virus	M. tuberculosis	Mycotic agents	Bacterial spores	Shelf life > 1 wk	Important characteristics Corrosive	Residue	Inactivated by organic matter	Skin irritant	Eye irritant	Respiratory irritant	Toxic
Isopropyl alcohol	60–95%	Low	+	+	−	+	+	−	+	−	−	+	−	+	−	+
Hydrogen peroxide	3–25%	CS/high	+	+	+	+	+	+	+	+	−	−	+	+	+	+
Formaldehyde	3–8%	High	+	+	+	+	+	−	+	−	+	−	+	+	+	+
Quaternary ammonium compounds	500–2500 pm quaternary	Low	+	+	−	−	±	−	+	−	−	+	+	+	−	+
Phenolic	700–2500 ppm phenol	Low	+	+	±	±	±	−	+	+	−	+	+	+	−	+
Chlorine	100–1000 ppm free chlorine	High/low	+	+	+	+	+	−	+	+	+	+	+	+	+	+
Iodophors	30–50 ppm free iodine	Low	+	+	±	±	−	+	+	+	+	+	+	−	+
Glutaraldehyde	2%	CS/high[c]	+	+	+	+	+	+	+	−	+	−	+	+	−	+

[a] Modified from Rutala WA: In: *Prevention and Control of Nosocomial Infections*. RP Wenzel, ed, Williams & Wilkins, Baltimore, 1987, pp 257–282.
[b] Inactivates all indicated microorganisms with a contact time of 30 min or less, except bacterial spores which require 6–10 hr contact time.
[c] CS = Chemosterilizer; + = yes; − = no; ± = variable.

HIV is much easier to kill than HBV. Although 70% isopropyl alcohol (contact time 10 min) is necessary to inactivate HBV, 35% isopropyl alcohol (contact time ≤ 10 min) will inactivate HIV (84). HBV is not sensitive to 70% ethyl alcohol (65). Because HBV is an important pathogen in the operating room setting, alcohol is not an appropriate agent for general disinfection. In one study the exposure of HBV positive blood to stainless steel surfaces at 25°C and 42% relative humidity resulted in only a 15 to 20% loss of antigenic activity (64). This suggests that much of the equipment and the instruments used by anesthesiologists are potential fomites for hepatitis B.

There is no evidence for the airborne transmission of HIV. If we accept that pulmonary secretions are similar to saliva, *there is little likelihood of transmitting HIV via blood-free secretions to an anesthesia machine*. Blood-tinged secretions from a patient infected with HIV can theoretically carry viruses in low concentrations, depending on the amount of blood in the secretions. Studies of aerosols suggest that following a cough, a large number of small particles (minimum diameter of 10 μm) are released (65). A filter capable of trapping small diameter aerosolized secretions should be sufficient to protect the anesthesia circuit. Some of the available filters (i.e., Pall HME filter) have a pore size of 0.2 μm, which traps even small blood-tinged aerosolized particles. Particles larger than 1 μm are physically removed by interception with the filter. Inertial impaction results in 0.5- to 1-μm particles colliding with the filter and being captured within its pores. Smaller particles undergo Brownian motion and are also retained by the filter membrane. To prevent contamination of the anesthetic circuit, the filter should be placed between the y-connector of the circle system and the patient (66). Isolation of viruses from respiratory equipment has not been described (67).

ANESTHESIA FOR THE HIV POSITIVE PATIENT

There have been a number of articles written on anesthesia for patients who are HIV positive. Most of these articles express poorly substantiated and contradictory medical opinions (68). Some caution against spinal or epidural anesthesia (69) and others against inhalational anesthetics (70). There are no studies that have investigated the immunomodulating effects of surgery and anesthesia in patients who are HIV positive. Because individuals infected with HIV have depressed immune systems, it may be reasonable to question whether anesthesia and surgery may further impair their immunodeficiency state and enhance the risk of new infection, dissemination of HIV, activation of HIV from its latent form, poor wound

healing, or cancer dissemination in the postoperative state. There is a large literature describing adverse immunologic consequences secondary to anesthesia and surgery in patients with normal immune systems. However, the alteration in immune parameters in patients with normal preoperative immune systems are transient and are rarely correlated with adverse clinical outcomes (68).

HIV affects multiple organ systems (71). *Respiratory complications* include pulmonary infection with *Pneumocystis carinii*, aspergillosis, tuberculosis, coccidiodomycosis, cytomegalovirus, oral and pharyngeal candidiasis, and herpetic infections. *Cardiac abnormalities* may be caused by endocarditis with associated valvular lesions and even congestive heart failure, particularly in association with intravenous drug abuse. *Gastrointestinal complications* including diarrhea and proctitis (frequently caused by cytomegalovirus); vomiting and loss of appetite are common. There are a number of *hematologic abnormalities* in patients with AIDS. Leukopenia occurs in over 60% of infected patients, thrombocytopenia in 70%, and anemia in 60%.

HIV is harbored within the central nervous system. *Neurologic complications* are common in persons infected with HIV. Approximately 10% of patients with AIDS present first with neurologic symptoms and signs; the most frequent presenting neurologic syndromes are aseptic meningitis or herpes zoster radiculitis (72). Progressive dementia of unexplained origin occurs in as many as 60% of patients with AIDS (73, 74). Clinical manifestations of common central neurologic disorders are presented in Table 34.7 and of peripheral nervous system complications in Table 34.8. These neurologic diseases may appear in the absence of immunologic abnormalities as the primary or only manifestation of the infection (75). HIV appears to infect the CNS early in the course of viral infection and before the development of AIDS-associated neurologic abnormalities. There are several studies in which infectious HIV has been isolated from CSF specimens of seropositive patients with and without neurologic symptoms (76, 77).

Vacuolar myelopathy is the most common spinal cord disorder seen in HIV-infected patients (75). A subacute or chronic progression of sensory disturbances, spasticity, and hyperreflexia is the usual clinical presentation. Paraparesis or quadriparesis, loss of sphincter control, and a spinal level of sensory loss may be seen in the more advanced stages. Patients with vacuolar myelopathy maintain their ankle reflexes but frequently have a Babinski response to plantar stimulation. Acute spinal cord myelopathies are uncommon but require immediate treatment. They may be due to spinal cord metastasis from systemic

Table 34.7
Clinical Manifestations of Common Central Nervous System Disorders in HIV Disorders in HIV-Infected Patients[a]

Neurologic Disorders	Estimated Frequency[b]	Clinical Manifestations
Opportunistic infections		
Toxoplasma gondii	+ + +	Cerebral mass lesions (i.e., encephalopathy and focal neurologic deficits)
Crytopococcal meningitis	+ + +	Headache, encephalopathy, cranial neuropathy
Aseptic meningitis	+ + +	Headache, frequent recurrence
Progressive multifocal leukoencephalopathy	+	Dementia, blindness, ataxia, hemiparesis
Miscellaneous viral encephalitis (cytomegalovirus, herpes simplex)	+ +	Encephalopathy, headache, seizures, focal deficits, rarely as myelopathy
Miscellaneous nonviral infections (mycobacteria, *Treponema pallidum, Candida*)	+ +	Variable (depending on the organism, may present as mass lesions, meningitis, or encephalitis)
Miscellaneous		
AIDS dementia complex	+ + + +	Dementia
Vacuolar myelopathy	+ + +	Spasticity, paresthesias, paraparesis
Primary central nervous system lymphoma	+ +	Similar to other cerebral mass lesions
Systemic lymphoma	+ +	Spinal cord compression, cranial neuropathy, and radiculopathy
Kaposi's sarcoma	+	Cerebral mass lesions
Stroke	+	Similar to stroke in the general population

[a] Reprinted by permission from So Y: Neurologic manifestations of AIDS. AIDS Clin Care 1:37–40, 1989.
[b] + + + to + + + + = very common; + + = uncommon; + = rare.

Table 34.8
Clinical Manifestations of Common Peripheral Nervous System Complications of HIV Infection[a]

Neurologic Disorders	Estimated Frequency[b]	Clinical Manifestations
Neuropathies		
Distal symmetric polyneuropathy	+ + +	Distal bilateral paresthesias, pain, loss of reflex
Demyelinating neuropathy	+	Weakness, sensory loss, loss of reflex
Mononeuropathy multiplex	+	Asymmetric weakness and sensory loss
Lumbosacral polyradiculopathy	+	Leg weakness and sensory loss, reflex loss, loss of sphincter control
Myopathies		
Myositis (some but not all are associated with AZT)	+	Symmetric proximal weakness in upper and lower extremities

[a] Reprinted by permission from So Y: Neurologic manifestations of AIDS. AIDS Clin Care 1:37–40, 1989.
[b] + + + = very common; + + = uncommon; + = rare.

lymphoma, tuberculous spinal abscess, and cord infection by cytomegalovirus or herpes virus.

There are several distinct neuropathy syndromes in HIV-infected patients (75). The most common is a distal symmetric polyneuropathy; this affects approximately one-third of AIDS patients with systemic symptoms. The neuropathy usually appears as numbness and tingling in a stocking or glove distribution. Burning dysesthesias, especially over the soles and the distal portion of the digits, are frequent presenting complaints. Clinical signs include depressed ankle reflex and impaired sensation to vibration in the toes.

Mononeuropathy multiplex and inflammatory demyelinating neuropathy have also been recognized in HIV-infected patients. They often occur in otherwise asymptomatic seropositive persons. These neuropathies tend to produce patchy motor and sensory deficits.

Lumbosacral polyradiculopathy is uncommon but carries a grave prognosis (75). It is primarily seen in patients with a long-standing history of systemic complications. There is a rapid progression of weakness and areflexia in the lower extremities, often accompanied by patchy sensory loss and sphincter dysfunction. The most common site of pathology appears to be in the cauda equina or lumbosacral roots. Cytomegalovirus is often found in the CSF of these patients.

There is no information to suggest that subarachnoid or epidural anesthesia is contraindicated in HIV-infected patients. However, lumbar puncture in patients with demonstrable mass lesions may be hazardous; lumbar puncture should be avoided in patients with a midline shift or localized ventricular dilation on computed tomography (CT) scan (78). *Because the neurologic manifestations of AIDS change rapidly, it is important to carefully evaluate and document neurologic deficits before performing anesthesia. In addition, coagulation function should be evaluated.*

There are reports of the successful use of an epidural blood patch for therapy of postdural puncture headache in HIV-positive males (79, 80). At issue is whether the injection of HIV-positive blood into the epidural space would increase the infectiousness of HIV in the CNS or would induce the formation of a Kaposi's sarcoma in the epidural space (79). There should be an adequate trial of conservative measures including intravenous hydration and intravenous caffeine therapy before proceeding to epidural blood patch (81). Some authors question whether intravenous infusion of epidural saline would have an advantage over epidural blood patch, and if an epidural blood patch is necessary, they ask whether it be performed with fresh HIV-negative blood from an appropriate donor (81).

A case of bilateral subdural hematoma following myelography performed with a 21-gauge needle has been reported (82). The diagnosis of subdural hematoma was not made until 2 months later at a time when the patient's platelet count was 60,000; the patient had persistent headaches since the myelogram.

CONCLUSION

As the epidemiology of HIV infection evolves, there will be more women of childbearing age with HIV infection—ranging from those with unrecognized infection to those in the terminal stages of AIDS. Devices and procedures are being developed to minimize the transmission of HIV between patients and health care workers and from mother to newborn. Unfortunately, many health care workers do not follow the universal precautions recommended by the Centers for Disease Control. If followed for *all* patients, these precautions greatly reduce the risk of transmission of HIV in the health care setting. If a health care worker or patient is exposed to HIV, the appropriate infection control authority should be

contacted to obtain the most current recommendations for management.

Currently, there are no published prospective or even retrospective studies of the effects of anesthesia on the progress of HIV infection. The choice of anesthetic should be determined by the patient's needs. The presence of HIV infection does not contraindicate epidural anesthesia. Rather, the patient should be evaluated for coagulopathy and mass lesions and any neurologic deficits should be documented.

References

1. Centers for Disease Control: AIDS in women—United States. MMWR 39:845–846, 1990.
2. Ellerbrock TV, Bush TJ, Chamberland ME, Oxtoby MJ: Epidemiology of women with AIDS in the United States, 1981 through 1990: A comparison with heterosexual men with AIDS. JAMA 265:2971–2975, 1991.
3. Chu SY, Buehler JW, Berkelman RL: Impact of the human immunodeficiency virus epidemic on mortality in women of reproductive age, United States. JAMA 264:225–229, 1990.
4. Barton JJ, O'Connor TM, Cannon MJ, Weldon-Linne CM: Prevalence of human immunodeficiency virus in a general prenatal population. Am J Obstet Gynecol 160:1316–1324, 1989.
5. Shapiro CN, Schulz SL, Lee NC, Dondero TJ: Review of human immunodeficiency virus in the United States. Obstet Gynecol 74:800–808, 1989.
6. Farzadegan H, Quinn T, Polk BF: Detecting antibodies to human immunodeficiency virus in dried blood on filter papers. J Infect Dis 155:1073–1074, 1987.
7. Mok JQ, De Rossi A, Ades AE, Giaquinto C, Grosch-Worner I, Peckham CS: Infants born to mothers seropositive for human immunodeficiency virus. Lancet 1:1164–1168, 1987.
8. Donegan SP, Edelin KC, Craven DE: HIV seroprevalence rate at the Boston City Hospital (letter). N Engl J Med 319:653, 1988.
9. Luk K-J, Darrow WW, Rutherford GW: A model-based estimate of the mean incubation period for AIDS in homosexual men. Science 240:1333–1335, 1988.
10. Rothenberg R, Woelfiel M, Stomeburner R, Milberg J, Parker R, Truman B: Survival with the acquired immunodeficiency syndrome: Experience with 5833 cases in New York City. N Engl J Med 317:1297–1302, 1987.
11. Sridama V, Pacini F, Yang SL, Moawad A, Reilly M, DeGroot: Decreased levels of helper T-cells: A possible cause of immunodeficiency in pregnancy. N Engl J Med 307:352–356, 1982.
12. Peckham CS, Senturia YD, Ades AE: Obstetric and perinatal consequences of human immunodeficiency virus (HIV) infection: A review. Br J Obstet Gynaecol 94:403–407, 1987.
13. Minkoff HL: Care of pregnant women infected with human immunodeficiency virus. JAMA 258:2714–2717, 1987.
14. Koonin LM, Ellerbrock TV, Atrash HK, Rogers MF, Smith JC, Hogue CJR, Harris MA, Chavkin W, Parker AL, Halpin GJ: Pregnancy-associated deaths due to AIDS in the United States. JAMA 261:1306–1309, 1989.
15. Jensen LP, O'Sullivan MJ, Gomez-del-Rio M, Setzer ES, Gaskin C, Penso C: Acquired immunodeficiency (AIDS) in pregnancy. Am J Obstet Gynecol 148:1145–1146, 1984.
16. Minkoff H, deRagt RH, Landesman S, Schwarz R: *Pneumocystis carinii* pneumonia associated with acquired immunodeficiency syndrome in pregnancy: A report of three maternal deaths. Obstet Gynecol 67:284–287, 1986.
17. Wetli CV, Roldan EO, Fojaco RM: Listeriosis as a cause of maternal death: An obstetric complication of the acquired immunodeficiency syndrome (AIDS). Am J Obstet Gynecol 147:7–9, 1983.

18. Antoine C, Morris M, Douglas D: Maternal and fetal mortality in acquired immunodeficiency syndrome. NY State J Med 86:443–445, 1986.
19. Rotmensch S, Rosenzweig BA, Phillippe M: The impact of the acquired immunodeficiency syndrome epidemic on the philosophy of childbirth. Am J Obstet Gynecol 161:855–856, 1989.
20. Centers for Disease Control: Recommendations for prevention of HIV transmission in health-care settings. MMWR 1 (suppl):18S, 1987.
21. Ho DD, Byington RE, Schooley RT, Flynn T, Rota TR, Hirsch MS: Infrequency of isolation of HTLV-III virus from saliva in AIDS. N Engl J. Med 313:1606, 1985.
22. Centers for Disease Control: Recommendations for prevention of HIV transmission in health-care settings. MMWR 37 (suppl):377–382, 1988.
23. Boucek CD: Blood in the mouth (letter). N Engl J Med 319:1607, 1988.
24. Matta H, Thompson AM, Rainey JB: Does wearing two pairs of gloves protect operating theatre staff from skin contamination? Br Med J 297:597–598, 1988.
25. Gerberding JL, Littell C, Tarkington A, Brown A, Schecter WP: Risk of exposure of surgical personnel to patients' blood during surgery at San Francisco General Hospital. N Engl J Med 322:1766–1793, 1990.
26. Doebbeling BN, Wenzel RP: The direct costs of universal precautions in a teaching hospital. JAMA 264:2083–2087, 1990.
27. Berry AJ: Prevention of blood-borne infections in anesthesia personnel (letter). Anesthesiology 68:164, 1988.
28. Despostio F, McSherry GD, Oleske JM: Blood products acquired HIV infection in children. Pediatr Ann 17:341–345, 1988.
29. Nanada D, Minkoff HL: HIV in pregnancy: Transmission and immune effects. Clin Obstet Gynecol 3:456–466, 1989.
30. European Collaborative Study: Children born to women with HIV-1 infection: Natural history and risk of transmission. Lancet 337:253–260, 1991.
31. Scott GB, Burke BE, Letterman JG, Bloom FL, Parks WP: Acquired immune deficiency syndrome in infants. N Engl J Med 310:76–81, 1984.
32. Terrangana A, De Maria, Sapietro F: Perinatal HIV infection: Evaluation of the risk for the mother and child. In *Abstracts of the IV International Conference on Acquired Immunodeficiency Syndrome, Stockholm, 1988.* US Dept of Health and Human Services and the World Health Organization, No. 4028.
33. Ryder RW, Nsa W, Behets F: Perinatal HIV transmission in two African hospitals: one year follow up. In *Abstracts of the IV International Conference on Acquired Immunodeficiency Syndrome, Stockholm, 1988.* US Dept of Health and Human Services and the World Health Organization, No. 4128.
34. Peutherer JF, Rebus S, Aw D, Smith I, Johnstone FD: Detection of HIV in the fetus: a study of six cases. *Abstracts of the IV International Conference on Acquired Immunodeficiency Syndrome, Stockholm, 1988.* US Dept of Health and Human Services and the World Health Organization, No. 7235.
35. Gianuinto C, DeRossi A, Elia RD: Natural history of pediatric HIV infection. Fourth International Conference on Aids. In *Abstracts of the IV International Conference on Acquired Immunodeficiency Syndrome, Stockholm, 1988.* US Dept of Health and Human Services and the World Health Organization, No 7227.
36. Cirara-Vigneron N, Nguyen TL, Bercau G: Prospective study for HIV infection among high risk pregnant women. In *Abstracts of the IV International Conference on Acquired Immunodeficiency Syndrome, Stockholm, 1988.* US Dept of Health and Human Services and the World Health Organization, No. 4629.
37. Blanche S, Rouzioux C, Moscato M-L G, Veber F, Mayaux M-J, Jacomet C, Tricoire J, Deveille A, Vial M, Firtion G, de Crepy A, Douard D, Robin M, Courpotin C, Ciraru-Vigneron N, le Deist F, Griscelli C: A prospective study of infants born to women seropositive for human immunodeficiency virus type 1. N Engl J Med 320:1643–1648, 1989.
38. Ryder RW, Nsa W, Hassig SE, Behets F, Rayfield M, Ekungola B, Nelson AM, Mulenda U, Francis H, Mwandagalirwa K, Davachi F, Rogers M, Nzilambi N, Greenberg A, Mann J, Quinn TC, Piot P, Curran JW: Perinatal transmission of the human immunodeficiency virus type 1 to infants of seropositive women in Zaire. N Engl J Med 320:1637–1642, 1989.
39. Marion RW, Wiznia AA, Hutcheon G, Rubinstein A: Human T cell lymphotrophic virus type III (HTLV-III) embryopathy: A new dysmorphia syndrome associated with intrauterine HTLV-III infection. Am J Dis Child 140:638–640, 1986.
40. Qazi QH, Sheikh TM, Fikrig S: Lack of evidence for craniofacial dysmorphism in perinatal HIV infection. J Pediatr 112:7–11, 1988.
41. Papointe N, Michaud J, Pekovic D, Chausseau JP, Dupuy JM: Transplacental transmission of HTLVIII virus. N Engl J Med 312:1325–1326, 1985.
42. Cowen MJ, Hellmar G, Chudwin D, Wara DW, Chang RS, Ammann A: Maternal transmission of acquired immune deficiency syndrome. Pediatrics 73:382–386, 1984.
43. Minkoff H, Nanda D, Menez R, Fikrig S: Pregnancies resulting in infants with acquired immunodeficiency syndrome or AIDS related complex. Obstet Gynecol 69:285–287, 1987.
44. Rutherford GW, Oliva GE, Grossman M, Green JR, Wara DW, Shaw NS, Echenberg DF, Wofsy CB, Weinstein DH, Stroud F: Guidelines for the control of perinatally transmitted human immunodeficiency virus infection and care of infected mothers, infants, and children. West J Med 147:104–108, 1987.
45. Swift EL: Acquired immunodeficiency syndrome and perinatal procedures (letter). Am J Obstet Gynecol 159:785, 1988.
46. Minkoff H, Feinkind L: Management of pregnancies of HIV-infected women. Clin Obstet Gynecol 32:467–476, 1989.
47. Pretlow RA: Hand-powered apparatus for aspiration of meconium from the airway. Pediatrics 79:642–643, 1987.
48. Minkoff H: Risk of AIDS from DeLee suctioning. JAMA 260:1622, 1988.
49. Mead PB: AIDS: Risk to the health profession. Clin Obstet Gynecol 32:485–496, 1989.
50. Centers for Disease Control: Update on hepatitis B prevention. MMWR 36:353–366, 1987.
51. Centers for Disease Control: AIDS and HIV update: AIDS and HIV infection among health care workers. MMWR 37:229–234, 1988.
52. Ho DD, Moudgil T, Alam M: Quantitation of human immunodeficiency virus type 1 in the blood of infected persons. N Engl J Med 321:1621–1625, 1989.
53. Henderson DK, Fahey BJ, Willy M, Schmitt JM, Carey K, Koziol DE, Lane HC, Fedio J, Saah AJ: Risk for occupational transmission of human immunodeficiency virus type 1 (HIV-1) associated with clinical exposures: A prospective evaluation. Ann Intern Med 113:740–746, 1990.
54. Napoli VM, McGowan JE Jr: How much blood in a needlestick? J Infect Dis 155:828, 1987.
55. Donegan E, Stuart M, Niland JC, Sacks HS, Azen SP, Dietrich SL, Faucett C, Fletcher MA, Kleinman SH, Operskalsk EA, Perkins HA, Pindyck J, Schiff ER, Stites DP, Tomasulo PA, Mosley JW, Transfusion Safety Group: Infection with human immunodeficiency virus type 1 (HIV-1) among recipients of antibody-positive blood donations. Ann Intern Med 113:733–739, 1990.
56. Marcus R, CDC Cooperative Needlestick Surveillance Group: Surveillance of health care workers exposed to blood from patients infected with the human immunodeficiency virus. N Engl J Med 319:1118–1123, 1988.
57. Gerberding JL, Bryant-LeBlanc CE, Nelson K, Moss AR, Osmond D, Chambers HF, Carlson JR, Drew WL, Levy JA, Sande MA: Risk of transmitting the human immunodeficiency virus, cytomegalovirus, and hepatitis B virus to health care workers exposed to patients with AIDS and AIDS-related conditions. J Infect Dis 156:1–7, 1987.
58. Elmslie K, O'Shaughnessy JV: National surveillance program on occupational exposure to HIV among health-care workers in Canada. Can Dis Wkly Rep 13:163–166, 1987.
59. Jagger J, Hunt EH, Brand-Elnaggar J, Pearson RD: Rates of

needle-stick injury caused by various devices in a university hospital. N Engl J Med 319:284–288, 1988.

60. Hein HAT, Reinhart BS, Wansbrough SR, Jantzen PAH, Giesecke AH Jr.: Recapping needles in anesthesia: Is it safe? Anesthesiology 67:A161, 1987.

61. AAS Task Force, AIDS and Orthopaedic Surgery: Recommendations for the prevention of human immunodeficiency virus (HIV) transmission in the practice of orthopaedic surgery. Am Acad Orthop Surg p 14, 1989.

62. Henderson DK, Gerberdling JL: AIDS commentary, Prophylactic zidovudine after occupational exposure to the human immunodeficiency virus: An interim analysis. J Infect Dis 160:321–327, 1989.

63. Looke DFM, Grove DI: Failed prophylactic zidovudine after needlestick injury. Lanet 339:1280–1281, 1990.

64. Favero H, Bond WW, Peterson NJ, Berquist KR, Maynard JE: Detection methods for study of the stability of hepatitis B antigen on surfaces. J Infect Dis 129:210–212, 1974.

65. du Moulin GC, Hedley-Whyte J: Hospital-associated viral infection and the anesthesiologist. Anesthesiology 59:51–65, 1983.

66. Berry AJ, Nolte FS: An alternative strategy for infection control of anesthesia breathing circuits: A laboratory assessment of the Pall HME filter. Anesth Analg 72:651–655, 1991.

67. Hovig B: Lower respiratory tract infections associated with respiratory therapy and anaesthesia equipment: Review article. J Hosp Infect 2:301–305, 1981.

68. Scannell KA: Surgery and the human immunodeficiency virus disease. J Acquir Immune Defic Syndr 2:43–53, 1989.

69. Green ER: Spinal and epidural anesthesia in patients with the acquired immunodeficiency syndrome. Anesth Analg 65:1090–1091, 1986.

70. Thomson DA: Anesthesia and the immune system. J Burn Care Rehab 8:483–487, 1987.

71. Frost EAM: Assessment of the patient with AIDS. Curr Rev Clin Anesth 11:65–72, 1990.

72. Levy RM, Bredesen DE, Rosenblum ML: Neurological manifestations of the acquired immunodeficiency syndrome (AIDS): Experience at UCSF and review of the literature. J Neurosurg 62:475–495, 1985.

73. Navia BA, Jordan BD, Price RW: The AIDS dementia complex. I. Clinical features. Ann Neurol 19:517–524, 1986.

74. Navia BA, Cho E-S, Petito CK, Price RW: The AIDS dementia complex. II. Neuropathology. Ann Neurol 19:525–535, 1986.

75. So Y: Neurologic manifestations of AIDS. AIDS Clin Care 1:37–40, 1989.

76. Hollander H, Levy JA: Neurologic abnormalities and recovery of human immunodeficiency virus from cerebrospinal fluid. Ann Intern Med 106:692–695, 1987.

77. Resnick L, Bergr JR, Shapshak P, Tourtellotte WW: Early penetration of the blood-brain barrier by HIV. Neurology 38:9–14, 1988.

78. Harris AA, Segreti J, Levin S: Central nervous system infections in patients with the acquired immune deficiency syndrome (AIDS). Clin Neuropharmacol 8:201–210, 1985.

79. Frame WA, Lightmann MW: Blood patch in the HIV-positive patient (letter). Anesthesiology 73:1297, 1990.

80. Bevacqua BK, Slucky AV: Epidural blood patch in a patient with HIV infection. Anesthesiology 74:952–953, 1991.

81. Gibbons JJ: Post-dural puncture headache in the HIV-positive patient (letter). Anesthesiology 74:953, 1991.

82. Manji H, Birley H: Subdural haematoma—A complication of myelography in a patient with AIDS. AIDS 4:698–700, 1990.

83. Goedert JJ, Duliège AM, Amos CI, Felton S, Biggar RJ and the International Registry of HIV-exposed twins: High risk of HIV-1 infection for first-born twins. Lancet 38:1471–1475, 1991.

84. Rutala WA: Draft guideline for selection and use of disinfectants. Am J Infect Control 17:24A–38A, 1989.

CHAPTER 35

Anesthesia and the Drug-Addicted Mother

Jan D. Vertommen, M.D.
Gershon Levinson, M.D.
Sol M. Shnider, M.D.

Anesthesiologists are confronted with the problems of maternal drug addiction when drug-addicted patients request analgesia for labor, require anesthesia for elective or emergency cesarean section, and when a drug-affected neonate requires resuscitation or suffers from withdrawal symptoms. Thus it is important for the anesthesiologist to be familiar with the consequences of the drugs most commonly abused by pregnant women. This chapter reviews the effects of the most popular illicit drugs in pregnant women and the repercussions on the fetus and/or neonate. In addition, the effects of other nonillicit substances, including alcohol, tobacco, and caffeine, will be discussed. Finally, some guidelines for the management of anesthesia in drug-addicted mothers are provided.

CURRENT CRISIS

The National Institute on Drug Abuse estimates that of 56 million American women in the childbearing age, 15% (or about 8 million) are currently substance abusers (1). The number of women who continue to abuse drugs once they become pregnant is unknown. However, the National Association for Perinatal Addiction Research and Education estimates that as many as 375,000 infants may be affected each year by their mothers' drug abuse during pregnancy. It is also estimated that 5% of the women of childbearing age can be considered "heavy" drinkers. Many women take multiple drugs and the combination of alcohol, cocaine, and marijuana is very popular (2). The simultaneous abuse of several substances makes it difficult to determine the effects of a particular drug. In addition, malnutrition, inadequate medical care, and infectious diseases can also be partially responsible for some of the adverse effects observed in drug addicts. Delayed diagnosis of pregnancy in drug-addicted women results in continued drug exposure in the fetus during the most

vulnerable stage (3). Most drugs that are abused readily cross the placenta. Often they are not only directly fetotoxic but have also indirect effects on the fetus. They disrupt normal maternal nutrition and may have maternal cardiovascular effects that interfere with normal placental blood supply. After birth, the neonate may still be under the influence of the drug and may develop withdrawal symptoms. Although congenital anatomic malformations are the most prominent features of many of these drugs used in pregnancy, behavioral teratology might even be more important (4). These effects are less obvious and can often escape detection. Drug and alcohol dependency in pregnancy is likely one of the most frequently missed diagnoses in obstetrics.

ALCOHOL

It is estimated that there are are 15.1 million alcohol-abusing individuals in the United States, and approximately 4.6 million are women (5). At least 1 million of these women are of childbearing age. Alcohol is usually involved in most cases of drug abuse (6). The best known abnormality associated with the abuse of alcohol during pregnancy is the "fetal alcohol syndrome" (FAS) (7). This syndrome includes a characteristic facies, growth retardation, microcephaly, and mental retardation. (Fig. 35.1) (Table 35.1). FAS occurs in about one-third of the infants born to mothers who drink 150 g or more of alcohol per day during pregnancy. However, a safe level of maternal alcohol consumption during pregnancy has never been defined (6). Children with complete FAS are usually born only to those women who consume large amounts of alcohol during pregnancy, but studies have reported neurobehavioral deficits, intrauterine growth retardation, and head and facial abnormalities in infants of moderate alcohol consumers (7–10). Most likely, heavy alcohol consumption throughout preg-

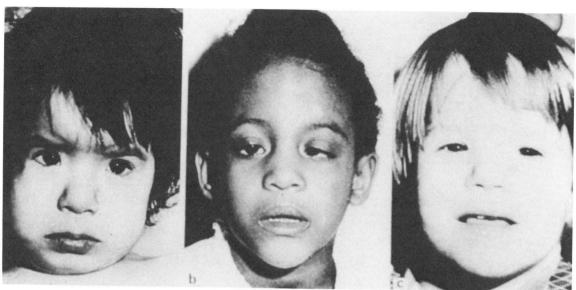

Figure 35.1. Fetal alcohol effects. Affected children of chronic alcoholic women at 1 year, 3 years and 9 months, and 2½ years. Note the short palpebral fissures for all children and strabismus and ptosis of the eyelid. (Reprinted by permission from James KL: *Smith's Recognizable Patterns of Human Malformation*, 4th ed. WB Saunders, Philadelphia, 1988, p 492.)

nancy produces the wide variety of effects characteristic of FAS, whereas episodic drinking produces partial expression of the syndrome according to the period of exposure.

When there is a history of alcohol abuse and not all the characteristics of FAS are present, the term "fetal alcohol effects" (FAE) is used. Mental retardation in later life has been one of the most common problems of alcohol exposure in utero and can be present in one-third of the infants without the more obvious signs of FAS. Ethanol appears to be responsible for FAS and FAE (11). Multiple mechanisms have been proposed for the fetal effects of maternal alcohol ingestion. First, ethanol can disrupt normal maternal nutrition by impairing intestinal absorption of nutrients and by disturbing liver function. Second, ethanol crosses the placenta and the primary metabolite of ethanol, acetaldehyde, is believed to have direct toxicity on the fetus. Third, ethanol (and/or acetaldehyde) may also be toxic to the placenta. Ethanol is teratogenic in a variety of animals, and the same anomalies are found in humans (12). Acute alcohol intoxication can also have distressing effects on the fetus and causes fetal tachycardia, decreased fetal heart rate variability, and late and variable decelerations (13). Studies in the rhesus monkey have shown that maternal ethanol levels of 200 to 300 mg/dL reduces umbilical blood flow and fetal oxygenation (Fig. 35.2) (14).

Anesthetic Considerations

Many problems face the anesthesiologist when taking care of an alcoholic because nearly all systems

in the body are affected (15). The main problems include hemodynamic instability and increased resistance to neuroleptics and analgesics (16). Cardiovascular disease is the leading case of death in alcoholics and cardiomyopathy should be considered in all cases of heavy alcohol abuse (17). The induction of general anesthesia should be a "rapid-sequence" induction, and is routine for every pregnant woman.

There is cross-tolerance with barbiturates and minor tranquilizers and with the usual anesthesic doses of inhalational agents; therefore induction doses of thiopental should be increased to a maximum of 6 mg/kg. However, during *acute* intoxication, ethanol and barbiturates produce a supraadditive effect. Even in *chronic* alcoholics, acute intoxication causes an increase in the half-life of barbiturates, and under this circumstance induction doses should be decreased.

Pregnant women pose a greater risk for acid aspiration syndrome than nonpregnant patients. When acutely intoxicated with alcohol, this risk is increased because alcohol is a potent stimulus to gastric acid secretion. In addition, there is a significant delay in gastric emptying caused by strong alcoholic beverages. Preoxygenation for 5 min should definitely not be omitted because cerebral tolerance to hypoxia is decreased significantly in the presence of only mild intoxication. Although most alcoholics require a larger induction dose of thiopental, due to tolerance and to an expanded plasma volume, routinely doubling the induction dose for alcoholics may be dangerous for those with hypoalbuminemia and

Table 35.1
Principal Features of Fetal Alcohol Syndrome Observed in 245 Affected Patients[a]

Feature	Manifestation (Expressed as Percentage of 245 Affected Patients)		
	>50%	26–50%	<25%
Facial characteristics			
Eyes	Short palpebral fissures	Ptosis; strabismus	Myopia; clinical microphthalmia, blepharophimosis
Nose	Short, upturned; hypoplastic philtrum		
Maxilla	Hypoplastic		
Mouth	Thinned upper vermilion; retrognathia in infancy; micrognathia or relative prognathia in adolescence	Prominent lateral palatine ridges	Cleft lip or cleft palate; small teeth with faulty enamel
Ears		Posterior rotation	Poorly formed concha
Central nervous system dysfunction			
Behavioral	Irritability in infancy; hyperactivity in childhood		
Intellectual	Mild to moderate mental retardation; microcephaly; poor coordination, hyptonia		
Neurologic			
Growth Deficiency:			
Prenatal	<2 SD for length and weight		
Postnatal	<2 SD for length and weight; disproportionately diminished adipose tissue		
Cardiac		Murmurs, especially in early childhood, usually atrial septal defect	Ventricular septal defect; great-vessel anomalies; tetralogy of Fallot
Renogenital		Labial hypoplasia	Hypospadias; small rotated kidneys; hydronephrosis
Cutaneous		Hemangiomas	Hirsutism in infancy
Skeletal		Aberrant palmar creases; pectus excavatum	Limited joint movements, especially fingers and elbows; nail hypoplasia, especially 5th finger, polydactyly; radioulnar synostosis; pectus carinatum; bifid xiphold; Klippel-Feil anomaly, scoliosis
Muscular			Hernias of diaphragm, umbilicus, or groin; diastasis recti

[a]Modified from Clarren SK, Smith DW: The fetal alcohol syndrome. N Engl J Med 298:1063–1067, 1978.

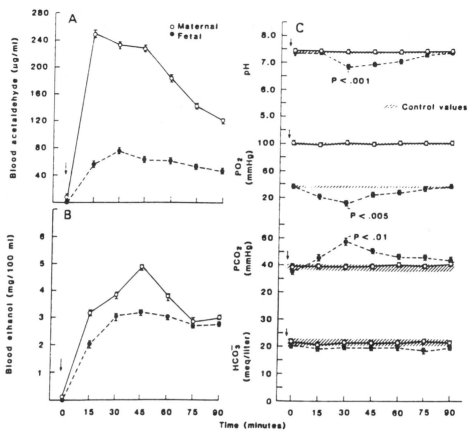

Figure 35.2.   Ethanol (*A*) and acetaldehyde (*B*) in maternal (O) and fetal (●) blood. Results are means ± standard deviation of the mean (*n* = 5). *C*, Maternal and fetal blood gas values. Results are means ± standard deviation of the mean (*n* = 5) and of the control groups (*n* = 4). The *shaded areas* represent normal control values. (Reprinted by permission from Mukherjee AB, Hodgen GD: Maternal ethanol exposure induces transient impairment of umbilical circulation and fetal hypoxia in monkeys. Science 218:700–702, 1982.)

cardiomyopathy (18). Similar findings of increased tolerance in the *chronic* alcoholic and the additive effect during *acute* intoxication have been described for propofol (19). Particular attention should be directed at the state of hydration and prevention of hypoglycemia. Maintenance of anesthesia is rarely a problem as long as one remembers that anesthetic requirements are usually increased unless acute intoxication is present. However, the postoperative period may be stormy due to alcohol withdrawal.

When the patient is not intoxicated, as for elective procedures, a withdrawal syndrome may occur. A minor withdrawal syndrome occurs in the majority of alcoholics within 6 to 8 hr of abstinence, and this is often the moment that elective interventions are started (20). This minor withdrawal syndrome is characterized by tremor, sweating, anorexia, vomiting, muscle weakness, and cramps. Autonomic imbalance also produces tachycardia, systolic hypertension, and dysrhythmias. Propranolol may control some of these symptoms, but pure β-blocking agents

may adversely affect the neonate's ability to adapt to the stress of delivery. Sedation is usually unnecessary, but small doses of diazepam (2.5 to 5 mg IV) may reduce autonomic hyperactivity without resulting in neonatal depression. Maintenance of anesthesia usually involves the administration of greater than normal amounts of anesthetic agents. Continued alcohol ingestion up until the time of surgery and intravenous alcohol in the immediate postoperative period have been recommended in nonpregnant patients.

Pulmonary and liver disease are frequent among alcoholics. As many as 66% may have abnormal chest x-ray findings (17). Succinylcholine activity may be prolonged by liver disease due to diminished cholinesterase activity. The action of nondepolarizing neuromuscular blocking agents may also be prolonged because of abnormal potassium or magnesium levels or, in fact, may be shortened in liver disease or malnutrition due to altered protein binding. Esophageal varices may make the insertion of nasogastric tubes, esophageal stethoscopes, and temperature probes hazardous, and extreme care must be exercised.

Regional anesthesia may be suitable in alcoholics but additional sedation may be required in the agitated alcoholic. Liver disease may produce coagulation defects, which may exclude the use of epidural and intrathecal techniques. Alcoholic neuropathy is not aggravated by or a medical contraindication to regional anesthesia, but it is medicolegally prudent to document preoperatively any signs or symptoms of peripheral neuropathy. Severe hypotension may result from dehydration, cardiomyopathy, or autonomic neuropathy.

MARIJUANA

Among illicit drugs, most experimentation occurs with marijuana (1). In 1985 approximately 31% of American women in their late teens and early 20s reported that they had used marijuana within the past year (21). Marijuana is most commonly used during the first trimester, probably because it reduces the incidence of nausea and vomiting. The main ingredient of marijuana, δ-9 tetrahydrocannabinol, rapidly crosses the placenta and accumulation of the drug in fat tissue makes elimination very slow, resulting in a long exposure (up to 30 days) in the fetus (22). Marijuana is harmful to the fetus in many ways. Marijuana is smoked and, as with cigarette smoking, it elevates the carbon monoxide levels in the blood resulting in less oxygen available for the fetus. Marijuana also increases the heart rate and blood pressure of the mother and reduces placental blood flow by increasing uterine vascular resistance, resulting in reduced fetal growth. In addition, marijuana use is associated with a significant reduction in the length of gestation and precipitate labor is significantly more frequent among women who reported using marijuana "at least once a month" (23). Interference with the production of progesterone and estrogen by marijuana may be partly responsible for some of the adverse effects (4).

There is an increased incidence of meconium in the amniotic fluid and resuscitation of the neonate is necessary more frequently when the mother has used marijuana close to the delivery. The babies exhibit signs of central nervous system excitation. Exposure to marijuana interrupts the fetus's sleep and may continue to interfere with the sleep pattern after birth (2). The reports on teratogenicity of cannabis extract and of δ-D-tetrahydrocannabinol are conflicting. Adminstration of cannabis to animals has proven to be toxic for mother and fetus. In humans, intrauterine growth retardation (21) has been found as

well as various neurological and morphological abnormalities (24, 25).

Anesthetic Considerations

Similar to cocaine and amphetamines discussed below, marijuana often results in tachycardia which may be treated with small doses of β-blockers (26). It is important to know that intraoperative tachycardia can be due to the marijuana and is not necessarily a sign of insufficient analgesia. The cardiovascular effects of marijuana may be potentiated by both epinephrine and atropine. However, the anticholinergic effect of marijuana results in decreased salivation and avoids the need for atropine. Addition of epinephrine to local anesthetic agents can potentiate marijuana-induced tachycardia (26). Marijuana increases the peripheral blood flow, from possible β-adrenergic stimulation, which may result in either hypo- or hypertension. Nevertheless, marijuana is a direct cardiac depressant and multiple ECG abnormalities have been noted. The duration of action of both ketamine and thiopental is prolonged, and during anesthesia there is an additive effect with volatile agents, which may result in severe cardiac depression (27, 28). Recent administration of marijuana may have additive effects with concomitantly administered sedatives (29). Marijuana also depresses the temperature-regulating mechanism. In addition, marijuana inhibits cholinesterase activity and may prolong the action of succinylcholine (30). Caution is recommended with the use of neostigmine. Postoperative hallucinations and disorientation can theoretically be treated with physostigmine, but is not recommended because this can result in severe depression. The depression, however, can be controlled with atropine.

NARCOTICS

Narcotic drug exposure during pregnancy produces intrauterine growth retardation, which in part might be explained by poor maternal nutrition (4). However, maternal undernutrition is not the only factor responsible for the growth retardation and narcotics also have a direct effect (3). In addition narcotic withdrawal in the last trimester of pregnancy can result in meconium staining, perinatal asphyxia, and neonatal death. The neonates of women addicted to narcotic drugs exhibit more respiratory distress, and there are reports of an increased incidence of sudden infant death syndrome among these infants. Due to the use of contaminated needles, women abusing heroin are particularly vulnerable to infectious complications, which may also affect the fetus (32). In one study almost 60% of heroin-exposed infants had features of antenatal infection or the mothers had evidence of an acute infection at the time of delivery (31). The currently most feared infection is AIDS, which is discussed in the previous chapter. Infants born to mothers on methadone maintenance weigh more at birth than the infants of mothers using heroin. For this reason heroin addicts are often switched to methadone. However, methadone also affects the unborn child (33) and will produce a more severe withdrawal syndrome in the newborn infant than does heroin (34).

Anesthetic Considerations

Cesarean section is required more often in drug-dependent women. The main reason is fetal distress. Intravenous induction using the usual rapid-sequence induction technique is usually smooth in narcotic addicts, although some authors have reported increased hypotension (29). Provided that their normal narcotic requirements are met, cross-tolerance is not a major problem during the maintenance phase of anesthesia.

Methadone may have an influence on the reactivity of the nonstress test and lead to unnecessary interventions (35). Fetal distress can originate from withdrawal, resulting in sympathetic hyperactivity and leading to fetal hypoxia (31). The symptoms of opiate withdrawal appear 8 to 12 hr after the last dose. Often meconium accumulation in the placenta has been found in heroin-addicted women and thought to be caused by withdrawal. To avoid withdrawal, it is important for an opiate addict to receive her regular daily dose (36). This dose must be considered as a physiologic requirement and should not be omitted if regional techniques are employed. However, the administration of narcotic agonist-antagonists, such as butorphanol, to patients addicted to narcotics should be avoided because they may result in withdrawal (37). There is a higher incidence of infectious disease in heroin-abusing patients, including endocarditis and infectious arthritis, which may exclude the use of regional techniques (38). Because opiate addicts and women under methadone maintenance have a 25% incidence of chronic anemia, replacement of blood loss must be considered (29). Establishing intravenous access can create major difficulties in the narcotic addict, and often a central venous line is the only possibility.

Another potential problem facing the anesthesiologist is a situation in which an addict takes an extra dose of narcotics before coming to the hospital because she was anxious or was attempting to provide her own analgesia. This may result in depression of the neonate's respiration. Naloxone, which is usually the drug of choice when respiration is depressed from narcotic abuse (39), should not be used in the pregnant woman or in the depressed newborn of a narcotic-addicted woman. Ventilation is the therapy of choice because naloxone can result in acute withdrawal symptoms in the newborn. Postoperative analgesia may be a problem. Intermittent injections of narcotics are likely to result in insufficient pain relief, and continuous infusions are preferred because they produce a more constant blood level of narcotic. However, there is always a possibility of abuse by the patient. The use of spinal and epidural opiates has not been sufficiently studied in this group of patients, but anecdotal experience would indicate it is safe and effective at the usual doses.

COCAINE

An estimated 10 million Americans have used cocaine at least once and 5 million use it on a regular basis (40, 41). Cocaine blocks the presynaptic reuptake of norepinephrine (42), which may result in severe hypertension. Case reports have linked rupture of intracranial aneurysms to cocaine abuse (43). Studies in animals have shown a decrease in uterine and placental perfusion and an increase in uterine contractility after cocaine (Fig. 35.3) (44–46). The spontaneous abortion rate is increased in cocaine-abusing women. Women who used cocaine in the third trimester reported feeling contractions and increased fetal activity within minutes of cocaine use (4). There is an increased incidence of spontaneous abortion among cocaine-using women (47), and the incidence of abruptio placentae is also increased, probably due to the hypertension and placental vasoconstriction caused by cocaine. In one report, four women experienced the onset of labor with abruptio placentae immediately after self-injection of cocaine (47). Maternal cocaine use may also cause fetal tachycardia and hypertension. Meconium staining of the amniotic fluid occurs more frequently, indicating fetal distress (48). Neonates born to cocaine-abusing mothers show transient signs of central nervous system irritability (49). Some infants have abnormal electroencephalograms during the first week of life. While signs of withdrawal after prenatal cocaine exposure are usually mild, they occur in a significant number of infants (48). Cerebral infarction has been reported in the infants of mothers who used cocaine just before labor and delivery (50). It is believed that cocaine produces intrauterine retardation and, in particular, a reduction in brain growth (49, 51). However, growth retardation has not been found in all studies (47). Cocaine-associated teratogenicity has also been reported (52, 53), and characteristic facies are shown in Figures 35.4 and 35.5.

Figure 35.3. Percentage of change in maternal mean arterial pressure (*MMAP*) and uterine blood flow (*UBF*) during cocaine administration to pregnant ewes ($n = 10$). Values are expressed as $\pm SD$. Changes are compared to baseline values with significance noted (* = $P < .05$). (Reprinted by permission from Vertommen JD, Hughes SC, Rosen MA, Shnider SM, Espinoza MI, Messer CP, Johnson JL, Parer JT: Hydralazine does not restore uterine blood flow during cocaine-induced hypertension in the pregnant ewe. Anesthesiology 76:580–587, 1992).

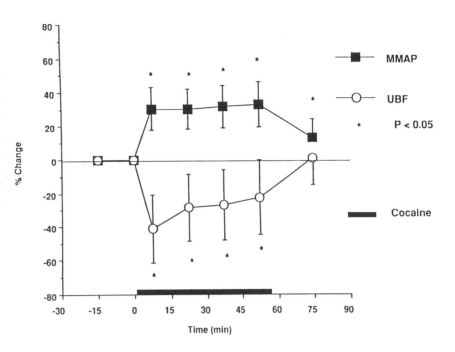

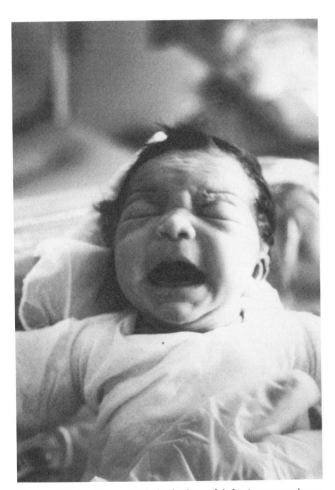

Figure 35.4. Characteristic facies of infant exposed prenatally to cocaine only. Note marked periorbital and eyelid edema, "double eyebrow" crease, short nose, lateral soft tissue nasal buildup, and neurologic irritability.

AMPHETAMINES

Traditionally, methamphetamine has been ingested as pills, "snorted," or injected intravenously. However, a new increasingly toxic preparation called "ice" can be smoked like marijuana or "crack." Amphetamines are particularly popular among women because, as an appetite suppressant, weight is lost quickly. Many women continue taking the drug while unknowingly pregnant. Amphetamines enhance the presynaptic release of norepinephrine, and in this respect have pharmacologic effects nearly identical to those of cocaine. In the 1950s obstetricians prescribed low oral doses of amphetamines to reduce weight gain in pregnancy. No structural abnormalities were found in those children. However, in a study from Sweden, there was an increase in the incidence of preterm labor, placental abruption, fetal distress, and postpartum hemorrhage (54). Thus both cocaine and amphetamine abuse seem to result in an increase in the incidence of placental abruption, intrauterine growth retardation, and preterm delivery with fetal distress (55). As with cocaine, infants born to mothers who abused amphetamines during pregnancy have a variety of symptoms including abnormal sleep patterns, tremors, hypertonia, high-pitched cry, poor or frantic sucking, vomiting, sneezing, and tachypnea (56). Many infants who were studied by ultrasonographic examination of the brain and who were otherwise entirely well had evidence of brain lesions. Amphetamine-exposed infants exhibit lethargy, poor feeding, poor alertness, and severe lassitude and most of the children have minor neurologic abnormalities. The data concerning congenital anatomical anom-

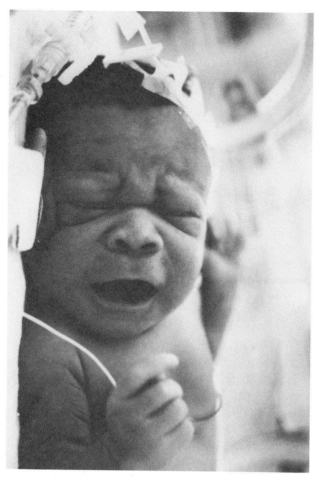

Figure 35.5. Facies of infant exposed prenatally to cocaine and alcohol. Note severe periorbital and eyelid edema "double eyebrow" crease, transverse nasal crease, lateral soft tissue nasal buildup, short nose, hirsuitism, and irritability. Features consistent with fetal alcohol exposure (long smooth philtrum, thin upper lip, bitemporal narrowing) are also recognizable.

alies are conflicting. Some studies report a significantly increased frequency of congenital anomalies (52), such as congenital heart disease (57). Other studies demonstrated no such increase (58).

Anesthetic Considerations

Both cocaine and amphetamine abuse results in the same problems of catecholamine excess during acute intoxication and catecholamine depletion in the chronic addict. The anesthesiologist can help minimize additional increases in uterine vascular resistance caused by an excess of catecholamines by reducing pain and anxiety during labor (59). Pain and anxiety during labor are associated with adrenergic stimulation leading to constriction of the uterine blood vessels. This additional constriction of the uterine blood vessels when the uterine blood flow is already compromised may be a critical factor resulting in

fetal distress and perinatal morbidity. Continuous epidural anesthesia is the most effective method of pain relief for labor and delivery. The use of epidural anesthesia may also avoid the need for narcotics and discourage the woman from providing her own analgesia.

Drug-addicted mothers often arrive at the hospital because labor has been induced by drugs, including cocaine and amphetamines. Severe hypertension and/or abruptio placentae may be present in these patients and require immediate intervention. The precise drugs of choice to treat the hypertension are as yet undefined. Hydralazine has been the standard drug of choice to treat hypertension in the pregnant patient but can lead to tachycardia, and this may be unacceptable in a patient who is already tachycardic from the abused drug (60). Other choices of treatment to consider include labetalol (61, 62) or esmolol (63). However, β-blocking agents are usually avoided in the pregnant patient. In addition, propranolol has been reported to result in severe hypertension when used during cocaine intoxication (64). Calcium channel-blocking agents (65) and neuroleptics (66) have also been advocated in cocaine intoxication. Short-term administration of nitroprusside may lower dangerously high blood pressures.

The anesthesiologist must be prepared to manage these maternal and fetal emergencies, often with immediate general anesthesia for cesarean section. Dramatic events, including cardiac arrest (67) and pulmonary edema (68), have been attributed to amphetamine abuse. The use of epidural anesthesia is not contraindicated for elective cesarean section in cocaine-abusing women, although the cocaine users seem to need more narcotic supplementation than nonabusing women. Extending an existing epidural block for labor analgesia to a T4 level is probably safe. However, in the presence of severe acute fetal distress, general anesthesia can be induced quickly.

In the presence of placental abruption with considerable blood loss, regional anesthesia is also relatively contraindicated. In the presence of hypotension, general anesthesia is preferably induced with ketamine or etomidate, and the anesthesiologist must be prepared to restore the circulating blood volume with infusions of blood, albumin, and/or balanced salt solution via large-bore intravenous cannulae. However, ketamine and halothane should be used very carefully. Ketamine may aggravate cocaine-induced hypertension. Halothane sensitizes the myocardium to the effects of catecholamines. Cocaine and amphetamines cause sympathetic hyperstimulation, and there is high risk of both cardiovascular and central nervous system effects, including cardiovascular collapse and convulsions.

A potentiation of the analgesic effect of opiates by cocaine has been reported. Chronic abusers may develop a depletion of catecholamines, whch may decrease their anesthetic needs. Chronic abuse results in catecholamine depletion, and this is the probable cause of the observed reduction in anesthetic requirements in chronic addicts and may be responsible for hypotension, which should be treated with directly acting vasopressors such as small doses of phenylephrine (20 to 40 µg). Halothane can safely be used in these patients, but a lower dose is recommended. In addition, because of catecholamine depletion, the recovery phase in these patients may be prolonged. Cocaine can also slightly prolong the action of succinylcholine and local ester-type anesthetics, but this is rarely clinically significant.

TOBACCO

There is currently no doubt concerning the adverse effects of tobacco on health. Nearly 2000 compounds have been identified in cigarette smoke and, in addition to nicotine, carbon monoxide and cyanide have been implicated in observed fetal effects (69). Nicotine causes an increase in maternal heart rate, systolic and diastolic blood pressure, and peripheral vasoconstriction (70). Infants born to mothers who smoke during pregnancy tend to be lighter in weight than infants born to nonsmokers. This can be explained by the vasoconstrictive effects of nicotine and the reduction of uteroplacental blood flow. Evidence exists that abruptio placentae and placenta previa are more common among women who smoke during pregnancy than among nonsmokers. The incidence of prematurity may double from 6 to 12% when the mother smokes at least 20 cigarettes per day. At birth these infants often have a higher hematocrit because the carbon monoxide is fixed to the hemoglobin of the fetus and the relative hypoxemia causes an increase in the erythropoiesis. Very often a syndrome with hyperexcitability, crying, and feeding difficulties has been observed without the need of treatment with sedatives. Also sleep disturbances and learning difficulties have been reported. Some studies suggest that the deleterious effects of nicotine on brain development extend for a period sufficient to cause long-lasting alterations that are eventually expressed as neurobehavioral teratogenic effects (71). Cigarette smoking causes a reduction in fetal breathing movements. Sudden infant death syndrome occurs twice as frequently in infants of mothers who smoke than of those who do not. The known effects of nicotine on fetal breathing may extend into the neonatal period. Perinatal mortality is also higher among infants born to smokers. A Swedish study has noted an increase of 50% in the risk of cancer in the infants of mothers who smoked at least 10 cigarettes per day (72).

Anesthetic Considerations

The longer a patient stops smoking before anesthesia, the better. A period of 48 hr should be sufficient for carboxyhemoglobin of all smokers to fall to a nonsmoker's level and to produce a rise in oxygen content and availability. This has been demonstrated in pregnant women, in whom smoking abstinence for 48 hr produced an 8% increase in available oxygen (73). Intraoperative and postoperative respiratory morbidity in smokers is increased by mucus hypersecretion, impairment of tracheobronchial clearance, and small airway narrowing. Acute bronchoconstriction is often treated with halogenated hydrocarbons or with β-mimetics such as terbutaline. Fewer cardiovascular problems are to be expected after 12 to 24 hr abstinence from carbon monoxide and nicotine elimination. Several days are required to improve ciliary function and 1 to 2 weeks to reduce the sputum volume. However, 4 to 6 weeks of abstinence are necessary to greatly decrease postoperative respiratory morbidity (74). Smoking has also been suggested to be responsible for increased gastric juice volume, placing smokers at higher risk for pulmonary aspiration (75).

CAFFEINE

The adverse effects of caffeine during pregnancy is a very controversial issue (76). Caffeine is a known teratogen in animals (77), and although it has been loosely linked to birth defects in humans, other researchers did not find this association (78). Caffeine may act directly on nucleic acids, since it is structurally similar to adenine and guanine, and in animals it results in chromosome aberrations. Major sources of caffeine are coffee, tea, chocolate/cocoa, and cola drinks; the largest source for most people is coffee (79). Several studies indicate an association of caffeine with spontaneous abortion, stillbirth, preterm delivery, and low birth weight (79, 81). Three cases of fetal arrhythmia resulting from excessive intake of caffeine by the mother during pregnancy have been reported (82). In two cases the arrhythmia resolved gradually over 3 days after birth without medical intervention. Caffeine may also act by an increase of catecholamines, which may reduce uteroplacental circulation through vasoconstriction and result in fetal hypoxia (80). There are reports of an association of caffeine with an increased risk of late first- and second-trimester spontaneous abortion. Some component of coffee other than caffeine may be responsible for some of the adverse effects.

Anesthetic Considerations

The main problem encountered in a patient with substantial coffee use is caffeine withdrawal in the postoperative period. The most consistent feature of caffeine withdrawal is headache (83), which is also an important side-effect of general anesthesia and spinal anesthesia or may occur after an inadvertent dural puncture during epidural anesthesia. Before performing a blood patch to relieve the symptoms of a "dural tap," it might be worthwhile to question the patient about her usual coffee intake.

CONCLUSIONS

Many other drugs can be added to this list of commonly abused drugs. None of them is harmless to mother or fetus, but most damage has already evolved before the anesthesiologist sees the patient. By knowing the most important pharmacologic actions of these drugs and by being prepared, the anesthesiologist may avoid some catastrophes during the last hours of pregnancy. Unfortunately, the current crisis of maternal drug addition is still intensifying, and more and more anesthesiologists will be confronted with the tragedy of the addicted mother, fetus, and neonate.

References

1. Silverman S: Scope, specifics of maternal drug use and effects on fetus are beginning to emerge from studies. JAMA 261:1688–1689, 1989.
2. Silverman S: Interaction of drug-abusing mother, fetus, types of drugs examined in numerous studies. JAMA 261:1689–1693, 1989.
3. Silverman S: Combinations of drugs taken by pregnant women add to problems in determining fetal damage. JAMA 261:1694, 1989.
4. Smith CG, Asch RH: Drug abuse and reproduction. Fertil Steril 48:355–373, 1987.
5. Williams GD, Grant BF, Harford TC, Noble BA: Population projections using DSM-III criteria: Alcohol abuse and dependence, 1990–2000. Alcohol Health Res World 13:366–370, 1989.
6. Becker CE: Alcohol and drug use: Is there a "safe" amount? West J Med 141:884–890, 1984.
7. Little RE, Asker RL, Sampson PD, Renwick JH: Fetal growth and moderate drinking in early pregnancy. Am J Epidemiol 123:270–278, 1986.
8. Coles CD, Smith IE, Lancaster JS, Falek A: Persistence over the first month of neurobehavioral differences in infants exposed to alcohol prenatally. Infant Behav Dev 10:23–37, 1987.
9. Russell M: Clinical implications of recent research on the fetal alcohol syndrome. Bull NY Acad Med 67:207–222, 1991.
10. Emhart CB, Sokol RJ, Martier S, Moron P, Nadler D, Ager JW, Wolf A: Alcohol teratogenicity in the human: A detailed assessment of specificity, critical period and threshold. Am J Obstet Gynecol 156:33–39, 1987.
11. Fisher SE, Karl PI: Maternal ethanol use and selective fetal malnutrition. Rec Dev Alcohol 6:277–289, 1988.
12. Clarren SK, Smith DW: The fetal alcohol syndrome. N Engl J Med 298:1063–1067, 1978.
13. Silva PD, Miller KD, Madden J, Keegan KA: Abnormal fetal heart rate pattern associated with severe intrapartum ethanol intoxication. J Reprod Med 32:144–146, 1987.
14. Mukherjee AB, Hodgen GD: Maternal ethanol exposure induces transient impairment of umbilical circulation and fetal hypoxia in monkeys. Science 218:700–702, 1982.
15. O'Daniel L: Anesthetic management of the alcoholic patient. AANA 48:445–451, 1980.
16. St. Haxholdt O, Krintel JJ, Johannson G: Pre-operative alcohol infusion. Anaesthesia 39:240–245, 1984.
17. Edwards R, Mosher VB: Alcohol abuse, anaesthesia and intensive care. Anaesthesia 35:474:489, 1980.
18. Bruce DL: Alcoholism and anesthesia. Anesth Analg 62:84–96, 1983.
19. du Cailar J, d'Athis F, Eledjam JJ, Bonnet MC: Propofol et éthylisme. Ann Fr Anesth Réanim 6:332–333, 1987.
20. Edwards R: Anaesthesia and alcohol. Br Med J 291:423–424, 1985.
21. Department of Health and Human Services: National household survey on drug abuse: Population estimates, 1985, (10 DHHS) Pub No 871539. Rockville, MD, Department of Health and Human Services, 1987.
22. Zuckerman B, Frank DA, Hingson R, Amaro H, Levenson SM, Kayne H, Parker S, Vinci R, Aboagye K, Fried LE, Cabral H, Timperi R, Bauchner H: Effects of maternal marijuana and cocaine use on fetal growth. N Engl J Med 320:762–768, 1989.
23. Greenland S, Staisch KJ, Brown N, Gross SJ: The effects of marijuana use during pregnancy. Am J Obstet Gynecol 143:408, 1982.
24. Qazi QH, Mariano E, Milman DH, Beller E, Crombleholme W: Abnormalities in offspring associated with prenatal marihuana exposure. Dev Pharmacol Ther 8:141–148, 1985.
25. Fried PA, Watkinson B, Willan A: Marijuana use during pregnancy and decreased length of gestation. Am J Obstet Gynecol 150:23–27, 1984.
26. Beaconsfield P, Ginsburg J, Rainsbury R: Marijuana smoking: Cardiovascular effects in man and possible mechanisms. N Engl J Med 287:209–212, 1972.
27. Stoelting RK, Martz RC, Gartner J, Creasser C, Brown DJ, Forney RB: Effects of delta 9-tetrahydrocannabinol on halothane MAC in dogs. Anesthesiology 38:521–524, 1973.
28. Vitez TS, Way WL, Miller RD, Eger EI II: Effects of delta 9-tetrahydrocannabinol on cycloprane MAC in the rat. Anesthesiology 38:525–527, 1973.
29. Wood PR, Soni N: Anaesthesia and substance abuse. Anaesthesia 44:672–680, 1989.
30. Ltasch L, Christ R: Probleme der Anaesthesie bei Drogenabhängigen. Anaesthesist 37:123–139, 1988.
31. Naeye RL, Blanc W, LeBlanc W, Khatamee MA: Fetal complications of maternal heroin addiction: Abnormal growth, infections and episodes of stress. J Pediatr 83:1055–1061, 1973.
32. Vassal TH, Pezzano M: Les complications médicales de l'héroïnomanie. La Revue du Practicien 37:1729–1734, 1987.
33. Finnegan LP: Effects of maternal opiate abuse on the newborn. Fed Proc 44:2314–2317, 1985.
34. Zelson C, Lee SJ, Casalino M: Neonatal narcotic addiction: Comparative effects of maternal intake of heroin and methadone. N Engl J Med 289:1216–1220, 1973.
35. Archie CL, Lee MI, Sokol RJ, Norman G: The effects of methadone treatment on the reactivity of the nonstress test. Obstet Gynecol 74:254–255, 1989.
36. Jage J: Anaesthesia und analgesie bei opiatabhängigen. Anaesthesist 37:470–482, 1988.
37. Weintraub SJ, Naulty JS: Acute abstinence syndrome after epidural injection of butorphanol. Anesth Analg 64:452–453, 1985.
38. Gomar C, Luis M, Nalda MA: Sacro-illitis in a heroin addict. Anaesthesia 39:167–170, 1984.
39. Bradberry JC, Raebel MA: Continuous infusion of naloxone in the treatment of narcotic overdose. Drug Intell Clin Pharm 15:945–950, 1981.
40. Abelson HI, Miller JD: A decade of trends in cocaine use in the household population. Natl Inst Drug Abus Res Mongr Ser 61:35–49, 1985.
41. Fishburn PM: National survey on drug abuse: Main findings, 1979, DHHS Pub No 80–976. National Inst Drug Abuse, Rockville, MD, 1980.

42. Ritchie JM, Green NM: Local anesthetics. In *The Pharmacological Basis of Therapeutics*, 7th ed. AG Gilman, LS Goodman, eds. Macmillan, New York, 1985, pp 309–310.

43. Henderson CE, Torbey M: Rupture of intracranial aneurysm associated with cocaine use during pregnancy. Am J Perinatol 5:142–143, 1988.

44. Woods JR, Plessinger MA, Clark KE: Effect of cocaine on uterine blood flow and fetal oxygenation. JAMA 257:957–961, 1987.

45. Moore TR, Sorg J, Miller L: Hemodynamic effects of intravenous cocaine on the pregnant ewe and fetus. Am J Obstet Gynecol 155:883–888, 1986.

46. Foutz SE, Kotelko DM, Shnider SM, Thigpen JW, Rosen MA, Brookshire GL, Koike M, Levinson G, Elias-Baker B: Placental transfer and effects of cocaine and uterine blood flow and the fetus. Anesthesiology 59:A442, 1983.

47. Chasnoff IJ, Burns WJ, Schnoll SH, Burns KA: Cocaine use in pregnancy. N Engl J Med 313:666–669, 1985.

48. Fulroth R, Phillips B, Durand DJ: Perinatal outcome of infants exposed to cocaine and/or heroin in utero. AJDC 143:905–910, 1989.

49. Dixon SD: Effects of transplacental exposure to cocaine and methamphetamine on the neonate. West J Med 150:436–442, 1989.

50. Tenorio GM, Nazvi M, Bickers GH, Hubbird RH: Intrauterine stroke and maternal polydrug use. Clin Pediatr 27:565–567, 1988.

51. Cherukuri R, Minkoff H, Feldman J, Parekh A, Glass L: A cohort study of alkaloidal cocaine ("crack") in pregnancy. Obstet Gynecol 72:147–151, 1988.

52. Nelson NM, Fofar JO: Associations between drugs administered during pregnancy and congenital abnormalities of the fetus. Br Med J 1:523–527, 1971.

53. Little BB, Snell LM, Klein VR, Gilstrap LC: Cocaine abuse during pregnancy: Maternal and fetal implications. Obstet Gynecol 73:157–160, 1989.

54. Erickson M, Larsson C, Windbladh B, Zetterström R: The influence of amphetamine addiction on pregnancy and the newborn infants. Acta Paediatr Scand 67:95–99, 1978.

55. Little BB, Snell LM, Gilstrap LC: Methamphetamine abuse during pregnancy: Outcome and fetal effects. Obstet Gynecol 72:541–544, 1988.

56. Oro AS, Dixon SD: Perinatal cocaine and methamphetamine exposure: Maternal and neonatal correlates. J Pediatr 111:571–578, 1987.

57. Nora JL, Vargo TA, Nora AH, Love KE, McNamara DG: Dexamphetamine: A possible environmental trigger in cardiovascular malformations. Lancet 1:1290, 1970.

58. Heinonen OP, Slone D, Shapiro S: *Birth Defects and Drugs in Pregnancy*. Publishing Sciences Group, Littleton, MA, 1977.

59. Hollmén A, Jouppila R, Jouppila P, Koivula A, Vierola H: Effect of extradural analgesia using bupivacaine and 2-chloroprocaine on intervillous blood flow during normal labour. Br J Anaesth 54:837–842, 1982.

60. Jouppila P, Kirkinen P, Koivula A, Ylikorkala O: Effects of dihydralazine infusion on the fetoplacental blood flow and maternal prostanoids. Obstet Gynecol 65:115–118, 1985.

61. Hughes SC, Vertommen JD, Rosen MA, Messer CP, Espinoza MI, Parer JT, Shnider SM: Cocaine-induced hypertension in the ewe and response to treatment with labetalol. Anesthesiology 75:A1075, 1991.

62. Gay RG, Loper KA: Control of cocaine-induced hypertension with labetalol. Anesth Analg 67:91–94, 1988.

63. Pollan S, Tadjziechy M: Esmolol in the management of epi-

nephrine- and cocaine-induced cardiovascular toxicity. Anesth Analg 69:663–664, 1989.

64. Ramoska E, Sacchetti AD: Propranolol-induced hypertension in treatment of cocaine intoxication. Ann Emerg Med 14:1112–1113, 1985.

65. Nahas G, Trouvé R, Demus JF, von Sitbon M: A calcium channel blocker as antidote to the cardiac effects of cocaine intoxication. N Engl J Med 313:519–520, 1985.

66. Catravas JD, Waters IW: Acute cocaine intoxication in the conscious dog: Studies on the mechanism of lethality. J Pharmacol Exp Ther 217:350–356, 1981.

67. Samuels IS, Maze A, Albright G: Cardiac arrest during cesarean section in a chronic amphetamine abuser. Anesth Analg 58:528–530, 1979.

68. Smith DS, Gutsche BB: Amphetamine abuse and obstetrical anesthesia. Anesth Analg 59:710–711, 1980.

68. Smith DS, Gutsche BB: Amphetamine abuse and obstetrical anesthesia. Anesth Analg 59:710–711, 1980.

69. Fried PA, O'Connell CM: A comparison of the effects of prenatal exposure to tobacco, alcohol, cannabis and caffeine on birth size and subsequent growth. Neurotoxicol Teratol 9:79–85, 1987.

70. Vert P, Lebrun F: Les nuissances toxiques pour le foetus: L'alcohol, les drogues psychoactives et le tabac. La Revue du Practicien 38:825–831, 1988.

71. Slotkin TA, Cho H, Whitmore WL: Effects of prenatal nicotine exposure on neuronal development. Selective actions on central and peripheral catecholaminergic pathways. Brain Res Bull 18:601–611, 1987.

72. Stjerfeldt M, Berglund K, Lindsten J, Ludvigsson J: Maternal smoking during pregnancy and risk of childhood cancer. Lancet 1:1350–1352, 1986.

73. Davies JM, Latto IP, Jones JG, Veale A, Wardrop CAJ: Effects of stopping smoking for 48 hours on oxygen availability from the blood: A study on pregnant women. Br Med J 2:355–356, 1979.

74. Pearse AC, Jones RM: Smoking and anesthesia: Preoperative abstinence and perioperative morbidity. Anesthesiology 61:576–584, 1984.

75. Wright DJ, Pandya A: Smoking and gastric juice volume in outpatients. Can Anaesth Soc J 26:328, 1979.

76. Leviton A: Caffeine consumption and the risk of reproductive hazards. J Reprod Med 33:175–178, 1988.

77. Smith SE, McElhatton PR, Sullivan FM: Effects of administering caffeine to pregnant rats either as a single daily dose or as divided doses four times a day. Food Chem Toxicol 25:125, 1987.

78. Linn S, Schoenbaum SC, Monson RR, Rosner B, Stubblefield PG, Ryan KJ: No association between coffee consumption and adverse outcomes of pregnancy. N Engl J Med 360:141–145, 1982.

79. Heller J: What do we know about the risks of caffeine consumption in pregnancy? Br J Addict 82:885–889, 1987.

80. Srisuphan W, Bracken MB: Caffeine consumption during pregnancy and association with late spontaneous abortion. Am J Obstet Gynecol 154:14–20, 1986.

81. Martin TR, Bracken MB: The association between low-birth weight and caffeine consumption during pregnancy. Am J Epidemiol 126:813–821, 1987.

82. Oei SG, Vosters RPK, van der Hagen NLJ: Fetal arrhythmia caused by excessive intake of caffeine by pregnant women. Br Med J 298:568, 1989.

83. Galletly DC, Fennelly M, Whitwam JG: Does caffeine withdrawal contribute to postanesthetic morbidity? Lancet 1:1335, 1989.

CHAPTER 36

Evaluation of the Fetus

Russell K. Laros, Jr., M.D.

A number of laboratory studies and tests are currently available that can be used to aid the clinician in assessing fetal well-being, function, and maturity. The obstetric anesthesiologist should be aware of the fetal status before undertaking care of the mother. Problems such as intrauterine growth retardation, prematurity, and fetal asphyxia will influence his or her choice of anesthesia. Fetuses at risk can now be identified with much greater precision than in the past. All available tests are not reviewed in this chapter; rather, discussion is limited to several techniques that have found the widest clinical acceptance. In each instance the physiologic basis for the particular study is briefly reviewed, and those clinical situations where it is of greatest value are indicated.

BIOCHEMICAL TESTS OF PLACENTAL AND FETAL FUNCTION

There has been an ongoing search for substances measurable in the maternal blood stream that are reflective of fetal and placental metabolic normalcy. Over the past decade tests of this type have been shown to be of little value. An exception is the maternal serum α-fetoprotein (MSAFP). Because some centers still use urinary and plasma estriol levels in managing pregnancy in a diabetic patient, we will also briefly discuss this assessment.

α-Fetoprotein

α-Fetoprotein is produced primarily in the fetal liver with lesser amounts coming from the yolk sac and the gastrointestinal tract. The fetal serum level reaches a maximum at 13 weeks' gestational age and declines thereafter, becoming virtually absent after the age of 2 years. Amniotic fluid levels parallel the fetal serum levels in a ratio of about 1:150, with the maximum occurring at 12 to 14 weeks' gestation. The maternal serum levels are lower than the fetal by a factor of 10,000. However, the maternal levels increase progressively until the 32nd week of pregnancy and then decline modestly to term. Normal values are usually defined at a given gestational age based on multiples of the median (MOM). Values greater than 2.5 MOM are considered abnormally high, and those less than 0.4 MOM are considered low (1, 2).

Screening programs aimed at detecting fetal neural tube defects are now a standard part of prenatal care. This approach takes advantage of the fact that amniotic fluid and maternal serum levels are substantially elevated if the fetus has an open neural tube defect. Women not at increased risk for carrying a fetus with a neural tube defect are offered serum screening at 16 to 18 weeks of gestation. Although the primary purpose of maternal serum screening is the detection of neural tube defects, there are a number of other fetal conditions associated with either an abnormally high or low level. Abnormally high or low MSAFP values must be carefully evaluated to rule in or out the various conditions listed in Table 36.1. Cases of unexplained, high MSAFP should have fetal surveillance carried out to term.

Urinary and Plasma Estrogens

During the first few weeks of pregnancy the corpus luteum produces most of the circulating estrogens.

Table 36.1
Conditions Associated with Abnormal Maternal α-Fetoprotein Levels

Elevated
Neural tube defects
Multiple gestations
Fetal death
Abdominal wall defects: omphalocele and gastroschisis
Esophageal and duodenal atresia
Congenital nephrosis
Cystic hygroma
Subsequent intrauterine growth retardation and poor fetal outcome
Renal anomalies
Sacrococcygeal teratoma
Underestimation of fetal age

Low
Chromosomal abnormalities (especially trisomies)
Fetal death
Overestimation of gestational age

With regression of the corpus luteum, maternal estrogens do not decrease, but rather there is a sharp rise in maternal plasma estrone (E_1) and estradiol (E_2). This rise is due to increased placental production of E_1 and E_2 using estrogen precursors. In the latter half of pregnancy approximately 90% of maternal E_3 arises from conversion of the fetal precursor 16-OH-DS by the placenta. The 16-OH-DS in turn

comes from conversion of DS produced by the fetal adrenal and the fetal liver (3). Serial E_3 determinations (either urinary or plasma) are valuable in assessing fetal well-being in diabetes mellitus (4). A significant fall in E_3 is that change that exceeds day-to-day variation. Either a downward trend or a precipitous fall in E_3 may be a sign of fetal deterioration. Prompt delivery should be considered in the context of the total clinical picture; that is, fetal maturity, cervical ripeness, and the underlying disease must be considered before reaching a decision for delivery or continuation of the pregnancy.

Other conditions besides fetal distress causing low E_3 values are summarized in Table 36.2.

Finally, the administration of antibiotics that decrease or eliminate normal intestinal flora can result in low E_3 values. The alteration in bacterial flora

Table 36.2
Causes of Low E_3 Other Than Placental Dysfunction

Fetal CNS abnormalities
Fetal adrenal disorders
Fetal liver dysfunction
Placental abnormalities
Maternal renal disease
Hepatointestinal circulation interruption

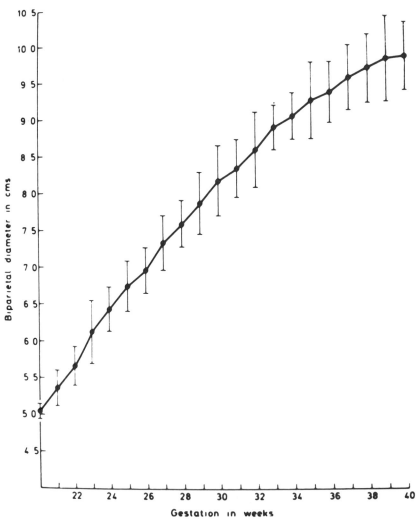

Figure 36.1. Fetal biparietal measurements for each week of gestation from 20 to 40 weeks (mean ± 2 SD). Measurements made using A-mode and B-mode ultrasonic techniques (Reprinted by permission from Campbell S: The prediction of fetal maturity by ultrasonic measurement of the biparietal diameter. J Obstet Gynaecol Br Commonw 76:603–609, 1969.)

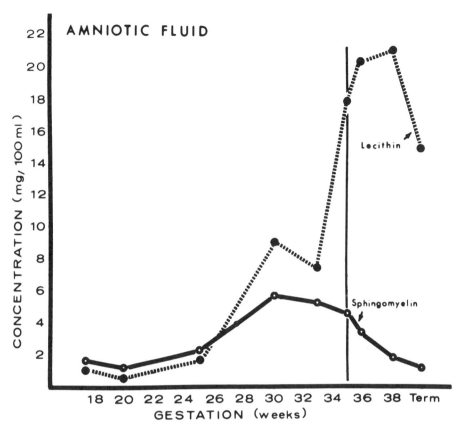

Figure 36.2. Levels of lecithin and sphingomyelin in amniotic fluid at increasing gestational ages. An acute rise in lecithin at 35 weeks marks pulmonary maturity. (Reprinted by permission from Gluck L, Kulovich MV, Borer RC Jr, Brenner PH, Anderson GG, Spellacy WN: The diagnosis of the respiratory distress syndrome (RDS) by amniocentesis. Am J Obstet Gynecol 109:440–445, 1971.)

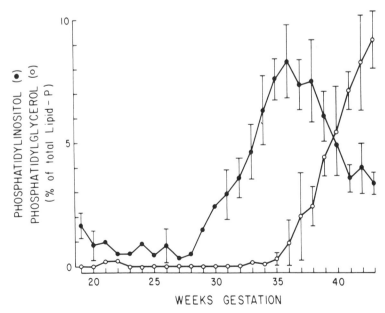

Figure 36.3. The content of PI (●) and PG (○) in amniotic fluid during normal gestation. The phospholipids were quantified by measuring the phosphorus (P) content and expressed as percentages of total lipid phosphorus. Means ± SD of three to five samples are shown for each *point*. (Reprinted by permission from Hallman M, Kulovich M, Kirkpatrick E, Sugarman RG, Gluck L: Phosphatidylinositol and phosphatidylglycerol in amniotic fluid: Indices of lung maturity. Am J Obstet Gynecol 125:613–623, 1976.)

decreases the rate of hydrolysis of E_3 conjugates, leading to an increased loss of E_3 in the stool rather than normal reabsorption into the maternal circulation (5).

ULTRASONOGRAPHY

In the last 20 years diagnostic ultrasound has rapidly established its place in clinical obstetrics. The apparatus consists of a piezoelectric crystal transducer that comes in direct contact with the maternal abdomen. When the crystal is excited by a pulsating electric current, it produces ultrasonic waves. As the sound waves pass through interfaces of different densities, echoes return to the crystal, where they are detected and translated into new electric signals.

Four types of ultrasound are now in clinical use. In the amplitude mode (A-mode) the presence and character of interface is studied. A second method is the brightness mode (B-mode), where the strength of the echoes determines the brightness of dots on an oscilloscope screen. The gray scale is simply on extension of the B-mode that allows more gradation of lightness or darkness. The motion mode (M-mode) is used to measure position and time for objects in motion. When an object's position changes in relation to the transducer, the position of the displayed echo will change correspondingly. Finally, a continuous beam or real-time device is available that pro-

duces a continuous moving image of the objects under the transducer. Real-time transducers are available for both abdominal and vaginal use and come as either linear array or sector scanners. Prospective study has shown that intrauterine diagnostic ultrasonography has no adverse effects on the fetus (6).

Although there are many uses for ultrasound during pregnancy, this discussion only considers assessment of fetal age, fetal growth, fetal weight, the presence of anomalies, definition of placental location, and Doppler flow.

Fetal Age

Fetal age can be determined quite accurately with ultrasound. Because all fetuses start at about the same size but vary widely in size as they approach term, the accuracy of an ultrasonic determination of age varies inversely with the age. Although a variety of structures can be measured and have been found to correlate well with fetal age, those most widely used are: the biparietal diameter (BPD) (Fig. 36.1), gestational sac diameter, crown-rump length, abdominal circumference, and femur length. The use of a combination of measurements will usually give a more reliable estimate of fetal age. Up to 20 weeks' gestation the accuracy of an ultrasonically determined gestational age is ± 1 week. A variety of normograms for calculating gestational age are available in standard texts (7–11).

Fetal Weight

There are now a number of reports presenting nomograms that allow estimation of fetal weight. The nomograms use BPD alone or in conjunction with other fetal measurements. Unfortunately, all current methods have large standard errors at either extreme of weight and are only precise over the middle weight range.

Fetal Growth

Sonography is frequently used to evaluate a fetus suspected of having intrauterine growth retardation (IUGR). As a first step, sonographic measurement of the BPD can confirm or assign a fetal age. Then serial sonography can be used to establish a BPD growth pattern. Other sonographic measurements of the fetus that alone or in combination may be useful in detecting IUGR are the abdominal circumference at the level of the umbilical vein and the intrauterine volume. Campbell and Wilkin (10), using a second-degree polynomial regression formula, were able to identify infants weighing less than 5% below their expected weight for gestational age with a 95% confidence at 32 weeks' gestation; this accuracy decreased to 63% at 38 weeks.

Table 36.3
Preparation of Tube Dilutions for a Rapid Test of Amniotic Fluid Surfactant

	Tube Dilutions (ml)		
	1/1	1/1.3	1/2
Amniotic fluid	1.0	0.75	0.50
NaCl	0.0	0.25	0.50
95% ethanol	1.0	1.0	1.0

Table 36.4
Risk of Developing Hyaline Membrane Disease (HMD) if Delivered within 24 Hr of Shake Test

Risk Group	Amniotic Fluid Dilution[a]			Incidence of HMD (%)
	1/1	1/1.3	1/2	
I	+	+	+	<1
II	+	+	±	10
	+	±	±	
III	+	±	−	25
	±	±	±	
IV	±	±	−	41
V	±	−	−	79
	−	−	−	

[a] + = positive; ± = intermediate; − = negative.

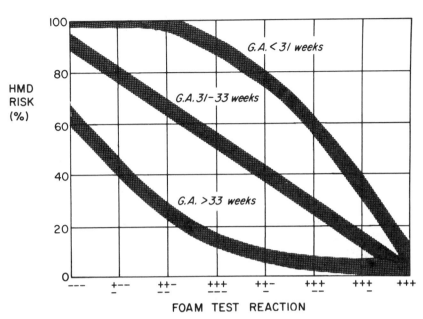

Figure 36.4. Scheme for antenatal prediction of hyaline membrane disease (*HMD*) from amniotic fluid foam test reaction plus gestational age. The risk is predicted from the *shaded band* appropriate for the gestational age. The width of each band approximates the error of the estimate. For example, with a foam test reaction of ± ± ± the risk of HMD is approximately 15% if gestational age is >33 weeks, 65% if the gestational age is 31 to 33 weeks, and approximately 90% if it is <31 weeks. (Reprinted by permission from Schleuter M, Phibbs RH, Creasy RK, Clements JA, Tooley WH: Antenatal prediction of graduated risk of hyaline membrane disease by amniotic fluid foam test for surfactant. Am J Obstet Gynecol 134:761–767, 1979.)

Their false-positive rate was just over 1% at all gestational ages. Unfortunately, recent studies have not been nearly as successful at defining IUGR and suggest a specificity and sensitivity of ultrasonic diagnoses of only 70% (11, 12, 13).

Both significant IUGR and macrosomia have clinical importance. IUGR may be asymmetric or symmetric. In the former, head growth is more normal than growth of either the abdomen or thorax. In the symmetric form the diminution of growth is proportionate in the head, thorax, and abdomen. When the estimated fetal weight (EFW) is below the 10th percentile for gestational age of the fetus, a careful consideration of causes of IUGR is undertaken and either delivery carried out or biweekly fetal surveillance begun. The decision for or against delivery is predicated on the probable cause for the IUGR, the gestational age, fetal lung maturity, and other evidence of fetal well-being (14).

Macrosomia is characterized either as a fetal weight above the 90th percentile or greater than 4000 or 4500 g. The absolute weight definition is used because of the increased incidence of birth trauma experienced by these very large infants. Macrosomia may be constitutional but also may be secondary to maternal glucose intolerance.

Placental Localization

Ultrasound can be used very effectively to locate the placenta. Such localization can be accomplished with 95% accuracy during the latter part of gestation and thus is very useful in the management of patients with antepartum hemorrhage. Additionally, placental localization is useful before amniocentesis and in managing patients with abnormal fetal lies (15).

Congenital Anomalies

Ultrasound can also be used to evaluate a fetus suspected of having a congenital anomaly. It is most useful in detecting hydramnios, fetal ascites, anencephaly, hydrocephaly, and anomalies of the fetal spine. Unfortunately, a negative finding does not definitively rule out these abnormalities.

Fetal Breathing

Finally, evaluation of fetal breathing using either real-time imaging or a special A-mode scanning device promises to be a sensitive indicator of intrauterine fetal hypoxia. In 1971 Boddy and Robinson described recording fetal chest wall movements in both lambs and human fetuses (16). These observations have been extended, and it is now recognized that there are distinct patterns of fetal breathing. These include times of low breathing activity (midnight,

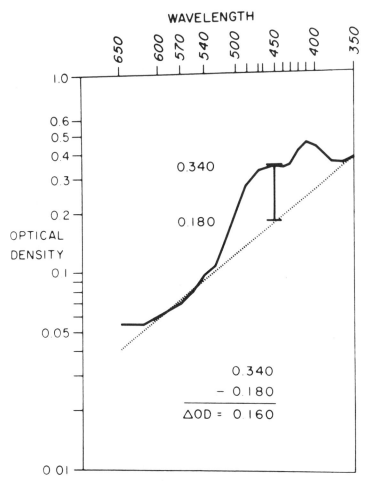

Figure 36.5. Determination of ΔOD 450 in amniotic fluid. An arbitrary *broken line* has been drawn connecting the spectrophotometric readings obtained at 375 and 600 nm. The *solid vertical line* represents the ΔOD at 450 nm. (Reprinted by permission from Merkatz IR, Aladjem S, Little B: The value of biochemical estimations on amniotic fluid in managment of the high-risk pregnancy. Clin Perinatol 1:301–319, 1974.)

8 AM, and 4 PM, with less than 10% of the fetuses breathing) and peaks of breathing rate (4 AM, noon, and 8 PM, with greater than 80% breathing) (17). Using A-scan technology, Boddy and Dawes (18) have noted patterns of prolonged apnea or gasping and apnea before fetal death. In contrast, the observation of normal fetal breathing patterns was a reassuring sign and correlated with normal fetal outcome (19).

AMNIOTIC FLUID ANALYSIS

Amniotic fluid can be obtained by transabdominal amniocentesis. It is most commonly used to assess fetal lung maturity. The hazards of delivering an immature infant are multiple and include difficulties in nutrition, problems in biochemical homeostasis, vulnerability of the immature fetal brain, and the development of idiopathic respiratory distress syndrome (IRDS) or hyaline membrane disease. Because IRDS leads to so much morbidity and mortality, its avoidance whenever possible is most desirable.

Amniotic Fluid Surfactant Determination

Gluck (20) has reviewed the pathophysiology of IRDS and the measurement of amniotic fluid surfactant activity in detail. In this discussion only several facets of clinical relevance are reviewed. The surfactant complex is made up primarily of phospholipids, the most abundant of which is lecithin. Lecithin is secreted by type II alveolar cells and is excreted into the fetal trachea and thence into the amniotic fluid. During early gestation only a small amount of surfactant activity is present; however, with maturation of the appropriate enzyme system between 34 and 36 weeks' of gestation, there is an abrupt rise in amniotic fluid surfactant activity (Fig. 36.2). This rise in activity above a critical level is accompanied by a virtual absence of IRDS in the neonate.

Surfactant activity can be measured directly using the amniotic fluid *foam test* or shake test described by Clements and associates (21) or by measuring the ratio of the major phospholipids lecithin and sphingomyelin (*L/S ratio*) as described by Gluck (22) and others. The L/S ratio is measured using thin-layer chromatography; a positive ratio is generally considered to be one greater than 2 to 3.5 and assures a very low risk that the fetus will develop IRDS. Additional information can be added by measuring the minor phospholipids *phosphatidylinositol (PI)* and *phosphatidylglycerol (PG)* (22, 23). The relative percentage of phospholipid represented by PI and PG at varying gestational ages is depicted in Figure 36.3. When the L/S ratio is less than 1, the PG and PI are vitually absent. PG, the unique phospholipid of lung surfactant, first appears when the L/S ratio exceeds

2 and indicates secretion of mature lung surfactant. Analysis of PG in amniotic fluid serves as an additional index of lung maturity and is especially useful when the specimen is contaminated by blood.

The foam test is based on the ability of lecithin to stabilize foam produced by mechanical agitation of a solution of amniotic fluid and alcohol. To perform the test, amniotic fluid in three dilutions with saline is mixed with 95% ethanol as indicated in Table 36.3. The test solution, having 47.5% volume fraction of ethanol, excludes interfering substances (protein, bile salts, fatty acids) from the surface of the amniotic fluid but permits double-chain phospholipids, such as lecithin, to compete for the surface film. When the solution is shaken with air, stable bubbles form if a sufficient number of double-chain phospholipids are present. The tubes are capped, shaken vigorously, placed in a rack, and left undisturbed for 15 min. The air-liquid interface of each tube is then examined for the presence of stable bubbles. A tube is recorded as positive when there are enough bubbles present to form a complete ring around the air-liquid interface. A tube is recorded as intermediate when small bubbles are present but not in sufficient numbers to form a complete ring, and negative when no bubbles are present. There is a progressive increase in incidence of hyaline membrane disease with decreasing reaction. Schlueter and associates (24) have defined five risk groups based on the degree of foam stability as outlined in Table 36.4. Infants at low risk (groups I and II) were heavier and more mature than those at high risk (groups III, IV, and V). However, among infants of equivalent gestational age or birth weight, the incidence of IRDS still correlated significantly with the foam test results (Fig. 36.4).

The advantage of the foam test is its rapidity and simplicity; the disadvantage is a high level of false-negative findings and the fact that it cannot be performed on specimens contaminated by meconium or

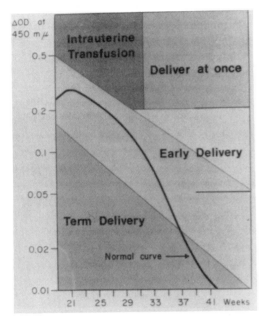

Figure 36.6. Suggested management of Rh-sensitized pregnancies based on level of ΔOD 450 and gestational age. (Reprinted by permission from Merkatz IR, Aladjem S, Little B: The value of biochemical estimations on amniotic fluid in management of the high-risk pregnancy. Clin Perinatol 1:301–319, 1974.)

Table 36.5
Scoring System for Evaluating the Nonstress Test[a]

Fetal Heart Rate Observation	Score		
	0	1	2
Baseline rate (beats/min)	<100 or >180	100–119 or 161–180	120–160
Fetal activity (movements/30 min)	0	1–4	≥5
Accelerations (per 30 min)	0	Periodic or 1–4 sporadic	≥5 sporadic
Baseline variability			
Oscillatory amplitude (beats/min)	<5	5–9 or >25	10–25
Oscillatory frequency (per min)	<3	3–6	>6
Decelerations	Severe variable or repetive late	Mild variable or non-repetitive late	None or early

[a]Reprinted by permission from Krebs HB, Petres RB: Clinical application of a scoring system for evaluation of antepartum fetal heart rate monitoring. Am J Obstet Gynecol 130:765–772, 1978.

empty

blood. The author has used the foam test as the first method of laboratory assessment of lung maturity. If the amniotic fluid is found to indicate risk group I, no further study is necessary. However, if the risk group is II or higher, an L/S ratio and PG level are performed on the fluid.

Measuring surfactant activity will aid the clinician in timing deliveries in a variety of situations. Hack and associates (25) found that 12% of all infants admitted to the intensive care nursery with IRDS were the products of elective interventions (cesarean sections or inductions). These findings suggest that some study of lung maturity should be used before elective repeat cesarean section or induction of labor in almost every case. This is especially true when there is the slightest doubt as to the actual fetal age.

Amniotic fluid analysis is also valuable in the early diagnosis of hereditary disorders and congenital anomalies and in managing fetuses with hemolytic disease.

Amniotic Cell Culture

Chromosomal abnormalities such as Down's syndrome, or trisomy 21, can be diagnosed from fetal cells obtained from the amniotic fluid and grown in culture (26). These cells may also be used to determine the enzyme deficiencies present in Tay-Sachs disease or galactosemia. Recently, the technique of chorionic villous biopsy has been described (27). A small catheter is passed into the uterus under ultrasonic guidance and a sample of chorion obtained by aspiration. Cell culture and analysis are then carried out similar to amniocentesis. The advantage of chorionic villous biopsy is that it is performed in the first trimester of pregnancy. In later pregnancy cordocentesis is required if rapid chromosomal analysis is needed. A small-gauge needle is passed into the umbilical cord at its insertion into the placenta under ultrasonic guidance. Fetal lymphocytes can then be cultured and chromosomal results made available within a few days. In addition to rapid karyotyping,

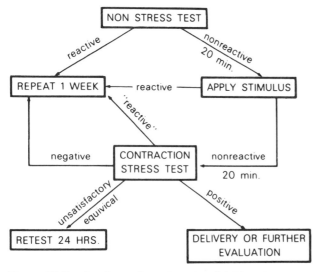

Figure 36.7. A schema for antepartum fetal heart rate testing using the nonstress test and contraction stress test. (Reprinted by permission from Everston LR, Gauthier RJ, Schifrin BS, Paul RH: Antepartum fetal heart rate testing. Am J Obstet Gynecol 133:29–33, 1979.)

Table 36.6
Scoring System for the Biophysical Profile[a]

Biophysical Variable	Normal (Score = 2)	Abnormal (Score = 0)
1. Fetal breathing movements	At least one episode of at least 30 sec duration in 30-min observation	Absent or no episode of ≥30 sec in 30 min
2. Gross body movement	At least three discrete body/limb movements in 30 min (episodes of active continuous movement considered as a single movement)	Two or fewer episodes of body/limb movements in 30 min
3. Fetal tone	At least one episode of active extension with return to flexion of fetal limb(s) or trunk. Opening and closing of hand considered normal tone	Either slow extension with return to partial flexion or movement of limb in full extension or absent fetal movement
4. Reactive fetal heart rate	At least two episodes of acceleration of ≥15 bpm and at least 15-sec duration associated with fetal movement in 30 min	Less than two accelerations or acceleration <15 bpm in 30 min
5. Qualitative amniotic fluid volume	At least one pocket of amniotic fluid that measures at least 1 cm in two perpendicular planes	Either no amniotic fluid pockets or a pocket <1 cm in two perpendicular planes

[a]Reprinted by permission from Manning FA, Morrison I, Lang IR, Harman C: Antepartum determination of fetal health: Composite biophysical profile scoring. Clin Perinatol 9:285–296, 1982.

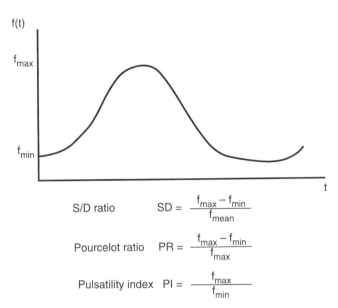

$$SD = \frac{f_{max} - f_{min}}{f_{mean}}$$

S/D ratio

$$PR = \frac{f_{max} - f_{min}}{f_{max}}$$

Pourcelot ratio

$$PI = \frac{f_{max}}{f_{min}}$$

Pulsatility index

Figure 36.8. Method of calculating the various indices of Doppler velocimetry.

cordocentesis is useful in the management of fetal anemia and thrombocytopenia and suspected intrauterine infection (28).

Fetal Hemolytic Anemia

Bilirubin is found in the amniotic fluid of normal pregnancies between the 12th and 36th week of gestation. The analysis for bilirubin is done spectrophotometrically by scanning the absorbance of amniotic fluid at wave lengths between 300 and 600 nm (29). The presence of bilirubin is indicated by increased optical density (OD) between 375 and 525 nm with a peak at 450 nm. The height of this peak is expressed as the ΔOD at 450 nm (Fig. 36.5). A ΔOD of less than 0.01 indicates fetal maturity.

The concentration of bilirubin in the amniotic fluid also accurately reflects the increased hemoglobin degradation found in erythroblastosis fetalis and thus serves as an index of the severity of the disease (29–31). The bilirubin level provides the indication for intrauterine fetal transfusion, early delivery, or no therapeutic intervention (29, 32–34) (Fig. 36.6).

A useful alternative to intraperitoneal transfusion is direct intravascular transfusion via cordocentesis. This approach has the advantage of allowing a pretransfusion and posttransfusion measurement of the fetal hematocrit and ensures that all of the transfused blood reaches the fetal circulation. Intravascular transfusion is the route of choice for all cases of fetal hydrops or when the fetal hematocrit concentration is less than 20%. The current approach to diagnosis and treatment should allow a woman with severe

isoimmunization an 80 to 90% chance of a successful fetal outcome (35–37).

FETAL ACTIVITY MONITORING

The pregnant woman herself has always been concerned by a decrease in or absence of fetal movement. Similarly, the absence of fetal movement in the presence of fetal heart activity has been thought to indicate a seriously ill fetus. However, it is only recently that the obstetrician has approached quantification of fetal activity in a systematic way.

The technique originally suggested by Sadovsky and associates requires extended periods of observation by the mother (38, 39). From their data it is clear that mothers could correctly interpret fetal movement approximately 90% of the time and that prolonged periods of counting are difficult for most women to carry out. "Kick counts" taken for 10 min once or twice per day are equally adequate. A woman carrying a normal, healthy fetus will detect 5 to 20 movements in 10 min. In instances of progressive fetal compromise there will be a rapid decline in the number of kicks over 2 to 3 days. The decline will be followed by 1 to 3 days of no detectable fetal movement, then fetal death will occur. This sequence of events should alert the physician to the need for nonstress or stress testing (39, 40).

In a prospective study, Moore and Piacquadio were able to gain 90% compliance by their patient population (41). Although the overall corrected perinatal mortality decreased from 5.9 per 1,000 to 1.6 per 1,000, the number of nonstress tests (NSTs) performed for decreased fetal movement increased by 58%. Fetal mortality for control mothers presenting to hospital because of decreased fetal movement was 44.5 per 1,000, as compared with 10.3 per 1,000 for mothers presenting for abnormal fetal activity counts.

STRESS AND NONSTRESS MONITORING

During a uterine contraction there is a significant fall in uteroplacental blood flow and thus a decrease in the amount of oxygen delivered to the fetus. The normal fetoplacental unit has sufficient respiratory reserve to withstand uterine contractions without production of transient episodes of fetal asphyxia. However, in situations of placental insufficiency, the added stress of contractions may cause transient asphyxia that is reflected by changes in the fetal heart rate pattern (Chapter 37).

The *contraction stress test* (CST) evolved from observation of periodic changes in the fetal heart rate noted with intrapartum monitoring. The test requires uterine contractions with a frequency of three in 10 min and each lasting 40 to 60 sec. Contractions can occur naturally or be provoked by oxytocin or manual nipple stimulation. The former is called an **oxytocin challenge test** (OCT) and the latter a **breast self-stimulation test** (BSST). An OCT is performed during the last trimester of pregnancy by stimulating uterine contractions with an intravenous infusion of dilute oxytocin solution. The uterine contractions and fetal heart rate are monitored with an external recording device. The method of performing an oxytocin challenge test has been detailed elsewhere (42). A positive OCT requires consistent and persistent hypoxic-type fetal heart rate patterns (late decelerations) occurring repeatedly with most uterine contractions (43–45). A BSST is performed by placing a warm, moist towel over one nipple and applying gentle massage (46).

The author wishes to emphasize the importance of obtaining adequate uterine activity, that is, at least three contractions of moderate intensity as determined by palpation, in a 10-min interval.

Indications for use of the contraction stress test or the nonstress test discussed below include hypertensive–renal disease, chronic hypertension, diabetes mellitus, cyanotic heart disease, hemoglobinopathy, hyperthyroidism, collagen disease, prolonged gestation (greater than 42 weeks), suspected IUGR, history of previous stillbirth, low E_3 excretion, decreased "kick counts," meconium-stained amniotic fluid, and Rh sensitization. Relative contraindications to a CST include previous classic cesarean section, placenta previa, and patients believed to be at risk for premature labor, that is, those with premature ruptured membranes, multiple pregnancies, or an incompetent cervix.

There now seems ample experience with the oxytocin challenge test to confirm that it does, in fact, allow rapid evaluation of placental respiratory function (44). A positive oxytocin challenge test may signify fetal compromise; however, there is an incidence of false-positive results of approximately 25%. Therefore the finding of a positive OCT dictates repetition of the study or the collection of other studies that allow evaluation of placental function, such as a biophysical profile, and analysis of the amniotic fluid for presence of meconium. In contrast, a negative OCT result is excellent evidence of continued fetal well-being for at least 7 days.

The use of the **nonstress test** (NST) also must be considered. In reviewing a large number of OCTs, Trierweiler and associates (47) concluded that variability of the fetal heart rate appeared to be characteristic of fetal well-being. Additionally, they supported the observation that a reactive fetus was characterized by acceleration of the fetal heart rate

in response to external stimuli or during fetal movement (48). The ability to derive equal information from observation of the fetal heart rate without the necessity of stimulating uterine contractions with oxytocin is obvious. Many authors have now confirmed the value of the nonstress test in high-risk patients (49–52). They were able to demonstrate a close correlation between nonstress patterns and neonatal outcome. Those fetuses with a reactive pattern (baseline variability greater than 6 beats/min and accelerations of at least 15 beats/min with fetal movement) had good outcomes. Krebs and Petres (52) have developed a scoring system for evaluation of the nonstress test that is summarized in Table 36.5. In their experience, a score of 9 to 12 was a reliable sign of fetal well-being and an OCT did not provide additional information. However, if the score was less than 9, an OCT should be performed.

The use of the **fetal acoustic stimulation test** (FAST) evolved from observations of fetal heart rate change in response to various stimuli, including sound (52). The sound stimulus most commonly used is an electronic artificial larynx, which generates sound levels averaging 82 dB. A stimulus is applied for ≤3 sec with repeated applications at 1-min intervals for a maximum of three times if no accelerations are noted after the initial application. Two or more accelerations of at least 15 bpm lasting 15 sec in a 10-min period constitutes a reactive test. The FAST test has fewer nonreactive tests initially, but the number of persistently nonreactive tests is about the same as with the NST (53–55).

An overall scheme for using both the nonstress and the stress test is depicted in Figure 36.7. This scheme allows one to use the simpler, less expensive nonstress test as a screening device without increasing the risk of having a false-negative study.

BIOPHYSICAL PROFILE

The biophysical profile (BPP) was developed because it was hoped that the assessment of multiple variables would better define fetal status (56–58). Five variables—fetal breathing movements, fetal movements, fetal tone, amniotic fluid volume, and the nonstress test—are measured in the same observation period. The scoring system devised by Manning and associates is shown in Table 36.6 (57). A score of 8 to 10 is normal, 4 to 6 is suspect and should be repeated in a matter of hours, and 0 to 2 indicates a very sick fetus that should be delivered immediately. The usefulness of the BPP has been validated by Manning and colleagues for both diabetic and postdate pregnancies. Although the above data suggest that the BPP has fewer false-positive test results, the author is not convinced that the routine use of the BPP offers any advantage over the systematic use of single evaluation tools, except in postdate pregnancies. In following the postdate pregnancy, the sonographic evaluation of the amniotic fluid is an important adjunct. The incidence of fetal bradycardia and variable decelerations increases as the volume of amniotic fluid decreases (61, 62).

DOPPLER VELOCIMETRY

The development of real-time ultrasound has provided new techniques for measuring maternal and fetal blood flow. Either a continuous or pulsed Doppler mode can be used. Several studies have shown no significant differences between the two techniques (63, 64). The pulsed doppler technique permits reliable vessel identification and appears to be gaining in popularity. Figure 36.8 depicts flow as a function of time and is the type of waveform seen in the umbilical artery. The systolic/diastolic (S/D) ratio, Pourcelot ratio and pulsatility index have all been evaluated in a variety of clinical conditions. Data have been accumulated on umbilical, uterine, and fetal carotid artery flow with the hope that they may provide a better physiologic understanding of the cause of abnormal growth in both singleton and multiple pregnancies (65–67). Devoe and colleagues examined the diagnostic value of NST, amniotic fluid volume, and umbilical artery velocimetry in 1000 high-risk patients (68). Unfortunately, Doppler velocimetry had the poorest sensitivity and the lowest positive predictive value. In our view, it is not yet useful for clinical decision making.

CONCLUSIONS

There are now available a number of studies that aid the clinician in management of both normal and abnormal pregnancies. Thoughtful use of these studies does improve perinatal outcome. As new studies are developed and those presently available (fetal breathing and nonstress monitoring) become better defined, even more accurate fetal surveillance and lower fetal morbidity and mortality can be anticipated.

References

1. Milunsky A, Flyate E: Prenatal diagnosis of neural tube defects: Problems and pitfalls—Analysis of 2495 cases using the α-fetoprotein assay, Obstet Gynecol 48:1–5, 1976.
2. Richard DS, Seeds JW, Katz VL, Lingley MS, Albright SG, Cefalo RC: Elevated maternal α-fetoprotein with normal ultrasound: Is amniocentesis always appropriate? A review of 20,069 screened patients. Obstet Gynecol 71:203–207, 1988.
3. Siiteri PK, MacDonald PC: Placental estrogen biosynthesis during human pregnancy. J Clin Endocrinol Metab 26:751–761, 1966.
4. Distler W, Gabbe SG, Freeman RK, Mestman JH, Goebelsmann V: Estriol in pregnancy. V. Unconjugated and total plasma estriol in management of pregnant diabetic patients. Am J Obstet Gynecol 130:424–431, 1978.
5. Boehm FM, DiPietro DL, Goss DA: The effect of ampicillin administration on urinary estriol and serum estradiol in the normal pregnant patient. Am J Obstet Gynecol 119:98–103, 1974.
6. Edmonds PD: Interactions of ultrasound and biological tissues. U.S. DWEW Publication (FDA) 73-8008. U.S. Food and Drug Administration, Washington, DC, 1972.
7. Campbell S: The prediction of fetal maturity by ultrasonic measurement of the biparietal diameter. J Obstet Gynaecol Br Commonw 76:603–609, 1969.
8. Sabbagha RE, Turner JH: Methodology of B-scan sonar cephalometry with electronic calipers and correlation with fetal birth weight. Obstet Gynecol 40:74–81, 1972.
9. Sabbagha RE, Tamura RK, Socol ML: The use of ultrasound in obstetrics. Clin Obstet Gynecol 25:735–752, 1982.
10. Campbell S, Wilkin D: Ultrasonic measurement of fetal abdominal circumference in the estimation of fetal weight. Br J Obstet Gynaecol 82:689–697, 1975.
11. Bowie JD, Andreotti RF: Estimating gestational age in utero. In Ultrasonography. PW Callen, ed. WB Saunders, Philadelphia, 1983, p 21.
12. Manning FA, Hill LM, Platt LD: Qualitative amniotic fluid volume determination by ultrasound: Antepartum detection of intrauterine growth retardation. Am J Obstet Gynecol 139:254–258, 1981.
13. Gross BH, Callen PW, Filly RA: The relationship of fetal transverse body diameter and biparietal diameter in the diagnosis of intrauterine growth retardation. J Ultrasound Med 1:361–365, 1982.
14. Grannum PAT: Ultrasonic measurement for diagnosis of intrauterine growth retardation. In Yearbook of Obstetrics and Gynecology. TL Gross, RJ Sokol, eds. Yearbook Medical Publishers, Chicago, 1989, p 123.
15. Kobayashi M, Hillman LM, Fillsti L: Placental localization. Am J Obstet Gynecol 106:279–285, 1970.
16. Boddy K, Robinson JS: External methods for detection of fetal breathing in utero. Lancet 2:1231–1235, 1971.
17. Fox HE, Hohler CW: Fetal evaluation by real-time imaging. Clin Obstet Gynecol 20:339–349, 1977.
18. Boddy K, Dawes GS: Fetal breathing. Br Med Bull 31:3–7, 1975.
19. Patrick J: Fetal breathing movements. Clin Obstet Gynecol 25:787–803, 1982.
20. Gluck L: Fetal maturity and amniotic fluid surfactant determinants. In Management of the High-Risk Pregnancy. WN Spellacy, ed. University Park Press, Baltimore, 1976, p 189.
21. Clements JA, Platzker ACG, Tierney DF, Hobel CJ, Creasy RK, Margolis AJ, Thibeault DW, Tooley WH, Oh W: Assessment of the risk of the respiratory distress syndrome by a rapid test for surfactant in amniotic fluid. N Engl J Med 286:1077–1081, 1972.
22. Hallman M, Kulovich M, Kirkpatrick E, Sugarman RG, Gluck L: Phosphatidylinositol and phosphatidylglycerol in amniotic fluid: Indices of lung maturity. Am J Obstet Gynecol 125:613–623, 1976.
23. Kulovich MV, Hallman MB, Gluck L: The lung profile. I. Normal lung. Am J Obstet Gynecol 135:57–63, 1979.
24. Schlueter M, Phibbs RH, Creasy RK, Clements JA, Tooley WH: Antenatal prediction of graduated risk of hyaline membrane disease by amniotic fluid foam test for surfactant. Am J Obstet Gynecol 134:761–767, 1979.
25. Hack M, Fanaroff AA, Klaus M, Mendelanity BD, Merkatz IR: Neonatal respiratory distress following elective delivery: A preventable disease? Am J Obstet Gynecol 126:43–47, 1976.
26. Golbus MS, Conte FA, Schneider EL, Epstein CJ: Intrauterine diagnosis of genetic defects, results, problems, and follow-up of 100 cases in a prenatal genetic detection center. Am J Obstet Gynecol 118:897–905, 1974.

27. Rhoads GG, Jackson LG, Schlesselman SE, de la Cruz FF, Desnick RJ, Goldbus MS, Ledbetter DH, Lubs HA, Mahoney MJ, Pergament E: The safety and efficacy of chorionic villus sampling for early prenatal diagnosis of cytogenetic abnormalities. N Engl J Med 320:609–617, 1989.

28. Weiner CP: Cordocentesis for diagnostic indications: Two years' experience. Obstet Gynecol 70:664–668, 1987.

29. Queenan JT: Amniotic fluid analysis. Clin Obstet Gynecol 14:505–536, 1971.

30. Bevis DCA: Blood pigment in haemolytic disease of the newborn. J Obstet Gynaecol Br Commonw 63:68–75, 1956.

31. Liley AW: Liquor amnii analysis in management of pregnancy complicated by Rhesus sensitization. Am J Obstet Gynecol 82:1359–1370, 1961.

32. Freda VJ: The Rh problem in obstetrics and a new concept of its management using amniocentesis and spectrophotometric scanning of amniotic fluid. Am J Obstet Gynecol 92:341–374, 1965.

33. Bowman JM: Management of Rh-isoimmunization. Obstet Gynecol 52:1–9, 1978.

34. Whitfield CR: A three year assessment of an action line method of timing intervention in rhesus isoimmunization. Am J Obstet Gynecol 108:1239–1244, 1970.

35. Rodeck CH, Letsky E: How the management of erythroblastosis fetalis has changed. Br J Obstet Gynaecol 96:759–763, 1989.

36. Harman CR, Bowman JM, Manning FA, Menticoglou SM: Intraperitoneal versus intravascular approach: A case-control comparison. Am J Obstet Gynecol 162:1053–1059, 1990.

37. Parer JT: Severe Rh isoimmunization: Current methods of in utero diagnosis and treatment. Am J Obstet Gynecol 158:1323–1329, 1988.

38. Sadovsky E, Polishuk WZ: Fetal movements in utero. Obstet Gynecol 50:49–55, 1977.

39. Sadovsky E: Fetal movements and fetal health. Semin Perinatol 5:131–143, 1981.

40. Harper RG, Greenberg M, Farahani G, Glassman I, Kierney CMP: Fetal movement, biochemical and biophysical parameters and the outcome of pregnancy. Am J Obstet Gynecol 141:39–42, 1981.

41. Moore T, Piacquadio K: A prospective evaluation of fetal movement screening to reduce the incidence of intrapartum fetal death. Am J Obstet Gynecol 160:1075–1081, 1989.

42. Ray M, Freeman R, Pine S, Hesselgesser R: Clinical experience with the oxytocin challenge test. Am J Obstet Gynecol 114:1–9, 1972.

43. Ewling D, Farina J, Otterson W: Clinical application of the oxytocin test. Obstet Gynecol 43:563–566, 1974.

44. Farahani G, Vasudeva K, Petric RH, Fenton, AN: Oxytocin challenge test in high risk pregnancy. Obstet Gynecol 47:159–168, 1976.

45. Freeman RK: The use of the oxytocin challenge test for antepartum clinical evaluation of respiratory function. Am J Obstet Gynecol 121:481–489, 1975.

46. Lenke R, Nemes J: Use of nipple stimulation to obtain contraction stress test. Obstet Gynecol 63:345–352, 1980.

47. Trierweiler MW, Freeman RK, James J: Baseline fetal heart rate characteristics as an indicator of fetal status during the antepartum period. Am J Obstet Gynecol 125:618–623, 1976.

48. Lee CY, DiLoreto FC, O'Lane JM: A study of fetal heart rate acceleration patterns. Obstet Gynecol 45:142–146, 1975.

49. Rochard F, Schifrin BS, Goupil F, Legrand H, Blottiere J, Sureau C: Nonstressed fetal heart rate monitoring in the antepartum period. Am J Obstet Gynecol 126:699–706, 1976.

50. Fox HE, Steinbrecher M, Ripton B: Antepartum fetal heart rate and uterine activity studies. Am J Obstet Gynecol 126:61–69, 1976.

51. Nichimson DJ, Turbeville JS, Terry JE, Petrie RH, Lundy LE: The non-stress test. Obstet Gynecol 51:419–421, 1978.

52. Krebs HB, Petres RB: Clinical application of a scoring system for evaluation of antepartum fetal heart rate monitoring. Am J Obstet Gynecol 130:765–772, 1978.

53. Read J, Miller F: Fetal heart rate accelerations in response to acoustic stimulation as a measure of fetal well being. Am J Obstet Gynecol 129:512–518, 1977.

54. Smith C, Phelan J, Paul R, Broussard P: Fetal acoustical stimulation testing: A retrospective experience with the fetal acoustic stimulation test. Am J Obstet Gynecol 153:567–571, 1985.

55. Smith C, Phelan J, Nguyen H, Jacobs N, Paul R: Continued experience with the fetal acoustic stimulation test. J Reprod Med 33:365–369, 1988.

56. Manning FA, Platt L, Sipos L: Antepartum fetal evaluation: Development of a fetal biophysical profile. Am J Obstet Gynecol 136:787–795, 1980.

57. Manning FA, Morrison I, Lange IR, Harman C: Antepartum determination of fetal health: Composite biophysical profile screening. Clin Perinatol 9:285–296, 1982.

58. Platt LD, Eglington GS, Sipos L, Boussard PM, Paul RH: Further experience with the biophysical profile. Obstet Gynecol 61:480–485, 1983.

59. Johnson J, Lange I, Harman C, Manning F: Biophysical profile scoring in the management of post term pregnancy: An analysis of 307 patients. Am J Obstet Gynecol 154:269–277, 1986.

60. Johnson J, Harman C, Lange I, Torchia M, Manning F: Biophysical profile scoring in the management of the diabetic pregnancy. Obstet Gynecol 72:841–846, 1988.

61. Phelan JP, Platt LD, Yeh SY, Broussard P, Paul R: The role of ultrasound assessment of amniotic fluid volume in the management of the postdates pregnancy. Am J Obstet Gynecol 151:304–308, 1985.

62. Rutherford S, Phelan JP, Smith C, Jacobs N: The four-quadrant assessment of amniotic fluid volume: An adjunct to antepartum fetal heart rate testing. Obstet Gynecol 70:353–357, 1987.

63. Brar H, Medearis A, Devore G, Platt L: Fetal umbilical velocimetry using continuous-wave doppler ultrasound in high-risk pregnancies: A comparison of systolic to diastolic ratios. Obstet Gynecol 72:607–612, 1988.

64. Mehalek K, Berkowitz G, Chitkara U, Rosenberg J, Berkowitz R: Comparison of continuous-wave and pulsed doppler S/D ratios of umbilical and uterine arteries. Obstet Gynecol 72:603–609, 1988.

65. Schulman H, Winter D, Farmakides G, Ducey J, Guzman E, Coury A, Penny B: Pregnancy surveillance with doppler velocimetry of uterine and umbilical arteries. Am J Obstet Gynecol 160:192–199, 1989.

66. Wladimiroff J, Wijngaard J, Degani S, Noordam M, v. Eyvk J, Tonge H: Cerebral and umbilical artery blood velocity waveforms in normal and growth retarded pregnancies. Obstet Gynecol 69:705–710, 1987.

67. Giles W, Trudinger B, Cook C, Connelly A: Umbilical artery blood flow velocity waveforms and twin pregnancy outcome. Obstet Gynecol 72:894–899, 1988.

68. Devoe L, Gardner P, Dear C, Castillo R: The diagnostic values of concurrent nonstress testing, amniotic fluid measurement, and doppler velocimetry in screening a general high-risk population. Am J Obstet Gynecol 163:1040–1050, 1990.

CHAPTER 37

Diagnosis and Management of Fetal Asphyxia

Julian T. Parer, M.D., Ph.D.

Intrauterine asphyxia is a common cause of still-births and newborn depression. Asphyxia can occur in the intrapartum period when transient decreases in uterine blood flow occur with each uterine contraction. A placenta with borderline function before the onset of contractions may be unable to provide adequate gas exchange during labor because uterine blood flow is an important determinant of placental function. Fetal asphyxia during pregnancy and labor can most effectively be predicted and therefore avoided by fetal monitoring. After approximately 20 years of clinical use, electronic fetal heart rate (FHR) monitoring is the most accurate screening technique currently available.

Initially, the interpretation of FHR patterns was purely empirical, with a pattern being described as abnormal when a depressed fetus resulted. Transient decelerations of fetal heart rate were noted in some cases with depressed fetuses (1, 2), whereas others noted that variability of fetal heart rate seemed to be a positive sign of fetal health (3). A major source of confusion in interpretation has been the fact that the so-called ominous patterns are actually associated with healthy fetuses in a significant number of cases (4, 5).

This difficulty was at least partially solved by the combination of electronic heart rate monitoring and fetal blood sampling during the intrapartum period. Scalp sampling was used to detect the false abnormal pattern (6–8). More recently there has been a heavier reliance on the presence of the FHR variability as an index of central nervous system (CNS) integrity. This has also enabled obstetricians to act conservatively in the case of what were previously considered "ominous" decelerations, and sometimes to avoid unnecessary invasive intervention (9, 10).

Despite the absence of a complete physiologic understanding of all of the various patterns, FHR monitoring is a valuable aid in diagnosing fetal asphyxia. The following approach to the interpretation of FHR patterns has been found valuable and is becoming widely accepted. It is admittedly still empirical, and its prime aims are: (a) to recognize the fetus that is becoming asphyxiated and that is at risk for physiologic decompensation, and (b) to minimize unnecessary obstetric interference for "fetal distress" except when it is, in fact, needed.

MECHANISMS OF FETAL ASPHYXIA

There are three major mechanisms by which the fetus can become asphyxiated: decreased maternal arterial oxygen tension, inadequate uterine blood flow, and inadequate umbilical blood flow.

Decreased Maternal Arterial Oxygen Tension

This can occur for example, in maternal apnea, pulmonary edema, amniotic fluid embolus, or severe asthma, but it is a relatively rare cause of fetal asphyxia in the intrapartum period.

Inadequate Uterine Blood Flow

Because uterine blood flow is one of the major determinants of oxygen exchange across the placenta, reduction below a certain level will result in inadequate fetal pickup of oxygen. This may occur acutely (e.g., abruptio placentae), chronically (e.g., in severe preeclampsia), or intermittently (with uterine contractions under certain conditions).

Inadequate Umbilical Blood Flow

Oxygen delivery from the fetal side of the placenta to the fetal body depends on an adequate fetal placental blood flow. When this is reduced with umbilical cord obstruction (e.g., during prolapse of the cord) or during severe bradycardia, there may be insufficient oxygen for basic fetal needs.

Variations on these mechanisms may occur. For example, if the fetal oxygen needs are increased in pyrexia resulting from chorioamnionitis, the uterine blood flow may be unable to supply baseline needs, particularly with reductions of uterine blood flow during contractions. Thus there is a relative insufficiency of blood flow.

Another variation may be fetal anemia (e.g., in fetal maternal bleeding or severe Rh isoimmunization). In this case umbilical blood flow may be normal, but there is a relative insufficiency of umbilical oxygen delivery for baseline fetal needs.

FETAL RESPONSES TO ASPHYXIA

There have been many recent studies on fetal responses to oxygen limitation provoked by various means, including reduced uterine and umbilical blood flows (11). It is becoming obvious that the most important protective response is the asphyxia-provoked redistribution of blood flow within the fetus, which favors certain vital organs. During fetal hypoxemia, the arterial venous oxygen concentration difference across the myocardial and cerebral circulation decreases and the respective blood flows increase; therefore oxygen consumption of the heart and brain remain constant (12, 13). In other organs and areas of the body, there is reduced blood flow and oxygen uptake, and metabolism is maintained in these beds by the less efficient anaerobic pathway. The end product, lactic acid, eventually accumulates in the blood, giving rise to a metabolic acidosis.

Numerous mechanisms responsible for these hemodynamic alterations have been identified. These include oxygen levels, carbon dioxide tension, α-adrenergic activity, β-adrenergic activity, arginine vasopressin, endogenous opioids, and prostaglandins (14). There are undoubtedly other as yet unidentified mechanisms.

When asphyxia becomes severe, these protective mechanisms are overwhelmed, and there is intense vasoconstriction of all vascular beds. At such degrees of hypoxia, oxygen consumption by all organs, including those previously favored, decreases. This stage preceeds the final bradycardia, hypotension, and death by a relatively short time period. It is thought that hypoxic organ damage occurs during this phase when physiologic decompensation occurs (15).

CLINICAL FETAL HEART RATE MONITORING

Technology

A number of commercial fetal heart rate monitors are available. They have two major components: a device for detecting each fetal cardiac cycle for processing of the beat-to-beat fetal heart rate and another component for detecting uterine activity. Each of these is displayed on a two-channel strip chart recorder.

Fetal heart rate can be detected invasively or noninvasively. In the invasive mode, an electrode is placed directly into the fetal scalp and a second pole is exposed to the mother's vaginal tissue. This detects the fetal heart beat. A cardiotachometer uses the peak or a threshold voltage of the fetal R wave to measure the period between fetal cardiac cycles. The data are processed and displayed on the chart as the instantaneous or beat-to-beat heart rate for each cardiac interval against time (Fig. 37.1).

The most commonly used device in the noninvasive mode is based on the Doppler principle and uses the frequency shift of an ultrasound wave directed toward the moving fetal heart for detection of cardiac cycles. The ultrasound device is placed on the mother's abdomen. Although it is convenient and

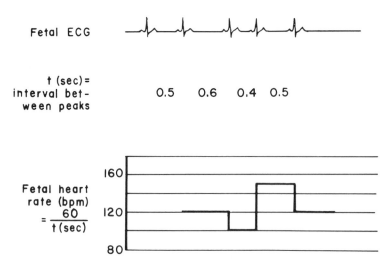

Figure 37.1. The operation of the cardiotachometer. The peaks of the R waves are detected and the time interval between them is measured. This is electronically divided into 60, and the resulting rate is traced on a strip chart recorder. This example shows the normal situation where there are slight differences in the intervals between adjacent heart beats, giving rise to heart rate "variability".

simple to apply, it has certain disadvantages. The Doppler detection of the cardiac cycle is not as discrete as is the detection of the fetal R wave. Thus some artifactual beat-to-beat variability may be displayed. Another disadvantage is that certain data may be lost in processing of the signal. For example, several machines use a running average of adjacent or several beats to compensate for the lack of discreteness of the signal or for missing data. This tends to disguise some of the beat-to-beat variability.

In the invasive mode for detection of uterine activity, a closed or open-ended fluid-filled catheter is placed transvaginally within the amniotic cavity. In this case intraamniotic pressure is detected and processed by a strain gauge transducer and displayed on a second channel of the strip chart recorder. This pressure can be directly quantitated in millimeters of mercury.

Adequate uterine activity is described as that which achieves acceptable cervical dilation per unit time, generally regarded as at least 1 cm/hr dilation in the active phase (9). When cervical dilation is less than this, uterine activity measurements can be used to determine whether such activity is adequate; if not, oxytocin augmentation may be used. Adequate uterine activity is generally described as approximately 250 to 300 Montevideo units, or contractions occurring every 2 or 3 min of 50- to 70-mm Hg intensity.

The noninvasive devise for detecting uterine activity is called the tocodynamometer. This is placed on the mother's abdomen over the uterus and detects the tightening that occurs with uterine contractions. Most commercially available tocodynamometers do not detect the intensity of the contraction, but simply the frequency and duration. Some types of tocodynamometers can be placed on the abdomen with a standard tension. These devices are at least partially quantifiable.

In the United States the almost universally accepted standard for scaling of the strip chart recorder in the above devices is as follows: (a) the paper speed is 3 cm/min on the horizontal scale; and (b) the fetal heart rate is displayed on the vertical scale at 30 beats/min/cm.

This scaling can be important in interpretation. For example, beat-to-beat variability, which is recognized as fluctuations of the recorder pen between adjacent or several beats, can be detected at the speed noted above. However, if a substantially slower speed is used (e.g., 1 cm/min) the beat-to-beat variability is obscured. The use of a slow paper speed tends to exaggerate the appearance of heart rate variability.

A second reason for the importance of scaling is that the heart rate patterns that are described below depend on the scaling. Thus people familiar with patterns at one scale will have difficulty translating the pattern recognition to a different scale with which they are not familiar.

FETAL BLOOD SAMPLING

Fetal blood sampling was introduced initially as an independent means of fetal surveillance during labor (16). Subsequently, an approach consisting of continuous FHR screening, with fetal blood sampling in the case of certain patterns, was introduced (6–8). The extensive list of indications for fetal blood sampling originally proposed has shortened in recent years, with the realization of the favorable prognostic significance of fetal heart rate variability (9, 10, 19).

Scalp sampling is carried out by placing an endoscope against the fetal presenting part and puncturing the fetal skin using a small blade device, until a droplet of blood wells up. This is collected anaerobically and analyzed for pH and P_{CO_2} (and other factors if necessary). The bicarbonate or base excess can be calculated by means of the Henderson-Hasselbalch equation. It has been noted that at pHs above 7.2 to 7.25 the fetus is generally vigorous at birth, whereas at pHs below 7.2 the fetus is usually depressed (6, 17, 18). However, there is a considerable overlap in the groups, and a single value such as 7.2 cannot be relied on entirely. Numerous other factors must be taken into account, such as the maternal acid-base status, the relationship of the sampling to uterine contractions, the permanence of the placental insult, the influence of in utero treatment, the type of acidosis (i.e., respiratory versus metabolic), the stage of labor, and the various other clinical aspects of the particular case.

The current integration of fetal blood sampling into FHR management is described more fully in discussions of management of various FHR patterns below.

TREATMENT OF THE FETUS IN UTERO

Only since the advent of heart rate monitoring and fetal blood sampling has it been possible to effectively treat the fetus undergoing asphyxial stress in utero. Previously such treatment could not be used rationally because there was no way of knowing whether the fetal condition improved.

Placental respiratory function is determined by adequacy of blood flow on each side of the placenta and adequate delivery of oxygen to and removal of carbon dioxide from the fetal circulation. Maneuvers used to treat the fetus in utero are directed toward correcting deficiencies in these functions. These treatments are listed in (Table 37.1) together with the supposed insult and the expected mechanism of correction of the defect.

Table 37.1
Treatment of the Fetus in Utero

Events Inciting Abnormal Patterns	Possible FHR Patterns	Corrective Maneuver	Mechanism
Hypotension (e.g., supine hypotension, conduction anesthesia)	Bradycardia; late decelerations	Intravenous fluids; position change; ephedrine	Restoration of uterine blood flow toward normal
Excessive uterine activity	Bradycardia; late decelerations	Decrease in oxytocin; lateral position	Restoration of uterine blood flow toward normal
Transient umbilical cord compression	Variable decelerations	Change in maternal position (e.g., left or right lateral, Trendelenburg)	Restoration of umbilical blood flow toward normal
Head compression in second stage	Variable decelerations	Discourage "pushing" efforts; and as above	Restoration of umbilical blood flow toward normal
Decreased uterine blood flow associated with uterine contraction below limits of fetal basal O_2 needs	Late decelerations	Change in maternal position (e.g., left lateral, Trendelenburg); establishment of maternal hyperoxia	Enhancement of uterine blood flow to optimum; increase in maternal-fetal O_2 gradient
		(?Tocolytic agents [e.g., ritodrine or terbutaline])	(Decrease in contractions, thus abolishing associated decrease of uterine blood flow)
Prolonged asphyxia	Decreasing FHR variability	Change in maternal position (e.g., left lateral position or Trendelenburg); establishment of maternal hyperoxia	Enhancement of uterine blood flow to optimum; increase in maternal fetal O_2 gradient

Characteristics of Fetal Heart Rate Tracings

BASELINE FEATURES

The baseline features of the heart rate are those predominant characteristics that can be recognized between uterine contractions. These consist of the following:

1. *Baseline rate.* The baseline fetal heart rate is conventionally considered to be between 120 and 160 beats/min. Values below 120 are termed bradycardia and those above 160, tachycardia.

2. *Fetal heart rate variability.* Two characteristics of fetal heart rate variability are clinically recognized. First, short-term variability is considered to be the beat-to-beat fluctuations in heart rate that arise from the slightly different period between R waves in the normal fetus. The second component is called long-term variability which can be described as either amplitude changes or frequency changes. These longer term unidirectional changes of fetal heart rate occupy a cycle of less than 1 min. In the United States, the most commonly accepted quantitation of long-term variability is the approximate bandwidth of the amplitude fluctuations in long-term variability. Frequency changes in long-term variability have gained little popularity for use in clinical practice.

PERIODIC PATTERNS

Periodic patterns are the alterations in fetal heart rate associated with uterine contractions. These con-sist of late decelerations, variable decelerations, and accelerations.

Normal Pattern

The normal fetal heart rate pattern (Fig. 37.2) has a predominant heart rate of 120 to 160 beats/min. Beat-to-beat variability is present, and long-term variability bandwidth is between 6 and 25 beats/min. There are no decelerative periodic changes, but there may be periodic accelerations.

It is widely accepted in clinical practice that the fetus born with this normal heart rate pattern is essentially "guaranteed" to be normally oxygenated if it is delivered when the normal heart rate pattern is traced. Of course, this will not hold should there be a subsequent traumatic delivery or a congenital anomaly inconsistent with extrauterine life.

In contrast to this high predictability of fetal normoxia with the normal pattern, there are a number of variant patterns that do not predict fetal asphyxia accurately. However, when placed in the context of the clinical case, the progressive change in the patterns, and the duration of the variant patterns, reasonable judgments can be made about the likelihood of fetal asphyxial decompensation. When this is used as a screening approach, impending intolerable fetal asphyxia can be presumed or, in certain cases, ruled out by the use of ancillary techniques such as the fetal stimulation test or fetal blood sampling.

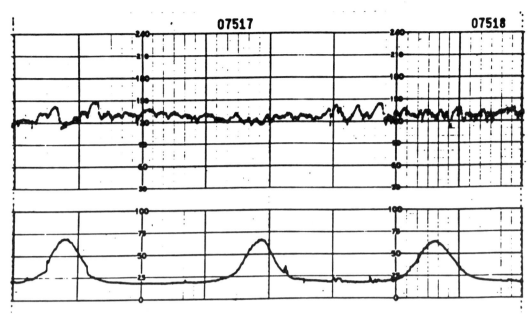

Figure 37.2. Normal fetal heart rate pattern with normal rate and variability and absence of periodic changes. This pattern illustrates a normally oxygenated fetus. Paper speed = 3 cm/min.

VARIANT FETAL HEART RATE PATTERNS

Rate Changes

BRADYCARDIA

The normal fetus initially responds to acute hypoxia or asphyxia with bradycardia (11). This statement contrasts with some earlier beliefs in which, under acutely operated or anesthetized conditions, fetal tachycardia was sometimes noted in response to acutely imposed hypoxia.

There are a number of nonasphyxial causes of bradycardia. These include the bradyarrhythmias (e.g., complete heart block), certain drugs (e.g., the β-blockers), or hypothermia. Other fetuses have a heart rate below 120 beats/min but are otherwise totally normal and simply represent a normal variation outside our arbitrarily set limits of normal heart rate.

Bradycardia is arbitrarily distinguished from the transient decelerations. A bradycardia represents a decrease in heart rate below 120 beats/min for 2 min or longer.

Prolonged bradycardia represents a prolonged stepwise decrease in fetal oxygenation (Fig. 37.3). This may be a consequence of fetal hypoxia resulting from vagal activity (and later, hypoxic myocardial decompression), or the bradycardia may eventually result in fetal hypoxia because of the fetus' inability to maintain a compensatory increase in stroke volume. The hypoxic fetus can increase stroke volume in response to bradycardia but loses this ability at severe decreases in heart rate such as below 60 beats/

min. Under these conditions, fetal cardiac output cannot be maintained, and therefore umbilical blood flow decreases. This results in insufficient oxygen transport from the fetal placenta to the fetal body and therefore in eventual fetal hypoxic decompensation. The decreased heart rate may result from a stepwise decrease in oxygenation such as occurs with maternal apnea or amniotic fluid embolus, a decrease in umbilical blood flow such as occurs with a prolapsed cord, or a decrease in uterine blood flow such as occurs with severe maternal hypotension.

TACHYCARDIA

Tachycardia is seen in some cases of fetal asphyxia but never alone. That is, in the presence of normal fetal heart rate variability and absent periodic changes, the tachycardia must be assumed to result from some cause other than hypoxia (11). Tachycardia is sometimes seen on recovery from asphyxia and probably represents catecholamine activity after increased sympathetic nervous or adrenal medullary activity in response to this asphyxial stress.

There are a number of nonasphyxial causes of tachycardia, the most common being maternal or fetal infections, especially chorioamnionitis. Drugs—including β-mimetic agents or parasympathetic blockers such as atropine—will cause tachycardia. Tachyarrythmias occasionally occur, and, at severe heart rate increases such as above 240 beats/min, they may cause fetal cardiac failure with subsequent hydrops.

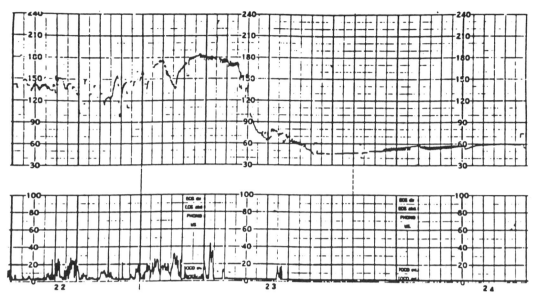

Figure 37.3. Sudden prolonged fetal bradycardia in a woman with an amniotic fluid embolus. There is immediate bradycardia to less than 60 beats/min with the onset of maternal cyanosis and pulmonary edema. There is also loss of fetal heart rate variability. (*Lower trace* = uterine activity.)

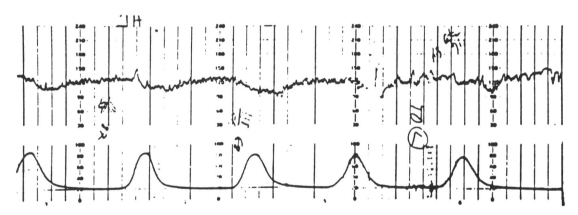

Figure 37.4. Reflex late decelerations. They are smooth and rounded in configuration and shifted to the right of the uterine contraction. Note the retention of fetal heart rate variability. (*Lower trace* = uterine contraction.)

Periodic Changes

LATE DECELERATIONS

Late decelerations have the following characteristics: They are smooth in configuration and are the mirror image of the contraction; their onset, nadir, and recovery are delayed 10 to 30 sec after the onset, apex, and resolution of the contraction; they are persistent, occurring with each contraction; and the depth of the dip is related to the intensity of the contraction (Fig. 37.4) (20).

There are two varieties of late decelerations (9). The first type, reflex late deceleration, is seen when a sudden acute insult (e.g., maternal hypotension) is superimposed on a previously normally oxygenated fetus. These late decelerations are caused by decreased uterine blood flow (with the uterine contraction) beyond the capacity of the fetus to extract sufficient oxygen. The deoxygenated blood is carried from the fetal placenta through the umbilical veins to the fetal heart and is distributed to the aorta, neck vessels, and head. Here, the low oxygen tension is sensed by chemoreceptors, and neuronal activity results in a vagal discharge, which causes the transient deceleration. The deceleration is presumed to be "late" because of the circulation time from the fetal placental site to the chemoreceptors. There may also be baroreceptor activity causing the vagal discharge (22, 23). Between contractions, oxygen delivery is adequate, so the heart rate is normal.

These late decelerations are accompanied by normal fetal heart rate variability, thus signify normal cerebral oxygenation (i.e., the fetus is physiologically "compensated" in the vital organs).

The second type of late deceleration results from the same initial mechanism, except that the deoxygenated bolus of blood from the placenta is insufficient to support myocardial action, so that for the period of the contraction there is direct myocardial hypoxic depression (or failure) as well as vagal activity (24). This variety is seen without variability (Fig. 37.5) signifying fetal "decompensation" (i.e., inadequate fetal cerebral and myocardial oxygenation). It is seen most commonly in states of decreased placental reserve (e.g., with preeclampsia or intrauterine growth retardation) or after prolonged asphyxial stresses, such as 30 min of severe late decelerations.

Severe late decelerations are those with a decrease of more that 45 beats/min below the baseline. There are heart rate and duration criteria for identifying mild and moderate late decelerations (Table 37.2) but they are mainly statistically, rather than clinically, important. The major factor to observe is retention of fetal heart rate variability. The fetus with the non-reflex type of late decelerations is considerably more acidotic than those with reflex late decelerations (Fig. 37.6).

When there are late decelerations, vigorous efforts should be made to eliminate them by optimizing placental blood flows and maternal hyperoxia. Vagal late decelerations, which result in most cases from an acute asphyxial episode, generally can be abolished. However, those caused by myocardial failure usually are seen when placental reserve is surpassed and the intermittent decreases in uterine blood flow with each contraction can no longer be tolerated.

Abolition of such late decelerations is unlikely, and rapid delivery is recommended.

VARIABLE DECELERATIONS

Variable decelerations (Fig. 37.7) have the following characteristics:

1. The appearance of the dip is variable in duration, profundity, and shape from contraction to contraction.

2. Variable decelerations are usually abrupt in onset and cessation, sometimes decreasing 60 beats/min in one or several beats. They are thus neurogenic (vagal) in origin.

3. They are described as severe when the decelerations are below 60 beats/min, 60 beats/min below baseline fetal heart rate, or longer than 60 sec in duration. Although other criteria have been proposed, those of Robert Goodlin's "Rule of 60s" as presented here are the most simple and practical.

4. Variable decelerations without the criteria listed in item 3 are classified as mild to moderate.

These abrupt heart rate decelerations represent the firing of the vagus nerve in response to certain stimuli, either umbilical cord compression (generally in the first stage of labor) or possibly substantial head compression (e.g., during pushing, late in the second stage of labor). Whether the fetus is still normoxic in the central tissues (i.e., physiologically compensated) can be determined by observation of the maintenance of fetal heart rate variability.

There are heart rate and duration criteria for mild and moderate variable decelerations, but these classifications are not important (Table 37.2). The major factor to observe is retention of baseline fetal heart rate variability.

When there are severe variable decelerations, vigorous efforts should be made to abolish them because it is likely that even the fetus with normal growth

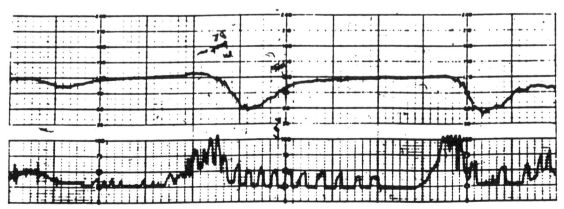

Figure 37.5. A sinister heart rate pattern with absent variability and severe late decelerations. Same patient as Figure 35.9, 11 hr later; 3340-g female with Apgar scores of 3 (1 min) and 4 (5 min). Cesarean section was considered contraindicated due to a severe maternal coagulopathy.

Table 37.2
Grading of Late and Variable Decelerations[a]

Deceleration	Mild	Moderate	Severe
Late	Drop in FHR of less than 15 beats/min	Drop in FHR of 15 to 45 beats/min	Drop in FHR of more than 45 beats/min
Variable	Duration shorter than 30 sec regardless of heart rate		
	or		
	Heart rate greater than 80 beats/min regardless of duration	Heart rate less than 70 beats/min with a duration of 30 to 60 sec	Heart rate less than 70 beats/min with a duration longer than 60 sec
	or	*or*	
	Heart rate greater than 70 beats/min with duration shorter than 60 sec	Heart rate greater than 70 beats/min with a duration of longer than 60 sec	

[a] Adapted from Kubli FW, Hon EH, Khazin AF, Takemura H: Observations on heart rate and pH in the human fetus during labor. Am J Obstet Gynecol 104:1190–1206, 1969.

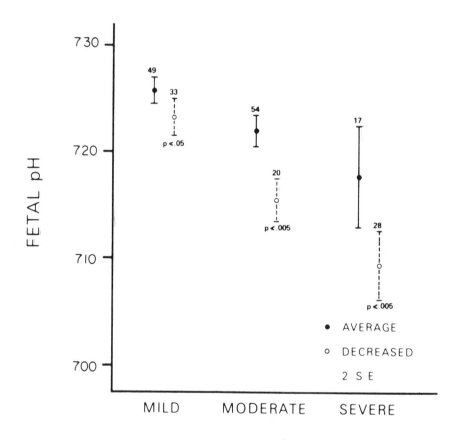

Figure 37.6. As late deceleration patterns become more marked, the mean pH value falls. However, when FHR variability is present in association with late deceleration patterns, the mean pH is consistently higher than when it is absent. (Reprinted by permission from Paul RH, Suidan AK, Yeh SY, Schifrin BS, Hon EH: Clinical fetal monitoring. VII. The evaluation and significance of intrapartum baseline FHR variability. Am J Obstet Gynecol 123:206-210, 1975.)

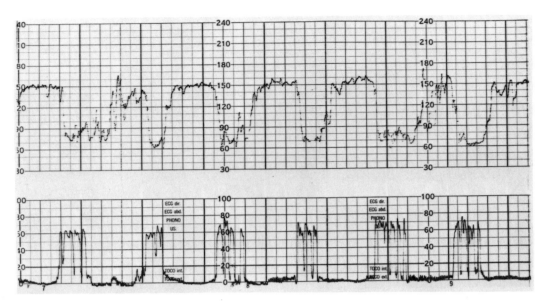

Figure 37.7. Variable decelerations. Intrapartum recording using fetal scalp electrode and tocodynamometer. The spikes on the uterine activity channel represent maternal pushing efforts in the second stage of labor. Note normal baseline variability between contractions. Paper speed = 3 cm/min.

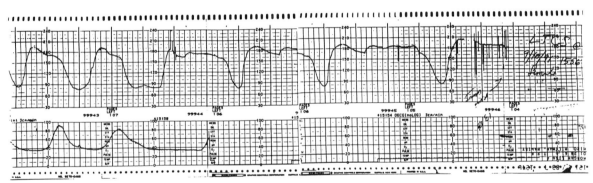

Figure 37.8. This fetal heart rate pattern of profound decelerations and absent fetal heart rate variability must be considered to represent serious asphyxia unless it can be ruled out by ancillary testing, such as fetal scalp sampling. Because the majority of such fetuses are, in fact, deeply asphyxiated, emergent delivery is recommended.

and placental function will eventually decompensate, although not usually before 30 min. However, the normal fetus can better tolerate mild or moderate variable decelerations for a prolonged period.

Some patterns are so severe that they must be considered to represent asphyxia unless it can be rapidly ruled out (Fig. 37.8). These consist of absent variability and profound decelerations, which at times are difficult to distinguish as late or variable. One cannot be certain whether such fetuses have already suffered cerebral damage, so rapid delivery is recommended.

ACCELERATIONS WITH CONTRACTIONS

Accelerations sometimes occur with uterine contractions and have no adverse prognostic significance (Fig 37.9). They are probably similar to the accelerations that are seen with fetal movements in the antepartum period and thus indicate a reactive and healthy fetus. Accelerations with contractions probably are the net result of greater sympathetic activity than parasympathetic activity during contractions with particular fetuses.

Fetal Heart Rate Variability Changes

Fetal heart rate variability is believed to represent an intact neurologic pathway that includes the fetal cerebral cortex, midbrain, vagus nerve, and cardiac conduction system (9). As noted previously, during asphyxia there is augmentation of blood flow to the brain and heart that matches the degree of hypoxemia such that there is constancy of oxygen uptake by these organs. However, at severe degrees of hypoxia these compensatory mechanisms break down and oxygen uptake can no longer be maintained by these organs. This decompensation may result from acute profound stepwise asphyxia or occur after prolonged

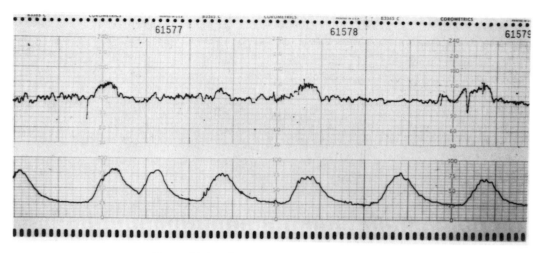

Figure 37.9. Accelerations with contractions.

Table 37.3
Nonasphyxic Causes of Decreased Variability

Drugs
  Central depressants (e.g., narcotics, tranquilizers)
  Parasympatholytics (e.g., atropine, scopolamine)
Tachycardia
Prematurity
"Sleep"
Bradyarrhythmias
Anencephaly

intermittent asphyxial stresses. This produces cumulative oxygen debt, which eventually prevents the fetus from maintaining oxygenation of the vital organs.

The current clinical approach is that, in the presence of bradycardias or a prolonged series of late or variable decelerations, when fetal heart rate variability decreases or is intermittently lost, one must assume that the fetus is becoming severely centrally asphyxiated, unless one can demonstrate otherwise by other techniques.

There are many other causes of decreased fetal heart rate variability besides asphyxia (Table 37.3) and part of the art of clinical management is determining when asphyxia is the cause and when it is unlikely to be the cause.

The most important concept is that decreased fetal heart rate variability resulting from asphyxia during the intrapartum period always follows the asphyxial stress patterns: bradycardia, late decelerations, or variable decelerations.

CURRENT MANAGEMENT RECOMMENDATIONS

These three asphyxial stress patterns are common during labor, but they rarely result in fetal neurologic damage. There is a substantial fetal resistance because of the physiologic mechanisms mentioned above. To clinically recognize asphyxial decompensation in the fetus, we note the persistence and time course of changes in the fetal heart rate pattern. Experience suggests that a previously normoxic baby can tolerate decelerations or severe variable decelerations for at least 30 min before decompensating.

The evolution of intrapartum fetal heart rate patterns during asphyxia is established, and it is known that fetal heart rate variability decreases and then disappears before substantial fetal depression or fetal death in utero. This decrease in fetal heart rate variability is considered to correlate clinically with decreased central nervous system function, which is presumed to precede central nervous system damage.

From the clinical management perspective, the approach above is important. It suggests that there is time for conservative management to alleviate the stress patterns before operative delivery is warranted. Thus, with uncorrectable decreased fetal heart rate variability in the presence of persistent asphyxial stress patterns, the fetus should be delivered immediately. With continued normal fetal heart rate variability with those stress patterns, one can conservatively await a vaginal delivery in selected cases.

Fetal blood sampling for acid-base measurement or fetal stimulation testing may be valuable in uncertain cases (26, 27). This approach implies the ability to rapidly "rescue" the fetus if the need arises, so decision-delivery times may need to be relatively short (i.e., 15 min or less).

Severe prolonged and sustained bradycardias are similar in some respects to the above. It has been noted that a bradycardia between 100 and 120 beats/min with normal fetal heart rate variability can be tolerated by most fetuses for essentially unlimited periods of time. In contrast, a fetal heart rate less than 60 beats/min (in the absence of heart block) is an obstetric emergency that necessitates immediate delivery. There is some evidence that neurologic damage may begin at 10 min in such cases. It is our current belief that a sustained fetal heart rate less than 80 beats/min also should be managed by immediate preparation for delivery, whereas rates of 80 to 100 beats/min can be handled more conservatively. In all of these cases, the presence of fetal heart rate variability has persistently been the most important prognostic sign of continued fetal central nervous system compensation.

FURTHER FETAL HEART RATE PATTERNS AND THEIR MANAGEMENT

Tachycardia

The most common cause of tachycardia is amnionitis, almost invariably seen with maternal fever. Fetal heart rate rarely exceeds 200 beats/min, and variability is retained, although there may be a tendency for it to decrease.

It is important to note that an uncomplicated tachycardia—that is, one with retention of FHR variability and without periodic changes—does not signify fetal asphyxia, in contrast to previously held beliefs. The infected fetus will have an increased oxygen need and may have relative hypoxia during labor, but this will show up as late decelerations.

Bradycardias

As noted previously, bradycardia is defined as a heart rate below 120 beats/min for 2 min or longer. This is to distinguish it from deceleration, which refers to a decrease in FHR below 120 beats/min for less than 2 min. These criteria are arbitrary and have been developed primarily for communication rather than being based strictly on a physiologic foundation.

Nomenclature has developed for the various bradycardias reflecting their appearance, occurrence, or presumed etiologic factors.

PROLONGED BRADYCARDIA

A moderate bradycardia (i.e., not below 100 beats/min) in the second stage of labor may represent continuous head compression and therefore vagal activity. Provided FHR variability is maintained the pattern is not associated with fetal acidosis.

Some fetuses with moderate bradycardia may in fact be totally normal, simply reflecting the fact that 120 beats/min may be too high as the lower limit of normal. The term *prolonged bradycardia* is generally applied to a sudden drop from a normal FHR to values below 120 beats/min, and especially below 80 beats/min. Bradycardia is the initial fetal response to

peripheral or central chemoreceptor activity. The asphyxial stimulus may be due to: (a) a decrease in maternal O_2 tension, such as during the apnea of a seizure; (b) a decrease in uterine blood flow, such as during excessive uterine contractions or acute maternal hypotension; (c) a decrease in umbilical blood flow (due to cord compression); or (d) loss of placental area (such as in abruptio placentae). The extent of bradycardia will depend on the degree of hypoxia. It may also be the baroreflex influence causing the bradycardia at more severe degrees of asphyxia.

In rare cases a prolonged bradycardia is the result of fetal hemorrhage, usually catastrophic, such as tearing of vasa previa or rupture of an anomalous fetal placental vessel in a velamentous umbilical cord insertion.

Immediately upon recognition of a bradycardia attempts should be made to optimize fetal oxygenation by methods outlined earlier (Table 37.1). There is rarely a need for grave concern if a moderate bradycardia is not abolished. However, if the bradycardia is below 100 beats/min, then more vigorous efforts should be made to alleviate it even in the presence of good FHR variability. A bradycardia below 60 beats/min will almost invariably result in fetal asphyxic decompensation eventually, and becomes an obstetric emergency to abolish it or deliver the baby before severe central asphyxia occurs.

Most of these sudden bradycardias tend to resolve spontaneously with various positional changes. Such bradycardias are particularly likely to occur in the postdates pregnancy. Such fetuses appear to be extremely responsive to various stimuli such as stimulation of the head during a vaginal examination, application of a scalp electrode, or even certain abrupt maternal positional changes. This has been ascribed to an excessively reactive vagus nerve in such fetuses. Generally these prolonged bradycardias are of sufficient concern that many women whose babies exhibit several of them are brought to the delivery room for labor and possible operative delivery, in case the FHR does not recover after one of them.

PROLONGED END-STAGE BRADYCARDIA

Prolonged end-stage bradycardia refers to a sudden prolonged deceleration, generally late in the second stage of labor in the presence of an otherwise normal FHR tracing. It is fairly common and will be seen much more frequently if one adopts the practice of taking the monitor to the delivery room and monitoring the fetus up until the time of delivery.

This is quite likely to be a vagal response to head compression as the head traverses the depths of the pelvis. It may be due to dural stimulation or brief local cerebral ischemia during head compression.

It has been observed that if the heart rate is at 80 beats/min or above, and the heart rate variability retained (which it usually is), fetuses can tolerate this condition for an almost unlimited amount of time. However, should the heart rate be persistently low and/or the heart rate variability lost, the author recommends termination of labor by delivery at this point. Since the vast majority of these patterns are seen with the head crowning, this is often simply a matter of cutting an episiotomy or applying outlet forceps. In other cases, delivery can be accomplished by encouraging voluntary maternal efforts.

Sometimes the decelerations in late second stage can be abolished by discouraging pushing with every other contraction. By this means the baby is allowed to "catch its breath" with each alternate push.

POSTPARACERVICAL BLOCK BRADYCARDIA

Postparacervical block bradycardia occurs on the average of 7 min after the paracervical block is administered and lasts an average of 8 min. The range in both of these values, the degree of bradycardia, and the associated FHR abnormalities are quite variable. Its incidence varies from 0 to 56% depending on the drug dosage and definition. An average incidence is 15%. Some fetal deaths have been associated with paracervical block bradycardia (28).

Although the etiologic factors are controversial, the most likely cause of the bradycardia is direct fetal toxicity by the local anesthetic drug, not necessarily by direct fetal injection but by rapid uptake by the fetus, possibly via the uterine arteries. The fetal level of the drugs can be quite high, although rarely higher than that of the mother. A further theory is that the local anesthetic agent causes a spasm of the uterine arteries, resulting in decreased uterine blood flow and hence fetal asphyxia. Acidosis has been demonstrated in these fetuses by blood sampling during the bradycardia (28).

Minimization of this undesirable side effect of paracervical block is assisted by using minimal quantities and volumes of drug. Careful technique to ensure that the drug is placed just submucosally will avoid accidental fetal injection. Paracervical block is considered to be contraindicated in the case of a fetus that already has an abnormal FHR pattern.

If the bradycardia does develop, supportive management is recommended (Table 37.1). If the pattern does resolve, and if the FHR returns to normal, no further evaluation is needed, but repeat paracervical injection should be avoided.

Except in rare and profoundly abnormal cases, delivery should be avoided during this bradycardia because the fetus is better able to get rid of the drug transplacentally than to detoxify it postnatally.

Dysrhythmias

A number of case reports have described numerous fetal dysrhythmias that have been diagnosed in utero. These include complete heart block, premature atrial contractions, premature ventricular contractions, bigeminy, supraventricular tachycardia, paroxysmal atrial tachycardia, blocked atrial premature beats, atrial flutter, and asystole of variable duration.

The FHR monitor detects and depicts the interval between beats and is thus a very sensitive dysrhythmia detector. Bradyarrhythmias are the most commonly reported. These appear as FHR tracings of approximately 50 to 60 beats/min, with virtually absent FHR variability. Bradycardias and tachycardias may be doubled or halved by the cardiotachometer, particularly in the Doppler mode. This artifact can almost always be ruled out by brief auscultation.

These dysrhythmias generally represent cardiac conduction defects, which have an anatomic or functional basis. The persistent types appear to have a worse prognosis than the intermittent ones, the latter often resolving in the newborn.

Complete heart block has an incidence of about 1 in 20,000 births, and approximately 30% of cases are associated with heart disease, often a cardiac structural abnormality. About 10% of newborns with congenital heart block die in early infancy.

The extreme tachycardias, generally above 240 beats/min, have sometimes been associated with hydrops, apparently because of intrauterine cardiac failure. There are case reports of in utero treatments with digoxin, β-adrenergic blocking agents, procainamide, or calcium channel blockers. In some cases there has been resolution of the hydrops.

A great deal of concern was experienced in the past over the fetus with a dysrhythmia. It has become obvious that only rarely are early interventions required and most of these infants can tolerate labor well. The author has investigated such cases with an attempted fetal ECG by external abdominal electrode, sonography, and echocardiography. The latter has been most helpful in diagnosing the condition and determining whether there are any obvious structural abnormalities before birth. The author has used internal fetal monitoring during labor with supplemental fetal blood sampling because of frequently bizarre FHR patterns.

Infants with heart block often have mothers with collagen vascular disease, particularly systemic lupus erythematosis, so such women should be screened appropriately.

The major problem in the fetus with dysrhythmia is generally in the newborn period. The author recommends that such infants be delivered in a tertiary care center with immediate access to pediatric cardiology care. Those with heart block may need cardiac pacing and those with a tachycardia may need digitalizing to prevent cardiac failure.

Sinusoidal Pattern

Sinusoidal pattern is a regular, smooth, sine wave-like baseline with a frequency of approximately 3 to 6/min and an amplitude range of up to 30 beats/min. The regularity of waves and lack of short-term variability distinguish the pattern from long-term variability complexes, which are crudely shaped and irregular.

The pattern was first described in a group of severely affected Rh-isoimmunized fetuses, but has subsequently been noted in association with fetuses that are anemic for other reasons, and in asphyxiated infants. It has also been described in cases of normal infants born without depression or acid-base abnormalities, although in the latter cases there is dispute about whether the patterns are truly sinusoidal or whether, because of the moderately irregular pattern, they are variants of long-term variability. Such patterns are also sometimes seen after administration of Butrophanol or nalbuphine to the mother. The author believes that an essential characteristic of the sinusoidal pattern is extreme regularity and smoothness.

If the sinusoidal pattern is seen in an Rh-sensitized patient with substantial hemolysis (as noted by the value of the change in optical density at 450 nm in amniotic fluid), this signifies a need for rapid intervention. This may take the form of delivery, or possibly intrauterine transfusion, depending on the gestational age and the preceding Rh data, treatment, and workup.

Management in the absence of Rh disease is somewhat more difficult to recommend. If the pattern is persistent, monotonously regular, and unaccompanied by short-term variability, and cannot be abolished by maneuvers as outlined above, fetal blood sampling is indicated. If fetal blood sampling is not available, delivery is recommended.

However, if the pattern is irregularly sinusoidal or "pseudosinusoidal," intermittently present, and not associated with intervening periodic decelerations, then it is very unlikely to indicate fetal compromise. Hence, immediate delivery is not warranted. Fetal blood sampling may assist in confirming normality in such cases.

Saltatory Pattern

Saltatory pattern consists of rapid variations in FHR with a frequency of 3 to 6/min, and amplitude range greater than 25 beats/min. It is qualitatively described as excessive variability, and the excessive swings have a strikingly bizarre appearance.

The saltatory pattern was associated with low Apgar scores in early discussions of FHR variability, but it was not possible to relate the time course of the pattern to the fetal depression (3). That is, fetuses with the pattern in the intrapartum period tended to have low Apgar scores, but it was not clear whether the pattern was present immediately before delivery or it preceded an evolution to a more serious FHR pattern.

Saltatory pattern is almost invariably seen during labor, rather than in the antepartum period. Because the author believes the fetus with this pattern is hemodynamically compensated (although it may be moderately asphyxically stressed), it is recommended that attempts be made to abolish it, by maneuvers such as the lateral position, avoidance of hypotension, avoidance of excessive uterine activity, and possibly maternal hyperoxia. The author does not know of such a pattern that has evolved into fetal decompensation; it probably has similar significance to mild or moderate variable decelerations.

THE PRETERM FETUS

Several investigators have examined both the antepartum and intrapartum FHR patterns of prematures, and their relationship to fetal blood acid-base status (29). There now seems little doubt that the same criteria used in the term fetus can be used for the premature. An important difference, however, is that prematures can quickly develop abnormal patterns, and that these patterns tend to progress much more rapidly in their severity than those in the term fetus.

There are some commonly held beliefs with regard to premature fetuses that are in error. The first is that prematures normally have a tachycardia. The second is that prematures have "flat baselines." In fact, the average FHR of the 28-week-old fetus is about 150 beats/min with a range of about 130 to 170—that is, only slightly above that of the term fetus. On the second point, most prematures have normal FHR variability, and with its disappearance or absence the management should be the same as that for a term fetus, even in the presence of a tachycardia. However, there is a tendency for prematures to have a smaller amplitude of variability.

CONGENITAL ANOMALIES

Except as described for the dysrhythmias, the vast majority of fetuses with congenital anomalies have normal FHR patterns and a response to asphyxia similar to that of the normal fetus (30). There are several exceptions, for example, in the case of complete heart block and anencephaly. Thus aneuploid fetuses such as those with Down's syndrome and trisomy 18, and those with aplastic lungs, meningomyelocele, hydrocephalus, and so on, may give no FHR warning of the defects. In one series it was noted that, although there was no pathognomonic pattern in such fetuses, the rate of cesarean section for fetal distress was significantly increased (24).

An important exception is seen with Potter's syndrome. Such fetuses are generally recognized as growth retarded because of the oligohydramnios, and in addition may have substantial variable decelerations, presumably for the same reason. That is, umbilical cord compression is more likely without the "padding" of adequate amniotic fluid. A number of such fetuses have been delivered by cesarean section for "fetal distress," with the tragic outcome of rapid neonatal death due to hypoplastic lungs.

There is no simple solution to the problem of emergency intervention (generally cesarean section) for the fetus who is destined to be severely defective or die in the neonatal period. Genetic evaluation in certain high risk groups may decrease the incidence of such problems, but in the case of a youthful primipara without significant family history of genetic disease, screening is not yet available, except possibly for open neural tube defects by α-fetoprotein measurements.

Even the advances in sonography for visualizing the fetus may be of borderline help during labor, because there are few defects that can definitely determine that a fetus should be "written off" at this stage. Such defects as severe hydrocephalus, severe meningomyelocele, and renal agenesis may fit this category, but many other defective fetuses, especially those with metabolic disorders or tracheal and certain other soft tissue abnormalities, often are not detected. In the case of asphyxic decompensation, such fetuses must be given the benefit of the doubt, and if necessary a cesarean section must be performed.

References

1. Hon EH: *An Atlas of Fetal Heart Rate Patterns.* Harty Press, New Haven, CT, 1968.
2. Caldeyro-Barcia R, Mendez-Bauer C, Poseiro JJ, Escarcena LA, Pose SV, Bieniarez J, Arnt I, Galin L, Althabe O: Control of human fetal heart rate during labor. In *The Heart and Circulation in the Newborn and Infant.* DE Cassels, ed. Grune & Stratton, New York, 1966, p 7.
3. Hammacher K, Huter KA, Bokelmann J, Werners PH: Foetal heart frequency and perinatal condition of the foetus and newborn. Gynaecologia 166:349-360, 1968.
4. Hon EH: Detection of fetal distress. In *Fifth World Congress of Gynecology and Obstetrics.* C Wood, ed. Butterworth, London, 1967, p 58.
5. Shifrin BS, Dame L: Fetal heart rate patterns: Prediction of Apgar score. JAMA 219:1322-1325, 1972.
6. Wood C, Newman W, Lumley L, Hammond J: Classification of fetal heart rate in relation to fetal scalp blood measurements and Apgar score. Am J Obstet Gynecol 105:942-948, 1969.
7. Beard RW, Filshie GM, Knight CA, Roberts GM: The significance of the changes in the continuous fetal heart rate in the first stage of labour. J Obstet Gynaecol Br Commonw 78:865-881, 1971.
8. Tejani N, Mann LI, Bhakthavathsalan C, Weiss RR: Correlation of fetal heart rate-uterine contraction patterns with fetal scalp blood pH. Obstet Gynecol 46:392-396, 1975.
9. Parer JT: *Handbook of Fetal Heart Rate Monitoring.* Saunders, Philadelphia, 1983.
10. Krebs HB, Petres RE, Dunn LE, Jordan HV, Segreti A: Intrapartum fetal heart rate monitoring. I. Classification and prognosis of fetal heart rate patterns. Am J Obstet Gynecol 133:762-772, 1979.
11. Court DJ, Parer JT: Experimental studies of fetal asphyxia and fetal heart rate interpretation. In *Research in Perinatal Medicine.* PW Nathanielsz, JT Parer, eds. Perinatology Press, New York, 1984, pp 113-169.
12. Fisher DJ, Heymann MA, Rudolph AM: Fetal myocardial and carbohydrate consumption during acutely induced hypoxia. Am J Physiol 242:H657-H661, 1982.
13. Jones MD, Sheldon RE, Peeters LL, Meschia G, Battaglia FC, Makowski EL: Fetal cerebral oxygen consumption at different levels of oxygenation. J Appl Physiol 43:1080-1084, 1977.
14. Auslender R, Arnold SA, Parer JT, Glosten B, Johnson J, Preston P: The effects of meclofenamate on fetal hemodynamics during hypoxia. *Proceeding of the International Symposium: Foetal and Neonatal Development.* CT Jones, ed. Perinatology Press, New York, 1988, pp 353-358.
15. Yaffe H, Parer JT, Block BS, Llanos AJ: Cardiorespiratory responses to graded reductions of uterine blood flow in the sheep fetus. J Dev Physiol 9:325-336, 1987.
16. Saling E, Scheider D: Biochemical supervision of the foetus during labour. J Obstet Gynaecol Br Commonw 74:799-811, 1967.
17. Beard RW, Morris ED, Clayton SG: pH of foetal capillary blood as an indicator of the condition of the foetus. J Obstet Gynaecol Br Commonw 74:812-822, 1967.
18. Mendez-Bauer C, Arnt IC, Gulin L, Escarcena L, Caldeyro-Barcia R: Relationship between blood pH and heart rate in the human fetus during labor. Am J Obstet Gynecol 97:530-545, 1967.
19. Paul RH, Suidan AK, Yeh SY, Schifrin BS, Hon EH: Clinical fetal monitoring. VIII. The evaluation and significance of intrapartum baseline FHR variability. Am J Obstet Gynecol 123:206-210, 1975.
20. Hon EH, Quilligan EJ: The classification of fetal heart rate. II. A revised working classification. Conn Med 31:779-784, 1967.
21. Parer JT, Krueger TR, Harris JL: Fetal oxygen consumption and mechanisms of heart rate response during artificially produced late deceleration of fetal heart rate in sheep. Am J Obstet Gynecol 136:478-482, 1980.
22. Martin CB Jr, DeHann J, van der Wildt B, Jongsma HW, Dieleman A, Arts THM: Mechanisms of late decelerations in the fetal heart rate: A study with autonomic blocking agents in fetal lambs. Eur J Obstet Gynaecol Reprod Biol 9:361-373, 1979.
23. Itskovitz J, Goetzman BW, Rudolph AM: The mechanisms of late deceleration of the heart rate and its relationship to oxygenation in normoxemic and chronically hypoxemic fetal lambs. Am J Obstet Gynecol 141:66-73, 1982.
24. Harris JL, Krueger TR, Parer JT: Mechanisms of late decelerations of the fetal heart rate during hypoxia. Am J Obstet Gynecol 144:491-496, 1982.
25. Kubli FW, Hon EH, Khazin AF, Takemura H: Observations on heart rate and pH in the human fetus during labor. Am J Obstet Gynecol 104:1190-1206, 1969.
26. Wood C, Ferguson R, Leeton J, Newman W, Walker A: Fetal heart rate and acid-base status in the assessment of fetal hypoxia. Am J Obstet Gynecol 98:62-70, 1967.
27. Clark SL, Gimovsky ML, Miller FC: The scalp stimulation test: A clinical alternative to fetal scalp blood sampling. Am J Obstet Gynecol 148:274-277, 1984.
28. Ralston DH, Shnider SM: The fetal and neonatal effects of regional anesthesia in obstetrics. Anesthesiology 48:34-64, 1978.
29. Bowes WA, Gabbe SG, Bowes C: Fetal heart rate monitoring in premature infants weighing 1500 grams or less. Am J Obstet Gynecol 137:791-796, 1980.
30. Garite TJ, Linzey EM, Freeman RK, Dorchester W: Fetal heart rate patterns and fetal distress in fetuses with congenital anomalies. Obstet Gynecol 53:716-720, 1979.

CHAPTER 38

Evaluation of the Neonate

Sheila E. Cohen, M.B., Ch.B., F.F.A.R.C.S.

Gershon Levinson, M.D.

Sol M. Shnider, M.D.

Evaluation of the fetus and neonate is of vital importance to detect and treat problems that result in increased perinatal morbidity and mortality. Factors that may modify infant outcome and survival include complications occurring during pregnancy or labor, perinatal asphyxia, anesthetic medications, and the presence of congenital abnormalities. Evaluation prior to delivery is primarily aimed at determining optimal obstetric management, whereas the importance of assessment immediately after birth lies in promptly identifying severely depressed infants who require active resuscitation. In the first hours of life it is imperative that infants who need special observation and therapy are identified and placed in intensive care nurseries. Such management has considerably reduced neonatal mortality, particularly with regard to premature infants. Further evaluation over the early days and months of life enables a prognosis to be formulated as to the long-term physical, neurologic, and psychologic well-being of the infant. In addition, most of these methods of evaluation are widely utilized to assess outcome in obstetric and anesthetic research.

EVALUATION OF THE NEONATE IN THE DELIVERY ROOM

Breathing Time, Crying Time, and Time to Sustained Respiration

After delivery, the infant's condition must be rapidly assessed to determine the need for immediate resuscitation. Before the introduction of the Apgar score, the time interval between delivery and the "first gasp" (breathing time) or "first cry" (crying time) was used to identify asphyxiated infants. The underlying hypothesis was that infants who breathed very shortly after birth (i.e., in the first 60 to 90 sec) were healthy and did not require resuscitation, whereas infants in whom respiration was delayed were asphyxiated. It was demonstrated subsequently by James et al. (1) that the mere onset of respiration

did not bear a constant relationship to oxygenation. In a group of 63 newborns with varying degrees of asphyxia, 26 had extremely low oxygen saturations or even a total absence of oxygen. In spite of this, 14 of these infants spontaneously initiated respiration or made respiratory efforts.

Although most infants who initiate respiration are healthy and will make satisfactory progress without resuscitation, some severely hypoxic infants who are moderately depressed will make initial respiratory efforts but will deteriorate in the absence of supplemental oxygen. Thus, as an index designed to discriminate which infants require resuscitation, the time of the first gasp or first cry is not wholly satisfactory. Because most severely depressed infants fail to breathe, this group usually can be identified as needing resuscitation. However, because of the expectant nature of the measurements, delay in intervention may occur. On the other hand, the time interval between delivery and the establishment of *sustained* respiration is used to identify the vigorous or depressed neonate. A time to sustained respiration greater than 90 sec invariably indicates a depressed or asphyxiated neonate and correlates well with an Apgar score of 6 or less.

Apgar Score

It was not until 1953, when Dr. Virginia Apgar developed her now universally accepted scoring system (2), that evaluation of the newborn immediately after birth was standardized into a simple, reproducible form that all personnel could easily be trained to perform. To ensure objectivity, it was intended that the score be performed by a pediatrician or some other individual not directly involved in care of the mother. The score was designed to clearly identify depressed infants requiring resuscitation and thereafter to follow their progress over the first minutes of life. The score directs the attendant's attention to five vital signs: heart rate, respiratory effort, muscle tone, reflex irritability, and color. Each sign is given a numeric value, as shown in Figure 38.1.

HEART RATE

Heart rate is determined by auscultation of the chest, or less commonly by observation of the epigastrium or precordium for visible heart beat or by palpation of the cord at the umbilicus. As with the fetus, the neonate at birth usually has a heart rate of over 100 beats/min. A heart rate less than this usually signifies asphyxia. Another very common cause in an otherwise healthy baby is reflex bradycardia from enthusiastic efforts to aspirate the pharynx or empty the stomach. Rarely, bradycardia is due to congenital heart block or propranolol therapy to the mother (3).

RESPIRATORY EFFORT

An infant who is breathing and crying lustily receives a 2 rating, whereas an apneic infant receives a score of 0. All other types of respiratory effort— such as irregular, shallow ventilation or weak cry— are scored 1. The respiratory rate, per se, is not considered, *only the quality of the respiratory efforts.*

MUSCLE TONE

A baby with active movement or spontaneously flexed arms and legs that resist extension is rated 2, whereas a completely flaccid infant receives a 0 score. Anything in between receives a value of 1. Some maternally administered drugs such as diazepam may selectively depress muscle tone without affecting circulation or respiration (4), whereas others, such as ketamine in large doses (>2 mg/kg), may increase tone while depressing respiration (5).

REFLEX IRRITABILITY

This is tested by either inserting a nasal catheter, flicking the soles of the feet, or drying the baby vig-

orously. A sneeze or lusty cry is scored 2, a grimace or weak cry 1, and no response 0.

COLOR

All infants are cyanotic at birth because of their high hemoglobin concentrations and low PaO_2. The disappearance of cyanosis is usually rapid when ventilation and circulation are normal. Many healthy, vigorous infants still have generalized or acrocyanosis at 1 min due in part to peripheral vasoconstriction in response to the cold delivery room. A completely pink baby receives a score of 2, a pale or blue baby a score of 0, and a neonate with acrocyanosis a score of 1. If an infant seems to be breathing well and does not become pink despite administration of 100% oxygen, the most common cause is acidosis and pulmonary vasoconstriction. Other causes include cyanotic congenital heart disease, methemoglobinemia, polycythemia, or pulmonary disease such as hypoplastic lungs. The very pale infant may be hypovolemic and hypotensive. Some maternally administered drugs such as alcohol or magnesium may cause peripheral vasodilation and a pink color in a hypotonic lethargic baby.

Evaluation of the Apgar Score

Of the five criteria in the Apgar score, heart rate and respiratory effort are most important in identifying a distressed newborn, and color is of least value. Modifications of this scoring system with relative weight values for each sign or elimination of the color evaluation have been suggested (6). However, the Apgar score as originally described has achieved its universal acceptance and popularity due in large part to its simplicity and reproducibility. The Apgar score has been claimed to have prognostic significance in regard to development of respiratory distress syn-

Score	A Appearance — Color	P Pulse — Heart Rate	G Grimace — Reflex Irritability	A Activity — Muscle Tone	R Respiration — Respiratory Effort
0	Blue, pale	Absent	No response	Limp	Absent
1	Body pink, Extremities blue	Below 100	Grimace	Some flexion of extremities	Slow, irregular
2	Completely pink	Over 100	Cough, sneeze, or cry	Active motion	Good, crying

Figure 38.1. Apgar score is based on five signs, each scored 0, 1, or 2.

drome (7), neurologic abnormalities (8), and indeed death (9). It quickly identifies those infants requiring active resuscitation, which, by its early initiation, will reduce neonatal morbidity and mortality.

The Apgar score is usually measured at 1 and 5 min after birth. If the infant's condition continues to change in response to resuscitative efforts, the score should be repeated at 10 and 20 min of life. In addition to its simplicity, this measure has the effect of forcing the birth attendants to focus attention on the neonate at a time when care of the mother may also be demanding their attention. Although it has been used for almost 30 years as an evaluative and prognostic tool, it is useful to review its value and limitations in light of knowledge acquired since its inception.

APGAR SCORE AND RESUSCITATION

On the basis of 1-min scores, neonates may be divided into three groups that relate to the degree of depression and, thus, to the need for active resuscitation. Several groups (10, 11) have found the Apgar score to correlate well with acid–base measurements performed immediately after birth: infants with scores greater than 7 had either normal values or, more commonly, a mild respiratory acidosis; infants with scores of 4 to 6 were moderately depressed, having a respiratory acidosis with some slight depression of buffer base; and those with low scores (0 to 3) usually had a combined metabolic and respiratory acidosis. This last group frequently had experienced a period of prolonged or severe asphyxia. This is similar to the relationship of fetal scalp samples taken just before delivery and Apgar scores at birth (Fig. 38.2) (12).

More recently, this relationship between Apgar score and the acid–base status has been challenged. In a prospective study of 1210 infants, Sykes et al. (13) found that, among babies with Apgar scores less than 7 at 1 and 5 min, only 21% and 19%, respectively, were severely acidotic (umbilical artery pH < 7.1 and base deficit > 13 mmol/liter). Conversely, of the babies with severe acidosis, 73% had Apgar scores over 7 at 1 min, and 86% had such scores at 5 min. The authors caution that the Apgar score should not be considered predictive of neonatal asphyxial damage.

Other investigators have also found a poor correlation between Apgar scores and acid–base status (14–20). Lauener et al. (14) found that the sensitivity of a 1-min Apgar score of less than 4 for an umbilical arterial pH less than 7.15 was 10.7%, whereas the specificity was 98.7%. This indicates that the score was very good at ruling out acidosis but could not be used to predict a low pH. In their study, of all

infants with Apgar scores less than 4, only 37% had an umbilical cord arterial pH less than 7.15. Similar results (i.e., poor positive predictive value but good negative predictive value) was also found in the relationship between lactic acidemia and Apgar scores (16) and Apgar scores less than 3 and umbilical cord arterial pH less than 7.21 in preterm infants (19).

As others (21, 22) have pointed out, newborn depression can result from a variety of factors, including maternally administered central nervous system depressants, birth trauma, or reflex bradycardia from excessively vigorous suctioning of the airway. Severe asphyxia can occur long before delivery, causing permanent damage in a baby whose acid–base status has completely recovered by birth (23). Alternatively, it can occur acutely, shortly before delivery in an otherwise healthy infant; such a baby may be born severely acidotic, but cries immediately, quickly restoring normal acid–base sta-

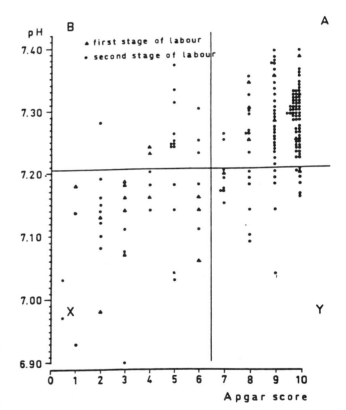

Figure 38.2. Relationship between fetal blood pH and Apgar score at 2 min. All samples were taken shortly before delivery. The diagram is arbitrarily divided, separating fetuses regarded as vigorous (Apgar score 7 or above) and those with "normal" pH (above 7.2). Note that there is a general relationship between the two variables (segments A and X) and also approximately 30% spillover into the false-normal and false-abnormal groups (B and Y). (Reprinted by permission from Beard RW, Morris ED, Clayton SG: pH of foetal capillary blood as an indicator of the condition of the foetus. J Obstet Gynaecol Br Commonw 74:812–822, 1967.)

tus. Recent studies indicate that the *combination* of either fetal heart rate monitoring or biophysical profile, cord blood pH, and Apgar score is better than any one parameter alone as an evaluation of neonatal status at delivery (24, 25).

Regardless of the cause of neonatal depression, the degree of intervention required during resuscitation relates to the extent to which the score is lowered. For example, essentially healthy neonates scoring 8 to 10 need no respiratory assistance, and mild to moderately depressed infants (scores 3 to 7) frequently improve rapidly in response to oxygen administered by mask (with positive pressure when necessary), whereas those who are severely depressed (scores 0 to 2) merit immediate active intervention, including endotracheal intubation and perhaps cardiac massage. A detailed description of resuscitation of the newborn based on the Apgar score is described in Chapter 39. A second evaluation of the score at 5 min (and subsequently at 5-min intervals until the score is greater than 7) forces the resuscitation team to assess their progress and better enables them to decide whether to continue their attempts. As a guide to identifying and treating the depressed neonate, the Apgar score has not yet been surpassed by any other index.

PROGNOSTIC VALUE OF THE APGAR SCORE

Apgar and James (26) and the Collaborative Study of Cerebral Palsy (27) investigated the correlation between neonatal mortality and Apgar score. The distribution of 1- and 5-min scores for the first 17,221 infants in the collaborative study is shown in Table 38.1. There was a strong positive correlation between Apgar scores and birth weight.

In Apgar's study the mortality in the first 28 days of life, in both full-term and premature infants, was inversely related to the score at 1 min. In very low birth weight infants, mortality tended to be high at all scores, although in all birth weight groups considered, there was a significant difference in survival in infants whose scores were poor (0 to 3), fair (4 to 6), or good (7 to 10) (26). In an attempt to establish a more accurate predictive index, the Collaborative Study evaluated scores at both 1 and 5 min. They

confirmed Apgar's results for 1-min scores, finding mortality in the first 27 days to be 23% for infants having scores of 0 or 1, decreasing to 0.1% for infants with 1-min scores of 10. The 27-day mortality of infants with 5-min scores of 0 or 1 was 49%; it decreased with increasing scores. The Collaborative Study also demonstrated that Apgar scores more accurately predicted mortality during the first 2 days of life, rather than the period from 2 to 27 days, and that the 5-min score was more useful in this respect (Fig. 38.3). In spite of a smaller incidence of low scores at 5 min, such scores were much more likely to be associated with increased mortality. When birth weight was considered in conjunction with Apgar score, the highest mortality occurred in infants with both low birth weight and low Apgar scores. There was also a trend to increased mortality in infants weighing over 4000 g, perhaps because these infants were the offspring of diabetic mothers or because they had sustained birth trauma during a difficult delivery.

In a continuation of these studies, the Collaborative Perinatal Project of the National Institute of Neurological and Communicative Disorders and Stroke (NCPP), reported data on 49,000 infants born between 1959 and 1966, further exploring the relationship between mortality and Apgar score (28). While low (0 to 3) 5-min Apgar scores were associated with a 10 to 15 fold greater mortality in the first year than were high scores (7 to 10), the persistence of a low score was the most significant factor. Among babies who still had a low score 20 min after birth, 59% of term infants and 96% of low birth weight (less than 2500 g) infants had died by the end of the first year.

LIMITATIONS OF THE APGAR SCORE

The Apgar score remains a useful general prognostic tool in predicting short-term mortality in groups of infants, particularly those of low birth weight. It has little value, however, when attempting to predict the likelihood of survival in any individual case.

Several problems become apparent when the Apgar score is critically examined as an evaluative index. The intended objectivity of the score may be threatened by lack of personnel available to measure it who are not involved with care of the patient. However, this criticism of subjectivity can be leveled equally justifiably at most other indices used to assess neonatal condition. Perhaps a more important limitation is the relative crudeness of the measurement, which looks only at the vital functions necessary to sustain life and continues observation for only a very brief period. Many serious neonatal problems do not present until after the infant has left the delivery room, and Apgar herself commented that

Table 38.1
Percentage Distribution of 1- and 5-Min-Apgar Scores[a]

Apgar Score	0–3	4–6	7–10
1 min	6.4	14.5	78.9
5 min	1.8	3.5	94.8

[a]Data from Drage JS, Kennedy C, Schwarz BK: The Apgar score as an index of neonatal mortality: A report from the Collaborative Study of Cerebral Palsy. Obstet Gynecol 24:222–230, 1964.

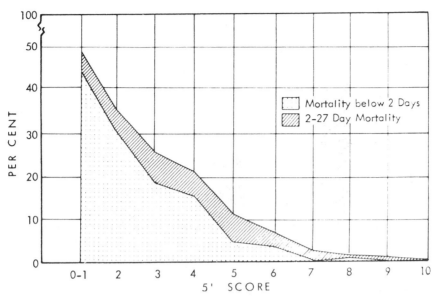

Figure 38.3. Percentage of neonatal mortality within each 5-min Apgar score. (Reprinted by permission from Drage JS, Berendes H: Apgar scores and outcome of the newborn. Pediatr Clin North Am 13:635–643, 1966.)

the score "is no substitute for a careful physical examination and careful observation over the first few hours of life." Because the infant has to be considerably affected to significantly lower the score, subtle effects of perinatal asphyxia or maternal medication may be missed entirely. Newer and more sophisticated techniques of examining the neurologic and behavioral aspects of the newborn have repeatedly demonstrated profound and sometimes prolonged depression in infants who have perfectly normal Apgar scores. Thus studies using this index as an outcome measure that have judged drug regimens as "safe" must be reinterpreted in the light of more recent data.

NEWBORN ASSESSMENT AND NEONATAL NEUROLOGIC INJURY

In addition to studying mortality, the same groups (8, 28) investigated the value of the Apgar score as a predictor of neonatal morbidity. Neurologic examinations were performed at 1 year of age and were related to 1- and 5-min Apgar scores and to birth weight (8). Of the 14,115 infants examined, 1.9% were discovered to have definite neurologic abnormalities. When considered in conjunction with Apgar scores at 1 min, an incidence of 3.6% of neurologically abnormal infants was found in the group who had scores of 0 to 3, whereas the incidence was only 1.6% in infants who had scored 7 to 10. When grouped according to 5-min score, the disparity was even greater; the incidence of abnormal infants in the "low score" group was four times as high as in the "high score" group. Again, birth weight was an extremely signif-

icant factor, with a more than sixfold increase in neurologic abnormalities in infants weighing 1001 to 2000 g at birth compared with those weighing over 2500 g (Figs. 38.4 and 38.5).

The Collaborative Project of the NCPP carefully screened children up to 7 years of age for cerebral palsy (CP), mental retardation, and more minor handicaps (28). Although the incidence of low Apgar scores was higher among infants with CP than among normal children, 73% of CP victims were born with Apgar scores above 7 (Fig. 38.6). This suggests that factors arising before or after birth are more significant with respect to the etiology of CP than those surrounding the birth process itself. However, prolonged neonatal depression (low Apgar score at 20 min) was closely correlated with morbidity, with 57% of surviving term infants subsequently developing severe CP. Surprisingly, the incidence of CP among low birth weight infants with prolonged depression was low. This is probably due to the very high mortality in this group and, among survivors, the resistance of the immature brain to asphyxial insults. In children free from CP, mental retardation and other disorders were not more commonly associated with low Apgar scores.

In spite of such data, health care professionals often are unduly pessimistic regarding the prognosis of low scoring infants (29, 30). This is ill deserved, as the vast majority (i.e., 95%) of infants with scores less than 3 who survive to age 7 have no neurologic deficit. The predictive accuracy of the Apgar score alone in this respect is poor; other factors, such as low birth weight, prematurity, and the presence of

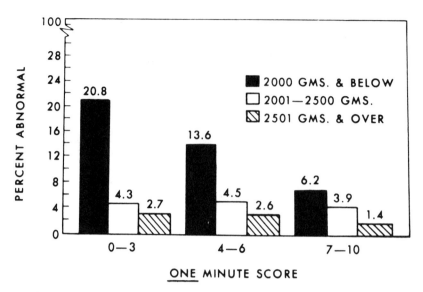

Figure 38.4. Percentage of neurologic abnormality at 1 year of age, by 1-min Apgar score and birth weight groups. (Modified from Drage JS, Kennedy C, Berendes H, Shwartz BK, Weiss W: The Apgar score as an index of infant morbidity. Dev Med Child Neurol 8:141–148, 1966.)

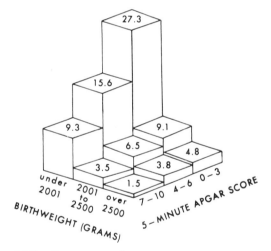

Figure 38.5. Percentage of neurologic abnormality at 1 year of age, by 5-min Apgar score and birth weight groups. (Modified from Drage JS, Kennedy C, Berendes H, Shwartz BK, Weiss W: The Apgar score as an index of infant morbidity. Dev Med Child Neurol 8:141–148, 1966.)

early neurologic deficit and seizures all must be taken into account. In addition, data obtained from the Collaborative Studies do not reflect the improvements in recent years in the availability and quality of neonatal intensive care. As yet, it is impossible to predict whether the increased survival that has been achieved among low birth weight infants will be associated with a higher, or lower, incidence of neurologic disability.

The association between perinatal asphyxia and cerebral palsy is weak (31), and the causes of most cases are unknown. Factors found more frequently than expected in babies with cerebral palsy were maternal proteinuria or mental retardation, breech presentation, major congenital malformation in the neonate not involving the central nervous system, and neonatal seizures. Most children (about 90%) with cerebral palsy are not asphyxiated at birth (32). In the approximately 10% of infants with cerebral palsy who were asphyxiated at birth, it is uncertain if the perinatal asphyxia caused the cerebral palsy or if the asphyxia was incidental or caused by a preexisting fetal abnormality. Similar to the poor correlation of a low Apgar score and cerebral palsy, numerous recent studies have shown no close association between umbilical cord metabolic acidosis and cerebral palsy (33–35).

The current consensus of opinion (36, 37) is that, to postulate a relationship between perinatal asphyxia and cerebral palsy in an individual patient, the following criteria must be present:

1. Profound umbilical artery metabolic or mixed acidemia (pH < 7)
2. Persistence of an Apgar score of 0 to 3 for longer than 5 min
3. Neonatal neurologic sequelae (e.g., seizures, coma, hypotonia)
4. Multiorgan system dysfunction (e.g., cardiovascular, gastrointestinal, hematologic, pulmonary, or renal)

Unless these characteristics are all present and other potential causes such as preexisting brain lesions eliminated, a link between the birth asphyxia and subsequent cerebral palsy is unlikely. It is noteworthy that the incidence of cerebral palsy in term infants (1 to 2/1000) has not changed despite the

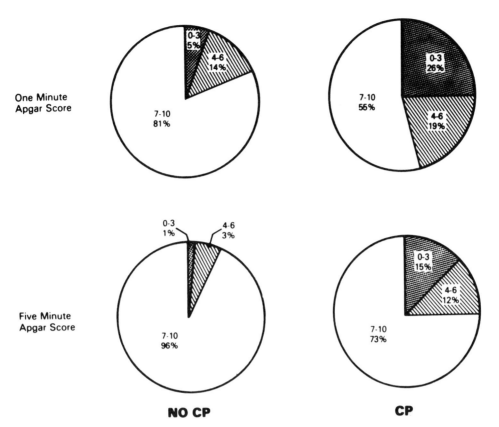

One Minute
Apgar Score

Five Minute
Apgar Score

NO CP   **CP**

Figure 38.6. Distribution of Apgar scores at 1 and 5 min in children with no later cerebral palsy (*CP*) (*left*), and in those with cerebral palsy (*right*). (Reprinted by permission from Nelson KB, Ellenberg JG: Apgar scores as predictors of chronic neurologic disability. Pediatrics 68:36–44, 1981.)

widespread use of fetal monitoring, the decreased use of forceps, the increased rate of cesarean sections for fetal indications, and improved neonatal resuscitation. The perception that birth asphyxia accounts for a significant portion of infants with cerebral palsy is clearly unwarranted.

LATER EVALUATION OF THE NEONATE

General Examination of the Newborn

As soon as the infant's condition has stabilized after delivery, a careful and thorough examination must be performed to look for abnormalities that may require special management. Developmental anomalies of the nervous system, such as spina bifida or myelomeningocele, are usually obvious, but congenital cardiac disease may be asymptomatic at this stage. An infant who remains cyanotic or whose lungs are difficult to inflate should immediately arouse suspicion of a diagnosis of diaphragmatic hernia, whereas the presence of bubbling secretions would suggest tracheoesophageal fistula. If either of the latter conditions is suspected, further diagnostic measures must be undertaken immediately. Examination of the mouth may reveal cleft lip or palate, a large tongue as in cretinism, or micrognathia as in the Pierre Robin syn-

drome. It is especially important to recognize these abnormalities because dangerous respiratory obstruction may develop, particularly during feeding.

Continued Observation of the Neonate

In most centers, for the first few hours of life the infant is intensively observed, regardless of whether it is "rooming in" or in a special nursery. During the first 24 hr the infant undergoes massive physiologic adjustments from intrauterine to extrauterine life. Desmond and associates (38) observed a number of physical signs during the first 10 hr of life in essentially healthy neonates (Fig. 38.7). A period of great activity is seen immediately after birth, which subsides after the first 30 min, giving way to sleep for subsequent hours. The infant then once more becomes active and aroused and may pass meconium and cry. Respiratory difficulties such as grunting or intercostal retraction, signifying the presence of respiratory distress syndrome, may not become obvious until this time. Central nervous system damage may manifest itself by irritability, "jitteriness," or seizures; in such cases, a full neurologic examination is indicated.

The biochemical status of the infant is also changing during this period. In normal infants the respi-

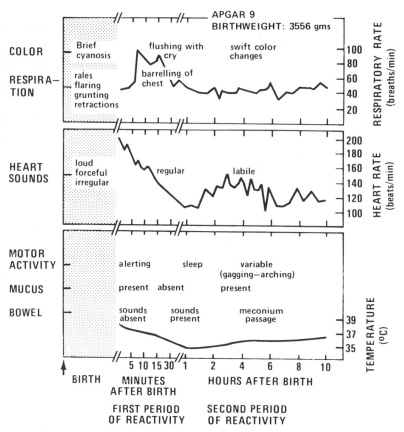

Figure 38.7. Physical findings noted during the first 10 hr of life in a high Apgar score infant delivered under spinal anesthesia without prior premedication. (Modified by permission from Desmond MM, Rudolph AJ, Phitaksphraiwan P: The transitional care nursery. Pediatr Clin North Am 13:651–668, 1966.)

ratory acidosis that is usually present at birth is rapidly corrected during the first hours of life, and by 24 hr, blood gases are similar to those found in utero (39). In sick neonates, serial evaluation of acid–base status using an umbilical arterial catheter may reveal abnormalities that point to the need for oxygen or bicarbonate therapy or ventilatory support. Asphyxiated infants or those severely depressed by anesthetic medication frequently demonstrate a prolonged respiratory acidosis in addition to a metabolic acidosis. The metabolic derangements in these and in premature infants resolve much more slowly than in healthy infants.

Assessment of Weight and Gestational Age

Morbidity and mortality are high in low–birth-weight infants. It is important to recognize that this group comprises two distinct subgroups: (a) infants who are small because they have been born prematurely and (b) infants who are of lower birth weight than would be expected from knowledge of their gestational age. Intrauterine growth standards have been constructed that permit classification of an infant as small, appropriate, or large for gestational-age (Fig.

38.8) (40). Deviation from normal growth occurs in a variety of pathologic conditions. Intrauterine growth retardation may occur in conjunction with chronic maternal hypertension, toxemia, placental insufficiency, cigarette smoking, alcoholism, or severe malnutrition. Frequently, the etiologic factor is unknown. The distinction between premature but appropriate-for-gestational-age infants and full-term infants of similar weight who are small for gestational age is important because different problems may be anticipated in each group. Premature infants are susceptible to respiratory distress, jaundice, hypothermia, intracranial hemorrhage, and retrolental fibroplasia. Small-for-gestational-age infants are more likely to suffer from hypoglycemia and infection, as well as requiring a greater caloric intake that is associated with a higher oxygen consumption (41). Congenital and chromosomal abnormalities occur more frequently in small-for-gestational-age infants.

The prognosis of small-for-gestational-age infants is generally poorer than premature appropriate-for-gestational-age infants of the same weight, as judged by the results of developmental testing. It can be postulated that the nutritional deficiency or chronic hypoxia that results in low birth weight is also responsible for poor neurologic development. Both morbidity and mortality in the newborn are related to gestational age, following a pattern similar to the relationship with birth weight, that is, rates are highest in infants of lowest birth weight and earliest gestational age and diminish as normal values are approached. Morbidity and mortality are also increased when excessive birth weight or postmaturity is present; large birth weight is often associated with maternal diabetes or difficult deliveries, and in postmaturity the fetus tends to have outgrown its placental supply. Consideration of gestational age with respect to birth weight is, of course, only possible if the former can be accurately determined. Although the date of the last menstrual period provides valuable information, bleeding early in pregnancy frequently cannot be distinguished from a normal period and, thus, the date of conception is unknown. Several schemes have been developed for assessing

gestational age that relate development to either the appearance of certain neurologic signs or to external characteristics in the newborn. Although either of these parameters gives a fair estimate of gestational age, the best approximation is provided by the Dubowitz score (42), which uses both sets of criteria. As modified by Ballard (Fig. 38.9), a graded score is awarded for the presence of six neurologic signs that predominantly reflect muscle tone and that are related to maturation of the nervous system. The signs selected are those least affected by the state of arousal of the infant or the presence of neurologic abnormality. Both of these factors had affected previous assessments based on neurologic criteria. Seven external characteristics (including skin texture, color and opacity, nipple formation, and ear form) are similarly considered, and a composite score is obtained. Dubowitz found that the total score could be reliably reproduced by different observers, could be performed at any time during the first 5 days of life, and

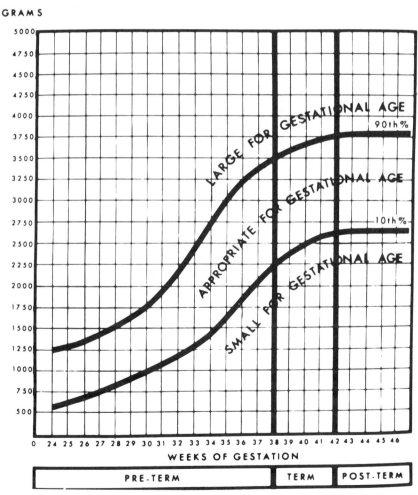

Figure 38.8. University of Colorado Medical Center classification of newborns by birth weight and gestational age. (Reprinted by permission from Lubchenco LO: Assessment of weight and gestational age. In *Neonatology*. GB Avery, ed. Lippincott, Philadelphia, 1975, p 127–148.)

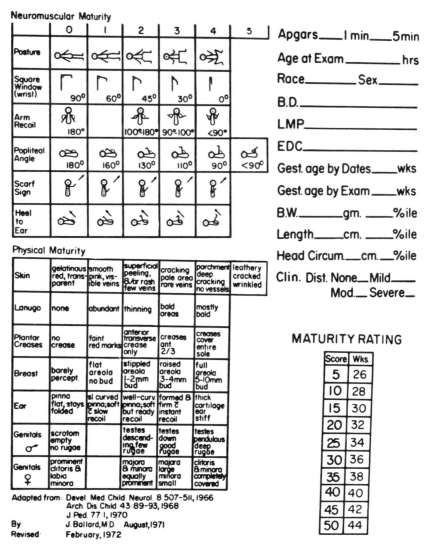

Figure 38.9. Assessment of gestational age. (Reprinted by permission from Sweet AY: Classification of the low-birth-weight infant. In *Care of the High Risk Neonate*. MH Klaus, AA Fanaroff, eds. Saunders, Philadelphia, 1973, p 47.)

was able to accurately assess gestational age to within 1 week.

Neurobehavioral Testing

The inability of the Apgar score to detect subtle or delayed effects of perinatal events led pediatricians, psychologists, and, more recently, anesthesiologists to seek more sensitive methods of evaluating the neonate. Although traditional neurologic examination is undoubtedly of diagnostic value in infants with frank neurologic problems, it is of limited value for recognizing the sequelae of lesser perinatal insults and for predicting their influence on future development. For a complete description of the neurologic examination of the neonate and the abnormalities associated with neurologic disorders, the reader is referred to Volpe's review of the subject (43).

Dissatisfaction with existing techniques has caused attention to be directed toward other aspects of newborn behavior. As far back as 1957, Graham and coworkers (44) correlated decreased performance in a series of neonatal behavior tests with the severity of perinatal hypoxia. Infants with a history of hypoxia could clearly be distinguished from a control group of "normal" infants. Drugs administered to the mother also may result in subtle and prolonged effects on the newborn, in spite of normal Apgar scores at birth.

Various neurobehavioral tests have been developed that have modified and extended the classic newborn neurologic examination. For many years the infant had been regarded as functioning only reflexively at a spinal or brain stem level. When subjected to closer scrutiny it was appreciated that the newborn is capable of quite organized behavior in the first days of life.

Brazelton (45) observed that maternal medication exaggerated and prolonged the period of relative disorganization that occurs for some period following "normal" delivery. This led him to develop a more exact way of quantitating the psychophysiologic adaptive changes occurring during the first week after birth. The Brazelton Neonatal Behavioral Assessment Scale (NBAS) (46) has formed the basis of many other such scales and examines various aspects of newborn behavior that are thought to involve the central nervous system (CNS) at a cortical level. Such functions include the newborn's ability to alter its state of arousal, suppress meaningless or intrusive stimuli, and respond appropriately to a spectrum of external events in its environment. CNS integrity is also evidenced by the newborn's motor behavior, both in initiating complex motor acts and in reflex motor responses. In the normal infant, smooth arcs of limb movements are present, whereas jerky, hypertonic activity signifies imbalance between flexor and extensor muscle groups and reflects a poorly organized CNS. The NBAS is a comprehensive evaluation of newborn behavior, but it is time consuming and must be performed by a trained observer.

Neonatal behavioral tests have proved sensitive in demonstrating depression of the neonate after perinatal asphyxia, illness, maternal medication, and a variety of other influences. Repeated assessments are most valuable because they allow recovery from such effects to be monitored and permit formulation of a long-term prognosis. The NBAS proved superior to routine neurologic examinations in predicting which infants would be neurologically abnormal at 7 years of age (47). Although both tests succeeded in identifying most of the infants who were ultimately considered to be impaired, the neurologic examination had a higher "false alarm" rate and mislabeled more normal children than the NBAS.

The obstetric anesthesiologist is, of course, most interested in the effects on the neonate of maternally administered drugs. Conway and Brackbill (48) claimed that both maternal analgesia and anesthesia could affect newborn behavior for as long as 4 weeks after birth, although it was difficult in their study to separate the effects of individual drugs, dosages, and anesthetic techniques. Behavioral effects have been correlated with electroencephalographic records of newborns and have confirmed that heavy maternal medication may cause transient CNS depression until the third day of life (49).

With the intention of studying primarily the effects on the neonate of maternal medication and anesthetic techniques, Scanlon and associates (50) devised a neurobehavioral test, the Early Neonatal Neurobehavioral Scale (ENNS), based on the Prechtl

and Beintema Neurological Examination (51) and the NBAS (Fig. 38.10). This examination has proved to be relatively simple and rapid to perform, with a high degree of reproducibility between observers. It was initially designed to assess infants during the first 8 to 12 hr of life, this period of time corresponding with the half-life of local anesthetics used for epidural anesthesia. The test must be conducted when the infant is awake but resting quietly in a room without other distracting influences. The observer assesses the infant's state of wakefulness on several occasions, reflex responses (rooting, sucking, Moro's maneuver), muscle tone and power, and responses to light, pinprick, and sound. Decrement behavior or "habituation" after repetition of these stimuli is also recorded. The ability of the infant to decrease and eventually abolish its response to stimuli that are meaningless to it seems to represent the earliest example of processing of information by the cerebral cortex, memory, and perhaps even learning. This property, commonly referred to as habituation, seems to be particularly sensitive to the effects of anesthetic drugs. Even small amounts of maternal systemic medication such as meperidine (50 mg), have been shown to depress such "higher" CNS functions, as reflected by a slower rate of habituation to a redundant sound stimulus. This parameter and responsiveness to external stimuli were found by Brackbill et al. (52) to be the most sensitive elements of a variety of evaluative tests.

Other investigators (53) consider alterations in motor tone to be more significant than habituation as indicators of neonatal CNS depression. With this in mind, Amiel-Tison, Barrier, and Shnider designed a neurobehavioral examination, the Neurologic and Adaptive Capacity Score (NACS) (53). This combines elements of the Amiel-Tison neurologic examination (54), the ENNS (50), and the NBAS (46). The NACS was specifically designed as a screening test to detect CNS depression caused by drugs and to distinguish it from that caused by perinatal asphyxia or birth trauma. Twenty criteria are tested and scored as 0, 1, or 2, encompassing five general areas: adaptive capacity, passive tone, active tone, primary reflexes, and alertness (Fig. 38.11). Tests of passive tone include the scarf sign (Fig. 38.12), recoil of elbows and lower limbs (Fig. 38.13), and measurement of the popliteal angle (Fig. 38.14). Tests of active tone include an assessment of the extensor and flexor muscles of the neck (Fig. 38.15), the response to traction (Fig. 38.16), and the supporting reaction (Fig. 38.17). Primary reflexes include the palmar grasp (Fig. 38.18), automatic walking (Fig. 38.19), the Moro reflex (Fig. 38.20), and the sucking reflex.

The emphasis on motor tone allows unilateral or

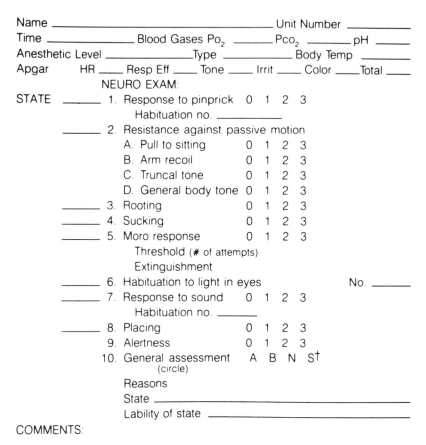

Figure 38.10. Protocol for Early Neonatal Neurobehavioral Scale (ENNS) or Scanlon Score. *A* = abnormal; *B* = borderline; *N* = normal; *S* = superior. (Reprinted by permission from Scanlon JW, Brown WU Jr, Weiss JB, Alper MH: Neurobehavioral responses of newborn infants after maternal epidural anesthesia. Anesthesiology 40:121–128, 1974.)

upper body hypotonus, which sometimes is indicative of mild birth trauma or asphyxia, to be distinguished from global motor depression, which is more likely to result from anesthetic depression. Hypertonus of neck extensors, which can accompany intracranial hypertension, merits a low score on the NACS, whereas it would be scored as 3, an optimal score, in the ENNS. In comparison with that score, less emphasis is placed on reflex activity, and habituation to noxious stimuli such as pinprick and repeated Moro maneuvers are avoided. The latter frequently prove distressing to the mother, who may be observing the examination. In the NACS, as in the NBAS, an optimal response is sought by encouraging the examiner to alter the sequence of the test according to the state of arousal of the infant, and by retesting items to ensure the best response. The NACS has high interobserver reliability, requires no special equipment, and takes only 3 to 4 min to perform (compared with 6 to 10 min for the ENNS and 45 min for the NBAS). A particular advantage of the NACS is that, as each item is progressively scored from 0 for a poor response to 2 for an optimal response, a total score can be compiled for each infant.

This enables easier statistical comparison of different treatment regimens than do other scales, which permit only comparison of numbers of infants with "high" or "low" scores for each specific variable. Arbitrarily, a score of 35 to 40 in the NACS has been designated as representing a neurologically vigorous neonate. When a group of newborns were examined with both the ENNS and NACS, 92% scored equally well on both examinations (53); this is hardly surprising given the similarity of the tests. Valid criticisms of both these scales relate to their subjective nature and the inability in any rapid simple test to evaluate all aspects of newborn behavior (55).

NEUROBEHAVIORAL EFFECTS OF ANESTHESIA

An increasing mass of information is accumulating that relates newborn behavior to the effects of anesthesia. This has been encouraged by the Food and Drug Administration's requirement that new drugs for use in the parturient be subjected to neurobehavioral testing in the neonate. Most of the studies that are discussed below have used either the ENNS, or more recently, the NACS.

NEUROLOGICAL AND ADAPTIVE CAPACITY SCORES

			0	1	2
Adaptive Capacity	1	Response to Sound	absent:	mild:	vigorous:
	2	Habituation to Sound	absent:	7-12 stimuli:	< 6 stimuli:
	3	Response to Light	absent:	mild:	brisk blink or startle:
	4	Habituation to Light	absent:	7-12 stimuli:	< 6 stimuli:
	5	Consolability	absent:	difficult:	easy:

TOTAL [ ]   ADAPTIVE CAPACITY

			0	1	2
Passive Tone	6	Scarf Sign	encircles the neck:	elbow slightly passes midline:	elbow does not reach midline:
	7	Recoil of Elbows	absent:	slow; weak:	brisk; reproducible:
	8	Popliteal Angle	>110°	100°-110°	< 90°
	9	Recoil of Lower Limbs	absent:	slow; weak:	brisk; reproducible:
Active Tone	10	Active Contraction of Neck Flexors	absent or abnormal:	difficult:	good; head is maintained in the axis of the body:
	11	Active Contraction of Neck Extensors (from leaning forward position)	absent or abnormal:	difficult:	good; head is maintained in the axis of the body:
	12	Palmar Grasp*	absent:	weak:	excellent; reproducible:
	13	Response to Traction (following palmar grasp)	absent:	Lifts part of the body weight:	lifts all of the body weight:
	14	Supporting Reaction (upright position)	absent:	incomplete; transitory:	Strong; supports all body weight:
*Primary Reflexes	15	Automatic Walking*	absent:	difficult to obtain:	perfect; reproducible:
	16	Moro Reflex*	absent:	weak; incomplete:	perfect; complete:
	17	Sucking*	absent:	weak:	perfect; synchronous with swallowing:
General Assessment	18	Alertness	coma:	lethargy:	normal:
	19	Crying	absent:	weak; high pitched; excessive:	normal:
	20	Motor Activity	absent or grossly excessive:	diminished or mildly excessive:	normal:

TOTAL [ ]   NEUROLOGICAL

TOTAL SCORE [ ] AT_____ MINUTES OF LIFE

Figure 38.11. Neurologic and Adaptive Capacity Scores (NACS). *Asterisks* signify primary reflexes. (Reprinted by permission from Amiel-Tison C, Barrier G, Shnider SM, Levinson G, Hughes SC, Stefani SJ: A new neurologic and adaptive capacity scoring system for evaluating obstetric medications in full-term newborns. Anesthesiology 56:340–350, 1982.)

Systemic Medications

In general, maternal administration of CNS depressants causes a transient depression of newborn behavior that appears to be related to the presence and quantity of drug in the neonatal circulation. Kron et al. (56) demonstrated that a single injection of 200 mg of secobarbital given to the mother immediately before delivery was associated with poorer sucking responses in the infant for as long as 4 days after birth. Brazelton (45) similarly found a lag of 2 days in the establishment of breastfeeding and 1 day in weight gain in babies of mothers who were heavily medicated in labor, as compared with those whose mothers were not. Visual attentiveness of the newborn also was depressed for as long as 4 days after the administration of narcotics or barbiturates to the mother within 1½ hr of delivery (57). Rolbin and coworkers (58) reported that diazepam, in doses of 2.5 to 10 mg, administered 30 to 55 min before cesarean section resulted in decreased muscle tone as detected

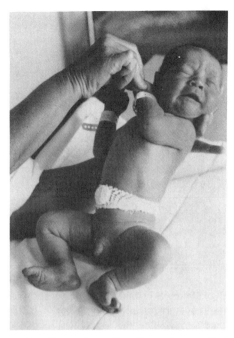

Figure 38.12. Scar sign. The elbow does not reach midline. (Reprinted by permission from Amiel-Tison C, Barrier G, Shnider SM, Levinson G, Hughes SC, Stefani SJ: A new neurologic and adaptive capacity scoring system for evaluating obstetric medications in full-term newborns. Anesthesiology 56:340–350, 1982.)

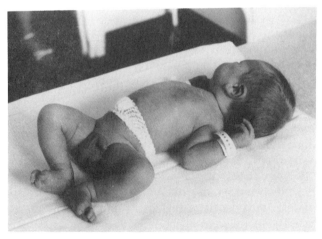

Figure 38.13. Posture and recoil. The infant is in a spontaneously flexed posture. Forearms and lower limbs return briskly to a position of flexion when extended. (Reprinted by permission from Amiel-Tison C, Barrier G, Shnider SM, Levinson G, Hughes SC, Stefani SJ: A new neurologic and adaptive capacity scoring system for evaluating obstetric medications in full-term newborns. Anesthesiology 56:340–350, 1982.)

by the ENNS at 4 hr of age. Other aspects of the test were normal, and tone had improved by 24 hr of age.

Numerous studies (59) have evaluated the neonatal effects of meperidine, which is perhaps the most commonly used narcotic for labor analgesia. Fifty to 100 mg of this agent, administered 1 to 3 hr before

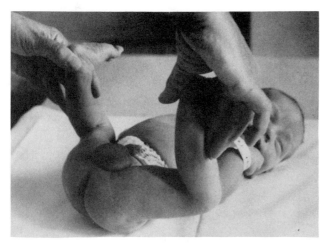

Figure 38.14. Popliteal angle. The angle between the leg and the thigh is the popliteal angle. (Reprinted by permission from Amiel-Tison C, Barrier G, Shnider SM, Levinson G, Hughes SC, Stefani SJ: A new neurologic and adaptive capacity scoring system for evaluating obstetric medications in full-term newborns. Anesthesiology 56:340–350, 1982.)

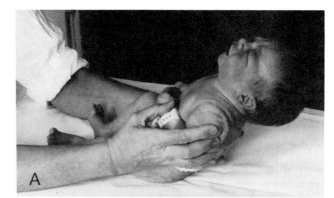

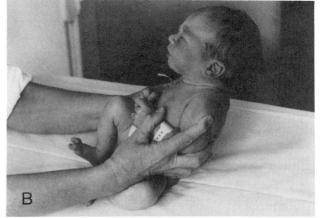

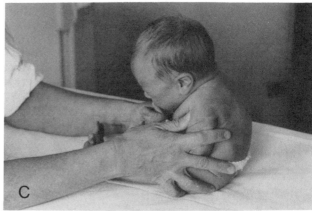

Figure 38.15. *A*, Note position of head in relation to trunk when infant is pulled from supine into sitting position. *B*, Extensor and flexor tone is balanced in the full-term infant. *C*, The head is maintained for a few seconds along the axis of the trunk before dropping forward. (Reprinted by permission from Amiel-Tison C, Barrier G, Shnider SM, Levinson G, Hughes SC, Stefani SJ: A new neurologic and adaptive capacity scoring system for evaluating obstetric medications in full-term newborns. Anesthesiology 56:340–350, 1982.)

delivery, does not usually lower Apgar scores, although it does adversely affect newborn behavior. In a large study of 920 term infants, Hodgkinson et al. (60) found that meperidine (50 to 150 mg) administered within 4 hr of delivery globally depressed the ENNS for the first 2 days of life; the degree of depression was dose related. Brackbill and co-workers (34), using the NBAS and a modification of the habituation test for an auditory stimulus, also reported lower scores in general, and delayed habituation in particular, following similar doses of meperidine. Brower et al. (61) studied neonatal electroencephalogram patterns following maternal meperidine administration and discovered that only the response to auditory stimuli was affected. Perhaps of more importance with respect to adverse effects is the finding by Kron et al. (56) of poorer sucking in infants exposed to moderate doses of this narcotic. Unfortunately, in most of the above investigations subjects were selected retrospectively, control groups were lacking, and patients were not differentiated according to socioeconomic status or obstetric complexity. In addition, many patients received a number of analgesic drugs. Leiberman and co-workers (62), in a well-controlled prospective study, compared 145 term infants whose mothers had received 100- to 150-mg doses of meperidine on demand with infants whose mothers had received epidural anesthesia with bupivacaine 0.375%. The only abnormality detected by repeated examinations (NBAS and Prechtl neonatal assessment) up to 42 days of age was decreased habituation to sound on day 3 in the meperidine group.

Fentanyl, a very popular opiate in labor, has not been studied extensively. Two studies (63, 64) indicate that intravenous fentanyl administration (mean dose 140 + 32 µg) has a minimal effect on the NACS. However, using patient-controlled intravenous analgesia for labor, it was found that nalbuphine in doses up to 42 mg produced lower NACS scores than did meperidine in doses up to 210 mg (65).

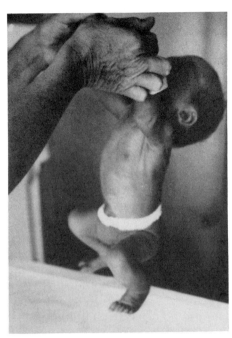

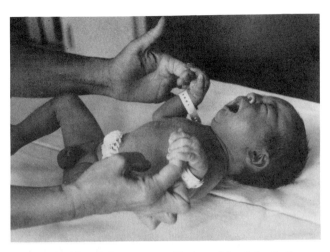

Figure 38.16. Response to traction. The contraction is spreading to flexor muscles of the upper limbs so that the infant can lift himself/herself completely. (Reprinted by permission from Amiel-Tison C, Barrier G, Shnider SM, Levinson G, Hughes SC, Stefani SJ: A new neurologic and adaptive capacity scoring system for evaluating obstetric medications in full-term newborns. Anesthesiology 56:340–350, 1982.)

Figure 38.18. Palmar grasp. Flexion of the infant's fingers onto the examiner's index fingers. (Reprinted by permission from Amiel-Tison C, Barrier G, Shnider SM, Levinson G, Hughes SC, Stefani SJ: A new neurologic and adaptive capacity scoring system for evaluating obstetric medications in full-term newborns. Anesthesiology 56:340–350, 1982.)

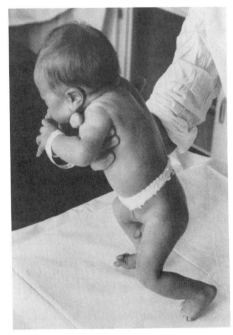

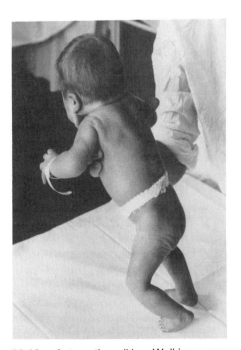

Figure 38.17. Supporting reaction. In the standing position, the legs straighten and the spinal muscles contract. (Reprinted by permission from Amiel-Tison C, Barrier G, Shnider SM, Levinson G, Hughes SC, Stefani SJ: A new neurologic and adaptive capacity scoring system for evaluating obstetric medications in full-term newborns. Anesthesiology 56:340–350, 1982.)

Figure 38.19. Automatic walking. Walking occurs when the supporting reaction is obtained. (Reprinted by permission from Amiel-Tison C, Barrier G, Shnider SM, Levinson G, Hughes SC, Stefani SJ: A new neurologic and adaptive capacity scoring system for evaluating obstetric medications in full-term newborns. Anesthesiology 56:340–350, 1982.)

686   SIX: FETUS AND NEWBORN

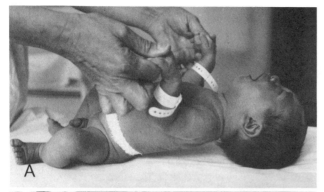

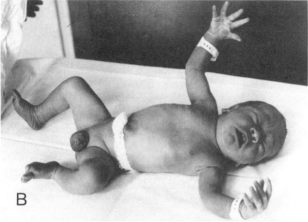

Figure 38.20. Moro reflex. *A*, To achieve neck and trunk angulation, the infant's shoulders are lifted a few centimeters off the table. *B*, The first part of the Moro reflex consists of a brisk abduction and extension of the arms and complete opening of the hands. (Reprinted by permission from Amiel-Tison C, Barrier G, Shnider SM, Levinson G, Hughes SC, Stefani SJ: A new neurologic and adaptive capacity scoring system for evaluating obstetric medications in full-term newborns. Anesthesiology 56:340–350, 1982.)

Butorphanol, a synthetic narcotic agonist/antagonist, has proved to be similar to meperidine with respect to neurobehavioral effects (66).

Several investigators (67, 68) have administered naloxone shortly before delivery to mothers who had received narcotics, in an attempt to prevent newborn depression. Disappointingly, benefit was either absent (67) or transient (68) in nature. Administration of naloxone directly to the neonate has proved more effective (69, 70). However, administration of naloxone to infants whose mothers have received narcotics cannot be advocated, except when respiratory or CNS depression is present. The naturally occurring endogenous opiates that are present in the neonate may be integral to the newborn's capacity for coping with stress.

Epidural Anesthesia

Scanlon et al. (50) reported that infants of mothers who received epidural anesthesia with either lido-

caine or mepivacaine had significantly lower scores than "nonepidural" infants on tests of muscle strength and tone, but behaved normally with respect to habituation to repetitive stimuli. They concluded that these infants were "floppy but alert," and that higher CNS functions had not been depressed by the medication. These effects were present only in the first 8 hr of life, which corresponds with the period during which significant concentrations of local anesthetics were found in the newborn circulation; lidocaine was detected in the neonatal bloodstream for 8 hr and mepivacaine for as long as 24 hr after birth (71). Subsequently, in two separate studies, the same authors found epidural anesthesia using bupivacaine (72) and chloroprocaine (73) to be free from the motor depression seen with lidocaine and mepivacaine. Bupivacaine is present only in very small amounts in the newborn circulation after epidural anesthesia and disappears much more rapidly from the fetal circulation than the other agents; chloroprocaine is rapidly metabolized by plasma cholinesterase. The mechanism by which local anesthetics might affect the newborn is unknown, although an effect on the neuromuscular junction has been postulated.

These studies have been criticized on several grounds: (*a*) the initial epidural group consisted of a mixture of patients, two-thirds of whom had received mepivacaine and only one-third lidocaine; (*b*) the number of infants exposed to lidocaine (i.e., 9) is too small to allow firm conclusions to be drawn; (*c*) the controls for the second and third studies were the same "nonepidural" babies that had formed the controls in the first study several years previously; and (*d*) approximately one-third of patients in the first study had received narcotics or barbiturates in the hours prior to delivery in addition to epidural anesthesia.

A number of studies have indicated that continuous epidural anesthesia with small ***intermittent bolus injections*** of all commonly used local anesthetics for labor and delivery, including lidocaine, bupivacaine, and chloroprocaine, have no adverse effects on the NACS. These studies with the NACS corroborated previous studies (74, 75) in which the Scanlon ENNS was used to study neurobehavior and *did not* agree with Scanlon's original report that lidocaine did indeed compromise neurobehavioral function in the neonate (50). Continuous infusion of local anesthetics, frequently employed for labor epidural analgesia, theoretically creates a risk for local anesthetic accumulation in the fetus. Using the NACS, no adverse affects of this continuous administration were found with bupivacaine, chloroprocaine, or lidocaine (76). One would expect that if local anesthetics adversely affected neonatal neurobehavior, the larger doses used for cesarean section would demonstrate these effects in both the NACS or ENNS.

Palahniuk et al. (77), in accordance with Scanlon's group, found transient neonatal hypotonia following epidural lidocaine administered for cesarean section. However, more recently, Abboud et al. (74, 78) administered lidocaine, chloroprocaine, and bupivacaine epidurally for labor or cesarean section and found that neonatal neurobehavioral depression was not present in any of the groups. Corroborating these findings, Kileff et al. (79), using the ENNS, compared infants of mothers having cesarean sections with epidural anesthesia using 2% lidocaine or 0.5% bupivacaine. Neonates in the lidocaine group scored as well as those in the bupivacaine group on all items of the ENNS. Kuhnert et al. (80), using the Brazelton Neonatal Behavioral Assessment Scale, compared neonates of mothers given chloroprocaine or lidocaine for vaginal delivery or cesarean section. Only very subtle changes were attributable to lidocaine. No babies had significant hypotonia. Although the differences in effects between the two drug groups were statistically significant, they were so small as to be clinically insignificant. Other investigators (81–83) have confirmed that lidocaine, bupivacaine, chloroprocaine, and etidocaine, even when administered in high dosage for cesarean section, are free from adverse neurobehavioral effects.

Epinephrine is commonly added to local anesthetics in epidural anesthesia in concentrations of 1:200,000 to 1:400,000 to decrease systemic absorption and peak blood levels of anesthetic, to provide a longer duration of action, and to intensify motor blockade (84–87). The use of epinephrine in obstetrics is controversial because of possible detrimental effects on uterine blood flow (88, 90) and activity (91, 95). Epinephrine that is slowly absorbed from the epidural space probably would not have clinically significant effects on uterine blood flow (96–99) and fetal well-being. These assumptions have been corroborated by the findings of no differences in the NACS whether or not epinephrine is added to 1.5% lidocaine (100), 0.5% bupivacaine (101), 2% chloroprocaine (102), or a mixture of bupivacaine 0.25%, butorphanol (1 mg), and epinephrine (103). Thus, for cesarean section in which larger doses of local anesthetic are used and more profound motor blockade is desired, the addition of epinephrine 1:200,000 to the local anesthetic solution may be advantageous and has no detrimental effects on the NACS.

In the United States, chloroprocaine (Nesacáine) has recently undergone a change in formulation. The sodium bisulfite has been removed as the antioxidant and replaced by EDTA. Studies of the new epidural bisulfite-free chloroprocaine with and without 1:300,000 epinephrine has had no detrimental effects on the NACS (104). These findings are similar to those using the old chloroprocaine formulation (102). Lidocaine, bupivacaine, and chloroprocaine are widely used in obstetric anesthesia and, in view of the above studies using the NACS and other neurobehavioral tests, appear to be safe drugs for the neonate when administered epidurally to the mother.

Spinal Anesthesia

McGuinness et al. (83) and Hodgkinson et al. (105) compared spinal anesthesia using tetracaine with epidural bupivacaine and with general anesthesia, respectively. Spinal anesthesia produced ENNS scores similar to those with bupivacaine, and significantly better scores than were associated with general anesthesia. The absence of neurobehavioral depression with spinal anesthesia is not surprising, given the extremely low dose of local anesthetic required to provide neural blockade.

Spinal and Epidural Opiates

The general concern of depressant effects of maternally administered narcotics on the newborn are always present. Concern for the newborn, in part, stimulated the initial interest in the use of *intraspinal narcotics*; it was thought that low-dose effective analgesia would pose less risk to the neonate. Hughes (106) found that newborns delivered of mothers who were given 2, 5, and 7.5 mg of epidural morphine had high Apgar and NACS scores and normal values for umbilical arterial and venous blood gas tension.

Abboud documented the safe use of intrathecal morphine with similar clinical data (107). With such low doses of 0.5 to 1 mg, this finding is not surprising. Intrathecal meperidine also does not depress the NACS (108). Dailey and co-workers (109) also found that a continuous maternal intravenous infusion of naloxone to decrease side effects such as severe itching did not adversely affect the infant's NACS. We have also found that epidural fentanyl (1 μg/kg) administered with local anesthetics for cesarean section has no adverse effects on the NACS (110), nor is the NACS adversely affected by the addition of fentanyl (50 to 100 μg), either administered in saline or mixed with bupivacaine for labor (111, 112). Use of epidural butorphanol with either bupivacaine (113) or lidocaine (114) for labor does not adversely affect the NACS. Epidural sufentanil for labor analgesia in doses of at least up to 30 μg, also does not depress the NACS (115).

Paracervical and Pudendal Block

The data relating to neurobehavioral effects of paracervical block are conflicting and difficult to interpret (59). The technique itself currently is little used because of the relatively high incidence of apparent fetal distress that accompanies it. Merkow et al. (116) reported that pudendal block with lidocaine, mepivacaine, and chloroprocaine did not result in neurobehavioral depression. In contrast to the neurobehavioral abnormalities found with epidurally administered mepivacaine (50), the habituation response was actually better in the infants who had been exposed to this agent via pudendal block. This difference probably relates to the significantly lower levels of mepivacaine identified following pudendal block, as compared with epidural block [0.1 μg/ml at 4 hr (116) versus 0.82 μg/ml at 8 hr (50)].

General Anesthesia

The effects of general anesthesia for elective cesarean section or vaginal delivery in normal pregnancies also have been studied. Infants whose mothers had undergone general rather than spinal anesthesia exhibited global depression of neurobehavioral performance, in spite of there being no difference in Apgar scores between the groups (105, 117). Palahniuk et al. (77) compared three anesthetic techniques for cesarean section: (a) methoxyflurane with high inspired oxygen, (b) nitrous oxide with low inspired oxygen, and (c) lumbar epidural anesthesia. Although all infants appeared clinically normal, those in the nitrous oxide group were less alert and had lower scores on neurobehavioral testing (ENNS) than the other groups for a period of 24 hr. A different study compared the results of the ENNS in infants whose mothers had received ketamine–nitrous oxide or thiopental–nitrous oxide general anesthesia or chloroprocaine epidural anesthesia for vaginal delivery (118). Epidural anesthesia was associated with the greatest percentage of high scores on the first and second days of life. The infants performed least well after thiopental, with ketamine producing an intermediate effect.

Halogenated anesthetics (halothane, enflurane, and isoflurane) administered at cesarean section in low concentrations to supplement nitrous oxide anesthesia and permit use of a high inspired oxygen concentration do not adversely affect acid–base status or Apgar scores (77), although some transient depression of the NACS has been noted (119) when the infants are compared to those born with spinal or epidural anesthesia. When analgesic concentrations of inhalation agents have been administered for labor, there have similarly been no adverse behavioral effects (120, 121).

SIGNIFICANCE OF NEUROBEHAVIORAL EFFECTS

It is appropriate at this juncture to question the significance, as regards well-being and future development, of abnormalities revealed by neurobehavioral testing. Tronick et al. (122) studied the effects of different analgesic regimens for labor on the behavior of normal neonates, attempting to control for other stress factors. Techniques included maternal local and regional anesthesia, and in some cases additional light systemic medication was administered. Only minimal effects were found in all groups. These proved to be transient, and all effects progressively improved over the first 10 days of life.

Similarly, most of the studies discussed in this chapter have found the effects of obstetric analgesia, as currently practiced, to either be absent or of short duration. In contrast, Standley et al (123) claimed that infants whose mothers had received either systemic analgesia or regional anesthetic blocks performed significantly less well in neurobehavioral examinations on the third day of life than infants whose mothers had no anesthesia. Infants exposed to local anesthetics were said to be most affected. However, this study can be faulted because of the multiplicity of drugs used and the inappropriate grouping together of different anesthetic techniques. Also, complicating obstetric factors were not adequately considered. Friedman et al. (124) have clearly demonstrated the correlation between dysfunctional labor or prolongation of the second stage and adverse neurobehavior. Forceps delivery and anesthesia are associated secondarily with these problems and may mistakenly be considered responsible for their consequences.

In a report that achieved great publicity, Kolata (125) quoted the work of Brackbill and Broman, who claimed that poorer physical and intellectual development persisted for up to 7 years in children of mothers who had received medication during childbirth. Although patients (who formed part of the Collaborative Perinatal Project in the 1950s) were claimed to be healthy, women with preeclampsia, difficult deliveries, and other obstetric complications were included. A panel of experts including statisticians, obstetricians, perinatologists, and anesthesiologists, and the Anesthetic and Life Support Committee of the Food and Drug Administration, carefully reviewed their data. Brackbill and Broman's conclusions subsequently were rejected on the grounds that their groups were not homogeneous, statistical analyses were poor, there was no control group, and the postpartum course of the children had not been taken into account (126). In two well-designed, controlled studies that carefully evaluated motor and cognitive abilities of children up to 4 (127, 128) and 5 (129) years of age using a number of tests, no correlation was found between maternal anesthetic technique and later development. As might have been anticipated, emergency cesarean section and peripartal asphyxia adversely affected subsequent development.

There is as yet no evidence that prolonged adverse effects are associated with neurobehavioral depression caused by maternal medication. However, the interaction between the newborn and its mother, "maternal-infant bonding" (130), and the environment in general is thought by many to be vital for the establishment of healthy behavior patterns. Inconsolability or excessive sleepiness may induce negative feelings in the mother toward her child, so that early bonding is impaired. On a more tangible level, it is easy to see that successful establishment of breastfeeding may be threatened by undue drowsiness in the infant. It is perhaps of greater prognostic significance when neurobehavioral depression occurs that cannot be attributed to medication and that, therefore, might be the result of perinatal asphyxia or brain damage. If the results of such assessments are to be used to predict further development, the history must be made known to the person interpreting the test.

Neurobehavioral assessment techniques have so far been used predominantly in the research area and are still probably too cumbersome to be applied routinely as a clinical diagnostic tool. Like most of the other evaluative indices, they can be criticized as being subjective and are regarded with scepticism by many as being less meaningful than "hard" scientific data. At the present time, neurobehavioral testing is only one method of evaluating the newborn and must not be used in isolation. It must take its place along with history, Apgar score, neurologic and biochemical investigations, and newer techniques such as evoked sensory potentials in the continuum of evaluation procedures in the newborn. Until further knowledge is gained of long-term effects of drug administration on the newborn, it is perhaps prudent to follow the recommendation of the Committee on Drugs of the American Academy of Pediatrics and to choose anesthetic or analgesic techniques that have the least observable effects, especially if their analgesic efficacy is indistinguishable from drugs with a more profound effect. With continuing efforts being directed toward assessing the effects of iatrogenic influences, not restricted to anesthesia, on the newborn, it is hoped that an improvement in perinatal care will result.

References

1. James LS, Weisbrot IM, Prince CE, Holaday DA, Apgar V: The acid-base status of human infants in relation to birth asphyxia and the onset of respiration. J Pediatr 52:379–394, 1958.
2. Apgar V: A proposal for a new method of evaluation of the newborn infant. Anesth Analg 32:260–267, 1953.
3. Gladstone GR, Hordof A, Gersony WM: Propranolol administration during pregnancy: Effects on the fetus. J Pediatr 86:962–964, 1975.
4. Flowers CE, Rudolph AJ, Desmond MM: Diazepam (Valium) as an adjunct in obstetric analgesia. Obstet Gynecol 34:68–81, 1969.
5. Little B, Chang T, Chucot L, Dill WA, Enrile LL, Glazko AJ, Janssani M, Kretchmer H, Sweet AY: Study of ketamine as an obstetric anesthetic agent. Am J Obstet Gynecol 113:247–260, 1972.
6. Crawford JS: Anaesthesia for caesarean section: A proposal for evaluation with analysis of a method. Br J Anaesth 34:179–195, 1962.
7. Rudolph AJ, Desmond MM, Pineda RG: Clinical diagnosis of respiratory difficulty in the newborn. Pediatr Clin North Am 13:669–692, 1966.
8. Drage JS, Kennedy C, Berendes H, Shwartz BK, Weiss W: The Apgar score as an index of infant morbidity. Dev Med Child Neurol 8:141–148, 1966.
9. Drage JS, Berendes H: Apgar scores and outcome of the newborn. Pediatr Clin North Am 13:635–643, 1966.
10. Crawford JS, Davies P, Pearson JE: Significance of the individual components of the Apgar score. Br J Anaesth 45:148–158, 1973.
11. Marx GF, Mahajan S, Miclat MN: Correlation of biochemical data with Apgar scores at birth and at one minute. Br J Anaesth 49:831–833, 1977.
12. Beard RW, Morris ED, Clayton SG: pH of foetal capillary blood as an indicator of the condition of the foetus. J Obstet Gynaecol Br Commonw 74:812–822, 1967.
13. Sykes GS, Molloy PM, Johnson P, Gu W, Ashworth F, Stirrat GM, Turnbull AC: Do Apgar scores indicate asphyxia? Lancet 1:494–496, 1982.
14. Lauener PA, Calame A, Janecek P, Bossart H, Monad JF: Systematic pH-measurements in the umbilical artery: Causes and predictive value of neonatal acidosis. J Perinat Med 11:278–285, 1983.
15. Fields LM, Entman SS, Boehm FH: Correlation of the one-minute Apgar score and the pH value of umbilical arterial blood. South Med J 76:1477–1479, 1983.
16. Suidan JS, Young BK: Outcome of fetuses with lactic acidemia. Am J Obstet Gynecol 150:33–37, 1984.
17. Boehm FH, Fields L, Entman SS, Vaughn WK: Correlation of the one minute Apgar score and umbilical cord acid-base status. South Med J 79:429–431, 1986.
18. Page PO, Martin J, Palmer S, Martin RW, Lucas JA, Meeks GR, Bucovaz ET, Morrison JC: Correlation of neonatal acid-base status with Apgar scores and fetal heart rate tracings. Am J Obstet Gynecol 154:1306–1311, 1986.
19. Luthy DA, Kirkwood KS, Strickland D, Wilson J, Bennett FC, Brown ZA, Benedetti TJ: Status of infants at birth and risk for adverse neonatal events and long-term sequelae: A study in low birth weight infants. Am J Obstet Gynecol 157:676–679, 1987.
20. Marrin M, Paes BA: Birth asphyxia: Does the Apgar score have diagnostic value? Obstet Gynecol 72:120–123, 1988.
21. Crawford JS: Apgar score and neonatal asphyxia. Lancet 1:684–685, 1982.
22. Hughes-Davies TH: Apgar score and neonatal asphyxia. Lancet 1:685, 1982.
23. Paul RH, Yonekura L, Cantrell CJ, Turkel S, Pavlova Z, Sipos L: Fetal injury prior to labor: Does it happen? Am J Obstet Gynecol 154:1187–1193, 1986.
24. Page FO, Martin JN, Palmer SM, Martin RW, Lucas JA, Meeks R, Bucovaz ET, Morrison JC: Correlation of neonatal acid-base status with Apgar scores and fetal heart rate tracings. Am J Obstet Gynecol 154:1306–1311, 1986.
25. Vintzileos AM, Gaffney SE, Salinger LM, Kontopoulos G, Campbell WA, Nochimson DJ: The relationships among the fetal biophysical profile, umbilical cord pH, and Apgar scores. Am J Obstet Gynecol 157:627–631, 1987.
26. Apgar V, James LS: Further observations on the newborn scoring system. Am J Dis Child 104:419–427, 1962.

27. Drage JS, Kennedy C, Schwarz BK: The Apgar score as an index of neonatal mortality: A report from the Collaborative Study of Cerebral Palsy. Obstet Gynecol 24:222–230, 1964.
28. Nelson KB, Ellenberg JH: Apgar scores as predictors of chronic neurologic disabilities. Pediatrics 68:36–44, 1981.
29. Scanlon JW: How is the baby? The Apgar score revisited. Clin Pediatr 12:61–63, 1973.
30. Paneth N, Fox HE: The relationship of Apgar score to neurologic handicaps: A survey of clinicians. Obstet Gynecol 61:547–550, 1983.
31. Nelson KB, Ellenberg JH: Antecedents of cerebral palsy: Multivariate analysis of risk. N Engl J Med 315:81–86, 1986.
32. Blair E, Stanley FJ: Intrapartum asphyxia: A rare cause of cerebral palsy. J Pediatr 112:515–519, 1988.
33. Ruth VJ, Raivio KO. Perinatal brain damage: Predictive value of metabolic acidosis and the Apgar score. Br Med J 297:24–27, 1988.
34. Fee S, Malee K, Deddish R, Minogue JP, Socol ML: Severe acidosis and subsequent neurologic status. Am J Obstet Gynecol 162:802–806, 1990.
35. Dennis J, Johnson A, Mutch L, Yudkin P, Johnson P: Acid-base status at birth and neurodevelopmental outcome at four and one-half years. Am J Obstet Gynecol 161:213–220, 1989.
36. Nelson KB: Perspective on the role of perinatal asphyxia in neurologic outcome: Its role in developmental deficits in children. Can Med Assoc J 141(Suppl):3–10, 1989.
37. Fetal and neonatal neurologic injury. ACOG Tech Bull 163:Jan, 1992.
38. Desmond MM, Rudolph AJ, Phitaksphraiwan P: The transitional care nursery. Pediatr Clin North Am 13:651–668, 1966.
39. Weisbrot IM, James LS, Prince CE, Holaday DA, Apgar V: Acid-base homeostasis of the newborn infant during the first 24 hours of life. J Pediatr 52:395–403, 1958.
40. Lubchenco LO: Assessment of weight and gestational age. In Neonatology. GB Avery, ed. Lippincott, Philadelphia, 1975, pp 127–148.
41. Brazelton TB, Paraker WB, Zuckerman B: Importance of behavioral assessment of the neonate. Curr Probl Pediatr 7:34–36, 1976.
42. Dubowitz LM, Dubowitz V, Goldberg C: Clinical assessment of gestational age in the newborn infant. J Pediatr 77:1–10, 1970.
43. Volpe JJ: Neurological disorders. In Neonatology. GB Avery, ed. Lippincott, Philadelphia, 1975, pp 729–796.
44. Graham FK, Pennoyer MM, Caldwell BM, Greenman M, Hartman AF: Relationship between clinical status and behavior test performance in a newborn group with histories suggesting anoxia. J Pediatr 50:177–189, 1957.
45. Brazelton TB: Psychophysiologic reactions in the neonate. II. Effect of maternal medication on the neonate and his behavior. J Pediatr 58:513–518, 1961.
46. Brazelton TB: Neonatal Behavioral Assessment Scale. Lippincott, Philadelphia, 1973.
47. Brazelton TB, Parker WB, Zuckerman B: Importance of behavioral assessment of the neonate. Curr Probl Pediatr 7:70–75, 1976.
48. Conway E, Brackbill Y: Delivery medication and infant outcome: An empirical study. Monogr Soc Res Child Dev 35:24–34, 1970.
49. Borgstedt AD, Rosen MG: Medication during labor correlated with behavior and EEG of the newborn. Am J Dis Child 115:21–24, 1968.
50. Scanlon JW, Brown WU Jr, Weiss JB, Alper MH: Neurobehavioral responses of newborn infants after maternal epidural anesthesia. Anesthesiology 40:121–128, 1974.
51. Prechtl H, Bientema D: The Neurological Examination of the Full-Term Newborn Infant. Little Club Clinics in Developmental Medicine, No 12. Spastics International Medical Publications, London, 1964.
52. Brackbill Y, Kane J, Manniello RL, Abramson D: Obstetric meperidine usage and assessment of neonatal status. Anesthesiology 40:116–120, 1974.

53. Amiel-Tison C, Barrier G, Shnider SM, Levinson G, Hughes SC, Stephani SJ: A new neurologic and adaptive capacity scoring system for evaluating obstetric medications in full-term newborns. Anesthesiology 56:340–350, 1982.
54. Amiel-Tison C: A method for neurological evaluation within the first year of life. Experience with full-term newborns. In Major Mental Handicap: Methods and Costs of Prevention. Ciba Foundation Symposium, No 59. Elsevier/Excerpta Medica/North Holland, Amsterdam, 1978, pp 107–126.
55. Tronick E: A critique of the Neonatal Neurologic Adaptive Capacity Score (NASC). Anesthesiology 56:338–339, 1982.
56. Kron RE, Stein M, Goddard KE: Newborn sucking behavior affected by obstetric sedation. Pediatrics 37:1012–1016, 1966.
57. Stechler G: Newborn attention as affected by medication during labor. Science 144:315–317, 1964.
58. Rolbin SH, Wright RG, Shnider SM, Levinson G, Roizen MF, Johnson J, Jones M: Diazepam during cesarean section—Effects on neonatal Apgar scores, acid-base status, neurobehavioral assessment and maternal and fetal plasma norepinephrine levels. In Abstracts of Scientific Papers, American Society of Anesthesiologists, New Orleans, 1977, p 449.
59. Dailey PA, Baysinger CL, Levinson G, Shnider SM: Neurobehavioral testing of the newborn infant—Effects of obstetric anesthesia. Clin Perinatol 9:191–214, 1982.
60. Hodgkinson R, Bhatt M, Wang CN: Double-blind comparison of the neurobehavior of neonates following administration of different doses of meperidine to the mother. Can Anaesth Soc J 25:405–411, 1978.
61. Brower KR, Crowell DH, Leung P, Cashman TM: Neonatal electroencephalographic patterns as affected by maternal drugs administered during labor and delivery. Anesth Analg 57:303–306, 1978.
62. Lieberman BA, Rosenblatt DB, Belsey E, Packer M, Redshaw M, Mills M, Caldwell J, Notarianni L, Smith RL, Williams M, Beard RW: The effects of maternally administered pethidine or epidural bupivacaine on the fetus and newborn. Br J Obstet Gynaecol 86:598–606, 1979.
63. Rayburn WF, Rathke A, Leuschen MP, Chleborad J, Weidner W: Fentanyl citrate during labor. Am J Obstet Gynecol 161:202–206, 1989.
64. Rayburn WF, Smith CV, Leuschen MP, Hoffman K: Comparison of patient-controlled and nurse-administered analgesia using intravenous fentanyl during labor. Anesth Rev 18:31–33, 1991.
65. Frank M, McAteer EJ, Cattermole R, Loughnan B, Stafford LB, Hitchoock AM: Nalbuphine for obstetric analgesia. Anaesthesia 42:697–703, 1987.
66. Hodgkinson R, Hugg RW, Hayashi RH, Husain FJ: Double-blind comparison of maternal analgesia and neonatal neurobehavior following intravenous butorphanol and meperidine. J Int Med Res 7:224–230, 1979.
67. Clark RB, Beard AG, Greifenstein FE, Barclay DL: Naloxone in the parturient and her infant. South Med J 69:570–575, 1976.
68. Hodgkinson R, Bhatt M, Grewal G, Marx GF: Neonatal neurobehavior in the first 48 hours of life: Effect of the administration of meperidine with and without naloxone in the mother. Pediatrics 62:294–298, 1978.
69. Bonta BW, Gagliardi JO, Williams V, Warshaw JB: Naloxone reversal of mild neurobehavioral depression in normal newborn infants after routine obstetric analgesia. J Pediatr 94:102–105, 1979.
70. Weiner PC, Hogg MI, Rosen M: Neonatal respiration, feeding and neurobehavioral state: Effects of intrapartum bupivacaine, pethidine and pethidine reversal by naloxone. Anaesthesia 34:996–1004, 1979.
71. Brown WU Jr, Bell GC, Lurie AO, Weiss JB, Scanlon JW, Alper MH: Newborn blood levels of lidocaine and mepivacaine in the first postnatal day following maternal epidural anesthesia. Anesthesiology 42:698–706, 1975.
72. Scanlon JW, Ostheimer GW, Lurie AO, Brown WU Jr, Weiss JB, Alper MH: Neurobehavioral responses and drug concen-

trations in newborns after maternal epidural anesthesia with bupivacaine. Anesthesiology 45:400–405, 1976.

73. Brown WU Jr: Guest discussion: In Hodgkinson R, Marx GF, Kim SS, et al: Neonatal neurobehavioral tests following vaginal delivery under ketamine, thiopental and extradural anesthesia. Anesth Analg 56:552–553, 1977.

74. Abboud TK, Khoo SS, Miller F, Duan T, Henriksen EH: Maternal, fetal, and neonatal responses after epidural anesthesia with bupivacaine, 2-chloroprocaine, or lidocaine. Anesth Analg 61:638–644, 1982.

75. Abboud TK, Sarkis F, Blikian A, Varakian L: Lack of adverse neurobehavioral effects of lidocaine. Anesthesiology 57:A404, 1982.

76. Abboud TK, Afrasiabi A, Sarkis F, Daftarian F, Nagappala S, Noueihid R, Kuhnert BR, Miller F: Continuous infusion epidural analgesia in parturients receiving bupivacaine, chloroprocaine, or lidocaine: Maternal, fetal and neonatal effects. Anesth Analg 63:421–428, 1984.

77. Deleted in proof.
78. Deleted in proof.

79. Kileff ME, James FM, Dewan DM, Floyd HM: Neonatal neurobehavioral responses after epidural anesthesia for cesarean section using lidocaine and bupivacaine. Anesth Analg 63:413–417, 1984.

80. Kuhnert BR, Harrison MJ, Linn PL, Kuhnert PM: Effect of maternal epidural anesthesia on neonatal behavior. Anesth Analg 63:301–308, 1984.

81. Datta S, Corke BC, Alper MH, Brown WU Jr, Ostheimer GW, Weiss JB: Epidural anesthesia for cesarean section: A comparison of bupivacaine, chloroprocaine, and etidocaine. Anesthesiology 52:48–51, 1980.

82. Lund PC, Cwik JC, Gannon RT, Vassalo HG: Etidocaine for caesarean section: Effects on mother and baby. Br J Anaesth 49:457–460, 1977.

83. McGuinness GA, Merkow AJ, Kennedy RL, Erenberg A: Epidural anesthesia with bupivacaine for cesarean section: Neonatal blood levels and neurobehavioral responses. Anesthesiology 49:270–273, 1978.

84. Bromage PR, Robson JG: Concentrations of lignocaine in the blood after intravenous, intramuscular, epidural and endotracheal administration. Anaesthesia 16:461, 1961.

85. Mather LE, Tucker GT, Murphy TM, Stanton-Hicks d'A, Bonica JJ: The effects of adding adrenaline to etidocaine and lignocaine in extradural anaesthesia. II. Pharmacokinetics. Br J Anaesth 48:989–994, 1976.

86. Scott DB, Jebson PRG, Braid DP, Örtengren B, Frisch P: Factors affecting plasma levels of lignocaine and prilocaine. Br J Anaesth 44:1040–1049, 1972.

87. Bromage PR: Physiology. In Epidural Analgesia. Saunders, Philadelphia, 1978, pp 357–360.

88. Rosenfeld CR, Barton MD, Meschia G: Effects of epinephrine on distribution of blood flow in the pregnant ewe. Am J Obstet Gynecol 124:156–163, 1976.

89. Wallis KL, Shnider SM, Hicks JS, Spivey HT: Epidural anesthesia in the normotensive pregnant ewe: Effects on uterine blood flow and fetal acid-base status. Anesthesiology 44:481–487, 1976.

90. Hood DD, Dewan DM, Rose JC, James FM III: Maternal and fetal effects of intravenous epinephrine containing solutions in gravid ewes. Anesthesiology 59:A393, 1983.

91. Rucker MP: The action of adrenalin on the pregnant uterus. South Med J 18:412, 1925.

92. Gunther RE, Bauman J: Obstetrical caudal anesthesia. I. A randomized study comparing 1% mepivacaine with 1% lidocaine plus epinephrine. Anesthesiology 31:5–19, 1969.

93. Gunther RE, Bellville JW: Obstetrical anesthesia. II. A randomized study comparing 1% mepivacaine with 1% mepivacaine plus epinephrine. Anesthesiology 37:288–298, 1972.

94. Matadial L, Cibils LA: The effect of epidural anesthesia on uterine activity and blood pressure. Am J Obstet Gynecol 125:846–854, 1976.

95. Zador G, Nilsson BA: Low-dose intermittent epidural anaesthesia with lidocaine for vaginal delivery. II. Influence on labour and foetal acid-base status. Acta Obstet Gynecol 34(Suppl):17–30, 1974.

96. Levinson G, Shnider SM, Krames E, Ring G: Epidural anesthesia for cesarean section: Effects of epinephrine in the local anesthetic solution. In Abstracts of Scientific Papers, American Society of Anesthesiologists, Chicago, 1975, p 285–286.

97. deRosayro AM, Hahrwold ML, Hill AB: Cardiovascular effects of epidural epinephrine in the pregnant sheep. Reg Anesth 6:4–7, 1981.

98. Albright GA, Jouppila R, Hollmén AL, Jouppila P, Vierola H, Koivula A: Epinephrine does not alter human intervillous blood flow during epidural anesthesia. Anesthesiology 54:131–135, 1981.

99. Craft JB Jr, Epstein BS, Coakley CS: Effect of lidocaine with epinephrine versus lidocaine (plain) on induced labor. Anesth Analg 51:243–246, 1972.

100. Abboud TK, David S, Nagappala S, Costandi J, Yanagi T, Haroutunian S, Yeh SU: Maternal, fetal and neonatal effects of lidocaine with and without epinephrine for epidural anesthesia in obstetrics. Anesth Analg 63:973–979, 1984.

101. Abboud TK, Sheik-Ol-Eslam A, Yanagi T, Murakawa K, Costandi J, Zakarian M, Hoffman D, Haroutunian S: Safety and efficacy of epinephrine added to bupivacaine for lumbar epidural analgesia in obstetrics. Anesth Analg 64:585–591, 1985.

102. Abboud TK, DerSarkissian L, Terrasi J, Murakawa K, Zhu J, Longhitano M: Comparative maternal, fetal and neonatal effects of chloroprocaine with and without epinephrine for epidural anesthesia in obstetrics. Anesth Analg 66:71–75, 1987.

103. Abboud TK, Afrasiabi A, Zhu J, Mantilla M, Reyes A, O'Onofrio L, Khoo N, Mosaad P, Steffens Z, Davidson J, Paul R: Bupivacaine/butorphanol/epinephrine for epidural anesthesia in obstetrics: Maternal and neonatal effects. Reg Anesth 14:219–224, 1989.

104. Abboud TK, Mosaad P, Maker A, Gangolly J, Dror A, Zhu J, Mantilla M, Zaki N, Davis H, Moore J, Swart F, Reyes A: Comparative maternal and neonatal effects of the new and the old formulations of 2-chloroprocaine. Reg Anesth 13:101–106, 1988.

105. Hodgkinson R, Bhatt M, Kim SS, Grewal G, Marx GF: Neonatal neurobehavioral tests following cesarean section under general and spinal anesthesia. Am J Obstet Gynecol 132:670–674, 1978.

106. Hughes SC, Rosen MA, Shnider SM, Abboud TK, Stefani SJ, Norton M: Maternal and neonatal effects of epidural morphine for labor and delivery. Anesth Analg 63:319–324, 1984.

107. Abboud TK, Shnider SM, Dailey PA, Raya JA, Sarkis N, Grobler M, Sadri S, Khoo SS, deSousa B, Baysinger CL, Miller F: Intrathecal administration of hyperbaric morphine for the relief of pain in labour. Br J Anaesth 56:1351–1359, 1984.

108. Talafre ML, Jacquinot P, Legagneux F, Jasson J, Conseiller C: Intrathecal administration of meperidine versus tetracaine for elective cesarean section. Anesthesiology 67:A620, 1987.

109. Dailey PA, Brookshire GL, Shnider SM, Abboud RK, Kotelko DM, Noueihid R, Thigpen JW, Khoo SS, Raya JA, Foutz SE, Brizgys RV, Goebelsmann UY, Lo M-W: The effects of naloxone associated with the intrathecal use of morphine in labor. Anesth Analg 64:658–666, 1985.

110. Preston P, Rosen M, Hughes SC, Glosten B, Ross BK, Daniels D, Shnider SM, Dailey PA: Epidural anesthesia with fentanyl and lidocaine for cesarean section: Maternal effects and neonatal outcome. Anesthesiology 68:938–943, 1988.

111. Murakawa K, Abboud TK, Yanagi T, Sarkis F, Sheikh-Ol-Eslam, Raya J, Yonekura ML: Clinical experience of epidural fentanyl for labor pain. J Anesthesia (Japan) 1:93–95, 1987.

112. Cohen SE, Tan S, Albright GA, Halpern J: Epidural fentanyl/bupivacaine mixtures for obstetric analgesia. Anesthesiology 67:403–407, 1987.

113. Abboud TK, Afrasiabi A, Zhu J, Mantilla M, Reyes A, D'Onofrio KL, Khoo N, Mossad P, Richardson M, Kalra M, Cheung M, Paul R: Epidural morphine or butorphanol augments bupivacaine analgesia during labor. Reg Anesth 14:115–120, 1989.

114. Zhu J, Abboud TK, Afrasiabi A, Reyes A, Sherman G, Vera Cruz R, Steffens Z: Epidural butorphanol augments lidocaine analgesia during labor. Anesthesiology 73:A979, 1990.

115. Little MS, McNitt JD, Choi HJ, Tremper KK: A pilot study of low dose epidural sufentanil and bupivacaine for labor anesthesia. Anesthesiology 67:A444, 1987.

116. Merkow AJ, McGuinness GA, Erenberg A, Kennedy RL: The neonatal neurobehavioral effects of bupivacaine, mepivacaine, and 2-chloroprocaine used for pudendal block. Anesthesiology 52:309–312, 1980.

117. Scanlon JW, Shea E, Alper MH: Neurobehavioral responses of newborn infants following general or spinal anesthesia for cesarean section. In *Abstracts of Scientific Papers*, American Society of Anesthesiologists, Chicago, 1975, p 91.

118. Hodgkinson R, Marx GF, Kim SS, Miclat NM: Neonatal neurobehavioral tests following vaginal delivery under ketamine, thiopental and extradural anesthesia. Anesth Analg 56:548–552, 1977.

119. Abboud TK, Nagappala S, Murakawa K, David S, Haroutunian S, Zakarian M, Yanagi T, Sheikh-Ol-Eslam A: Comparison of the effects of general and regional anesthesia for cesarean section on neonatal neurologic and adaptive capacity scores. Anesth Analg 64:996–1000, 1985.

120. Stefani SJ, Hughes SC, Shnider SM, Levinson G, Abboud TK, Henriksen EH, Williams V, Johnson J: Neonatal neurobehavioral effects of inhalation analgesia for delivery. Anesthesiology 56:351–355, 1982.

121. Abboud TK, Gangolly J, Mossaad P, Crowell D: Isoflurane in obstetrics. Anesth Analg 68:388–391, 1989.

122. Tronick E, Wise S, Als H, Adamson L, Scanlon J, Brazelton TB: Regional obstetric anesthesia and newborn behavior: Effects over the first ten days of life. Pediatrics 58:95–100, 1976.

123. Standley K, Soule AB, Duchowny MS: Local-regional anesthesia during childbirth: Effect on newborn behaviors. Science 186:634–635, 1974.

124. Friedman EA, Sachtleben MR, Bresky PA: Dysfunctional labor. XII. Long-term effects on infants. Am J Obstet Gynecol 127:779–783, 1977.

125. Kolata GB: Behavioral teratology: Birth defects of the mind. Science 202:732–734, 1978.

126. Kolata GB: Scientists attack report that obstetrical medications endanger children: But natural childbirth advocates rally to its defense. Science 204:391–392, 1979.

127. Ounsted M, Scott A, Moar V: Delivery and development: To what extent can one associate cause and effect? J R Soc Med 73:786–792, 1980.

128. Ounsted M: Pain relief during childbirth and development at 4 years. J R Soc Med 74:629–630, 1981.

129. Van den Berg BJ, Levinson G, Shnider SM, Hughes SC, Stefani SJ: Evaluation of long term effects of obstetric medication on clinical development. In *Abstracts of Scientific Papers, Society for Obstetric Anesthesia and Perinatology*, Boston, 1980, p 52.

130. Klaus MH, Kennell JH: *Maternal-Infant Bonding*. CV Mosby, St Louis. 1976.

CHAPTER 39

Resuscitation of the Newborn

Gershon Levinson, M.D.

Sol M. Shnider, M.D.

George A. Gregory, M.D.

Immediately after delivery, as the fetus becomes a neonate, major changes in the pulmonary and circulatory systems must occur. The lungs must now assume the role of the placenta in the exchange of oxygen and carbon dioxide. This requires pulmonary expansion, aeration, and perfusion. In the vast majority of instances these changes occur spontaneously. Some infants, however, require resuscitation to make the transition from dependent fetal to independent neonatal existence. This chapter discusses the normal changes at birth, pathophysiology of asphyxia, and recommended techniques for resuscitation of the newborn.

CHANGES AT BIRTH

In utero, blood is oxygenated in the placenta and returns to the fetal heart via the umbilical vein, hepatic veins, the ductus venosus, and the inferior vena cava (1, 2) (see Fig. 5.9). At the junction of the inferior vena cava and right atrium the caval blood divides into two streams. Approximately 40% enters the right heart, where it mixes with venous blood returning via the superior vena cava from the upper part of the body. This blood is ejected by the right ventricle into the pulmonary arteries. However, because the pulmonary vascular resistance is so high, only 5 to 10% actually perfuses the fetal lungs, the remainder being shunted across the ductus arteriosus into the thoracic aorta. About 60% of the well-oxygenated blood returning via the inferior vena cava is deflected by the crista dividens through the foramen ovale into the left atrium. Although this blood undergoes admixture with the small amount of venous blood returning from the lungs, it is relatively well oxygenated and provides the heart and brain with somewhat better oxygenation than the lower half of the body.

With clamping of the cord and vasoconstriction of the umbilical vessels at birth, systemic vascular resistance increases markedly, left artrial pressure rises, and flow through the foramen ovale ceases; the lungs expand, pulmonary vascular resistance falls, and 90 to 100% of the right ventricular output now perfuses the lungs (3, 4).

As arterial oxygen and pH rise, the pulmonary vessels dilate, pulmonary vascular resistance falls further, pulmonary blood pressure falls below systemic, and right-to-left shunting of blood through the ductus arteriosus ceases. In the normal newborn the rise in arterial oxygen to above 60 torr will cause vasoconstriction of the ductus arteriosus and aid in functional closure (5, 6).

ASPHYXIA

If immediately after birth adequate ventilation is not established, then the ensuing hypoxemia and respiratory and metabolic acidosis will prevent establishment of a normal adult circulation. Pulmonary vascular resistance will remain high and pulmonary blood flow low, and the ductus arteriosus and foramen ovale will remain widely patent with a large right-to-left shunt through both. With progressive hypoxemia and acidosis, myocardial failure and brain damage will occur.

In the extreme case when no pulmonary ventilation occurs in a newborn mammal, by 5 min the PaO_2 will fall to under 2 torr, the $PaCO_2$ will rise to 100 torr, and the pH will fall to 7 or less units (Fig. 39.1) (1). Heart rate and blood pressure will fall and, after a period of gasping, apnea will occur. In the monkey, by 7 min there will be irreversible brain damage. After the cessation of gasping, nothing will reinitiate breathing other than artificial ventilation.

ESTABLISHMENT OF VENTILATION

In utero, the fetal lung is filled with an ultrafiltrate of plasma, approximately 30 ml/kg of body weight (7, 8). This fluid produced in the lungs must be removed during and immediately after birth. During a vaginal delivery the thorax of the fetus is squeezed while passing through the birth canal. This helps push out approximately two-thirds of the fluid from

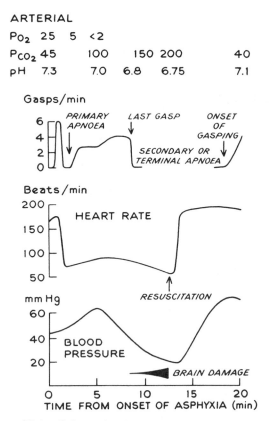

ARTERIAL

PO_2	25	5	<2		
PCO_2	45	100	150 200		40
pH	7.3	7.0	6.8 6.75		7.1

Figure 39.1. Schematic diagram of changes in Rhesus monkeys during asphyxia and resuscitation by positive pressure ventilation. Brain damage was assessed by histologic examination some weeks or months later. (Reprinted by permission from Dawes GS: *Foetal and Neonatal Physiology.* Year Book Medical Publishers, Chicago, 1968, pp 141–157.)

the lung, and the remainder is removed after birth by capillaries and lymphatics (9). Infants delivered by cesarean section do not benefit from the vaginal squeeze, which may account for their increased difficulty in establishing normal ventilation (10).

Normal infants make their first respiratory movements within seconds of delivery of the thorax. This is due in part to the elastic recoil of the chest wall following expulsion. During the first breath a negative pressure of 60 to 100 cm H_2O is generated and up to 80 ml of air inspired (Fig. 39.2) (11). The breath is generally held for about 2 sec and then partly exhaled. Approximately 75% of the first breath is retained in the lung as part of the developing functional residual capacity. The next few breaths are similar to the first, with lesser amounts of air retained each time. Once ventilation is established the normal mature infant has a tidal volume of 10 to 30 ml, a vital capacity of over 100 ml, a breathing frequency of 30 to 60 times/min, a minute ventilation of over 500 ml, and a lung compliance of 5 ml/cm H_2O (11).

By 90 sec after delivery most infants have begun rhythmic respirations. Initiation of breathing de-

pends on the condition of the respiratory center, including peripheral chemoreceptors responsive to low pH and low PO_2.

CAUSES OF NEONATAL DEPRESSION

A number of factors may depress the respiratory center of the neonate, including drugs administered to the mother—such as anesthetics, narcotics, barbiturates, and magnesium—severe intrauterine fetal hypoxia and acidosis, high or low environmental temperature, or central nervous system trauma associated with the birth process. In addition, certain congenital anomalies may make adaptation to extrauterine life difficult or impossible. Some of these are listed in Table 39.1.

There are also various situation in which serious neonatal morbidity may occur. Identifying these high-risk fetuses prior to birth allows the anesthesiologist, obstetrician, and neonatologist to prepare for immediate resuscitation of the newborn. Some of the factors that should alert the anesthesiologist that the fetus is at high risk are listed in Table 39.2.

The mechanism for the adverse effect on the neonate is obvious in conditions like preeclampsia and anemia, which are associated with decreased uteroplacental blood flow or oxygenation. In conditions such as diabetes mellitus, neonatal morbidity and mortality are very high but the precise etiologic factors are not known. Nevertheless, in all these conditions aggressive management of the newborn is indicated.

UMBILICAL CORD BLOOD SAMPLING

At delivery the acid-base status and oxygenation of the fetus may be easily ascertained by sampling from a doubly clamped segment of umbilical cord. Babies who have demonstrated fetal distress in utero or who are clinically depressed at 1 min of age should be studied. Some favor routinely measuring umbilical cord blood acid-base status at all deliveries (12). This approach has been discussed fully in the preceding chapter. Blood is drawn separately with heparinized syringes from both an umbilical artery and the umbilical vein. It should be recalled that the umbilical vein blood is the best oxygenated blood. The normal blood gas values are shown in Table 39.3 (13). If both umbilical venous and umbilical artery blood show low PO_2 and high PCO_2, then uteroplacental insufficiency was present. If umbilical artery blood shows signs of asphyxia but umbilical venous blood is relatively normal—that is, a wide venous-arterial difference exists, then umbilical cord compression has likely occurred during delivery. With partial compression of the umbilical cord or in conditions with severe low fetal cardiac output, the transit time

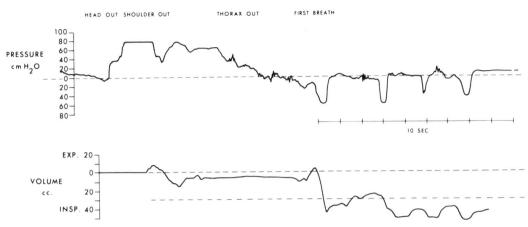

Figure 39.2. Intrathoracic pressures during and immediately after delivery. (Reprinted by permission from Karlberg P: The adaptive changes in the immediate postnatal period, with particular reference to respiration. J Pediatr 56:585–604, 1960.)

Table 39.1
Other Causes of Neonatal Depression in the Delivery Room

Congenital defects of the respiratory system
  Nose: choanal stenosis and atresia
  Upper airway: micrognathia (Pierre Robin syndrome)
  Larynx
    Webs
    Fusions
    Atresia
    Vocal cord paralysis
    Subglottic stenosis
  Trachea
    Tracheal agenesis
    Tracheal rings
    Cartilage
  Vascular
    Hemangiomas
    Webs
    Tumors
  Bronchi
    Congenital bronchial stenosis
Diaphragmatic hernia
Esophageal atresia and tracheoesophageal fistula
Congenital heart disease
Central nervous system dysfunction (congenital/acquired)
Fetal sepsis

Table 39.2
Factors that May Help to Identify High Risk Fetuses

Maternal conditions
  Preeclampsia-eclampsia
  Chronic hypertension
  Diabetes mellitus
  Chronic renal disease
  Maternal malnutrition or severe obesity
  Sickle cell disease
  Anemia (< 9 g hemoglobin)
  Rh or ABO incompatibility
  Heart disease
  Pulmonary disease
  Third-trimester bleeding
  Drug therapy (e.g., lithium carbonate, magnesium, adrenergic-blocking drugs)
  Drug or ethanol abuse
  Maternal infection
  Uterine or pelvic anatomic abnormalities
  Prolonged rupture of membranes
  Previous fetal or neonatal deaths
Fetal conditions: antepartum
  Premature delivery
  Postmaturity (> 43 weeks)
  Intrauterine growth retardation
  Multiple births
  Oligo- or polyhydramnios
Labor and delivery conditions
  Breech or other abnormal presentations
  Forceps delivery (other than low elective)
  Cesarean section
  Prolapsed umbilical cord
  Nuchal cord
  Prolonged general anesthesia
  Excessive sedation or analgesia
  Anesthetic complications (such as untreated hypotension or hypoxia)
  Prolonged or precipitous labor
  Uterine hypertonus (spontaneous/oxytocin induced)
  Abnormal fetal heart rate or rhythm
  Meconium-stained amniotic fluid

of fetal blood through the placenta is increased, thus allowing more time for equilibration with the maternal blood. The umbilical venous blood becomes well oxygenated, but, because of the obstruction of blood flow from the placenta to the fetus, an inadequate amount of oxygen is delivered to the fetal tissues and the umbilical arterial blood will demonstrate a low PO_2 and pH. A depressed neonate with normal umbilical venous oxygen and acid-base values may, in fact, be asphyxiated. It is obvious, therefore, that both the umbilical vein and artery blood

Table 39.3
Normal Values for Umbilical Cord Blood[a,b]

Cord Blood	pH	Pco₂ (mm Hg)	Po₂ (mm Hg)	Bicarbonate (mEq/L)
Arterial	7.28 ± 0.05 (7.15 − 7.43)	49.2 ± 8.4 (31.1 − 74.3)	18.0 ± 6.2 (3.8 − 33.8)	22.3 ± 2.5 (13.3 − 27.5)
Venous	7.35 ± 0.05 (7.24 − 7.49)	38.2 ± 5.6 (23.2 − 49.2)	29.2 ± 5.9 (15.4 − 48.2)	20.4 ± 2.1 (15.9 − 24.7)

[a] Yeomans ER, Hauth JC, Gilstrap LC III, Strickland DM: Umbilical cord pH, Pco₂ and bicarbonate following uncomplicated term vaginal deliveries. Am J Obstet Gynecol 151:798–800, 1985.
[b] Results are for 146 newborns after uncomplicated labor and vaginal delivery at 37 to 42 weeks of gestation. Values are mean ± standard deviation; ranges are given in parentheses.

should be analyzed for correct diagnosis of etiology and significance of depression. If umbilical cord blood gases are normal but the neonate is depressed at birth, common causes include drug depression, sepsis, acute birth trauma, or other factors listed in Table 39.1.

IMMEDIATE CARE OF THE NEWBORN

Equipment for Resuscitation

Each delivery room should contain the basic equipment for resuscitating the depressed newborn (Table 39.4). This includes infant laryngoscope, supply of batteries and bulbs, endotracheal tubes, infant airways, and suction bulbs and catheters. In addition, each room should have a mobile or portable (delivery room to nursery) resuscitation crib. This apparatus should provide a simple but sufficiently large, nonslippery surface on which to place the baby with easy access to oxygen and suction, and it should be adaptable to various modes of resuscitation, including simultaneous positive pressure ventilation and placement of umbilical vessel catheters for acid-base control and blood sampling. A source of radiant heat should be mounted above each resuscitation unit. The energy output should be servocontrolled by a sensor taped to the infant's abdomen.

In addition, a special neonatal treatment room located immediately adjacent to the delivery room is desirable for intensive care of the immature or severely asphyxiated newborn in need of prolonged resuscitation. More sophisticated ventilatory and monitoring equipment and a variety of cardiac emergency drugs should be immediately available.

Establishment of an Airway

As the infant's head is delivered, the mouth and nose are gently suctioned to remove the lung fluid as well as amniotic fluid, blood, mucus, and meconium that might be in the pharynx (Figure 39.3). Babies born through meconium require more extensive airway management as will be described subsequently. The infant is placed in the head-down position to allow gravity drainage of this fluid. Suctioning of the pharynx and nose should be brief and gentle, because prolonged or too vigorous suctioning may produce breath holding, laryngospasm, or profound bradycardia and other arrhythmias. In addition to removing debris from the airway with nasal suctioning, anatomic abnormalities such as choanal atresia may be noted. Babies are nasal breathers and will often develop severe hypoxia if unable to breathe through their nose.

Routine Tracheal Suctioning for Meconium

Meconium aspiration pneumonitis is the leading respiratory cause of death in the full-term newborn. Treatment of meconium aspiration should begin in the delivery room. With suctioning of the airways there is a significant reduction in morbidity and mortality rates (Fig. 39.4) (14–17). Infants who aspirate blood, mucus, meconium, or cells in utero often have airway obstruction and severe asphyxia after birth. The best studied example is the meconium aspiration syndrome.

Meconium is the breakdown product of swallowed amniotic fluid, gastrointestinal cells, and intestinal secretions. Aspiration of meconium is uncommon in fetuses of less than 34 weeks' gestation, but increasingly common after 42 weeks' gestation. Older fetuses respond to stress (hypoxia) with increased gut motility, relaxation of the anal sphincters, defecation (1, 2), and gasping. Normal fetal breathing results in inhalation of about 1 ml of fluid; gasping leads to as much as 60 ml of amniotic fluid and debris being inhaled. Most of the aspirated material is in the mouth, trachea, and mainstem bronchi. If birth is delayed 24 hr, the aspirated material is broken down by the lung fluid and expelled from the lungs by the continuous production of lung fluid. If birth occurs within 12 to 24 hr of aspiration, the meconium in the major airways will move progressively into the periphery of the lung with initiation and maintenance of air breathing. This causes ob-

Table 39.4
Equipment for Neonatal Resuscitation

Basic Equipment
  Radiantly heated, mobile resuscitation crib
  Suction devices: sterile bulb suction *or* DeLee suction
    trap, meconium aspirator and vacuum suction with
    sterile catheters (6, 8, 10 French)
  Stethoscope
  Oxygen source with flowmeter and tubing
  Infant resuscitation bag with a pressure-release valve or
    pressure gauge. The bag must be capable of deliver-
    ing 90 to 100% oxygen
  Infant face masks (newborn and premature sizes)
  Infant oropharyngeal airways (newborn and premature
    sizes)
  Laryngoscope with straight blades (No 0 and 1)
    (extra bulbs and batteries for laryngoscope)
  Sterile endotracheal tubes sizes (2, 2.5, 3, 3.5 and
    4 mm) with stylets
  Sterile umbilical vessel catheterization tray including 3.5
    and 5 French umbilical vessel catheters
  Drug tray including:
    Epinephrine 1:10,000
    Naloxone 0.4 mg/ml or 1 mg/ml
    Sodium bicarbonate 4.2%
    Dextrose 10%
    Sterile water
    Normal saline
    Volume expanders: either albumin 5% solution, normal
      saline or Ringer's lactate solution
    Dopamine
  Syringes: 1, 3, 5, 10, 20, and 50 ml
  Needles: 18, 21, and 25 gauge
  Sterile gloves, scissors, adhesive tape, alcohol sponges,
    and three-way stopcocks
For Special Neonatal Treatment Room: All of the above
plus:
  Oscillometric or Doppler device for neonatal blood pres-
    sure
  Source of oxygen *and* air with oxygen-air blender
  Heated nebulizer
  Anaeroid manometer for observing airway pressures dur-
    ing controlled ventilation
  Oxygen analyzer
  Pulse oximeter
  Pressure transducers and monitor for intraarterial and
    venous pressures
  ECG and heart rate monitor
  Blood gas and pH electrodes and machine readily
    available
  Thoracocentesis tray including size 10 to 16 French red,
    rubber catheters for treatment of pneumothorax

struction of small airways which leads to mismatch-ing of ventilation and perfusion. Respiration becomes rapid (100 to 150 breaths/min) and shallow, and lung compliance decreases to levels seen in infants with hyaline membrane disease (0.8 ml/cm H_2O).

The precise management of neonates born through meconium is controversial. *All agree that the mouth and nose of all these neonates should be suctioned by the obstetrician as soon as the head is out but before the shoulders are delivered and the infant starts breathing.* Subsequent endotracheal intubation and suctioning is somewhat controversial and is discussed extensively in a recent review (17). Most neonatalogists recommend endotracheal intubation and suctioning of all meconium-stained neonates. Some suggest that intubation is only necessary if thick, particulate, "pea-soup" meconium is present. In the presence of thin, watery, yellow-tinged meconium-stained amniotic fluid with no visible particles, they believe no special management is required. Others examine the oropharynx with a laryngoscope and only intubate if meconium is present in the oro-pharynx or at the vocal cords. Finally, some believe that, regardless of the nature of the meconium, if the infant is vigorous (Apgar score of 8 or more), intubation is not necessary.

We believe that the respiratory failure induced by meconium aspiration can be prevented in most cases by removing the meconium from the lung and large airways before it can obstruct small airways. All infants, regardless of vigor, who are born through thick meconium should therefore undergo endotracheal suction. We do not believe examination of the oro-pharynx is reliable. Babies born through thin meconium probably do not require special management, but the clinical judgment of the resuscitator in evaluating the nature of the meconium is crucial. If uncertain, intubation is advised. Similarly, the depressed neonate born through thin meconium may benefit from endotracheal intubation and suction (18, 19). It must be emphasized that, despite appropriate management, some infants will still develop meconium aspiration syndrome, respiratory failure, and death.

To remove thick meconium (Fig. 39.5), a 3-mm endotracheal tube is inserted, and suction is applied to the tube by a suction device specially designed for this purpose (Fig. 39.6; see Fig. 34.4). As the suction is applied, the tube is withdrawn from the trachea. Meconium withdrawn into the tube is immediately expelled from the tube, and the trachea is reintubated to repeat the procedure. If meconium is not recovered, the trachea is not reintubated. In either case the infant is then allowed to breathe or is ventilated with oxygen as required. The trachea can then be reintubated if meconium was obtained during the second period of suctioning. Excessive airway pressures must be avoided because pulmonary gas leaks are common following meconium aspiration (14) and can occur any time during the first 3 days of life. If the above procedure is followed, the mortality from meconium aspiration is only 0.06 per 1000 live births, compared to 2.2 per 1000 live births when no suc-

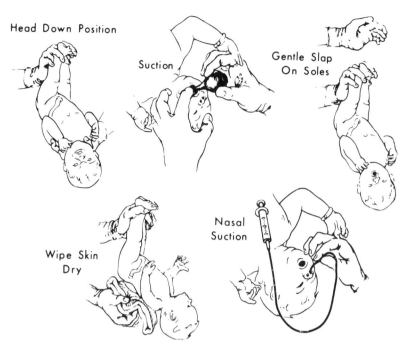

Head Down Position

Suction

Gentle Slap
On Soles

Wipe Skin
Dry

Nasal
Suction

Figure 39.3. Establishment of patency of upper airway by gravity drainage, suctioning, and stimulation to cry by rubbing the infant with a towel. (Reprinted by permission from Gregory

GA: Cardiopulmonary resuscitation of the newborn. In *The Anesthesiologist, Mother and Newborn.* SM Shnider, F Moya, eds. Williams & Wilkins, Baltimore, 1974, p 20.)

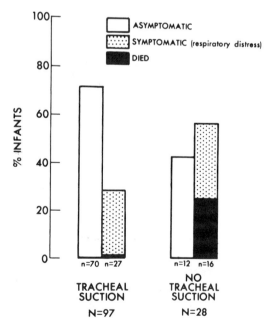

Figure 39.4. Comparison of percentage of incidence of respiratory distress and percentage of mortality in 97 infants who received tracheal suction in the delivery room and 28 infants who did not (numbers of infants below columns); note that 1 infant died in the tracheal suction group and 7 died in the no tracheal suction group. (Reprinted by permission from Ting P, Brady JP: Tracheal suction in meconium aspiration. Am J Obstet Gynecol 122:767–771, 1975.)

tioning is applied. Infants whose tracheas are suctioned seldom require assisted ventilation following meconium aspiration. However, as previously stated, there will always be some infants who develop respiratory failure despite suctioning.

If the airway is not suctioned and the meconium is allowed to obstruct the airway, cyanosis, retractions, tachypnea, and grunting respiration develop. The PaO_2 falls below 50 mm Hg ($FIO_2 = 0.21$) and the $PaCO_2$ often falls below 30 mm Hg. Similar to patients with asthma, a rise in $PaCO_2$ indicates impending severe respiratory failure. Hypoxia should be treated with oxygen. If, despite breathing 80% oxygen, PaO_2 remains below 50 mm Hg, an endotracheal tube should be inserted and 3 to 5 cm H_2O continuous positive airway pressure applied. If the PaO_2 still remains below 50 mm Hg, mechanical ventilation should be instituted and 3 to 5 cm H_2O positive end-expiratory pressure applied. One should use the lowest ventilatory pressures possible because approximately 50% of meconium-stained, mechanically ventilated infants develop a pneumothorax (21). Infants with meconium aspiration should be hydrated; they should also receive chest physiotherapy every 30 min for the first 2 hr and hourly for the next 6 hr.

Infants with meconium aspiration and respiratory

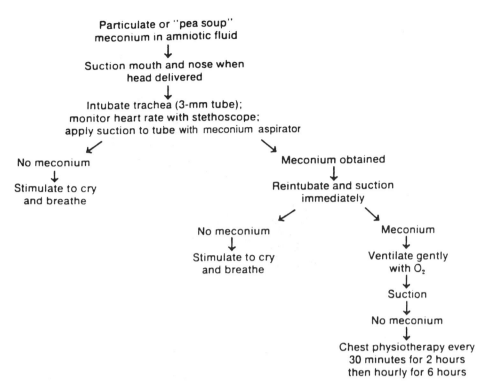

Figure 39.5. Treatment of meconium aspiration.

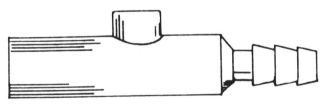

Figure 39.6. An example of a disposable mechanical meconium aspirator. Wall suction is connected to the smaller end with the barbed fitting. Wall suction is set at 80 mm Hg. After the patient is intubated, the larger end (15 mm ID) of the meconium aspirator is connected to the endotracheal tube adapter. The suction control port on top of the aspirator is occluded to regulate suction and remove meconium.

distress frequently develop pulmonary hypertension and right-to-left shunting of blood through the foramen ovale and ductus arteriosus. The cause of the hypertension is unknown. Its diagnosis is made by observing a higher PaO_2 in the right radial artery (radial > umbilical) than in the descending aorta or by detecting shunting of blood through the foramen ovale by echocardiogram. Treatment of pulmonary hypertension includes mechanical ventilation, hyperventilation ($PaCO_2$ 20 to 25 mm Hg; pH 7.55 to 7.65), pulmonary vasodilation with tolazoline (Priscoline), and fluid replacement (20). It is often necessary to infuse more than 20 μg/kg/min of dopamine to maintain a mean arterial pressure of 50 to 60 mm Hg

during tolazoline administration. About 80% of patients treated this way survive.

Tactile Stimulation of the Baby

Many babies must be stimulated at birth to arouse them sufficiently to breathe effectively. This may be accomplished by drying the baby's skin with a warm towel. This maneuver not only stimulates respiration but also reduces heat loss from the infant due to evaporation. Gently flicking the soles of the feet may also produce a cry and rhythmic respiration. Vigorous slapping of the feet, buttocks, and costovertebral angles may cause ecchymoses and kidney and adrenal damage.

Maintenance of Body Temperature

Immediately after birth particular attention must be given to the prevention of heat loss by the infant. The naked, wet baby delivered into a room at 25°C will rapidly lose heat by conduction, convection, evaporation, and radiation. Catecholamine-mediated, nonshivering thermogenesis by metabolism of brown fat is the principal mechanism utilized by the neonate in his/her usually futile attempt to maintain normal body temperature (22–24). This leads to a dramatic increase in oxygen consumption (Fig. 39.7) (25). If the neonate's temperature falls, his/her pulmonary vessels constrict, there is an increased right-

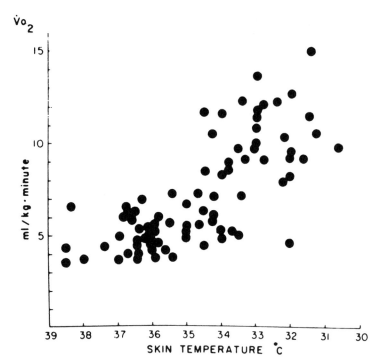

Figure 39.7. The relationship between oxygen consumption and skin temperature of newborn infants under a variety of thermal environmental conditions. (Reprinted by permission from Adamsons K Jr, Gandy GM, James LS: The influence of thermal factors upon oxygen consumption of the newborn infant. J Pediatr 66:495–508, 1965.)

to-left shunt, and hypoxemia, metabolic acidosis, tachypnea, and grunting occur.

Heat conservation techniques must be used. In addition to drying the skin, the baby should be placed under a radiant heater, preferably one servocontrolled by a sensor placed on the baby's skin.

Clinical Assessment of the Neonate

The most widely used method for evaluating the condition of the infant in the delivery room is a score devised by Virginia Apgar in 1953 (26, 27). It is fully described in Chapter 36. This easily performed assessment is usually made 1 and 5 min after birth. There are five signs: heart rate, respiratory effort, muscle tone, response to stimulation, and skin color. A score of 0, 1, or 2 is assigned according to the presence or absence of each of the signs.

A popular scheme of resuscitation of the newborn based on the 1-min Apgar score is described here. However, when an infant is known to be severely asphyxiated or depressed, active resuscitation should always be started without waiting for 1 min to elapse.

VIGOROUS NEONATES (APGAR SCORE 8 TO 10)

The vast majority of newborns fall into this category. They require only the usual upper airway suctioning, drying of the skin, and a warm ambient environment. Occasionally a baby vigorous at 1 min of age will deteriorate shortly thereafter. Possible causes are drug depression becoming apparent after stim-

ulation of the baby ceases, persistent nasopharyngeal suctioning resulting in reflex bradycardia and laryngospasm, hypoxia due to spontaneous pneumothorax, regurgitation and aspiration of gastric contents, or congenital anomalies such as a diaphragmatic hernia, which makes adaptation to extrauterine life difficult. A brief physical examination for obvious congenital anomalies should be performed on every newborn. Ideally, this includes a measurement of blood pressure with an external device. Normal systolic pressure in a full-term baby is 65 to 75 mm Hg (24). A pressure below 50 mm Hg is considered hypotensive.

Aspiration and measurement of gastric contents is often also included in the routine examination. This procedure will prevent aspiration of gastric contents in the immediate neonatal period and help in the diagnosis of choanal atresia, esophageal atresia, and small bowel obstruction. A soft plastic catheter (8 French) is passed into the stomach. Its position **must** be confirmed by injecting 2 to 3 ml of air while auscultating or palpating the left upper abdominal quadrant. It is possible to aspirate a small amount of fluid from an esophageal pouch of an atretic esophagus and fail to diagnose the anomaly. The volume of gastric contents should be measured. The average amount is 4 to 8 ml, but larger quantities are frequently found after cesarean sections. If 25 to 50 ml of fluid are present, a small bowel obstruction should be suspected; amounts greater than 50 ml indicate the need for immediate x-ray examination of the abdomen (29).

MILDLY DEPRESSED NEONATES (APGAR SCORE 5 TO 7)

These infants are minimally depressed either from a brief episode of birth asphyxia or from slight drug depression. They usually respond to a combination of tactile stimulation and oxygen-enriched air to breathe. After they become vigorous they are managed as described above. If the baby does not rapidly improve with oxygen blown over the face, then oxygen should be administered by positive pressure (Fig. 39.8).

MODERATELY DEPRESSED NEONATES (APGAR SCORE 3 TO 4)

These babies are usually more hypoxic and acidotic or have received a larger amount of depressing drugs than the babies who score 5 to 7. They require oxygen by positive pressure ventilation. This can usually be accomplished with a face mask and rebreathing bag, providing the upper airway is clear and an adequate mask fit can be obtained. The infant's head should be in a neutral position, and care must be taken not to occlude the trachea with the fingers supporting the mandible. A small oral airway may be helpful in preventing upper airway obstruction by the tongue. Pressures of 25 to 30 cm H_2O administered for 1 to 2 sec are usually necessary. Higher pressures may rupture the lungs. Once the lungs have been inflated, pressures of 10 to 15 cm H_2O are usually sufficient to deliver an adequate volume. As with the adult, positive pressure ventilation via a face mask may result in gaseous distension of the stomach, ocular damage due to pressure applied to the eyes, or abrasions to the face. Gastric distension can be prevented by maintaining an open airway, placement of a nasogastric tube with the upper end open to the atmosphere, or gentle manual pressure

in the left upper quadrant during controlled ventilation. In addition to correcting hypoxia, positive pressure ventilation may stimulate sensitive stretch receptors in the pulmonary tree and initiate a gasp (30).

If there is no immediate improvement in the clinical condition of the neonate then positive pressure with the face mask is likely ineffective and prompt endotracheal intubation for ventilation is indicated.

SEVERELY DEPRESSED NEONATES (APGAR SCORE 0 TO 2)

These infants are usually severely hypoxic, acidotic, and apneic. They require immediate ventilation with oxygen via an endotracheal tube. The infant's head should be placed in the neutral "sniffing position" rather than hyperextended. The larynx of the neonate is more anterior than in the adult and at the level of the second cervical vertebra rather than the sixth. Thus a small straight blade, such as a Miller 0 to 1, provides the best visualization of the larynx. As the laryngoscope is introduced into the right-hand corner of the mouth, the tongue is moved toward the left and the epiglottis is located (Fig. 39.9). Gentle pressure over the hyoid bone with the little finger of the hand holding the laryngoscope will move the larynx posteriorly to help expose the epiglottis. The tip of the laryngoscope blade may either be placed in the vallecula or posterior to the epiglottis, and with gentle upward pressure the cords are visualized. If unable to visualize the larynx or insert the endotracheal tube after 24 sec of trying, the neonate should be ventilated with a bag and mask before a subsequent attempt.

The sterile endotracheal tube should be of such a size that with positive pressure ventilation there is a small air leak. Too large a tube may cause subglotic stenosis, and too small a tube will not permit adequate ventilation and may become plugged easily. Depending on the size of the neonate, a size 2 to 4

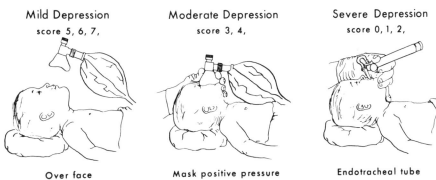

Mild Depression
score 5, 6, 7,
Over face

Moderate Depression
score 3, 4,
Mask positive pressure

Severe Depression
score 0, 1, 2,
Endotracheal tube

Figure 39.8. A plan for oxygen delivery during resuscitation of the newborn. (Reprinted by permission from SM Shnider (ed): *Obstetrical Anesthesia: Current Concepts and Practice.* Williams & Wilkins, 1970, p 223.)

mm is chosen. The tube should be inserted about 2 cm past the cords, and ventilation with 100% oxygen should be begun. Although a pressure of 25 to 30 cm H_2O is usually sufficient to ventilate most asphyxiated infants, those with low compliance, as is found in erythroblastosis or pulmonary hypoplasia, may require higher pressures.

The correct placement of the endotracheal tube, and the adequacy of ventilation must be immediately ascertained (Fig. 39.10). This is done by observation and auscultation of the chest. Both sides of the chest

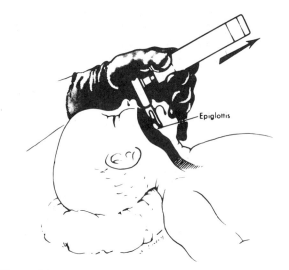

Figure 39.9. Technique for laryngoscopy. Left hand holds the laryngoscope and steadies the head and the little finger depresses the hyoid bone to help bring the larynx into view. (Reprinted by permission from Gregory GA: Resuscitation of the newborn. Anesthesiology 43:225–237, 1975.)

should seem to expand equally, breath sounds auscultated in the midaxillary line should be equal bilaterally and louder over the chest than the stomach, and the heart rate, color, and body tone should improve. Inadvertent esophageal or endobronchial intubations may occur and must be immediately recognized. Esophageal ventilation will also produce chest movement and sounds. However, the sounds will be louder over the abdomen than the chest, and no chest movement will occur at the apices. Clinically the infant will continue to deteriorate. An endobronchial intubation may be recognized by asymmetric movement of the chest and absent or decreased breath sounds over the unventilated lung. It is noteworthy that auscultation for breath sounds even by the experienced resuscitator may be misleading, because sound is well transmitted in these small infants. Thus relying on this sign alone for diagnosis of correct placement of the endotracheal tube is dangerous.

If despite adequate ventilation with 100% oxygen the infant fails to improve and has an Apgar score of 2 or less at 2 min or 5 or less at 5 min then umbilical artery catheterization is indicated. This will allow measurement of oxygenation, acid–base status, and systemic blood pressure and will permit administration of fluids, blood, or appropriate drugs.

Umbilical Vessel Catheterization

Using sterile technique a 3.5 or 5 French catheter is inserted into the umbilical artery at the stump of the umbilical cord (31). The catheter is advanced 2 cm beyond the point at which blood can first be

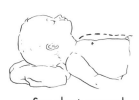

See chest expand

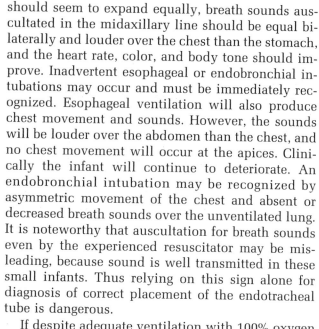

Hear bilateral breath sounds

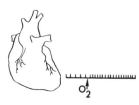

Hear pulse rate increase

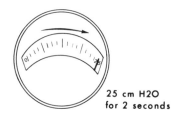

25 cm H2O
for 2 seconds

Avoid excessive pressures

Figure 39.10. Means of determining adequacy of ventilation clinically. (Reprinted by permission from SM Shnider (ed): *Obstetrical Anesthesia: Current Concepts and Practice.* Williams & Wilkins, Baltimore, 1970, p 225.)

aspirated. This should place the tip of the catheter just above the bifurcation of the aorta and below the celiac, renal, and mesenteric arteries. The location of the catheter tip is important because improper placement may be associated with thrombosis or embolism in these major aortic tributaries. Immediately after catheterization blood is sampled for PO_2, PCO_2, and pH, and blood pressure is measured with an appropriate strain gauge.

The umbilical vein is larger and easier to cannulate than the artery. However, using this vessel will not permit assessment of oxygenation or systemic blood pressure. In addition, administration of drugs or hypertonic solutions through this catheter may be hazardous. The catheter can become wedged in a venous radicle of the liver or enter the portal vein. The wedged catheter tip may cause hepatic injury or portal vein thrombosis (32). Consequently, before injecting a drug through the umbilical vein, the catheter tip must be advanced through the ductus venosus into the inferior vena cava near the right atrium. The precise location of the catheter should be checked by x-ray. It is possible, however, to determine whether the catheter tip has bypassed the liver and is above the diaphragm by noting that the venous pressure decreases with each spontaneous inspiration (31).

Correction of Acidosis

Severe acidosis, that is, a pH less than 7 or a base deficit of 15 mEq/liter or more, should be promptly corrected by alkali administration to assure normal pulmonary perfusion and oxygenation (3). If the base excess is known then the dose of sodium bicarbonate needed can be calculated by the formula:

$$\text{mEq of NaHCO}_3 = 0.6 \times \text{weight (kg)}$$
$$\times \text{ base excess in mEq/liter}$$

Usually one-fourth of the calculated dose is administered and blood gases are reevaluated. Subsequent doses are administered as necessary. The rate of bicarbonate administration should be slow. *A 4.2% solution (0.5 mEq/ml) is given at a rate of 1 mEq/kg/min or slower.* If blood gas analysis is not readily available and the neonate is severely depressed with an Apgar score of 5 or less at 5 min despite endotracheal oxygenation, then a dose of bicarbonate of 2 to 3 mEq/kg may be given at the rate described above.

Recent investigations have suggested that there is an association between intracranial hemorrhage and sodium bicarbonate administration (33). Because intracranial hemorrhage is a common finding in very small, premature infants, particularly those with asphyxia, it is not clear whether the high incidence of intracranial hemorrhage reported following *rapid* bicarbonate administration was due to an acute in-

crease in osmolarity, a rise in arterial PCO_2, or the asphyxia for which the bicarbonate was given. Others have reported that if bicarbonate administration is slow and ventilation is controlled, a rapid improvement in neonatal oxygenation can be expected to occur with no neonatal complications (34).

Sodium bicarbonate should not be infused unless metabolic acidosis or neonatal depression is severe and then only if the bicarbonate is slowly administered and the infant is being effectively ventilated. Moderate or mild metabolic and respiratory acidosis—that is, a pH between 7.05 and 7.3 and a base deficit of 5 to 15 mEq/liter—will usually be corrected spontaneously or by assisted ventilation and volume expansion if indicated.

Treatment of Shock

The most common cause of shock in the newly born infant is hypovolemia. It frequently follows severe intrapartum asphyxia during which a greater than normal portion of fetal blood is shunted to the placenta and remains there following cord clamping and delivery (35). Hypovolemia is also commonly associated with umbilical cord compression in vertex and especially breech vaginal deliveries. Aside from the consequences of asphyxia, acute compression of the umbilical cord during delivery may result in trapping of fetal blood in the placenta due to occlusion of the compliant umbilical vein when there is flow through the more rigid and muscular umbilical arteries. Ruptured placental or umbilical vessels, although occurring far less frequently than intrapartum asphyxia and cord compression, may result in severe hypovolemic shock.

Hypovolemia should be suspected if the neonate is pale and has poor capillary refill, tachycardia, and tachypnea. Precise diagnosis and treatment require constant monitoring of arterial and central venous pressures and heart rate and repeated measurements of PaO_2, $PaCO_2$, pH, and hematocrit. Normal aortic blood pressure measured with the umbilical artery catheter varies with birth weight (29). Figure 39.11 shows the normal mean arterial blood pressure for each birth weight and the 95% confidence limits of this relationship. Newborns with blood pressures below the lower confidence line are hypotensive and most likely hypovolemic. Intrathoracic venous pressures measured with the umbilical venous catheter are normally 5 to 12 cm H_2O when measured at end expiration (31). If pressure is less than 5 cm H_2O, hypovolemia is likely.

Hypovolemic shock requires immediate therapy. Because whole blood (O-negative blood, cross-matched with the mother's blood) is not always immediately available, an infusion of normal saline or Ringer's lactate solution (10 ml/kg body weight over a 5- to

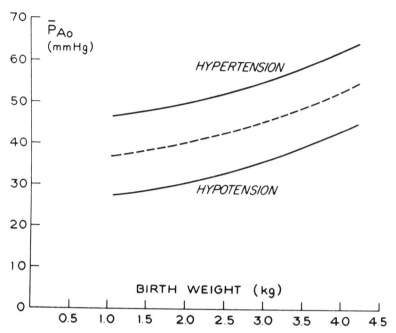

Figure 39.11. Mean aortic blood pressure obtained from an umbilical artery catheter. The *dashed line* is the average blood pressure at each birth weight, and the *solid lines* represent the 95% confidence limits. (Reprinted by permission from Kitterman JA, Phibbs RH, Tooley WH: Aortic blood pressure in normal newborn infants during the first 12 hours of life. Pediatrics 44:959–968, 1969.)

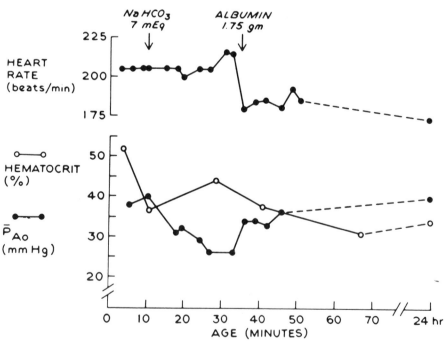

Figure 39.12. Heart rate, hematocrit, and mean aortic pressure in a 1370-g, 30-weeks' gestation infant with asphyxia at birth and respiratory distress. At 12 min of age severe metabolic acidosis was treated with $NaHCO_3$. Hypovolemia then became apparent by the progressive fall in blood pressure. Albumin administration restored blood pressure and alleviated tachycardia. (Reprinted by permission from Phibbs RH: What is the evidence that blood pressure monitoring is useful? In *Problems of Neonatal Intensive Care Units. Report of 59th Ross Conference on Pediatric Research.* JF Lucey, ed. Ross Laboratories. Columbus, 1969, p 81.)

10-min period) should be given and the response evaluated to determine whether the dose should be repeated immediately. A 5% albumin/saline solution (or other plasma substitute)) may also be used. Repeated infusions of fluid or whole blood should be given as needed to establish and maintain adequate intravascular pressure.

Frequently a hypovolemic asphyxiated neonate will have a relatively normal arterial blood pressure and hematocrit due to intense peripheral vasoconstriction. When the acidosis is corrected with bicarbonate and hyperventilation the blood vessels dilate and hypotension occurs, unmasking the presence of hypovolemia (Fig. 39.12). Alternately, when severe hy-

povolemia is corrected a marked metabolic acidemia may reappear after systemic circulatory status and peripheral perfusion improves.

With persistent signs of hypovolemia, the presence of metabolic acidosis and the need for sodium bicarbonate should be considered. With persistent hypotension, the administration of dopamine should also be considered (Table 39.5).

Treatment of Hypoglycemia

Infants with intrauterine growth retardation (postmature), or with diabetic mothers, or born following severe intrapartum asphyxia may be hypoglycemic (less than 30 mg/100 ml in full-sized infant and less

Table 39.5
Medications for Resuscitation of the Newborn[a]

Medication	Concentration to Administer	Preparation	Dosage/Route*	Indications for Use	Rate/Precautions
Epinephrine	1:10,000	1 ml	0.1–0.3 ml/kg IV[b] or ET[c]	1. No detectable heart beat 2. Heart rate <80/min despite 30 sec of ventilation and chest compression	Give rapidly
Volume Expanders	Whole blood 5% Albumin Normal saline Ringer's lactate solution	40 ml	10 ml/kg IV	1. Evidence of acute bleeding 2. Signs of hypovolemia	Give over 5 to 10 min
Sodium Bicarbonate	0.5 mEq/ml (4.2% solution)	20 ml or two 10-ml prefilled syringes	2 mEq/kg IV	Documented or assumed metabolic acidosis	Give *slowly*, over at least 2 min Give only if infant being effectively ventilated
Naloxone	0.4 mg/ml 1.0 mg/ml	1 ml 1 ml	0.1 mg/kg (0.25 ml/kg) IV, ET, IM,[d] SQ[e] 0.1 mg/kg (0.1 ml/kg) IV, ET, IM, SQ	Severe respiratory depression *and* maternal narcotic administration within the past 4 hr	Give rapidly IV, ET preferred IM, SQ acceptable
Dopamine	$6 \times \dfrac{\text{weight (kg)} \times \text{desired dose } (\mu g/kg/min)}{\text{desired fluid (ml/hr)}}$	mg of dopamine per 100 ml of solution	Begin at 5 μg/kg/min (may increase to 20 μg/kg/min if necessary) IV	Infant shows evidence of shock and poor peripheral perfusion after giving epinephrine, volume expander, and sodium bicarbonate	Give as a continuous infusion using an infusion pump Monitor HR and BP closely Seek consultation

[a]Modified from Bloom RS, Cropley C: *Textbook of Neonatal Resuscitation* © 1987, 1990 American Heart Association.
[b]*IV* = Intravenous.
[c]*ET* = Endotracheal.
[d]*IM* = Intramuscular.
[e]*SQ* = Subcutaneous.

than 20 mg/100 ml in low–birth-weight infant). Hypoglycemia results in reduced cardiac output, hypotension, and, when severe, tremors, convulsions, and apnea. It should be treated with 5 to 10 ml/kg body weight of 10% dextrose administered slowly.

Treatment of Cardiac Arrest

If after 15 to 30 sec of positive pressure ventilation the heart beat is absent or barely detectable with a rate less than 80 beats/min, closed-chest cardiac massage should be started. Both thumbs are placed on the sternum at the junction of the lower and middle thirds, and the back is supported with the fingers (Fig. 39.13) (36). The sternum should be compressed to a depth of ½ to ¾ inch at a rate of 120/min. Ventilation should occur at a rate of 40 to 60/min.

An alternate technique is shown in Figure 39.14. The tips of the middle finger and either the index or ring finger of one hand are used for compression. The two fingers should be positioned perpendicular to the chest and only the two fingertips should rest on the chest. The other hand can be used to support the infant's back so that the heart is more effectively compressed.

An adequate cardiac output with massage can be ascertained by an improvement in the neonate's color, constriction of the pupils, and palpable arterial pulses. Drug administration, as previously described and listed in Table 39.5, should be immediately initiated. Umbilical vessels should be catheterized immediately, and an electrocardiogram should be obtained to monitor heart rate and rhythm.

SPECIAL PROBLEMS IN RESUSCITATION
Narcotic Depression

When narcotics are administered for pain relief during labor and delivery, the infant may be born mildly to moderately depressed. As with the adult, the usual sign of narcotic depression in a neonate is hypoventilation and poor response to stimuli. If respiratory depression is thought to be due to narcotic overdose, these infants should be oxygenated and then treated with a narcotic antagonist. Naloxone, 0.1 mg/kg, is the antagonist of choice. If the mother is a narcotic addict, the use of naloxone is contraindicated in the neonate because acute withdrawal symptoms may be precipitated.

Magnesium Intoxication

Babies born to parturients treated with large doses of magnesium for toxemia of pregnancy may display signs of hypermagnesemia. These infants are peripherally vasodilated, pink, hypotensive, and hypotonic. Calcium chloride is an effective antidote.

Local Anesthetic Toxicity

Fetal intoxication with local anesthetics may occasionally occur inadvertently during the maternal administration of caudal or paracervical blocks (37, 38). The infants are severely depressed with bradycardia, hypotension, apnea, hypotonia, and convulsions. Careful examination of the baby's head often discloses the needle puncture site. In addition to the usual resuscitation of a severely depressed neonate,

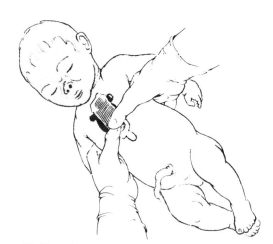

Figure 39.13. Closed-chest cardiac massage in the newborn. Location of the thumbs for sternal compression in the infant. For simplification, ventilation of the infant is not shown. (Reprinted by permission from Gregory GA: Cardiopulmonary resuscitation of the newborn. In *The Anesthesiologist, Mother and Newborn*, SM Shnider, F Moya, eds. Williams & Wilkins, Baltimore, 1974, p 207.)

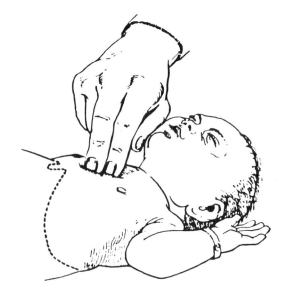

Figure 39.14. Two-finger method for performing chest compressions. (Reprinted by permission from Moya F, James LS, Burnard ED, Hanks EC: Cardiac massage in the newborn infant through the intact chest. Am J Obstet Gynecol 84:798–803, 1962.)

Overview of
Resuscitation in the Delivery Room

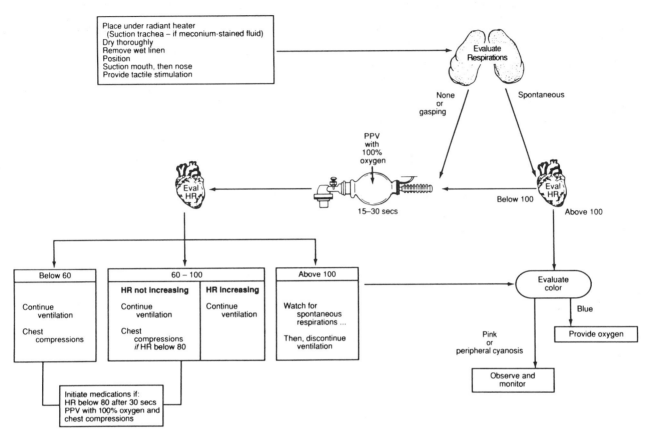

Figure 39.15. Overview of resuscitation of the newborn. (Reprinted by permission from Bloom RS, Cropley C: *Textbook of Neonatal Resuscitation.* American Heart Association and American Academy of Pediatrics, Dallas, 1987, 1990, p 1–5.)

usual resuscitation of a severely depressed neonate, these babies should be detoxified by gastric lavage with isotonic saline and exchange transfusion.

Pneumothorax

Pneumothorax in the delivery room may occur spontaneously, often associated with meconium aspiration (in which ball–valve air trapping occurs) or with other diseases associated with poor lung compliance (such as diaphragmatic hernia and pulmonary hypoplasia). When it occurs in a normal lung it is usually caused by excessive airway pressures administered in the resuscitation of a depressed newborn. Tension pneumothorax, in which high intrapleural pressure prevents venous return to the heart, is catastrophic and life-threatening. When the diagnosis is suspected, a 22-gauge needle connected to a three-way stopcock and syringe is inserted in the second intercostal space in the midclavicular line. If air is aspirated then the needle should be replaced

by an adequately sized catheter (10 to 16 French) and connected to underwater seal and continuous suction.

CONCLUSION

Rapid, organized, and skillful resuscitation of the depressed newborn is mandatory. The obstetrician, anesthesiologist, and neonatologist must work as a team in evaluating the newborn, establishing a patent airway, providing adequate ventilation, and restoring normal blood volume, cardiac output, and acid-base status. An overview of resuscitation of the newborn in the delivery room, as recommended by the American Heart Association and the American Academy of Pediatrics, is shown in Figure 39.15.

References

1. Dawes GS: *Foetal and Neonatal Physiology.* Year Book Medical Publishers, Chicago, 1968, pp 91–105.
2. Rudolph AM, Heymann MA: Fetal and neonatal circulation and respiration. Ann Rev Physiol 36:187–207, 1974.

3. Rudolph AM, Yuen S: Response of the pulmonary vasculature to hypoxia and H$^+$ ion concentration changes. J Clin Invest 45:399–411, 1966.
4. Cassen S, Dawes GS, Mott JC, Ross BB, Strong LB: The vascular resistance of the foetal and newly ventilated lung of the lamb. J Physiol 171:61–79, 1964.
5. Assali NS, Morris JA, Smith EW, Manson WA: Studies on ductus arteriosus circulation. Circ Res 13:478–489, 1963.
6. Boreus LO, Malmfors T, McMurphy DM, Olson L: Demonstration of adrenergic receptor function and innervation in the ductus arteriosus of the human fetus. Acta Physiol Scand 77:316–321, 1969.
7. Adams FH, Moss AJ, Fagan L: The tracheal fluid of the foetal lamb. Biol Neonate 5:151–158, 1963.
8. Ross BB: Comparison of foetal pulmonary fluid with foetal plasma and amniotic fluid. Nature 199:1100, 1963.
9. Karlberg P: The adaptive changes in the immediate postnatal period, with particular reference to respiration. J Pediatr 56:585–604, 1960.
10. Usher RH, Allen AC, McLean FH: Risk of respiratory distress syndrome related to gestational age, role of delivery and maternal diabetes. Am J Obstet Gynecol 111:826–832, 1971.
11. Karlberg P: The breaths of life. In *Modern Perinatal Medicine*. L Gluck, ed. Year Book Medical Publishers, Chicago, 1974, pp 391–408.
12. Johnson JWC, Richards DS, Wagaman RA: The case for routine umbilical blood acid-base studies at delivery. Am J Obstet Gynecol 162:621–625, 1990.
13. Yeomans ER, Hauth JC, Gilstrap LC III, Strickland DM: Umbilical cord pH, P_{CO_2} and bicarbonate following uncomplicated term vaginal deliveries. Am J Obstet Gynecol 151:798–800, 1985.
14. Gregory GA, Gooding C, Phibbs RH, Tooley WH: Meconium aspiration: A prospective study. J Pediatr 85:848–852, 1974.
15. Ting P, Brady JP: Tracheal suction in meconium aspiration. Am J Obstet Gynecol 122:767–771, 1975.
16. Carson BS, Losey RW, Bowes WA Jr, Simmons MA: Combined obstetric and pediatric approach to prevent meconium aspiration syndrome. Am J Obstet Gynecol 126:712–715, 1976.
17. Wiswell TE, Tuggle JM, Turner BS: Meconium aspiration syndrome: Have we made a difference? Pediatrics 85:715–721, 1990.
18. Hageman JR, Conley M, Francis K, Stenske J, Wolf I, Santi V, Farrell EE: Delivery room management of meconium staining of the amniotic fluid and the development of meconium aspiration syndrome. J Perinatol 8:127–131, 1988.
19. Yeh TF, Harris V, Srinivasan G, Lilien L, Pyati S, Pildes RS: Roentgenographic findings in infants with meconium aspiration syndrome. JAMA 242:60–63, 1979.
20. Levin DL, Heymann MA, Kitterman JA, Gregory GA, Phibbs RH, Rudolph AM: Persistent pulmonary hypertension in the newborn. J Pediatr 89:626–630, 1976.
21. Steele RW, Metz JR, Bass JW, DuBois JJ: Pneumothorax and pneumomediastinum in the newborn. Radiology 98:629–632, 1971.
22. Aherne W, Hull D: The site of heat production in the newborn infant. Proc R Soc Med 57:1172–1173, 1964.
23. Karlberg P, Moore RE, Oliver TK: The thermogenic response of the newborn infant to noradrenaline. Acta Paediatr Scand 51:284–292, 1962.
24. Dawkins MJR, Scopes JW: Non-shivering thermogenesis and brown adipose tissue in the human newborn infant. Nature 206:201–202, 1965.
25. Adamsons K Jr, Gandy GM, James LS: The influence of thermal factors upon oxygen consumption of the newborn infant. J Pediatr 66:495–508, 1965.
26. Apgar V: A proposal for a new method of evaluation of the newborn infant. Anesth Analg (Curr Res) 32:260–267, 1953.
27. Apgar V, James LS: Further observations on the newborn scoring system. Am J Dis Child 104:419–428, 1962.
28. Kitterman JA, Phibbs RH, Tooley WH: Aortic blood pressure in normal newborn infants during the first 12 hours of life. Pediatrics 44:959–968, 1969.
29. Moya F, Apgar V, James LS, Berrien C: Hydramnios and congenital anomalies. JAMA 173:1552–1556, 1960.
30. Cross K, Klaus M, Tooley WH, Weisser K: The response of the newborn baby to inflation of the lungs. J Physiol 151:551–565, 1960.
31. Kitterman JA, Phibbs RH, Tooley WH: Catheterization of umbilical vessels in newborn infants. Pediatr Clin North Am 17:895–912, 1970.
32. Erkan V, Blankenship W, Stahlman MT: The complications of chronic umbilical vessel catheterization. Pediatr Res 2:317, 1968.
33. Simmons MA, Adcock EW, Bard H, Battaglia FC: Hypernatremia and intracranial hemorrhage in neonates. N Engl J Med 291:6–10, 1974.
34. Tooley WH: Alkali therapy in the asphyxiated newborn infant. In *Obstetrical Anesthesia*. SM Shnider, ed. Williams & Wilkins, Baltimore, 1970, p 230.
35. Ballard R, Kitterman JR, Phibbs RH, Simpson H, Tooley WH: Observations on hypovolemia in the newborn. Clin Res 20:278, 1972.
36. Gregory GA: Cardiopulmonary resuscitation of the newborn. In *The Anesthesiologist, Mother and Newborn*. SM Shnider, F Moya, eds. Williams & Wilkins, Baltimore, 1974, p 20.
37. Finster M, Poppers PJ, Sinclair JC, Morishima HO, Daniel SS: Accidental intoxication of the fetus with local anesthetic drug during caudal anesthesia. Am J Obstet Gynecol 92:922–924, 1965.
38. Dodson WE, Hillman RE, Hillman LS: Brain tissue levels in a fatal case of neonatal mepivacaine poisoning. J Pediatr 86:624–627, 1975.

Fetal and Neonatal Effects of Maternally Administered Drugs

Richard G. Wright, M.D.
Sol M. Shnider, M.D.
Craig J. Fong, M.D.

It has been estimated that an average of four of every five pregnant women take some form of medication during pregnancy. Hill et al. (131) have reported on the drug use of 231 women during pregnancy. If labor and delivery are excluded, the number of drug preparations taken per patient was reported as 9.6. Prescription drugs accounted for a mean of 6.4 drugs per patient. In addition, many parturients receive some medication during labor and delivery to relieve pain or anxiety. When obstetric complications arise, patients may require substantial doses of several drugs to ensure a safe outcome.

It is probable that all maternally administered drugs cross the placenta to some extent. Movement is primarily by passive diffusion. Both a large transplacental drug gradient and a high diffusion constant facilitate movement across the placental membrane. Drugs with a high diffusion constant are those of low molecular weight and high lipid solubility which exist primarily in the non-ionized unbound form.

When administered during the first trimester, the period of organogenesis, certain drugs may modify development of fetal tissues with resultant congenital anomalies. However, drugs are not the sole factor which may have an adverse effect on fetal tissue organization and development. In fact, the cause of most malformations is not known. Only a small percentage are directly attributable to known hereditary and environmental factors (the latter including infection, irradiation and drug use). Organogenesis is complete by the end of the first trimester, with important exceptions being the teeth, genital system and central nervous system. The vast majority of congenital malformations arise during the first trimester of pregnancy when organ systems are developing and embryonic cells are rapidly dividing. The teratogenic effects of a drug are both dose and time related. The timing of a teratogenic influence is crucial in determining the system affected. In humans, for example, the period of greatest development and organization of the cardiovascular system is between 20 and 40 days after conception, that of the limbs is from 24 to 46 days, and that of the nervous system is from 15 to 25 days. Exposure to an appropriate teratogen between 15 and 25 days after conception may, for example, result in nervous system but not skeletal anomalies. It is possible that teratogenic drugs exert their effects on development within the first 2 weeks of conception—before the woman knows that she is pregnant. However, from the time of fertilization until implantation of the blastocyst, most deleterious drugs abort the conception rather than deform it.

Only three types of drugs are definitely known to be teratogenic in humans: certain antimetabolites, thalidomide and steroid hormones with androgenic activity. Epidemiologic surveys have been undertaken to examine the possible association between maternal drug ingestion and congenital defects in the infant. Most studies are difficult to interpret. Associations are loose, and it is usually impossible to differentiate the effects of a drug from those of the maternal disease for which the medication was prescribed. From these studies it seems that many drugs are highly suspect for inducing fetal abnormalities but that the risk is often relatively low. Although considerable work has been done on teratogenicity in animals, it should be stressed that little, if any, parallel exists between the ability to induce abnormalities in a particular species of animal and that in humans.

Drugs administered at any time during pregnancy or labor may modify fetal and newborn physiology. Such changes are usually of no clinical relevance, but, on occasion, they may be either detrimental or beneficial.

Analgesic or anesthetic drugs administered to the

mother prior to delivery may depress the fetus and lessen the reserve of the newborn for adapting to extrauterine life. The most widely used method for evaluating the condition of the infant in the delivery room is the Apgar score. There are five signs: heart rate, respiratory effort, muscle tone, response to stimulation and skin color. A score of 0, 1 or 2 is assigned to the presence or absence of each sign. Apgar scoring quickly identifies those infants with significant depression of vital function. Maternally administered drugs may reduce neonatal vigor and subsequently result in lower Apgar scores. Such drug-induced depression is infrequent in uncomplicated well conducted obstetrics but may occur, for instance, with general anesthesia for cesarean section. When drug depression does occur, it is in the form of respiratory depression, and ventilation may require support for a short period of time.

Although the Apgar score is useful in identifying those infants requiring active resuscitation, it fails to detect both subtle drug effects and those extending past the immediate newborn period. Scanlon et al. (271) and Amiel-Tison et al. (9) have developed simple, rapid and reproducible techniques of assessing certain aspects of behavior in the first few hours of life. The examinations are an adaptation of standard neurological and behavioral testing of newborns as developed by Prechtl and Beintema (240), Beintema (26), and Brazelton et al. (40). Neonates who are vigorous as assessed by Apgar score may score low on the neurobehavioral examination in the first hours of life. These neurobehavioral changes are transient, and their clinical significance, if any, is not known.

The following table lists some of the more frequently used drugs with their possible effects on the fetus and newborn. Comments and references are included where appropriate.

Drug	Effects	Comments	References
Analgesics (narcotics)			
	Small for gestational age	With chronic abuse	147
	Lung maturation	Reported acceleration of appearance of mature L/S ratio in heroin addicts	102, 107
	Decreased incidence of neonatal jaundice	Heroin reported to induce fetal hepatic enzymes	13, 213, 230
	or		
	Increased incidence of neonatal jaundice	Reported with methadone only; mechanism unknown	349
	Intrauterine death	Associated with maternal narcotic withdrawal	50, 248
	Neonatal withdrawal syndrome	With chronic abuse	103, 129, 151, 158, 261, 349
	Neonatal depression	Inappropriate doses during labor, morphine most depressant	296
Analgesics (non-narcotic)			
Acetaminophen	Possible interstitial nephritis	One case report	131
	Spontaneous abortions	Associated with toxic maternal ingestions and late *N*-acetylcysteine treatment	253
	Fetal hepatotoxicity and neonatal coagulopathy	One case report	159
Indomethacin	Possible pulmonary hypertension in newborn period	Large doses, prostaglandin synthetase inhibition may allow ductus arteriosus constriction in utero	169, 170, 182, 139, 205
	Hydrops fetalis with stillbirth reported		
Propoxyphene (Darvon)	Neonatal withdrawal syndrome	Chronic abuse	86
Salicylates	Suspicion of congenital anomalies	Low index of suspicion	216, 251, 303
	Possibly small for gestational age and increased incidence of stillbirths	Conflicting data in patients consuming large amounts	290, 326
	Possible increased incidence of postdate deliveries	Data conflict; the postulated mechanism is via prostaglandin synthesis inhibition	172, 290
	Increased unbound bilirubin with increased risk of kernicterus	Competes with bilirubin for albumin	131
	Possibility of increased hemorrhagic phenomenon, including intracranial hemorrhage in low–birth-weight newborns	Platelet dysfunction and decreased factor XII	33, 263
	Possible pulmonary hypertension in newborn period	Large doses, prostaglandin synthetase inhibition may allow ductus arteriosus constriction in utero	169 170, 182
Anticholinergics			
Atropine	Fetal tachycardia, decreased beat-to-beat variability, elimination of variable and early decelerations	Anticholinergic effect following placental transfer with large doses, little or no effect with modest clinical doses	2, 4, 135, 190
Glycopyrrolate	No effect on fetal heart rate	Quaternary ammonium compound does not readily cross biologic membranes	

Drug	Effects	Comments	References
Anticoagulants			
Coumadin (Dicumarol)	Intracranial hemorrhage, fetal death	Most significant during third trimester and labor	35, 92, 110
	Conradi disease, with nasal hypoplasia and generalized bony abnormalities	Teratogenic	19, 25, 58, 154, 232, 236, 291, 292, 333
	Central nervous system problems including mental retardation, hydrocephalus		
	Possible ophthalmologic abnormalities		
Heparin	No increase in incidence of abnormalities in offspring of heparin-treated mothers	Does not cross the placenta	329
Anticonvulsants			
Diphenylhydantoin	Fetal hydantoin syndrome with microcephaly, mental and growth retardation, peculiar facies, skeletal anomalies, occasional facial cleft or congential heart disease,	Epileptic state itself is associated with an increased risk of anomalies. Incidence of the complete syndrome is probably 5 to 10%, 30% incidence of the incomplete syndrome	6, 30, 79, 89, 109, 117, 118, 132, 133, 179, 190, 198, 202, 206, 218, 308, 309, 336, 348
	Neuroblastoma		
	Hemorrhagic disease	Vitamin-K depletion by induced liver microsomal enzymes	
Valproic acid	Spina bifida, meningomyelocele	One study shows 1% probability of this defect if drug use in first trimester	47
Phenobarbital	Low to no teratogenic potential	One case report of an epileptic mother on high doses of phenobarbital giving birth to two children with fetal hydantoin-like syndrome	29, 89, 197, 285, 289
	Drug withdrawal reported in newborns of mothers receiving barbiturates during pregnancy		34, 74
	Sedation reported in breastfeeding infants		215
Trimethadione (Tridione)	Fetal trimethadione syndrome, as well as isolated defects, reported	Appears to be teratogenic	91, 98, 257, 347, 105
Magnesium sulfate	Neonatal depression	Effect of high neonatal blood levels associated with the therapy of preeclampsia	5, 82, 175, 268
	Hypotonia		
	Hypotension		
Antidepressants			
Amphetamines	Suspicion of congenital heart disease, congenital biliary atresia, oral clefts	Considerable conflicting evidence	171, 195, 220
	Neonate may initially show signs of intoxication, later withdrawal		84, 226, 245
Lithium	Suspicion of cardiovascular anomalies (especially Ebstein's anomaly)	Alternate therapy strongly recommended, especially during first trimester	42, 71, 194, 219, 278, 279, 280, 311, 341
	Meningomyelocele, spina bifida, hydrocephalus		
	Bradycardia, arrhythmias, cardiomegaly		

Drug	Effects	Comments	References
Tricyclics, e.g., imipramine (Tofranil)	Goiter, hyperthyroidism Hypotonia Suspicion of craniofacial and central nervous system anomalies	Possible association	18, 138, 188, 242, 338
	Limb reduction defects	Possible association shown in Australia, not confirmed in American study	
	Neonatal intoxication and/or withdrawal		
Antiemetics			
Bendectin	Pyloric stenosis	Conflicting studies; if a causative factor, weak association	7, 85, 203
	Limb reduction defects, encephalocele, esophageal atresia	If causal association, risk is extremely small	63, 204, 195
	Oral clefts, cardiac defects	Probably no causal association	
		No longer available in North America	
Thalidomide	Congenital limb defects (amelia, phocomelia), possible cardiovascular and uterovaginal anomalies	Proven, no longer available	134, 168, 187, 320
Antihypertensives			
Angiotensin-converting enzyme inhibitors	Fetal renal tubular dysgenesis and hypocalvaria	Two case reports	20
	Oligohydramnios, renal failure, fetal death	Second and third trimester exposure	283
Chlorothiazide	Hypokalemia		11
	Hyponatremia		8
	Acute pancreatitis		201
	Hypoglycemia		286
	Thrombocytopenia		149
Diazoxide (Hyperstat)	Hyperglycemia	May occur with acute intravenous use	199, 221
	Alopecia		
	Hypertrichosis laruginosa	May follow weeks of oral use	
	Decreased bone age		
Ethacrynic acid (Edecrin); Thiazides	Neonatal deafness	Potential cited	93, 150, 255
	Hyponatremia		
	Thrombocytopenia		
Ganglionic blockers, e.g., trimethaphan (Arfonad) pentolinium, trimethidinium, hexamethionium, mecamylamine	Neonatal ileus		115
Propranolol (Inderal)	Possibly associated with intrauterine growth retardation	Associated with chronic use	101, 113, 246, 327
	Bradycardia		
	Hypoglycemia		
	Abnormally long time to sustained respiration	Follows 1 mg intravenously minutes prior to delivery	325
Reserpine (Serpasil)	Nasal obstruction	Accompanies late pregnancy use	44, 73, 306, 344
	Lethargy		
	Anorexia		
	Respiratory depression		

Drug	Effects	Comments	References
Sodium nitroprusside (Nipride)	Impairment of nonshivering thermogenesis Potential for cyanide intoxication	Not present with modest doses used for short periods; higher doses for longer periods may present a problem	252
Antimetabolites			
Folic acid analogs, e.g., methotrexate, aminopterin	Dextrocardia, malformation of bones of skull and face, CNS malformations Aminopterin syndrome	Proven teratogens	81, 156, 191, 200, 293, 322
Natural products, e.g., vinca alkaloids, vincristine, vinblastine	One normal infant reported with mother taking vinblastine throughout pregnancy	Mostly animal studies available with several different anomalies	15
Purine analogs, e.g., azathioprine (Imuran)	Possible intrauterine growth retardation Pulmonary valvular stenosis	Several successful pregnancies in renal transplant patients	108, 156, 282
Pyrimidine analogs, e.g., cytosine arabinoside		Only animal studies available	233, 241
Antiproliferative-Immunosuppressive Drugs			
Alkylating agents			
Chlorambucil	Strong suspicion of major malformations		39, 75, 112, 282, 299, 307, 315
Cyclophosphamide (Cytoxan)	Intrauterine growth retardation		
Busulfan (Myleran)			
Antimicrobials			
Aminoglycosides	Deafness	Potential exists throughout pregnancy, streptomycin is the only one extensively investigated	56, 60, 254, 339, 77
Chloramphenicol (Chloromycetin)	"Grey baby syndrome"	Risk when administered close to delivery, more likely when hepatic and renal function immature	45, 55, 153, 284
Quinine	Suspicion of congenital anomalies of the central nervous and skeletal systems Deafness Optic nerve hypoplasia Thrombocytopenia Hemolysis	Associated with GGPD deficiency in newborn	131, 184, 328 104
Sulfonamides	Increased unbound bilirubin with increased risk of kernicterus	Drug competes with bilirubin for albumin binding, relevant when administered near delivery, especially when long-acting drug used or infant premature	148, 300
	Hemolytic anemia and possible hydrops fetalis	More likely if GGPD deficient	234
Tetracycline	Dental discoloration Enamel hypoplasia Diminished growth of long bones	Mechanism is through the chelation of calcium	55, 56, 57, 249, 324
	Cataracts	Possible association	120
	Possibly increased risk of inguinal hernia, hypospadias	Studies conflicting	67, 80, 125

Drug	Effects	Comments	References
Antithyroid medication			
Iodide	Goiter ± hypothyroidism	A large goiter occasionally results in cephalopelvic disproportion or ischeal compression in the newborn; these goiters are due to fetal thyroid inhibition with secondary compensatory hypertrophy	46, 96
Radioactive iodine (^{131}I)	Hypoplastic or absent thyroid giving rise to hypothyroid state with possible mental retardation	Destruction of fetal thyroid most likely to occur if the medication is administered after the fetal thyroid develops iodide concentrating ability (about the 74th day of gestation)	46, 94, 111, 312
	Carcinoma of the thyroid	Potential carcinogenic effect with a long latent period	
Methimazole (Tapazole)	Suspicion of causing aplasia cutis		211
Propylthiouracil	Goiter ± hypothyroidism	Goiter is not a common occurrence, and when it does occur, the gland is not extremely large; hypothyroidism is less common and not clearly related to drug therapy; the drug readily crosses the placenta; presumably sufficient maternal thyroid hormone crosses to meet fetal needs in most instances	46, 143, 193
Bronchodilators			
Terbutaline	Neonatal hypoglycemia reported	Case report when drug used for tocolysis	83
Theophylline	Tachycardia, neonatal irritability reported	Associated with therapeutic drug level in mother	16
	Neonatal withdrawal reported		136
Environmental toxins			
Carbon Monoxide	CNS injury with retardation, convulsions	Occurs with toxic exposure to mother. Chronic low-level exposure may be harmful	178
Lead	Small for gestational age. Failure to thrive. Spasticity. Mental retardation	Possible neonatal problem with maternal levels often thought to be nontoxic	131, 27
Mercury	Cerebral palsy. Mental retardation. Convulsions. Involuntary movements. Defective vision		10, 119, 131
Polychlorinated biphenyls (PCBs)	Low birth weight, disporportionately small head size. Developmental delay	Problems generally follow high level exposure	90, 256
Inhalation anesthetics			
Halothane, cyclopropane, nitrous oxide, enflurane, isoflurane	Dose-related neonatal depression		210, 335
	Suspicion of spontaneous	A possible effect of exposure;	12, 21, 305

Drug	Effects	Comments	References
	abortion, congenital anomalies	only work is in animals; human studies available do not show strong correlation	
Operating room environment	Increased incidence of spontaneous abortion	A possible effect of chronic operating room exposure; potential sources include trace anesthetic gases, irradiation, stress, and infection	53, 61, 62, 265
Local anesthetics			
Chloroprocaine, bupivacaine	No effect on Apgar or neurobehavioral scores	No difference from neonates not exposed to drugs	137, 243, 272
Lidocaine, mepivacaine	Decreased neonatal Apgar scores	Rare with conventional uncomplicated anesthesia	207, 297
	No effect on neurobehavioral scores	Initial effect reported in small population not seen with further studies	1, 3, 271
	Seizures, cardiovascular collapse	With high toxic levels such as follow direct injection into the fetus	223, 301
Oral hypoglycemics			
Chlorpropamide (Diabinese)	One study reported high combined perinatal mortality	Diabetic statistics alone associated with a higher than normal incidence of congenital anomalies	140, 316
		Although in one study, high doses of chlorpropamide gave more than double the incidence of perinatal mortality as compared with tolbutamide therapy, subsequent studies have suggested much of the mortality was related to the diabetic state	
Tolbutamide (Orinase)	Conflicting data but possible low incidence of multiple congenital anomalies	Anomalies are possibly unrelated to drug ingestion but rather to the diabetic state per se	165, 166, 275, 310, 237
Oxytocics, myometrial depressants			
Oxytocin	Increased incidence of neonatal hyperbilirubinemia	Consensus of somewhat conflicting data	23, 24, 49, 69, 99, 227, 323, 343
	Asphyxia	Uterine hypertonus from overdose	
Isoxsuprine (Vasodilan)	Tachycardia	β-Adrenergic effect following placental transfer	41, 48, 167, 295
Ritodrine	Hyperglycemia, hypoglycemia		
Sedatives, hypnotics			
Barbiturates	Neonatal depression	Result of inappropriately large doses in labor or for induction maintenance of general anesthesia for delivery	157, 262
	Decreased serum bilirubin	Chronic use induces hepatic enzymes	185, 244
	Hemorrhagic disease of the newborn	Rare case reports with decreased Stuart-Prower factor with chronic use	281
	Neonatal withdrawal syndrome	Chronic exposure	34, 74, 89, 285, 289
	Low or no incidence of anomalies	Possible fetal hydantoin-like syndrome with very high doses	125

Drug	Effects	Comments	References
Bromide-containing sedatives	Acneiform rash Lethargy High-pitched cry Feeding problems Anomalies including cardiac and small cranium Intrauterine growth retardation	Sporadic isolated reports	131, 224 239
Glutethimide (Doriden)	Neonatal withdrawal syndrome	Possible association with chronic use	
Meprobamate (Miltown, Equanil)	Suspicion of congenital anomalies		122, 197
Skeletal muscle relaxants	No clinical effect during routine general anesthesia	Quaternary ammonium compounds do not cross the placenta in clinically significant amounts, with the possible exception of gallamine	209
Social and illicit drugs (See Chapter 35) Alcohol	Fetal alcohol syndrome (includes small for gestational age with persisting growth lag, craniofacial, cardiovascular, and possibly renal abnormalities, mental and psychomotor retardation)	Proven with chronic abuse and may be among commonest causes of mental retardation. May not be alcohol per se but poor diet, alcohol contaminants, etc.	72, 116, 117, 144, 163, 212, 228, 230, 314, 321
	Neonatal depression, hypoglycemia, increased heat loss	Acute overdose in premature	331
	Neonatal withdrawal syndrome	Chronic abuse	131
Caffeine	Most studies show little or no effect with modest intake		68, 174, 208, 258
Cannabis (marijuana)	Only isolated reports of congenital anomalies	No pattern of abnormalities in these case reports. Possibly not a significant teratogen	123, 217, 156
	Prematurity, intrauterine growth retardation		
Cocaine	Preliminary works suggest not a major teratogen	Most users exposed to other drugs	156
	Perinatal cerebral infarction	Secondary to acute intoxication	51
	Placental abruption		181, 225
	Prematurity, intrauterine growth retardation		
	Acute withdrawal	Occasionally occurs	52
	Neurobehavior changes		52
Lysergic acid diethylamide (LSD)	Chromosomal breaks, possible skeletal malformations	Many feel probably not a major teratogen	54, 156, 177, 189, 273, 304
Tobacco	Small for gestation age	Chronic abuse	131, 164
	Spontaneous abortion	Chronic abuse	155
	Decreased fetal breathing	Induced by two cigarettes, significance unknown	183
	Lower neonatal bilirubin levels	Possible transplacental induction of hepatic enzymes with cyanide from tobacco	131

Drug	Effects	Comments	References
	Increased incidence of placental abruption		164
Steroids			
17 δ-hydroxyprogesterone	Possibility of strabismus, premature cranial suture closure	Isolated case reports, very possibly due to coincidence	247, 287
	Masculinization of female fetus	Rare (2/1500) report of clitoral hypertrophy	
Betamethasone	Lung maturation	Induces surfactant production	173
	Hypoglycemia		231
Cortisone	Suspicion of cleft palate, abortion, fetal death	Effects due to drug or disease per se?	38, 76, 121, 288, 332, 334
Diethylstilbesterol (Stilbesterol) (DES)	Clitoral hypertrophy in female newborns		37, 126, 222
	Benign adenosis of vagina		
	Adenocarcinoma of vagina and cervix	Proven transplacental carcinogen with a long latent period	100, 127
	Epididymal, testicular, or spermatozoal abnormalities but generally no malignancies in males		
	Case report of a seminoma		59
Estrogens	Suspicion of increased incidence of cardiovascular defects, perhaps others	Evidence is conflicting	124, 106, 235, 260
Hydrocortisone	As with cortisone, cleft palates	Incidence of adverse effects is low	
		Mostly from animal work	14, 146, 238
Prednisone	Neonatal hypoadrenalism	Poor placental transfer makes the incidence low	38, 152, 250, 344
	Possibly greater incidence of stillbirth		337
Progestins	Masculinization of the female fetus: labial fusion early, clitoral hypertrophy late		37, 141, 145, 341, 345
Tranquilizers			
Major			
Phenothiazines	Suspicion of congenital anomalies, especially cardiovascular and respiratory	Not all studies show difference from control; some suggest anomalies, more likely with the 3-carbon aliphatic side chain, (e.g., chlorpromazine)	64, 195, 264, 302, 318, 330
	Neonatal withdrawal syndrome extrapyramidal signs		130, 319
Chlorpromazine (Thorazine)	Possible retinopathy	Due to affinity of the drug for melanin	128
	Those listed above, plus possibly ileus	Case report	87
	Hypotension		43
Minor			
Benzodiazepines Chlordiazepoxide (Librium)	Suspicion of congenital anomalies	The cause-and-effect relationship of minor tranquilizers and congenital anomalies is not proved, but the Food and Drug Administration recommends that these drugs not be used in the first trimester	97, 122, 125, 197

Drug	Effects	Comments	References
	Neonatal withdrawal syndrome	Chronic exposure	17, 32
Diazepam (Valium)	Suspicion of cleft lip and/or palate	The cause-and-effect relationship of minor tranquilizers and congenital anomalies is not proven but the food and Drug Administration recommends that these drugs not be used in the first trimester	22, 66, 160, 161, 266, 267, 269, 270
	Neonatal withdrawal	Chronic exposure	186
	Decreased Apgar scores	Large doses in labor	95
	Decreased neonatal muscle tone	Large doses in labor	65, 95
	Decreased ability to withstand cold stress		65, 229
	Decreased fetal heart rate beat-to-beat variability	Lessens diagnostic capabilities of fetal heart rate monitoring	274, 346
	Bilirubin displacement from albumin	Due to sodium benzoate preservative, unlikely of clinical significance unless administered directly to the neonate	214, 276
Flumazenil (antagonist)	No embryotoxic or teratogenic effect noted	Animal studies only	277
Vasopressors			
Ephedrine	Increased fetal heart rate variability	Direct placental transfer	342
Centrally acting pressors (ephedrine, mephentermine)	As therapy of spinal hypotension, prevents fetal asphyxia	Returns uterine blood flow toward control with correction of spinal hypotension	142, 298
Peripherally acting pressors (methoxamine, phenylephrine)	As therapy of spinal hypotension, does not prevent fetal asphyxia	Uterine blood flow does not recover with correction of spinal hypotension	142
Vitamins			
Hypervitaminosis A	Possible urogenital anomaly	Isolated case reports	28, 88
Vitamin A analog Isotretinoin (Accutane)	Spontaneous abortions, multiple congenital malformations possible including small, malformed or absent ears, cleft palate, congenital heart disease (especially anomalies of the great vessels), central nervous system abnormalities (especially hydrocephal, posterior fossa cysts)	Proven Incidence may be 100% if taken in second month of gestation	114, 162
Vitamin D	Congenital supravalvular aortic stenosis Mental retardation Hypercalcemia	Excessive intake	131
Vitamin K	Increased incidence of hyperbilirubinemia and risk of kernicterus	Water-soluble analogs with prematurity	180

References

1. Abboud TK et al.: Anesth Analg 61:638, 1982.
2. Abboud TK et al.: Anesth Analg 62:426, 1983.
3. Abboud TK et al.: Anesth Analg 62:473, 1983.
4. Abboud TK et al.: Obstet Gynecol 57:224, 1981.
5. Aldrete JA: In *The Anesthesiologist, Mother and Newborn.* Williams & Wilkins, Baltimore, 1974, p 133.
6. Allen RWJ Jr et al.: JAMA 244:1464, 1980.
7. Alselton P et al.: Am J Epidemiol 120:251, 1984.
8. Alstatt LB: J Pediatr 66:985, 1965.
9. Amiel-Tison C, Barrier G, Shnider SM et al.: Anesthesiology 56:340, 1982.
10. Amin-Zakil et al.: J Appl Toxicol 1:210, 1981.
11. Anderson GG, Hanson TM: Obstet Gynecol 44:896, 1974.
12. Anderson NB: Anesthesiology 29:113, 1968.
13. Annunziato D: Pediatrics 47:787, 1971.
14. Aoyama T et al.: Oyo Yakuri 8:1037, 1974.
15. Armstrong JG et al.: Science 143:703, 1964.
16. Arwood LL et al.: Pediatrics 63:844, 1979.
17. Athinarayanan P, Pierog SH, Nigam SK et al.: Am J Obstet Gynecol 124:212, 1976.
18. Banister P et al.: Lancet 1:838, 1972.
19. Barr M, Burdi AR: Teratology 14:129, 1976.
20. Barr M Jr et al.: Teratology 44:485, 1991.
21. Basford AB, Fink BR: Anesthesiology 29:1167, 1968.
22. Beall JR: Can Med Assoc J 106:1061, 1972.
23. Beazley J, Alderman B: Br J Obstet Gynecol 82:265, 1975.
24. Beazley JM, Alderman B: Lancet 1:45, 1975.
25. Becker MH, Genieser NB, Finegold M: Am J Dis Child 129:356, 1975.
26. Beintema DJ: Clin Dev Med 28, 1968.
27. Bellinger D et al.: N Engl J Med 316:1037, 1987.
28. Bernhardt IB, Dorsey DJ: Obstet Gynecol 43:750, 1974.
29. Bethenod M, Frederich A: (French) Pediatrie 30:227, 1975.
30. Biale Y, Lewenthal H, Aderet NG: Obstet Gynecol 45:439, 1975.
31. Bingol N et al.: J Pediatr 110:93, 1987.
32. Bitnum S: Can Med Assoc J 100:351, 1969.
33. Bleyer WA, Breckenridge RT: JAMA 213:2049, 1970.
34. Bleyer WA, Marshall RE: JAMA 221:185, 1972.
35. Bloomfield DK: Am J Obstet Gynecol 107:883, 1970.
36. Deleted in proof.
37. Bongiovanni AM, DiGeorge Am, Grumach MM: J Clin Endocrinol 19:1004, 1959.
38. Bongiovanni AM, McPadden AJ: Fertil Steril 11:181, 1960.
39. Boros SJ, Reynolds JW: Am J Obstet Gynecol 129:111, 1977.
40. Brazelton TB, Robey TS, Lother GA: Pediatrics 44:275, 1969.
41. Brettes JP, Renaud R, Gandar R: Am J Obstet Gynecol 124:164, 1976.
42. Briggs GG et al.: In *Drugs in Pregnancy and Lactation.* Williams & Wilkins, Baltimore, MD, 1986, p 42.
43. Bryans C Jr et al.: Am J Obstet Gynecol 77:406, 1959.
44. Budnick IJ, Leiken S, Hoeck LE: Am J Dis Child 90:286, 1955.
45. Burns LE, Hodgman JE, Cass AB: N Engl J Med 261:1318, 1959.
46. Burrow GN: N Engl J Med 298:150, 1978.
47. Center for Disease Control: MMWR 31:565, 1982.
48. Caritis SN et al.: Am J Obstet Gynecol 147:752, 1983.
49. Chalmers I, Campbell H, Turnbull AC: Br Med J 2:116, 1975.
50. Chappel JN: JAMA 221:1516, 1972.
51. Chasnoff IJ et al.: J Pediatr 108:456, 1986.
52. Chasnoff IJ et al.: N Engl J Med 313:666, 1985.
53. Cohen EN, Bellville JW, Brown BW: Anesthesiology 35:343, 1971.
54. Cohen MM, Hirschhorn K, Verbo S et al.: Pediatr Res 2:486, 1968.
55. Cohlan SQ, Bevelander G, Tiamsic T: Am J Dis Child 105:453, 1963.
56. Cohlan SQ: NY J Med 64:493, 1964.
57. Cohlan SQ: Teratology 15:127, 1977.
58. Collins P, Olufs R, Kravitz H et al.: Am J Obstet Gynecol 127:4, 1977.
59. Conley GR et al.: JAMA 249:1325, 1983.
60. Conway N, Birt BD: Br Med J 2:260, 1965.
61. Corbett TH, Cornell RG, Lieding K: Anesthesiology 38:260, 1973.
62. Corbett TH, Cornell RG, Endres JL et al.: Anesthesiology 41:341, 1974.
63. Cordero JF et al.: JAMA 245:2307, 1981.
64. Corner BD: Med J Southwest 77:284, 1962.
65. Cree JE, Meyer J, Hailey DM: Br Med J 4:251, 1973.
66. Crombie DL et al.: N Engl J Med 293:198, 1975.
67. Cullshaw JA: Br Med J 2:924, 1962.
68. Curatolo PW, Robertson D: Ann Intern Med 98:641, 1983.
69. Davidson DC, Ford JA, McIntosh W: Br Med J 4:106, 1973.
70. Day HJ, Conrad FG, Moore JE: Am J Med Sci 236:475, 1958.
71. De La Torre R, Krompotic E: Teratology 13:131, 1976.
72. DeBeukelaer MM, Randall CL, Stroud DR: J Pediatr 91:759, 1977.
73. Desmond MM, Rogers SF, Lindley JE et al.: Obstet Gynecol 10:140, 1957.
74. Desmond MM, Schwanecke RP, Wilson GS et al.: J Pediatr 80:190, 1972.
75. Diamond I et al.: Pediatrics 25:85, 1960.
76. Doig RK, Coltman OM: Lancet 2:730, 1956.
77. Donald PR, Sellars SL: S Afr Med J 60:316, 1981.
78. Done AK: Clin Pharmacol Ther 5:432, 1964.
79. Ehrenbard JT, Chaganti RSK: Lancet 2:97, 1981.
80. Elder HA et al.: Am J Obstet Gynecol 111:441, 1971.
81. Emerson DJ: Am J Obstet Gynecol 84:356, 1962.
82. Engel RR, Elin RJ: J Pediatr 77:631, 1970.
83. Epstein MF et al.: J Pediatr 94:449, 1979.
84. Eriksson M, et al.: Acta Paediatr Scand 67:95, 1978.
85. Eskenazi B, Bracken MB: Am J Obstet Gynecol 144:919, 1982.
86. FDA Drug Bull 8:14, 1978.
87. Falterman CG et al.: J Pediatr 97:308, 1980.
88. Fantel AG et al.: Teratology 15:65, 1977.
89. Fedrick J: Br Med J 2:442, 1973.
90. Fein GG et al.: J Pediatr 105:315, 1984.
91. Feldman GL, Weaver DD, Lovrien EW: Am J Dis Child 131:1389, 1977.
92. Fillmore SJ, McDevitt E: Ann Intern Med 73:731, 1970.
93. Finnerty F: Clin Obstet Gynecol 18:145, 1975.
94. Fisher WD, Voorhess ML, Gardner LI: J Pediatr 62:132, 1963.
95. Flowers CE, Rudolph AJ, Desmond MM: Obstet Gynecol 34:68, 1971.
96. Galina MP et al.: N Engl J Med 267:1124, 1962.
97. Geber WF et al.: Teratology 21:39A, 1980.
98. German J, Kowal A, Ehlers KH: Teratology 3:349, 1970.
99. Ghosh A, Hudson FP: Br Med J 3:636, 1973.
100. Gill WB: J Reprod Med 16:147, 1976.
101. Gladstone GR: J Pediatr 86:962, 1975.
102. Glass L, Rajegowda BK, Evans HE: Lancet 2:685, 1971.
103. Glass L, Rajegowda BK, Kahn EJ et al.: N Engl J Med 286:746, 1972.
104. Glass L: Pediatrics 82:734, 1973.
105. Goldman AS et al.: Teratology 17:103, 1978.
106. Gonjard J et al.: Lancet 1:482, 1977.
107. Gluck L, Kulovich MV: Am J Obstet Gynecol 115:539, 1973.
108. Goldby M: Transplantation 10:201, 1970.
109. Goodman RM, Katznelson MB, Hertz M et al.: Am J Dis Child 130:884, 1976.
110. Gordon RR, Dean T: Br Med J 2:719, 1955.
111. Green HG et al.: Am J Dis Child 122:247, 1971.
112. Greenberg LH, Tanaka KR: JAMA 188:423, 1964.
113. Habib A, McCarthy JS: J Pediatr 91:808, 1977.
114. Hall JG: J Pediatr 105:583, 1984.
115. Hallum JL: Arch Dis Child 29:354, 1954.
116. Hanson JW et al.: J Pediatr 92:457, 1978.
117. Hanson JW, Jones KL, Smith DW: JAMA 235:1458, 1976.
118. Hanson JW, Myrianthopoulos NC, Harvey MAS et al.: J Pediatr 89:662, 1976.
119. Harada M: Teratology 18:285, 1978.
120. Harley JD, Farrar JF, Gray JB et al.: Lancet 1:472, 1964.
121. Harris JWS, Ross IP: Lancet 1:1045, 1956.

122. Hartz SC, Heinonen OP, Shapiro S et al.: N Engl J Med 292:726, 1975.
123. Hecht F et al.: Lancet 2:1087, 1968.
124. Heinonen OP, Slone D, Monson RR et al.: N Engl J Med 296:67, 1977.
125. Heinonen OP et al.: *Birth Defects and Drugs in Pregnancy.* PSG Publishing, Littleton, MA, 1977.
126. Herbst AL et al.: N Engl J Med 292:334, 1975.
127. Herbst AL, Ulfelder H, Poskanzer DC: N Engl J Med 284:878, 1971.
128. Herxheimer A: Lancet 1:448, 1971.
129. Herzlinder RA, Kandall SR, Vaughan HG: J Pediatr 91:638, 1977.
130. Hill RM et al.: J Pediatr 69:589, 1966.
131. Hill RM, Craig JP, Chaney MD et al.: Clin Obstet Gynecol 20:381, 1977.
132. Hill RM, Vernaiud WH: Am J Dis Child 127:645, 1974.
133. Hill RM: Am J Dis Child 130:923, 1976.
134. Hoffmann W, Grospietsch G, Kuhn W: Lancet 2:794, 1976.
135. Hon EH et al.: Am J Obstet Gynecol 82:291, 1961.
136. Horowitz DA et al.: Am J Dis Child 136:73, 1982.
137. Hyman MD, Shnider SM: Anesthesiology 34:81, 1971.
138. Idanpaan-Heikkila J: Lancet 2:282, 1973.
134. Itskovitz J et al.: J Reprod Med 24:137, 1980.
140. Jackson WPU, Campbell GD, Notelovitz MB, et al.: Diabetes 11(suppl):98, 1962.
141. Jacobson BD: Am J Obstet Gynecol 84:962, 1962.
142. James FM, Greiss FC, Kemp RA: Anesthesiology 33:25, 1970.
143. Javett SN, Senior B, Braudo JL et al.: Pediatrics 24:65, 1959.
144. Jones KL, Smith DW: Teratology 12:1, 1975.
145. Jost A: Harvey Lect 55:201, 1961.
146. Kalter H, Froger FC: Nature 169:665, 1952.
147. Kandall SR, Albin S, Lowinson J et al.: Pediatrics 58:681, 1976.
148. Kantor HI et al.: Obstet Gynecol 17:494, 1961.
149. Karpatkin S et al.: Am J Med 52:776, 1972.
150. Kelly JV: Clin Obstet Gynecol 20:395, 1977.
151. Kendall SR, Gartner LM: Pediatr Res 7:92, 1973.
152. Kenny FM, Preeyasombat C, Spaulding JS et al.: Pediatrics 37:960, 1966.
153. Kent SP, Wideman GL: JAMA 171:1199, 1959.
154. Kerber IJ, Warr OS, Richardson C: JAMA 203:223, 1968.
155. Kline J, Stein ZA, Susser M et al.: N Engl J Med 297:793, 1977.
156. Koren G: *Maternal-Fetal Toxicology.* Marcel Dekker Inc, New York, 1990.
157. Kosaka Y, Takahashi T, Mark LC: Anesthesiology 31:489, 1969.
158. Kron RF, Litt M, Finnegan LP: Pediatr Res 7:64, 1973.
159. Kurzel RB: South Med J 83:953, 1990.
160. Laegreid L et al.: J Pediatr 114:126, 1989.
161. Laegreid L: Devel Pharm Therapeutics 15:186, 1990.
162. Lammer EJ et al.: N Engl J Med 313:837, 1985.
163. Landesman-Dwyer S et al.: Alcoholism. Clin Exp Res 2:171, 1978.
164. Landesman-Dwyer S, Emanuel I: Teratology 19:119, 1979.
165. Larsson Y, Sterkey G: Lancet 2:1424, 1960.
166. Lazarus SS, Volk BW: J Clin Endocrinol 23:597, 1963.
167. Leake RD et al.: Clin Res 28:90A, 1980.
168. Lenz W, Knapp K: Dtsch Med Wochenschr 87:1232, 1962.
169. Levin D, Fixler D, Morriss F et al.: J Pediatr 92:478, 1978.
170. Levin D, Hyman A, Heymann MA et al.: J Pediatr 92:265, 1978.
171. Levin JN: J Pediatr 79:130, 1971.
172. Lewis RM, Schulman JD: Lancet 2:338, 1975.
173. Liggins GC, Howie RN: Pediatrics 50:515, 1972.
174. Linn S et al.: N Engl J Med 306:141, 1982.
175. Lipeltz PJ: Pediatrics 39:401, 1968.
176. Deleted in proof.
177. Long S: Teratology 6:75, 1972.
178. Longo LD: Am J Obstet Gynecol 129:69, 1977.
179. Lowe CR: Lancet 1;9, 1973.
180. Lucey JF, Dolan RG: Pediatrics 23:553, 1959.

181. Madden JD et al.: Pediatrics 77:209, 1986.
182. Manchester D, Margolis HS, Sheldon RE: Am J Obstet Gynecol 126:467, 1976.
183. Manning F, Winpugh E, Boddy K: Br Med J 1:552, 1975.
184. Matz GJ, Nauntan RF: Arch Otolaryngol 88:370, 1968.
185. Mauer HM, Wolff JA, Finster M et al.: Lancet 2:122, 1968.
186. Mazzi E: Am J Obstet Gynecol 129:586, 1977.
186. McBride WG: Lancet 2:1358, 1961.
187. McBride WG: Med J Aust 1:492, 1972.
188. McBride WG: Med J Aust 1:492, 1972.
189. McGlothlin WH, Sparkes RS, Arnold DO: JAMA 212:1483, 1970.
190. Meadow SR: Proc R Soc Med 63:48, 1970.
191. Meltzer HJ: JAMA 161:1253, 1956.
192. Mendez-Bauer C et al.: Am J Obstet Gynecol 85:1033, 1963.
193. Milham S, Elledge W: Teratology 5:125, 1972.
194. Milkovich L, van den Berg BJ: Am J Dis Child 131:924, 1977.
195. Milkovich L, van den Berg BJ: Am J Obstet Gynecol 125:244, 1976.
196. Milkovich L, van den Berg BJ: Am J Obstet Gynecol 129:637, 1977.
197. Milkovich L, van den Berg BJ: N Engl J Med 291:1268, 1974.
198. Millar JHD, Nevin NC: Lancet 1:328, 1973.
199. Milner RD, Chouksey SK: Arch Dis Child 47:537, 1972.
200. Milunsky A et al.: J Pediatr 72:790, 1968.
201. Minkowitz S et al.: Obstet Gynecol 24:337, 1964.
202. Mirkin BL: J Pediatr 78:329, 1971.
203. Mitchell AA et al.: Am J Obstet Gynecol 147:737, 1983.
204. Mitchell AA et al.: JAMA 245:2311, 1981.
205. Mogilner BM et al.: Acta Obstet Gynecol Scand 61:183, 1982.
206. Monson RR, Rosenberg L, Hartz SC et al.: N Engl J Med 289:1049, 1973.
207. Morishima HO, Daniel SS, Finster M et al.: Anesthesiology 27:147, 1966.
208. Morris MB, Weinstein L: Am J Obstet Gynecol 140:607, 1981.
209. Moya F, Thorndike V: Clin Pharmacol Ther 4:628, 1963.
210. Moya F: NY J Med 62:2169, 1962.
211. Mujtaba Q, Burrow GN: Obstet Gynecol 46:282, 1975.
212. Mulvihill J, Klimas JT, Stokes DC: Am J Obstet Gynecol 125:937, 1976.
213. Nathenson G, Cohen MI, Litt IF: J Pediatr 81:899, 1972.
214. Nathenson G, Cohen MI, McNamara H: J Pediatr 86:799, 1975.
215. Nau H et al.: Clin Phamaco Kinet 7:508, 1982.
216. Nelson MM, Forfar JO: Br Med J 1:523, 1971.
217. Neu RL et al.: Lancet 1:675, 1969.
218. Niswander JD, Wertelecki W: Lancet 2:1962, 1973.
219. Nora JJ et al.: Lancet 2:594, 1974.
220. Nora JJ, Vargo TA, Nora AH et al.: Lancet 1:1290, 1970.
221. Nuwayhid B, Brinkman CR, Katchen B et al.: Obstet Gynecol 46:197, 1975.
222. O'Brien PC et al.: Obstet Gynecol 53:300, 1979.
223. O'Meara OP, Brazie JV: N Engl J Med 278:1127, 1968.
224. Opitz JM et al.: Lancet 1:91, 1972.
225. Oro AS, Dixon SD: J Pediatr 111:571, 1987.
226. Oro AS et al.: J Pediatr 111:571, 1987.
227. Oski FA: Am J Dis Child 129:1139, 1975.
228. Ouellette EM, Rosett HL, Rosman NP et al.: N Engl J Med 297:528, 1977.
229. Owen JR, Irani SF, Blair AW: Arch Dis Child 47:107, 1972.
230. Palmer RH, Ouellette EM, Warner L: Pediatrics 53:490, 1974.
231. Papageorgiou AN et al.: Pediatrics 63:73, 1979.
232. Pauli RM, Madden JD et al.: J Pediatr 88:506, 1976.
233. Percy DH: Teratology 11:103, 1975.
234. Perkins RP: Am J Obstet Gynecol 111:379, 1971.
235. Peterson WF: Obstet Gynecol 34:363, 1969.
236. Pettitior JM, Benson R: J Pediatr 86:459, 1975.
237. Piacquadio K et al.: Lancet 338:866, 1991.
238. Pinsky L, DiGeorge AM: Science 147:402, 1965.
239. Pleasure JR et al.: Pediatrics 55:503, 1975.
240. Prechtl HFR, Beintema D: Clin Dev Med 12, 1974.
241. Puchkov VF: Bull Exp Biol 7:99, 1967.
242. Rachelefsky GS et al.: Lancet 1:838, 1972.
243. Ralston DH, Shnider SM: Anesthesiology 48:34, 1978.

244. Ramboer C, Thompson RPH, Williams R: Lancet 1:966, 1969.
245. Ramer CM: Clin Pediatr 13:596, 1974.
246. Reed RL, Cheney CB, Fearon RE et al.: Anesth Analg 53:214, 1974.
247. Reifenstein ED: Ann NY Acad SCi 71:762, 1958.
248. Rementeria JL, Nunag NN: Am J Obstet Gynecol 116:1152, 1973.
249. Rendle-Short TJ: Lancet 1:1188, 1962.
250. Renisch JM et al.: Science 202:4236, 1978.
251. Richards ID: Br J Prev Soc Med 23:218, 1969.
252. Ring G, Krames E, Shnider S et al.: Obstet Gynecol 50:598, 1977.
253. Riggs BS et al.: Obstet Gynecol 74:247, 1989.
254. Robinson GC, Cambon KG: N Engl J Med 271:949, 1964.
255. Rodriguez SU, Leikin SL, Hiller MC: N Engl J Med 270:881, 1964.
256. Rogan WJ et al.: Science 241:334, 1988.
257. Rosen RC, Lightner ES: J Pediatr 92:240, 1978.
258. Rosenberg L et al.: JAMA 247:1429, 1982.
259. Rothman KJ et al.: Am J Epidemiol 109:433, 1979.
260. Rothman KJ et al.: N Engl J Med 299:522, 1978.
261. Rothstein P, Gould JM: Pediatr Clin North Am 21:307, 1974.
262. Rucker E: J Med Assoc State Ala 23:59, 1953.
263. Rumack CM et al.: Obstet Gynecol 58(suppl):525, 1981.
264. Rumeau-Rouquette C, Goujaro J, Huel G: Teratology 15:57, 1977.
265. Rushton DI: Lancet 2:141, 1976.
266. Safra MJ, Oakley GP: Lancet 2:478, 1975.
267. Safra ML, Oakley GP: Cleft Palate J 13:198, 1976.
268. Savory J, Monif GRG: Am J Obstet Gynecol 110:556, 1971.
269. Saxen I, Saxen L: Lancet 2:498, 1975.
270. Saxen I: Int J Epid 4:37, 1975.
271. Scanlon JW, Brown WU, Weiss JB et al.: Anesthesiology 40:121, 1974.
272. Scanlon JW, Ostheimer GW, Lurie AO et al.: Anesthesiology 45:400, 1976.
273. Schardein JL: *Chemically Induced Birth Defects*. Marcel Dekker, New York, 1985, p 273.
274. Scher J: J Obstet Gynecol Br Commow 79:635, 1972.
275. Schiff D, Aranda JV, Stern L: J Pediatr 77:457, 1970.
276. Schiff D, Chan G, Stern L: Pediatrics 48:139, 1971.
277. Schlappi B et al.: Arzneimittel-Forschung 38:247, 1988.
278. Schou M, Goldfield MD, Weinstein MR et al.: Obstet Gynecol Surv 28:794, 1973.
279. Schou M et al.: Br Med J 2:135, 1973.
280. Schou M: Acta Psychiatr Scand 54:193, 1976.
281. Schulz J, van Creveld S: Etudes Neo-Natales 7:133, 1958.
282. Scott JR: Am J Obstet Gynecol 128:668, 1977.
283. Scott AA et al.: Am J Obstet Gynecol 160:1223, 1989.
284. Scott WC, Warner RF: JAMA 142:1331, 1950.
285. Seip M: Acta Paediatr Scand 65:617, 1976.
286. Senior B et al.: Lancet 2:377, 1976.
287. Serment H, Ruf H: Bull Fed Soc Gynecol Obstet Lang Fr 20:69, 1968.
288. Serment H, Ruf H: Bull Fed Soc Gynecol Obstet Lang Fr 20:77, 1968.
289. Shapiro S et al.: Lancet 1:272, 1976.
290. Shapiro S, Siskind V, Monson RR et al.: Lancet 1:1375, 1976.
291. Shaul WL, Emergy H, Hall JG: Am J Dis Child 129:360, 1975.
292. Shaul WL, Hall JG: Am J Obstet Gynecol 127:191, 1977.
293. Shaw EB, Steinbach HL: Am J Dis Child 115:477, 1968.
294. Shaw EB: Am J Dis Child 124:93, 1972.
295. Shenker L: Obstet Gynecol 26:104, 1965.
296. Shnider SM, Moya F: Am J Obstet Gynecol 89:1009, 1964.
297. Shnider SM, Way EL: Anesthesiology 29:951, 1968.
298. Shnider SM, deLorimier AA, Holl JW et al.: Am J Obstet Gynecol 102:911, 1968.
299. Shotton D, Monie IW: Jama 186:74, 1963.
300. Silverman WA, Anderson DH, Blank WA et al.: Pediatrics 18:614, 1956.
301. Sinclair JC, Fox HA, Lentz JF: N Engl J Med 273:1173, 1965.
302. Slone D, Siskind V, Heinonen OP et al.: Am J Obstet Gynecol 128:486, 1977.
303. Slone D, Siskind V, Heinonen OP et al.: Lancet 1:1373, 1976.
304. Smart RG, Bateman K: Can Med Assoc J 99:805, 1968.
305. Smith BE, Gaub ML, Moya F: Anesthesiology 26:260, 1965.
306. Sobel DE: Arch Gen Psychiatry 2:606, 1960.
307. Sokal JE, Lessmann EM: JAMA 172:1765, 1960.
308. South J: Lancet 2:1154, 1972.
309. Speidel BD, Meadow SR: Lancet 2:839, 1972.
310. Sterne J: Lancet 1:1165, 1963.
311. Stevens D, Burman D, Midwinter A: Lancet 2:595, 1974.
312. Stoffer SS, Hamburger JI: J Nucl Med 17:146, 1976.
313. Deleted in proof.
314. Streissguth AP, Herman CS, Smith DW: J Pediatr 92:363, 1978.
315. Stutzman L, Sokal JE: Clin Obstet Gynecol 11:416, 1968.
316. Sutherland HW et al.: Arch Dis Child 49:283, 1974.
317. Sutherland JM, Keller WH: Am J Dis Child 101:447, 1961.
318. Szabo KT, Brent RL: Lancet 1:565, 1974.
319. Tamer A et al.: J Pediatr 75:479, 1969.
320. Taussig HB: JAMA 180:1106, 1962.
321. Tenbrinck MS, Buchin SY: JAMA 232:1144, 1975.
322. Thiersch JB: Am J Obstet Gynecol 63:1298, 1952.
323. Thiery M, De Hemptinne D, Schuddinck L et al.: Lancet 1:161, 1975.
324. Toaff R, Ravid R: In *Drug Induced Diseases*. Excerpta Medica Foundation, Amsterdam, 1968, p 113.
325. Tunstall ME: Br J Anaesth 41:792, 1969.
326. Turner G, Collins E: Lancet 2:338, 1975.
327. Turner GM, Oakley CM, Dixon HG: Br Med J 4:281, 1968.
328. Uhlig H: Arzenim Forsch 12:61, 1957.
329. Villasanta U: Am J Obstet Gynecol 93:142, 1965.
330. Vince DJ: Can Med Assoc J 100:223, 1969.
331. Wagner L, Wagner G, Guerrero J: Am J Obstet Gynecol 108:308, 1970.
332. Walker B: Teratology 4:39, 1971.
333. Warkany J: Teratology 14:205, 1976.
334. Warrell DW, Taylor R: Lancet 1:117, 1968.
335. Warren TM et al.: Anesth Analg 62:516, 1983.
336. Waziri M, Lonasescu V, Zellweger H: Am J Dis Child 130:1022, 1976.
337. Warrel DW, Taylor R: Lancet 1:117, 1968.
338. Webster PAC: Lancet 2:318, 1973.
339. Weinstein L, Dalton C: N Engl J Med 279:526, 1968.
340. Deleted in proof.
341. Wilkins L: JAMA 172:1028, 1960.
342. Wright RG et al.: Am J Obstet Gynecol 57:734, 1981.
343. Wynne J, Milner AD, Hodson AK: Arch Dis Child 50:331, 1975.
344. Yaffe SJ, Stern L: In *Perinatal Pharmacology and Therapeutics*. Academic Press, New York, 1976, p 355.
345. Yaffe SJ: Can Med Assoc J 98:301, 1968.
346. Yeh SY, Paul RH, Cordero L et al.: Obstet Gynecol 43:363, 1974.
347. Zackai EH, Mellman WJ, Neiderer B et al.: J Pediatr 87:280, 1975.
348. Zellweger H: Clin Pediatr 13:338, 1974.
349. Zelson C: N Engl J Med 288:1393, 1973.
350. Zelson C, Rubin E, Wasserman E: Pediatrics 48:178, 1971.

Index

Page numbers in italics denote figures; those followed by "t" denote tables.

Surgery during pregnancy—*continued*
  maternal safety of anesthesia for, 259–
    264
  neurosurgery, 551–560. *See also* Neuro-
    surgery during pregnancy
  open-heart, 515
  pain threshold, 259–260, *263–264*
  patient preparation for, 276
  physiologic changes affecting anesthetic
    requirements, 259, *260–262*
  preventing preterm labor during, 275
  teratogenicity of anesthetics for, 264–
    272
  urgent, 276
Syncytiotrophoblast, 19
Systemic drugs, 115–131
  antagonists, 130–131
  dissociative, 128–129
  narcotics, 119–128
  neonatal neurobehavioral effects of,
    683–686
  neuroleptanalgesia, 129–130
  sedative-tranquilizers, 115–119
  teratogenicity of, 264–266
    in animals, 264–265
    in humans, 265–266
Systemic lupus erythematosus, 603–605
  anesthetic management of patient with,
    604–605
  cardiac effects of, 604
  cesarean section for patient with, 605
  coagulation defects in, 604
  fetal effects of, 604
  nephritis in, 604
  neurologic complications of, 604
  signs and symptoms of, 604
  treatment during pregnancy, 604
  vaginal delivery of patient with, 605
Systemic vascular resistance
  in aortic coarctation, 505
  in aortic insufficiency, 496
  in asymmetric septal hypertrophy, 512
  at birth, 693
  in Eisenmenger's syndrome, 504
  in mitral insufficiency, 493
  in mitral stenosis, 491
  in mitral valve prolapse, 494
  during open-heart surgery, 515
  in patent ductus arteriosus, 501, 502
  postpartum, 486
  in preeclampsia, 307, 308t
  in pulmonary hypertension, 508
  in pulmonic stenosis, 506–507
  ritodrine effect on, 343
  in tetralogy of Fallot, 502–503
  in ventricular septal defect, 499, 500

Tachycardia
  drug-induced, 491
  due to β-adrenergic tocolytic therapy,
    344, 348
  fetal, 660–661, 667
  marijuana-induced, 637
  paroxysmal atrial, 516
  in patient with mitral valve prolapse,
    494
Talwin. *See* Pentazocine
Tapazole. *See* Methimazole
Temporomandibular joint, 601–602
Teratogenicity, *264–265, 264–272,* 555,
    709
  of aminophylline, 528

animal studies of, 266–268
  cyclopropane, 267
  diethyl ether, 267
  enflurane, 267
  fluroxene, 267
  halothane, 267
  isoflurane, 267
  local anesthetics, 268
  methoxyflurane, 267
  muscle relaxants, 268
  nitrous oxide, 266–267, *267*
of anticonvulsants, 566
behavioral teratology, *271,* 271–272
of cocaine, 638
of corticosteroids, 528
of ethanol, 634
human studies of, 268–270, 269t, *270*
of maternal emotional stress and trauma,
    271
related to arterial blood gas alterations,
    270–271
related to timing of organ development,
    264, *265*
of sedatives, 528
of systemic medications, 264–266
  animal studies of, 264–265
  human studies of, 265–266
of tetrahydrocannabinol, 637
transplacental carcinogenesis, 272
Terbutaline, 339, 341, 349. *See also* β-
    Adrenergic agents
  for asthma, 528, 529
  for diabetic mother, 544
  effect on progress of labor, 531
  fetal/neonatal effects of, 715
Test dose, 137–141
  air injection for, 140–141
  choice of local anesthetic for, 139
  criteria for, 139
  epinephrine in, 139–140
  function of, 137–139
  of local anesthetic for cesarean section,
    219
Tetracaine
  for spinal anesthesia, 148
  structure of, *84*
  for subarachnoid block for cesarean sec-
    tion, 217
Tetracycline, 714
Tetrahydrocannabinol, 637
Tetralogy of Fallot, 502–503
  anesthesia for vaginal delivery/cesarean
    section in patient with, 503
  anesthetic considerations in patient
    with, 502–503
  clinical manifestations of, 502
  maternal/fetal mortality related to, 502,
    503
  pathophysiology of, 502
  pregnancy effects on, 502
Thalassemias, 370–371, 372t
  α-thalassemia, 370–371
    diagnosis of, 371
    hemoglobin H disease, 370–371
    minor, 371
  β-thalassemia, 370–371
    minor, 371
  prenatal diagnosis of, 371
Thalidomide, 264, *265,* 713
Theophylline, 529, 715
Thiamylal, 264
Thiopental, 229–232, *231*
  in breast milk, 255

effects on uterine blood flow, 32, *32*
lack of neonatal depression from, 229,
    232
placental transfer of, 229
for postpartum sterilization surgery, 252
to prevent local anesthetic-induced con-
    vulsions, 142
use in alcohol-abusing mother, 634
use in asthmatic patient, 533
use in patient with mitral stenosis, 491
use in patient with multiple sclerosis,
    572
Thorazine. *See* Chlorpromazine
Thrombin time, 367, 367t
Thrombocytopenia, 368–369
  in preeclampsia, 311–313, 312t–313t
Thromboxane, preeclampsia related to,
    306, *307*
Thyroid hormones, 14
Tidal volume, 259, *260*
Time to sustained respiration, 671
Tobacco use, 641, 717
Tocodynamometer, 53, 659
Tocolytic therapy. *See also* specific drugs
  β-adrenergic agents for, 341–349
  calcium channel blockers for, 353–354
  contraindications to, 339
  cost effectiveness of, 337, *338*
  criteria for use of, 339t
  for diabetic mother, 544
  efficacy of, 340
  ethanol for, 341
  fetal/neonatal effects of, 716
  goals of, 339
  magnesium sulfate for, 349–350
  prostaglandin synthetase inhibitors for,
    350–353
  side effects of, 339, 340t
  site of action of drugs used for, *341*
  use during fetal therapeutic procedures,
    291–292
Tofranil. *See* Imipramine
Tolbutamide, 716
Total lung capacity, 259, *261*
Traction response, 681, *685*
Tranquilizers. *See* Sedative-tranquilizers
Transcutaneous electrical nerve stimula-
    tion, 108–110, *109*
  clinical experience with, 109–110
  electrode placement for, 109, *109*
  mechanism of action of, 108–109
  technique for, 109–110
Transfusion
  due to blood loss at delivery, 7–8
  exchange, for sickle cell anemia, 372,
    372t
  intrauterine, 281, 653
  for patient with abruptio placentae, 391
Transplantation
  cardiac, 515
  renal, 607–609
Transtracheal jet ventilation system, 228,
    228
Trendelenburg position
  effect on aortocaval compression, 11
  for patient with total spinal anesthesia,
    142
  for regional anesthesia-induced hypoten-
    sion, 135, 137
Trichloroethylene, 202, 272
Trimethadione (Tridione), 712
Trimethaphan, 328t
  for acute postpartum hypertension, 143